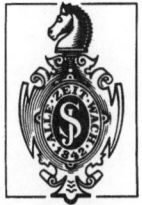

Werner Hacke (Ed.)

Neurocritical Care

Coeditors
Daniel F. Hanley, Baltimore
Karl M. Einhäupl, Berlin
Thomas P. Bleck, Charlottesville
Michael N. Diringer, St. Louis

Guest Editor
Allan H. Ropper, Boston

Neuroradiological Advisor
Klaus Sartor, Heidelberg

With Contributions by Numerous International Authors
from North America and Europe

Springer-Verlag
Berlin Heidelberg New York
London Paris Tokyo
Hong Kong Barcelona
Budapest

With 125 Figures, 3 in Colour and 248 Tables

ISBN 978-3-642-87604-2   ISBN 978-3-642-87602-8 (eBook)
DOI 10.1007/978-3-642-87602-8

Library of Congress Cataloging-in-Publication Data. Neurocritial care / Werner Hacke, ed.; coeditors, Daniel F. Hanley ... [et al.]; guest editor, Allan Ropper; neuroradiological advisor, Klaus Sartor; with contributions by numerous international authors from North America and Europe. p. cm. Includes bibliographical references and index. ISBN-13: 978-3-642-87604-2   1. Neurological intensive care. I. Hacke, W. (Werner), 1948– . [DNLM: 1. Nervous System Diseases – therapy. 2. Critical Care. 3. Intensive Care Units. WL 100 N492 1992] RC350.N49N44 1994 616.8'0428 – dc20 DNLM/DLC for Library of Congress 93-48232

Typesetting: Best-set Typesetter Ltd., Hong Kong

SPIN: 10048741   19/3130/SPS – 5 4 3 2 1 0 – Printed on acid-free paper

Editor

WERNER HACKE, M.D.
Professor and Chairman
Department of Neurology
Ruprecht-Karls-University
Im Neuenheimer Feld 400
69120 Heidelberg, Germany

Coeditors

DANIEL F. HANLEY, M.D.
Associate Professor
Department of Neurology
Director Neuroscience Critical
Johns Hopkins Hospital
600 North Wall Street
Baltimore, MD 21205, USA

KARL M. EINHÄUPL, M.D.
Professor and Chairman
Department of Neurology
Charité
Humboldt University Berlin
Schumannstr. 20/21
10117 Berlin, Germany

MICHAEL N. DIRINGER, M.D.
Assistant Professor
Department of Neurology
Washington University
Medical Center
P.O. Box 8111
660 South Euclid Avenue
St. Louis, MO 63110, USA

THOMAS P. BLECK, M.D.
Associate Professor
Department of Neurology
University of Virginia
Medical Center
Box 394
Charlottesville, VA 22908, USA

Guest Editor

ALLAN H. ROPPER, M.D.
Professor of Neurology
St. Elizabeth's Hospital
Department of Neurology
32 Fruit Street
Boston, MA 02114, USA

Neuroradiological Advisor

KLAUS SARTOR, M.D.
Professor and Chairman
Department of Neuroradiology
Ruprecht-Karls-University
Im Neuenheimer Feld 400
69120 Heidelberg, Germany

Preface

Neurological critical care medicine is one of the fastest growing fields in clinical neurology. Recent developments in the pathophysiology, diagnosis, and treatment of severe neurological diseases have resulted in maximal care for patients.

Patients with severe neurological diseases are frequently treated in general medical and cardiac intensive care units or on neurosurgical wards. The number of specialized neurocritical care units, however, is increasing. In North America, neurocritical care units are often combined neurological-neurosurgical-neuroanesthesiology units directed by neurologists, neurosurgeons, and anesthesiologists. In Germany, separate neurocritical care units are common, with about 50 such units nationwide. Specialized neurocritical care units have some unique special features. These include (a) a team approach consisting of nurses, physical therapists, social workers, and physicians, (b) a high percentage of patients requiring long term artificial ventilation and (c) unique problems of critical care in patients with damage to the most precious human organ – the brain.

Physicians working in the field of neurocritical care have assembled several national and international organizations such as the German Arbeitsgemeinschaft Neurologische Intensivmedizin (ANIM), the section on Neurological Critical Care in the American Academy of Neurology (AAN), and the Research Group on Neurological Intensive Care in the World Federation of Neurology (WFN). Neurocritical care, like other critical care specialties, depends heavily on close professional cooperation. Internists, anesthesiologists, infectious disease specialists, and physical therapists are frequent advisers in all neurocritical care units. There is daily collaboration with neurosurgeons and neuroradiologists. Without this cooperation, the growth and development of neurocritical care would not have been possible. This fact is reflected in this textbook. About one third of the authors are non-neurologists and include neurosurgeons, anesthesiologists, internists, hematologists, and other specialists.

There are a number of excellent neurocritical care textbooks, some larger, some smaller, such as those by Sakman (1980), Ropper (1993; 1989 together with Kennedy), and those in German by Hacke (1986, 1988), Stöhr, Einhäupl, and Brandt (1990), and Jörg (1989). These books can be recommended without reservation. Why, then, is there a need for another textbook on neurocritical care? One reason is the rapid growth of knowledge in this field. We felt that a new up-to-date textbook was needed to present new information. Secondly, most other books represent the views of a single author or of a team of authors from one or only a few institutions. Individual, local, regional, or national biases are inevitable with this approach.

In this book, we have tried to get around this problem: the almost 100 chapters are written by 130 authors from more than 50 institutions in 8 North American and European countries. Only a few short chapters are written by a single author or have more than one author from the same institution. Most of the chapters are co-authored by scientists from both sides of the Atlantic Ocean. This created an enormous organizational and editorial burden. The design of the book forced colleagues, who in many instances had not previously collaborated, to seek a consensus and create a common manuscript. In some instances, different views from different countries are mentioned. The chapters by single authors were edited by a section editor from the other continent. The respective section editor's name is listed on the first page of each chapter.

Because of the growing importance and complexity of neuroradiology, all the chapters that included neuroradiological statements were reviewed by our neuroradiological adviser, Dr. Klaus Sartor, Heidelberg, formerly with the Malincrodt Institute in St. Louis, MO. Dr. Sartor is very familiar with both European and North American approaches in neuroradiology and their occasional differences.

This book has been published less than two years after the first letters of invitation were sent to the contributing authors, a remarkably short time given the transcontinental collaboration. The editors wish to thank all the authors for the effort, dedication, and professionalism they showed by almost always meeting the deadlines. We also wish to thank our guest editor, Dr. Allan Ropper, for his pleasant and creative cooperation.

The main editorial and organizational work on the book was carried out in Heidelberg. We would like to express our sincerest thanks to all the secretaries involved, especially Mrs. Marion Wilczek and Mrs. Petra Günter in Heidelberg. Their perfect secretarial assistance and documentation, coordination of manuscripts that were sent and faxed back and forth, writing of letters to the authors, exchange of information, and reminding of deadlines were crucial for the success of this endeavor. Dr. Michael DeGeorgia, from Ann Arbor, MI, currently a clinical fellow at the Department of Neurology in Heidelberg, was kind enough to accept the task of language editing the chapters without American coauthors.

Both parties to the project of publishing this book are accepting a challenge. Springer-Verlag agreed to take the risk of publishing this book without the guarantees of any sponsorship by companies; its' staff, represented by Victor P. Oehm, was extremely helpful and cooperative throughout this project. The other party, the authors and editors, are also making a sacrifice. In order to keep this 1000 page volume inexpensive, they are foregoing any honoria or other compensation for their work.

We hope that this book will serve its aim, namely to give practical, unbiased, and easy-to-read information to neurologists and other specialists encountering problems of critically ill patients with neurological diseases. This book is not meant to be a complete reference source or a detailed exhaustive volume, rather it is meant to provide useful advise that is readily available in the form of tables (with exact doses of medications). In order to improve readability, the authors were asked not to cite references within the text, a format that some readers from North America may not be familiar with. References for suggested reading are found at the end of each chapter. For further details, especially on pathophysiology and basic science, the reader should refer to more detailed monographs. The authors and editors encourage readers to send their comments, additions, and criticisms, which will be used to improve the second edition.

WERNER HACKE, Heidelberg, Germany
DANIEL F. HANLEY, Baltimore, MD, USA
KARL M. EINHÄUPL, Berlin, Germany
THOMAS P. BLECK, Charlotesville, VA, USA
MICHAEL N. DIRINGER, St. Louis, MO, USA

Contents

General Treatment Strategies

Part II Differential Diagnosis of Symptoms and Signs

Part III Neurocritical Care for Defined Diseases

Inflammatory Diseases: Bacterial Infections

Neurotrauma

*Central Nervous System Neoplasms, Metastases, and
Carcinomatous Meningitis*

Part IV Neurological Manifestations of Internal Diseases

List of Contributors

Eric Aldrich, M.D.
Johns Hopkins Medical Institutions, Dept. of Pathology 509,
600 North Wolfe Street, Baltimore, MD 21287, USA

Heinz Angstwurm, M.D.
Neurologischer Konsiliardienst, Ziemsenstr. 1,
D-80336 München, Germany

Alfred A. Aschoff, M.D.
Neurochirurgische Univ.-Klinik, Im Neuenheimer Feld 400,
D-69120 Heidelberg, Germany

William A. Baumgartner, M.D.
Johns Hopkins Medical Institutions, Dept. of Neurology,
Meyer 6-113, 600 North Wolfe Street, Baltimore, MD 21205, USA

Peter Berlit, M.D.
Alfried Krupp v. Bohlen Krankenhaus, Alfried Krupp Str. 21,
D-45131 Essen, Germany

Michael P. Biber, M.D.
1400 Center Street, Newton Center, MA 02159, USA

Rolf Biniek, M.D.
Neurologische Univ.-Klinik, Klinikum der RWTH Aachen,
Pauwelsstrasse, D-52074 Aachen, Germany

Thomas P. Bleck, M.D.
Associate Professor, University of Virginia School of Medicine,
Dept. of Neurology, Box 394, Charlottesville, VA 22908, USA

Matthias Blumenstein, M.D.
Medizinische Klinik I, Klinikum Großhadern, Marchioninistr. 15,
D-81377 München, Germany

Wolfgang J. Bock, M.D.
Neurochirurgische-Univ.-Klinik Düsseldorf, Moorenstr. 5,
D-40225 Düsseldorf, Germany

Ulrich Bogdahn, M.D.
Neurologische Univ.-Klinik, Josef-Schneider-Str. 11,
D-97080 Würzburg, Germany

Hubert Böhrer, M.D.
Anaesthesiologische Univ.-Klinik, Im Neuenheimer Feld 110,
D-69120 Heidelberg, Germany

Charles F. Bolton, MD., F.R.C.P. (C)
Victoria Hospital, Dept. of Clinical Neurological Sciences,
375 South Street, London-Ontario N6A 4G5/Canada

Cecil Borel, M.D.
Associate Professor, Dept. of Anesthesiology, Duke University
Medical Center, 105 Baher House, Box 3094, Durham, NC 27710,
USA

Dennis L. Bourke, M.D.
Associate Professor, Johns Hopkins Medical Institutions,
Dept. of Anesthesiology/Critical Care Medicine, Osler 303,
600 North Wolfe Street, Baltimore, MD 21205, USA

Marie-Germaine Bousser, M.D.
Hopital Sain Antoine, Service de Neurologie, 184, rue du Faubourg,
Saint-Antoine, F-Paris, Cedex 12, France

Johannes Brachmann, M.D.
Medizinische Univ.-Klinik, Abt. Innere Medizin III,
Bergheimer Str. 58, D-69115 Heidelberg, Germany

Alexander Brawanski, M.D.
Neurochirurgische Klinik, Franz Josef Strauss Allee,
D-93053 Regensburg, Germany

Josef Briegel, M.D.
Anästhesie, Klinikum Großhadern, Marchioninistr. 15,
D-81377 München 15, Germany

Thomas Brott, M.D.
Department of Neurology, University of Cincinnati,
4010 Medical Sciences Building, 231 Bethesda Avenue, Cincinnati,
OH, USA

Helmut Buchner, M.D.
Neurologische Univ.-Klinik, Klinikum der RWTH Aachen,
Pauwelsstrasse, D-52074 Aachen, Germany

Otto Busse, M.D.
Neurologische Klinik, Friedrichstr. 17, D-32427 Minden, Germany

David R. Cornblath, M.D.
Johns Hopkins Medical Institutions, Dept. of Neurology, Pathology
625, 600 North Wolfe Street, Baltimore, MD 21205, USA

Gerald Dal Pan, M.D.
Fellow, AIDS Division, Johns Hopkins Medical Institution,
Dept. of Neurology, Meyer 6-109, 600 North Wolfe Street,
Baltimore, MD 21287-7609, USA

James N. Davis, M.D.
Chairman, Dept. of Neurology T 12-020-HSC, State University of
New York, at Suny-Stony Brook, Stony Brook, NY, USA

Larry E. Davis, M.D.
Professor and Chairman, Department of Neurology, Medical Center,
2100 Ridgecrest Drive SE, Albuquerque, NM 87108, USA

Michael A. DeGeorgia, M.D.
Neurologische Universitäts-Klinik, Im Neuenheimer Feld 400,
D-69120 Heidelberg, Germany

Petra Denzler, M.D.
Klinik Berlin, Neurologische Rehabilitation, Kladower Damm 221,
D-14089 Berlin, Germany

Anna Mae Diehl, M.D.
Associate Professor, Johns Hopkins Medical Institutions, GI
Division, Ross Building, Rm 918, 1830 Monument Street, Baltimore,
MD 21205, USA

Marianne Dieterich, M.D.
Neurologische Poliklinik, Klinikum Großhadern, Marchioninistr. 15,
D-81377 München 15, Germany

Michael N. Diringer, M.D.
Associate Professor, Dept. of Neurology, Washington University
Medical Center, Box 8111, 660 South Euclid Avenue, St. Louis,
MO 63110, USA

Eric R. Eggenberger, M.D.
Dept. of Neurology, Neuroscience Critical Care Unit,
600 North Wall Street, Baltimore, MD 21205, USA

Karl M. Einhäupl, M.D.
Neurologische Univ.-Klinik, Medizinische Fakultät Charité,
Schumannstr. 20/21, D-10117 Berlin, Germany

Wolfgang Enzensberger, M.D.
Neurologische Univ.-Klinik, Schleusenweg 2-16,
D-60528 Frankfurt, Germany

Andreas Ferbert, M.D.
Neurologische Klinik der Städtischen Kliniken, Mönchebergstrasse,
D-34125 Kassel, Germany

Cesare Fieschi, M.D.
Universita Degli Studi di Roma, "La Sapienza", Dipartimento di
Scienze Neurologiche, V.le dell' Universito, 30, I-00185 Roma, Italy

Matthew E. Fink, M.D.
Director, Division of Neurology, Beth Israel Hospital, 317E, 17th
Street, New York, NY 10003, USA

Michael Forsting, M.D.
Neurologische Univ.-Klinik, Abt. Neuroradiologie,
Im Neuenheimer Feld 400, D-69120 Heidelberg, Germany

Jeffrey I. Frank, M.D.
Neurosurgical Intensive Care Unit, The Cleveland Clinic
Foundation, 9500 Euclid Ave, Cleveland, OH 44195, USA

Anthony J. Furlan, M.D.
Dept. of Neurology, Cleveland Clinic Foundation,
9500 Euclid Avenue, Cleveland, OH 44106, USA

Berthilde Ganz, R.N.
Neurologische Univ.-Klinik, Im Neuenheimer Feld 400,
D-69120 Heidelberg, Germany

Christoph Garner, M.D.
Stift Rottal, Max-Köhler-Str. 3, 94086 Griesbach, Germany

Heinrich K. Geiss, M.D.
Hygiene-Institut, Im Neuenheimer Feld 324,
D-69120 Heidelberg, Germany

Jonathan Greenberg, M.D.
Associate Professor, University of Miami, c/o Physician Services, 73
Underwood Street, Orlando, FL 32806, USA

Diane E. Griffin, M.D.
Professor, Internal Medicine and Neurology, Johns Hopkins Medical
Institutions, Dept. of Neurology, Meyer 6-181, 600 North Wolfe
Street, Baltimore, MD 21205, USA

Roman Haberl, M.D.
Neurologische Klinik, Klinikum Großhadern, Marchioninistr. 15,
D-81377 München 15, Germany

Werner Hacke, M.D.
Neurologische Univ.-Klinik, Im Neuenheimer Feld 400,
D-69120 Heidelberg, Germany

Markus S. von Haken, M.D.
The University of Chicago, Dept. of Surgery, Section of
Neurosurgery, MC 3026, 5841 South Maryland Avenue, Chicago,
IL 60637, USA

Daniel F. Hanley, M.D.
Associate Professor, Johns Hopkins Medical Institutions, Dept. of
Neurology, Meyer 8-139, 600 North Wolfe Street, Baltimore,
MD 21205, USA

Alexander Hartmann, M.D.
Neurologische Univ.-Klinik, Sigmund Freud Str. 25,
D-53127 Bonn, Germany

Hans-Peter Hartung, M.D.
Neurologische Univ.-Klinik, Josef-Schneider-Str. 11,
D-97080 Würzburg, Germany

Richard Herrmann, M.D.
Leiter der Abteilung für Onkologie, Dept. f. Innere Medizin,
Kantonsspital Basel, Petersgraben 4, CH-4031 Basel, Switzerland

William W. Hofmann, M.D.
Dept. of Neurology, Stanford University, School of Medicine,
300 Pasteur Drive, Palo Alto, CA 94305, USA

Reinhard Hohlfeld, M.D.
Neurologische Klinik, Klinikum Großhadern, Marchioninistr. 15,
D-81377 München 15, Germany

Volker Hömberg, M.D.
Neurologisches Therapiezentrum, Heinrich-Heine Universität,
Hohensandweg 37, D-40591 Düsseldorf, Germany

Manfred Hörmann, M.D.
Karlsplatz 3/V, D-81377 München, Germany

Ernst F. Hund, M.D.
Neurologische Univ.-Klinik, Im Neuenheimer Feld 400,
D-69120 Heidelberg, Germany

Martin Hutschenreuter, M.D.
Schmiedgasse 1, D-94065 Waldkirchen, Germany

Rudolf W. Ch. Janzen, M.D.
Neurologische Klinik, Krankenhaus Nordwest,
Steinbacher Hohl 2-26, D-60488 Frankfurt, Germany

Johannes Jörg, M.D.
Neurologische Klinik, Klinikum Barmen, Heusnerstr. 40,
D-42283 Wuppertal, Germany

Robert W. Katz, M.D.
Department of Veterans Affairs, Medical Center,
2100 Ridgecrest Drive SE, Albuquerque, NM 87108, USA

Detlef Kömpf, M.D.
Neurologische Univ.-Klinik, Ratzeburger Allee 160,
D-23562 Lübeck, Germany

Paul Kremer, M.D.
Neurochirurgische Univ.-Klinik, Im Neuenheimer Feld 400,
D-69120 Heidelberg, Germany

Derk Krieger, M.D.
Neurologische Univ.-Klinik, Im Neuenheimer Feld 400,
D-69120 Heidelberg, Germany

Rüdiger von Kummer, M.D.
Abt. Neuroradiologie, Neurologische Univ.-Klinik,
Im Neuenheimer Feld 400, D-69120 Heidelberg, Germany

Ralph W. Kuncl, M.D.
Associate Professor, Johns Hopkins Medical Institutions,
Dept. of Neurology, Meyer 5-119, 600 North Wolfe Street,
Baltimore, MD 21205, USA

Klaus Kunze, M.D.
Neurologische Univ.-Klinik Eppendorf, Martinistr. 52,
D-20251 Hamburg-Eppendorf 20, Germany

Ellen S. Lathi, M.D.
St. Elizabeth's Hospital, Division of Neurology,
736 Cambridge Street, Boston, MA 02135, USA

Frank Lehmann-Hom, M.D.
Abt. f. Angewandte Physiologie, Universität Ulm,
Albert-Einstein-Allee 11, D-89081 Ulm, Germany

Ronald B. Lesser, M.D.
Johns Hopkins Medical Institutions, Dept. of Neurology,
Meyer 1-130, 600 North Wolfe Street, Baltimore, MD 21205, USA

Judith Ski Lower, RN, MSN, CCRN, CNRN
Nurse Manager, Neurosciences Critical Care Unit, Johns Hopkins
Hospital, 600 North Wolfe Street, Baltimore, MD 21287-7700, USA

Ken Marek, M.D., Ph.D.
Assistant Professor of Neurology, Yale University School of
Medicine, 333 Cedar Street,
New Haven, CT 06511, USA

Luis Marsano, M.D.
Johns Hopkins Medical Institutions, GI Division, Ross Building,
Rm 918, 1830 Monument Street, Baltimore, MD 21205, USA

Eike Martin, M.D.
Anaesthesiologische Univ.-Klinik Heidelberg,
Im Neuenheimer Feld 110, D-69120 Heidelberg, Germany

Karl-Heinz Mauritz, M.D.
Klinik Berlin, Neurologische Rehabilitation, Kladower Damm 221,
D-14089 Berlin, Germany

Hans-Michael Meinck, M.D.
Neurologische Univ.-Klinik, Im Neuenheimer Feld 400,
D-69120 Heidelberg, Germany

Uta Meyding-Lamadé, M.D.
Neurologische Univ.-Klinik, Im Neuenheimer Feld 400,
D-69120 Heidelberg, Germany

Neil R. Miller, M.D.
Johns Hopkins Medical Institutions, Dept. of Opthalmology, B107
Maumenee, 600 North Wolfe Street, Baltimore, MD 21205, USA

Laurie Moore, M.D.
Johns Hopkins University, Meyer 8-139, 600 North Wolfe Street,
Baltimore, MA 21205, USA

Patricia M. Moore, M.D.
Dept. of Neurology, 4201 St. Anotine, University Health Center 6E,
Detroit, MI 48201, USA

Wolfgang Müllges, M.D.
Neurologische Univ.-Klinik, Josef-Schneider-Str. 22,
D-97080 Würzburg, Germany

Marc Nuwer, M.D.
University of California at Los Angeles, Reed Neurological Research
Center, 710 Westwood Plaza, Los Angeles, CA 90024, USA

Wolfgang Oertel, M.D.
Neurologische Klinik, Klinikum Großhadern, Marchioninistr. 15,
D-81377 München, Germany

Wolfgang Pankl, M.D.
Neurolog. Abteilung, Klinikum Rosenhü gel, A-1130 Wien, Austria

Shreyas V. Patel, M.D.
St. Elizabeth's Hospital, Division of Neurology,
736 Cambridge Street, Boston, MA 02135, USA

Michael S. Pessin, M.D.
Dept. of Neurology, Tufts-New England Medical Ctr.,
750 Washington Street, Boston, MA 02111, USA

Hans Walter Pfister, M.D.
Neurologische Klinik, Klinikum Großhadern, Marchioninistr. 15,
D-81377 München, Germany

Jürgen Piek, M.D.
Neurochirurgische Klinik, Ernst-Moritz-Arndt Universität
Greifswald, Fleischmannstrasse, Bettenhaus 1, Ebene 5,
D-17487 Greifswald, Germany

Klaus Poeck, M.D.
Königstr. 73, D-53115 Bonn, Germany

Werner Poewe, M.D.
Universitätsklinikum Rudolf Virchow, Abt. für Neurologie,
Augustenburger Platz 1, D-13353 Berlin, Germany

Hilmar Prange, M.D.
Neurologische Univ.-Klinik, Robert Koch Str. 40,
D-37075 Göttingen, Germany

C. George Ray, M.D.
Member, Fred Hutchinson Cancer Research Center, Director,
Diagnostic Virology Laboratory, Professor of Pathobiology,
University of Washington, 1124 Columbia Street, Seattle,
WA 98104-2092, USA

Alex Razumovsky, Ph.D.
Research Assoc., Johns Hopkins Medical Institutions, Head,
Neurocirculatory Physiology Lab, Meyer 841,
600 North Wolfe Street, Baltimore, MD 21205, USA

Klaus Rieke, M.D.
Neurologische Univ.-Klinik, Im Neuenheimer Feld 400,
D-69120 Heidelberg, Germany

Erick Bernd Ringelstein, M.D.
Neurologische Univ.-Klinik Münster, Albert-Schweitzer-Str. 33,
D-48149 Münster, Germany

Ulrich Roelcke, M.D.
Paul Scherrer Institut, Med. PET, CH-5232 Villingen PSI,
Switzerland

Karen L. Roos, M.D.
Dept. of Neurology, Indiana University, Indianapolis, IN, USA

Allan H. Ropper, M.D.
Dept. of Neurology, St. Elizabeth's Hospital, Dept. of Neurology,
32 Fruit Street, Boston, MA 02114, USA

Friedrich von Rosen, M.D.
Innenstadt Klinik, Psychiatrische Abteilung, Nußbaumstr. 7,
D-80336 München, Germany

Walter Royal, M.D.
Johns Hopkins Hospital, Dept. of Neurology, 600 North Wolfe
Street, Meyer 6-109, Baltimore, MD 21205-9977, USA

Martin Schabet, M.D.
Neurologische Univ.-Klinik, Hoppe-Seyler-Str. 3,
D-72076 Tübingen, Germany

G. Schmitz-Schackert, M.D.
Neurochirurgische Universitätsklinik, Technische Universität,
Fetscherstr. 74, D-01307 Dresden, Germany

Mark S. Schnitzer, M.D.
Johns Hopkins Medical Institution, Dept. of Neurology,
Meyer 8-139, 600 North Wolfe Street, Baltimore, MD 21205, USA

Volker Schuchardt, M.D.
Neurologische Univ.-Klinik, Im Neuenheimer Feld 400,
D-69120 Heidelberg, Germany

Tricia Schultz, MS, RD, LD
Dept. of Nutrition, CMSC B-100cal Care Unit, Johns Hopkins
Hospital, 600 North Wolfe Street, Baltimore, MD 21287-3051, USA

Erich Schmutzhard, M.D.
Neurologische Univ.-Klinik, Anichstr. 35, A-6020 Innsbruck,
Austria

Hans-Peter Schuster, M.D.
Medizinische Klinik I, Städt. Krankenhaus Hildesheim, Weinberg 1,
D-31134 Hildesheim, Germany

Hansgeorg Schultz
Neurologische Klinik, Am Städt. Klinikum Frankfurt-Hoechst,
Gotenstr. 6-8, D-65929 Frankfurt-Hoechst, Germany

Stefan Schwab, M.D.
Neurologische Univ.-Klinik, Im Neuenheimer Feld 400,
D-69120 Heidelberg, Germany

Birgit Sköldenberg, M.D.
Associate Professor of Infection Diseases, Institution of Infectious
Diseases, Karolinska Institute at Danderyd Hospital, Stockholm,
Sweden

Klaus Spitzer, M.D.
Abteilung für Medizinische Informatik, Universität Heidelberg,
Im Neuenheimer Feld 400, D-69120 Heidelberg, Germany

Matthias Spranger, M.D.
Neurologische Univ.-Klinik, Im Neuenheimer Feld 400,
D-69120 Heidelberg, Germany

Hermann Stefan, M.D.
Neurologische Univ.-Klinik, Schwabachanlage 6,
D-91054 Erlangen, Germany

Hans-Herbert Steiner, M.D.
Neurochirurgische Univ.-Klinik, Im Neuenheimer Feld 400,
D-69120 Heidelberg, Germany

Thorsten Steiner, M.D.
Klinikum der Univ. Heidelberg, Neurologische Klinik, Im
Neuenheimer Feld 400, D-69120 Heidelberg, Germany

Robert Stingele, M.D.
Dept. of Neurology, Johns Hopkins Hospital,
600 North Wolfe Street, Baltimore, MD 21287, USA

Brigitte Storch-Hagenlocher, M.D.
Neurologische Univ.-Klinik, Im Neuenheimer Feld 400,
D-69120 Heidelberg, Germany

Frank Tiecks, M.D.
Neurologische Klinik, Klinikum Großhadern, Marchioninistr. 15,
D-81377 München, Germany

Klaus V. Toyka, M.D.
Neurologische Univ.-Klinik, Josef-Schneider-Str. 11,
D-97080 Würzburg, Germany

Ronald J. Tusa, M.D., Ph.D.
Johns Hopkins Medical Institution, Dept. of Neurology, Meyer 2-
147, 600 North Wolfe Street, Baltimore, MD 21205, USA

John A. Ulatowski, M.D.
Johns Hopkins Medical Institutions, Dept. of Anesthesiology/
Critical Care Medicine, Meyer 8-134A, 600 North Wolfe Street,
Baltimore, MD 21205, USA

Klaus Unertl, M.D.
Neurologische Univ.-Klinik, Klinikum Großhadern, Marchioninistr.
15, D-81377 München, Germany

Philip A. Villanueva, M.D.
Dept. of Neurological Surgery, Director Neurosurgical Intensive
Care, University of Miami, Dept. of Neurological Surgery D4-6,
1501 N.W. 9th Ave., Miami, FL 33136, USA

Arno Villringer, M.D.
Neurologische Klinik, Charité Berlin, Humboldt Universität,
Schumannstrasse, D-10117 Berlin, Germany

Dennis G. Vollmer, M.D.
Washington University School of Medicine, Dept. of Neurology and
Neurological Surgery, Box 8057, 660 South Euclid Avenue,
St. Louis, MO 63110, USA

Karin Weißenborn, M.D.
Medizinische Hochschule, Konstanty-Gutschow-Str. 8,
D-30625 Hannover, Germany

Christian Werner, M.D.
Anästhesiologische Universitätsklinik, Martinistrasse,
D-20251 Hamburg, Germany

Brigitte Wildemann, M.D.
Neurologische Univ.-Klinik, Im Neuenheimer Feld 400,
D-69120 Heidelberg, Germany

Christian Wüster, M.D.
Abt. Endokrinologie, Ludolf-Krehl-Klinik, Bergheimer Str. 56,
D-69115 Heidelberg, Germany

G. Bryan Young, MD, FRCPC
Victoria Hospital, Dept. of Clinical Neurological Sciences,
375 South Street, London-Ontario, Canada N6A 4G5

Josef F. Zander, M.D.
Abt. für Anaesthesie, Univ.-Klinikum Münster,
Albert-Schweitzer-Str. 33, D-48149 Münster, Germany

Rainer Zimmermann, M.D.
Stiftung Rehabilitation, Bonhoeffer Strasse,
D-69123 Heidelberg-Wieblingen, Germany

Gregory J. del Zoppo, M.D.
Department of Molecular and Experimental Medicine, The Scripps
Research Institute, 10666 North Torrey Pines Road, La Jolla,
CA 92037, USA

Part I
General Approaches to Neurocritical Care

Intensive Care and Monitoring

Chapter 1

General Assessment and Care of the New Patient

KLAUS RIEKE, JOHN A. ULATOWSKI, and WERNER HACKE

Introduction

Advances in the diagnosis and treatment of neurological disease have recently led to a dramatic increase in neurocritical care units. As most patients with acute life-threatening neurological diseases have systemic disease, the critical care unit facilitates an interdisciplinary approach to patient care that involves neurology, neurosurgery, anesthesiology, and internal medicine. Patients should receive neurocritical care if they have signs of increased intracranial pressure, coma, or neurological disease associated with respiratory or cardiovascular failure. Other patients who may benefit from neurocritical care include those with subarachnoid hemorrhage (all grades), space-occupying hemorrhage or stroke, meningitis, encephalitis, status epilepticus, and progressive muscular weakness (especially involving the respiratory muscles; Table 1). Patients receiving

Section Editors: Karl M. Einhäupl and Werner Hacke

thrombolytic therapy and plasmapheresis or those undergoing interventional neuroradiological procedures may also benefit from neurocritical care (high- or low-acuity monitoring).

Patients with less acute disease that is not life-threatening (for example, those with instability of only one organ system) should be admitted to intermediate care units ("step down units") where they can be closely observed and transferred to the neurocritical care unit if necessary. Ideally, the two units should be located close to one another. In some centers, patients with head injuries are admitted to neurocritical care units, but more often they are treated in neurosurgical units or trauma units.

Initial Treatment of Patients in the Neurocritical Care Unit

On admission, a brief but accurate history should be elicited from patients or their relatives. This history should focus on both disease onset and progression (acute or chronic), as well as the presence of trauma, headache,

Table 1. Signs and conditions that indicate treatment or observation in a neurocritical care unit

Increased intracranial pressure
Coma, reduced level of consciousness
Cardiopulmonary and respiratory failure
Subarachnoid hemorrhage (all grades)
Space-occupying cerebellar hemorrhage or stroke
Space-occupying cerebral hemorrhage or stroke
Progressive stroke
Meningitis (bacterial meningitis)
Encephalitis (especially herpetic encephalitis)
Status epilepticus, intractable series of seizures
Progressive weakness of the extremities with involvement of respiratory muscles

Manipulation of the cerebral vessels (interventional neuroradiology)
Aggressive neurological treatment (thrombolysis, plasma exchange, immunosuppression)

Head injuries

seizures, neurological deficits, vascular risk factors (diabetes mellitus, hypertension), and history of cardiovascular disease. A thorough drug history should also be elicited. The initial neurological examination should focus on the level of consciousness (specifically, the stimulus necessary to elicit a response, such as voice, light touch, pain, and so on), pupil size and response to light, and reflexes. Whenever possible, patients should be examined before sedatives or neuromuscular blocking drugs are given.

Respiratory status should be evaluated in all patients, especially in those with unprotected airways. Oxygenation can be assessed noninvasively by pulse oximetry or invasively by arterial blood gas analysis. Ventilation can be assessed by measuring forced vital capacity (FVC), and negative inspiratory force (NIF).

These measurements can be helpful in both the acute setting and for monitoring disease. Patients require assisted ventilation if $PO_2 \leq 50$ mmHg, $PCO_2 \geq 50$ mmHg, FVC <15 ml/kg body weight, and NIF ≤ -20 mmHg. Those with impaired function of caudal cranial nerves may also need to be intubated (see Chap. 2). Cardiovascular status can be monitored with frequent blood pressure and heart rate measurements.

Adequate end organ perfusion is the primary goal of resuscitation in critical care. Cerebral perfusion pressure (CPP), the difference between mean arterial pressure and intracranial pressure, should be kept ≥ 50 mmHg (the usual lower limit of autoregulation). In patients with hypotension, volume status should be assessed immediately (invasive monitoring of central venous pressure or pulmonary capillary wedge pressure may be indicated). Plasma expanders, such as normal saline, serum protein fractions, or Hetastarch, should be given if hypovolemia is present (blood products can be used instead of plasma expanders in those with anemia or coagulopathy). If hypotension persists despite fluid challenge, treatment with vasopressor drugs should be started while the underlying cause of hypotension is determined (that is, low cardiac output versus low systemic resistance). Initially, dopamine, a vasoconstrictor and inotropic agent (dosage 5–20 μg/kg per minute) or dobutamine, a potent inotropic agent (dosage 5–10 μg/kg per minute) is usually used. Although both are β-1 agonists, dobutamine also has β-2 agonist properties and can provide some afterload reduction. Phenylephrine, a direct α-agonist, may be especially useful in patients with low systemic resistance but normal cardiac output, e.g., patients with septic shock or end-stage liver disease (dosage 10–60 μg/kg per minute). Catecholamines, because of their potent inotropic properties, are beneficial to those with low cardiac output. Central venous access and invasive arterial blood pressure monitoring are recommended in patients with cardiovascular instability and in those requiring vasopressor drugs (see Chap. 2).

Patients with increased intracranial pressure may develop reflex bradycardia (sinus bradycardia, junctional rhythm, or heart block), hypertension, or both. Often, treatment of the underlying increased intracranial pressure is sufficient to control dysrythmias and hypertension. In general, patients with sinus bradycardia, junctional rhythm, or Möbitz type I AV [Atrioventricular] block who are symptomatic (hypotensive) should be treated with atropine (0.5–1.0 mg in adults, 20 μg/kg in children). The dose can be repeated every 5 min until a total of 2 mg in adults or 1 mg in children has been reached. Patients refractory to atropine should be treated with a tempory pacemaker or isoproterenol infusion (2–10 μg/kg per minute in adults, 0.1–0.2 μg/kg per minute in children). Patients with Möbitz type II or third degree AV block require a pacemaker regardless of symptoms. Patients with severe ischemic stroke may benefit from treatment of bradycardia earlier to improve cerebral perfusion.

Because rapid reduction of blood pressure can aggravate cerebral ischemia, pharmacological treatment, when deemed necessary, should be carried out cautiously so that the CPP is maintained at or above 50 mmHg. In most patients, blood pressure should be decreased initially to 160 ± 10 mmHg (MAP < 120 mmHg). In the presence of intracerebral hemorrhage, blood pressure should be maintained in the normal range (systolic blood pressure 100–140 mmHg, MAP < 100 mmHg). Treatment of hypertension can be difficult in patients with acute ischemic stroke (see Chap. 56). In general, direct vasodilators should be avoided because of the risk of increasing cerebral blood flow and making intracranial hypertension worse. However, hydralazine (2–20 mg) and sodium nitoprusside (0.5–8 μg/kg per minute) may be used if intracranial pressure is closely monitored or if the dura has been opened and intracranial pressure can be controlled. The preferred drugs for treatment of hypertension in patients with acute stroke are β-blockers (esmolol HCl, metoprolol tartrate, propranolol HCl), α-blockers (clonidine HCl, methyldopa, phentolamine mesylate, urapidil), mixed α- and β-blockers (labetalol HCl), and calcium channel blockers (nifedipine and verapamil HCl).

After stabilization of airway, breathing, and circulation, all patients presenting with decreased levels of consciousness should first have blood samples taken for determination of glucose concentration and should then be given a bolus of 50–100 ml 20%–40% glucose solution. Thiamine (50–100 mg) should always be given simultaneously because of the risk of precipitating Wernicke's encephalopathy in thiamine-deficient patients. Blood and urine should be analyzed for drugs. Patients with suspected narcotic overdoses should be given naloxone in divided doses (0.4–2 mg initially, 10 mg total). This should be done cautiously in those with known cardiovascular disease because the reversal of narcotic effects may worsen cardiac ischemia. All patients with signs of increased intracranial pressure or deteriorating clinical condition should be treated immediately.

Trauma should always be considered in patients presenting with decreased levels of consciousness. A firm cervical collar should be used until cervical X-rays exclude a fracture or dislocation. The possibility of an intracranial mass or an extracranial surgical condition should also be considered. Further diagnostic studies, such as computed tomographic scanning, should be done after basic vital functions have been stabilized.

Initial Neurological Examination of Alert Patients

The initial neurological examination should be brief and focused and is important primarily for triaging patients. A more complete examination can be done later and is important as a reference for other health care workers and consultants and as a baseline for future reference. In patients who are alert and awake, the initial examination does not differ from the routine examination and includes a detailed mental status exam, testing of cranial nerves, reflexes, motor and sensory function, and co-ordination. In patients with depressed consciousness, observation and elicitable neurological signs play a greater role. The Glasgow Coma Scale (GCS) is a common and simple scale that can be used in the early evaluation of comatose patients.

Consciousness can be depressed as a result of bilateral hemispheric dysfunction or brainstem dysfunction. Meningismus may be seen in those with meningitis, meningoencephalitis, and subdural and subarachnoid hemorrhages (patients with cervical trauma can also have meningismus). In severe cases, patients may have hyperextension of head and back (opisthotonus). Other signs of a generalized cerebral process include generalized seizures, myoclonus, asterixis, confusion, disturbances of mood, and perseveration. It is important not to miss focal signs, such as aphasia, in these patients. Abnormal posturing of the extremities usually indicates functional or structural damage to the brainstem.

The presence of focal signs is important when determining an anatomical diagnosis. For example, a language deficit suggests damage to the dominant hemisphere. Hemianopsia suggests damage to the contralateral hemisphere. Eye or head deviation may suggest either a focal hemispheric lesion or a brainstem lesion. A flaccid, externally rotated leg, fisted arm, and unilateral hyperreflexia suggest hemiparesis. Focal motor or sensory seizures have the same anatomical value. Loss of sensory functions (stereoagnosis, two-point discrimination, graphesthesia, topographical localization, double simultaneous stimulation) on one side suggest a lesion in the contralateral parietal cortex. Focal signs in comatose patients with trauma usually indicate a surgically correctable lesion.

Mental Status Exam

Many terms can be used to describe patients with decreased levels of consciousness, but for simplicity we use the following four descriptions: (1) *Alert* patients are awake and oriented with their eyes open, though they are sometimes sleepy. They respond normally when spoken to. (2) *Somnolent* patients are sleepy and often have difficulty keeping their eyes open. They usually respond to a loud voice or a gentle shake. Spontaneous speech is decreased and concentration and attention are usually poor (the term "lethargy" is often used in the US for this level, whereas "somnolence" is more commonly used in Europe). (3) *Stuporous* patients do not respond when called and require vigorous physical stimulation to arouse. They have no spontaneous speech. Focal neurological signs may be present. (4) *Comatose* patients cannot be aroused by voice or physical stimulation. Deep pain may elicit only movements of the extremities. Abnormal movements, such as extensor (decerebrate) or flexor (decorticate) posturing, and cranial nerve abnormalities are common.

Plum and Posner conceptualized depression of consciousness secondary to supratentorial lesions as a continuum of dysfunction beginning in the diencephalon and progressing to the midbrain (mesencephalon), pons, and medulla. Patients with diencephalic dysfunction typically are lethargic or stuporous and have Cheyne-Stokes breathing patterns. Pupil function and eye movements are normal. Motor response to pain includes withdrawal and flexor posturing. Coma is usually still reversible at this point.

Patients with midbrain dysfunction have central hyperventilation and fixed pupils. The oculocephalic reflex ("doll's eyes") remains intact as long as the oculomotor nerve (third cranial nerve) and nucleus are spared. The oculovestibular reflex ("cold calorics") also remains intact. Extensor posturing to pain occurs when the red nucleus is damaged, though some patients may show extensor posturing spontaneously when mesencephalic dysfunction is severe. Patients with pontine and upper medullary dysfunction have loss of oculocephalic and oculovestibular reflexes and have flaccid motor tone or only triple flexion responses in the legs on stimulation. The medullary stage is also marked by loss of remaining brainstem functions, that is, patients initially have deep gasping (agonal) respirations, hypotension, dysrhythmias, and ultimately apnea and asystole. A detailed description of different levels consciousness may be found in Chap. 24.

Mental functions attributed to global cerebral processes include orientation, attention, memory, reasoning, and judgement. Patients with acute confusion or delirium have deficits of these mental functions and often require neurocritical care because of serious underlying medical conditions. Dementia generally develops gradually and patients rarely require neurocritical care. Focal lesions, such as those causing dysphasia, dyslexia, and hemianopsia, can also result in abnormal mental function (for example, because of difficulty communicating). Focal lesions are helpful when determining an anatomical diagnosis.

Cranial Nerves

Patients with lesions in the inferior frontal lobes or floor of the frontal fossa may present with anosmia. The *olfactory nerve* (first cranial nerve) can be tested with a variety of aromas. Although irritating vapors, such as ammonia, may be used as a stimulus for arousal, they may also stimulate the trigeminal nerve and should not be used simply for olfactory nerve testing. The *optic nerve* (second cranial nerve) can be tested by assessing visual acuity, visual fields, pupillary response to light (afferent component), and by direct observation with ophthalmoscopy. Visual acuity can be measured with a miniature Snellen chart printed on a card (refractive error can be eliminated by having patients look through a pin hole). Visual fields can be tested by confrontation, using the examiner's visual fields for comparison or by visual threat in patients with impaired consciousness. Direct observation of the optic nerve with ophthalmoscopy may reveal specific diseases, such as vascular or inflammatory diseases, or signs of increased intracranial pressure (papilledema). *The pupils should never be pharmacologically dilated in patients with impaired consciousness since further observation of pupil size and response to light is then hindered.*

The pupillary response to light should generally be assessed as part of the evaluation of intrinsic eye muscles. To distinguish asymmetries, pupils should be examined individually (direct light reflex) and then together (consensual light reflex). Pupil size is determined by the tonic input of two opposing systems: constriction is mediated by the parasympathetic nervous system and dilatation is mediated by the sympathetic nervous system. Axons of the retinal ganglion cell, running in the optic nerve and optic tract, synapse in the pretectal nucleus of the midbrain. From there, nerve fibers synapse in the Edinger-Westphal nucleus and run in the oculomotor nerve (third cranial nerve) to the ciliary ganglion. Short ciliary nerves innervate the iris sphincter muscles. Pupils constrict in response to light and convergence. Failure of pupils to constrict in response to light may be caused by either an afferent defect or an efferent defect. Lesions of the optic nerve cause afferent defects; neither pupil constricts when light is shown in the abnormal eye (since impulses from the retina are not carried to the pretectal nucleus, i.e., the direct light reflex is impaired), while both pupils constrict when light is shown in the normal eye (since the afferent limb from that eye and the efferent limb to both eyes are functioning, i.e., the consensual light reflex is normal). Lesions of the oculomotor nerve cause efferent defects; the abnormal eye constricts neither when light is shown in it nor when light is shown in the normal eye (since, although impulses are carried to the pretectal nucleus, they cannot be projected back out to the iris sphinctor muscles, i.e., both direct and consensual light reflexes are impaired). An abnormally dilated eye indicates injury to the oculomotor nucleus or nerve in the brainstem or inhibition of the normal neuromuscular transmission at the iris.

Pupillary dilatation is controlled by the sympathetic nervous system. Sympathetic neurons descend from the hypothalamus (down the neuraxis) to the thoracic cord where they join the peripheral sympathetic chain. They follow the internal carotid artery into the cavernous sinus and enter the orbit as the long ciliary nerve. A variety of stimuli can affect the central sympathetic nervous system. Alternatively, peripheral autonomic reflexes bypass the brainstem (ciliospinal reflex). For example, an afferent stimulus (such as pain in the face, neck, or shoulder) is carried to the peripheral sympathetic chain in the spinal cord. The reflex arc is completed with the efferent response causing pupillary dilatation (usually ipsilaterally, occasionally bilaterally in drowsy or stuporous patients). Damage to the central sympathetic pathway causes ipsilateral miosis, ptosis, and anhydrosis of the face (Horner's syndrome). Miosis and ptosis without anhydrosis likely indicate a peripheral lesion (of the postganglionic fibers) distal to the bifurcation of the common carotid artery. Pharmacological tests may be needed to distinguish between central (preganglionic) and peripheral (postganglionic) lesions. With central lesions, neither the normal nor the Horner pupil dilates with instillation of epinephrine 1:1000; however, both pupils dilate with instillation of cocaine 4%. With peripheral lesions, only the Horner pupil dilates to epinephrine and only the normal pupil dilates to cocaine. Miotic pupils should always be examined in a dimly lit room with a magnifying glass.

Limitation of eye movements may be caused by lesions in the cortical or brainstem gaze centers, cranial nerves or nuclei, neuromuscular junction, or by local muscle entrapment or dysfunction. Examination of extrinsic eye muscles individually and in each eye aids in determining the anatomical diagnosis. The lateral rectus muscle, innervated by the *abducens nerve* (sixth cranial nerve), abducts the eye and the medial rectus muscle, innervated by the *Oculomotor* (third cranial nerve), adducts the eye. When the eye is abducted, the superior rectus muscle is the strongest elevator and the inferior rectus muscle is the strongest depressor. When the eye is adducted, the inferior oblique muscle is the strongest elevator and the superior oblique muscle is the strongest depressor. The oculomotor nerve (third cranial nerve) innervates the superior rectus, inferior rectus, and inferior oblique muscles as well as the eyelid levator muscle. The trochlear nerve innervates the superior oblique muscle. Diplopia is the most common complaint of patients with isolated ocular muscle weakness.

In general, oculomotor dysfunction without associated cerebral, brainstem, or sensorimotor long tract signs usually indicates an isolated cranial nerve or nuclear lesion or an abnormality of the peripheral components controlling eye movements. Local trauma or entrapment can be deduced from forced movements of the eye within the orbit. The examination of eye movements gives information about visual, acoustic, cerebellar, and sensory pathways. The assessment of the oculomotor system begins by observing the spontaneous position of the eyes (normally conjugate). Awake patients are asked to move their eyes in all directions of gaze, which tests ocular muscles, slow smooth pursuit movements (of a target), and quick saccadic movements (between targets). The stimulus for conjugate eye movements begins in the cortex and travels to the brainstem gaze centers via the corticobulbar tracts. The brainstem center for horizontal gaze is the pontine paramedian reticular formation (PPRF) and the brainstem center for vertical gaze is the rostral interstitial nucleus of the medial longitudinal fasiculus (riMLF). Eye movements are connected by the medial longitudinal fasiculus (MLF) within the brainstem. If the cortical gaze center is damaged (for example, in patients with hemispheric strokes), input to the contralateral PPRF is decreased. The normal tonic input that draws the eyes to that side is lost and the eyes are pulled to the other side by the other PPRF (that is, to the same side as the stroke). If the cortical gaze center is activated (for example, in patients with a seizure focus), input to the contralateral PPRF is increased and the eyes are tonically pulled to that side (that is, to opposite the side of the seizure focus). In patients with coma from bilateral lesions, the eyes maintain their conjugate orientation either in neutral gaze or in roving lateral movements. Normally, the conjugate position of the eyes may be lost during sleep but is quickly regained once arousal occurs.

The brainstem gaze centers also receive information from the labyrinths which allows the eyes to remain fixed on a target despite head movements. This can be supressed by the cortex. In comatose patients, brainstem and cranial nerve integrity can be assessed with the oculocephalic and vestibulo ocular reflexes. The oculocephalic reflex can be elicited by rotating the head horizontally and vertically. Normally, the eyes remain conjugate and fixed on some point in the environment (teleologically, on some danger). This indicates intact cranial nerve innervation to the eyes and communication between cranial nerve nuclei in the brainstem. The test should not be performed if there is a possibility of cervical trauma. To elicit the vestibulo ocular reflex, patients should be positioned at 30° head elevation and more potent stimulus to the vestibular apparatus – cold water or air – is introduced to the external auditory canal. The cold stimulus sets up convection currents in the lateral semicircular canal that go away from the cupola, thereby inhibiting it. The contralateral semicircular canal then pushes the eyes toward the cold stimulus. In an awake person, there is a corrective jerk, controlled by the cortex, in the opposite direction to keep the eyes in the direction willed by the person. The initial deviation is referred to as the slow component of nystagmus and the corrective jerk is referred to as the fast component. In comatose patients (from cortical lesions), this corrective jerk is lost and the eyes remain deviated to the side of the cold stimulus. The test should be repeated in the other ear if the response is unclear. Lesions affecting the abducens nucleus or PPRF cause local interruption of transmission from higher cortical centers or the vestibular apparatus and result in conjugate gaze away from the lesion. A more cephalic lesion in the brainstem, involving the riMLF, oculomotor nucleus, or dorasal midbrain (Parinaud's syndrome), results in conjugate upgaze paralysis.

Dysconjugate gaze may occur from lesions in the peripheral components of the oculomotor apparatus (cranial nerve, neuromuscular junction, or muscle) or lesions in the brainstem including the cranial nuclei and the pathways connecting them. The anatomical differential diagnosis is narrowed by looking for associated signs elsewhere in the nervous system. Examining each eye individually helps determine whether a monocular or binocular problem (brainstem lesion) is present. Patients with dysconjugate gaze as a result of an oculomotor nerve lesion usually have ptosis and pupillary dysfunction. Patients with an oculomotor nuclear lesion present with bilateral oculomotor signs or associated brainstem dysfunction and long tract signs. Skew deviation is usually a result of lesions in the brainstem (pons) and is dysconjugate gaze in the vertical plane. In contrast to cranial nerve palsies, skew deviation occurs in all directions of gaze (albeit variably).

Unilateral injury to the MLF causes internuclear ophthalmoplegia (INO) secondary to interruption of the connecting mechanism between the abducens nucleus on one side and the oculomotor nucleus on the other. The stimulus for lateral gaze arrives at the pons first (abducens nucleus), then travels across the brainstem to ascend in the contralateral MLF to the oculomotor nucleus. This pathway allows simultaneous stimulation of the lateral rectus muscle and the contralateral medial rectus muscle to result in lateral conjugate gaze. If the PPRF and abducens nucleus are intact, abduction of the eye is normal. An MLF lesion, however, prevents the stimulus from reaching the oculomotor nucleus. Therefore, INO appears as if the patient has an isolated medial rectal palsy on the side of the adducting eye. Nystagmus in the abducting eye is a common concurrent finding. A lesion in the rostral MLF (near the midbrain convergence center) causes INO associated with inability to converge. A lesion in the caudal MLF (pons) usually spares convergence (a finding that also excludes a medial rectus palsy).

The *trigeminal nerve* (fifth cranial nerve) motor function is tested by having patients open (pterygoid muscle) and close (masseter and temporalis muscles) their jaws. Sensory innervation of the face and mouth is also carried by the trigeminal nerve: the ophthalmic division (cranial nerve V_1) over the forehead and cornea, the maxillary division (V_2) over the cheek and upper lip, and the mandibular division (V_3) over the jaw and mentum (sparing the angle of the jaw). Because these divisions converge from a wide area of distribution to form the gasserian ganglion, each may be injured individually (for example, V_1 in the superior orbital fissure or the cavernous sinus). The trigeminal nerve can be tested in comatose patients by eliciting the jaw jerk reflex. Increased masseter tone (trismus) is a sign of tetanus. The *facial nerve* (seventh cranial nerve) innervates all facial muscles controlling the furrowing of the brow, eye closure, grimacing, and smiling. Because both sides of the brain control the forehead muscles, only a peripheral lesion (nuclear or distal) can paralyze the entire face on one side. A unilateral supranuclear lesion results in contralateral lower facial muscle paralysis. Because the facial nerve carries other fibers, facial nerve lesions may be associated with loss of hearing and taste or hyperacusis. The corneal reflex can be elicited by touching the cornea with a wisp of cotton. Normally, there is a brisk, ipsilateral closure of the eyelid (contraction of the periorbital muscle). It is a useful test in coma because, if present, it verifies function of two cranial nerves and the brainstem between their nuclei (trigeminal nerve for the efferent component). Patients with peripheral facial nerve lesions may have diminished or absent corneal reflexes. The reflex should be elicited and compared bilaterally.

Injury to the *acoustic nerve* (eighth cranial nerve) results in decreased hearing and dysequilibrium. The Weber and Rinne tests, bedside tests for examination of hearing, are generally crude and of little benefit for patients in a neurocritical care setting. Formal audiometry and evoked potentials are generally recommended. In awake patients, vestibular function can be evaluated with provocative testing on a tilt table, in a Barany chair, or with electronystagmography. These tests are usually not applicable to patients in the neurocritical care unit. Distinguishing between nystagmus of peripheral (labyrinthine) or central origin (brainstem or cerebellum) is sometimes difficult. Upbeat or downbeat nystagmus (especially in neutral gaze) and coarse or pendular horizontal nystagmus usually indicate a central lesion. Fine horizontal nystagmus may be either peripheral or central in origin. In general, nystagmus that is peripheral in origin is fatigable upon repeat motion, can be overridden by willful fixation on an object, and occurs in the same direction even when the eyes are moved in a variety of directions. Nystagmus from a peripheral lesion (labyrinth) is greatest when looking away from the lesion and that from a central lesion (cerebellum) is greatest when looking towards the lesion. Opticokinetic nystagmus allows one to count a series of objects passing rapidly across the visual field. It is normal in awake individuals. Eliciting opticokinetic nystagmus tests several anatomical areas of visual function including recognition, tracking, and saccadic conjugate eye movements. Testing vestibular function in coma has been described with eye movements.

The *glossopharyngeal nerve* (ninth cranial nerve) provides taste from the posterior tongue and touch from the pharynx to the level of the glottis. The *vagus nerve* (tenth cranial nerve), in addition to being the major effector of the parasympathetic nervous system in the chest and abdomen, provides motor control of the soft palate, pharynx, and esophagus and sensory innervation to the airway below the glottis. The afferent component of the gag reflex is carried by the glossopharyngeal nerve and the efferent component is carried by the vagus nerve (which also carries the afferent component of the cough reflex). The *spinal accessory nerve* (eleventh cranial nerve) innervates the sternocleidomastoid muscle (tested by head rotation or flexion) and trapezius muscle (tested by shoulder elevation). Testing this nerve evaluates the caudal brainstem, peripheral nerve, and muscles, but adds little to the evaluation of cerebral processes. The *hypoglossal nerve* (twelfth cranial nerve) innervates the tongue. Each nerve is responsible for protruding the tongue to the opposite cheek. Testing the hypoglossal nerve evaluates caudal brainstem and cranial nerve function and is important when evaluating patients with lower motor neuron diseases (associated with muscle wasting and fasciculations).

Motor Function

Evaluation of motor function begins by testing pyramidal and extrapyramidal systems and ends with the examination of the muscles. The primary motor neuron, or upper motor neuron, begins in the motor cortex and descends through the cerebral peduncles to synapse with the secondary motor neuron, or lower motor neuron, in the brainstem (cranial nerve nuclei) or spinal cord (anterior horn cells). Motor impulses then travel to the muscles in peripheral nerves (cranial or spinal) along side sensory fibers coming from the periphery. Complex and coordinated movements are modified by the basal ganglia and the cerebellum.

Weakness is the most common complaint and finding in patients with disease of the motor system. Establishing an anatomical differential diagnosis first greatly reduces what sometimes seems like an endless list of possible causes of weakness. Patients with upper motor neuron lesions present with increased muscle tone (spasticity or rigidity), hyperreflexia, and extensor plantar responses (Babinski's sign). These features may not be present early in the course and may be fluctuating. An anatomical diagnosis is facilitated because upper motor neurons are only in the brain, brainstem, and spinal cord. Upper motor neuron type weakness associated with signs of cerebral dysfunction usually indicates a lesion above the foramen magnum. Patients with lower motor neuron lesions present with decreased muscle tone and bulk, hyporeflexia, and flexor plantar responses. Signs of lower motor neuron type weakness place the lesion along the root, plexus, peripheral nerve, or neuromuscular junction. A combination of upper motor neuron type weakness in the arms and legs and lower motor neuron signs, such as a cranial nerve palsy, suggests a lesion in the brainstem at the level of that cranial nerve. Similarly, upper motor nerve signs in the legs and lower motor nerve signs in the arms suggests a lesion at the cervical spinal cord level. Upper motor nerve signs in the legs but normal motor function of the head and arms localize the lesion to the thoracic or lumbar spinal cord level. Therefore, lower motor neuron lesions associated with more caudal upper motor neuron findings are signposts along the rostral-caudal pathway of the primary motor neuron which aid in the diagnosis. Injury to the root, plexus, and nerve is usually associated with sensory findings in the same distribution. Abnormalities of the neuromuscular junction are characterized by motor weakness that fluctuates with repetitive stimulation. In difficult cases, electrodiagnostic studies of the muscles and nerves may be necessary to determine the anatomical diagnosis.

Tendon reflexes are sensitive markers for hemiparesis and radicular lesions and should be assessed in all patients. Although an isolated finding of generally diminished reflexes may not be diagnostic, loss of reflexes over the course of an illness suggests an inflammatory polyneuropathy (Guillain-Barré syndrome). Similarly, progressive paralysis associated with development of hyperreflexia may in-

14   K. Rieke et al.

dicate a mass lesion or transverse myelitis.

Sensory Function

Examination of sensory function may assist in confirming the location of a lesion. However, because of the subjective nature of sensory testing, findings may be misleading or unobtainable in patients with impaired consciousness. Primary sensory modalities of pain, temperature, touch, and vibration may be affected anywhere along the sensory pathway, whereas secondary sensory modalities, such as two-point discrimination, topographical localization, simultaneous stimulation, graphesthesia, and stereoagnosis, are affected only with parietal lobe dysfunction. Patients must be able to perceive primary sensory modalities before they can perceive secondary sensory modalities. A "sensory level," below which there is loss of feeling, is an important anatomical sign of spinal cord injury. Discrete sensory loss in the distribution of a nerve or dermatome may assist in distinguishing between a nerve or root lesion. Sensory abnormalities may help to exclude pure motor processes, such as myopathy, myasthenia gravis, and motor neuron disease.

Assessment of Comatose Patients

A complete neurological examination is not always possible in comatose patients and a short, accurate examination is preferable. The Glasgow Coma Scale (GCS) is a simple screening system that is often used. It is heavily weighted toward motor function. After assessing level of consciousness, neck, muscle tone should be carefully assessed. Meningismus is seen with meningitis, menigoencephalitis, subdural and subarachnoid hemorrhages, and cervical spine trauma. Before movement of the neck, the possibility of trauma to the cervical spine must be excluded.

The examination of cranial nerves in comatose patients is limited. Pupil size and response to light (both directly and consensually) is one of the most significant parts of the examination and should be repeated frequently. Dilated pupils and asymmetries in size or response to light suggest increased intracranial pressure or a mass. *Pharmacological pupillary dilatation should never be done in unconscious patients*. Assessment of eye movements is more difficult in unconscious patients. Brainstem and oculomotor nerve integrity can be tested by eliciting the oculocephalic reflex (in which normally the eyes remain conjugate and seemingly fixed on a point in the environment) and the vestibulo ocular reflex (in which normally the eyes conjugately move toward the side of the cold stimulus). Skew deviation (dysconjugate gaze in the vertical plane) suggests a pontine lesion. In contrast to cranial nerve palsies, skew deviation occurs in all directions of gaze, albeit variably.

The integrity of the trigeminal nerve and facial nerve can be tested by eliciting the corneal reflex. Asymmetrical or absent responses may indicate hemiparesis. The trigeminal nerve can also be tested by eliciting the jaw jerk reflex and the glossopharyngeal and vagus nerves can be tested by eliciting the gag and cough reflexes. Tendon reflexes may be markers for hemiparesis and radicular lesions. Although isolated diminished reflexes may not be diagnostic, loss of reflexes over the course of an illness (especially when combined with rapidly progressive paralysis) suggests an acute inflammatory polyneuropathy (Guillain-Barré syndrome). Progressive paralysis associated with hyperreflexia suggests a mass lesion or transverse myelitis. Unilateral hyperreflexia and extensor plantar responses suggest hemiparesis, though these features may not be present early in the course or may be fluctuating.

Assessment of motor function in comatose patients usually requires observing the response to painful stimuli. For example, using the Glasgow Coma Scale, response to verbal or painful stimuli is described (from best to worst) as obeys, localizes, withdraws, abnormal flexion, abnormal extension, or absent response. Details about evaluation of comatose patients can be found in Chap. 3.

Conclusion

The initial evaluation of critically ill patients requires attention to vital functions and quick assessment of the disease with physical examination and diagnostic tests. An anatomical differential diagnosis together with the course of the disease help narrow the pathological differential diagnosis which may save valuable time spent "chasing zebras."

Suggested Reading

Adams RD, Victor M (eds) (1989) Principles of neurology. McGraw-Hill, New York
Hacke W (eds) (1988) Neurologische Intensivmedizin. Perimed, Erlangen
Leigh RJ, Zee DS (eds) (1991) The neurology of eye movements. Davis, Philadelphia
Margulies S (1987) Everyday doctoring: a new approach to the logic and reasoning of neurology and medicine. Panda, Baltimore
Patten J (1987) Neurological differential diagnosis. Springer, New York Berlin Heidelberg
Plum F, Posner JB (1982) The diagnosis of stupor and coma. Davis, Philadelphia
Ropper AH, Kennedy SK (eds) (1988) Neurological and neurosurgical intensive care. Aspen, Rockville
Stöhr M, Brandt T, Einhäupl KM (1990) Neurologische Syndrome in der Intensivmedizin. Kohlhammer, Stuttgart

Chapter 2

Standard Management and Prophylaxis

KLAUS RIEKE and JOHN A. ULATOWSKI

This chapter reviews standard management protocols for patients with acute neurological diseases and may serve as a brief summary for physicians in the emergency department or in the neurocritical care unit. Most of the topics described are discussed in detail in other chapters.

Admission

In general, patients with acute neurological diseases should be transported to the hospital as quickly and as safely as possible. All patients should be stabilized first before transfer. Rapid transportation by helicopter may be beneficial in most critically ill patients, but it is expensive and may cause great anxiety in some patients. Transferring patients between hospitals requires careful planning and direct communication between physicans. To be more time-efficient, information about the patient should always be communicated to the receiving physician, since

appropriate therapy can often be started before or during the transfer. On admission, vital signs should be assessed and patients should be stabilized with regard to airway, breathing, and circulation. A brief examination should be done; a more complete examination can be done later. General protocols are helpful to stipulate the tasks required of members of the accepting team and what kinds of imaging and laboratory tests should be performed. The personal needs of patients and their family members should always be considered; patient dignity should be respected at all times and routine care should be delayed, if possible, until after the initial triage period. All major caretakers should be present when patients arrive so that needless repetition can be avoided. Although sedation and analgesia should be given when necessary, the neurological examination may be obscured and intracranial pressure may be adversely affected (because of respiratory depression). Thus, short-acting, reversible agents are always preferred. Sleep patterns are frequently disrupted in critical care units and many

Section Editor: Werner Hacke

patients experience fatigue and depression. Activity should be limited to the daytime as much as possible. Treatment with antidepressant drugs 1 h before sleep may also be beneficial. Adequate hydration and nutrition are extremely important as the caloric needs of critically ill patients are often 1.5–2 times baseline.

Airway Protection and Assisted Ventilation

Alteration of the respiratory system is a frequent indication for neurocritical care. Patients with central respiratory disturbances and neuromuscular disorders can develop respiratory failure and pneumonia (including aspiration pneumonia). Thus, the first step in resuscitation is establishing an adequate airway. Upper airway occlusion often occurs as a result of decreased muscle tone of the pharynx or a relapsing tongue. This can be prevented with an oral or nasal airway stent. Respiratory status (oxygenation and ventilation) should be assessed in all patients. Arterial blood gas analysis is the best way to assess oxygenation and also provides additional information about acid base status. Oxygenation can be assessed noninvasively with pulse oximetry. Ventilatory status can be assessed with spirometry and end-tidal CO_2 analysis.

Early intubation is recommended in patients with severe hypoxemia or hypercarbia, coma (with or without cranial nerve disturbances), and in those with pathological breathing patterns. In emergencies, orotracheal intubation provides rapid control of the airway and is generally the preferred approach. Blind nasotracheal and fiberoptically guided intubation can also be done in spontaneously ventilating patients. Nasotracheal intubation may be less uncomfortable for patients who require long-term intubation and may make nursing care of the mouth easier, but it is associated with a higher risk of sinusitis. Patients who are not severely hypoxemic or who do not have pathological breathing patterns should be given oxygen by nasal cannula.

Patients should be intubated electively and under optimal conditions whenever possible. They should be monitored with electrocardiography (ECG), blood pressure cuff, pulse oximetry, and capnography. Two laryngoscopes, two sources of suction, and two stiletted endotracheal tubes should be available. Patients should be placed supine with head extended and chin protruded ("sniffing position"). If there is a risk of aspiration, pressure should be applied to the cricoid cartilage to occlude the esophagus ("Sellick maneuver"). General anesthesia blunts the stress response of manipulating the airway and can be attained with thiopental (2–4 mg/kg), etomidate (0.3–0.4 mg/kg), midazolam HCl (0.1–0.3 mg/kg), and propofol (1.0–2.5 mg/kg). These agents should be used cautiously because some patients may suffer exaggerated cardiovascular effects (especially when high doses are used). Fentanyl (3–7 mg/kg) or lidocaine (1–2 mg/kg) can be given to blunt the cardiovascular effects of intubation. Anticholinergic drugs (atropine), routinely given to children before intubation because of their susceptibility to bradycardia, should be used cautiously in adults because of the possibility of concomitant coronary artery disease.

Treatment with neuromuscular blocking drugs can facilitate rapid intubation. Agents with rapid onset and short duration, such as the nondepolarizing neuromuscular blocker succinylcholine (1–2 mg/kg), are usually preferred (especially in patients at risk of aspiration, such as those with a full stomach). When using succinylcholine, two aspects are important. First, there is a transient increase in intracranial pressure after the injection that can be prevented by prior hyperventilation or induction of general anesthesia. Second, patients with injury to the brain, spinal cord, or peripheral nervous system may be at risk for hyperkalemia. Other nondepolarizing agents, such as vecuronium bromide and atracurium, can also be used; however, higher doses may be needed to achieve the same rapid onset (which may cause prolonged apnea and may obscure the neurological examination).

The endotracheal tube should be positioned in the trachea so that the balloon cuff is just below the vocal cords. Proper positioning should be confirmed by hearing symmetrical breath sounds bilaterally on auscultation, assessing the presence of end-tidal CO_2 from the tube, and palpation of the balloon cuff in the suprasternal notch. A chest X-ray should also be used to document the position of the tube in the trachea below the glottis and above the carina. The tube should be secured to the skin overlying the maxilla. We recommend volume-controlled assisted ventilation with 100% oxygen initially until ventilation and oxygenation requirements are known. Weaning can be facilitated with pulse oximetry or blood gas analysis.

Hemodynamic Monitoring

Hemodynamic monitoring is necessary for most critically ill patients, especially for those with vascular disease. Extensive monitoring is often needed in patients with circulatory failure (myocardial infarction or shock). Blood pressure should be monitored either with an intra-arterial cannula or a blood pressure cuff (dynamometry). Intra-arterial cannulas provide beat-to-beat measurements and easy access for arterial blood sampling. They are placed in superficial arteries using the Seldinger technique. The radial artery of the wrist is most often used because it is an end artery with collateral circulation from the ulnar artery (adequate collateral circulation should be confirmed with the Allen test before puncture). The brachial artery or dorsalis pedis artery can also be used. Use of the femoral artery is associated with a high risk of infection and arteriovenous fistula formation. ECG monitoring provides continuous analysis of heart rate, ryhthm, and S-T segments.

With central venous pressure (CVP) monitoring, volume status, cardiac function, and venous compliance can be assessed. Central catheters provide easy venous access and also serve as a route for fluids, nutrition, and medications. Venous air can be aspirated from central catheters in patients with air emboli. Peripheral placement of central catheters (for example, through the basilic vein in the antecubital fossa) are the safest approaches with the lowest risk to pneumothorax and hemothorax. Occasionally, the catheter may not be long enough to reach the superior vena cava or may coil in the axillary vein, go up the jugular vein, cross the chest via the contralateral subclavian vein, or pass into the inferior vena cava. A chest X-ray should always be obtained to confirm correct positioning of the catheter and to exclude pneumothorax. The femoral vein can be easily and rapidly cannulated as a route for giving fluids (especially concentrated fluids and vasoactive substances). This route is generally not recommended, however, because of the higher risk of infection and less reliable CVP measurements (secondary to confounding abdominal pressure). Direct placement of catheters into the neck veins (for example, the internal jugular or subclavian veins) can be used when peripheral routes are not possible. Although the risk of pneumothorax is less with the internal jugular approach, venous drainage from the brain can be impaired (especially in those with increased intracranial pressure) and there is a risk of jugular venous thrombosis. Therefore, the subclavian approach is often preferred. Double or triple lumen catheters should be used in patients who require fluids, multiple medications, vasopressors, or parenteral nutrition. This allows uninterrupted therapy and simultaneous measurement of the CVP.

The normal CVP is $1-8\,\text{mmHg}$ or $2-10\,\text{cmH}_2\text{O}$. As an estimate of intravascular volume, use of the CVP is limited because it is composed of four components: volume in the central veins, right atrial and ventricular contractility, tone of central veins (capacitance), and intrathoracic pressure. Unless normal, isolated measurements of CVP are usually not helpful. Serial measurements of CVP are better. In general, however, when intrathoracic pressure is stable, there is a good correlation between CVP and the response of the systemic blood pressure to fluid challenges.

For a more accurate assessment of volume status and cardiac function, pulmonary artery catheterization with a Swan-Ganz catheter is recommended. The pulmonary artery pressure (PAP) (normal $10-20\,\text{mmHg}$) is a reflection of right ventricular contractility, left-to-right shunting, and pulmonary vascular resisitance. The pulmonary capillary wedge pressure (PCWP) is a reflection of left ventricular end-diastolic pressure (normal $5-12\,\text{mmHg}$). Cardiac output and systemic vascular resistance can also be estimated. The Swan-Ganz catheter is placed using the Seldinger technique, usually through the right internal jugular vein or left subclavian vein, but any central venous access can be used. The position of the tip of the catheter should be confirmed daily by chest X-rays and pressure tracings. Complications include pulmonary artery infarction and rupture.

Transesophageal echocardiography (TEE) is an adjunct to transthoracic echocardiography. It can be done in awake patients under local anesthesia, sedated patients, or comatose patients. Two-dimensional images allow assessment of chamber volume, valvular function, and myocardial wall motion. Color flow Doppler ultrasonography can be used to detect right-to-left shunts. It may also be possible to measure cardiac output with this technique.

Treatment of Increased Intracranial Pressure

All patients with signs of increased intracranial pressure, such as headache, vomiting, hiccoughs, dizziness, or impaired consciousness, require neurocritical care. To facilitate venous drainage, patients should be positioned with 30° head elevation. Physical examination and diagnostic and therapeutic procedures should be performed as far as possible in this position. The first line of treatment of increased intracranial pressure is hyperventilation, although this may be less beneficial when given over a long period. Hyperosmolar treatment can also be used. In Europe, the agent of first choice is glycerine 10% (250 ml four times daily). Glycerine is hepatically metabolized and rebound increases in intracranial pressure with prolonged treatment are less severe than with other agents. Because it has a slow onset of action, patients who require more rapid reduction of intracranial pressure (for example, those with signs of transtentorial herniation) should be treated with mannitol 20% (0.25–1.0 g/kg). Both agents work primarily by removing water from normal brain areas. Thus, they must be used cautiously in patients with subdural and epidural hemorrhages because rapid reduction of intracranial volume may enlarge the hemorrhage. Treatment with osmotic agents is often complicated by intravascular dehydration and other approaches, such as hypertonic solutions and tris-hydroxymethyl-aminomethane (THAM) buffer solution, have recently been introduced as alternatives to osmotic agents. Corticosteroids should be reserved for patients with vasogenic edema (intracranial tumor or abscess) or spinal cord trauma. Dexamethasone can be given intravenously at a dose of 10–20 mg (100 mg in some centers) followed by 4 mg every 6 h. A detailed review of treatment of increased intracranial pressure can be found in Chap. 9.

Treatment of Seizures

Seizures can occur in several settings including trauma, intoxication, delirium, encephalitis, thrombosis of intracranial veins or sinuses, intracranial tumors, hemorrhages, hypoglycemia, or hypoxemia. Focal seizures (including those that generalize) are usually caused by structural lesions, and generalized seizures are usually caused by metabolic abnormalities or are idiopathic. Adults who present with focal seizures should undergo computed tomography or magnetic resonance imaging to exclude structural lesions.

All patients with seizures should be stabilized first with regard to airway, breathing, and circulation. Patients with a single seizure do not necessarily need antiseizure treatment. Reversible causes, such as hypoxemia, hypoglycemia, or narcosis, should be sought and treated. Antiseizure treatment should be started in those with more than one seizure and those with status epilepticus (continuous seizures or failure to regain consciousness between seizures). Benzodiazepines (clonazepam, diazepam, lorazepam, or midazolam HCl) are the drugs of first choice because of their ease of administration and their rapid onset. Side effects include sedation and increased endotracheal secretions. Phenytoin can also be given intravenously (15–20 mg/kg loading dose, 5 mg/kg per day maintenance) and causes little sedation. It should be mixed with saline solution to prevent precipitation and should not be given faster than 50 mg/min (1 mg/kg per minute in children) to avoid hypotension and dysrhythmias. Patients should be subjected to continuous ECG monitoring. Both classes of drugs should be used in patients with status epilepticus.

Second line treatment of seizures includes phenobarbital (15–20 mg/kg loading dose, 1–3 mg/kg per day maintenance). For rapid control of seizures, phenobarbital is usually given at a rate of 50–100 mg/min (slower in children), titrating the rate to effect. Side effects include hypotension, sedation, and respiratory depression (and may be additive to side effects of other antiseizure drugs). Patients should be intubated at this point if this has not already been done. If seizure activity is still not controlled, treatment with valproic acid may be considered (given by nasogastric or rectal route at a dosage of 600–1200 mg four times daily). For continuing partial status epilepticus, carbamazepine (100–300 mg four times daily) is often added, although it has the disadvantage of requiring oral administration. In patients with refractory, prolonged status epilepticus, general anesthesia should be induced. In the neurocritical care unit, thiopental or etomidate treatment can be easily started in combination with neuromuscular blocking drugs (for example, pancuronium bromide). Continuous EEG recording is sug-gested in this situation. Status epilepticus is reviewed in detail in Chap. 66.

Treatment of Pneumonia

Nosocomial pneumonia is common in critically ill patients. In general, broad-spectrum antibiotics should initially be used to cover the most likely organisms. Once the organism has been identified and sensitivities are known, the antibiotic regimen can be narrowed. Duration of treatment depends on clinical response to treatment, including resolving signs of inflammation, decreasing leukocytosis, and absence of fever for more than 3 days. If patients have persistent fever, leukocytosis, and purulent secretions after 5 days of antibiotic treatment, then the antibiotic coverage should be broadened or changed. If patients then still continue to have signs of inflammation, stopping antibiotics may be considered in order to obtain new cultures. Nonbacterial pathogens should also be considered.

Oral antifungal agents are often used for gastrointestinal prophylaxis in patients receiving prolonged treatment with broad-spectrum antibiotics. Systemic antifungal treatment should only be started, however, in those with documented fungal infections (by culture or by serology). Fluconazole (200 mg/day) is often the drug of first choice and may be given orally or intravenously for a least 3–4 weeks. Amphotericin B and fluocytosine, because of their side effects, should be used only if fluconazole treatment fails.

Prophylaxis in Neurocritical Care

Pneumonia prophylaxis includes breathing exercises (incentive spirometry, deep breathing, and coughing) at least twice daily. These exercises should be continued in patients who develop pneumonia. Immobilized patients should be repositioned every 2 h. In some centers, surveillance cultures of the sputum are performed twice weekly. Some centers have begun giving intratracheal or intragastric antibiotics to intubated patients; although preliminary data are encouraging, the cost/benefit ratio requires further study. In general, systemic antibiotics should not be given prophylactically. Because of the close quarters in most neurocritical care units, strict antisepsis is crucial.

Decubitus ulcers should be prevented by frequent turning of patients, adequate nutrition, and use of soft care mattresses. Ulcers usually respond to cleaning and local antibiotics. Deep venous thrombosis prophylaxis should be started in all patients in the neurocritical care unit and should include fitted elastic compression stockings and either subcutaneous heparin or intermittent pneumatic compression. Full-dose heparinization is frequently used in patients with Guillain-Barré syndrome. Early ambulation should be encouraged and bedside physical therapy should be started as soon as possible. A detailed review of deep venous thrombosis prophylaxis can be found in Chap. 13.

Suggested Reading

Blitt CD (ed) (1990) Monitoring in anesthesia and critical care medicine. Churchill Livingstone, New York

Hall JB, Schmidt GA, Wood LDH (eds) (1992) Principles of critical care. McGraw-Hill, New York

Larsen R (1987) Anaesthesie. Urban and Schwarzenberg, Munich

Rogers MC, Tinker JH, Covino BG, Longnecker DE (eds) (1992) Principles and practice of anesthesiology. Mosby-Yearbook, St Louis

Salcman M (ed) (1990) Neurologic emergencies. Raven, New York

Weiner WJ (1992) Emergent and urgent neurology. Lippincott, Philadelphia

Chapter 3

How to Approach an Unconscious Patient

Eric Aldrich and Rolf Biniek

Introduction

The unconscious patient presents a challenging emergency in the intensive care unit. This is a dangerous time for the patient; patient evaluation and treatment must occur simultaneously. Clinical circumstances with immediate therapeutic consequences, such as hypoxia or hypoglycemia, must be identified and treated quickly. Then, as the patient's condition is being stabilized, a working diagnosis must be made and a treatment plan formulated. Lengthy diagnostic procedures, such as angiography and magnetic resonance imaging, should be considered only after these initial steps are taken.

The approach to evaluating an unconscious patient should begin before an emergency situation actually occurs. Organization and planning will help ensure that the first few ·crucial minutes are utilized efficiently. Some points to keep in mind are:

- Be sure that the patient is never left unattended until a proper

Section Editor: Werner Hacke

airway can be maintained. Furthermore, the patient must be monitored closely for any acute changes.

- Proper back-up should already be in place if you encounter a situation you cannot deal with on your own. Never be reluctant to call for assistance.

- Universal precautions should be observed at all times, even in an emergency situation. Assume that *all* patients are infected with HIV and/or hepatitis until proven otherwise.

A flow chart summarizing the sequence of actions is given in Fig. 1.

ABC and Vital Signs

The first priority in evaluating an unconscious patient is to make sure that the patient will survive the next few minutes. Airway, breathing, and circulation (ABCs) must be established immediately (see flow chart in Fig. 1). Check respiration, pulse, and blood pressure and then decide whether cardiopulmonary resuscitation (CPR),

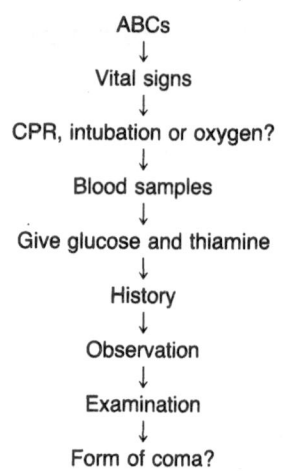

ABCs
↓
Vital signs
↓
CPR, intubation or oxygen?
↓
Blood samples
↓
Give glucose and thiamine
↓
History
↓
Observation
↓
Examination
↓
Form of coma?

Fig. 1. Flow chart for sequence of action on emergency admission of an unconscious patient. ABCs, Airway breathing and circulation; CPR, Cardiopulmonary resuscitation

intubation and/or artificial ventilation are indicated.

Intubation in neurological diseases is often performed much earlier than in other clinical situations. Do not feel safe if the respiratory rate is sufficient and the patient is able to cough. The unconscious patient may vomit suddenly, and changes in the level of consciousness can occur quickly. Therefore, it is appropriate to intubate patients for airway protection to avoid aspiration, even if respiratory function is sufficient for proper oxygenation and ventilation. However, intubation may require sedation and thus eliminate the opportunity for a neurological examination. In cases when there is no need for immediate CPR, intubation can be delayed briefly while a short physical and neurological examination are performed.

Supplemental oxygen is the next priority. An arterial blood gas sample should be sent for analysis, but do not wait for the results to begin oxygen

therapy. Pulse oximetry can be useful because it provides immediate information regarding arterial oxygen saturation.

Glucose and Thiamine

Once the ABCs have been addressed intravenous access should be established and blood samples collected – preferably by someone else while you continue with the assessment. Hypoglycemia is a frequent cause of decreased level of consciousness; thus glucose should be given intravenously immediately – *before* the results of the blood tests are available. One ampoule of D50W (25 g glucose as a 50% solution) given intravenously with 100 mg thiamine is a good start for the average adult.

There are several reasons for such empiric treatment. Brain tissue is dependent on glucose as its energy source and is intolerant of prolonged hypoglycemia. Furthermore, even if *hyper*glycemia is the underlying cause of the altered mental status, a transient further increase of the blood sugar will do less harm to the patient than extended hypoglycemia. In addition, thiamine *always* should be given with the intravenous glucose because glucose given alone in a thiamine-deficient patient can lead to a quick depletion of the thiamine stores and produce Wernicke's encephalopathy. Also, a thiamine deficiency itself may be the cause for the decreased level of consciousness.

History

In many cases it is difficult to get an adequate history, especially when the patient has been "found down" and his or her identity is unknown. Nevertheless, it is important to interview the person(s) who found the patient about the specific circumstances in which he or she was discovered, including:

- Witnessed events – head trauma, tonic-clonic activity, specific aspects of a motor vehicle accident, or simply the detail "found down".
- Development of clinical signs – acute or delayed onset, progressive or recurrent paresis, headache, fever.
- Recent medical history – surgical procedures, infections, current medications.
- Past medical history – psychiatric therapy, depression, epileptic seizures, head trauma, drug or alcohol abuse, stroke(s), diabetes, hypertension, cancer.

Keep in mind that the patient's condition should be stabilized before a complete history is taken. Often it is better to ask someone else to take the history while you attend to the patient.

Physical Examination

Observation

After checking the patient's vital signs, take a moment to inspect the patient. A great deal of information can be obtained by simple observation. Remove all sheets, blankets, and the patient's clothes for a proper assessment.

- *General appearance.* Look carefully for lacerations, abrasions, contusions, or other signs of trauma. Notice whether the patient is cachectic – indicating a possible consuming cancer or AIDS. If the patient is unkempt, consider drug/alcohol abuse or psychiatric illness.
- *Breathing.* Respiratory pattern can provide information concerning the depth of the coma and its possible causes. Smell the patient's breath. Uremia and hepatic dysfunction produce distinctive breath odors.
- *Skin color and appearance.* Be sensitive to the dusky blue of cyanosis, the icteric yellow of hepatic failure, or the ashen, cold, clammy appearance of shock. Remember that a fresh and pink appearance ("cherry red") actually can be due to carbon monoxide intoxication. In reality, such patients are severely hypoxic despite a "normal" PaO_2 on routine blood gas analysis. Skin bubbles are seen in barbiturate intoxication, splinter hemorrhages in endocarditis and sepsis. Needle "tracks" and injection points, especially in atypical locations (feet, neck, between the toes), are indicative of intravenous drug abuse.
- *Body posture.* If the patient is lying in a natural comfortable position, as though in natural sleep, the level of consciousness is probably not very depressed. Yawning and swallowing have the same significance. Jaw and lid tone are also

indicative of the degree of uncon-sciousness; open lids and a hanging jaw are indicative of a severely depressed mental status. An opisthotonic posture can indicate severe paravertebral muscle spasm, signaling meningeal irritation. Such patients have a tendency to lie on their side with an extended back.

- *Hemiparesis.* Hemiparesis can often also be detected by simple observation of the posture. Older spastic hemiparesis shows the typical pattern of flexion of the arm and extension of the leg. In contrast, acute hemiparesis is flaccid; the limbs of one side are either lying flat on the stretcher or there is asymmetry in the positioning of the limbs, such as external rotation of the lower extremity or finger flexion of the upper extremity.
- *Spontaneous movements of the extremities.* Lack of movement or asymmetry of degree of spontaneous movement may indicate trauma, fracture, or hemiparesis. Look for the striking rhythmic movements of seizures, the isolated jerks of myoclonus or singultus (hiccups).
- *Body fluids.* Look for traces of blood that may indicate trauma or a seizure with a tongue injury. Evidence of urination or defecation also suggests seizures. Vomit should raise concerns regarding raised intracranial pressure, drug intoxication, or hypoxia secondary to aspiration.

These points are only a few examples of what can be learned by simply observing the patient.

The physical examination comes next. A brief, directed general examination is conducted first. The head should be inspected for evidence of trauma, then the neck, keeping in the mind the possibility of cervical fracture or instability. Cervical spine films should be considered if there is any history or evidence of trauma. Cardiac, pulmonary, and abdominal examinations should be directed towards detecting trauma or a severe, acute process. One should then quickly move on to the neurologic examination, proceeding in a standardized, systematic fashion. This can be accomplished within minutes and without any special instruments. The following points should be checked:

- Level of alertness
- Response to verbal commands
- Motor responses to (noxious) stimuli
- Respiratory pattern
- Size and reactivity of pupils
- Spontaneous and induced eye movements
- Corneal reflex
- Neck/meningismus
- Muscle tone
- Spontaneous motor activities

Level of Consciousness

Consciousness may be defined as awareness of one's self and one's environment. It is a function of both the level of arousal and higher cognitive abilities. It runs a continuum from full alertness to total unresponsiveness. In clinical practice, decreased level of consciousness has been subdivided into stages in several ways. However, as there is much confusion about the different coma scales, it is often best simply to describe the clinical findings. Note the patient's best reaction to verbal commands, verbal stimuli, and noxious stimuli. The sentence "No reaction to loud commands and abnormal extension to pain" gives much more information than "coma grade 4." Some physicians, however, prefer to use the terms "somnolence," "stupor," "light coma," and "deep coma":

- *Somnolence*. A state characterized by the presence of the ability to respond to verbal commands and the presence of "fending-off" movements induced by painful stimuli.
- *Stupor*. An incomplete arousal to painful stimuli. It is characterized by inconsistent and ambiguous responses to verbal commands. No verbal responses can be evoked at all. The best motor response to noxious stimuli is only "fending-off" movements.
- *Light coma*. Primitive and disorganized motor responses to noxious stimuli.
- *Deep coma*. No purposeful response is obtained even to the most painful stimuli. Stereotyped motor responses such as decerebrate or decorticate posturing may be noted.

One standardized and widely used coma scale is the Glasgow Coma Scale (GCS). The GCS was actually designed to describe patients with acute head trauma patients, but it is often applied to any patient with an alteration in mental status. It is a "responsiveness" scale, and as such it has both advantages and disadvantages. One disadvantage is that it does not specifically test brain stem reflexes. Also,

an aphasic patient would be scored as more "comatose" than a patient with a similar-sized lesion in the nondominant hemisphere. The advantage of this scale is that it is simple, standardized, and reproducible – allowing paramedical and medical staff to communicate accurately and rapidly.

The GCS score is obtained by assigning points in the categories of eye opening, best motor response, and best verbal response. The minimum stimulus required to elicit opening one or both eyes is scored from 1 to 4. The best motor response in either the upper or lower extremities is rated on a scale of 1 to 6. Before scoring 1 (no response), spinal cord injury and inadequate stimuli must be excluded. The best verbal response receives from 1 to 5 points. To score the full 5 points, the patient must be able to give his or her name, location, the year and month, and converse with others. If there is any disorientation 4 points are assigned. "Verbalization" (3 points) refers to intelligible words that are disorganized or used in an exclamatory fashion. "Vocalization" (2 points) indicates the uttering of sounds like a moan or groan which are unrecognizable as words.

The Glasgow Coma Scale is generally used by emergency rescue teams in the field and upon presentation to the Emergency Department. In the hospital a description of the clinical findings is preferred.

Best Reaction to Verbal Commands

To assess the level of consciousness, first call the name of the patient and observe the reaction. Be sure that you are loud enough. If the patient does not react, clap your hands just beside each of the patient's ears. If there is still no reaction, apply some tactile stimuli to the face, followed by loud claps in front of the face and by calling aloud "Hello!" or the patient's name.

Sometimes a patient may open his or her eyes yet not look in the direction of the examiner. If you have the impression that the patient is searching only a portion of his or her visual field, move to the other side and repeat the examination. It is possible you may have detected a hemianopsia. In the case of a visible hemiparesis, the examination should be performed from the nonparetic side to ensure that the examiner is in the patient's visual field.

If the patient opens his or her eyes and fixates, try to communicate. Check for orientation to person, place, and time. Use simple questions concerning pain, nausea, etc. With a somnolent patient it is wise to pardon yourself in advance for your "stupid questions," otherwise the patient may feel bewildered and stop communicating. If the patient tries to communicate, note fluency and articulation as well as signs of aphasia or dysarthria. A patient who tries to communicate but is unable to produce any noise is "anarthric" and may have a stroke in the dominant hemisphere.

If the patient opens his or her eyes in response to verbal commands and tries to communicate, he or she may be sufficiently conscious to cooperate for a standard neurologic examination.

Best Motor Reaction

If there is no response or an incomplete reaction to verbal stimuli, it is necessary to apply a noxious stimulus. The preferred site for application of painful stimuli is the medial side of the arms or legs. It is important to use the *medial* side of the limb to differentiate a localization of pain response versus abnormal flexor or extensor posturing. If the patient's motion is *toward* the medially applied noxious stimulus, it would be inconsistent with a localization response because the patient would naturally move his or her limb away from a painful stimulus. A laterally applied noxious stimulus thus would be more difficult to interpret.

Make sure that an *adequate* noxious stimulus is applied. You need not worry about black-and-blue marks. Sometimes, especially if the patient has been treated in an intensive care unit for several days, the skin has been treated with lotion for skin protection and it is not easy to pinch the skin adequately. In such cases, press the fingernail bed with a pen. Other noxious stimuli include rubbing the patient's sternum with your knuckles or applying thumb pressure to the supraorbital notch. Pressure to ocular bulbi to produce pain should be avoided. Such pressure has been known to result in excessive vagal stimulation with subsequent cardiac arrhythmia in patients with acute polyneuropathy and other dysautonomic syndromes.

While applying a noxious stimulus, observe the patient's reaction. The motor response to noxious stimuli can be classified into the following categories:

- Fending-off movements with localization of pain
- Fending-off movements without localization of pain

- Abnormal flexion
- Abnormal extension
- No response

By watching the pattern of withdrawal a great deal can be learned about focal abnormalities. The patient need not be conscious to provide helpful diagnostic information. A patient with a major motor hemiparesis will withdraw the unaffected side more significantly, regardless of the side of stimulus application. In the case of a sensory hemiparesis, withdrawal of both sides occurs following a unilateral painful stimulus. Contralateral withdrawal only and no reaction to pain on the nonparetic side may indicate a spinal cord injury with a Brown-Sequard syndrome. Regarding the lower extremities, a "normal" withdrawal of the legs is a quick, brief flexion of the hip and knee. This should not be confused with the "triple-flexion reflex", which is a slower, more tonic and repeatable response. The triple-flexion reflex consists of the contraction of the tensor fascia lata, flexion of the hip and knee, dorsiflexion of the ankle and great toes with dorsiflexion and fanning of the small toes. This reflex is a profound upper motor neuron injury response (i.e., an exaggerated Babinski reflex).

"Abnormal extension" refers to extension and pronation of the arm with adduction and internal rotation of the shoulder. The leg extends and internally rotates and the foot plantar flexes.

Each extremity should be examined separately and the patient's response described in the chart. As with the description of level of consciousness, general terms such as "decorticate state" should be avoided in lieu of simple descriptions such as "withdrawal," "flexion," or "extension."

As is true of any aspect of the neurologic examination, a patient's motor function can change and evolve as a pathologic process continues unabated. In a patient with a hemispheric lesion with secondary progressive brain stem dysfunction, one can observe a decline of the motor responses from initial fending-off movements, to flexion of the arms and extension of legs, to abnormal extension of all extremities and finally no reaction at all. However, in a primary infratentorial lesion this regular decline is not usually seen.

Respiratory Pattern

The patient's respiratory pattern is helpful in determining the site of injury, and in certain instances suggests the nature of the underlying pathologic process. Respiratory function is controlled by both voluntary and involuntary mechanisms. The involuntary respiratory control has an important metabolic function – maintaining normal oxygenation and acid-base balance. These classic respiratory centers are located in the reticular formation of the lower brain stem, between the mid-pons and the cervical-medullary junction. Voluntary control of the respiratory pattern is necessary for speech, and is mediated via pre-pontine structures and the forebrain. The two controlling systems are largely integrated at the lower brain stem and spinal cord.

There are three breathing patterns that one should be aware of when treating an unconscious patient: Cheyne-Stokes respiration, central neurogenic hyperventilation, and ataxic or Biot's breathing. Each can reveal information concerning the location of brain dysfunction, and a change from one form to the next can indicate worsening of the patient's condition.

Cheyne-Stokes Respiration

Cheyne-Stokes respiration is a pattern of periodic breathing characterized by a hyperpneic phase of slowly increasing then decreasing respiratory rate, followed by an apneic phase. This apneic phase is usually shorter than the hyperpneic phase. Cheyne-Stokes respiration is the result of an abnormally increased ventilatory response to rising PCO_2 causing hyperventilation, followed by an abnormally decreased forebrain response resulting in post-hyperventilation apnea. It can be observed in bilateral damage of descending pathways anywhere from forebrain to upper pons. It is seen frequently in patients with bilateral cerebral infarction, hypertensive encephalopathy, metabolic derangements such as uremia, or even hypoxia from profound heart failure.

Central Neurogenic Hyperventilation

Rapid, extended, and deep ventilation in a regular rhythm is referred to as "central neurogenic hyperventilation." It is known to occur in patients with rostral brain stem tegmentum dysfunction. Regularity rather than rate is the prognostic sign to pay attention to; increasing regularity correlates with increasing depth of coma. However, because many unconscious patients hyperventilate, hyperventilation itself has no specific localizing significance. For example, hypoxia should be excluded quickly before it is concluded that the hyperventilation is of neurogenic origin.

Ataxic (Biot's) Breathing

Ataxic breathing is characterized by a generally slow, irregular pattern of breaths of variable size which rapidly can progress to compete apnea. These patients need complete respiratory assistance at once, as they can run into respiratory arrest at any moment. This pattern is due to lesions in the reticular formation in the dorsomedial medulla, where respiratory cycles are generated. It is a very poor prognostic sign.

Hiccups

Hiccups (singultus), like vomiting, are a gastrointestinal reflex involving the respiratory muscles. Most hiccups are the result of thoracoabdominal disease or drugs. Neurologic causes may be lesions within the medulla oblongata, or lesions that surround or compress the medulla such as neoplasms, hematomas, or bleeding into the fourth ventricle.

Size and Reactivity of Pupils

The next step is to assess pupil size and reactivity. Note pupil size and roundness, comparing both sides, then pupil reactivity (the ambient light in an emergency room is sufficient to generate some degree of pupillary constriction). Remember to look for signs of prior ophthalmologic procedures or injury. Both eyes must be checked separately. This can be done by covering one eye with one hand and watching the reaction of the pupil after opening the other eyelid. The consensual light reflex also should be checked.

Normally reactive pupils indicate an intact midbrain. Midposition nonreactive pupils are evidence of midbrain damage. Bilateral small reactive pupils may signify pontine damage, but narcotic intoxication also can produce profound pupillary constriction. In fact, many drugs have effects on pupil size, producing miosis or mydriasis. Therefore, it is important to consider the possible effects of medications patients may have in their system before judging the clinical significance of the pupillary examination.

A unilateral dilated and unreactive pupil in a comatose patient is a sign of third nerve compression, which can be secondary to a posterior cerebral artery aneurysm or to temporal lobe (uncal) herniation. Other signs of third nerve dysfunction (drooping of eyelid, abduction of the eye) may be present or develop later. Midbrain damage less frequently results in a unilateral, dilated, non-reactive pupil.

Unilateral pupil constriction may indicate Horner's syndrome. Be careful to look for the other associated signs such as ptosis, anhidrosis, and enophthalmos. Contralateral hemiparesis and Horner's syndrome are signs of an internal carotid artery dissection – a neurologic emergency. These signs result from dysfunction of the sympathetic nerves surrounding the internal carotid itself.

Spontaneous
and Induced Eye Movements

After checking pupil size and reactivity, observe the relative position of the eyes and any spontaneous eye movements. Note the position of the eyes in primary position (at rest) as well as the eye movement characteristics – either spontaneous or induced during the examination. Observe whether the eyes move as a yoked pair (conjugate), or at times asymmetrically (disconjugate). Also note the presence of nystagmus – either at rest or at the extremes of gaze.

There are many types of spontaneous eye movements, both normal and abnormal. The abnormal eye movement disorders often result from brain stem or frontal lobe lesions. This large topic is discussed at length elsewhere, but a few types should always be kept in mind during the initial assessment:

- *Roving eye movements.* This term refers to slow, random deviations much like the eye movements of light sleep in normal persons. They can be both conjugate and disconjugate. Horizontal movements are more frequent, but vertical movements also may occur. Roving eye movements are slower than the conjugate rapid eye movements (REM) of sleep. Because roving eye movements cannot be mimicked voluntarily, they rule out psychogenic unconsciousness. Decreased roving movements indicate depressed brain stem function.

- *Conjugate deviation.* Conjugate horizontal deviation can occur as a result of infratentorial or supratentorial lesions. With pontine lesions the eyes deviate toward the hemiparetic side. In contrast, acute damage to one hemisphere can produce a deviation looking *away* from the hemiparesis. Epileptic seizures involving the frontal lobe classically generate conjugate eye deviation away from the focus. Downward conjugate deviation of the eyes may be seen in thalamic lesions, or as a part of the dorsal midbrain syndrome (Parinaud's syndrome). Transient upward deviation is often seen with drug intoxication, especially with neuroleptics.

- *Disconjugate eye deviation.* This phenomenon may reflect palsies of the third, fourth, or sixth cranial nerves or brain stem parenchymal lesions. A skew deviation (one eye "looking" up, the other down) is due to a disturbance of prenuclear inputs and indicates a brain stem lesion. A slight divergence of the bulbi can be seen in patients who are asleep or with moderately depressed level of consciousness (e.g., narcotic intoxication). This phenomenon is due to the decreased tone of the extraocular muscles, and is of little significance in a comatose patient.
- *Nystagmus.* Spontaneous nystagmus is uncommon in coma because the quick phase depends upon the influence of the cerebral cortex upon the oculovestibular system. If the influence of the cortex is reduced or absent, fast-beating nystagmus would be expected to disappear. Unilateral nystagmus, however, accompanies severe midpons to lower pontine damage.

In addition to spontaneous eye movements, eye movements can be induced using the oculocephalic reflex. Such induced responses are a powerful diagnostic tool in assessing the unconscious patient. Before testing these movements, you should examine the neck to ensure that your patient has not sustained trauma sufficient to cause a cervical fracture or dislocation. To examine the oculocephalic reflex (OCR), or doll's eyes phenomenon, one holds the patient's eyelids open and rotates the head from one side to the other. This can be done by smoothly rocking the head side to side or with more brisk motions. Both lateral directions should be tested, and if necessary vertical eye movements as well. If the OCR is intact (a *positive* response), head rotation will result in contraversive conjugate eye deviation. For example, if the head is rotated to the right, the eyes deviate to the left. The head may be flexed and extended in a similar fashion to induce vertical eye movements (vertical OCR).

Conscious patients usually inhibit the OCR via higher cortical gaze centers. That is, they are able to fixate, making the OCR absent or inconsistent. Therefore, the OCR is negative in a conscious patient. In an unconscious patient with an intact brain stem, there is no cortical suppression and head rotation will induce compensatory contraversive eye movements – a positive OCR. Using the OCR it is possible to test all of the extraocular eye movements in a comatose patient just as with a conscious patient. Cranial nerve deficits or brain stem lesions can still be detected. In deep coma, however, the OCR will diminish and become difficult to elicit. Therefore, a negative OCR in a comatose patient must be interpreted with caution. Many common drugs (ototoxic antibiotics, sedatives, neuromuscular blockers) or pre-existing vestibular disease also may reduce the OCR.

Impairment of eye movements to one side is seen with ipsilateral lesions in the region of the parapontine reticular formation, just adjacent to each abducens nucleus. Impaired abduction of a single eye may indicate a unilateral sixth nerve palsy. Impaired adduction is seen in third nerve palsy, or in an ipsilateral lesion of the medial longitudinal fasciculus (internuclear ophthalmoplegia). An isolated fourth nerve palsy is rare, and is characterized by a deficit of inward torsional movement. The vertical OCR is impaired by midbrain lesions, especially in the region of the posterior commissure, or in a bilateral internuclear ophthalmoplegia. Downward vertical gaze palsy can result from lesions at the cervicomedullary junction.

In the absence of an OCR, eye movements still can be tested using caloric stimulation. This is a time-consuming procedure and is not a part of the standard emergency examination. In a potentially brain-dead patient, however, cold water caloric stimulation is an essential part of the examination to determine if any brain stem function exists.

Corneal and Blink Reflexes

In the unresponsive patient, the eye lids usually remain shut by a tonic contraction of the orbicularis oculi muscle. Spontaneous blinking implies an intact pontine reticular formation in the unresponsive patient. Blinking in response to bright light or a sudden loud noise indicates some preservation of the visual or auditory pathways. Blinking to a threatening movement

towards both eyes from only one side may indicate a homonymous hemianopia.

The corneal reflex can be tested by gauging the response to a cotton wisp drawn across the cornea and is recorded as present or absent for each eye. A common mistake of the inexperienced examiner is to stimulate only the sclera. The cornea itself must be touched with the cotton wisp to truly determine the presence or absence of the reflex. With deep sedation corneal pressure may be required to elicit a response as this reflex can be suppressed. The normal response is a unilateral or bilateral protective reflex of full eyelid closure or at least a reproducible movement of the eye lids. A difference between sides can be due to dysfunction of either the afferent fifth nerve pathway or the efferent seventh nerve pathway. To localize the lesion further, simply compare one side to the other as well as the bilateral response.

Neck and Meningismus

As previously noted, diagnostic movements of the neck and head should be done only after excluding traumatic injury to the cervical spine. Meningismus can be tested by flexing the patient's head with one hand. Normally, it is possible to flex the head far enough to touch the chin to the sternum without resistance. In older patients with degenerative osteoarthritis of the cervical spine, this flexion is no longer possible. To differentiate from meningismus, rotate the head from side to side, as there is often resistance to this motion with arthritis. Another potential pitfall is that meningismus can fade appreciably in deep coma. Therefore, in deep coma the absence of meningismus never rules out acute meningitis.

Muscle Tone and Deep Tendon Reflexes

The patient's muscle tone should be recorded for all extremities as normal, paratonic, spastic or flaccid.

- *Paratonia (gegenhalten)*. A bilateral, plastic-like increase in resistance to all passive movements throughout the range of motions. It occurs in response to slow or quick motions. Paratonia indicates diffuse forebrain dysfunction and is seen in dementia.
- *Spasticity*. Spastic tone refers to an increased tone to *quick* passive movements of the extremities. The muscle responds differently to fast and to slow passive motion of the limb. For example, when a spastic leg is raised slowly by lifting from behind the knee, the foot will drag along the bed. When lifted abruptly, however, the same leg will remain stiff and the foot will be lifted directly off the bed. Spasticity is a sign of upper motor neuron injury, and is a common finding in both supra- and infratentorial lesions.
- *Flaccid tone*. Essentially a limp limb, flaccid tone can be due to a lower motor neuron lesion. However, acute *upper* motor neuron lesions also present as flaccidity. Spasticity develops later, typically several days after the initial injury.

Deep tendon reflexes (DTRs) require an intact sensory nerve and motor

Table 1. Summary of physical examination

1. Best reaction to loud command:
   Verbal reactions: oriented, confused, aphasic, no reaction
   Opening eyes: fixate on examiner, no fixation, no reaction
2. Best motor reaction to noxious stimuli:
   Fending-off movements with localization of pain
   Fending-off movements without localization
   Abnormal flexion
   Abnormal extension
   No response
3. Respiratory pattern:
   Normal respiration
   Cheyne-Stokes breathing
   Central neurogenic hyperventilation
   Ataxic breathing
   Hiccup
4. Size and reaction of pupils:
   Size
   Equal vs. unequal
   Reactivity to light
5. Spontaneous and induced eye movements:
   Primary position
   Conjugate vs. disconjugate gaze
   Gaze deviation
   Isolated gaze palsies
   Spontaneous eye movements:
     Roving eye movements
     Ping-pong gaze
     Refractory nystagmus
     Convergence nystagmus
     Ocular bobbing
     "Seesaw" nystagmus
   Induced eye movements (oculocephalic reflex)
6. Corneal and blink reflex:
   Blinking:
     Spontaneous
     In response to bright light or loud noise
     In response to threatening movements
   Corneal reflex:
     Normal on both eyes
     Decreased or absent on one eye
     Decreased or absent on both eyes
7. Neck and meningismus
8. Muscle tone and deep tendon reflexes

nerve, as well as the corresponding spinal cord level. DTRs are tonically inhibited by cortical projections. Therefore any interruption of that suppression, at any point rostral to the spinal cord level, will result in hyper-reflexia. Hyporeflexia or areflexia indicates either a lower motor neuron lesion at the corresponding spinal cord level or damage to the peripheral nerves. Motor nerve injury profoundly affects DTRs, but sensory nerve injury typically must be more severe to produce a detectable reduction in a DTR. One should be particularly interested in asymmetry of reflexes. Depressed yet symmetric reflexes can be a normal variant, while asymmetric reflexes imply pathology.

The Babinski sign is checked by scratching the lateral sole of the feet. If an conventional instrument is not available a key can be used for this purpose. To avoid ambiguity, it is best to describe the patient's response as extensor or flexor, or, better yet, as upgoing or downgoing. Table 1 summarizes the physical examination.

Next Diagnostic Steps

After the examination is complete one can classify the patient into one of five forms of coma:

1. Simple coma (metabolic coma, intoxication, hypoxia)

2. Coma with hemiparesis including face (stroke, trauma, encephalitis, subarachnoid hemorrhage)
3. Coma with brain stem involvement (basilar artery thrombosis, trauma, parenchymal hemorrhage)
4. Coma with multiple focal signs (multiple strokes, endocarditis)
5. Coma with meningitis (meningitis, endocarditis, encephalitis, subarachnoid hemorrhage)

This classification can be done relatively quickly at the bedside using the approach just described. These five forms of coma are very general, yet they are helpful in identifying the underlying pathologic process and in formulating a working diagnosis. When time is precious and any movement of the patient to a diagnostic test potentially destabilizing, it is essential to make an accurate assessment as soon as possible. Only at that point are you best prepared to decide which diagnostic and therapeutic steps will benefit the patient most.

Suggested Reading

Plum F, Posner JB (1984) The diagnosis of stupor and coma. Davis, Philadelphia
Stohr M, Brandt T, Einhäupl KM (1990) Neurologische Syndrom in der Intensivmedizin. Kohlhammer, Stuttgart

Decisions to Implement and Withdraw Therapy in the Neurologic Intensive Care Unit

Michael N. Diringer and Rudolf W.Ch. Janzen

Introduction

Fulfilling the claims of dignity and humanity during the course of a disease is the challenge of ethics in medicine. In the Neurologic Intensive Care Unit (NICU) this concept is sometimes difficult to maintain. Often the acuteness and severity of the central nervous system (CNS) dysfunction may become so extreme that the patient's family need a long time and repeated explanations before they appreciate the gravity of the situation and the dismal prognosis. In addition, despite great advances in therapeutic interventions, our ability to predict which patients will respond favorably is limited. Thus, uncertainty regarding prognosis often makes it difficult to define an appropriate care plan.

A global generally accepted body of ethical and legal aspects of the decision to implement and withdraw therapy in critically ill neurologic patients has not been achieved, and therefore the ethics and legal implications of various approaches to man-

agement vary widely. These factors influence not only this special situation, but are relevant in every decision in the NICU. This chapter will present some guidelines for implementation and withdrawal of therapy for critically ill neurologic patients based on medical ethics and legal considerations.

Identification of Patients Best Served by Neurologic Intensive Care Units

NICUs are specialized intensive care units established to care for patients who are seriously ill due to a dysfunction of the CNS, peripheral nervous system (PNS), or muscles. These units provide an environment with expertise in clinical assessment, neuromonitoring, and treatment of nervous system disease as well as the basic systemic supports necessary to treat critically ill patients. The patient best served by such a unit is one who would benefit from this unique combination of skills. Such patients include those with acute deteriorations due to nervous system failure, those patients

---

Section Editor: Werner Hacke

who require expectant monitoring of nervous system performance, and patients with systemic disease in which nervous system dysfunction is a prominent component.

Early identification of appropriate patients, in some case prior to their arrival in the hospital, is an important component of providing intensive care for neurologically impaired patients. Those in the prodromal stage of an acute illness, e.g., crescendo transient ischemic attacks prior to basilar artery occlusion or respiratory compromise in myasthenia gravis, should be admitted to an NICU. Rapid identification of appropriate patients in the Emergency Department and transfer to the NICU for definitive care is essential.

Allocation and appropriate use of available intensive care resources require admission criteria to determine which patients are best cared for in an NICU. These criteria should reflect the overall intensive care structure of each individual institution. In general, priority categories are defined and patients in the higher priority group are admitted preferentially. The following priority categories are useful in determining which patients should be admitted to an NICU.

Table 1. Conditions in which intensive therapeutic interventions would be expected to be efficacious

A. Acute dysfunction with respiratory depression
1. Peripheral nervous system
Guillain-Barré syndrome
myasthenia gravis
polymyositis
myopathy (e.g., Pompe's disease)
2. Central nervous system
tetanus
myoclonic/tetanic brain stem syndromes
pontine myelolysis
status epilepticus
cervical spine or medullary compression
B. Progressive intracranial mass lesions
1. Hemorrhage
ventricular
intracerebral
intracerebellar
subarachnoid
subdural
epidural
2. Traumatic contusions/hematomas
3. Space occupying infarcts
hemispheric
cerebellar
4. Tumor
5. Abscess
6. Other space-occupying lesions
C. Acute central/peripheral nervous system infections
Encephalitis
Ventriculitis
Meningitis
Abscess
Associated complications
D. Pre-/postsurgical instability

Category 1: Patients who are critically ill and unstable due to an acute deterioration of nervous system function in whom intensive therapeutic interventions are efficacious or are expected to be efficacious (Table 1). This category includes:

1. Acutely deteriorating patients with signs and symptoms of mass lesions in the intracranial or in-

traspinal spaces; e.g., the patient whose condition is deteriorating due to an intracranial hemorrhage who would be a candidate for medical or surgical treatment.

2. Acutely deteriorating patients with dysfunctions of the CNS or PNS requiring immediate support and who can uniquely be cared for in the NICU; e.g., the patient with

motor impairment of ventilatory function requiring mechanical ventilation.

3. Patients who have undergone intracranial or intraspinal procedures and are unstable in the postoperative period; e.g., a patient whose condition is acutely deteriorating due to intracranial hypertension, who has undergone a craniotomy, and in whom further treatment of the condition is either expected and/or needed.

4. Patients with neurologic and/or severe systemic compromise due to acute CNS infections, e.g., the patient with encephalitis, meningitis, or ventriculitis.

Category 2: Patients who are not critically ill at the time of admission but who require the sophisticated expectant neurologic monitoring available in the NICU. These patients would benefit from monitoring when there is a defined treatment based on the monitored variable. They are at risk for requiring immmediate intensive treatments and would be expected to benefit from intervention. The category consists of a diverse group of patients who have in common the need for expectant monitoring. Priority should be given to those patients requiring monitoring of multiple physiological modalities such as intracranial pressure, EEG, evoked potentials, blood pressure, pulmonary artery pressure, central venous pressure, and/or cardiac rhythm.

Category 3: Critically ill, unstable neurologic/neurosurgical patients in need of intensive treatments due to a non-neurologic deterioration in function where intensive therapeutic inter-ventions are expected to be efficacious. Such patients would include those on the neurologic/neurosurgical service with an acute deterioration of cardiac or pulmonary function unrelated to CNS or PNS disease. Such patients could include those whose unstable condition is due to infection or aspiration.

When patients are likely to require sophisticated interventions routinely performed in other ICUs, admission should be sought in those units. Examples include: cardiac pacing or balloon pump, abdominal surgery, or cardiac surgery.

Category 4: Critically ill patients whose previous state of health, underlying disease, or acute illness, either alone or in combination, severely reduces the likelihood of benefit from treatment in an NICU.

Patients in categories 1–3 should always be aggressively treated initially, with no limitations on therapy. As the clinical situation evolves, a lack of response to therapy or a deterioration in the patient's clinical condition due to progression of the underlying disease or unavoidable complications may suggest that the level of care should be reduced. Category 4 patients may also receive limited care; the level of care for these patients should be clearly defined at the time of admission.

When to Reduce Maximal Care

Medicine and society now consider it, under certain circumstances, acceptable to withdraw life-sustaining interventions when they are considered futile. The definition of which patients fit into this category and which interventions may be withdrawn continues to evolve. One broad definition considers a futile life-sustaining intervention as any intervention which serves merely to preserve life without reversing the underlying medical condition. Another definition considers interventions futile if they merely sustain a permanent state of unconsciousness, vegatative state, or permanent dependence on intensive care. On the other hand, some persons argue that the mere preservation of life without regard to quality or expected duration of life is a worthy goal and therefore no therapy could be considered futile. The final determination of what is considered futile for an individual patient now rests with the patient. It usually reflects their feeling about what constitutes a meaningful existence. If a patient loses decision-making capacity, the authority to make these decisions is, under certain circumstances, shifted to a surrogate. The attempts of the American legal system to define these circumstances are discussed below.

Central to a decision about withdrawal of care is being able to provide clear information about eventual outcome. Ideally one would determine whether a patient will survive an illness and with what quality of life. Currently, in many situations, this determination is based on clinical judgement with limited support from the literature or data banks. There have been many attempts to define outcome in severely neurologically impaired patients on the basis of clinical, electrophysiologic, radiologic, and metabolic criteria. These studies have been able to define a group of severely affected patients for whom there is an

almost certain likelihood that they will progress to cerebral death or survive in a persistent vegetative state. Examples of such circumstances include patients in coma 24 h after cardiac arrest who have absent corneal or pupillary reflexes, or patients after severe head injury with absent cortical responses to somatosensory evoked potentials bilaterally. A spectrum of additional findings may contribute to the prediction of poor outcome: burst-suppression-EEG in anoxic coma, increased CK-BB lactate, increased ICP $> 60\,\mathrm{mmHg}$ for more than 30 min, flat EEG, absence of brainstem function. Withdrawing treatment is a syndrome-related process adjusted to the individual situation of the patient.

At the other end of the spectrum, patients who do well and improve quickly are easily identified and in these the withdrawal of support is never considered. This leaves a group of seriously ill patients receiving aggressive, expensive medical therapies for whom it is not possible to reliably determine whether they will ever improve. Several systems have been developed in an attempt to improve determination of prognosis for patients in ICUs. Physiologic data from multiple organ systems are scored and the likelihood of discharge alive from the hospital predicted from this (e.g., APACHE III). Unfortunately, the applicability of such systems to neurologic patients is limited since the outcome in these patients is primarily determined by one organ system. Until better criteria are developed for the prediction of outcome for critically ill neurologic patients in the acute phase of the underlying disease, decisions regarding withdrawal of therapy will be difficult ones. In general, if uncertainty exists regarding prognosis, maximal therapy should be continued. The situation should continually be reassessed and the level of care modified appropriately.

Even when prognosis can be established, decisions regarding reduction in therapy are not easily made. Until recently medicine has considered the preservation of life to be paramount. Improvements in technology have created a situation in which this goal needs to be reassessed. Redefinition of the ultimate goals of medicine involves both ethical and legal considerations.

Ethical Principles

Several fundamental ethical principles are important in making decisions about withdrawal of therapy. They include beneficence, nonmaleficence, patient autonomy, and social justice.

The principles of beneficence and nonmaleficence require physicians to act to benefit patients and to do no harm. They have been the driving force behind medical practice for centuries and the justification for continuing medical treatment under any circumstances. However, aggressive medical care can also be considered a burden on the patient. Defining whether the care provides benefit is difficult and is based on the patient's (or surrogate's) definition of quality of life. The patient's capability to adapt to the presumed final outcome should be explored carefully and repeatedly. Conflict arises when the health care team's definition differs from that of

the patient (or surrogate). In general the patient's (surrogate's) definition should be respected.

Patient autonomy – the right of patients to determine their medical care – has increasingly gained acceptance in North America and Europe. This principle requires that physicians respect a competent patient's decision to forego any medical treatment, even when this will hasten the patient's death. The limits of this principle have been recently explored in the courts (see below).

The principle of social justice requires the allocation of medical resources fairly and according to medical need. As resources become more and more limited this principle will necessarily impact on clinical decision making.

Legal Considerations

Several recent legal cases have addressed the principle of patient autonomy. They dealt with questions of which therapies a patient may refuse and the right of the family to request withdrawal of treatment when the patient's wishes had not been previously expressed.

The *Quinlan* case addressed the question of withdrawal of *ventilation* from a patient in a persistent vegetative state. The New Jersey Supreme Count ruled that "the state's interest [in preserving life] weakens and the individual's right to privacy grows as the degree of bodily invasion increases and the prognosis dims." The court invoked "substituted judgement" to justify allowing the patient's family to make decisions regarding continued care when the patient had not expressed her wishes.

The question of withdrawal of *feeding* and *nutrition* was addressed in a later case. In California, two physicians were charged with murder for withdrawing feeding and hydration which led to the death of a patient with severe brain damage. The physicians were acquitted and the court felt that feeding and hydration should be considered as any other medical procedure. In the *Brophy* case, the Massachusetts Supreme Judicial Court ruled that feeding did not constitute ordinary care and could be withdrawn so that a patient in a persistent vegetative state could be allowed to die. The right of conscious patients to refuse feeding was upheld in the *Bouvia* case, where the court allowed a conscious patient without a terminal disease to refuse feeding. In many other countries feeding, hydration, and mechanical ventilation are considered a basic component of patient care in all subjects unless the patient or family refuse them.

While the right of a patient to refuse any therapy, including feeding and hydration, is now established, controversy exists when patients can no longer express their wishes and have not previously done so. In the Quinlan case the court gave the patient's father the authority to decide if ventilation should be removed. On the other hand, in the *Cruzan* case, the Missouri court felt that life-sustaining therapies could not be withdrawn at the family's request unless the patient had provided "clear and convincing" evidence stating that life-sustaining measures should be withheld. In Germany relatives are not allowed to make decisions for unconscious patients unless they have been appointed legal guardian by the court.

These cases have all dealt with the circumstance that a patient or surrogate has requested the withdrawal of therapy and the medical care team has resisted that request. In the *Wanglie* case, the patient's husband insisted that ventilatory support be continued for a patient in a vegetative state despite the recommendations of the health care team. The court supported continued ventilation since, in the family's view, the mere maintenance of life was a worthy goal and the ventilator was essential to achieve that goal.

Advance Directives

To avoid these conflicts the concept of a "living will" has evolved in the United States. In this document the patient clearly states his or her wishes regarding withdrawal of therapy in the event of a terminal illness. In addition, a recently enacted US federal law, the Patient Self-Determination Act, requires health care providers to discuss advance directives with all patients. In Europe, the patient's requests are handled in a similar fashion.

Unfortunately, in practice, the execution of these documents is only helpful in a limited number of situations. The documents generally only address the situation of a terminal illness and are usually drawn up at a time when the patient and family have little understanding of the disease process or the interventions required to maintain seriously ill patients. An alternative which deals with these limitations is the execution of durable power-of-attorney for health care. In this situation the patient executes a document which designates a surrogate to make health care decisions if the patient loses decision-making capacity. This allows the surrogate to make decisions in all situations based on their understanding of the patient's wishes.

Practical Principles

Ideally, when patients explore their wishes regarding medical care with family and physician, a care plan can be developed which respects those wishes. An advance directive (living will, durable power-of-attorney, or, preferably, both) should be executed by all patients prior to the stressful situation associated with serious illness. This should be actively encouraged by the medical and legal communities. As awareness grows this practice should become more commonplace.

When no advance directive is available the following course of action can facilitate decision making regarding the withdrawal of therapies.

1. The principle of patient autonomy should always be respected when questions arise regarding withdrawal of therapy. Effective communication between health care workers, patients, and families will help establish and respect patient autonomy. In the critical care setting stress, fear, intimidation, and unfamiliarity with the situation can compromise attempts at communication. It therefore becomes important that health care providers not only *attempt* but take measures to *ensure* effective communication. This process can be assisted by the use of a facilitator, e.g., a social worker, chaplain, or psycho therapist. Use of a quiet, unpressured environment is important to encourage meaningful communication. The physician should recognize that the reasoning ability of patients and families is often impaired by stress. Discussion should take place in clear straightforward language and questions should be encouraged.

2. An important aspect of these discussions is the early determination, and ongoing review, of individual quality of life values. Each patient has a *unique perspective* on what he or she considers an acceptable quality of life. In addition, as the clinical condition evolves this perspective may change. It is important that health care providers avoid making assumptions regarding this perspective and avoid imposing their values on the patient.

3. Unanimity among the members of the health care team should be sought to ensure that all members of the team are comfortable with the recommendations. This will help avoid inconsistent communications with the family.

4. When there is uncertainty or disagreement within the family, decision making should not be rushed. Ample time should be allowed for discussions within the family, with health care providers, and with others who could facilitate decision making. Often establishing a defined period of

treatment and then assessing concrete milestones that herald improvement or failure helps to alleviate confusion or guilt.

5. When there is disagreement between the patient (or surrogate) and the health care team the following measures may be useful:

   (a) Attempt resolution by having additional discussions between the health care team and the patient (surrogate). These discussions could make use of facilitators such as clergy, social workers, or psychotherapists.

   (b) Utilize institutional dispute resolution mechanisms such as an ethics committee.

   (c) Transfer the care of the patient to a physician who can accept the patient's (surrogate's) desires.

   (d) Utilize the courts only as a last resort.

The "Do Not Resuscitate" Patient

In all cases, decisions about reduction of level of care or withdrawal of therapy should be made jointly by the primary physician and the NICU team. Once the decision has been made to reduce maximal support the new level of care needs to be clearly defined. The reduction in level of care may simply be withholding cardiopulmonary resuscitation (CPR) in the event of cardiopulmonary arrest, or complete cessation of all interventions that would prolong the dying process. The determination of the new level of care should be made by the health care

team guided by the expressed wishes of the patient (surrogate). This will allow the patient or family to define the direction of care without burdening them with the responsibility for deciding the details of care. While this will result in an individualized care plan, the reduced level of care usually fits into one of the three categories listed below. As the process evolves the appropriateness of the do-not-resuscitate order should be periodically assessed and the patient may move from one category to another.

1. One option is to continue maximal therapy but refrain from performing CPR if it is needed. This option is particularly applicable to patients with a terminal illness who wish to be aggressively treated in order to slow the progression of the disease but do not wish to be maintained on "life support" in the event of a cardiac arrest or when the disease has progressed to the point where they require mechanical ventilation to stay alive. An exception is those patients with respiratory failure desirous of home ventilation. This approach is also appropriate in situations where CPR has been shown to be of no medical benefit, such as in patients with advanced cancer, sepsis, or gastrointestinal hemorrhage.

2. A second option is to continue the level of care that the patient is receiving but not to increase the level of care. This option is useful in situations where, given the current level of support, the patient may recover, but if he should deteriorate further interventions would be considered futile, and

thus the addition of new, more aggressive therapies such as mechanical ventilation or administration of vasopressors is not undertaken. These patients are generally not candidates for continued care in the ICU.

3. The third option is the reorientation of the patient's care from treatment of an illness to treatment directed exclusively toward patient comfort. In this situation it is agreed that any further treatment is futile and would merely prolong the dying process. Therefore it is appropriate to withdraw all therapy that is of no benefit to the patient but remains a source of pain and discomfort and interferes with the patient's ability to die with dignity. This should include discontinuing all therapies and medications that are not specifically directed toward patient comfort, discontinuing all painful procedures, including blood drawing, and providing nursing measures designed for comfort such as turning, suctioning, treatment of fever, and physiotherapy. In these cases, weaning off mechanical ventilation and discontinuing feeding and hydration are appropriate.

Weaning off mechanical ventilation remains controversial and continues to be a source of unease to many physicians. If the patient is breathing spontaneously then ventilatory support can easily be withdrawn. On the other extreme, if the patient meets the criteria for brain death then ventilation should be discontinued since the patient is legally dead. Difficulty arises when the patient is not brain dead and requires mechanical support to maintain ventilation. Some physicians do not feel it is appropriate to reduce ventilation since this will hasten death. Others are comfortable reducing or discontinuing ventilation when there is no possibility of recovery. These measures should only be undertaken if they represent the expressed will of the patient or surrogate and after discussing the implications with the family. Similarly in spontaneously breathing intubated patients, the decision to remove the endotracheal tube, which may result in airway obstruction, should be undertaken only after discussion with the family. Some physicians will use potent analgesics (including opiates) as appropriate to assure the absence of pain or discomfort, while others avoid the use of such agents since they can further embarrass respiratory function. However, since the focus of care has shifted from maintenance of life to provision of comfort, use of these drugs is appropriate. Ample opportunity should be provided for visits from family and clergy.

Suggested Reading

ACCP/SCCM Consensus Panel (1990) Ethical and moral guidelines for the initiation, continuation and withdrawal of intensive care. Chest 97:949–958

Blackhall LJ (1987) Must we always use CPR? N Engl J Med 318:1281–1285

Greco PJ, Schulman KA, Lavizzo-Mourey R, Hansen-Flaschen J (1991) The patient self-determination act and the future of advance directives. Ann Intern Med 115:639–643

Ruark JE, Raffin TA, Stanford Committee of Ethics (1988) Initiating and withdrawing life support. N Engl J Med 318:25–30

Schneiderman LJ, Jecker NS, Jonsen AR (1990) Medical futility: its meaning and ethical implications. Ann Intern Med 112:949–954

Sprung CL (1990) Changing attitudes and practices in forgoing life-sustaining treatments. JAMA 263:2211–2215

Younger SJ, Landefeld S, Coulton C, Juknialis BW, Leary M (1989) Brain death and organ retrieval: a cross-sectional survey of knowledge and concepts among health professionals. JAMA 261:2205–2210

Chapter 5

Documentation and Scores

Klaus Spitzer and Erich Schmutzhard

Introduction

Neurological scoring systems are used to assess the severity of illness in patients with neurological diseases. Their use in clinical trials has resulted in increased precision and patient description as well as in improved reliability and validity of results. They can be used to monitor clinical course, to document complications of therapy, to record findings for data banks, and to help identify prognostic factors. Computer-aided documentation in neurocritical care is less helpful when these standardized scoring systems are not used.

Problems of Quantitation of Neurological Disease

Assessing the severity of neurological disease has proven difficult to standardize for many reasons: (1) many controlled treatment trials choose vague, arbitrary definitions such as "improved, stable, worsened, or death" to monitor clinical course, and there is no consistency or common language among trials; (2) most scoring systems are disease specific (for example, systems for patients with multiple sclerosis cannot be used for those with acute stroke); (3) it is often difficult to use one system for different types of the same disease (for example, systems for patients with hemispheric infarcts cannot be used for those with brain-stem infarcts); (4) most scoring systems have not been assessed for inter-rater reliability; (5) frequently, the same scoring system is used to assess initial severity and outcome, rather than one system for the initial assessment (reflecting prognostic features of the examination) and another system for outcome (reflecting treatment differences); (6) finally, most scoring systems are not corrected for limitations in applicability (for example, assessment of sensory deficits in patients with aphasia or coma).

Section Editor: Michael N. Diringer

Requirements for Neurological Scoring Systems

A standardized neurological scoring system should be comprehensive, reliable, valid, brief, and practical. It should include only those parameters relevant to diagnosis, treatment, and prognosis. It should be written with simple, unambiguous definitions and should be easy to use for people with different degrees of medical training. The number of grades for each parameter should be minimized for better reliability. It should be sensitive enough to detect clinical changes and to reflect clinical outcome. A standardized neurological scoring system that is generally accepted would create a common language for all clinical investigators. Unfortunately, such a system does not exist at this time.

The extent of agreement among observers, or reliability, reflects the feasibility of using a scoring system. Many systems have been studied for inter-rater reliability. The kappa value (κ) is defined as the difference between the observed proportional agreements (P_o, number of all pairwise agreements divided by the number of all possible agreements) and the proportion of agreements expected by chance (P_c), divided by one minus proportion of agreements expected by chance; that is, $[P_o - P_c]/[1 - P_c]$. The kappa value reflects inter-rater agreement of variables scored on a nominal scale, such that κ of 0 = poor agreement, $0-0.2$ = slight agreement, $0.21-0.40$ = fair agreement, $0.41-0.80$ = substantial agreement, $0.81-0.99$ = almost perfect agreement, and 1.00 = perfect agreement.

Neurological Scores and Functional Scores

Two types of scoring systems are commonly used: neurological scoring systems, to quantitate neurological deficits ("N scores"), and functional scoring systems, to characterize patients' abilities to perform activites of daily living ("ADL scores", used to quantitate the functional outcome with and without therapy). Some "mixed" scales include both N scores and ADL scores. In most cases, N scores are used during the initial assessment and ADL scores are used for the outcome assessment.

N Scores

The Glasgow Coma Scale (GCS) is a neurological scoring system that is commonly used in critical care units (Table 1). It is often used as part of an initial rating for estimating prognosis

Table 1. Glasgow Coma Scale

Item	Factor	Score
Best motor response	Obeys	6
	Localizes	5
	Withdraws (flexion)	4
	Abnormal flexion	3
	Extensor response	2
	Nil	1
Verbal response	Oriented	5
	Confused conversation	4
	Inappropriate words	3
	Incomprehensible sounds	2
	Nil	1
Eye opening	Spontaneous	4
	To speech	3
	To pain	2
	Nil	1

Table 2. Oxbury Score (Mathew et al. 1972), modified (Prescott et al. 1982)

Item	Factor	Score
Consciousness	Fully conscious	6
	Somnolent, can be awakened to full consciousness	4
	Reacts to verbal command, but is not fully conscious	2
Eye movements	No gaze palsy	4
	Gaze palsy present	2
	Conjugate eye deviation	0
Arm, motor power (assessed only on affected side)	Raises arm with normal strength	6
	Raises arm with reduced strength	5
	Raises arm with flexion in elbow	4
	Can move, but not against gravity	2
	Paralysis	0
Hand, motor power (assessed only on affected side)	Normal strength	6
	Reduced strength in full range	4
	Some movement, fingertips do not reach palm	2
	Paralysis	0
Leg, motor power (assessed only on affected side)	Normal strength	6
	Raises straight leg with reduced strength	5
	Raises leg with flexion of knee	4
	Can move, but not against gravity	2
	Paralysis	0
Orientation	Correct for time, place and person	6
	Two of these	4
	One of these	2
	Completetely disorientated	0
Speech	No aphasia	10
	Limited vocabulary or incoherent speech	6
	More than yes/no, but not longer sentences	3
	Only yes/no or less	0
Facial palsy	None/dubious	2
	Present	0
Gait	Walks 5 m without aids	12
	Walks with aids	9
	Walks with help of another person	6
	Sits without support	3
	Bedridden/wheelchair	0

and functional outcome. Scoring is fast and reliable, and many of the scores used in some of the newer treatment studies are derived from the GCS.

The first neurological scoring system published was the Oxbury scale, developed to predict outcome from stroke. As with most initial assessment scales, no ADL parameters are included. A modified Oxbury scale was used in the Scandinavian Multicenter Trial of Hemodilution in Ischemic Stroke (Table 2). Another scale, the Orgogozo scale (Table 3),

Table 3. Orgogozo Scale

Item	Factor	Score
Consciousness	Normal	0
	Somnolent	1
	Stuporous	2
	Comatose	3
Mental confusion	Absent	0
	Partial	1
	Severe	2
Communication	Normal	0
	Disturbed	1
	Impossible	2
Visual function	Normal	0
	Partial visual loss	1
	Hemianopia or quadrianopia	2
Conjugate deviation of eyes	Absent	0
	Moderate	1
	Severe	2
Facial weakness	Absent	0
	Mild or moderate	1
	Severe or complete	2
Movement of upper limb	Normal	0
	Movement against resistance	1
	Movement against gravity or less	2
Function of hand	Normal	0
	Restricted	1
	Possible	2
	Impossible	3
Tone of upper limb	Normal	0
	Spastic	1
	Flaccid	2
Movement of lower limb	Normal	0
	Movement against resistance	1
	Movement against gravity	2
	Minimal movement or less	3
Tone of lower limb	Normal	0
	Spastic	1
	Flaccid	2
Disturbance of sensation	Absent	0
	Minimal or moderate	1
	Severe or complete	2
Urinary incontinence	Absent	0
	Occasionally	1
	Frequent or constant	2

Table 4. Canadian Neurological Score

Item	Factor	Score
Mentation	Alert	3
Level of consciousness	Drowsy	1.5
Orientation	Oriented	1
	Disoriented or not applicable	0
Speech	Normal	1
	Expressive deficit	0.5
	Receptive deficit	0
Motor fuctions	No comprehension deficit → section A1	
	Comprehension deficit → section A2	
→ Section A1		
Weakness		
– face	None	0.5
	Present	0
– arm, proximal	None	1.5
	Mild	1
	Significant	0.5
	Total	0
– arm, distal	None	1.5
	Mild	1
	Significant	0.5
	Total	0
– leg	None	1.5
	Mild	1
	Significant	0.5
	Total	0
→ Section A2		
Motor response		
– face	Symmetrical	0.5
	Asymmetrical	0
– arms	Equal	1.5
	Unequal	0
– legs	Equal	1.5
	Unequal	0

includes 13 parameters, although some, such as "mental confusion," "visual field," and "sensory disorders," have been associated with poor inter-rater agreement.

Scoring motor functions may be impossible in comatose patients or in those with impaired comprehension. The Canadian Neurological Scale (Table 4) was designed to take this into account and includes two sections: one for those with impaired comprehension and one for those without. It is both reliable and valid. The Mathew scale (Table 5) has been used in many stroke studies, such as those evaluating glycerol therapy in acute stroke and many of the nimodipine trials. It

Table 5. Mathew Scale

Item	Factor	Score
Mentation		
Level of consciousness	Fully conscious	8
	Lethargic but mentally intact	6
	Obtundent	4
	Stuporous	2
	Comatose	0
Orientation	Oriented × 3	6
	Oriented × 2	4
	Oriented × 1	2
	Disoriented	0
Speech	Normal	23
(Reitan test)	Incoherent words	15
	Expressive or impressive words	10
	Speechless	0
Cranial nerves		
Homonymous hemianopsia	Intact	3
	Mild	2
	Moderate	1
	Severe	0
Conjugate deviation of eyes	Intact	3
	Mild	2
	Moderate	1
	Severe	0
Facial weakness	Intact	3
	Mild	2
	Moderate	1
	Severe	0
Motor power (each limb separately)	Normal strength	5
	Contracts against resistance	4
	Elevates against gravity	3
	Gravity eliminated	2
	Flicker	1
	No movements	0
Performance or disability status scale	Normal	28
	Mild impairment	21
	Moderate impairment	14
	Severe impairment	7
	Death	0
Reflexes	Normal	3
	Asymmetrical or pathological reflexes	2
	Clonus	1
	No reflexes elicited	0
Sensation	Normal	3
	Mild sensory abnormality	2
	Severe sensory abnormality	1
	No response to pain	0

Table 6. NIH Stroke Scale

Item	Factor	Score
Level of consciousness	Alert, keenly responsive	0
	Drowsy, but arousable by minor stimulation to obey, answer, or respond	1
	Requires repeated stimulation to attend, or is lethargic or obtundent, requiring strong or painful stimulation to make movements (not stereotyped)	2
	Responds only with reflex motor or autonomic effects, or is totally unresponsive, flaccid, reflexless	3
Level of consciousness questions (the patient is asked the month and his or her age; only the initial answer is graded)	Answers both correctly	0
	Answers one correctly	1
	Answers both incorrectly or is unable to speak	2
Level of consciousness commands (the patient is instructed to open or close his or her hand or eyes; only initial responses are graded; credit is given if an unequivocal attempt is made but not completed)	Obeys both correctly	0
	Obeys one correctly	1
	Incorrect	2
Extraocular movements	Normal	0
	Partial gaze palsy; score is given when gaze is abnormal in one or both eyes; but where forced deviation or total gaze paresis is not present	1
	Forced deviation or total gaze paresis not overcome by the oculocephalic maneuver	2
Visual fields (test for hemianopia using moving or confrontation with both of patient's eyes open; double simultaneous stimulation is also performed; use visual threat where level of consciousness or comprehension limit testing, but score 1 only if clear-cut asymmetry is found; complete hemianopia [score of 2] is recorded for dense loss extending to within 5 to 10 degrees of fixation)	No visual loss	0
	Partial hemianopia	1
	Complete hemianopia	2
Facial palsy	Normal	0
	Minor	1
	Partial	2
	Complete	3
Motor arm (patient is examined with arms out-stretched at 90° if sitting, or at 45° if supine; request full effort for 10 s; if consciousness or comprehension are abnormal, cue the patient by actively lifting his or her arms into position as the request for effort is orally given)	Limb holds for 90° for full 10 s	0
	Limb holds 90°-position but drifts before full 10 s	1
	Limb cannot hold 90°-position for full 10 s, but there is some effort against gravity	2
	Limb falls, no effort against gravity	3

Table 6. *Continued*

Item	Factor	Score
Motor leg (while supine, patient is asked to maintain weaker leg at 30° for 5 s; if consciousness or comprehension are abnormal, cue the patient by actively lifting the leg into position as the request for effort is orally given)	Leg holds 30°-position for 5-s period	0
	Leg falls to intermediate position by the end of the 5-s period	1
	Leg falls to bed by 5 s, but there is some effort against gravity	2
	Leg falls to bed immediately with no effort against gravity	3
Limb ataxia (finger-to-nose and heel-to-shin tests are performed; ataxia is scored only if clearly out of proportion to weakness; limb ataxia would be "absent" in the hemiplegic, not untestable)	Absent	0
	Ataxia is present in one limb	1
	Ataxia is present in two limbs	2
Sensory (test with pin; when consciousness or comprehension are abnormal, score sensory normal unless deficit is clearly recognized [e.g., by clear-cut grimace asymmetry, withdrawal asymmetry]; only hemisensory losses are counted as abnormal)	Normal, no sensation loss	0
	Mild to moderate; patient feels pinprick is less sharp or is dull on the affected side; or there is a loss of superficial pain with pinprick but patient is aware of being touched	1
	Severe-to-total sensation loss; the patient is not aware of being touched	2
Neglect	No neglect	0
	Visual, tactile, or auditory hemi-inattention	1
	Profound inattention to more than one modality	2
Dysarthria	Normal	0
	Mild to moderate; patient slurs at least some words and, at worst, can be understood with some difficulty	1
	Patient's speech is so slurred as to be unintelligible (in absence of, or out of proportion to, any dysphasia)	2
Language (the patient is asked to name the items on the naming sheet and then is asked to read from the reading sheet; comprehension is judged from response to all of the commauds in the preceding general neurologic examination)	Normal	0
	Mild to moderate, as follows: naming crrors, word-finding errors, paraphasias, and/or impairment of comprehension or expression disability	1
	Severe: fully developed Broca's or Wernicke's aphasia (or variant)	2
	Mute or global aphasia	3

has both N score and ADL score features. Interobserver variability was studied by Gelmers in 1988. The NIH Stoke Scale, first developed by Adams and Biller, is used in many current stroke studies (Table 6). Inter-rater agreement has been found to be moderate to substantial for nine of 13 items.

Special scores in neurocritical care have been developed to predict outcome at an early stage of treatment.

Table 7. Rankin Scale

Factor	Score
No symptoms at all	0
No significant disability despite symptoms: able to carry out all usual duties and activities	1
Slight disability: unable to carry out all previous activities but able to look after own affairs without assistance	2
Moderate disability: requiring some help, but able to walk without assistance	3
Moderately severe disability: unable to walk without assistance, and unable to attend to own bodily needs without assistance	4
Severe disability: bedridden, incontinent, and requiring constant nursing care and attention	5

The Innsbruck Coma Scale is highly accurate in predicting nonsurvival in patients with severe head injuries and has been shown to be more accurate than other scales, such as the Apache II. The Leeds prognostic score, based on the Glasgow Coma Scale, also takes into account age, pupil reaction, intracranial pressure, blood pressure, CT (computerized tomography) findings, and other extracranial injuries.

ADL Scores

The Rankin Scale, developed in 1957, has only five ADL parameters (Table 7). Its validity has been assessed. In

Table 8. Barthel Index

Item	Factor	Score
All categories	Unable to perform task	0
Feeding	Independent	10
	Needs help	5
Bathing	Performs without assistance	5
Personal toilet (grooming)	Washes face, combs hair, brushes teeth, shaves	5
Dressing	Independent	10
	Needs help	5
Bowel control	No accidents	10
	Occasional accidents	5
Bladder control	No accidents	10
	Occasional accidents	5
Toilet	Independent	10
	Needs help	5
Chair/bed transfers	Independent	15
	Minimum assistance	10
	Able to sit but needs maximum assistance to transfer	5
Ambulation	Independent for 45 m	15
	With help for 45 m	10
	Wheelchair for 45 m	5
Stair climbing	Independent	10
	Needs help	5

1988, a slightly modified Rankin Scale was used in the Dutch TIA trial and the UK-TIA trial. The Barthel Scale is a similar functional scale that is simple and has high inter-rater reliability. It contains items that directly reflect disability in all daily activites: feeding, bathing, toileting, dressing, bowel and bladder control, transfers, walking, and stair climbing (Table 8). The Barthel Scale can be used both for initial assessment and for outcome. It has been validated and is used in most studies on recovery from stroke. The Expanded Disability Status Scale (EDSS) is the most detailed and specific functional scale available. It is based on functional systems (pyramidal, cerebellar, brain-stem, sensory, bowel and bladder, visual, mental, and other). Although it was initially used for assessment of soldiers in the Second World War, today it is mainly used for patients with multiple sclerosis. Nevertheless, it has limited applicability for patients requiring neurocritical care.

Other Scales

Some other common scales not described in detail here are the Garraway Score, Smith Outcome Score, and Katz Scale. Scales for assessment of patients with Parkinson's disease include the Hoehn-Yahr staging, Webster Rating Scale, and Minimental Status exam. The latter scale can also be used for patients with Alzheimer's dementia. For those with amyotrophic lateral sclerosis or multiple sclerosis, the EDSS, Neurological Rating System, and Illness Severity Score can be used.

Suggested Reading

Adams HP, Olinger CP, Barsan WG (1986) A dose-escalation study of large doses of naloxone for the treatment of patients with acute cerebral ischemia. Stroke 17: 404–409

Adams RJ, Meador KJ, Sethi KD, Grotta JC, Thomson-DS (1987) Graded neurologic scale for use in acute hemispheric stroke treatment protocols. Stroke 18:665–669

Asplund K (1987) Clinimetrics in stroke research. Stroke 18:528–530

Benzer A, Mitterschiffthaler G, Marosi M, Luef G, Pühringer F, de la Renotiere K, Lehner H, Schmutzhard E (1991) Prediction of non-survival after trauma: The Innsbuck Coma Scale. Lancet 338:977–978

Biller J, Massey EW, Adams HP (1987) A dose-escalation study of ORG 10172 in the treatment of acute cerebral infarction. Ann Neurol 22:159

Brott T, Adams HP, Olinger CP, Marler JR, Barsan WG, Biller J, Spilker J, Holleran R, Eberle R, Hertzberg V, Rorick M, Moomaw CJ, Walker M (1989) Measurements of acute cerebral infarction: a clinical examination scale. Stroke 20:864–870

Cote R, Hachinski VC, Shurvell BL, Norris JW, Wolfson C (1986) The Canadian Neurological Scale: a preliminary study in acute stroke. Stroke 17:731–737

Cote R, Battista RN, Wolfson C, Boucher J, Adam J, Hachinski V (1989) The Canadian Neurological Scale: validation and reliability assessment. Neurology 39:638–643

Feldman Z, Contant CF, Robertson CS, Narayan RK, Grossman RG (1991) Evaluation of the Leeds prognostic score for severe head injury. Lancet 337:1451–1453

Fleiss JL (1971) Measuring nominal scale agreement among many raters. Psychol Bull 76:378–382

Fleiss JL, Nee JCM, Landis JR (1979) Large sample variance of kappa in the case of different scts of raters. Psychol Bull 86: 974–977

Marks RJ, Simons RS, Blizzard RA, Browne DRG (1991) Predicting outcome in intensive therapy units – a comparison of Apache II with subjective assessments. Intensive Care Med 17:159–163

Fujitsu K, Muramoto M, Ikeda Y, Inada Y, Kim I, Kuwabara T (1990) Indications for surgical treatment of putaminal hemor-rhage, Comparative study based on serial CT and time-course analysis. J Neurosurg 73:518–525

Garraway WM, Akhtar AJ, Gore SM, Prescott RJ, Smith RG (1976) Observer variation in the clinical assessment of stroke. Age Aging 5:233–240

Gelmers HJ, Gorter K, de Weerdt CJ, Wiezer HJ (1988) A controlled trial of nimodipine in acute ischemic stroke. N Engl J Med 318:203–207

Gelmers HJ, Gorter K, de Weerdt CJ, Wiezer HJA (1988) Assessment of interobserver variability in a Dutch multicenter study on acute ischemic stroke. Stroke 19:709–711

Gelmers HJ, Hennerici M (1990) Effect of nimodipine on acute ischemic stroke. Pooled results from five randomized trials. Stroke 21:81–84

Gensemer IB, Smith JL, Walker JC, McMurry F, Indeck M, Brotman S (1989) Psychological consequences of blunt head trauma and relation to other indices of severity of injury. Ann Emerg Med 18:9–12

Goldstein LB, Bertels C, Davis JN (1989) Interrater reliability of the NIH Stroke Scale. Arch Neurol 46:660–662

Hacke W (1986) Neurologische Intensivmedizin, Notfallmedizin, vol 15. Perimed Fachbuch-Verlagsgesellschaft, Erlangen

Katz S, Akpom CA (1976) A measure of primary sociobiological functions. Int J Health Serv 6:493–507

Katz S, Ford AB, Moskowitz RW, Jackson BA, Jaffe MW (1963) Studies of illness in the aged. JAMA 185:914–919

K-TIA Study Group (1988) United Kingdom transient ischaemic attack (UK-TIA) aspirin trial: interim results. Br Med J 296:316–320

Kurtzke JF (1955) A new scale for evaluating disability in multiple sclerosis. Neurology 5:580–583

Kurtzke JF (1983) Rating neurologic impairment in multiple sclerosis: an expanded disability status scale (EDSS). Neurology 33:1444–1452

Mahoney FI, Barthel DW (1965) Functional evaluation: the Barthel Index. Maryland State Med J 14:61–65

Mathew NT, Meyer JS, Rivera VM, Charney JZ, Hartmann A (1972) Double-blind evaluation of glycerol therapy in acute cerebral infarction. Lancet 2:1327–1333

Olsen TS (1991) Outcome following occlusion of the middle cerebral artery. Acta Neurol Scand 83:254–258

Orgogozo JM, Capildeo R, Anagnostou CN, Juge O, Pere JJ, dar tigues JF, Steiner TF, Yotis A, Clifford Rose F (1983) A new stroke skale. Presse Med 12:3039–3044

Oxbury JM, Greenhall RCD, Grainger KMR (1975) Predicting the outcome of stroke: acute stage after cerebral infarction. Br Med J 3:125–127

Prescott RJ, Garraway WM, Akhtar AH (1982) Predicting functional outcome following acute stroke using a standard clinical examination. Stroke 13:641–647

Rankin J (1957) Cerebral vascular accidents in patients over the age of 60, 2. Prognosis. Scott Med J 2:200–215

Ropper AH, Griswold K, McKenna D, Souder D (1981) Computer-guided neurologic assessment in the neurologic intensive care unit. Heart Lung 10:54–60

Scandinavian Stroke Study Group (1985) Multicenter trial of hemodilution in ischemic stroke – background and study protocol. Stroke 16:885–890

Skilbeck CE, Wade DT, Hewer RL, Wood VA (1983) Recovery after stroke. J Neurol Neurosurg Psychiatry 46:5–8

Smith ME, Garraway WM, Akhtar AJ, Andrews CJA (1977) An assessment unit for measuring the outcome of stroke rehabilitation. Br J Occ Ther 40:51–53

Spence JD, Donner AD (1982) Problems in design of stroke treatment trials. Stroke 13:94–99

The Dutch TIA Trial (1988) protective effects of low-dose aspirin and atenolol in patients with transient ischemic attacks or non-disabling stroke. Stroke 19:512–517

Tourtellote WW, Syndulko K (1989) Quantifying the neurologic examination: principles, constraints, and opportunities. In: Munsat TL (ed) Quantification of neurologic deficit. Butterworths, Boston, pp 7–16

Tuhrim S, Dambrosia JM, Price TR, Mohr JP, Wolf PA, Heyman A, Kase CS (1988) Prediction of intracerebral hemorrhage survival. Ann Neurol 24:258–263

van Swieten JC, Koudstaal PJ, Visser MC, Schouten HJ, van Gijn J (1988) Interobserver agreement for the assessment of handicap in stroke patients. Stroke 19:604–607

General Monitoring

Chapter 6 | # Electrophysiologic Monitoring

DERK KRIEGER, MARC NUWER, and HELMUT BUCHNER

Introduction

The main goals of electrophysiologic monitoring techniques – electroencephalography (EEG) and evoked potentials (EP) – in the intensive care unit and operating room are to evaluate central nervous system (CNS) function in unresponsive patients and forecast neurological deficit. Monitoring CNS function by objective variables is of particular interest in artificially paralyzed or anesthetized patients, since clinical neurological assessment is very limited. Monitoring is achieved by continuous or sequential assessment of various nervous functions in order to detect spontaneous or induced changes in the patient's condition. In principle, EEG reflects cortical electrical activity deriving from synergy of cortical and subcortical structures, whereas EP consist of the summation of electrical responses at various levels of the neuraxis within a sensory pathway following repetitive distal stimulation. In practice, monitoring CNS

function using electrophysiologic techniques in intensive care unit patients is subject to several limitations: (a) data aquisition requires well-trained staff, (b) signal processing and analysis requires sophisticated computers and software, (c) the specificity of any EEG and EP signal pattern is low, and (d) the signal-to-noise ratio has to be low.

Monitoring EEG and EP signal pattern variation may assist in early detection of deterioration of CNS functioning. For example, by the time temporal lobe herniation has reached the stage of third cranial nerve compression with pupillary dilatation, it may already be too late for any useful intervention, since substantial irreparable damage has already occurred. Or, in the case of cerebral vasospasm, hours can pass between the onset of cerebral ischemia and clear demonstration of a focal neurological deficit. In regard to prompt therapeutic intervention in such patients, it is of paramount importance to have instruments that are able to detect subtle alteration of central nervous function. Thus, continuous EEG may become an important adjunct in monitoring

Section Editor: Michael N. Diringer

neurocritical care patients. Since analog EEG recordings generate huge amounts of complex information, raw data processing strategies have been developed to simplify interpretation. While anecdotal reports have shown that continuous EEG monitoring on neurointensive care units is helpful, it has not been studied prospectively in most disorders prevalent in neurocritical care. Thus, other than in standard analog EEG recordings, normative data and clinical correlations remain poorly defined. Furthermore, the effect of intercurrent abnormalities on the patient's EEG, such as hypotension, sepsis, hypoxemia, and numerous simultaneously administered drugs has yet to be established. Nor has it been proven that EEG changes beyond a given threshold call for clinical intervention.

Current interest focuses on the diagnostic and monitoring capabilities of EP because they are resistant to alteration by anything except structural pathology and are closely tied to anatomical structures, thus testing the integrity of sensory pathways. Subcortical potentials, brainstem auditory evoked potentials (BAEP) waves I–V and primary cortical responses of somatosensory evoked potentials (SSEP) peak N20, remain essentially unchanged in deep anesthesia; however, later cortical components (VEP peak P75, SSEP components following N20) vary considerably according to the depth of anesthesia. Since amplitudes of EP usually do not exceed $10\,\mu V$, signal processing requires averaging of numerous sweeps and at least two reproduced trials. Thus, for monitoring purposes, it has to be stressed that real-time monitoring as with conventional EEG is not possible

using EP. Subtle changes of wave patterns, not necessarily leading to interpeak latency increases, may escape recognition. Presently, analysis of EP primarily relies on heuristic methods, such as determination of latency and amplitude of reproduced signals. The principal disadvantage of this routine is that it requires wave pattern recognition and thus depends mainly on the investigator's experience. Attempts to augment the significance of EP monitoring include alternative concepts of signal processing and analysis. Considerable effort has been directed to developing methods that improve event-related signal detection and EP estimation. Although recent progress in digital filtering techniques such as time-varying filters or Wiener filtering seems promising, their practical usefulness has not been established. Standard averaging is still the state of the art in EP processing, but is limited in its ability to detect instant changes during continuous EP monitoring. Potential options include increasing the stimulus rate above 300/s for median nerve SSEP and above 1500/s for BAEP by delivering encoded stimuli at pseudorandomized interstimulus intervals. The recorded overlapped evoked response is thereafter corrected for the submitted stimulus sequence. In addition, presentation of various stimulus rates might disclose alterations in the nervous system's response, in particular in global encephalopathic states or under general anesthesia.

For further analysis of serial or continuous neuroelectric potentials, EP feature extraction and data standardization are essential. Traditional heuristic methods involve recognition of certain wave form patterns which are easily identified in healthy subjects but can be difficult, if not impossible, to recognize in patients with severe CNS dysfunction. Although subjective methods of EP interpretation are adequate for many clinical questions, there are shortcomings in evaluating comatose patients. Statistical methods of EP data processing, such as cross-correlation analysis, condense the amount of data generated by primary averaging, but do not depend on subjective interpretation of EP wave forms. Cross-correlation analysis assesses the similarity of two signals and quantifies the congruence of reproduced trials, thus detecting subtle changes. Computerized calculation of mean absolute amplitude of the averaged trials may serve as an alternative method to ensure the presence of a valid stimulus locked signal.

EEG Monitoring[1]

EEG activity represents the spatial and temporal summation of post-synaptic excitatory and inhibitory potentials arising from neurons occupying layers III and V of the pyramidal cortex. These neurons are influenced by afferent activity of subcortical origin. The presence, level of activity, and interaction of these post-synaptic potentials reflect the cerebral metabolism. Since pyramidal cells of layers III and V within the cortical gray matter are selectively vulnerable to hypoxia and ischemia, EEG may serve as a sensitive cerebral monitor. Although studies have confirmed that

the International 10/20 Electrode Placement System does establish a consistent relationship between electrode scalp placement and underlying cerebral topography, EEG cannot provide the anatomical resolution of imaging studies. However, the crucial factor that makes electrophysiologic techniques so valuable for cerebral monitoring purposes is that both EEG and EP become abnormal before irreversible cell injury occurs. EEG deteriorates prior to cell membrane failure and reduction of tissue concentration of adenosine triphosphate. In cerebral ischemia, EEG and EP abnormalities occur when cerebral blood flow drops to 30 ml/100 g per minute. Burst and suppression pattern and isoelectric EEG are found with flows between 12 and 18 ml/100 g per minute.

In neurocritical care patients EEG monitoring is helpful in predicting the severity of cortical dysfunction in encephalopathies. However, it cannot distinguish between the various possible etiologies: metabolic, anoxic, toxic, infectious, or degenerative. EEG changes may predate the clinical findings, especially in metabolic encephalopathies, but EEG improvement may lag several weeks or more behind clinical improvement, especially if the EEG abnormality was severe. Only in a few instances can EEG features be suggestive of a specific etiology, such as subacute sclerosing panencephalitis (SSPE), Creutzfeldt-Jakob disease (CJD), or herpes simplex encephalitis (HSE). Toxicity in an obtunded patient whose EEG contains prominent frontal β-activity is likely to originate from a barbiturate or benzodiazepine. Psychogenic unresponsiveness can easily be distinguished

---

[1] For reviews see Prior (1979) and Chiappa (1988).

from organic states. Nonconvulsive status epilepticus can be recognized and treated. Diffuse bilateral EEG changes are associated with an altered level of consciousness. Confusion and impaired cognition, often with lethargy, is associated with slowing of the background rhythms to θ. Intermittent rhythmic δ-activity, usually frontal in adults and occipital in children, is then seen.

Bilateral synchronous paroxysmal EEG discharges are seen in diffuse cortical and subcortical grey matter disease but not in patients with predominant cortical grey matter involvement. When grey and white matter are involved, continuous polymorphic δ-activity and bilateral synchronous paroxysmal EEG discharges were seen. Periodic paroxysmal discharges are predominantly found in SSPE, CJD, and HSE.

Triphasic waves were initially described in the EEG of patients in hepatic coma but can also be seen in other metabolic and anoxic encephalopathies. Triphasic waves have an initial negative sharp component, a positive component, and then a slow negative component. They are seen with deteriorating levels of consciousness and indicate a grave prognosis. It has been proposed that triphasic waves are generated by the same thalamocortical volleys that normally induce sleep spindles.

EEG in Coma

The onset of coma is associated with high-voltage polymorphic δ activity and marked decrease of faster frequencies. Use of computerized EEG frequency analysis, compressed spec-

tral array (CSA), has proven prognostically helpful in comatose patients. Those with sustained, slow, and monotonous rhythms die or enter vegetative states, in contrast to those who demonstrate modulation of physiologic sleep activity. A better outcome has been reported in association with variable EEG patterns. To study spontaneous alteration of EEG and sleep patterns in comatose patients adequately it is necessary to record the EEG in combination with other physiological parameters such as blood pressure, heart rate, eye movements, and chin electromyogram over an extended period of time (>6h). Several studies have revealed differences in the EEG activity recorded during the day and at night in comatose patients. Some showed typical EEG sleep patterns even with a normal circadian cycle, others demonstrated disorganized circadian rhythms or reported abnormal, stimulus-related slow-wave arousal responses in comatose patients. It was also found that diazepam medication did not increase EEG fast activity in comatose subjects with poor outcome, and hyperventilation increased faster frequencies in those patients with a more favorable outcome.

The magnitude of EEG changes is closely related to the severity of outcome in hypoxic encephalopathy. The EEG should be obtained no sooner than 8h after the hypoxic episode. Electrocerebral silence and burst suppression are usually associated with a fatal outcome. Bilateral periodic sharp-wave activity at approximately 1 Hz associated with myoclonic jerks may be found. Otherwise, there tends to be a poor electrographic correlation with clinical seizures. Unilateral or bilaterally independent, periodic lateralized epileptic discharges (PLEDs) are also seen in a variety of severe encephalopathies. The specific pattern of "α-coma" is a rhythm resembling normal α-activity, that usually appears after an anoxic episode and carries an almost invariably fatal prognosis. The neuropathologic correlate of α-coma is widespread diffuse neuronal loss within the entire brain. It is sometimes difficult to distinguish this rhythm from medication-induced fast activity or a normal α-rhythm, which is occasionlly seen in comatose patients. Using CSA "α-rhythm coma" can be distinguished from physiologic α-activity by a broader spread of power over the 8- to 13-Hz band, frequency instability, and progressive decline in amplitude over several days. It also must be distinguished from the occipitally dominant α seen in the locked-in syndrome, in which the patient is mute and paralyzed due to an extended bilateral pontine infarct sparing the tegmentum. These individuals are alert and show normal waking and sleeping patterns. There is no specific EEG pattern attributed to patients with persistent vegetative states; however, EEG pattern is unresponsive to external stimuli in most of these patients.

Infections of the central nervous system produce alterations of the EEG, from mild slowing of background rhythms in approximately half of patients with aseptic meningitis to marked diffuse slowing with polymorphic δ-activity in purulent meningitis. Epileptiform activity is seen occasionly, mainly in patients with clinical seizures. Encephalitis is almost always associated with an abnormal EEG recording demonstrating diffuse polymorphic δ-activity. Focal slowing or attenuation in one temporal lobe, often associated with periodic sharp waves or PLEDs, is characteristic of HSE.

Continuous EEG monitoring in patients with elevated intracranial pressure (ICP) has been used mainly to guide intravenous barbiturate therapy. While some authors recommend doses to suppress all EEG activity, others recommend achieving either a burst suppression pattern or titrating the dose to therapeutic efficacy. Attempts to correlate ICP levels to particular EEG patterns have failed. However, when elevated ICP is stable, without pressure waves, the EEG contains regular high-voltage slow waves, while an alternating EEG is mainly seen in patients whose ICP tracing contain Lundberg B waves.

EEG in Status Epilepticus

In cases where generalized convulsive status epilepticus is refractory to standard therapy, barbiturate-induced coma has been recommended. Several protocols have suggested the use of different doses, ranging from the minimal dose needed to interrupt clinical seizures to induction of deep anesthesia with electrocerebral inactivity. Continuous EEG monitoring is necessary in order to detect persistent or recurrent seizure activity, since clinical assessment is unreliable. Status epilepticus may be considered to be the underlying cause of continuing coma in a previously seizuring patient, or in the presence of unusual movements in a comatose patient. Intermittent or continuous spike-and-wave EEG activity was found in more than two-thirds of comatose patients with rhythmic clonic movements; however,

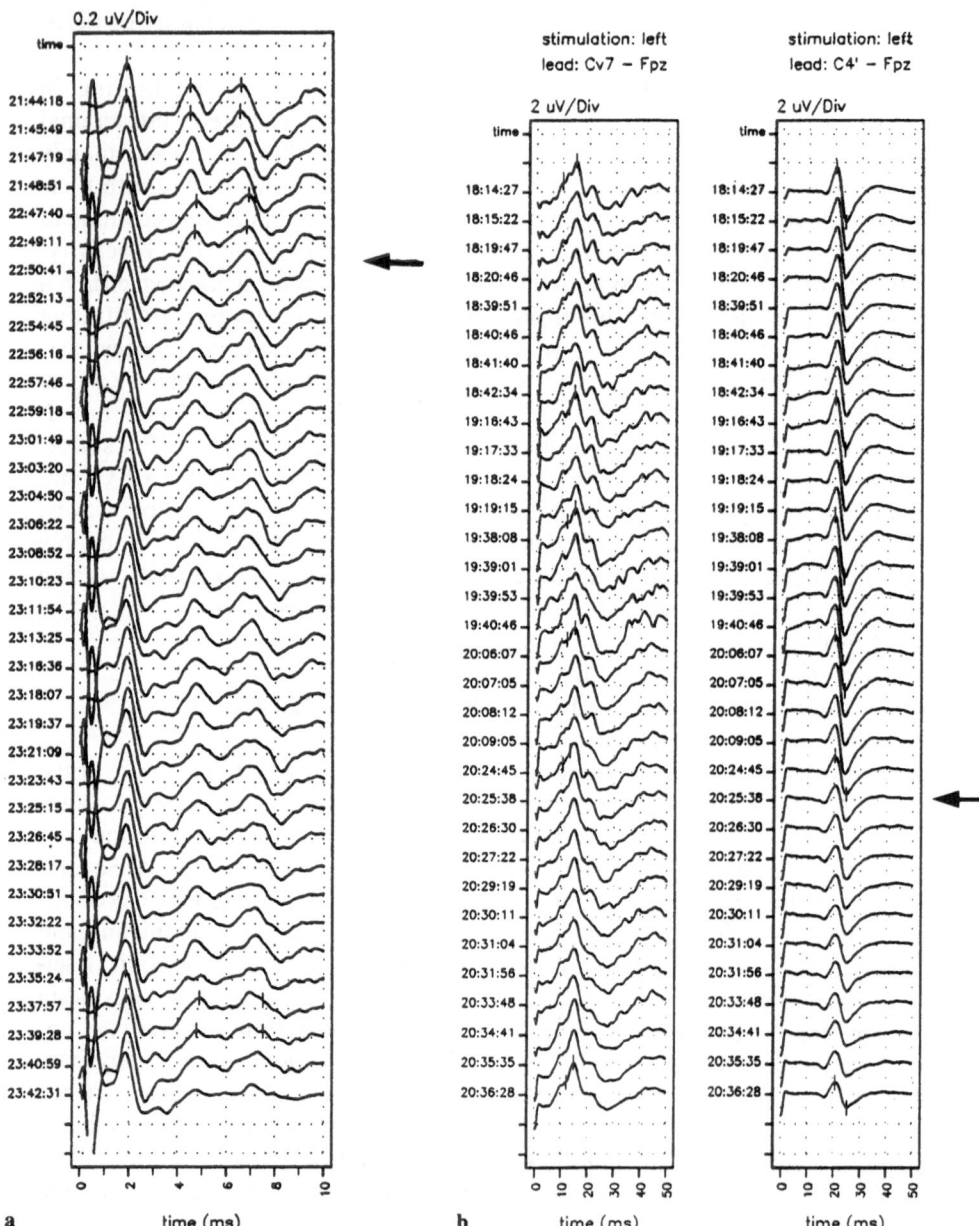

stimulation: right
alternating clicks
lead: M2 − Fpz

0.2 uV/Div

stimulation: left
lead: Cv7 − Fpz

2 uV/Div

stimulation: left
lead: C4' − Fpz

2 uV/Div

a   time (ms)
b   time (ms)
             time (ms)

Fig. 1a,b. Continuous monitoring of brainstem auditory evoked potentials (BAEP; **a**) and somato-sensory evoked potentials (SSEP; **b**) in two patients with clinical signs of transtentorial herniation. A A 22-year-old man with a massive subarachnoid hemorrhage (SAH) from a giant basilar aneurysm not suitable for surgery. Continuous BAEP monitoring for brainstem ischemia was performed after several thrombogenic metal coils were introduced into the aneurysm in an attempt of obliteration. The intubated and artificially ventilated patient developed acute severe hypertension and bilaterally eccentric, enlarged, nonreactive pupils shortly after the procedure (22:49, *arrow*). Autopsy revealed massive SAH from the ruptured basilar aneurysm. **b** A 57-year-old woman suffering from a massive a few patients showed EEG seizures without any clinical evidence of seizures. These findings raise the question whether nonconvulsive status epilepticus may be more common than was previously thought among unconscious neurointensive care patients. Prospective studies on continuous EEG monitoring in unconscious individuals, in particular those with anoxic-ischemic coma, are required to resolve the issue.

Evoked Potential Monitoring[2]

Intensive Care Electrophysiologic Monitoring

EP monitoring with BAEP, SSEP, visual evoked potentials (VEP), and motor evoked potentials (MEP) has been mainly used for predicting the outcome of neurologic catastrophes, in particular following global ischemia and head trauma.

Prognosis on the basis of BAEP is sometimes hampered by the absence of wave I because of sensorineural hearing loss or hematotympanon. Additionally, due to the location of BAEP wave generators, auditory pathway monitoring focuses on intrinsic brain-

---

[2] For review see Chiappa (1989).

stem processes, brainstem compression secondary to posterior fossa-expanding lesions, and supratentorial mass lesions producing tissue shifts at the transtentorial notch. Clinical signs of brainstem dysfunction and basilar artery occlusion level in brainstem infarction have been correlated with specific BAEP wave patterns. Bilateral abnormal BAEP imply a poor prognosis in patients with proven basilar artery thrombosis. Normal or unilateral abnormal BAEP are less helpful, because they can be associated with persistent coma or vegetative state. The diagnostic yield of BAEP in intrinsic brainstem disease seems low compared to that of magnetic resonance imaging. Serial BAEP recordings are helpful in assessing the clinical course in patients with brainstem compression due to supratentorial and infratentorial mass lesions. However, the variation of BAEP and SSEP signals may be quite unapparent in profound clinical deterioration. As a consequence, serial recordings must be performed within short intervals and analysis must relate to wave form rather than interpeak latencies (Fig. 1). Serial BAEP studies are valuable in cerebellar mass lesions with secondary brainstem compression (Fig. 2). BAEP changes reflect restoration of brainstem function following decompressive surgery. It seems that pro-

---

left hemispheric infarction due to severe vasospasm following SAH of an anterior communicating artery aneurysm. In the presence of generalized severe vasospasm her condition deteriorated and was subsequently intubated and artificially ventilated prior to continuous SSEP monitoring. Maximal medical antiedema procedures were carried out since she was not a candidate for surgical decompression. Shortly after, she too developed acute hypertension and bilaterally eccentric, enlarged, nonreactive pupils during continous SSEP monitoring (20:25, *arrow*). *Note:* Interpeak latency determination does not reveal any change during neurologic deterioration, but variation in signal pattern is obvious

66   D. Krieger et al.

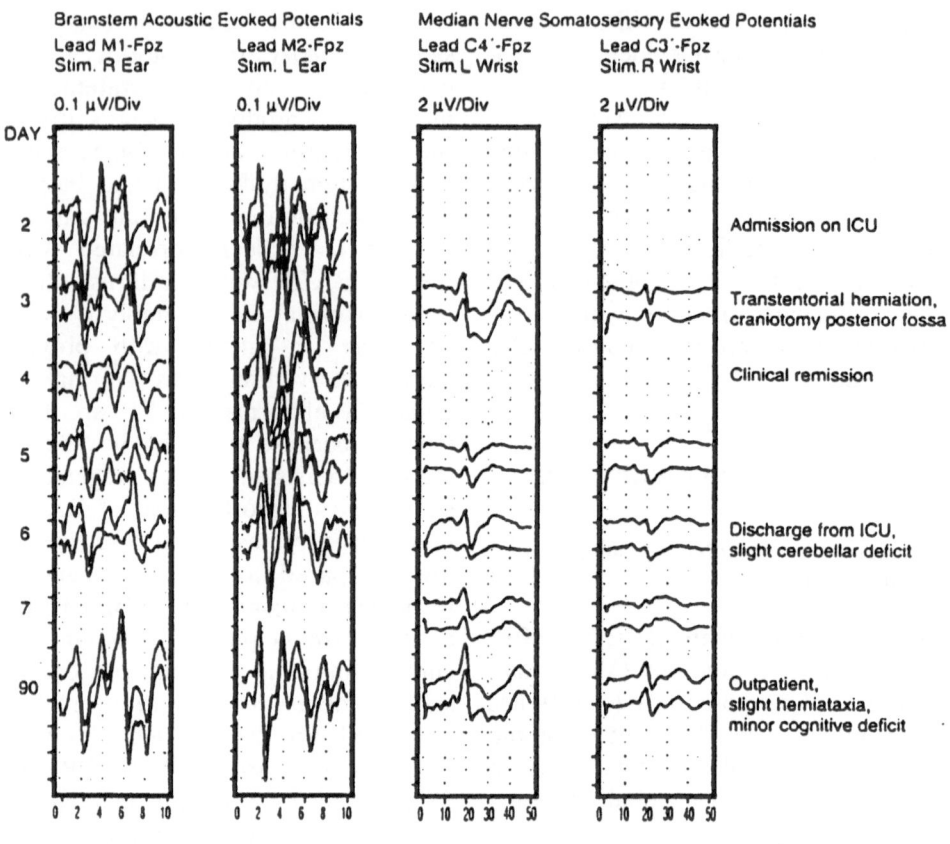

Fig. 2. a Serial recordings of BAEP in a 35-year-old female patient with bilateral cerebellar infarctions in the territory of the superior cerebellar artery.
October 21, 1989: Admission to ICU in a deeply stuporous state
October 22, 1989: Neurological deterioration, decompressive surgery
October 23–November 6, 1989: Clinical remission, discharge with slight cerebellar deficit
April 7, 1990: Slight hemiataxia, minor cognitive deficit

gressive desynchronization of waves IV and V indicates severe brainstem compression and calls for immediate decompressive surgery, but presence of wave III is a prerequisite for survival.

In a recent comparative study on 100 patients with severe head injury, the superior prognostic value of SSEP testing over EEG analysis was demonstrated. Several studies revealed that in neurologic catastrophes, with a few exceptions, early bilateral absence of cortical SSEP following median nerve (N20/P25 complex) and tibial nerve stimulation (N35/P40 complex) are associated with death or an otherwise poor outcome. In contrast, preservation of cortical waves does not assure a good outcome, but comatose patients with both cortical potentials preserved probably have the potential for recovery. Currently, the use of SSEP in

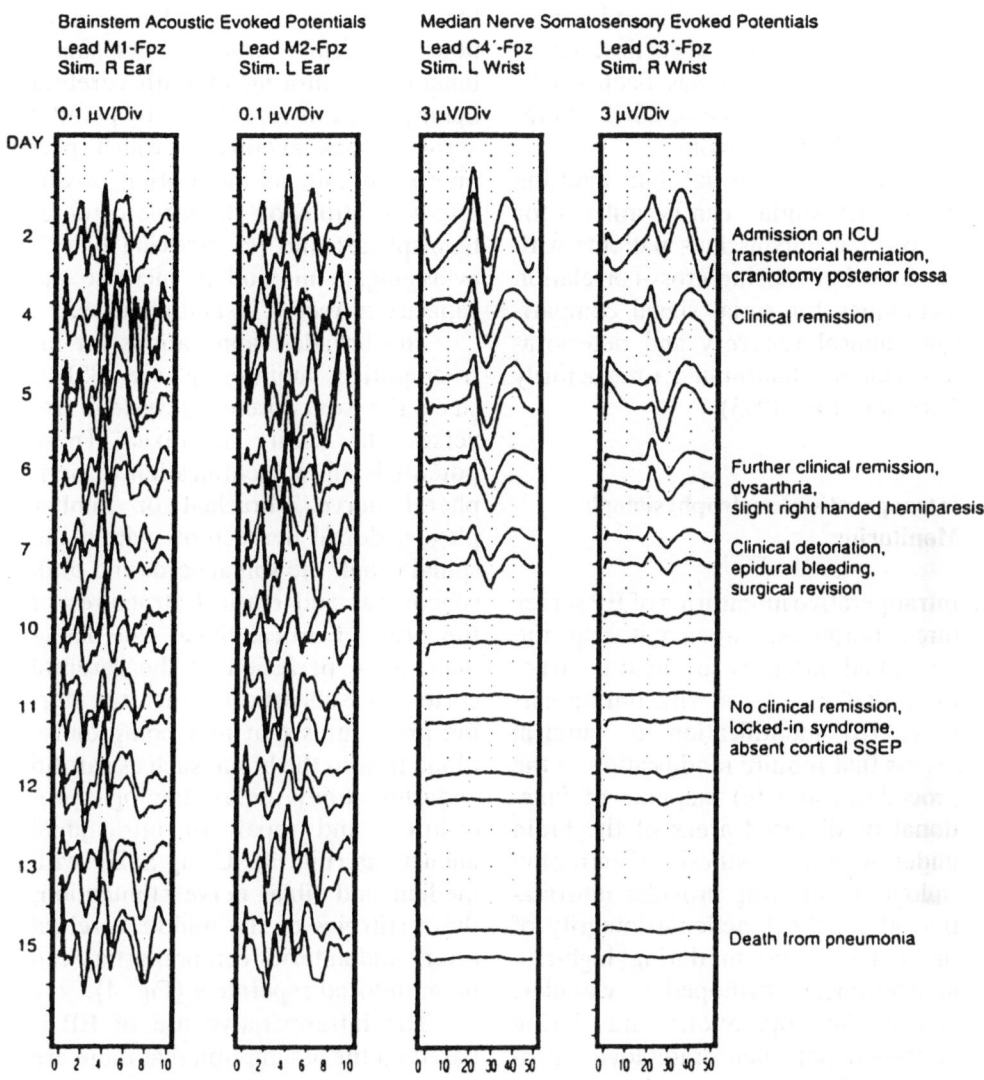

b   Time (ms) after Stimulus Onset

Fig. 2. b Serial recordings of BAEP in a 64-year-old male patient with bilateral cerebellar infarctions in the territory of the posterior inferior cerebellar artery.
September 13, 1989: Admission to ICU a deeply stuporous state
September 13, 1989, a few hours after admission: Neurological deterioration, decompressive surgery
September 14 16, 1989: Clinical remission, dysarthria, slight right-sided hemiparesis
September 17, 1989: Clinical deterioration, epidural rebleeding, surgical revision
September 18–25, 1989: No further clinical remission, locked-in syndrome
(Both from Rieke et al. 1993)

comatose patients is limited since, except in the absence of cortical potentials, no correlation has been established between degree of SSEP alteration and clinical outcome.

Additionally, serial light emitting diode-VEP studies can be utilized for monitoring unconscious patients with elevated ICP. Using cross-correlation techniques for serial signal comparison, clinical recovery and deterioration can be determined satisfactorily (Krieger et al. 1993).

Intraoperative Electrophysiologic Monitoring[3]

Intraoperative monitoring of EP serves three purposes: (a) monitoring the functional integrity of neural structures that may be at risk during surgery, (b) identification of surgical events that require modification of the procedure, and (c) mapping of functional or diseased areas of the brain under general anesthesia. Electrophysiologic monitoring provides information about the functional integrity of the nervous system during high-risk neurosurgical, orthopedic, vascular, and cardiac operations and during interventional neuroradiologic procedures. During the monitoring procedure, distinctions must be made between EP alterations that reflect threats to the functional integrity of vital neural structures and changes that are due to technical difficulties or reversible pharmacologic or physiologic manipulations.

Currently, three variations of standard averaging technique are available

for routine use: (a) parallel synchronous averaging, which allows simultaneous monitoring of both cerebral hemispheres in real time; (b) parallel asynchronous averaging, which permits simultaneous monitoring of different locations on the same cerebral hemisphere; and (c) "moving block" averaging, a method to increase the capacity to record instant changes.

The broadest applications for intraoperative monitoring are SSEP, since the somatosensory system traverses the entire neuraxis. These potentials allow identification of peripheral nerves, brachial or lumbar plexus, dorsal nerve roots within the spinal canal, the spinal cord, and both subcortical and cortical structures of the brain. Cortical SSEP can detect inadequate perfusion of the cerebral cortex or subcortical structures during procedures that may compromise blood flow to the brain, such as carotid endarterectomy, neuroradiologic procedures, and repair of intracranial aneurysms (Fig. 3). Using SSEP with median and tibial nerve stimulation, the territories of the middle cerebral artery and anterior cerebral artery can be monitored seperately (Fig. 4).

The intraoperative use of EP is based on the assumption that there are relationships between the brain's evoked electrical activity and ischemia. Recent work has suggested that a prolonged period of time spent below the level of functional threshold for preservation of EP may be sufficient to produce an infarct. In clinical practice, the key measurement for SSEP remains the determination of the central conduction time. For continuous intraoperative monitoring, the magnitude and duration of EP changes that may be reversible are yet not well defined.

---

[3] For review see Grundy (1986), Nuwer (1989), and Hacke (1989).

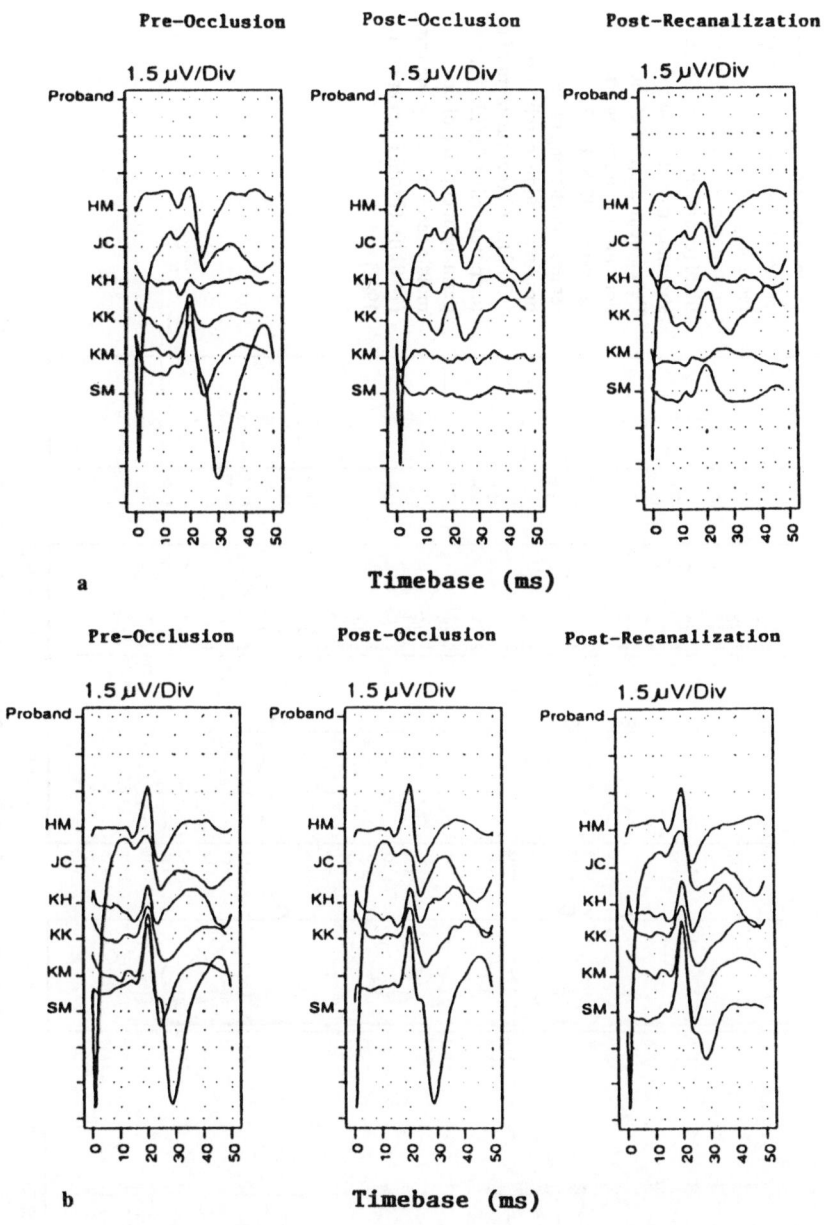

Fig. 3a,b. Cortical SSEP following median nerve stimulation in six patients undergoing transient occlusion of the middle cerebral artery during surgical aneurysm repair. **a** Ipsilateral leads: In three patients (H.M., J.C., K.K.) normal SSEP were recorded throughout the occlusion period and no postoperative deficit occurred. In two patients (K.M., S.M.) SSEP disappeared shortly after currently clipping and recovered only in patient S.M. after removal of the clip. K.M. suffered from moderate to severe hemiparesis postoperatively. K.H. presented with abnormal SSEP prior to surgery, resulting from an intracerebral hemorrhage due to the ruptured aneurysm; this demonstrates the limitations of intraoperative neuromonitoring in patients with preexisting damage of the neural pathway. **b** Contralateral leads: Almost identical SSEP were recorded throughout the occlusion period on the contralateral side

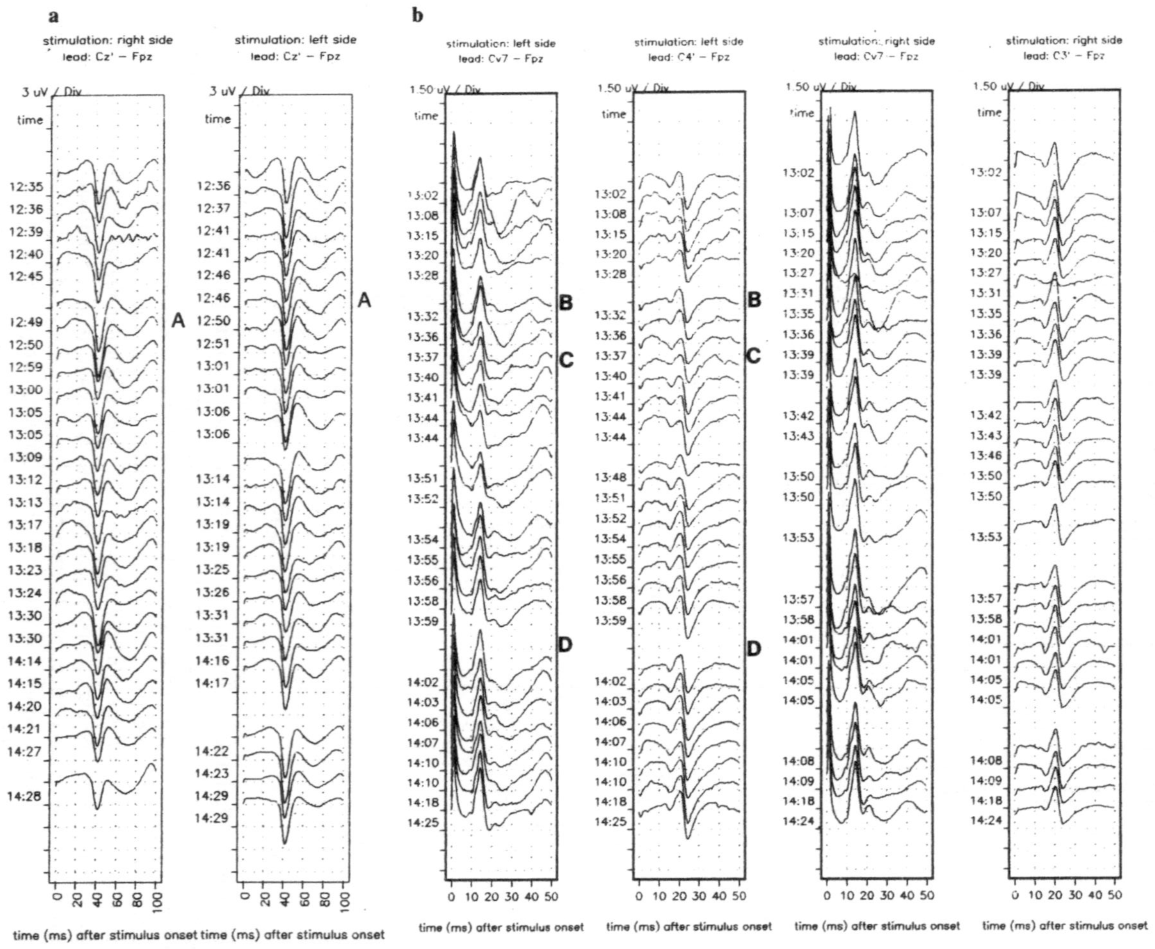

Fig. 4a–d. Cortical SSEP following tibial (**a**) and spinal and cortical SSEP following median nerve (**b**) stimulation during surgery. Intraoperative events are listed parallel to the recordings (*A–D*). Postoperative SSEP following tibial (**c**) and median nerve (**d**) stimulation on day 2 and 7. *A*, Permanent clipping of the anterior comunicating artery aneurysm (12:50h); *B*, temporary clipping of the proximal middle cerebral artery (13:32h); *C*, readjustment of the temporary clip (*B*) (13:39h); *D*, permanent clipping of the middle cerebral artery aneurysm (14:01h). (From Krieger et al. 1992)

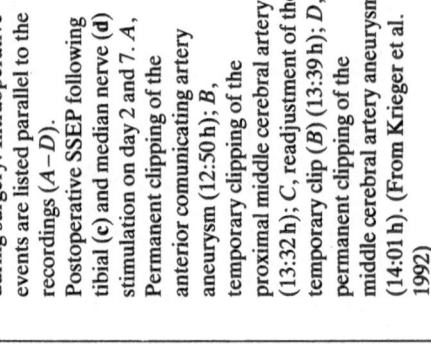

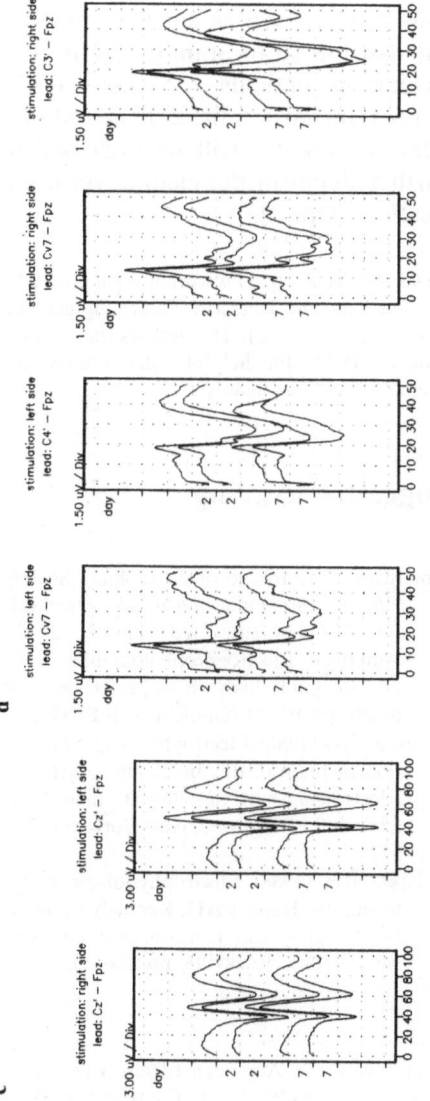

Thus, reports on correlations between intraoperative EP findings and neurologic outcomes are mainly descriptive in character. However, the beneficial effect of intraoperative BAEP monitoring could be demonstrated in a large series of patients with cerebello-pontine angle tumors, comparing preservation of hearing before and after introduction of continuous intraoperative monitoring. Currently, false positives (loss of EP without neurologic deficit) are mostly attributed to technical mishaps; and, false negatives can be related to events that occur while the patient is not being electrophysiologically monitored or the deficit occurs in silent regions. To increase the validity of intraoperative SSEP procedures, patients should, whenever possible, be monitored before induction of anesthesia and until complete responsiveness is reattained in the recovery room. Multimodal EP monitoring may enhance sensitivity by increasing the coverage of tissue at risk. Using advanced wave form analysis techniques, such as pattern recognition strategies or statistical rather than heuristic data analysis, more information can be extracted from the EP.

Intraoperative monitoring of BAEP is most frequently employed for monitoring the eighth nerve and brainstem during operations in the posterior fossa, particularly for cerebellopontine angle tumors. Other indications include microvascular decompression of cranial nerves in the posterior fossa and monitoring brainstem function during resections of arteriovenous malformations in the posterior fossa or interventional neuroradiological procedures. Damage to the eighth cranial nerve or the brainstem auditory pathway can result from ischemia or retraction. Reversible changes, including transient loss of the potential, do not necessarily indicate postoperative hearing impairment; BAEP signal recovery times of more than 3 h have been reported.

Motor evoked potentials are not yet usable for central motor pathway monitoring, using either transcranial electric or magnetic stimulation. Under routine general anesthesia cortically evoked muscular responses are virtually abolished. In magnetic stimulation area 4 pyramidal tract neurons are activated via interneurons. All narcotic drugs in doses used for general anesthesia suppress cortical neuronal activity, thus preventing magnetoelectric excitation. For single shock electric stimulation, membrane potential propagation at the spinal motoneuron level is prevented. However, by combining transcranial electric stimulation of the cortex and a well-timed peripheral stimulus, reproducible muscle responses can be elicited under general anesthesia. Cortical magnetic stimulation appears to be superior to SSEP monitoring in awake patients presenting with severe polyneuropathies. Recent reports using cortically applied low-intensity electric stimuli trains seem more promising, but the technique requires craniotomy and central motorstrip mapping techniques.

Flash-evoked VEP were the first modality used for intraoperative monitoring purposes. The limiting factor of VEP for intraoperative use is their sensitivity to the effects of general anesthetics.

Electrophysiologic Evaluation of Brain Death[4]

The demonstration of electrocerebral inactivity in patients with brain death syndrome was first reported by Fischgold and Mathis (1959). Since that time, technical and interpretative aspects have been addressed in many studies and guidelines for recording and analysis established.

We conclude that evoked potentials can be used as ancillary tools in the assessment of brain death, in particular in patients to whom CNS-depressant drugs have been administered, and this will be discussed in further detail in the chapter on brain death (Chap. 21).

Acknowledgements. This work was supported by a grant from the Deutsche Forschungsgemeinschaft (Ha 1394/3–2). The authors thank H.-P. Adams, DIM, for helpful collaboration and preparation of the figures.

Suggested Reading

American Electroencephalographic Society (1980) Minimum technical standards for EEG in suspected cerebral death. American Electroencepholographic Society, for guide lines, in suspected cerebral death. pp 19–22 (Guidelines in EEG 4)

Chatrian GE (1986) Electrophysiologic evaluation of brain death. In: Aminoff MJ (ed) Electrodiagnosis in clinical neurology. Churchill Livingstone, New York, pp 525–572

Chiappa KH (1988) Electrophysiologic monitoring. In: Ropper AH, Kennedy SK (eds) Neurological and neurosurgical intensive care. Aspen, Rockville, pp 129–155

---

[4] For review see American Electro-Encephalographic Society (1980), and Chatrian (1986).

Chiappa KH (1989) Evoked potentials in clinical medicine. Raven, New York

Fischgold H, Mathis P (1959) Obnubilations, comas et stupeurs. Electroencephalogr Clin Neurophysiol 11 [Suppl]:125

Grundy B (1986) Intraoperative monitoring by evoked potential techniques. In: Aminoff MJ (ed) Electrodiagnosis in clinical neurology. Churchill Livingstone, New York, pp 597–634

Hacke W (1989) Neuromonitoring during neuroradiological procedures. In: Desmedt JE (ed) Neuromonitoring in surgery. Elsevier, Amsterdam, pp 597–634

Krieger D, Adams H-P, Albert F, von Haken M, Hacke W (1992) Pure motor hemiparesis with stable somatosensory evoked potential monitoring during aneurysm surgery. Case report. Neurosurgery 31:145–150

Krieger D, Adams H-P, Rieke K, Hacke W (1993) Monitoring therapeutic efficacy of decompressive craniotomy in space occupying cerebellar infarcts using brain-stem auditory evoked potentials. Electroencephalogr Clin Neurophysiol 88:261–270

Nuwer MR (1989) Evoked potential monitoring in the operating room. Raven, New York

Prior PF (1979) Monitoring cerebral function. Elsevier, Amsterdam

Rieke K, Krieger D, Adams H-P, Aschoff A, Meyding-Lamadé U, Hacke W (1993) Management of acute cerebellar stroke. Cerebrovasc Dis 3:45–55

Chapter 7

Doppler Ultrasound Monitoring

Erich Bernd Ringelstein, Christian Werner, and
Alex Razumovsky

Introduction

Due to its unique temporal resolution
in the range of milliseconds, Doppler
ultrasound has become one of the
clinically and scientifically most fruitful
and innovative noninvasive techniques
for the investigation of the cerebral
circulation. This refers to extracranial
continuous-wave Doppler sonography
(ECD) of the extracranial brain arteries, transcranial Doppler sonography of the large basal intracranial
brain arteries, and transcranial color-
coded Duplex scanning (TC-Duplex)
with low-frequency (approximately 2
MHz) pulsed ultrasound. Particularly,
transcranial Doppler sonography
(TCD) has a great impact on ultrasound
monitoring in neurocritical care. It can
be administered as frequently and for
as long as desired. With simple provocative stimuli, it also permits a
number of functional tests of the
cerebral circulation. TCD provides a
quantitative estimate of the true blood
flow volume. Mean flow velocity of the
blood column, if compared intraindi-

vidually, closely reflects the true
volume flow when compared with elec-
tromagnetic or CBF measurements.

The term "monitoring" may be
interpreted in two different ways,
namely as a *continuous* or as an *intermittent* surveillance of key functions.
Both types of monitoring will be
addressed here.

Monitoring in neurocritical care
refers to the evaluation of neurophysiological and/or circulatory parameters of the brain in order to detect
otherwise obscure alterations in the
patient's cerebral condition, particularly if the desired information cannot
be acquired with more commonly used
methods. This is why monitoring techniques are predominantly applied with
noncooperative or comatose patients.
The underlying idea is that monitoring
can deliver immediate information
about the effectiveness or potential
hazards of interventions and may thus
rapidly modify and guide treatment.

Electrophysiological parameters
have certain disadvantages, such as
difficulties in their formal interpretation under general anesthesia and
their inability to differentiate between
reversible and irreversible brain

Section Editor: Werner Hacke

damage. Furthermore, due to time delay for data acquisition, the information received may no longer reflect the actual state of the brain. Transcranial Doppler sonography compensates for some of these shortcomings, in that it immediately reflects the true circulatory conditions within the insonated arteries. Doppler monitoring is of particular interest in the surveillance of cerebrovascular interventions, since the ultrasound abnormalities precede both functional disturbances as well as definite structural damage of the brain, thus increasing the time span for preventative interventions.

Technical equipment

Most of the pioneering studies have been performed with hand-held probes during interventions and at critical stages of life-threatening diseases. Meanwhile, a much more comfortable surveillance of intracranial blood flow velocity has become possible with the help of flat probes, mounted on a helmet-like holder or glued on the temporal plane. TCD monitoring can also be performed bilaterally, and flow signals will be available from various sites of the cerebral vasculature and in combination with electrophysiological and other circulatory parameters.

Technique

Probe positioning depends on the vascular territory under study. So far, we have used predominantly the transtemporal approach via which all major cerebral brain arteries and components of the circle of Willis can be insonated except for the vertebrobasilar artery. During TCD monitoring, interest is focused mainly on the proximal stem (= M1 segment) of the middle cerebral artery (MCA), the characteristic insonation depth of which is 45–55 mm, with a slightly rostral angulation of the beam. Continuous vertebrobasilar TCD monitoring is technically difficult but possible; intermittent monitoring is preferable here.

Pre- and Intraoperative Monitoring of MCA Flow Velocity During Open Heart Surgery

During cardiopulmonary bypass, extracorporeal oxygenation of the blood requires a pumping technology which severely alters physiological blood flow. During mechanical maintenance of the arterial circulation, low-flow induced hypoxic brain damage, hyperperfusion-related brain edema, and showers of gaseous or solid microemboli with subsequent ischemic encephalopathy may occur. The potentials of TCD monitoring during open heart surgery are manifold: (a) to analyze the presumed dissociation of the flow-metabolism junction, (b) to identify accidental hypo- or hyperperfusion, (c) to maintain sufficient MCA flow velocities known to be on the safe side of a critial perfusion pressure, (d) to empirically evaluate the lower limit of a still tolerable flow reduction at a certain body temperature, and (e) to identify and quantify microemboli. Showers of gas bubbles and solid material (thrombi, platelet aggregates, cholesterol cristals, plaque debris,

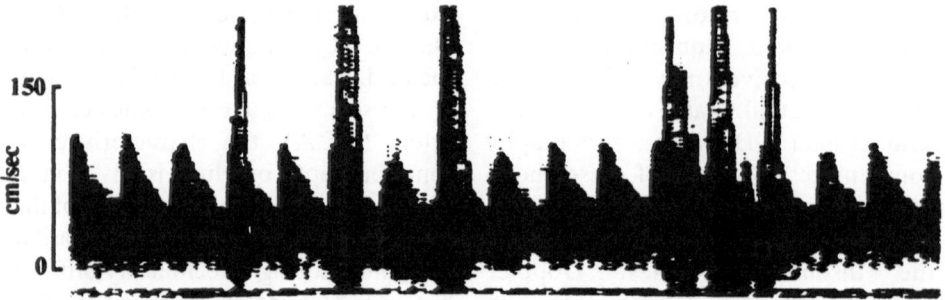

Fig. 1. High-amplitude flow disturbance signals in the MCA during carotid endarterectomy, representing gaseous or solid embolic material passing the MCA during carotid reflooding immediately after removal of clamps

etc.) are presumably the main causative factor for postoperative encephalopathy (Fig. 1).

TCD will allow for a more precise adaptation of the heart-lung machine to the patient's demands. Lundar and colleagues (1985) observed various kinds of flow impairment during cardiopulmonary bypass. Initially, *hyper*perfusion of the brain was a common finding; a complete loss of cerebral autoregulation was found during subsequent phases of the operative procedure. Von Reutern et al. also favored the idea that severe postoperative encephalopathy could best be explained by accidental *hyper*perfusion of the brain rather than by critical low flow.

Preoperatively, TCD helps to identify patients at high risk for ischemic brain damage due to occlusive disease in the neck. With the help of a CO_2 inhalation test or by intravenous injection of 1 g acetazolamide, the autoregulatory capacity of the brain arterioles can easily be assessed. Physiological testing with hypocapnia also has considerable prognostic impact in blunt head trauma and other severe brain diseases (see section on CO_2, below).

Transcranial Doppler Montioring During Carotid Endarterectomy

Monitoring during carotid endarterectomy (CEA) has two major aspects. First, it helps the vascular surgeon, during carotid clamping, to decide whether a shunt is necessary or not. This is important, since shunting has its own intrinsic morbidity. A recent international cooperative study of a large cohort clearly demonstrated the lowest incidence of perioperative ischemic accidents when shunting was performed highly selectively, based on the TCD findings during ICA clamping.

The effect of preoperative, tentative manual compression of the common carotid artery on MCA blood flow velocity is predictive of the intraoperative flow reduction during cross-clamping of the exposed carotid bifurcation. From the authors' own experience, a mean flow velocity drop of less than 66% or a residual mean MCA flow velocity of 15 cm/s does not require a shunt. This threshold corresponds to approximately 20 ml/100 g cerebral blood flow per minute, and even a lower perfusion has been tolerated in individual cases. Changes in TCD blood flow velocity were also closely related to changes in amplitude and latency of somatosensory-evoked potentials (SEP) during temporary unilateral internal carotid ligation. Velocities of less than 60% from baseline were defined as the ischemic threshold. Discrepancies may be explained by different sensitivities of TCD, EEG, and SEP in detecting regionally critical falls in cerebral perfusion or deterioration of brain function. Also, TCD provided a less critical margin of error with percentage MCA blood flow velocity decreases than with stump pressure measurement.

The second aspect of TCD monitoring during CEA is the detection of emboli. Several studies are underway to monitor the influx of embolic material into the cerebral arteries during the various stages of carotid endarterectomy (see section on embolus detection, below). The final goal of these investigations is to identify certain manipulations and surgical procedures which bear a particularly great danger of embolism, and to identify patients or certain types of lesions at particularly high risk of intraoperative embolic complications. So far, we know that microembolism during carotid endarterectomy is frequent, but its clinical impact is still to be evaluated.

It is surprising that the period during which most cerebrovascular accidents occur is generally not monitored with Doppler techniques. This is the time immediately after the end of the surgical procedure when the patient is "parked" in a side room until he wakes up. Circulatory and neurophysiological monitoring during this phase would presumably deliver further clues for avoiding perioperative complications in the future.

TCD Monitoring of Vasospasm

The risk of delayed ischemia and cerebral infarction after aneurysmal subarachnoid hemorrhage (SAH) is dependent on rebleeding, vasospasm, acute hydrocephalus, and edema following neurosurgical operation. Vasospasm remains a major complication, and delayed ischemic deficit occurs in 30% of these cases. As opposed to angiography, TCD sonography permits noninvasive and repeated measurement of the increase in blood flow velocities (BFV) associated with asymptomatic or symptomatic vasospasm after aneurysmal SAH or following head trauma. In the majority of publications, the increase in BFV in the MCA was used as a TCD determinant of the site and severity of vasospasm, since BFV is often asymmetrically increased and higher on the side of the aneurysmal rupture. In some cases, however, the BFV may be higher on the side opposite to the ruptured aneurysm. A BFV asymmetry in the C1 segment of the ICA from day 3 on proved to be a sensitive and early indicator of developing vasospasm. Grosset et al. (1993) analyzed a variety of TCD parameters in 121 patients with SAH caused by rupture of an aneurysm, but only the rise in BFV was found to correlate with clinical findings and outcome. An increase of more than $50 \text{ cm s}^{-1} 24 \text{ h}^{-1}$ identifies those patients who are most likely to develop delayed ischemic deficit, a finding first described by Harders and Gilsbach in 1987. Thus, recording the daily TCD changes in BFV during the first 2 weeks after SAH can help predict which patients are at risk for developing delayed ischemic deficit and should thus be treated prophylactically.

CO₂ Reactivity of the Cerebral Vasculature and Cerebral Autoregulation

CO₂ reactivity refers to the ability of the cerebral arterioles (so-called resistance vessels) to promptly react to hyper- and hypocapnia with vasodilation or vasoconstriction, respectively. In contrast, the diameter of the large basal cerebral arteries is not significantly affected by pCO_2, and BFV can be assumed to linearly reflect changes in cerebral blood flow due to the capnic modification of the tone of the resistance vessels. The term *cerebral autoregulation* refers to the vasomotor response following changes in cerebral perfusion pressure, e.g., vasodilation, to compensate for a low perfusion pressure. As a rule, the CO₂ reactivity and the cerebral autoregulation parallel each other, although in the so-called postischemic reperfusion period a dissociation may occur. Since a rigorous modification of the systemic arterial blood pressure in critically ill patients for diagnostic or prognostic purposes is ethically unacceptable, we have to confine ourselves to capnic stimuli. Opiates and volatile anesthetics may modify the CO₂ reactivity but do not compromise it.

Hypercapnic stimulation is an adequate provocative test in patients with reduced cerebral perfusion pressure, e.g., in high-grade extracranial occlusive carotid lesions, aortic arch dissections, or valvular heart disease with low output. The critically ill patient with severe cerebral disease, however, can be tested only with hypocapnic stimuli induced by hyperventilation. Hypercapnia bears the risk of considerably increasing the intracranial pressure.

Various techniques of hypercapnic testing have been used. Only a severe reduction of more than 3 standard deviations below normal mean value or complete loss of the CO₂ reactivity of the cerebral vasculature is indicative of ischemic compromise to the brain, particularly during pressure-lowering procedures.

The more important test during neurocritical care is to measure BFV reduction during hypocapnia. Sander and Klingelhöfer (1992) have shown that the more reduced the vasoconstrictor capacity of the cerebral vasculature, the worse was the outcome in patients with severe brain injuries (Fig. 2). The concomitant loss of autoregulation can be so complete that cerebral BFV fluctuates rhythmically with the changes of the intracranial pressure (ICP) induced by artificial respiration. Surprisingly, the prognostic impact of this parameter was independent of the type of brain lesion.

Elevated Intracranial Pressure and Cerebral Circulatory Arrest

Brain death is generally accepted to indicate an individual's death, i.e., irreversibly fatal outcome, even if re-

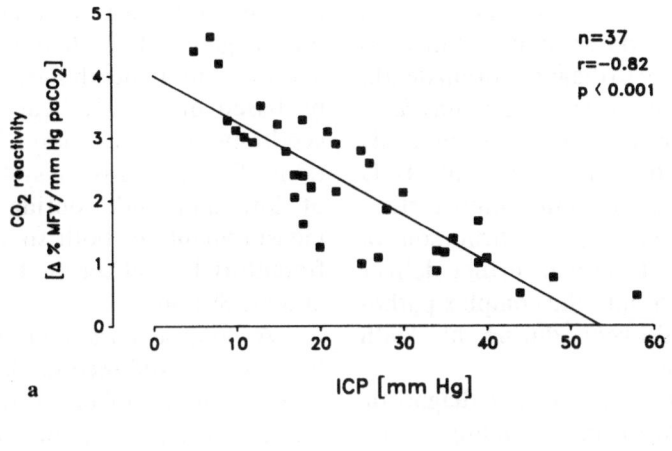

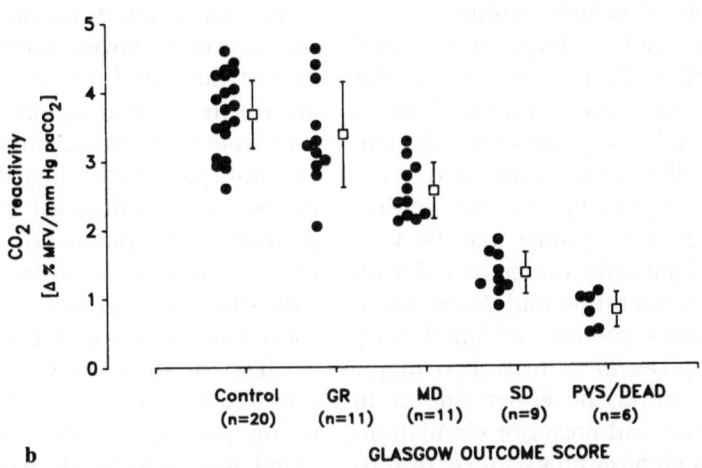

Fig. 2a,b. Relationship between hypocapnic CO_2 reactivity and intracranial pressure (*ICP*) or outcome in patients with severe head injury. **a** Linear regression analysis (*n* = 37) between CO_2 reactivity and ICP revealed a strong negative correlation (*r* = −0.82; *p* < 0.001). *MFV*, Mean flow velocity within the middle cerebral artery. **b** With decreasing CO_2 reactivity in patients with severe brain injuries, the Glasgow Outcome Score and clinical outcome worsened dramatically. *GR*, Good recovery; *MD*, moderate disability; *SD*, severe disability; *PVS*, persistent vegetative state or death. (Courtesy of Drs. D. Sander and J. Klingelhöfer)

spiration and extracerebral circulation are still preserved. This delicate situation has important implications for organ transplantation, ethical limitations of intensive care treatment, and costs of advanced life support. From a legal point of view, at least in

Germany, aortography is not allowed as a diagnostic means of proving a presumed brain death if not performed for other reasons. Transcranial Doppler ultrasound can be used to diagnose cessation of the intracranial circulation. Since findings depend on the examiner's experience, TCD should not be accepted as a standard method or the sole way to diagnose brain death, but should be used as an *ancillary*, *confirmatory* technique in clinically suggestive situations. Meanwhile TCD has been inserted into some institutional protocols for confirmation of brain death. TCD will further deliver deeper insight into the complex pathophysiological events during the death struggle (Fig. 3).

The characteristic and diagnostic phenomenon of an impending or definite arrest of cerebral perfusion is an oscillating "to-and-fro" movement of the blood column within the extracranial and/or large intracranial arteries (Fig. 4). The plane under the early systolic, spiky "forward" curve nearly equals the plane under the late systolic, flattened "backward" excursion. Depending on the cardiac output, the flow profile may be very sharp and pulsatile, or dampened, with sluggish acceleration and deceleration of the blood column, or small early systolic spikes in at least two major cerebral arteries on either side or in the anterior and posterior circulation. Transient biphasic flow patterns or zero flow may also occur during percutaneous transluminal aortic valvuloplasty or in patients with intra-aortic ballon pumps. Hassler et al. (1988) found a transient, sometimes unilateral reversal of diastolic flow immediately following bleeding in SAH or angioma patients, but this phenomenon never lasted longer than 30 min if not associated with clinical signs of brain death. In contrast, in brain-dead patients with posterior fossa masses, during ventricular drainage, or after traumatic cerebral edema has been relieved, a nearly normal diastolic forward flow may be recorded in the MCAs, thus providing false-negative TCD findings. The diagnosis of brain death should therefore be based only on a clear-cut clinical syndrome in conjunction with bidirectional flow patterns or systolic spikes of low amplitude during repetitive measurements in both supra- and infratentorial basal cerebral arteries for at least 30 min.

As long as an antegrade diastolic blood flow is still recordable, the brain tissue in the periphery of the vascular tree is still perfused. As soon as cerebral perfusion pressure falls below intracranial pressure, tissue perfusion stops, and a reflux phenomen during late systole following antegrade ejection of the blood into the large brain arteries is the pathognomonic finding for cerebral circulatory arrest (Fig. 4). For more pathophysiological details see Aaslid and Lindegaard (1986). The gradual development of circulatory arrest within the brain in conjunction with the concomitant EEG power spectra is documented in Fig. 3.

The diastolic flow velocity is a sensitive parameter of cerebral perfusion pressure, in that the diastolic blood flow velocity decreases as ICP increases. Animal experiments also suggest a close correlation between cortical or brain-stem electrical activity and the diastolic flow velocity pattern with or without concomitant decreases of the peak flow velocity. Increases in ICP beyond the level of diastolic arterial blood pressure reduce the diastolic flow velocity to zero. The underlying pathophysiological mechanism remains controversal. Either the ICP-induced increase in transmural pressure generates consecutive capillary collapse, or increases in ICP reduce the pressure drop along the still patent

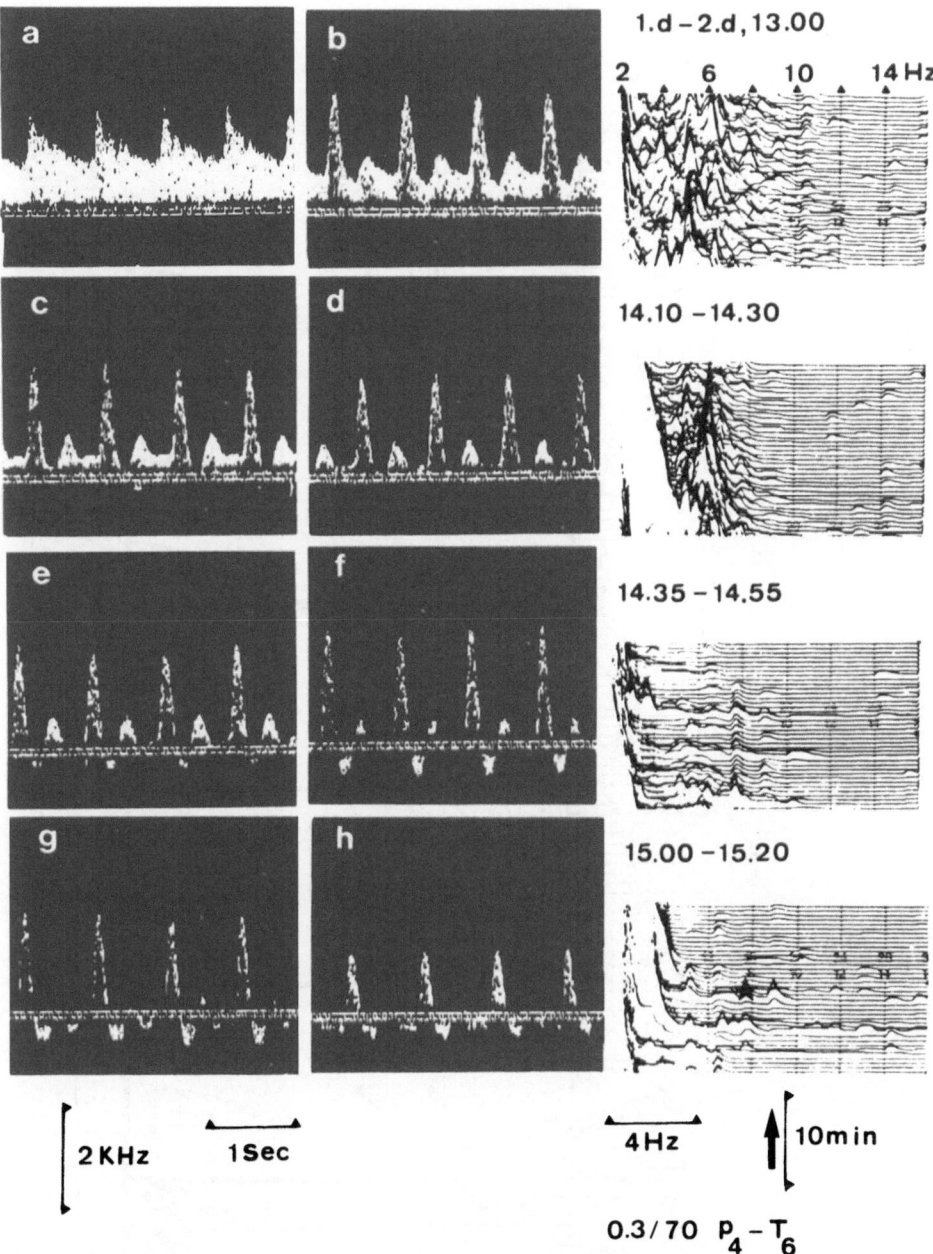

Fig. 3. Cessation of cerebral blood flow and subsequent brain death due to intracranial hemorrhage. *Left*: The gradual development of a reverberatory blood flow within the MCA is recorded in six steps over a period of 2 days. *Right*: At the same time, EEG power spectrum deteriorated and showed burst suppression pattern or isoelectricity as soon as the movement of the blood column became bidirectional. Numbers indicate time p.m. on the second day. (From Ringelstein 1986)

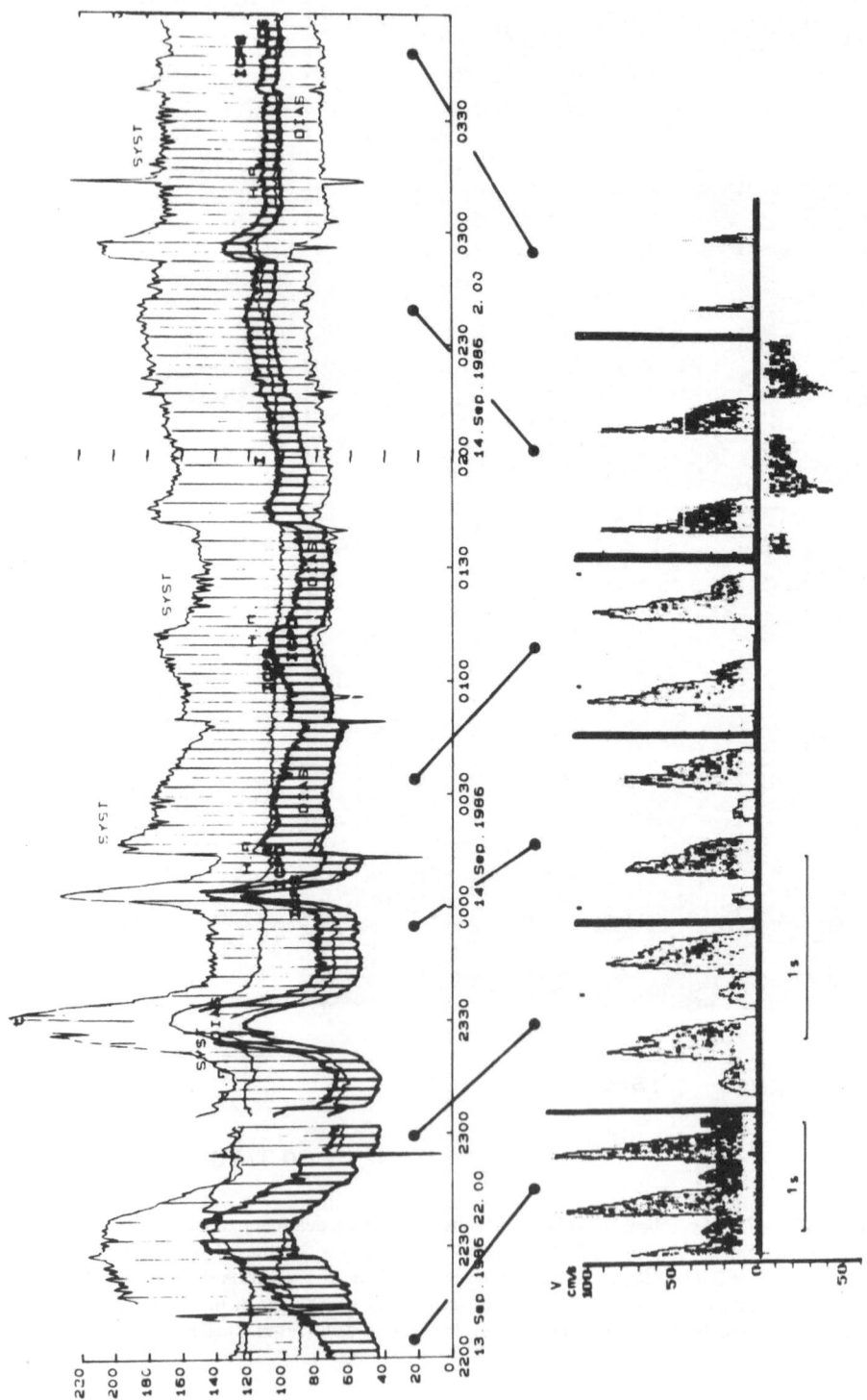

vascular bed. A deterioration of the diastolic blood flow velocity pattern strongly suggests a critical cerebral blood flow and ischemic neuronal threat due to decreased cerebral perfusion pressure. Continuous diastolic blood flow velocity recordings by TCD bear therapeutic options, particularly in patients in whom direct measurement of ICP is impossible (e.g., hepatic coma).

With increasing ICP, preventive treatment is possible only before cerebral circulatory arrest has occurred. Aaslid and Lindegaard (1986) have proposed a refined method of analyzing pulse-wave dynamics by subjecting the velocity waveform to a Fourier analysis using up to five harmonics, and comparing its deviations from the systemic arterial pulse wave. They evaluated this parameter as an indirect measure of the ICP in patients with an intraventricular catheter. Their formula was:

$$CPP^1 = \frac{ABP_1 \times V_{MCA0}}{V_{MCA1}}$$

where ABP_1 is the first harmonic of the arterial blood pressure wave at the arm, V_{MCA1} is the first harmonic of the velocity wave within the middle cer-

---

[1] Cerebral pesfusion pressure, defined as mean arterial pressure (MAP) minus ICP.

ebral artery, and V_{MCA0} is the mean of the MCA flow velocity. They succeeded in demonstrating a very good correlation coefficient of $r = 0.89$ between the calculated CPP and its measured value. A prototype of this machine is already in clinical use for testing (Multidop X, DWL, Laengerach, Germany). This type of computer-aided analysis would considerably improve monitoring of the critically ill in neurosurgery, neurology and anesthesiology, since most of these patients are threatened by an increased ICP. A monitoring-based and computer-controlled dosage of anti-ICP compounds such as mannitol, glycerol, etc., could perhaps improve the prognosis of these life-threatening conditions. Clinically sufficient experience, however, is still lacking.

Monitoring of Cerebral Ischemia

Cerebral ischemia may frequently occur in the perioperative period and during neurocritical care. Ischemic insults may be due to therapeutic or accidental occlusion of brain-supplying arteries, low cardiac output or cardiac arrest, elevated ICP, and/or showers of cerebral emboli.

Fig. 4. Transcranial Doppler ultrasonograms showing flow velocity in the middle cerebral artery (*below*) related to the continuous registration (*above*) of systemic arterial blood pressure (SAP) and intracranial pressure (ICP) in a head-injured patient with severe brain swelling. On the computer-generated printout (above) the light hatches connect the curves of systolic and diastolic SAP (*SYST, DIAS*) and the dark hatches connect systolic and diastolic ICP. *H.R.*, Heart rate. Diastolic flow velocity becomes zero when diastolic ICP reaches diastolic SAP. With ICP ranging between systolic and diastolic SAP, biphasic patterns occur. Later, only small systolic spikes remain detectable, corresponding with brain death and angiographic intracranial circulatory arrest. (From Hassler et al. 1988)

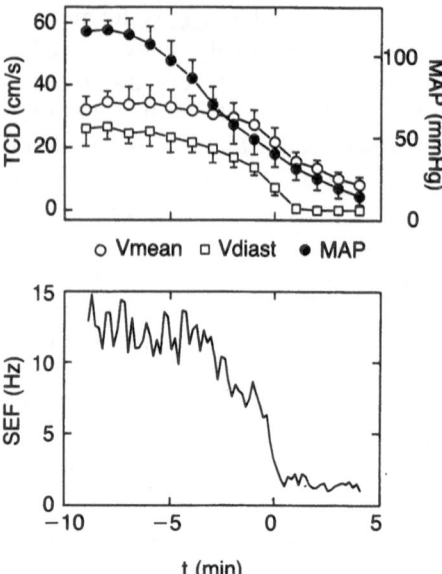

o Vmean □ Vdiast ● MAP

Fig. 5. Changes in mean (*Vmean,cm/s*) and diastolic blood flow (*Vdiast,cm/s*) and EEG (*SEF*: spectral edge frequency) during hemorrhagic hypotension in dogs. TCD and EEG did not change within the mean arterial blood pressure (*MAP*) range of 115 ± 7–49 ± 9 mmHg. Below 49 ± 9 mmHg, decreases of the TCD signal were associated with a shift of the EEG to lower frequencies. Brain electrical silence occurred at a MAP of 31 ± 7 mmHg, paralleled by a loss of the diastolic flow velocity pattern (mean ± SD). (From Werner et al. 1992b)

The blood flow velocity pattern associated with loss of neuronal function due to systemic hypotension has characteristic features. Changes in MCA blood flow velocity and EEG spectral edge frequency (SEF) due to decreasing mean arterial blood pressure (MAP) in fentanyl/N$_2$O anesthetized dogs are shown in Fig. 5. V$_{mean}$ and SEF did not change within an MAP range of 115 ± 7–49 ± 9 mmHg, suggesting preserved autoregulation. Below 49 ± 9 mmHg, decreases in mean and diastolic blood flow velocity were associated with lower EEG frequencies, and brain electrical silence occurred at an MAP of 31 ± 7 mmHg, paralleled by a 20 ± 6 cm mean flow velocity and a loss of diastolic flow during TCD. Deterioration of the *diastolic* flow pattern is a more sensitive parameter for the detection of cerebral ischemia than absolute or relative changes in mean blood flow velocity. Its monitoring may improve the management of patients at risk to develop ischemic neuronal injury. This is particularly true in situations of maximal brain electrical suppression (e.g., burst-suppression EEG pattern induced by anesthetics, trauma, or intoxication) where the threshold of CPP for ischemia fluctuates.

Monitoring of the Recanalization of Occluded Brain Arteries

The timing of spontaneous or therapeutically induced recanalization of an embolically occluded middle cerebral artery (MCA) is generally unknown, as is modification of the size of the infarct and the clinical course by the rapidity and degree of reperfusion. Ringelstein and co-workers (1992) have meanwhile investigated a series of 76 consecutive patients with acute stroke and forebrain infarction due to embolic occlusion of the MCA. Flow renewal following acute MCA occlusion was investigated by means of close-meshed repetitive transcranial Doppler sonography studies, cerebral arteriography, brain imaging on CT, and clinical tests to analyze the time course of MCA recanalization and its impact on infarct size and prognosis. They also investigated the influence of the origin of the

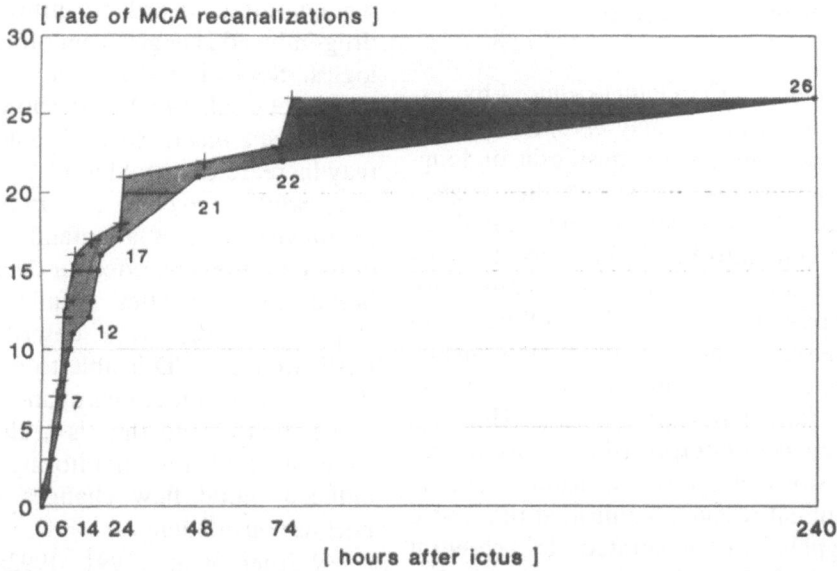

Fig. 6. Frequency of MCA recanalization versus time ($n = 34$). The hatched zone indicates the recanalization period, i.e., the time span within which reopening of the MCA must have occurred. The majority of cases (21/34) experienced MCA recanalization within the first 48 h. (From Ringelstein et al. 1992)

embolic material on the rapidity of recanalization by considering subgroups of patients with proven arterio-arterial or cardiogenic embolism. Recanalization of the MCA over time showed an exponential curve, with a 66% reopening rate after 72 h and a plateauing after weeks in the 80–90% range (Fig. 6). Only very early recanalization within the first 8 h in combination with a good leptomeningeal collateral blood flow during early arteriography predicted a smaller infarct size and a significantly better clinical outcome than later recanalization and/or poor transcortical collateralization. In another subgroup of 33 patients investigated within the first 8 h after stroke, they demonstrated that cardiogenic emboli lyse significantly more rapidly than arterio-arterial emboli from the carotid bifurcation

(Ringelstein and co-workers, unpublished data).

This type of very close-meshed, intermittent monitoring of acute stroke patients proves the decisive importance of very early arterial recanalization for the reduction of damaged brain tissue and stroke-related sequelae and handicaps. It will also clarify whether fibrinolytic compounds are able to really accelerate recanalization of the embolically occluded MCA if administered within the first few hours after stroke. Such studies will also help shed light on the relation between arterial recanalization and hemorrhagic transformation or major bleeding into infarcts. They would also permit the investigation of reperfusion injury in man and what it means in terms of clinical deterioration, infarct size, and outcome.

Embolus Detection

Ischemic EEG changes caused by cerebral embolism may escape detection in patients under anesthesia or long-term sedation. Recent studies suggest that TCD can detect cerebral emboli. TCD monitoring during carotid endarterectomy or during cardiopulmonary bypass revealed high-amplitude and high-frequency signals of flow disturbances during implantation of shunts or cannulation of the aorta (Fig. 1); they were interpreted as ultrasonic reflexions of air or particulate matter. Animal research confirmed that these signals are generated by cerebral emboli. Russell (1992) has shown that injection of air or particulate matter produces material-specific high-amplitude flow disturbance signals. Further studies have suggested that the Doppler characteristics may even identify size and volume of emboli. Meanwhile, TCD is already being used routinely as a sensitive detector of embolic material during surgery and in neurocritical care. This type of TCD monitoring provides further insight into the mechanisms of embolic stroke and, as an early-warning system for cerebral ischemia, may guide early therapeutic interventions.

Effects of Opioids, Intravenous Anesthetics, and Narcotics on Cerebral Blood Flow Velocities

Anesthesia and long-term analgesic sedation produce drug-specific and dose-dependent changes in CBF and cerebral metabolism. It is clinically important to monitor cerebral hemo-dynamic effects in order to differentiate drug-induced changes from other etiologies. Several studies (for a review see Thiel et al. 1992) have shown that *volatile anesthetics* such as halothane may increase cerebral blood flow velocity, while *narcotics or intravenous anesthetics* such as alfentanil or propofol either had no effect or decreased blood flow velocities. Similar drug-response curves were described in CBF studies. TCD is able to evaluate the hemodynamic effects of anesthetics and narcotics and thus is a clinically valuable tool for monitoring drug-induced blood flow changes in the unconscious patient.

Werner et al. (1991, 1992a) and Kochs et al. (1992) investigated the effects of the intravenous anesthetics and sedative propofol, the volatile anesthetic isoflurane, and the new narcotic sufentanil on CBF, MCA blood flow velocity, EEG, cerebral oxygen consumption ($CMRO_2$), and ICP in dogs. The effects of 0.8 mg/kg/min propofol on CBF, EEG, and V_{mean} are shown in Fig. 7. Propofol significantly reduced CBF, V_{mean}, and $CMRO_2$ from baseline values with a hysteresis, in that these parameters remained reduced after recovery (recovery time: 50–80 min). Changes in CBF and V_{mean} were closely correlated ($r = 0.86$). The reduction in CBF and V_{mean} was paralleled by a strong decrease in ICP, indicating that a propofol-induced decrease in CBF is associated with a reduction in cerebral blood volume. Significant and closely correlated ($r = 0.81$, $p < 0.01$) increases in CBF, V_{mean}, and ICP during incremental end-tidal concentrations of isoflurane (1%, 2%, and 3%) are also shown in Fig. 7. This was associated with decreases in $CMRO_2$.

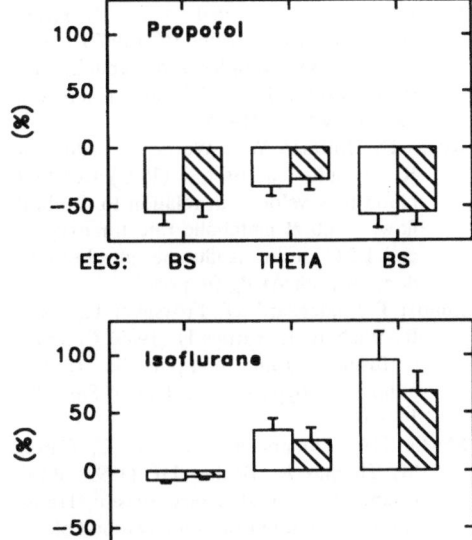

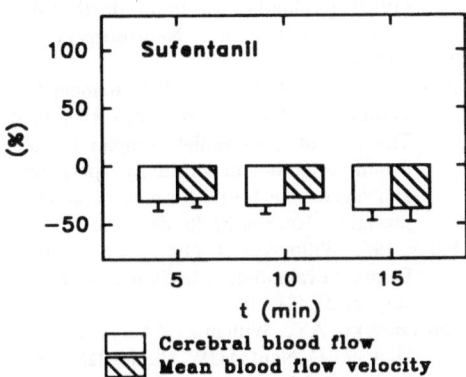

☐ Cerebral blood flow
▨ Mean blood flow velocity

Fig. 7. Changes in MCA mean blood flow velocity and cerebral blood flow (in % from baseline) during infusion of *propofol, isoflurane,* or *sufentanil*. BS, Burst suppression; mean ± SD. (From Werner et al. 1992a)

Isoflurane increases both CBF and cerebral blood volume with an un-coupling of the cerebral metabolism/CBF ratio (Kochs et al. 1992). Sufentanil in a dosage of $20\,\mu g/$ kg decreased CBF and V_{mean} consistently ($r = 0.82$), but ICP did not

change over time. The decrease in CBF is interpreted as a consequence of decreased metabolism. In conclusion, the striking parallelism of CBF and velocity changes indicates that TCD is a good noninvasive technique for continuously measuring relative changes in CBF during administration of anesthetics and narcotics. Propofol and sufentanil can be used safely for sedation and analgesia during neuro-critical care, whereas isoflurane is a cerebral metabolic depressant but increases CBF and ICP at higher concentrations due to uncoupling of the flow/metabolism ratio.

Suggested Reading

Aaslid R, Lindegaard KF (1986) Cerebral hemodynamics. In: Aaslid R (ed) Transcranial Doppler sonography. Springer, Vienna New York, pp 60–85

Aaslid R, Lindegaard K-F, Sorteberg W, Nornes H (1989) Cerebral autoregulation dynamics in humans. Stroke 20:45–52

Becker G, Greiner K, Kaune B, Winkler J, Brawanski A, Warmuth-Metz M, Bogdahn U (1991) Diagnosis and monitoring of subarachnoid hemorrhage by transcranial color-coded real-time sonography. Neurosurgery 28:814–820

Benugin L, Wahl D, Albin M (1991) Estimation of embolic air volume in the middle cerebral artery (MCA) using transcranial sonography. Anesthesiology 75:A471

Chan KW, Dearden MN, Miller D (1992) The significance of post-traumatic increase in cerebral blood flow velocity: a transcranial Doppler ultrasound study. Neurosurgery 30:697–700

Edelmann R, Ringelstein EB, Richert F (1986) Transcranial Doppler sonography for monitoring the middle cerebral artery blood flow veocity during carotid endarterectomy. Rev Bras Angiol Circ Vasc 16:96–100

Ferguson GG (1982) Intraoperative monitoring and internal shunts: are they necessary in carotid endarterectomy? Stroke 13:287–289

Giller CA, Bowman G, Dyer H, Mootz L, Krippner W (1993) Cerebral arterial diameters during changes in blood pressure and CO_2 during craniotomy. Neurosurgery (in press)

Greenfield JC, Tiendall GT (1965) Effect of acute increase in intracranial pressure on blood flow in the internal carotid artery. J Clin Invest 44:1343–1351

Grosset DG, Straton J, McDonald I, Cockburn M, Bullock P (1993) Use of transcranial Doppler sonography to predict development of a delayed ischemic deficit after subarachnoid hemorrhage. J Neurosurg 78:183–187

Grote E, Hassler W (1988) The critical first minutes after subarachnoid hemorrhage. Neurosurgery 22:654

Halsey JH Jr, McDowell HA, Gelmon S, Morawetz RB (1989) Blood velocity in the middle cerebral artery and regional cerebral blood flow during carotid endarterectomy. Stroke 20:53–58

Halsey JH Jr (1992) Risks and benefits of shunting in carotid and arterectomy. Stroke 23:1583–1587

Harders AG, Gilsbach JM (1987) Time course of blood velocity changes related to vasospasm in the circle of Willis measured by transcranial Doppler ultrasound. J Neurosurg 66:718–728

Hassler W, Steinmetz H, Gawlowski J (1988) Transcranial Doppler ultrasonography in raised intracranial pressure and in intracranial circulatory arrest. J Neurosurg 68:745–751

Hassler W, Steinmetz H, Pirschel J (1989) Transcranial Doppler study of intracranial circulatory arrest. J Neurosurg 71:195–201

Henriksen L, Hjems E, Lindburgh T (1983) Brain hyperperfusion during cardiac operations: cerebral blood flow measured in man by intra-arterial injection of xenon 133: evidence suggestive of intraoperative microembolism. Thorac Cardiovasc Surg 86:202–211

Jacobs LA, Brinkmann SD, Morrell RM, Shirley JG, Ganji S (1983) Long-latency somatosensory evoked potentials during carotid endarterectomy. Am Surg 49:338–344

Karnik R, Valentin A, Bonner G, Ziegler B, Slany J (1990) Transcranial Doppler monitoring during percutaneous transluminal aortic valvuloplasty. Angiology 41:106–111

Kirkham FJ, Levin SC, Padayachee TS, Kyme MC, Nevill BG, Gosling RG (1987) Transcranial pulsed Doppler ultrasound findings in brain-stem death. J Neurol Neurosurg Psychiatry 50:1504–1513

Kochs E, Hoffman WE, Werner C, Albrecht RF, Schulte am Esch J (1992) Cerebral blood flow velocity in relation to cerebral flow, cerebral metabolic rate for oxygen, and EEG during isoflurane anesthesia in dogs. Anesth Analg (in press)

Lundar T, Lindegaard KF, Fröysaker T, Aaslid R, Wieberg J, Nornes H (1985) Cerebral perfusion during non-pulsatile cardiopulmonary bypass. Ann Thorac Surg 40:144–148

Martin NA, Doberstein C, Zane C, Caron M, Thomas K, Becker DP (1992) Post-traumatic cerebral artery spasm: Transcranial Doppler ultrasound, cerebral blood flow, and angiographic findings. J Neurosurg 77:575–583

Newell DW, Grady MS, Sirotta P, Winn HR (1989) Evaluation of brain death using transcranial Doppler. Neurosurgery 24:509–513

Petty GW, Mohr JP, Pedley TA, Tatemichi TK, Lennihan L, Duterte DI, Sacco RL (1990) The role of transcranial Doppler in confirming brain death: sensitivity, specificity, and suggestions for performance and interpretation. Neurology 40:300–303

Pillay PK, Willberger J (1989) Transcranial Doppler evaluation of brain death. Neurosurgery 25:481–482

Razumovsky AY, Williams MA, A Lee A, Danchev D, Nauta HJW, Hanley DF (1993) Patterns of linear blood flow asymmetry following subarachnoid hemorrhage. In: Findlay JM (ed) Proceedings of the 5th international conference on cerebral vasospasm 1993. Elsevier, Amsterdam (in press)

Ries F, Moskopp D (1989) Value of the transcranial Doppler ultrasound technique (TCD) for the determination of brain death. Neurosurg Rev 12 [suppl 1]:302–306

Ringelstein EB (1986) Transcranial Doppler monitoring. In: Aaslid R (ed) Transcranial Doppler sonography. Springer, Vienna New York, pp 147–163

Ringelstein EB (1988) A practical guide to transcranial Doppler sonography. In: Weinberger J (ed) Noninvasive assessment of the cerebral circulation in cerebrovascular disease. Frontiers of clinical neuroscience theories. Liss, New York, pp 75–121

Ringelstein EB, Sievers C, Ecker S, Schneider PA, Otis SM (1988) Noninvasive assessment of CO_2-induced cerebral vasomotor response in normal individuals and patients with internal carotid artery occlusions. Stroke 19:963–969

Ringelstein EB, Biniek R, Weiller C, Ammeling B, Nolte PN, Thron A (1992) Type and extent of hemispheric brain infarctions and clinical outcome in early and delayed middle cerebral artery recanalization. Neurology 42:289–298

Ropper AH, Kehne SM, Wechsler L (1987) Trancranial Doppler in brain death. Neurology 37:1733–1735

Russell D (1992) The detection of cerebral emboli using Doppler ultrasound. Theoretical, experimental and clinical aspects. In: Newell DW, Aaslid R (eds) Transcranial Doppler. Raven, New York, pp 207–214

Sander D, Klingelhöfer J (1992) Doppler CO_2 test as an indicator of cerebral vasoreactivity and prognosis in severe intracranial hemorrhages. Stroke 23:962–966

Schmidt-Kastner R, Ophoff BG, Hossmann K-A (1987) Delayed recovery of CO_2 reactivity after one hour's complete ischemia of cat brain. J Neurol 233:367–369

Sloan MA, Haley EC Jr, Kassel HF, Henry ML, Stewart SR, Beskin RR, Sevilla EA, Torner JC (1989) Sensitivity ad specifity of transcranial Doppler ultrasonography in the diagnosis of vasospasm following subarachnoid hemorrhage. Neurology 39:1514–1518

Spencer MP (1992) Detection of cerebral arterial emboli. In: Newell DW, Aaslid R (eds) Transcranial Doppler. Raven, New York, pp 215–230

Spencer MP, Thomas GI, Moehring MA (1992) Relation between middle cerebral artery blood flow velocity and stump pressure during carotid endarterectomy. Stroke 23:1439–1445

Thiel A, Russ W, Zeiler D, Dapper F, Hempelmann G (1990) Transcranial Doppler sonography and somatosensory evoked potential monitoring in carotid surgery. Eur J Vasc Surg 4:597–602

Thiel A, Zickmann B, Zimmermann R, Hempelmann G (1992) Transcranial

Doppler sonography: effects of halothane, enflurane and isoflurane on blood flow velocity in the middle cerebral artery. Br J Anaesth 68:388–393

Torner JC, Kassel HF, Haley EC (1990) The timing of surgery and vasospasm. Neurosurg Clin North Am 1:335–347

Van der Linden JH, Casimir-Ahn H (1991) When do cerebral emboli appear during open heart operations? A transcranial Doppler study. Ann Thorac Surg 51:237–241

von Reutern GM, Hetzel A, Birnbaum D, Schlosser V (1988) Transcranial Doppler ultrasonography during cardiopulmonary bypass in patients with severe carotid stenosis or occlusion. Stroke 19:674–680

Werner C, Kochs E, Rau M, Schulte am Esch J (1990) Transcranial Doppler as a supplement in the detection of cerebral circulatory arrest. J Neurosurg Anesth 3:159–165

Werner C, Hoffman WE, Baughman VL, Albrecht RF, Schulte am Esch J (1991) Effects of sufentanil on cerebral blood flow, cerebral blood flow velocity and metabolism in dogs. Anesth Analg 72:177–181

Werner C, Hoffman WE, Kochs E, Albrecht RF, Schulte am Esch J (1992a) The effects of propofol on cerebral blood flow in correlation to cerebral blood flow velocity in dogs. J Neurosurg Anesth 4:41–46

Werner C, Hoffman WE, Kochs E, Albrecht RF, Schulte am Esch J (1992b) Transcranial Doppler sonography indicates critical brain perfusion during haemorrhagic hypotension in dogs. Anesth Analg 74:347

Widder B, Paulat K, Hackspacher I, Mayr E (1986) Transcranial Doppler CO_2 test for the detection of hemodynamically critical carotid artery stenoses and occlusions. Eur Arch Psychiatr Neurol Sci 236:162–168

Williams MA, Razumovsky AY, Diringer MN, Hanley DF (1993) Transcranial Doppler ultrasonography in the intensive care unit. In: Babikian VL, Wechsler LR (eds) Transcranial Doppler ultrasonography. Mosby, St Louis, pp 175–189

Yoneda YS, Nichimoto A, Nukada T (1974) To-and-fro movement and external escape of carotid arterial blood in brain death cases. A Doppler ultrasonic study. Stroke 5:707–713

Chapter 8

Intracranial Pressure Monitoring

MARK S. SCHNITZER and ALFRED A. ASCHOFF

Introduction

History

Recognition of the unique nature of the cranial contents and the motivation for monitoring the pressure in the cranium can be traced back to 1783 and Alexander Monro (Secundus)' monograph, "Observations on the Structure and Functions of the Nervous System." Monro writes:

For being enclosed in a case of bone the blood must be continually flowing out of the veins, that room may be given to the blood which is entering by the arteries. For as the substance of the brain, like that of other solids of our body, is nearly incompressible, the quantity of blood within the head must be the same, or very nearly the same, at all times, whether in health or disease, in life or after death, those cases only excepted in which water or other matter is effused, or secreted, from the blood vessels; for in these, a quantity of blood, equal in bulk to the effused matter, will be pressed out of the cranium.

George Kellie, a student of Monro's, published similar conclusions in 1824, after performing extensive

autopsy studies, still without reference to cerebrospinal fluid as a normal constituent of the cranial vault. Francois Magendie, in his landmark publication of 1825, first described CSF as a physiological substance required for the normal functioning of the nervous system, although he did not attempt to modify the doctrine of Monro and Kellie. George Burrows, an English physician, is credited with modifying the Monro-Kellie doctrine to include the cerebrospinal fluid. Through his experiments he deduced that the blood and CSF volumes were variable and related to one another in a reciprocal fashion. In 1875, Key and Retzius reported on extensive anatomical studies using intrathecal injections of a colored tracer. They commented upon the pressure of the CSF during lumbar puncture in their experimental animals, and they observed the one-way flow through the pacchionian granulations when the dye they injected was infused with sufficient force. Lumbar spinal puncture was introduced into clinical use in 1891 by Quincke. With a technique not substantially different from that in use today, he measured CSF pressure as well as hematological and

Section Editor: Werner Hacke

chemical parameters of the fluid. The interested reader is invited to see also the germinal works of Pagenstecher, Duret, and von Bergman, all of whom contributed to the study of intracranial dynamics in the late nineteenth century.

Anatomical and Physiological Preconditions

The craniospinal cavity is divided into four anatomically distinct compartments by the falx, tentorium, and foramen magnum. Of the 1500–1900 cc total volume of the cranium, approximately 85% is occupied by brain, 10% by CSF, and 5–10% by blood volume. Under normal conditions, where flow of CSF is unhindered, the intracranial pressure is uniform throughout the craniospinal axis, apart from any hydrostatic differences. Under pathological conditions such as acute mass lesions or obstruction of CSF pathways, the pressure in the different compartments varies, with obvious implications. A volume increase in any single compartment produces a pressure gradient towards the other compartments. Until the gradient is dispersed, a mass movement of brain tissue results, with ensuing incarceration in the narrows between compartments.

In order to record meaningful values of intracranial pressure, the effect of hydrostatic level of measurement differences must be carefully considered. To eliminate errors resulting from these differences, convention has chosen the intraventricular foramina as the hydrostatic reference point. Deviation from this point, as may be seen in movement of the head or changing position in the bed, is one of the most common causes of ICP measurement error.

Indications for ICP Monitoring

Normal intracranial pressure in human beings is about 10 mmHg or 135 mm CSF, and intracranial hypertension is defined as a pressure exceeding 20 mmHg (270 mm CSF). The close correlation between intracranial pressure and outcome has been the object of numerous studies over the past quarter century. Primary damage to brain tissue, while irreparable, is seldom fatal and the subsequent morbidity and mortality are compounded by secondary insult to the damaged brain tissue. This secondary injury, which occurs with depletion of volume-buffering capacity, arises as a consequence of compromised cerebral perfusion and shifts of intracranial contents. The severity of the secondary injury depends on the length of time the insult goes unrecognized and thus untreated. Clinical examination, often suppressed further by therapy, can be insensitive to severe intracranial pathology. Thus monitoring the intracranial pressure as an index of secondary cerebral injury serves to (a) facilitate earlier diagnosis, (b) minimize morbidity and mortality associated with persistent untreated intracranial hypertension, and (c) monitor the effectiveness of therapy. Intracranial pressure monitoring finds application in trauma, nontraumatic coma, and pre- and postoperative care. The mean (average) value of the intracranial pressure may, in some circumstances, be a relatively late indicator of secondary brain injury; therefore, the data obtained from such monitoring may be used to identify the cerebral perfusion pressure or the compliance of the cranial vault.

Methods

Noninvasive

A variety of noninvasive techniques exist to estimate intracranial pressure, or at least to serve as alternative indices of the degree of secondary brain injury. The neurological examination, though often obscured by therapy as well as by the brain injury, is of great value in following the clinical course of the brain-injured patient. Fundoscopy should be performed, though papilledema, while reliable, is a slow indicator of intracranial hypertension. CT scanning, as it is often performed on trauma patients prior to notification of the neurosurgical consultant, is particularly worthy of note. The appearance of normal basal cisterns on the first CT scan in trauma patients has been identified as a good early predictor of low risk for development of significant ICP increase, though the relationship to outcome is unsettled. Endeavors to produce a practical equation for estimation of intracranial pressure by the appearance of the cranial CT have resulted in an equation in five variables with a statistically significant multiple regression coefficient $R = 0.8$. Unfortunately, the error increases with increasing ICP, such as to make it unreliable for pressures over 30–40 mmHg. This is not too surprising, given the exponential nature of the pressure-volume relationship. Naturally, imaging is a static representation of a dynamic process and frequent CT scans are expensive and too slow to follow therapy. Additionally, transport to the CT scanner may be hazardous for critically ill, unstable patients.

Transcranial Doppler ultrasound allows continuous and sequential assessment of blood flow velocity through major intracranial vessels. Various manipulations of the data so obtained yield a variety of indicators variably suited to assess the state of cerebral hemodynamics. Two of these, the Pourcelot resistive index (RI) and the pulsatility index, have recently been studied in neonates and in adults with respect to intracranial hypertension. In both cases, the indices were found to vary linearly with the intracranial pressure, though the correlation was better at the extremes than at the threshold. Unfortunately, space-occupying lesions which alter the course of the intracranial vessels may lead to significant errors by introducing an unpredictable change in the sonographic angle. Additionally, a number of unrelated conditions may affect the blood-flow velocity, such as cardiac decompensation, pneumothorax, GI bleeding, and seizure. Furthermore, the wide range of normal values and significant overlap of abnormal values preclude standardization and utilization as an objective measure of intracranial pressure. Nonetheless, these techniques may prove useful in following the course of an individual patient.

In neonates, the intracranial pressure can be estimated accurately and safely by application of a transducer to the anterior fontanelle. The uncharacterized and variable frequency characteristics of the fontanelle lead to pressure damping, which results in inaccuracies and underestimation of high ICP. Furthermore, a high degree of clinical experience with the technique as well as availability of devices with applanation rings and mechanisms for standardized applanation are preferred. Therefore, this technique finds use in situations requiring continuous monitoring of neonates in circumstances where ICP is not expected to change rapidly from baseline.

Finally, two other methods may prove particularly useful in following patients with hydrocephalus. In one retrospective study of MRI, variations of the signal intensity of the CSF in the ventricular system allowed for differentiation between normal and increased ICP. MRI shares the limitations of CT scanning and, in addition, the strong magnetic field may cause difficulty with ventilation, monitoring, retained metal foreign bodies (bullets), and implanted devices (pacemakers, Swan-Ganz catheters, etc.). Another study utilized the transmission of ICP through the cochlear aqueduct to the cochlear perilymph. Perilymph pressure can be indirectly assessed by observing the displacement of the tympanic membrane during reflex contraction of the stapedius muscle elicited by a loud sound. As with transcranial Doppler and MRI, this method may prove useful in serial measurements, but it does not reveal the true intracranial pressure.

Invasive

Under normal anatomical conditions, the supra- and infratentorial fossae can be considered as a single compartment. This equilibrium may become radically altered by occlusions of the basilar cisterns, herniations, or surgery resulting in secondary brain injury. Recognizing the need to minimize the effects of secondary injury and monitor the effects of therapy, many clinicians choose to measure intracranial pressure directly. This decision is based upon several factors, not the least of which includes the clinician's level of comfort in dealing with the information so obtained. In general, the decision to monitor directly is based upon the presence of any or all of the following: inability to perform or follow serial clinical examinations, absent or compressed basal cisterns on initial head CT, GCS < 8, hypotension, abnormal posturing, associated severe pulmonary injury, barbiturate therapy, or post-op trauma patients with brain swelling. Once the decision to directly monitor intracranial pressure is made, the decision as to which type of device to use remains.

Direct measurement of the intracranial pressure is obtained by transducing (a) directly from CSF-filled cavities, (b) along a vector normal (perpendicular) to enveloping membranes, or (c) from within the brain tissue proper. Various methods have been devised to access these sites, all placing slightly different weight on the significance of: risk of infection, stability, feasibility of calibration, temperature insensitivity, ease of implantation, accuracy, resistance to corrosion by tissue fluids, and sensitivity to atmospheric pressure, as well as the constraints imposed by the desired location of placement.

The so-called gold standard of intracranial pressure measurement was introduced into clinical practice by Guillaume and Janny (1951) and Lundberg (1960), whereby a fluid-filled catheter, positioned in the lateral ventricle, transmits the intraventricular pressure to an external transducer. As the CSF can be considered a Newtonian fluid, that is to say, there is a linear relationship between the applied shear stress and the rate of angular deformation, the pressure will be uniform throughout the communicating CSF spaces. For this reason, the ventricular CSF pressure may be considered representative of the global intracranial pressure. This method is preferred in circumstances requiring therapeutic drainage to circumvent an obstruction. What is frequently overlooked, however, is the fact that the properties of the entire measuring chain contribute to the observed waveform. Considerable artifacts are introduced by fluid-filled catheters, which become more apparent as the catheters become longer, thinner, and more rigid. Thus small transducers affixed to the head by short catheters of sufficient diameter minimize both the artifact introduced by movement and that of hydrostatic errors. Additional errors can be introduced when such a device is simultaneously used to record and to treat intracranial hypertension by draining CSF. It is well known that introduction of a low-outflow resistance into a pressurized system introduces a pressure drop proportional to the flow rate. This naturally introduces a marked discrepancy between the actual ICP and the recorded ICP. Furthermore, collapse of the ventricular system about a drainage catheter results in serious underestimation of intracranial pressure, as insufficient fluid remains to maintain a fluid column to the transducer. However, the consequences of obvious failure of registration are minor compared with the danger of partially shifted ICP registration in dislocated or obliterated tubes. The transluminal transfer of the pressure in surrounding brain tissue can produce a damped signal which is significantly lower than the true ICP, while continuing to show a waveform mimicking adequate function. These ICP surrogates are extremely difficult to identify, as they are often reversible and occur most often during periods of very high ICP. Thus, some investigators consider intraventricular ICP monitoring a "fair-weather" technique, for during the "stormy phase" of ICP crisis or in the presence of slit ventricles the failure rate increases.

Techniques for measuring intracranial pressure upon enveloping membranes rely on the principle of coplanarity, as described by Schettini and Walsh (1974). This principle explains, in effect, how an externally applied transducer can negate the effects of tension within the membrane (dura, arachnoid, pia) while accurately indicating the intracavitary pressure of the brain, simply by being placed flat (e.g., parallel) against the tensile force in the membrane, which results in a position normal (e.g., perpendicular) to the pressure in the brain. Essentially, this method entails creation of an incompressible fluid column between the enveloping membrane and an external transducer by means of a hollow bolt or sensing balloon placed through a burr hole. Further issues relating to the use of fluid-filled systems with externally placed transducers include the seemingly trivial issue of maintaining the correct level of the transducer, which in fact is extremely difficult and can result in errors of ± 10 cm H_2O (± 7 mmHg).

Techniques for recording pressure from within brain tissue proper, known for nearly 2 decades, are currently enjoying renewed interest. Originally, this was accomplished by the insertion of a fluid-filled catheter into the brain parenchyma, with a wick of cotton attached to protect the catheter tip from occlusion by tissue debris. Electronic miniaturization has allowed introduction of a piezoresistive microtransducer, applied to the tip of a catheter, for monitoring of cerebral tissue pressure. Even more recent is the development of a fiberoptic system utilizing solid-state electronics to sense changes in the light reflected from a pressure-sensitive diaphragm at the tip of a fiberoptic catheter. These tip transducers avoid many of the problems of waveform transmission and work well in the presence of compressed ventricles or in the subdural space, but they are expensive, sensitive to mechanical stress, and have no mechanism for in vivo calibration.

Finally, it is essential to note the evolving development of telemetric ICP monitoring devices. Essentially a variable tuned circuit, once implanted, changes in intracranial pressure result in unambiguous changes in the transducer's resonance frequency. An externally applied impedance measuring device is electromagnetically coupled, converting the resonance frequency into a pressure analogous voltage. These devices have been designed for intraventricular and epidural implantation. Without continuous external connections, these devices are ideal for long-term monitoring, even in the outpatient setting. However, as with the other internal transducer systems described, once they are implanted, re-zeroing and re-calibrating are impossible in situ. Furthermore, compatibility with modern imaging techniques is not yet assured.

Risks

Benefits of monitoring intracranial pressure have to be weighed against the potential risks and complications. Risks of invasive monitoring are related to: the degree of invasiveness, location, duration, concurrent sites of infection or systemic infection, the need to restrict patient movement, and the requirement for multiple monitors. Potential complications include: infection, hematoma, epilepsy, cerebral puncture, cranial nerve palsies, and CSF leaks, with the incidence of complications particularly infection, ranging up to 27%. Infection is the major factor limiting the duration of nontelemetric, invasive ICP monitoring, particularly if flushing or sampling are required. The cumulative incidence of infection rises such that by 3–5 days it is no longer acceptable. Since brain edema is seldom controlled in this brief interval, some argue that monitors must be replaced regularly until no longer needed. Still others argue that the cumulative incidence does not reveal whether or not a subsequent infection will occur if the monitor is left in place, and it is well known that the risk of infection is greatest at the time of insertion. In a recent retrospective study the risk of subsequent infection tended to fall after 6 days and remained zero after day 11, thus arguing for retention of an existing device until no longer needed or until the appearance of signs of infection, thereby minimizing the hazard of re-exposure to contamination.

Suggested Reading

Aaslid R, Markwalder T-M, Nornes H (1982) Noninvasive transcranial Doppler ultrasound recording of flow velocity in basal cerebral arteries. J Neurosurg 57:769–774

Belopavlovic M, Buchthal A, Beks JW, Journée HL (1981) Some principles of postoperative epidural pressure monitoring. Acta Neurochir (Wien) 55:227–245

Bouma GJ, Muizelaar JP, Bandoh K, Marmarou A (1992) Blood pressure and intracranial pressure-volume dynamics in severe head injury: relationship with cerebral blood flow. J Neurosurg 77:15–19

Bullock R, Golek J, Blake G (1989) Traumatic intracerebral hematoma – which patients should undergo surgical evacuation? CT scan features and ICP monitoring as a basis for decision making. Surg Neurol 32: 181–187

Burrows FA, Hillier SC, McLeod ME, Iron KS, Taylor MJ (1990) Anterior fontanel pressure and visual evoked potentials in neonates and infants undergoing profound hypothermic circulatory arrest. Anesthesiology 73:632–636

Chambers IR, Mendelow AD, Sinar EJ, Modha P (1990) A clinical evaluation of the Camino subdural screw and ventricular monitoring kits. Neurosurgery 26:421–423

Chan K, Miller JD, Dearden NM, Andrews PJD, Midgley S (1992) The effect of changes in cerebral perfusion pressure upon middle cerebral artery blood flow velocity and jugular bulb venous oxygen saturation after severe brain injury. J Neurosurg 77:55–61

Clark WC, Muhlbauer MS, Lowrey R, Hartman M, Ray MW, Watridge CB (1989) Complications of intracranial pressure monitoring in trauma patients. Neurosurgery 25:20–24

Colditz PB, Williams GL, Berry AB, Symonds PJ (1988) Fontanelle pressure and cerebral perfusion pressure: continuous measurement in neonates. Crit Care Med 16:876–879

Constantini S, Cotev S, Rappaport ZH, Pomeranz S, Shalit MN (1988) Intracranial pressure monitoring after elective intracranial surgery. J Neurosurg 69:540–544

Crutchfield JS, Narayan RK, Robertson CS, Michael LH (1990) Evaluation of a fiberoptic intracranial pressure monitor. J Neurosurg 72:482–487

Gaab MR, Heissler HE, Bruce DA (1984) ICP monitoring. Crit Rev Biomed Eng 11: 189–250

Garcia-Merino A, Garcia-Sola R, Vela L, Martin-Gonzales E (1990) Intracranial pressure monitoring in acute disseminated encephalomyelitis in childhood. Crit Care Med 18:1481–1483

Go KG (1991) Cerebral pathophysiology: an integral approach with some emphasis on clinical implications. Elsevier, Amsterdam

Guillaume J, Janny P (1951) Manometrie intracranienne continue: interet de la methode et premiers resultats. Rev Neurol 84:131–142

Hara M, Kadowaki C, Watanabe H, Shiogai T, Numoto M, Takeuchi K (1988) Necessity for ICP monitoring to supplement GCS in head trauma cases. Neurochirurgia (Stuttg) 31:39–44

Kanter PK, Weiner LB, Patti AM, Robson LK (1985) Infectious complications and duration of intracranial pressure monitoring. Crit Care Med 13:837–839

Kawahara N, Sasaki M, Mii K, Tsuzuki M, Takakura K (1989) Sequential changes of auditory brain stem responses in relation to intracranial and cerebral perfusion pressure and initiation of secondary brain-stem damage. Acta Neurochir (Wien) 100: 142–149

Kosteljanetz M (1987) Intracranial pressure: cerebrospinal fluid dynamics and pressure-volume relations. Acta Neurol Scand [Suppl] 111:1–23

Lorig RJ, Cheng EM, Ko WH (1976) Systems for the long-term monitoring of intraventricular pressure in neurosurgery. In: Flemming DG, Ko WH, Neuman MR (eds) Indwelling and implantable pressure transducers. CRC Press, Cleveland, pp 79–84

Lundberg N (1960) Continuous recording and control of ventricular fluid pressure in neurosurgical practice. Acta Psychiatr Neurol Scand [Suppl] 49:1–193

Lundberg N (1983) The saga of the Monro-Kellie doctrine. In: Ishii S, Nagai H, Brock M (eds) Intracranial pressure V. Springer, Berlin Heidelberg New York, pp 68–76

Lyons MK, Meyer FB (1990) Cerebrospinal fluid physiology and the management of increased intracranial pressure. Mayo Clin Proc 65:684–707

Maas AI, de Jong DA (1986) The Rotterdam Teletransducer: state of the device. Acta Neurochir (Wien) 79:5–12

Marmarou A, Anderson RL, Ward JD et al. (1991) NINDS traumatic coma data bank: intracranial pressure monitoring methodology. J Neurosurg 75:s21–s27

Maset AL, Marmarou A, Ward JD et al. (1987) Pressure-volume index in head injury. J Neurosurg 67:832–840

Mizutani T, Manaka S, Tsutsumi H (1990) Estimation of intracranial pressure using computed tomography scan findings in patients with severe head injury. Surg Neurol 33:178–184

Nordby HK, Gunnerod N (1985) Epidural monitoring of the intracranial pressure in severe head injury characterized by non-localizing motor response. Acta Neurochir (Wien) 74:21–26

Ohara S, Nagai H, Matsumoto T, Banno T (1988) MR imaging of CSF pulsatory flow and its relation to intracranial pressure. J Neurosurg 69:675–682

Pfenninger EG, Reith A, Breitig D, Grunert A, Ahnefeld FW (1989) Early changes of intracranial pressure, perfusion pressure, and blood flow after acute head injury. 1. An experimental study of the underlying pathophysiology. J Neurosurg 70:774–779

Piek J, Kosub B, Kuch F, Bock WJ (1987) A practical technique for continuous monitoring of cerebral tissue pressure in neurosurgical patients. Preliminary results. Acta Neurochir (Wien) 87:144–149

Reid A, Marchbanks RJ, Bateman DE et al. (1989) Mean intracranial pressure monitoring by a noninvasive audiological technique: a pilot study. J Neurol Neurosurg Psychiatry 52:610–612

Robertson CS, Narayan RK, Contant CF et al. (1989) Clinical experience with a continuous monitor of intracranial compliance. J Neurosurg 71:673–680

Rosenwasser RH, Kleiner LI, Krzeminski JP, Buchheit WA (1989) Intracranial pressure monitoring in the posterior fossa: a preliminary report. J Neurosurg 71:503–505

Schettini A, Walsh EK (1974) Experimental identification of the subarachnoid and subpial compartments by intracranial pressure measurements. J Neurosurg 40:609–616

Seibert JJ, McCowan TC, Chadduck WM et al. (1989) Duplex pulsed doppler US versus intracranial pressure in the neonate: clinical and experimental studies. Radiology 171:155–159

Takeuchi S, Koike T, Sasaki O, Kamada K, Tanaka R, Arai H (1989) Intracranial extradural pressure monitoring after direct operation on ruptured cerebral aneurysms. Neurosurgery 24:878–883

Tasker RC, Matthew DJ, Helms P, Dinwiddie R, Boyd S (1988) Monitoring in non-traumatic coma. I. Invasive intracranial measurements. Arch Dis Child 63:888–894

Tasker RC, Boyd S, Harden A, Matthew DJ (1988) Monitoring in non-traumatic coma. II. Electroencephalography. Arch Dis Child 63:895–899

Walker AE, Viernstein LJ, Chubbuck JG (1976) Intracranial pressure monitoring in neurosurgery. In: Flemming DG, Ko WH, Neuman MR (eds) Indwelling and implantable pressure transducers. CRC Press, Cleveland, pp 69–77

Wilkinson HA, Yarzebski J, Wilkinson EC, Anderson FA (1989) Erroneous measurement of intracranial pressure caused by simultaneous ventricular drainage: a hydrodynamic model study. Neurosurgery 24:348–354

Yano M, Ikeda Y, Kobayashi S, Otsuka T (1987) Intracranial pressure in head-injured patients with various intracranial lesions is identical throughout the supratentorial intracranial compartment. Neurosurgery 21:688–692

General Treatment Strategies

Chapter 9

General Treatment Strategies for Elevated Intracerebral Pressure

ALEXANDER HARTMANN, ROBERT STINGELE, and MARK SCHNITZER

Pathophysiology

Intracerebral Pressure and Compliance

Since the brain is largely entrapped by the skull, it has only a limited volume in which to expand and a limited capacity to compensate for increases of total volume. The physiologic compartments contained within the skull are brain tissue, intravascular blood, and cerebrospinal fluid (CSF). If one of these compartments is increased in volume by tumors, intracranial or intracerebral bleeding, impairment of CSF flow, or development of brain edema, the Monro-Kellie doctrine requires a compensatory decrease of the other compartments. However, after this compensatory mechanism fails, intracranial pressure increases rapidly (Fig. 1). The normal ICP is 5–10 mmHg, depending on body position, and ICP is considered to be definitely increased beyond 15 mmHg. The compensatory capacity depends on the amount of intracranial mass,

the rapidity of volume increase, and the regional anatomy of the dural compartments. Since about 1 ml of CSF can be expressed from the intradural space per minute, a slow increase of brain or lesion volume below this level is tolerated without an elevation of the ICP. An atrophic brain with enlarged sulci filled with CSF may tolerate mass expansion much better than a brain with small sulci and proportionally less CSF. Figure 1 shows the increase of CSF pressure in a patient during intrathecal infusion of fluid. The change from the initial flat portion of the compliance curve to the steeper portion is reflected by the approximately exponential rise of CSF pressure.

Intracranial pressure is a dynamic phenomenon, both because it oscillates periodically with systemic arterial blood pressure and with respiration (Fig. 2), and because various perturbations alter the compliance (the shape of the pressure-volume relationship) mainly by changes in the buffering capacity of intracranial blood volume.

Section Editor: Daniel F. Hanley

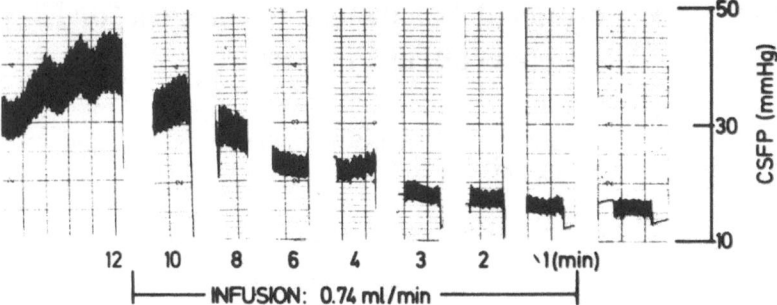

Fig. 1. Increase of intracranial pressure (ICP, here: cerebrospinal fluid pressure, *CSFP*) during intraspinal infusion of artifical CSF. The curve reads *from right to left*. With increasing amounts of added volume, CSFP, as well as the amplitude, rises, indicating reduction of compliance. CSFP was recorded by a thin polyethylene catheter introduced into the lumbar subarachnoid space

Brain Edema

Brain edema is the most frequent consequence of acute brain-tissue damage. Water transport across the glial and neuronal cell membranes depends largely on normal electrolyte concentrations, particularly that of sodium. If active transport of Na^+ across the membrane is damaged, Na^+ enters the cell freely, accompanied by water. This overloading of the cell with water leads to cytotoxic brain edema (Fig. 3). Since swelling of astrocytes is limited and is primarily due to shifting of water from the extracellular to the intracellular space, this type of edema theoretically is not accompanied by increased ICP but by a reduction of the extracellular tissue space. However, an increase of ICP may be observed when destruction of macromolecules and accumulation of lactate lead to an increase of brain-tissue osmolarity. The resulting osmolarity gradient attracts more water from the vascular compartment, resulting in an increase of ICP.

Depending on the type of process, disruption of the blood-brain barrier eventually occurs, with opening of endothelial tight junctions. A cell-free plasma filtrate, including macromolecules, can then pass into the intercellular space and increase the total intracranial volume, a condition termed vasogenic edema, because of the associated disruption of the vascular endothelial lining (Fig. 3).

Cytotoxic edema appears after hypoxia (cardiac arrest, pulmonary insufficiency), in the early state of acute cerebral ischemia, with water intoxication, hepatic and renal encephalopathy, hemodilutional hyponatremic encephalopathy, inappropriate secretion of ADH, and Reye's syndrome in children. Vasogenic edema occurs in cerebral mass lesions of any kind, including encephalitis, trauma, cerebral hemorrhage, cerebral infarction, and lead encephalopathy, and after brain radiation. The edema of diabetic coma is probably of a mixed nature.

Interstitial or hydrostatic edema results from obstructive or communi-

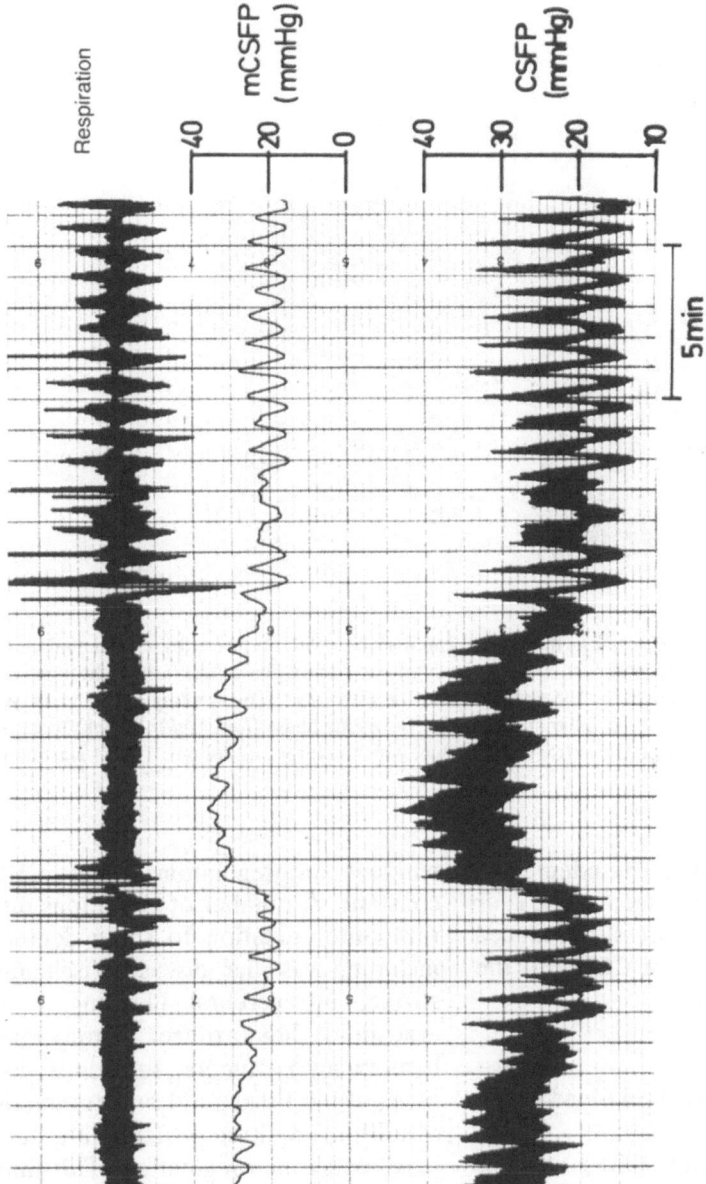

Fig. 2. Change of intracranial pressure (ICP, here: cerebrospinal fluid pressure *CSFP*) during alteration of breathing pattern and plateau waves. The curve reads *from right to left*. Depending on the Cheyne-Stokes breathing pattern, CSFP changes periodically. During start of a plateau wave CSFP rises, and the amplitude as well. The increase of the amplitude indicates the reduction of compliance. The patient suffers from a subarachnoid hemorrhage with acute extraventricular obstructing hydrocephalus. *CSFP* and *mCSFP*, Cerebrospinal fluid pressure and mean CSFP; breathing pattern by impedance technique

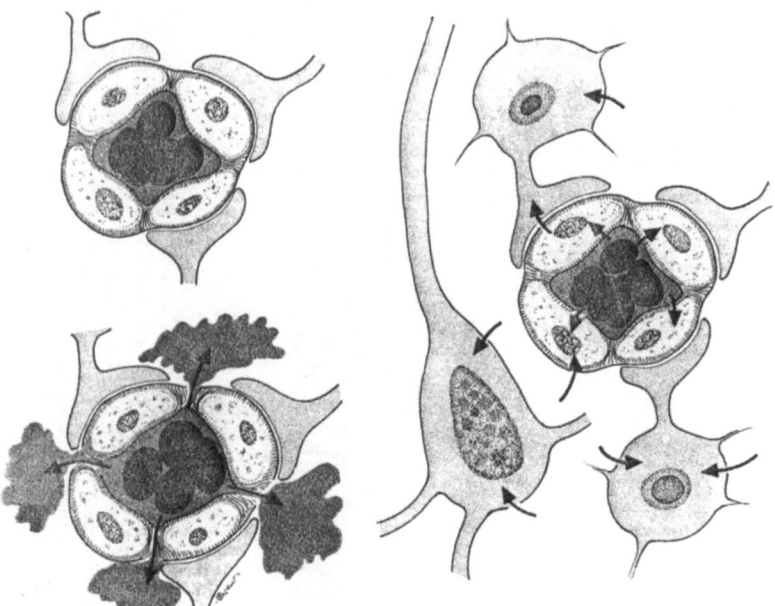

Fig. 3. Edema formation. *Upper left*: the normal capillary bed with erythrocytes, endothelial lining with tight junctions and astrocyte feet. During the cytotoxic edema phase (*right*) the tight junctions are preserved and water moves via the endothel into the astrocytes. The swelling of the astroctyes results in narrowing of the extracellular space. In the vasogenic phase (*lower left*) the tight junction opens and fluid can move into the extracellular space, which enlarges its volume. (From Hartmann and Wassmann 1987)

cating hydrocephalus. The edematous white matter can be seen on CT or MRI as a result of pressure-induced transependymal flow of CSF into the periventricular space.

Effects of ICP on Cerebral Blood Flow

Cerebral blood flow (CBF) remains essentially constant through a mechanism of autoregulation for cerebral perfusion pressures (CPP) between approximately 60 and 180 mmHg. Cerebral perfusion pressure is defined as the difference between mean arterial blood pressure (MABP) and ICP. With increasing ICP, the cerebral perfusion pressure drops, but in a limited window autoregulation keeps CBF constant. A number of conditions disrupt autoregulation to some degree, including vascular diseases (ischemic stroke, intracerebral bleeding, subarachnoid hemorrhage, intracranial hemorrhage), tumors, infectious diseases of the tissue, and post-traumatic conditions, and the postepileptic state may reduce autoregulation. This may affect the whole brain or remain localized to a single vascular territory. In regions of impaired autoregulation, CBF follows changes in arterial pressure passively. Even mild hypotension, in these circumstances, can provoke a reduction of tissue perfusion. Conversely, any increase in intracranial volume is more prone to reduce CBF in regions of impaired autoregulation. In patients with long-standing arterial hypertension the limits of autoregulation are thought to be shifted towards higher blood pressure levels: reduction of perfusion pressure is then poorly tolerated, while increased perfusion pressure is well tolerated. Furthermore, the impairment of autoregulation may not be permanent. In patients with ischemic stroke it may recover after a few days or weeks. The biochemical and systemic features of brain dysfunction in relation to head injury are discussed in detail in Chap. 61.

Clinical Syndromes, Symptoms, and Signs

The clinical consequences of increased ICP are eventually due to the reduction of CBF and manifest as symptoms of generalized reduced brain function, the extreme of which is brain death. If increased ICP is compartmentalized, displacement of tissue away from the mass occurs, leading to compression of parts of the brain at a distance from the mass. Depending on the brain region entrapped in an adjacent compartment, several types of herniation can be distinguished.

Cingulate Herniation/Subfalcine Herniation

A lesion localized to the parietal or frontal lobes of one hemisphere may push brain tissue beneath the free edge of the falx, with resulting herniation of the ipsilateral supracallosal gyrus or compression of the corpus callosum. The third ventricle is bulged medially, and the pericallosal branch of the anterior cerebral artery is shifted to the contralateral side. The flow through this artery may be impaired due to entrapment at the falcine edge, leading to infarction of the medial frontal lobe. The cingulate gyrus is compressed by the falx, resulting in local hemorrhagic necrosis.

Uncal and Medial Temporal Lobe Herniation

Space-occupying mass lesions in the temporal lobe may displace the uncus into the tentorial incisura. The medial temporal lobe, particularly the parahippocampal gyrus on the side of the mass, is thought to move across the tentorial incisura, thus compressing the midbrain. The contralateral cerebral peduncle is simultaneously compressed against the ipsilateral tentorial edge (Kernohan's notch phenomenon). Since the third cranial nerve passes across the tentorial incisura it may be compressed by the prolapsing tissue or stretched as the midbrain is displaced horizontally, resulting in an ipsilateral third nerve palsy, typically beginning with an initial mydriasis often preceded by a sluggish pupillary reaction to light, sometimes with ptosis. The final consequence of midbrain compression by the temporal lobe is a midbrain syndrome with diminished consciousness and focal lesions of the descending tracts and oculomotor nuclei. Recently, the role of herniation per se in causing midbrain compression has been questioned, and predominantly horizontal shift with compression above the tentorial plane has been postulated to cause drowsiness and stupor.

Central Transtentorial Herniation

This situation is characterized by a downward displacement of midline structures through the tentorial notch. The first signs classically relate to the diencephalic level: alteration of alertness, Cheyne-Stokes respiration, or deep yawns interrupting a regular pattern, small reactive pupils, but preserved oculocephalic movements and usually Babinski's sign. Later on in the diencephalic stage stupor occurs. The final stage is marked by decorticate posturing. Subsequent clinical signs of central transtentorial herniation follow the rostrocaudal arrangement of the functional centers in the brain stem: in the midbrain-upper pons syndrome, the respiratory pattern evolves from Cheyne-Stoke's type to tachypnea, pupils dilate and fix in mid position (5 mm), oculovestibular reflexes are sluggish or absent, and eye movements may become disconjugate. There is often bilateral extensor rigidity. A few patients have diabetes insipidus due to downward traction of the pituitary stalk and the hypothalamus. Hypothalamic damage is further indicated by wide ranges of measured body temperature. The downward movement may cause stretching of the anterior choroidal and posterior cerebral arteries with subsequent infarction in the occipital lobe, hippocampus, and thalamus. The lower pontine-medullary syndrome is characterized by slowing of tachypnea, changing to ratchet-type breathing or cluster breathing, absent oculovestibular response, and midsize fixed pupils. The medullary syndrome indicates a terminal state with a low chance for recovery. Tachypnea of shallow volume alternates with brief or even long episodes of apnea. Blood pressure drops and, finally, breathing ceases.

Upward Transtentorial Herniation

Space-occupying lesions of the posterior fossa lead to upward displacement and subsequent herniation of the superior vermis cerebelli, which then compresses the hippocampal gyrus and the posterior wall of the third ventricle. The superior cerebellar arteries may be stretched or compressed, resulting in ischemia of the superior parts of the cerebellum. If the aqueduct is distorted obstructive hydrocephalus with further rapid increase of ICP occurs. Obstruction of the vein of Galen may complicate the clinical picture.

Tonsillar Cerebellar Herniation Through the Foramen Magnum

If the ICP in the posterior fossa displaces the tonsils of the cerebellum downward the cisterna magna may be obliterated and the medulla compressed. Pathologically, the cerebellum and the medulla display impressions of the bony foramen magnum margin. Clinical signs are irregular breathing, apnea and fall of the blood pressure, sometimes preceded by brief hypertension.

Symptoms and Signs

Headache due to increased ICP may be minor or severe. Sometimes it awakens the patient at night due to the additional increase of intracranial volume. Valsalva's maneuver and coughing or sneezing intensify the pain.

It is rather difficult to determine from the side of the pain the localization of the space-occupying mass. Since the trigeminal nerve supplies the frontal part of the dura, stretching of that part by a frontal tumor projects the pain behind the eye or into the frontal aspect of the skull. On the other hand, masses in the posterior fossa very often lead to pain radiating down the neck and between the shoulders. A rapidly expanding intracranial mass often leads to headache, whereas a slowly developing mass (chronic subdural hematoma) may result in headache and focal signs only in the terminal stage. Neck stiffness, when a sign of increased ICP, usually indicates cerebellar tonsillar impaction.

Hiccups may appear as a sign of raised pressure in the posterior fossa or distortion of the medulla by a mass. Particularly in children, compression of the brain stem may cause vomiting, sometimes violent and projectile but without preceding nausea. Changing the head position provokes vomiting in some patients.

Impairment of vision is one of the most frequent signs of chronically increased ICP but is not common in acute situations. Peripheral fields constrict and the blind spot enlarges due to sustained papilledema.

Cushing's reflex is an increase of systemic blood pressure accompanied by decrease of heart rate, both provoked by increase of ICP and apparently due to reduction of perfusion or distortion of the medullary baroreceptor and vasoregulator centers. Various irregular respiratory patterns that follow Cheyne-Stokes patterns have been attributed to specific brain-stem levels, but they occur infrequently, and few have such a consistent relation-ship in clinical practice (see Chap. 60). Neurogenic pulmonary edema may be a consequence of high ICP and medullary distortion. Autonomic disturbances are the basis of this phenomenon.

Treatment

Criteria for Admission to an ICU and Indications for ICP Monitoring

In general, triage of a patient with an intracranial mass to an ICU is based upon the presence or anticipation of any of the following: inability to perform or follow serial clinical examinations, impairment of consciousness, generally with Glasgow Coma Scale under 8, absent or compressed basal cisterns on initial head CT, hypotension, abnormal posturing, associated pulmonary injury, barbiturate therapy, or postoperative brain swelling. Clinical examinations, often obscured further by therapy such as barbiturates, sedatives, or anticonvulsants, are often insensitive to changes in intracranial pathology. Thus monitoring the intracranial pressure as an index of secondary cerebral injury serves to (a) facilitate earlier diagnosis of increasing ICP, (b) minimize morbidity and mortality associated with persistent untreated intracranial hypertension, (c) monitor the effectiveness of therapy, and (d) recognize iatrogenic causes of raised ICP such as respiratory pressure, inadvertent free water administration, or excessive blood pressure changes. Recognizing the need to minimize the effects of secondary injury and monitor the effects of therapy, many clinicians choose to measure intracranial pressure directly. This decision is based upon several factors, not the least of which includes the clinician's level of comfort in dealing with the information obtained and the device used for pressure measurements.

Supportive Measures

Maintenance of Airway, Breathing, and Circulation

It almost goes without saying that maintenance of an airway and treatment of shock are the first priorities in any patient in extremis. Thought must be given to how other therapies will affect the patient's ability to protect his airway and maintain blood pressure.

Positioning, Analgesia, Sedation, and Muscle Relaxation

Coughing or increases of intra-abdominal pressure normally produce considerable increases of ICP. In patients with raised ICP these events potentially can precipitate dangerous plateau waves. Therefore, an important point in anti-ICP therapy is to keep the patient calm and sedated. Nursing procedures such as turning, endotracheal suction, and enemas have been shown to raise ICP considerably. Often, sedation and mechanical ventilation are necessary to protect the patient, potent analgesics such as fentanyl can be used in combination with midazolam (e.g., fentanyl/midazolam; dosage: 0.15–0.3 mg fentanyl/h; 5–15 mg midazolam/h). An alternative for sedation is propofol, which has been shown to have favorable effects on ICP. Care must be taken to recognize hypotension following propofol administration in some patients, and parenteral nutrition has to be adapted with propofol sedation because of its high fat content. Ketamine should not be used because of its adverse effect on ICP. Short-acting, reversible agents are preferred to allow for frequent examinations.

The patient should generally be maintained in a 30° upright position with the head not turned to either side. This point has been controversial and depends in part on whether ICP alone or net perfusion pressure is optimized. The ideal posture in bed is found if ICP monitoring is available. Unnecessary invasive procedures should be avoided, and before interventional procedures are undertaken, the level of sedation must be adjusted to avoid pain and anxiety.

Endocrine/Metabolic Concerns

Fever in a patient stimulates increased cerebral blood flow, and in patients with a mass, raised ICP. Antipyretics should therefore be used liberally. Some concern arises if a cooling blanket is needed, since shivering has been associated with raised ICP.

Glucocorticoids are useful in the treatment of the vasogenic edema associated with brain tumors; however, the use of steroids in treatment of traumatic brain injury is unsupported. Regarding their use in cerebral hemorrhage, some controversy remains, but most evidence does not support it. The mineralocorticoid effects of dexamethasone are much less than with hydrocortisone; this favors the former. The treatment scheme should start with a loading dose of 0.2–0.25 mg/kg body weight, followed by repeated doses every 6 h up to a total daily dosage of 0.40–0.50 mg/kg BW. In severe edema, higher doses up to 0.75 mg/kg BW/day may be given. The clinical effect may be observed within 1–4 h but usually not before 12 h. The effect on brain edema appearance on CT is delayed compared with the clinical improvement, but the effect on ICP, particularly the reduction of the pressure waves, is seen early and indicates the effect in the individual patient.

Contraindications such as gastric ulcer or even gastritis, tuberculosis, and severe diabetes mellitus must be regarded. If dexamethasone is given, blood sugar must be followed closely. If steroids are given in the presence of an infection or in intracerebral infectious diseases such as abscesses, tuberculosis, or encephalitis, maximum vigilance is required. With antituberculosis therapy the treatment of severe edema due to an intracerebral tuberculoma is safe and sometimes the only way to overcome the problems of increased ICP. The effect of steroids may be accelerated by administration of furosemide, but the additional benefit is minimal.

Prevention of Seizures

Seizures are the most common repercussion of head trauma. Roughly 5% of patients who sustain closed head injuries and 50% of those with open head injuries will experience at least one seizure. Deliberate cerebral cortical injury (e.g., surgery) can also result in a seizure focus. Insofar as seizures can result in breath-holding (hypercarbia) and Valsalva, as well as in a tremendous increase in the metabolic, and therefore blood flow, requirements of the brain, they should

be anticipated in appropriate circumstances and suppressed with phenytoin or barbiturates in patients with raised ICP.

Specific Measures

Controlled Hyperventilation

Arterial tension of carbon dioxide ($PaCO_2$) has a major effect on the diameter of cerebral vessels. Reducing $PaCO_2$ constricts cerebral vessels with a preserved ability to respond and reduces cerebral blood volume and therefore ICP. The mechanism responsible for CO_2 reactivity seems to be independent of autoregulation to systemic blood pressure, but both are often disrupted in the same region. This is suggested by the fact that further vasodilation can be induced by an increase of $PaCO_2$ in vessels that are maximally dilated in response to hypotension.

Cerebral vasoconstriction is not maintained with prolonged hyperventilation because CSF pH returns to normal values even if $PaCO_2$ remains low. With prolonged hyperventilation, responsiveness of cerebral vessels to changes in $PaCO_2$ increases; i.e., minute changes in $PaCO_2$ produce large increases of vessel diameter. This is due to a low concentration of bicarbonate in the CSF, leading to a decrease in buffering capacity. This may also lead to a rebound phenomenon if normoventilation is resumed too rapidly. Although controlled hyperventilation is a powerful tool for achieving short-term reduction of ICP, exaggerated hyperventilation may reduce CBF below ischemic thresholds in some regions of the brain as demonstrated by greatly reduced jugular venous oxygen saturation, and prolonged hyperventilation may lead to a rebound phenomenon if normoventilation is acutely restored. Therefore, it is preferable to use hyperventilation for intervention in acutely elevated ICP (e.g., to truncate A-pressure waves). In addition, $PaCO_2$ should not be brought to below 28 mmHg in adults in order to prevent ischemia.

Diuretics and Hypertonic Solutions

Low-mol.-wt. hypertonic solutions such as mannitol, sorbitol, and glycerol are used to reduce brain water. They produce an osmolar gradient between blood and brain tissue, thus provoking water movement from the brain tissue into the vascular compartment. A gradient of 35 mosmol/l is sufficient, and a serum osmolarity of 340 mosmol/l should generally not be surmounted. The integrity of the blood-brain barrier is required for this therapeutic effect. The theoretical possibility of paradoxically exaggerating herniation by shrinking normal brain has not yet been observed in practice. Another potential problem is a rebound phenomenon due to diffusion of the solutions into the area of destroyed blood-brain barrier, resulting in water attraction to this region and a delayed increased ICP. The rebound phenomenon has been less frequent with oral glycerol than with sorbitol. Since high-concentration solutions of glucose or levulose (50%) and urea are able to penetrate the intact blood-brain barrier an associated rebound phenomenon may be prominent. These solutions are therefore not used for therapy of increased ICP. In our experience, the duration of the ICP reduction with mannitol

lasts up to 6–9 h, with sorbitol up to 3 h, and with intravenous glycerol up to 10 h. Since i.v. glycerol can be given only slowly (10% as 500 ml over 3–4 h) the initial ICP reduction appears only slowly (Fig. 4). Mannitol as a 20% solution and sorbitol as a 40% solution can be given as 250 ml over 10–20 min and act more quickly (Fig. 5). It may be better to administer frequent small doses (3–4 × 80–125 ml/day) of mannitol than to give one large dose. Mannitol is excreted renally and sorbitol is metabolized in the liver. Fructose intolerance has been reported in rare cases after sorbitol infusion. It has been argued that mannitol might also alter vascular diameter and thus CBF, thereby influencing intracranial compliance and ICP directly. Pulmonary edema can be avoided by administration of the above-mentioned frequent small doses. If mannitol is not excreted by the kidney in renal insufficiency it may lead to intravascular hypervolemia. Furthermore, if these solutions are used for several days (more than 3) brain tissue osmolarity increases slowly, thus reducing the effect of the osmotherapeutics. Therefore, these solutions should be given only when a mass has been proven by cranial CT or when the clinical situation worsens due to brain edema. Prophylactic therapy in anticipation of raised ICP is ineffective. Sorbitol acts very quickly (within minutes) and briefly, whereas mannitol begins more slowly (10–20 min) but has prolonged activity, and glycerol, due to its slow infusion limitations, takes about 1 h for a significant ICP-reducing effect, which then may last for several hours. Sorbitol irritates the veins; therefore, a central venous catheter is preferred in cases in which the clinical condition

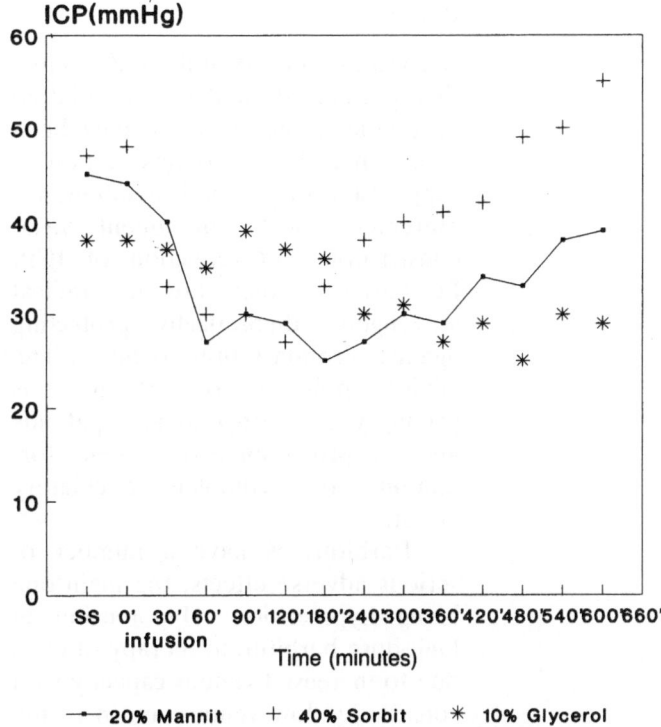

Fig. 4. Effect of hyperosmolar solutions on cerebrospinal fluid pressure in intracranial tumors. In six patients of each group CSFP was recorded for a minimum of 11 h. Each solution was given as 200 ml over 60 min (0–60). It became evident that sorbitol (*Sorbit*) acted faster than both others but had a shorter duration of effect. Glycerol had the slowest but most consistent effect. Values are mean values for six patients; standard deviations are not given for clear identification of the curves, but they changed significantly between individual patients

permits the time to introduce it. Glycerol may cause hemolysis if infused too rapidly (faster than 500 ml of a 10% solution within 4 h). All osmotic agents are capable of producing excessive dehydration and hypernatremia, as well as hypokalemia.

THAM

Tris–hydroxy–methyl–aminomethane (THAM) leads to vasoconstriction and decreased ICP after i.v. administration. For clinical purposes, it has been tried only if all other maneuvers, particularly controlled hyperventilation, have failed. THAM as a dose of 60 mmol in 100 ml 5% glucose may be administered i.v. over 45 min. If ICP falls by 10–15 mmHg after this initial dosage it may be infused at a rate of 3 mmol/h. Blood gases must be checked hourly to limit base excess to +6 mEq and a pH below 7.55. Since THAM may depress respiration by its alkalotic effect it can be used only in ventilated patients and should not be used for prolonged periods. As soon as ICP is controlled, THAM should be stopped since it is nephro- and hepatotoxic.

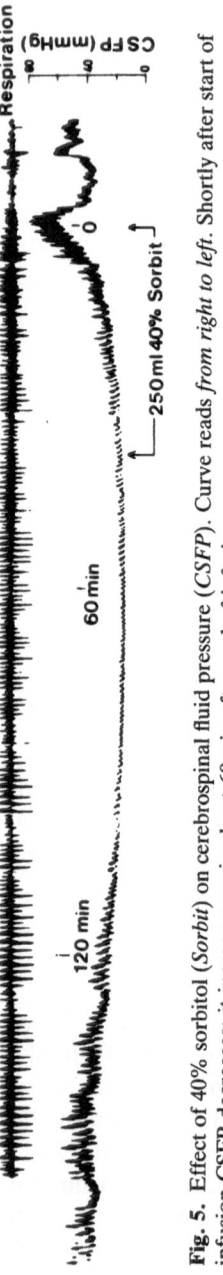

Fig. 5. Effect of 40% sorbitol (*Sorbit*) on cerebrospinal fluid pressure (*CSFP*). Curve reads *from right to left*. Shortly after start of infusion CSFP decreases; it increases again about 60 min after end of infusion

Barbiturates

Barbiturates may be utilized if osmotic therapy, steroids, and hyperventilation have failed. Clinical results have been conflicting. Their primary action is suppression of cerebral metabolic requirements with subsequent vasoconstriction and reduction of ICP. Furthermore, they are free-radical scavengers, theoretically protecting against secondary brain damage. The clinical application of barbiturates is primarily in post-traumatic patients and for protection from edema formation after complete circulatory arrest.

Barbiturates have a number of serious adverse effects, the main one being hypotension. Hypotension in high-dose barbiturate therapy often is due to increased venous capacity with consecutive low venous return to the heart. This effect is pronounced in patients with dehydration due to mannitol therapy. Depression of myocardial function may also occur. Therefore, volume expansion with colloids may be required. If this is not effective, systemic blood pressure can be increased with catecholamines to prevent ischemia due to low CPP. The dosage of a test bolus injection with thiopental is 250–500 mg over a few minutes while monitoring blood pressure, followed by a continuous infusion of thiopental (5 mg/kg/h) or intermittent boluses. EEG monitoring may be used but is not required, since the medication can be titrated to its effect on ICP and blood pressure.

Surgical Intervention

In consideration of surgical intervention for treatment of elevated intracranial pressure, mention of the effects of anesthesia must be made. Anesthetics reduce cerebral blood volume, arterial blood pressure, and central venous pressure. Additionally, they may affect the dynamics of cerebrospinal fluid. For induction of general anesthesia, thiopentone and most other i.v. hypnotics reduce ICP, presumably by decreasing cerebral blood flow and cerebral blood volume. Of this class of agent, only ketamine increases cerebral blood flow and increases ICP. Nitrous oxide and barbiturates are not recommended for induction purposes, as the former causes cerebral vasodilation directly and the latter by respiratory depression and hypercapnia, the end result being a further increase in intracranial pressure. Inhalational agents are generally employed for the maintenance of general anesthesia. Nitrous oxide causes only a minimal increase in ICP, while enflurane and isoflurane result in a moderate, brief increase as a result of vasodilation. The vasodilatory effects of halothane, trichloroethylene, and methoxyflurane may result in considerable elevations in ICP. Of interest is the observation that hyperventilation counters the vasodilatory effects of isoflurane and halothane; however, with the latter, hyperventilation must precede administration. With regard to the effects on CSF dynamics, halothane decreases the formation rate of CSF, while enflurane increases it and isoflurane has no effect. Additionally, resistance to absorption is increased in the presence of halothane and enflurane but decreased by isoflurane.

Surgery is the preferred treatment for accessible intracranial mass lesions in appropriate candidates. Emergency surgery is the treatment of choice for extra-axial hematomas with resultant mass effect and elevation of intracranial pressure and, depending on the location, size, and mass effect, parenchymal hematomas may also come to surgical attention. In the face of generalized cerebral edema and ICP elevations that are refractory to all nonsurgical therapy, carefully selected patients are considered for a lobectomy or a hemicraniectomy. In selected cases of acute ischemic stroke with prominent edema and elevated ICP, hemicraniectomy may be life-saving. Favorable conditions for hemicraniectomy include a lesion in the nondominant hemisphere, young age, and incomplete neurological deficit on admission. Once failure of conservative therapy is recognized, heparin anticoagulation is discontinued, but it may be resumed 12 h after decompression. After craniectomy, compression on the side of surgery has to be avoided; often the 30° elevation of the head results in ICP levels higher than those encountered in the supine position because, with the skull bone removed, the weight of the hemisphere itself compresses deeper brain structures. Palpation of the exposed hemisphere often is a more reliable indicator of ICP than the transducer values.

Serial early acoustic and median-nerve-evoked potentials may be of particular value in following patients with cerebellar infarction. In patients with normal evoked potentials and a compressed fourth ventricle, osmotherapy is performed. If electrophysiology suggests beginning brain-stem compression (prolonged interpeak latencies of the early auditory responses, usually normal median-nerve-evoked potentials) a CT scan is done. If the CT scan reveals hydrocephalus or brain-stem compression, a ventriculostomy is done and osmotherapy is instituted. If the basal cisterns are compressed by edema and evoked potentials reveal pathological responses with both modalities, surgical decompression of the posterior fossa and ventriculostomy are performed.

Suggested Reading

Christensen MS (1974) Acid-base changes in cerebrospinal fluid and blood, and blood volume changes following prolonged hyperventilation in man. Br J Anaesth 46:348

Delashaw JB, Broaddus WC, Kassell NF, Haley EC, Pendleto GA, Vollmer DG, Maggio WW, Grady MS (1990) Treatment of right hemispheric cerebral infarction by hemicraniectomy. Stroke 21:874–881

Eisenberg HM, Frankowski RF, Contant CF, Marshall LF, Walker MD (1988) High-dose barbiturate control of elevated intracranial pressure in patients with severe head injury. J Neurosurg 69:15–23

Foldes FF, Arrowood JG (1948) Changes in cerebrospinal fluid pressure under the influence of continuous subarachnoid infusion of normal saline. J Clin Invest 27:346–351

Gaab M, Knoblich OE, Spohr A, Boneke H, Fuhrmeister U (1980) Effect of THAM on ICP, EEG and tissue edema parameters in experimental and clinical brain edema. In: Shulman K, Marmarou A, Miller JD, Becker DP, Hochwald GM, Brock M (eds) Intracranial pressure, IV. Springer, Berlin Heidelberg New York, pp 664–668

Gaab MR, Heissler HE (1984) ICP monitoring. Crit Rev Biomed Eng 11(3):189–250

Gaab MR, Rittierodt M, Lorenz M, Heissler HE (1990) Traumatic brain swelling and operative decompression: a prospective investigation. Acta Neurochir Suppl (Wien) 51:326–328

Go KG (1991) Cerebral pathophysiology. Elsevier, Amsterdam, pp 173–207

Hartmann A, Wassmann H (eds) (1987) Hirninfarkt. Urban and Schwarzenberg, Munich, p 55

Inao S, Kuchiwaki H, Wachi A et al. (1990) Effect of mannitol on intracranial pressure volume status and cerebral haemodynamics in brain oedema. Acta Neurochir Suppl (Wien) 51:401–403

Ivamoto H, Numoto M, Donaghy R (1974) Surgical decompression for cerebral and cerebellar infarcts. Stroke 5:365–370

Kaieda R, Todd MM, Weeks JB, Warner DS (1989) A comparison of the effects of halothane, isoflurane, and pentobarbital anesthesia on intracranial pressure and cerebral edema formation following brain injury in rabbits. Anesthesiology 71:571–579

Langfitt TW (1982) Increased intracranial pressure and cerebral circulation. In: Youmans (ed) Neurological surgery, vol 2, 2nd edn. Saunders, Philadelphia, pp 846–930

Lundberg N (1960) Continuous recordings and control of intraventricular pressure in neurosurgical practice. Acta Psychiatry Scand 36[Suppl 149]:1–193

Marshall LF, Shapiro HM (1980) Barbiturates for intracranial hypertension: a ten-year perspective. In: Shulman K, Marmarou A, Miller JD, Becker DP, Hochwald GM, Brock M (eds) Intracranial pressure, IV. Springer, Berlin Heidelberg New York, pp 627–629

Matsuoka Y, Hossmann K-A (1981) Corticosteroid therapy of experimental tumor edema. Neurosurg Rev 4:185–190

Mendelow AD, Russel T, Patterson J, Teasdale G (1983) The effects of mannitol on intracranial pressure, cerebral perfusion pressure and cerebral blood flow in head injury. In: Ishii S, Nagai H, Brock M (eds) Intracranial pressure, V. Springer, Berlin Heidelberg New York, pp 746–750

Muizelaar JP, van der Poel HG (1989) Cerebral vasoconstriction is not maintained with prolonged hyperventilation. In: Hoff JT, Betz AL (eds) Intracranial pressure, VII. Springer, Berlin Heidelberg New York, pp 899–903

Narayan RK, Becker DP (1985) Selection of patients for ICP monitoring. J Neurosurg 62:624–625

Node Y, Nakazawa S (1990) Clinical study of mannitol and glycerol on raised intracranial pressure and on their rebound phenomenon. Adv Neurol 52:359–363

Plum F, Brown HW (1963) The effect on respiration of central nervous system disease. Ann NY Acad Sci 109:915

Razumovsky AY, Hanley DF (1992) Intracranial pressure measurement/cranial vault mechanics: clinical and experimental observations. Curr Opin Neurol Neurosurg 5:818–825

Rockoff MA, Marshall LF, Shapiro HM (1979) High-dose barbiturate therapy in humans. A clinical review of 60 patients. Ann Neurol 6:194–199

Rosner MJ, Becker DP (1984) Origin and evolution of plateau waves. Experimental observations and a theoretical model. J Neurosurg 50:312–324

Smith HP, Kelly DL, McWhorter JM et al. (1986) Comparison of mannitol regimens in patients with severe head injury undergoing intracranial monitoring. J Neurosurg 65:820–824

Weed LH, McKibben PS (1919) Pressure changes in cerbrospinal fluid following intravenous injection of solutions of various concentrations. Am J Physiol 48:512–530

Wise BL, Cater N (1962) The value of hypertonic mannitol solution in decreasing brain mass and lowering cerebrospinal fluid pressure. J Neurosurg 19:1038–1043

Chapter 10 | **Pain Relief and Sedation**

Josef F. Zander and Dennis L. Bourke

Introduction

Patients in the critical care environment are exposed to a number of influences that produce excessive anxiety and stress, thereby causing impairment of both central and peripheral nervous system function. The end result can be significant increases in morbidity and mortality. These factors can be of either exogenous or endogenous origin and can be considered under the following broad categories:

Environmental factors	Auditory
	Visual
	Temperature
Psychological factors	Anxiety disorder
	Sleep disturbances and deprivation
	Psychological trauma
	Post-aggression syndrome
Medical factors	Respiratory failure
	Pain
	Endocrine disorders
	Infection

Section Editor: Daniel F. Hanley

Sepsis and sepsis
  syndrome
Cardiovascular
  impairment
Hypoxemia
Drug effects

Almost all of these factors, taken singly or in combination, result in anxiety and stress – the most common complications of confinement to an ICU; only rarely is the underlying cause a psychiatric disorder. The incidence and type of psychiatric symptoms depends both on the type of ICU and the nature of the patients who are treated. For example, the most frequent diagnosis in a cardiac ICU is anxiety; in a surgical or respiratory ICU it is delirium. There is also a predictable progression of psychiatric symptoms during the course of a disease.

Pain is the second important factor that must be treated in ICU patients. Untreated pain will lead to anxiety and stress and frequently to behavioral disturbances. Almost every patient in the critical care setting will experience pain during some stage of his disease. Inadequate analgesia and sedation can cause post-aggression syndrome, thereby increasing metabolic rate and oxygen consumption and promoting hemodynamic instability. In patients with pulmonary failure, the post-aggression syndrome may make effective ventilation impossible despite the use of modern pressure-supported ventilation techniques. Furthermore, agitation may lead to problems in nursing care as well as to the risk of self-injury.

Although the above problems are well known, no simple, clear-cut techniques for ideal analgesia and sedation are known. Moreover, there is no single ideal drug for any of these goals. As a result, many different drugs and multiple combinations of drugs are used more or less pragmatically. Additionally, drug dosage cannot always be determined by simple pharmacological principles. Criteria for the ideal drug for sedation and analgesia include the following: a short duration of effects, minimal or no interactions with other drugs, and no effect on organ system and immune functions. Its metabolism should be independent of disturbed organ function, and it should be inexpensive and easy to use. No such drug is yet available.

Pharmacology

Sedation

Sedation and anxiolysis must be provided for the ICU patient to protect him from the myriad of constant external stimuli as well as from the deleterious effects of his own internal anxiety and stress. In extreme cases heavy sedation to the point of near anesthesia will be necessary. Two important points should be borne in mind: Mechanical ventilation does not always require heavy sedation, and sedation is never an appropriate substitute for adequate analgesia.

Benzodiazepines

Benzodiazepines, at the usual clinical doses, have anxiolytic, antiepileptic, and amnesiac properties. They also decrease muscle tone, an effect mediated at glycine receptors. In higher doses, benzodiazepines have a primary sedative effect and may cause respiratory depression. Benzodiazepines act by augmenting the effect of endogenous GABA on $GABA_A$-receptors. As a result, benzodiazepines have a ceiling effect. Benzodiazepines, however, do not act at all GABA receptors. Many other drugs such as ethyl alcohol and the barbiturates can have agonistic actions at the GABA receptor and thereby produce effects additive to the benzodiazepines.

A primary consideration when choosing among the benzodiazepines is the beta half-life, but this is not the only criterion to be considered. Receptor binding, active metabolites, and the potential for rebound phenomena are also important.

The prototype of benzodiazepines is diazepam. Because the metabolites are also active, effects last for a relatively long time and accumulation is possible.

Midazolam has several advantages for use in the ICU setting when compared with other benzodiazepines. It is water soluble, making it useful for i.v. administration, and it has only one weakly active metabolite. The onset of action is as rapid, and recovery after continuous infusion is usually faster than with other benzodiazepines. At comparable anxiolytic doses the sedative effect is stronger than that of diazepam. Therefore, midazolam has become the most widely used sedative drug in the intensive care setting. Despite its favorable pharmacokinetic properties, midazolam may not reach a steady state effect in critically ill patients. There are circumstances where it can accumulate.

Lorazepam is very similar to diazepam in its pharmacodynamic properties. It distributes extensively in the central nervous system. Though it has a long half-life, there is little accumulation. However, because of its binding properties and distribution in the brain, the clinical action is longer than expected on the basis of serum half-life.

Some patients demonstrate an acute tolerance to benzodiazepines, so that an increased dosage is necessary. However, in other patients even high doses do not provide sufficient sedation. In these instances, a second sedative should be combined with the benzodiazepine or an alternative drug selected (e.g., a barbiturate or propofol).

Finally, some patients show an as yet unexplained paradoxical reaction to benzodiazepines. The therapy of choice is either the addition of a phenothiazine or the use of a benzodiazepine antagonist such as flumazenil.

Neuroleptics

Two classes of neuroleptic drugs are commonly used for critically ill patients: butyrophenones and phenothiazines. The butyrophenones used most often are haloperidol and dehydrobenzperidol. These drugs are especially indicated for patients who do not have significant pain or anxiety but who react strongly to sensory stimuli. These patients should receive the lowest dose possible to put them in an apparent stage of indifference.

In addition to their neuroleptic effects, both agents have alpha-antagonistic effects. Hypotension may occur if the patient is hypovolemic or if a rapid bolus of the drug is administered. The antidopaminergic effect of the butyrophenones does not cause impairment of renal function. Additionally, butyrophenones have a strong antiemetic effect.

Butyrophenones have strong antipsychotic and antidelirium effects and produce a sedation that appears vegetative in character. Butyrophenones can be administered orally or intravenously. They are particularly effective in controlling agitation. The butyrophenones frequently cause dose-and time-dependent extrapyramidal side effects. For this reason they are often given in combination with a benzodiazepine or phenothiazine in order to reduce the dose. Haloperidol is the most commonly used butyrophenone; the initial intravenous dose is 2–10 mg, which can be repeated after 20–30 min. Dehydrobenzperidol, with its shorter half-life, is more suited to continuous infusions; the initial dose is similar to that for haloperidol. Extrapyramidal side effects of the butyrophenones can be antagonized with biperiden; however, biperiden should be used with caution since it may itself induce delirium and has a high potential for addiction.

Phenothiazines have a smaller neuroleptic effect but are better sedatives than butyrophenones. They also have an antihistaminic effect. Phenothiazines are best used in combination with analgesics or with butyrophenones to enhance sedative effects.

Barbiturates

In contrast to benzodiazepines, barbiturates act on excitatory mechanisms of the brain as well as the $GABA_A$. As a result, there is no ceiling effect; an increase in dosage always leads to increased drug effects. Thiopental and methohexital are both effective given as continuous infusions. Thiopental impairs granulocyte function, can induce liver enzymes, and because of its relatively slow metabolism may accumulate. Methohexital has a shorter half-life, a nonhepatic-dependent metabolism, and the advantage of stimulating the adenosine system.

Other Drugs

In recent years, alpha-2-adrenergic agonists such as clonidine have been used more frequently in intensive care settings. They augment the analgesic and sedative effects of other drugs, cause an increase in the level of endorphins, and reduce sympathetic tone.

Propofol is being increasingly used for sedation in the ICU. It is rapidly metabolized and demonstrates minimal accumulation. It is always given as a continuous infusion. The advantage of using propofol is that even after prolonged sedation, patients awaken a few minutes after the drug is discontinued. Disadvantages include the lack of widespread assessment of side effects and clinical risks in the ICU setting.

Occasionally, ketamine, in combination with a benzodiazepine, is used. It is advantageous in asthmatic patients for whom other therapeutic methods have failed. Ketamine causes sedation, analgesia, and, at increased doses, anesthesia. Because it can induce hypertension and a subsequent rise in intracranial pressure, ketamine should not be used in patients with decreased cerebral compliance or raised intracranial pressure. It can have advantages, however, in asthmatic patients for whom other therapeutic procedures have failed.

Delirium in an ICU patient can arise from a number of causes including alcohol withdrawal, side effects of other drugs used in treatment, or an absolute or relative deficiency of acetylcholine in the CNS. In the latter case, 2 mg of physostigmine, the anticholinesterase that crosses the blood-brain barrier, can be dramatically effective. Pretreatment with 0.5 mg atropine will prevent bradycardia.

Analgesia

Analgesia can be produced in three general ways: at the nociceptive site (prostaglandin inhibitors, local anesthetics), by interruption of nociceptive transmission (epidural or intrathecal opioids, local anesthetics, α-2 agonists), or in the brain (opioids).

Opioids

Opioids act at endogenous receptors. The most important are the μ, κ, and σ receptors. The σ receptor mediates analgesia, respiratory depression, and some sedation. The most prominent effect of the κ receptor is sedation. The μ receptor mediates primarily analgesia and respiratory depression.

The most useful pure agonists have primarily μ and κ activity. There is a wide range of pharmacokinetic and pharmodynamic properties among the clinically available opioids, and the choice of a specific opioid should be made with regard to these properties, as well as in consideration of their side effects.

Opioids should not be used as sedatives, since sedation occurs only at high doses. However, the synergism between sedatives and opioids can be exploited to reduce doses and side effects of both drugs. Typical side effects of opioids are respiratory depression, decreased chest wall compliance, inhibition of gastrointestinal function, and increased tone of the bile duct. Side effects vary among the agents but are generally dose dependent. All patients treated with opioids must be monitored with regard to respiratory function. The choice of an opioid should be made as rationally as the choice of a sedative drug.

Morphine

Morphine as the prototype opioid agonist is still the gold standard of analgesia. Although it acts primarily on μ receptors, it can cause histamine release. Furthermore, morphine clearance is impaired in renal and in hepatic failure. Hemodynamics in critically ill patients are not always as stable with morphine as with alternative opioids.

Fentanyl

Fentanyl has an analgesic potency 75 to 125 times that of morphine, but it has less sedative action. Being highly lipid soluble, it easily crosses the blood-brain barrier and is widely distributed in all tissues. This wide distribution and its relatively slow metabolism account for its long duration of action when used in larger doses or over a long period of time. Fentanyl has minimal cardiovascular or other side effects. For these reasons it is an excellent analgesic for mechanically ventilated patients.

Alfentanil

Alfentanil is approximately 25 times as potent as morphine. Its advantage with respect to fentanyl is its short redistribution half-life (about 11 min) and its short elimination half-life (about 94 min). Termination of its effect depends mainly on hepatic clearance, not on redistribution. Alfentanil, however, is expensive and therfore may not be the first choice for prolonged analgesia.

Piritramid

Piritramid has a slightly smaller analgesic effect than morphine. However, it has significantly fewer side effects, such as nausea and vomiting. It can be used alone just for analgesia, or, like the other opioids, it can be used with benzodiazepines or barbiturates. In smaller dosages, it can also be given as an analgesic drug for spontaneously breathing patients. (Piritramid is not currently vailable in the USA.)

Meperidine

Meperidine should be used only for short-term or single-dose analgesia. It has adverse effects on thermoregulation, can cause histamine release, and can cause excessive sedation and respiratory depression when used in combination with sedatives. Normeperidine, a metabolite, has opioid activity and a prolonged half-life, and it can cause myoclonic convulsions, particularly in patients with renal failure. Meperidine should not be used for patients taking MAO inhibitors.

Muscle Relaxants

Muscle relaxants are rarely necessary in the ICU. The flexibility of modern ventilation techniques, combined with the intelligent use of opioids, sedatives, and hyperventilation, is usually sufficient to provide adequate conditions for patient management. Only in the critical phase of a disease or in those patients with severe pulmonary failure, requiring high levels of PEEP or inverse ventilation ratios, is the use of muscle relaxants still necessary. Relaxants should be given in intermittent boluses to keep the dose as low as possible. Continuous administration may lead to down-regulation of acetylcholine receptors. Muscle relaxants

should be avoided, if possible, in patients with neurological diseases affecting the muscles. When muscle relaxants are used in these patients, the dosage must be carefully titrated. It should be remembered that muscle relaxants provide no analgesia, sedation, or amnesia.

Drug Combinations

Combinations of sedatives and analgesics (see Table 1) in the ICU should be administered intravenously to avoid problems with absorption from the gastrointestinal tract.

Clinical Assessment and Management

The main problem in providing drug therapy to intensive care patients is the difference in pharmacokinetics and pharmacodynamics compared with healthy patients. Disease-induced alterations in hepatic function, renal

Table 1. Combinations of sedative and analgesic drugs used in the intensive care unit

	Sedative		Analgesic	
	Drug	Route	Drug	Route
Combined analgesia	Midazolam	C	Piritramid	C or I
and sedation	Midazolam	C	Fentanyl	C
	Midazolam	C	Alfentanil	C
	Butyrophenone	I	Opioid	I
	Butyrophenone and midazolam	C	Opioid	C
	Propofol	C	Opioid	I
	Barbiturate	C	Opioid	I
Analgesia only	–	–	Opioid	I
Sedation/anxiolysis only	Midazolam	C or I	–	–

C, Continuous infusion; I, intermittent bolus doses.

function, cardiovascular dynamics, plasma proteins, and various other physiological variables dramatically complicate the calculation of appropriate drug doses.

Electrophysiological monitoring of analgesia and sedation is not always reliable. Therefore, in most cases a subjective clinical scale is valuable in establishing the level of sedation. The scale ranges from 1 to 6 points. A value of 1 is assigned to the obviously agitated, combative patient and a value of 6 to the unresponsive patient. This scale can be very helpful in the clinical setting to establish the effects of endogenous and exogenous influences on the central nervous system and to permit data to be compared inter- and intraindividually. With this simple numerical scale it is possible to adjust a patient's drug dosage to achieve the desired degree of sedation. Pain as a source of agitation is frequently difficult to assess, and a trial of an analgesic should always be considered in the patient who is difficult to sedate.

The patient's neurological status should be determined daily, including the directed use of imaging, EEG, or other neurophysiological methods such as SEP or AEP. This is especially important in patients who are deeply sedated or who are being treated with muscle relaxants. This should be done when deterioration of the neurological status is suspected.

Flumazenil can be given to antagonize benzodiazepines, and naloxone can be given to antagonize opioids. Antagonists should be given with care to avoid precipitating an acute crisis. It should also be remembered that both antagonists have relatively short half-lives compared with most of their agonists.

Considerations for Patients with Neurological Disease

Continuous monitoring of cerebral function is especially important in patients with neurological disease. Measurement of blood levels of sedatives or analgesic drugs does not always correlate with clinical effects. The serial use of simple numerical scales is invaluable in assessing patients' status. However, when severe side effects are detected, blood levels should be determined to be certain that plasma levels are not excessively high, due to impaired organ function. Accumulation of active metabolites should also be considered.

Neurotrauma

Barbiturates lower intracranial pressure by vasoconstriction and consequent reduction of the intracranial blood volume. In addition, they have a potent anticonvulsive effect (see Chap. 9).

Benzodiazepines can be useful in neurotrauma, since they reduce the brain's metabolic rate and have anticonvulsive effects. Propofol also lowers intracranial pressure. Because of its possible hypotensive action, it must be administered very cautiously. Whether the propofol solvent, a 10% fat emulsion, has any negative effects on the brain is yet unknown.

In most neurotrauma cases it becomes necessary to monitor both ICP and cerebral perfusion pressure. Perfusion pressure must be maintained with pressors if necessary.

Guillan-Barré Syndrome

Pain, a common problem for patients with Guillan-Barré syndrome, is due to partial involvement of sensory nerves in the enervating process. For cases where it does not respond to systemic analgesics, epidural opioids have been recommended. Whether morphine or a more lipid-soluble opioid is preferable has not been determined. In ventilated GBS patients, the above-described combinations of opioids and sedatives are frequently used. In many cases, very long treatment duration may lead to tolerance and may make it difficult to reach an adequate analgo-sedative effect.

Tetanus

Generalized tetanus triggers severe muscle spasms, especially of the neck and trunk. Any sensory stimulus can precipitate a severe attack. To prevent and control the spasms the patient should be sedated and, in some cases, treated with a muscle relaxant. Benzodiazepines are the drugs of choice. Since they cause both sedation and diminished muscle tone, tolerance develops and the effect decreases over a period of time. As an alternative a combination of barbiturates and opioid can be used.

Alcohol and Drug Withdrawal (for extended coverage see Chap. 77)

Delirium can be treated with alcohol agonists, such as benzodiazepines or clomethiazol. In many cases butyrophenones will be added to the bezodiazepines. Autonomic symptoms may require an alpha-2 agonist such as clonidine. Daily doses of 3 mg or more of clonidine are not unusual in the acute phase of delirium. Bradycardia, usually the only side effect, can be treated with intravenous atropine. Intravenous clometiazol is available only in Europe. It may cause bronchial oversecretion and respiratory depression.

Continuous administration of benzodiazepines leads to a deregulation of the intrinsic GABA mechanisms and to a down-regulation of GABA receptors. An abrupt discontinuation of benzodiazepines results in a deficit of GABA in the brain. As a result there is an excess of excitatory influences. The degree and the time course of this effect depend on the pharmacokinetics of the particular benzodiazepine used. Treatment is reinstitution of the drug, followed by careful detoxification. Refractory cases are treated symptomatically using neuroleptics.

Conclusion

Sedation and analgesia are important aspects of care in intensive care settings. The indications for sedation and analgesia must be considered individually for every patient and re-evaluated with each phase of the disease. Careful attention to side effects and interactions are important for the proper selection of drugs and doses. The amount of the drug given should produce only the degree of sedation and analgesia that is necessary. Physical dependency can develop and must be considered if the patient demonstrates vegetative signs when the dosage of the drug is decreased.

Psychological dependency, however, is rarely a problem. New methods should be investigated to produce better and more continuous control over patient sedation. During prolonged drug administration patients should be closely monitored and frequently re-evaluated. Unanticipated new side effects, such as cortisol suppression by etomidate, may go unnoticed without careful evaluation. Continued research will produce drugs with more continuous sedation and analgesia as well as fewer side effects.

Suggested Reading

Baumgartner GR, Rowen RC (1987) Clonidine vs chlordiazepoxide in the management of acute alcohol withdrawal syndrome. Arch Intern Med 147:1223

Bion J, Logan B, Newman P, Brodie M, Oliver J, Aitchinson T, Ledigham IM (1986) Sedation in intensive care: morphine and renal function. Intensive Care Med 12: 359–365

Bodenham A, Shelly M, Park G (1988) The altered pharmacokinetics and pharmacodynamics of drugs used in critically ill patients. Clinical Pharmacokinet 14:347–373

Bovill J (1987) Which potent opioid? Important criteria for selection. Drugs 33:520–530

Dlin B, Rosen H, Dickstein K, Syons J, Fischer H (1971) The problems of sleep and rest in the intensive care unit. Psychosomatics 12:155–163

Editorial (1981) Paralyzed with fear. Lancet II:427

Harris CE, Grounds RM, Murray AM, Lumley J, Royston D, Morgan M (1990) Propofol for long-term sedation in the intensive care unit. Anaesthesia 45:366–372

Lipowski Z (1989) Delirium in the elderly patient. N Engl J Med 320:95–97

Loper K, Butler S, Nessly M, Wild L (1989) Terror in the ICU: Paralyzed with pain. Anaesth Analg 68:S170

Merrimann H (1981) The techniques used to sedate ventilated patients. A survey of methods used in 34 ICUs in Great Britain. Intensive Care Med 8:217–224

Nolop K, Natow A (1985) Unprecedented sedative requirements during delirium tremens. Crit Care Med 13:246–247

O'Sullivan G, Park G (1990) The assessment of sedation in critically ill patients. Clin Intensive Care 1:116–122

Rie MA, Wilson RS (1978) Morphine therapy control of autonomic hyperactivity in tetanus. Ann Intern Med 88:653

Robinson BJ, Robinson GM, Maling TJ, Johnson RH (1989) Is clonidine useful in the treatment of alcohol withdrawal? Alcohol Clin Exp Res 13:95–98

Rosenfeld B, Borel C, Hanley D (1986) Epidural morphine treatment of pain in Guillain-Barré Syndrome. Arch Neurol 43:1194–1196

Secor JW, Schenker S (1987) Drug metabolism in patients with liver disease. Adv Intern Med 32:379–406

Shetty G, Kelsall P, Ryan D (1986) Long-term ketamine infusion. Anaesthesia 41:1262

Chapter 11 | # Nutrition

TRICIA SCHULTZ and ERNST F. HUND

Introduction

Severe brain injury, whether from trauma or stroke, constitutes a massive metabolic insult. There is a consensus in the literature that patients with acute neurologic injury are hypermetabolic (increased energy expenditure) and hypercatabolic (increased protein degradation). This hypermetabolism is evidenced by increased oxygen consumption which peaks within 5–12 days and generally resolves thereafter unless there are infectious complications, continued steroid administration, persistent seizure activity, or decerebrate posturing. These will all prolong the hypermetabolic response. Correlations have been shown between severity of brain injury and energy requirements. The mechanism of the hypermetabolic response following neurologic injury has been only partially defined. It is now believed that the primary mediators of this hypermetabolic/hypercatabolic response are the catecholamines, gluco-

corticoids, glucagon, and the now more recently identified cytokines. Release of these counterregulatory hormones is markedly increased. Circulating levels of insulin also tend to be high in the stressed state, although tissue responsiveness is severly blunted as a result of insulin resistance caused by the other hormones. The most evident metabolic change is a shift from storage to utilization of protein, fat, and glycogen reserves. It is important to keep in mind that the metabolically stressed patient does not exhibit the normal adaptation to starvation because of the changes in the hormonal milieu. The typical 70 kg man has approximately 225 g of glycogen stores in the liver and muscle, which will be exhausted in less than 24 h of fasting. After this, the nonstressed individual begins to break down adipose tissue preferentially to spare tissue protein and significantly reduces the need for glucose. The stressed patient, on the other hand, continues to use glucose as a primary source of energy, catabolizing muscle protein to provide substrate for gluconeogenesis. Glucose is the major fuel used by injured tissues and by the

Section Editor: Daniel F. Hanley

cells involved in repair and immune processes. Adipose tissue is also mobilized at an accelerated rate under stressed states, with free fatty acids providing a significant fuel source for the liver and skeletal muscle.

As an index of stress, nitrogen excretion is increased to levels comparable to, and often greater than, those in the patient with multiple trauma or thermal injuries. There is broad agreement that the increase in nitrogen excretion reflects the breakdown and mobilization of amino acids from skeletal muscle to meet the increased demands for tissue fuel and synthesis of acute-phase proteins. If no nutrition is provided and if no metabolic adaptation occurs, this leads to a progressive erosion of lean body mass and a progressive depletion of circulating proteins. The resulting protein-calorie deficits can be factors determining the outcome following brain injury. The use of protein is very costly to the body as there are no protein "reserves", so any significant loss of body protein can have important clinical consequences. Acute loss of approximately 15% body weight is associated with a protein loss of around 20% and will likely result in significant impairment of organ mass and function (Table 1). Loss of 40% body weight can be lethal. Nutritional support itself does not reverse the hypermetabolic/hypercatabolic state and prevent the autocannibalism, but it can offset the losses by tipping the balance in favor of protein synthesis. Only when the mediator of the stress response has resolved do the hormone levels return to normal.

Many factors will determine the extent and duration of this stress response and the response to nutritional

Table 1. Clinical impact of protein-calorie malnutrition on organ mass and function

Brain
  Increased lethargy
  Decreased mental alertness
  Increased confusion
Respiratory system
  Deterioration in vital capacity, respiratory rate, and tidal volume
  Decreased sensitivity of oxygen receptors to hypoxic stimuli
  Marked blunting of respiratory response to hypercapnia
Gastrointestinal system
  Atrophy and thinning of gastrointestinal tract mucosa
  Possible translocation of bacteria into the systemic circulation
  Blunting of mucosal villi and brush border enzyme activity
Liver
  Decreased liver mass
  Impaired protein synthesis
Cardiac system
  Cardiac mass depletion proportional to body weight loss
  Potential for congestive heart failure with refeeding
Renal system
  Decreased rate of glomerular filtration and acid excretion
  Decreased response to ADH
Skin
  Impaired would healing
  Formation of decubital ulcers
Immune system
  Reduced lymphocyte count
  Reduced phagocytosis
  Impaired immunoglobulin and antibody production

intervention in the critical care unit. Not only are there wide individual variations to similar neurologic insults; there may also be significant differences among types of neurologic illnesses, co-morbidities, medical management, and drug therapies that may influence nutrient requirements. The goals of nutrition support in the critical care unit are: (a) to maintain organ structure and function by minimizing endogenous protein catabolism and muscle wasting, while supporting synthesis of acute-phase reactants and other secretory proteins; (b) to facilitate management of fluid and electrolyte balance; (c) to maintain immunocompetence.

Nutrition Assessment

Nutrition assessment is a tool used to detect the presence of malnutrition. Standards set from a healthy population are used to determine the extent of nutrient deficits. Nutrition assessment parameters checked serially can be used to assess the efficacy of nutrition support therapy. The initial evaluation of a patient's nutritional status includes a basic physical examination, height and weight history, baseline laboratory data, and a diet history, if possible. Physical examination will show whether patients are obviously overweight or underweight, or if they appear average weight for height, but it will tell very little else about a person's actual nutritional status. A closer physical exam may produce findings that are suggestive of vitamin, mineral, and/or protein-calorie deficiencies; however, most of the signs are not specific for individual nutrient deficiencies and must be integrated with the patient's history and laboratory data to form a diagnosis.

Patients admitted to a neurologic critical care unit (NCCU) are generally of two types. One group are the previously healthy individuals admitted without any apparent nutritional deficits who suffer an acute neurologic injury. They usually have adequate adipose tissue, somatic protein, and visceral protein stores, and are unlikely to suffer from vitamin or mineral deficiencies. The second group includes individuals who, for many reasons, have had impaired nutrient intake or utilization prior to their hospitalization. This group may consist of patients who have had dysphagia from a progressive neuromuscular or neurodegenerative disease, those with brain tumors resulting in impaired intake combined with increased nutrient demands, alcohol or drug abusers, or the elderly. These patients will often present with some degree of protein-calorie malnutrition and quite possibly with micronutrient deficiencies (vitamins and trace minerals), although the latter are more difficult to detect.

Anthropometrics

Anthropometrics are tools to help determine body composition. The most common measurements are height, body weight (including actual weight, usual weight, and ideal weight), triceps skin fold (TSF), and mid-arm muscle circumference (MAMC). In the intensive care unit, the TSF and MAMC are not usually valid due to changes in interstitial fluid status. Height and weight measurements can serve as a preliminary assessment of lean body mass (LBM) when they are compared with ideal weight for height tables and the percent deficit is calculated. Since height/weight tables are derived from populations, they should be used as only a rough guide for individuals. Actual body weight as a percent of usual weight is more useful (Table 2).

Table 2. Clinical assessment of nutritional status in the NCCU

Anthropometrics
  Actual weight
  Usual weight/% usual weight
  Ideal or desirable body weight/% ideal
    weight
  Height
Laboratory data
  Albumin
  Transferrin
  Prealbumin
  Total lymphocyte count
  24-h urine for urea nitrogen
  24° urine for creatinine

Weight should be measured precisely on admission and the premorbid weight and length of illness recorded.

Weight parameters known to impact nutrition status are: weight <20% ideal body weight (IBW); weight loss >10% of usual weight in <6-month period (associated with significant depletion of protein, fat, vitamins, and minerals). The major difficulty in interpreting body weight in a hospitalized patient, especially in the ICU, is in distinguishing between lean and fluid compartments. Fluid retention into the interstitial space can mask loss of fat and somatic protein stores. On the other hand, weight loss due to a reduction in LBM is often mistaken for fluid diuresis. The medical management of the patient and the appropriateness/adequacy of nutritional support must be considered. Body weight usually reflects true changes in body composition when measured over time. Acute changes generally reflect a change in fluid status.

Although weight loss and low body weight are usually emphasized in identifying patients at nutritional risk, the obese individual may also be at risk because of the attitude that these patients are overnourished and can endure long periods without being fed. A patient who is grossly overweight may suffer extreme protein malnutrition, and the protein requirements of such patients are often overlooked. During critical illness, weight reduction does not usually need to be a primary goal. Without nutritional support, the weight loss that does occur will be primarily from muscle protein rather than adipose tissue.

Laboratory Data

Many routine laboratory tests are useful in assessing nutritional status. Baseline data, either directly upon admission or preadmission, are most beneficial. Large volumes of intravenous fluid, surgery, and many other types of therapy will acutely alter laboratory values, rendering most of the traditional parameters invalid for assessing nutritional status. It is often not possible to obtain such data, however, due to the urgent nature of many admissions to the intensive care unit.

Visceral Proteins. The visceral protein depot is located in internal organs such as the liver, kidney, heart, and gastrointestinal tract. Measurement of the actual mass of these organs is not possible during life, but an estimate of the visceral compartment can be obtained by measuring the synthesis of protein by the liver. In the absence of primary liver disease, plasma protein concentrations will be affected by substrate availability, rates of synthesis and utilization, intravascular-extravascular transfer, catabolism, excretion, and hydration. During acute stress, the liver shifts from synthesis of homeostatic proteins such as albumin, transferrin, and prealbumin to the synthesis of acute-phase proteins such as C-reactive protein, alpha-1 glycoprotein, and fibrinogen to support the stress response.

Albumin. Albumin is a transport protein necessary for maintaining plasma oncotic pressure. The $T\frac{1}{2}$ is approximately 21 days, so albumin is relatively insensitive as an indicator of early protein malnutrition or of protein repletion. Serum concentrations decrease rapidly with acute catabolic stress and stay depressed until the anabolic phase begins. Levels can usually return to normal within several weeks of nutritional rehabilitation and are useful in gauging the adequacy of the nutrition support regimen when used in conjunction with other parameters such as nitrogen balance studies. If whole blood or plasma products have recently been given or the patient is undergoing plasmapheresis, serum albumin levels are not reflective of liver synthesis. Data consistently indicate a positive correlation between depressed albumin levels and poor clinical outcome: normal value = 3.5–5.0 g/dl; mild depletion = 2.9–3.4 g/dl; moderate depletion = 2.1–2.8 g/dl; severe depletion = <2.1 g/dl.

Transferrin. Transferrin is the transport protein for iron. It is a more sensitive index of protein nutriture than albumin, as the $T\frac{1}{2}$ is 8–10 days, so it will change more rapidly with changes in protein status. Caution must be exercised in interpreting transferrin, as levels are often markedly increased in iron deficiency anemia: normal value = 200–400 mg/dl; mild depletion = 160–199 mg/dl; moderate depletion = 120–159 mg/dl; severe depletion = <120 mg/dl.

Prealbumin. Also termed thyroxin-binding prealbumin, this serum protein plays a major role in the transport of thyroxin; it also functions as a carrier protein for retinol-binding protein. The $T\frac{1}{2}$ is approximately 2 days, so prealbumin is very sensitive to changes in protein status. Any sudden demand for increased protein synthesis, such as trauma or infection, will rapidly depress prealbumin. Low levels during stress must therefore be interpreted cautiously: normal value = 8–31 mg/dl.

Total Lymphocyte Count. Depressed total lymphocyte count (TLC) suggests impaired cellular defense mechanisms and is often present with protein-calorie malnutrition (PCM). Interpretation of results should take into consideration the presence of immune deficiency diseases or use of immunosuppressive therapy: normal value = >1500 mm³; mild depletion = 1200–1499 mm³; moderate depletion = 900–1199 mm³; severe depletion = <900 mm³.

Urinary Urea Nitrogen. Nitrogen balance studies are useful in determining the extent of protein catabolism and the amount of protein required to maintain nitrogen equilibrium or to achieve a positive nitrogen balance. Nitrogen balance studies measure the net protein loss/gain. Interpretation of the results must take into account the patient's caloric intake, as studies conducted in the face of inadequate caloric intake will primarily reflect the use of protein as an energy substrate. Renal insufficiency or failure will also invalidate the results. Nitrogen balance may be calculated from the following formula:

$$N_{balance} = N_{intake} - (N_{output} + 4.0\,g)$$

N_{intake} is calculated from a 24-h intake record and should include all oral, enteral, and intravenous protein sources. The N_2 content is determined by dividing grams protein by 6.25. Ideally, the patient's protein intake should be fairly constant for a few days before the measurement.

N_{output} is determined by a 24-h urine collection for urea nitrogen (UUN) in grams per day. To the net output is added a factor to account for insensible losses (skin, gastrointestinal, and nonurea urinary N_2 sources). The above formula may thus also be written as:

$$N_{balance} = \frac{\text{Protein intake}}{6.25} - (\text{UUN} + 4.0)$$

Nitrogen equilibrium is 0–1 g/day and indicates maintenance of total body protein. A *Positive nitrogen balance* signifies a net increase in body protein but does not indicate the site of retention. A gain of +3–6 g/day is the goal for nutritional repletion. A *negative nitrogen balance* indicates a net loss of body protein. The level of N_2 excretion is a good index of the degree of metabolic stress. When at least 150 g of carbohydrate are provided, a negative balance is associated with catabolism as follows: 5–10 g/day = mild catabolism; 10–15 g/day = moderate catabolism; 15 or more g/day = severe catabolism.

Injured or septic patients will have large obligatory N_2 losses during the early phase that cannot be prevented by providing more than adequate amounts of exogenous protein and energy. During this period, it may be possible only to offset the N_2 losses rather than to achieve a positive N_2 balance. The increased urea excretion is derived primarily from skeletal muscle. After spinal cord injury, nitrogen balance will be negative for up to 2 months due to disuse atrophy. Guillain-Barré patients will experience similar losses which cannot be regained until function begins to return. For patients with chronic sepsis or multiple organ failure, persistent negative balances may contribute to morbidity and mortality.

Urinary Creatinine Excretion (Creatinine Height Index). Creatinine is a normal metabolite of skeletal muscle catabolism, and its 24-h excretion may serve as an indicator of lean body mass (LBM). When renal function is normal, a predictable amount of urinary creatinine is excreted daily. As LBM decreases, creatinine excretion will fall. Likewise, as LBM is accrued, creatinine excretion should rise. These data can be used to provide information on changes in body composition during the course of hospitalization. Values of 80–100% of predicted indicate adequate muscle mass, 60–80% of predicted is associated with a moderate deficit, and values <60% are correlated with a severe deficit of muscle mass.

The creatinine height index (CHI) can be calculated from the following formula:

$$CHI = \frac{\text{actual 24-h urinary creatinine (mg)} \times 100}{\text{predicted 24-h urinary creatinine (mg)}}$$

Table 3. Predicted 24-h urinary creatinine excretion in adults (after Long et al. 1977)

Men			Women		
Height		Predicted creatinine (mg/24 h)	Height		Predicted creatinine (mg/24 h)
5′2″	157.5 cm	1288	4′10″	147.3 cm	830
5′3″	160.0 cm	1325	4′11″	149.9 cm	851
5′4″	162.6 cm	1359	5′0″	152.4 cm	875
5′5″	165.1 cm	1386	5′1″	154.9 cm	900
5′6″	167.6 cm	1426	5′2″	157.5 cm	925
5′7″	170.2 cm	1467	5′3″	160.0 cm	949
5′8″	172.7 cm	1513	5′4″	162.6 cm	977
5′9″	175.3 cm	1555	5′5″	165.1 cm	1006
5′10″	177.8 cm	1596	5′6″	167.6 cm	1044
5′11″	180.3 cm	1642	5′7″	170.2 cm	1076
6′0″	182.9 cm	1691	5′8″	172.7 cm	1109
6′1″	185.4 cm	1739	5′9″	175.3 cm	1141
6′2″	188.0 cm	1785	5′10″	177.8 cm	1174
6′3″	190.5 cm	1831	5′11″	180.3 cm	1206
6′4″	193.0 cm	1891	6′0″	182.9 cm	1240

For this formula, values for predicted 24-h urinary creatinine excretion can be taken from Table 3. Expected 24-h creatinine excretion can also be estimated based on body weight using the following calculations:

$$\text{Expected 24-h creatinine excretion (men)} = \frac{23\,\text{mg/kg}}{\text{of IBW}}$$

$$\text{Expected 24-h creatinine excretion (women)} = \frac{18\,\text{mg/kg}}{\text{of IBW}}$$

Electrolytes. Many patients in an NCCU will receive steroids, diuretics, or hypervolemic therapy. These modalities result in increased excretion and requirements for PO_4, Mg^{++}, K^+, and Ca^{++}. Daily supplementation is often needed to maintain normal values. It is also very important to monitor these parameters daily if a patient is malnourished upon admission and is started on a feeding re-gimen that exceeds their previous intake. The sudden shift from utilization of endogenous fat stores as a primary energy source to predominantly carbohydrates drives the electrolytes intracellularly and may result in severe serum deficits.

Glucose. Hyperglycemia is a hallmark of the stress response. Infection and steroids exacerbate this problem. Glucose intake should not exceed 5 mg/kg/minute but should not go below 2 mg/kg/minute. The goal appears to be 3–4 mg/kg/minute. If this goal is met, and serum glucose remains high, glucose needs to be controlled with exogenous insulin.

Guidelines for laboratory assessment of nutrition status:

Serum albumin and transferrin	Weekly
Serum Ca^{++}, PO_4, Mg^{++}, K^+	Daily until stable, then 2 times a week

24-h UUN and   Weekly
   creatinine

Calorie Requirements

Ideally, calorie requirements should be determined by indirect calorimetry (IC). Since the body consumes oxygen in proportion to its metabolic rate, calorie requirements can be calculated by measuring oxygen consumption. Indirect calorimetry measures the amounts of CO_2 produced and O_2 consumed. This provides a measure of the resting energy expenditure (REE). The ratio of CO_2 and O_2 consumed reflects the net substrate utilization and is referred to as the respiratory quotient (RQ), where RQ = V_{CO_2}/V_{O_2}.

RQ = 0.7 for fat utilization
RQ = 0.85 for mixed fuel
        oxidation
RQ = 1.0 for carbohydrate
        oxidation
RQ = >1.0 for lipogenesis

An RQ in the range of 0.80–0.90 is desirable. An RQ close to 0.7 may reflect inadequate feeding, whereas as RQ > 1.0 may indicate overfeeding. If IC is not available, other methods are available to estimate calorie requirements. The Harris-Benedict equation can be used to estimate a patient's basal energy expenditure (BEE):

BEE (men) = 66.47 + 13.75W
              + 5.00H − 6.76A
BEE (women) = 655.10 + 9.56W
                + 1.85H
                − 4.68A

where W = weight in kg, H = height in cm, and A = age in years.

Estimated total calorie requirements are then determined by multiplying BEE by a factor that accounts for the stress of the illness. In the ICU, multiplying the BEE by a factor of 1.4–1.6 will approximate the actual energy expenditure of a large percentage of patients. Patients with severe head injuries and those with severe Guillan-Barré syndrome have been shown to require up to 2.0 × BEE. If all the factors for the above equation are not available, calorie needs can be estimated based on weight alone. Most ICU patients require 35–40 kcal/kg actual body weight. Those with more severe injuries may require up to 50 kcal/kg, which is in the range of needs of patients with thermal injury. Caution must be used with this method in the morbidly obese patient.

Many factors can influence calorie needs in an individual patient. Persistant fevers will further increase energy needs. For each degree centigrade, calorie needs increase by approximately 13%, for each degree Fahrenheit by 7%. Persistent seizure activity, posturing to pain, and steroid administration may also increase caloric expenditure. There is some evidence that patients who are comatose, whether this is drug-induced or from other causes, have slightly reduced caloric needs. Pentobarbitol coma reduces cerebral metabolism and possibly total body cellular demands. Patients with spinal cord injuries have also been shown to have energy needs lower than those of other trauma patients because of reduced metabolic activity of denervated muscle. The higher the lesion, the lower the energy expenditure. Although it is important to provide adequate calories, overfeeding of calories can be detrimental, leading to respiratory distress and hyperglycemia.

Protein Requirements

Acutely ill patients almost always require higher protein intakes than do healthy, nonstressed individuals. The recommended daily allowance (RDA) for healthy adult persons is approximately 0.8 g/kg. Metabolically stressed patients often require a minimum of 1.2 g/kg and may require as high as 2.5 g/kg. Starting with a goal of 1.2–1.5 g/kg is prudent, adjusting as needed based on UUN results. If N_2 excretion exceeds the protein equivalent of around 2.5 g/kg, higher protein intakes will not likely promote N_2 retention, but will instead drive ureagenesis. Attempts to improve nitrogen balance by administration of anabolic steroids usually reveal only slight reductions in nitrogen loss, and appropriately controlled studies were unable to document significant effects on body weight and muscle strength.

Protein requirements can also be estimated by the percentage of total calorie intake. A healthy, nonstressed individual requires 10–12% of calories from protein, increasing up to 25% of calorie intake with physiologic stress. Put another way, the ratio of calories to nitrogen ($Cal:N_2$) suggested for mild stress is $150:1$ ($=16\%$ of calories), decreasing to $100:1$ ($=25\%$ of calories) for more severe stress.

Routes of Feeding

Oral

Patients with neurologic impairment, especially those in an NCCU, often cannot take oral nutrition because of depressed levels of conciousness, impaired swallowing function, or the use of mechanical ventilation. In the case where a patient is able to tolerate oral feeding, strict calorie counts should be obtained to assure adequate intake. If intake consistently falls below 50–75% of nutrient goals for 5–7 days, supplemental nutritional support should be initiated. The longer the deficits are allowed to persist, the longer the rehabilitation phase will be.

Enteral

The enteral route is preferred when the patient is unable to eat or takes insufficient quantities of food. Enteral nutrition has the advantages of utilizing the normal physiologic action of digestion and absorption and maintaining the integrity of the intestinal mucosa. There is a growing body of evidence pointing to the fact that disuse of the gastrointestinal tract may exacerbate the stress response by means of translocation of gut bacteria into the bloodstream, thereby increasing the secretion of catabolic hormones. Delaying enteral nutrition is associated with loss of GI mucosal mass, decreased tolerance to enteral feedings, and increased energy expenditure. Other advantages of enteral feeding over parenteral feeding are lower risk of sepsis, lower cost, and the ability to better stay within fluid allowances. Ideally, feeding should begin within the first 48h of injury. Once the choice has been made to feed a patient enterally, the site and route of nutrient delivery must be decided upon. The risk of aspiration and the anticipated length of time the patient will require tube feedings are pivotal.

If the patient has good bowel sounds and is not at high aspiration risk, nasogastric feeding can be used safely. Gastric residuals should be checked every 4h, holding the feeding if the residual is >1.5 times the infusion rate. The patient should also be monitored for abdominal distension, nausea, and/or vomiting. Generally, patients who do not have severe injuries can be fed with a nasogastric tube. Continuous infusion feeding with the use of gastric motility stimulants has been successful. Because of sedation with narcotics, the use of barbiturates, or prolonged post-injury ileus, some patients will not tolerate gastric feedings. In these cases, postpyloric feeding may be successful. These tubes can be placed at bedside by endoscopy.

Conventional wisdom has been that critically ill patients better tolerate feeding delivered via continuous pump-assisted infusion. This method is certainly required for intestinal feeding but has not been proven to reduce aspiration risk or minimize other gastrointestinal complications with gastric feeding. In spite of a lack of clear evidence against intermittent or bolus feedings, it still seems prudent to use continuous feeding in this patient population. Continuous feeding, however, has been reported to promote better glucose control, to lower carbon dioxide production, and to slightly reduce calorie requirements (due to less thermic effect of food). Bolus feedings are usually limited to the more stable, mobile patient.

Nasogastric or nasoduodenal/nasojejunal tubes are for short-term enteral nutrition. Patients who will require enteral feeding on a long-term basis should have a gastrostomy or gastrojejunostomy tube placed. The percutaneous endoscopic gastrostomy (PEG) tube has advantages over the surgical G-tubes, in that it does not require general anesthesia, is less costly, the feeding can be initiated in less than 24h after placement, and it can be placed at bedside, which is a major advantage in the intensive care unit.

Enteral Formula Selection

The development of commercial enteral formulas began in the 1960s. Over the past several years there has been a marked growth in the availability and variety of these formulas, with over 100 different formulas now on the market. Because of this, selection of the right formula can seem confusing. Appropriate formula choices need be based on only limited criteria, as many of the features promoted have minimal known physiologic value.

The first consideration should be caloric density. Caloric density determines the amount of calories, protein, and other nutrients delivered per liter. Most commercial formulas have a caloric density ranging from 1.0 to 2.0 cal/cc. For the majority of patients, a 1.0-cal/cc product is suggested, advancing to a rate that meets the patients estimated calorie needs. Patients requiring fluid restriction may need a formula providing 1.5–2.0 cal/cc. Fluid and electrolyte balance need to be closely monitored in patients receiving concentrated formulas to prevent severe dehydration. Next, the protein requirements of a patient must be considered. Formulas provide varying levels of protein/l and varying cal/N_2 ratios (see section on protein requirements).

The osmolality of the formula should not usually be a significant factor. As a general rule, gastric feeding can be initiated at full strength, regardless of the osmolality, unless there is delayed gastric emptying, the feeding is a transition from an extended course of NPO and parenteral nutrition, and/or the patient presents with severe protein-calorie malnutrition. In these cases, an isotonic formula is recommended initially. Post-pyloric feeding is best accomplished starting with isotonic strength, advancing to full strength as tolerated. It must be kept in mind that diluting formulas to 1/4 or 1/2 strength reduces the nutrient intake and may give a false sense that the patient's nutritional requirements are being met. Diluting some formulas to approximately 1/2 strength to achieve isotonicity should be done no longer than about 2 days. One-quarter strength dilution is never necessary. In all cases, feeding should be initiated at a low rate (20–30 ml/h), advancing slowly as tolerated to the goal infusion rate.

The large majority of patients in a neurologic ICU have a normally functioning gastrointestinal tract; therefore, the use of intact nutrient formulas is indicated for most patients who can tolerate enteral feedings. Hydrolyzed, "elemental" formulas are appropriate only when there is known impairment of digestion or absorption.

Complications of Enteral Feeding

Diarrhea

Diarrhea is a common problem in acutely ill patients and appears to be most often related to severity of illness and medications, rather than being a direct result of tube feeding. One of the most common causes of diarrhea is alteration of colonic flora by broad-spectrum antibiotics. Patients should be tested for infectious sources and the medication list reviewed. Administration of hyperosmolar oral electrolyte solutions may contribute to diarrhea. To minimize the possibility of tube-feeding-related diarrhea, feeding should be initiated at a low rate and advanced slowly as tolerated, especially after an extended NPO period. Antidiarrheals should be administered only after all known causes have been ruled out.

Gastric Retention and Pulmonary Aspiration

The primary concern with gastric retention of feedings is the risk of regurgitation and subsequent aspiration. Gastric emptying may be delayed with sepsis, severe head injury, peritonitis, pancreatitis, abdominal surgery, and protein-calorie malnutrition, and with the use of narcotics, sedatives, barbiturates, and gastric secretion blockers.

Gastric residuals should be checked every 4 h and the head of the bed should remain elevated 30–45°. Gastric motility stimulants should be tried first. If residuals remain high, either post-pyloric feeding or parenteral nutrition will be required.

Metabolic Complications

Hyperglycemia is a common problem in critically ill patients. Excessive calorie and carbohydrate intake may contribute to this. The feeding formula should be assessed for carbohydrate content, formulas being changed if intake is excessive. The patients caloric goal should also not be exceeded (see section on calorie requirements and serum glucose). Electrolyte abnormalities may also occur in patients receiving enteral feedings. Hypokalemia, hypophosphatemia, and hypomagnesemia may develop upon refeeding after a period of inadequate intake (see section on laboratory data).

Parenteral Nutrition

Parenteral nutrition (PN) or intravenous (i.v.) feeding may be indicated when a patient's gastrointestinal tract is unable to tolerate oral or enteral feeding for at least 5–7 days. In the NCCU, PN may be necessary for patients with prolonged ileus (commonly seen with severe head injury, barbiturate coma, or use of high-dose narcotics), or when access to the GI tract is unavailable after head or neck trauma. PN can be delivered through either a central or a peripheral vein. The length of time that the patient

is expected to receive PN and the nutrient requirements and fluid tolerances of the patient must be considered. Patients expected to receive PN for >7 days should receive central venous nutrition (CVN), whereas peripheral venous nutrition (PVN or PPN) is generally suggested for expected duration <7 days.

Central Venous Nutrition

To meet most patients' calorie and protein requirements without giving excess fluid volume, solutions must be given in a concentrated from. The hyperosmolar nature of these formulas (up to 1800 mOsm/kg water) is very irritating to the venous epithelium, so they must be infused into a central vein where they are rapidly diluted by high blood flow. Even with the most concentrated solutions, most patients will require at least 1.5 l fluid/day to meet total nutrient needs. Most institutions offer a variety of formulas providing varying concentrations of dextrose, protein (in the form of crystalline amino acids), and fat (as lipid emulsions). Lipid emulsions must be provided at least 2 times a week to prevent essential fatty acid (EFA) deficiency. Daily use of lipids, however, is more physiologic, lowers the osmolality of the solutions, may improve glucose control, and provides a major source of nonprotein calories. Lipid emulsions can be admixed with the dextrose and amino acids in 3-in-1 or total nutrient admixture (TNA) in a variety of concentrations, as long as certain guidelines are adhered to. Some institutions allow CVN to be individually tailored to a patient's specific nutrient needs, whereas others offer a "menu" of formula choices. Most often electrolytes, vitamin and mineral supplements, and some medications can be individualized. Standard parenteral vitamin and mineral preparations are usually provided.

Peripheral Venous Nutrition

For short-term PN, use of peripheral veins to administer solution is suggested. Even with a final dextrose concentration of 10%, the osmolality of these formulas is 900–1100 mOsm/kg water, resulting in fairly short periods of vein patency. To increase the calorie concentration, i.v. lipids must be infused daily to compensate for the dilute dextrose. Total volumes of 2.5–3.0 l or greater are usually required to meet a patient's calorie needs, and this exceeds the tolerance of some patients.

Complications of Parenteral Nutrition

Serious complications can usually be avoided by careful patient management and by observing general guidelines.

Metabolic

Hyperglycemia is common in critically ill patients. To minimize the effect of PN, start the solution at a low rate, advancing to the goal in 2–3 days. Insulin can be added to the solution and daily lipids should be used, unless contraindicated, to meet up to 60% of nonprotein calorie needs. Hypogly-

cemia may occur if PN is inadvertently interrupted or abruptly discontinued. This problem is unlikely to occur if the formula is tapered off slowly. It is also less likely to occur if insulin has been added to the solution.

Electrolyte abnormalities can occur, and requirements may change significantly from day to day, depending upon the patient's underlying illness and course of therapy. The electrolyte complications of refeeding may be more pronounced with the use of PN. Malnourished patients should be monitored very closely for hypophosphatemia, hypokalemia, and hypomagnesemia (see section on laboratory data). PN solutions should be adjusted daily according to laboratory data. If more urgent correction is needed, appropriate i.v. fluids can be administered via a peripheral vein.

Liver function abnormalities are fairly common in patients receiving PN. Mild to moderate elevations of alkaline phosphatase, AST, ALT, LDH, and bilirubin may be seen and are usually benign and self-limited. More pronounced elevations may signify another cause.

Infectious

Catheter sepsis is often a result of a break in the aseptic catheter care technique. This can usually be avoided if careful guidelines are adhered to. Triple-lumen catheters should be replaced 1–2 times a week using a sterile technique. Skin contaminants are the usual offending organisms, but gram-negative bacteria may also be a source in the hospitalized patient. Catheter sepsis usually requires removal of the catheter.

Technical

The most common technical complications are pneumothorax and hemothorax. These can usually be prevented with careful line insertion by an experienced physician.

Suggested Reading

Alpers DH, Clouse RE, Stenson WF (eds) (1983) Manual of nutritional therapuetics. Little Brown, Boston

Annis K, Ott L, Kearney PA (1991) Nutritional support of the severe head-injured patient. Nutr Clin Prac 6:245–250

Clifton GL, Robertson CS, Gross RG et al. (1984) The metabolic response to severe head injury. J Neurosurg 60:687–696

Dempsey DT, Guenter P, Mullen JL et al. (1985) Energy expenditure in acute trauma to the head with and without barbiturate coma. Surg Gynecol Obstet 160:128–134

Gadisseux P, Ward JD, Young HF et al. (1984) Nutrition and the neurosurgical patient. J Neurosurg 60:219–232

Kaufman HH, Rowlands BJ, Stein DK et al. (1985) General metabolism in patients with acute paraplegia and quadraplegia. Neurosurgery 16:309–313

Long CL, Schaffel N, Geiger JW et al. (1979) Metabolic response to injury and illness: estimation of protein and energy needs from indirect calorimetry and nitrogen balance. JPEN 3:452–456

Ott L, Young B (1991) Nutrition in the neurologically injured patient. Nutr Clin Prac 6:223–229

Rombeau JL, Caldwell MD (eds) (1986) Parenteral nutrition, vol 2. Saunders, Philadelphia

Rombeau JL, Caldwell MD (eds) (1990) Clinical nutrition, enteral and tube feedings, 2nd edn. Saunders, Philadelphia

Weinsier RL, Heimburger DC, Butterworth CE (eds) (1989) Handbook of clinical nutrition, 2nd edn. Mosby, St Louis

Young B, Ott L, Twyman D et al. (1987) The effect of nutritional support on outcome from severe head injury. J Neurosurg 67:668–676

Respiratory Management in Neurological Critical Care: Basics and Techniques of Artificial Ventilation

CECIL BOREL and JOSEF BRIEGEL

Introduction

Acute respiratory care, including management of mechanical ventilation, is the primary reason for the development of critical care units. Although the use of life-support machinery to maintain respiration crosses the boundaries of all intensive care units, the modalities of respiratory management have evolved in many specialty care units to meet the needs of specific diseases. An evolution and refinement of respiratory management has taken place in the neurologic critical care areas as well. Historically, the development of mechanical ventilation and respiratory care originated in the early neurointensive care units with the acute ventilatory management of neuromuscular diseases and the polio epidemics of the late 1940s and early 1950s. Neurointensive care units still manage patients with acute neuromuscular ventilatory failure, such as patients with Guillain-Barré syndrome and myasthenia gravis. However, the usefulness of respiratory supportive

care and ventilator management has been extended to virtually all of the acute life-threatening illnesses found in the neurologic critical care units today. Furthermore, advances in artificial airway management facilitated long-term mechanical ventilation in patients with chronic ventilatory failure such as neuromuscular diseases and restrictive chest wall. For selected patients intermittent and chronic mechanical ventilation at home has become a therapeutic advance and contributes to improved prognosis and quality of life.

This review focuses on the basics of respiratory care and ventilator management applied to patients commonly found in the neurointensive care unit. It also covers the selection of patients for long-term and at-home mechanical ventilation.

Pathophysiology

Respiratory failure is a major cause of death in patients with neurologic disorders ranging from cerebral injuries to myopathic disorders of respiratory

---

Section Editor: Daniel F. Hanley

Table 1. Ventilatory failure in neurointensive care

Pathophysiology	Underlying disorder	Assessment
Ventilatory drive ↓	Opioids, sedatives, relaxants Cerebral injuries Brain-stem disorders Hypercarbia Ondine's curse, brain death	Respiratory rate Blood gasses Pulse oximetry End-tidal CO_2
Ventilatory drive ↑	Muscle weakness, drug withdrawal, ARDS	$P\,0.1$
Upper airway obstruction	Neuromuscular diseases Vocal cord paresis Artificial airway obstruction	Laryngoscopy Flow-volume loop
Aspiration	Dysphagia Brain-stem disorders Artificial airway and supine position	Gag, swallow, cough reflex Chest X-ray CCT, NMR
Muscular failure Weakness Fatigue	Neuromuscular diseases Cervical spine injuries Intensive care polyneuropathy Sepsis, sepsis syndrome	Vt, FVC, Plmax, PEmax Respiratory rate $P\,0.1$ EMG high/low ratio Respiratory alternans Abdominal paradox
Work of breathing Lung compliance Chest-wall compl. Lower airway obstruction	Pneumonia, pulmonary edema, atelectasis Adult respiratory distress syndrome Neuromuscular diseases, paraplegia Chronic obstructive pulmonary diseases	Chest X-ray Pressure-volume integral Compliance calculations FEV1 indirect calorimetry

muscles (Table 1). Respiratory gas exchange hinges on the mechanics of ventilation, which in turn depend on pulmonary secretion clearance, a clear airway, effective ventilatory muscle activity, and adequate ventilatory drive. Regardless of the disease, patients with respiratory impairment predictably evolve from poor secretion clearance and inadequate airway protection to insufficient ventilatory muscle performance and decreased ventilatory drive. When respiratory impairment is acute, rapid assessment of essential respiratory functions such as airway patency, gas exchange, and cough assume the highest priority in patients with life-threatening neurologic illness. Initiation of therapy must always proceed rapidly when tissue oxygen delivery is threatened. Some interventions may be tailored to the specific nature of ventilatory compromise and may be successful in preventing evolution of ventilatory failure. Mechanical ventilatory support should be started whenever ventilation is insufficient for metabolic needs.

Airway

Patients presenting with serious cerebral injuries often require control of the upper airway as the initial therapeutic intervention. Secondary neurologic damage from cerebral anoxia or raised ICP can be minimized by preventing hypoxemia, hypercarbia, and acidosis, and by initiating hyperventilation early. A decreased level of consciousness (e.g., Glasgow Coma Score <9) is associated with a decreased ability to protect the upper airway and suggests that there may be additional potential benefit from mechanical hyperventilation to control raised ICP. Airway management should be considered for any patient, regardless of the disease process, who does not open his eyes to voice and who postures to pain. Cerebral injuries with brainstem involvement impair airway reflexes, coughing, and ventilatory drive. When cervical spine injury is present, ventilatory muscle dysfunction adds the risk of hypoventilation. Aspiration of gastric contents is a constant risk in all patients with deteriorating neurologic status.

When airway muscles are weakened, recurrent and "silent" aspiration and upper airway obstruction become major forms of morbidity. Airway muscles include those of the tongue, jaw, pharynx, glottis, and larynx. These muscles may be affected by any disease process that effects respiratory muscles, such as acute polyneuropathies, neuromuscular junction disorders, and myopathies. The ninth, tenth, and twelfth cranial nerves supply most of the motor innervation to the airway, while sensory stimuli are mediated though the ninth and tenth cranial nerves. A unilateral lesion of the vagus nerve leads to difficulty in coughing, clearing the voice, and swallowing. Bilateral lesions of the vagus nerves result in difficulty swallowing, regurgitation of food, and positional airway obstruction. Injury to one of the recurrent laryngeal nerves of the vagus causes vocal cord paresis and results in hoarseness; bilateral injury produces stridor. The glossopharyngeal and vagus nerves supply the afferent fibers of touch and pain senses to the mucosa of the posterior part of the soft palate, pharynx, larynx, and trachea. The gag reflex results in constriction and elevation of the pharynx, and is mediated by the sensory fibers of the glossopharyngeal nerve synapsing in the nucleus ambiguous, which sends efferent fibers to the striated muscles of the pharynx. Loss of the gag reflex due to decreased sensation in the pharynx leads to recurrent aspiration of pharyngeal contents.

Breathing

Ventilation depends entirely on the stimulation of respiratory muscles by the central nervous system. Chemoreceptors and mechanoreceptors convey information to the brain stem and spinal cord regarding carbon dioxide and oxygen tension and the expansion of the lung. The brain stem respiratory centers are located in the medulla. The duration of inspiration and expiration is controlled by two medullary centers. They integrate input from the cerebral cortex, reticular formation, and the spinal cord to modify automatic ventilatory rhythm. When the need for ventilation increases, the tidal volume rises first, followed by an increase in respiratory rate. When respiratory rate increases, the time between breaths (expiratory time) shortens more than the inspiratory time, increasing the relative proportion of time spent in inspiration (Ti/Ttot ↑). Control of inspiratory time, expiratory time, and tidal volume allows fine tuning of mechanical performance to maintain minute ventilation at the lowest possible work of breathing.

Ventilation requires muscle activity for inspiration. Negative intrathoracic pressure (relative to atmospheric pressure) is generated mainly by the contraction of diaphragm and intercostal muscles. Expiration is independent of muscle contraction because expiratory forces are generated from the elastic recoil of the lung tissue itself and from the thin film of surfactant that lines the alveolar units. After forced inspiration the elastic recoil of the chest wall also contributes to expiration. Gas exchange, particularly excretion of CO_2, is dependent on alveolar air flow which is a function of both minute ventilation and the dead-space-to-tidal-volume ratio. Dead space is the portion of tidal volume necessary to fill the parts of the respiratory system not participating in gas exchange, and is a fixed volume. As tidal volume decreases during ventilatory failure, the proportion of dead space increases relative to the decreasing alveolar ventilation, limiting the ability to excrete CO_2.

When inspiratory effort is compromised the initial result is an insidious loss of ability to increase minute ventilation at times of increased demand. Sepsis, fever, starvation-refeeding, and increased alveolar dead space all demand an increase in minute ventilation. As demands are increased, partially weakened inspiratory musculature begins to fatigue as a consequence of overuse, leading to further exacerbation of ventilatory insufficiency. A sustained decrease in the high/low-frequency ratios of a diaphragmatic electromyogram denotes the development of muscle fatigue. Tachypnea is usually the first clinical response to unfulfilled ventilatory demand. Unfortunately, tachypnea increases the proportion of dead space ventilation to tidal volume and the

relative amount of time spent in inspiration. Since diaphragmatic nutrient blood flow occurs in expiration, increasing the time spent in inspiration may exacerbate the fatigue of compromised inspiratory musculature. Patients sometimes rest fatiguing inspiratory musculature by alternating patterns of breathing between weakened and accessory groups (respiratory alternans), even at the expense of decreased tidal volume and CO_2 clearance. The loss of diaphragmatic strength and efficiency results in a paradoxical inward motion of the abdomen in inspiration. Finally the patient's ability to excrete carbon dioxide will be lost.

Though expiration is a passive process resulting from the elastic recoil of the stretched lungs and chest wall to expel air, active forced exhalation is crucial to clearing secretions and foreign objects from the respiratory tract. Weakening the muscles of forced exhalation results in an impaired ability to cough. When cough is impaired, secretions accumulate in the most dependent portion of the lung, leading to collapse of alveoli, subsegments, and even entire lobes. Collapsed segments are not ventilated. Hypoxic pulmonary vasoconstriction may decrease perfusion to the unventilated segments, but this compensation is incomplete. Oxygen in unventilated alveoli is absorbed quickly, so that further perfusion of blood through these regions cannot load oxygen. The result is dilution of oxygenated blood from ventilated alveoli with blood from collapsed alveoli low in oxygen. The dilution process lowers the total oxygen content of arterial blood and is described as the process of intrapulmonary shunt. Alveolar collapse may progress to hypoxemia and death. Retained airway secretions are fertile media for bacterial colonization and pneumonia. Infection leads to further alveolar congestion, shunting, and hypoxemia. The decreased ability to cough has profound implications for recovery from ventilatory failure.

Assessment

Ventilatory failure is the inability to maintain minute ventilation, oxygenation, or airway integrity. Patients who meet criteria for ventilatory failure should be transferred to a critical care unit, undergo endotracheal intubation, and begin mechanical ventilation. When ventilatory insufficiency evolves more slowly, admission to a closely monitored area and initiation of other forms of medical therapy may suffice.

Airway

Airway integrity depends on the level of consciousness and the gag, swallow, and cough reflexes. The level of consciousness is assessed using the Glasgow Coma Score; a GCS < 9 predicts the need for intubation. The gag reflex is assessed by stimulating the pharynx with a cotton-tipped applicator and observing the elevation of the uvula in response. The swallow reflex is induced by application of 20 ml of water into the pharynx. Cough is stimulated by the passage of a suction catheter via the nasopharynx through the vocal cords. Whenever the gag, swallow, or cough reflexes are diminished, related to either level of consciousness or decreased reflex responsiveness, maintaining a competent airway is at risk. The inability to maintain airway integrity leads to airway obstruction, or to aspiration of pharyngeal or gastric contents.

Breathing

Paradoxical movement of the abdomen and rib cage, use of the accessory muscles of ventilation, and an increase in the respiratory rate portend ventilatory failure due to respiratory muscle weakness. Bedside spirometry measures respiratory volumes and pressures and provides indirect measurements of respiratory muscle strength. Tidal volume (Vt), forced vital capacity (FVC), inspiratory force (PImax), and expiratory force (PEmax) are among the values obtained. A forced vital capacity of 10–15 ml/kg, or an inspiratory force or expiratory force of greater than 25 cm H_2O generally correlates with adequate ventilatory strength. Daily measurements are used to track changes in respiratory muscle function.

The inability to oxygenate is an early manifestation of compromised gas exchange. Arterial blood gasses and pulse oximetry offer a means of monitoring oxygenation, and are important assessments when ventilatory function is compromised. Chest X-ray reveals the presence of atelectasis or infiltrate which may worsen hypoxemia. Neurologic manifestations of hypoxemia are late indicators of ventilatory insufficiency.

Ventilatory drive must be assessed in all patients requiring mechanical ventilation. Insensitivity to rising PCO_2 or falling PO_2 makes weaning from mechanical ventilation difficult and dangerous. Altered ventilatory drive responses do not always correlate with sedative administration, alkalosis, or duration of controlled ventilation. The simplest technique for assessing drive is to observe the rate and tidal volume response to stopping mechanical ventilation while monitoring oxygen saturation and end-tidal CO_2. Airway occlusion for 100 ms ($P_{0.1}$) has also been used to measure central ventilatory output.

Management

Acute Airway Management

Airway management for patients in neurologic critical care units is often complicated by underlying diseases. Airway management and intubation should be attempted only by the most skilled and experienced individuals. Endotracheal intubation should be performed expeditiously, with awareness of the potential for increasing neurologic injury during the intubation procedure. No technique is free of risk. Laryngoscopy, hypoventilation, struggling, and the use of succinylcholine without defasciculation have been shown to raise ICP. Inadequate control of hemodynamic responses to laryngoscopy and intubation may result in bleeding from intracranial vascular abnormalities. Cervical spine injury can be exacerbated by moving the neck to facilitate visualization of vocal cords. The ever-present risk of aspiration of gastric contents requires support of airway reflexes and the prevention of passive regurgitation at all times during intubation. Depolarizing

Table 2. Nondepolarizing muscle relaxants (adapted from Miller and Savarese (1990))

Drug	Potency factor	Intubation
Pancuronium	1	0.06–0.08
Metocurine	4	0.3–0.4
d-Tubocurarine	7	0.5–0.6
Gallamine	40	3.0–4.0
Alcuronium	3	0.3
Fazadinium	20	1.5
Atracurium	4	0.4–0.5
Vecuronium	0.9	0.07–0.10
Mivacurium	1.6	0.18
Pipecuronium	0.9	0.10
Doxacurium	0.4	0.06

Dosages are in mg/kg.

relaxants used for endotracheal intubation, such as succinylcholine, may cause pathologic muscle contracture and lethal hyperkalemia in patients with neuropathic muscle denervation. The intensity and duration of nondepolarizing relaxants used for intubation, (Table 2), such as pancuronium, is enhanced in patients with abnormalities of the neuromuscular junction, particularly myasthenia gravis. In patients with malignant hyperthermia and other congenital myopathies, abnormal contracture of facial and respiratory musculature in response to depolarizing agents may make orotracheal intubation impossible, impair mechanical ventilatory efforts, and trigger a hyperthermic reaction.

Long-term Airway Management

The indications for tracheostomy vary and the appropriate duration of endotracheal intubation has not been defined. Major risks of long-term endotracheal intubation are laryngotracheal injuries, nosocomial infections, and recurrent aspiration of gastric contents to the lower airways. The risk of severe tracheal injuries such as tracheal stenosis and tracheomalacia has been markedly reduced using tubes made of soft materials with high-volume/low-pressure cuffs and pressure equilibration. The topical application of gentamicin and polymyxin B sufficiently prevents the bacterial colonization of the oropharynx and stomach and decreases the risk of nosocomial pneumonia. Changing the body position from supine to semirecumbent is a simple prophylactic measure which markedly reduces the aspiration of gastric contents.

We prefer to proceed to tracheostomy when we believe the patient will need mechanical ventilation or airway protection for more than 14–30 days. Tracheostomy offers advantages in allowing easier pulmonary toilet, negative pressure ventilation, and avoidance of the risks of long-term endotracheal intubation. Cuffed tracheostomy tubes are used to reduce aspiration. Uncuffed tubes are adequate for patients with sufficient airway reflexes to manage oral fluids, who require long-term secretion management or negative-pressure ventilation.

The ability to protect upper airways and to fulfill ventilatory demands is required before removing the artificial airway. Artificial airway devices should be removed in a controlled environment. Endotracheal tubes are removed by personnel experienced in intubation. The trachea and pharynx are suctioned. Then the cuff is deflated. Following a deep breath, the tube is quickly removed and the patient is encouraged to cough. We use a similar process to remove cuffed tracheos-

tomy tubes. The risks of removal of these devices include aspiration, laryngospasm, and tracheal collapse secondary to tracheomalacia.

Physical Therapy

In ventilated patients secretion management requires airway suctioning, coughing, and deep breathing. Frequent changing of the body position contributes markedly to mobilization and expectoration of pulmonary secretions. The use of mucolytics is still a subject of controversy for mechanically ventilated patients. Tracheal lavage with either saline, diluted mucolytics, or bicarbonate is useful if secretions are tenacious. Atelectasis is usually treated by positioning, percussion, and positive-pressure breathing. Atelactasis resistant to physiotherapy requires bronchoscopic guided reinflation.

After disconnection of mechanical ventilation, sustained maximal inspiration maneuvers with incentive spirometers sufficiently ventilate dependent parts of the lungs and prevent atelectasis formation. In patients with muscle weakness who appear to need prolonged pulmonary toilet, prophylactic percussion and intermittent positive-pressure breathing (IPPB) are useful. Two or three percussions daily may be effective in clearing secretions from infiltrates. Postural percussion and drainage of dependent lobes is reserved for patients with infiltrates or atelectasis who lack adequate ability to cough.

Mechanical Ventilation

Modern ventilators incorporate micro-processor technology to offer different modes of mechanical ventilation. This new technology has markedly improved patients' ventilatory security due to meticulous monitoring of breathing parameters (i.e., minute volume, breathing frequency and airway pressures), limiting peak inspiratory pressure (<40 cm H_2O), and apneic ventilation modes. Synchronization of spontaneous breathing and mechanical support has contributed to patient comfort during the weaning period as well as during long-term mechanical ventilation.

All modes of mechanical ventilation may operate in an assisted or controlled fashion. The utility of these various modes is based on the particular need of the patient. Controlled modes imply that the breathing frequency of the ventilator is set to a value determined by the physician. In assisted modes the frequency of breathing is determined by the patient.

Pressure-cycled ventilatory modes are set to a target inspiratory airway pressure and continue air flow until the predetermined inspiratory pressure is achieved. This target pressure is usually added to the end-expiratory pressure (PEEP), so that the final airway pressure will equal inspiratory pressure plus PEEP. The tidal volume that is delivered by a pressure-cycled ventilator depends on the inspiratory pressure as well as on the compliance of the entire respiratory system. Sudden changes in compliance due to pulmonary edema, secretions, or even kinking of the endotracheal tube may dramatically decrease the delivered tidal volume.

Pressure-controlled ventilation (PCV) offers the advantage of adjusting peak airway pressure to peak alveolar pressure, thereby reducing the risk of barotrauma such as pneumothorax or pulmonary interstitial emphysema. The tidal volume is delivered with a decelerating flow pattern, which provides a better gas distribution within the alveolar units than constant flow patterns. This reduces alveolar dead space and the required alveolar ventilation compared with volume cycled modes (see Fig. 1). The same tidal volume is achieved by lower transpulmonary pressures. Some ventilators generate initial peak flow rates which exceed physiological flow rates and may damage lung tissue by generating shear forces in the airways.

For pressure-assisted modes, such as pressure-support ventilation (PSV), the delivered tidal volume also depends on the patient's inspiratory effort. The final tidal volume for each breath will depend on the inspiratory pressure delivered by the ventilator and the inspiratory effort expended by the patient during the breath. The minute ventilation during PSV will depend on the inspiratory pressure set on the ventilator, the additional inspiratory effort from the patient, and the frequency of breathing determined by the patient. Due to the low impedance of the trigger mechanism in modern ventilators, PSV does not interfere with diaphragm movements. Because the contraction of the diaphragm shifts ventilation towards the lung bases, PSV contributes to a more uniform intrapulmonary gas distribution and improved gas exchange.

The main problem with this ventilation mode is the correct titration of pressure support depending on the

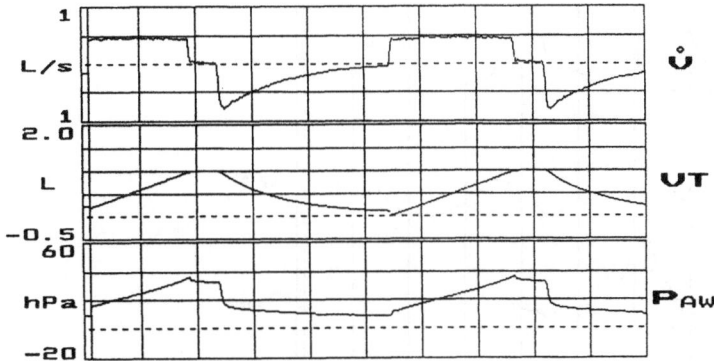

Fig. 1. Control mode ventilation

patient's particular need. We titrate pressure support starting from 5 cm H_2O until the abdominal paradox and the use of accessory inspiratory muscles are excluded. This procedure is repeated twice a day with the goal of reducing pressure support. Prior to extubation we maintain a pressure support of 5–10 cm H_2O to overcome system-derived inspiratory impedance.

Volume-cycled ventilatory modes are set to deliver a predetermined tidal volume independent (within limits) of the pressure necessary to deliver the breath. Volume-cycled ventilatory modes will reliably deliver minute ventilation in spite of changes in lung compliance. However, if peak inspiratory pressure exceeds the preset pressure limitation the delivered tidal and minute volume will decrease. If a patient is to do any of his own breathing work, it must be independent of the volume-cycled breath provided by the ventilator. Volume-cycled breaths perform all of the work of breathing.

Controlled-mode ventilation (CMV) (Fig. 1) delivers a preset tidal volume at a preset frequency and is suitable for patients who are apneic due to brain injury, paralysis, or drugs.

Assist-control-mode ventilation (AMV or SCMV) allows the patient to trigger the ventilator to deliver a volume-cycled tidal volume. The preset breathing frequency guarantees the minimum minute volume. Since no breathing effort is necessary in the AC mode, less muscular work is performed during inspiration. The AC mode qualifies as an "assisted" mode of ventilation because the patient determines the frequency of breathing. Intermittent mandatory ventilation (IMV) is a mode of volume-cycled controlled ventilation that allows the patient to breath independently of machine support between volume-cycled breaths. SIMV allows synchronization of the IMV breath to coincide with one of the patient's spontaneous breathing efforts (Fig. 2). Although the effort to trigger the machine requires a small amount of inspiratory muscle work, the breath itself is delivered without further patient effort. Unlike PSV, the delivered tidal volume in the AMV and IMV modes does not depend on patient effort. The pitfall of assisted-volume-cycled modes is an inappropriately low peak inspiratory flow despite the patient's

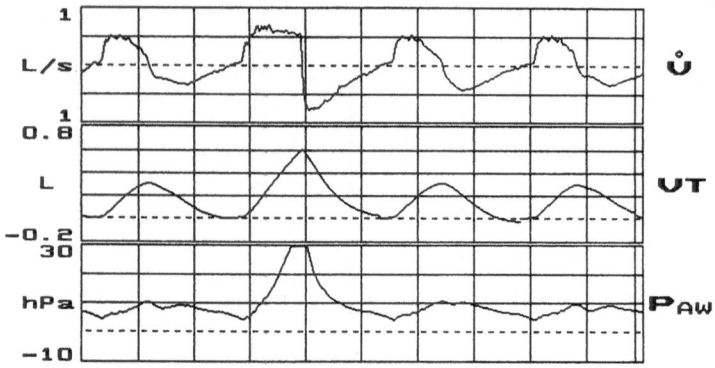

Fig. 2. Synchronous intermittent mandatory ventilation

need. This results in negative airway pressures, worsens the gas exchange, and contributes to atelectasis formation.

Weaning from Mechanical Ventilation

We use both PSV and SIMV modes to wean from mechanical ventilation. Weaning failures are usually related to muscle weakness and fatigue, and not to method of support. Consequently, we withdraw ventilatory support in either mode in proportion to the return of ventilatory performance. The patient is rested if clinical signs of fatigue or CO_2 retention are encountered.

In patients with an intact ventilatory drive, we prefer the PSV of mechanical ventilation (Figs 3 and 4). We adjust ventilatory assistance to an inspiratory pressure until the abdominal paradox and the use of accessory inspiratory muscles are excluded. Increasing pressure support can be used to ease tachypnea, increase tidal volume, and reduce the resistance of the airway circuit to the patient. In practice, we titrate pressure support

starting from 5 cm H_2O to 25 cm H_2O to achieve a respiratory rate of less than 25 breaths/min and a tidal volume of greater than 5 ml/kg. We usually add 5–8 cm H_2O of PEEP to facilitate trigger efforts and to prevent atelectasis. The triggering pressure for assisted breaths should be easily attained, ranging between 1 and 2 cm H_2O. Once the patient is stable on the above regimen, we wean by reducing the pressure support to 2–5 cm H_2O and observing respiratory rate and tidal volume response. We follow the same parameters to assess the need for rest periods. Pressure support is raised 2–10 mmHg to allow rest and encourage sleep. Atelectasis is treated by a combination of chest PT, increased PEEP, and increased pressure support. When a pressure support of 5 cm H_2O is tolerated well, the patient no longer needs ventilatory assistance. Arterial blood gasses are monitored as needed. If arterial access is limited, pulse oximetry and end-tidal CO_2 monitors usually suffice. We have found that this method of weaning is quite comfortable for patients. It allows for inspiratory muscle training continuously by encouraging inspira-

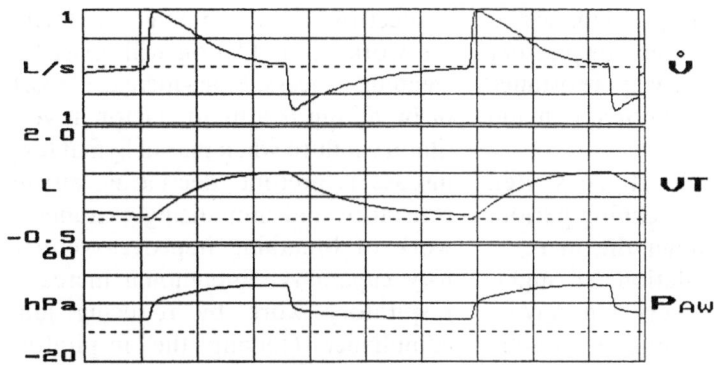

Fig. 3. Pressure-controlled ventilation

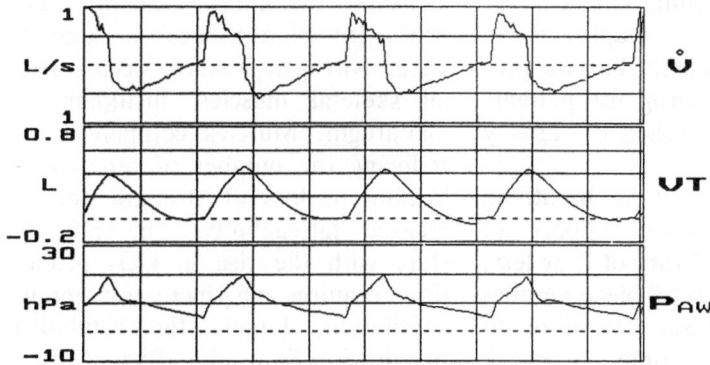

Fig. 4. Pressure-support ventilation

tory muscle effort. The major problems with this method are the correct titration of pressure support depending on the patient's particular need, the inability to trigger breaths due to weakness, changes in lung compliance, and ventilatory drive dysfunction.

Intermittent mandatory ventilation is an important mode of mechanical ventilation and may be used in conjunction with pressure-support ventilation. Patients who lack sufficient ventilatory drive need this mode of mechanical ventilatory support to prevent hypercarbia. We wean from IMV by gradually decreasing the daytime rate and allowing nocturnal rest.

Normocarbia is maintained. End-expiratory pressure is generally set at 5 cm H_2O and adjusted as clinically indicated by degree of atelectasis, shunting, or arterial hypoxemia. Pressure support may be added to overcome the resistance of the airway circuit during spontaneous breathing. We generally wean the IMV rate to less than 4 breaths/min before weaning pressure support. IMV weaning suffers from two disadvantages. Patients may "buck" the volume-cycled breaths, raising peak airway pressures and risking barotrauma and patient discomfort, or the unassisted breaths may be inefficient and rapidly lead to ventilatory muscle fatigue. Unassisted breaths require a high inspiratory force to overcome airway resistance and trigger the ventilator's demand valve.

Ventilatory muscle fatigue is often a problem during the weaning period. Nocturnal rest, through the increase of mechanical ventilation at night, allows sleep and recovery and may be used throughout weaning. Diaphragmatic and accessory muscle training with appropriate rest periods are also helpful in increasing respiratory muscle strength. Aminophylline has been reported to increase diaphragmatic strength and endurance, but we presently reserve this drug for patients with concurrent reactive airway problems.

When the patient is breathing easily on a pressure support of 5 mmHg or an IMV rate of 2 or less, we attempt a trial of T-piece ventilation. Various indexes are used to predict weaning outcome. A PEEP value of 2.5–7.5 cm H_2O may be added to maintain expiratory lung volumes and prevent atelectasis. Respiratory rate and clinical signs of respiratory distress are used as indicators of success or failure. Arterial blood gas measurements or pulse oximetry and end-tidal CO_2 are monitored. We generally monitor long-term ventilatory failure patients for signs of respiratory distress for at least 24 h after the discontinuation of mechanical ventilation.

Medical Management

Medical management involves treatment of underlying lung pathology, infection, malnutrition, and correction of electrolyte abnormalities. Reducing the work of ventilation will assist the weaning process. Since increased work of breathing is a major factor in ventilatory failure when parenchymal lung disease is present, decreasing airway resistance and minimizing extraneous work of breathing improves ventilatory capability. Pneumonia increases respiratory work by reducing lung compliance (forcing the inspiratory muscles to develop more force to generate the same tidal volume).

The treatment of any infection will assist the weaning process in several ways. Infection induces a catabolic state. Nitrogen wasting occurs from all skeletal muscles, including the diaphragm. Muscles compensate by reducing the number of sarcomeres, leading to loss of strength and increased fatiguability. The catabolic state with the rise in CO_2 production requires an increased minute ventilation. Finally the catabolism of infection limits the efficient use of nutrients.

Nutritional support is important in maintaining muscle strength and structure. The changes described in muscle during infection also occur during starvation. Autopsy studies show a reduction in diaphragmatic mass which correlates with body weight. Maintaining adequate nitrogen intake will correct and reverse this process. Routine measurements of 24-h urinary nitrogen excretion are useful in adjusting protein intake to account for nitrogen utilization. Both commercial and modular enteral feeding preparations will achieve a positive nitrogen balance. If enteral delivery of protein is not tolerated or is insufficient, we use parenteral nutrition to satisfy nutrient requirements.

Electrolyte imbalance and deficiency states can also contribute to muscle weakness and weaning difficulties. Hypophosphatemia is a common problem in nutritionally depleted patients and a well-documented cause of reversible muscle weakness. Hypomagnesemia has also been reported to cause mild respiratory weakness. Although iron and potassium depletion have not been reported to cause diaphragmatic weakness, they have been reported to cause limb muscle weakness. Routine monitoring and supplementation will avoid these problems.

We attempt to augment normal ventilatory drive. Sedatives and narcotics are decreased as much as possible. Abnormalities of blood pH are corrected, especially metabolic alkalosis, because the compensatory respiratory acidosis is achieved by hypoventilation. We correct metabolic alkalosis by replacing chloride and removing bicarbonate and acetate from intravenous and nutritional fluids. If this is unsuccessful, volume expansion with chloride and diuresis with acetazolamide are used to induce mild metabolic acidosis. In order to avoid compensation for either hyper- or hypocarbia, normocapnia is maintained by appropriate minute ventilation.

Chronic Ventilatory Failure and Out Hospital Chronic Ventilation

Much of the clinical experience gained during the poliomyelitis era provided the historical basis for long-term mechanical ventilation. Mechanical ventilation soon became a therapeutic alternative in conditions with chronic ventilatory failure other than poliomyelitis, i.e., tetraplegia due to high cervical spinal cord injuries and neuromuscular disorders. At-home chronic ventilation was the natural consequence. During the past 2 decades respiratory muscle weakness has been recognized as playing an essential pathophysiologic role in both acute and chronic respiratory failure. Based on the hypothesis that the rest of the respiratory muscles would improve their strength and endurance, intermittent mechanical ventilation became a new concept in the treatment of neuromuscular disorders. This approach, initially provided by cuirass or by positive-pressure ventilation via tracheostomy, was made easier by new medical practices and devices: Portable ventilators, easy to handle and with integrated oxygen concentrators, have been designed and constructed for home care. The custom-made nasal masks has reduced the complications of the artifical airway and has proved to be an efficient, safe, and well-accepted method for intermittent nocturnal mechanical ventilation. Despite these medical and technical improvements, physicians and patients are faced with a lack of public health care services providing comprehensive surveillance of at-home chronic ventilation. In various countries of the western world efforts have been made to develop home care programs, which presently are best realized in France.

Chronic Ventilatory Failure in Neurologic Disorders (Fig. 5)

In principle, chronic ventilatory failure results from disorders of automatic re-

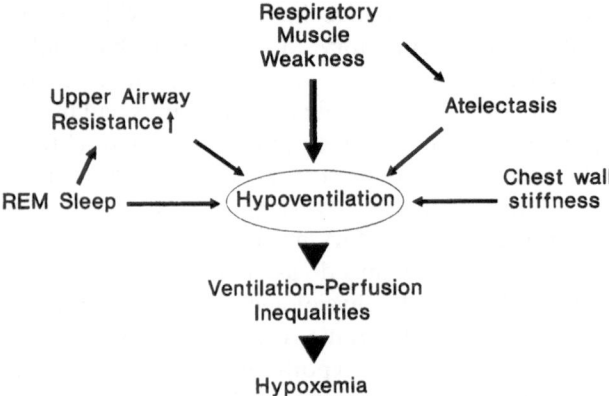

Fig. 5. Factors contributing to respiratory failure in neuromuscular disorders

spiratory control mechanisms and from muscular weakness. Depending on the location, spinal cord disorders involve different pathways, i.e., complete loss of respiratory control or loss of muscular function. Patients who suffer from neuromuscular diseases develop progressive ventilatory pump dysfunction due mainly to muscular weakness. Usually, weakness of respiratory muscles becomes evident during the later stages of a well-diagnosed disease. In some cases, however, respiratory muscle may already be involved in the absence of any other symptom or dyspnea. The long-standing weakness of respiratory muscles lead to a loss of lung volume that will be enhanced by a generalized decrease in the elastic properties of the lung. The reduced lung compliance and the accompanying chest wall stiffness increase the work of breathing. However, a stiff rib cage may also stabilize the intrathoracic volume, thereby preventing loss of lung volume and paradoxical thoracic inward movement during inspiration. Therefore, the net effect of chest wall stiffness in chronic respiratory pump failure is not

yet clear; it may also be beneficial. It was also hypothesized that the loss of the elastic properties of the lung and chest wall stiffness, combined with an impaired clearance of bronchial secretions, contributes to atelectasis formation, enhancing ventilatory disturbances.

All these factors, with respiratory muscle weakness predominating, result in alveolar hypoventilation. Depending on the functional integrity of hypoxic pulmonary vasoconstriction, hypoventilation induces ventilation-perfusion inhomogeneities resulting in hypoxemia (Fig. 4). If chronic hypoventilation persists over years, fixed pulmonary hypertension may develop, worsening the cardiorespiratory function. Despite severe hypoventilation patients have usually little or no feeling of dyspnea. It is not yet clear whether this results from blunting of peripheral and central respiratory chemoreceptor response, or whether it is an integrative central nervous mechanism of optimizing the pattern of breathing to prevent muscular fatigue. During REM sleep hypoventilation may be enhanced by increased resistance and intermittent obstruction of the upper airways and by depressed central respiratory drive. Episodes of severe oxygen desaturation in response to nocturnal hypoventilation are a regular consequence. Since the protective function of the upper airways may be compromised during sleep, patients are usually rehospitalized for acute respiratory failure due to aspiration and respiratory infection. Generally, they can be successfully treated and disconnected from mechanical ventilation. However, earlier diagnosis of progressive ventilatory failure is desirable. The therapeutic goal is either to select the patients for specific training programs of respiratory muscles (i.e., in cervical cord injuries) or to consider them for intermittent positive-pressure ventilation at home.

Selection of Patients for Out-Hospital Chronic Ventilation

Restless sleep, early morning headaches, and drowsiness are the first symptoms of chronic ventilatory failure due to nocturnal hypoventilation. This may result either from sleep apnea or from respiratory muscle weakness. Commonly, the diaphragm, the most powerful inspiratory pressure generator, is already affected in this early stage. Typical clinical signs of diaphragmatic weakness are the dissociation of lower rib cage and abdomen motions, and the paradoxical inward movement of the abdomen on inspiration or sniff. If diaphragm weakness is less severe and other respiratory muscles are affected, these signs may be absent. Thus daytime blood gas tensions may be normal in mild neuro-

muscular disorders. However, hypercarbia, indicating chronic alveolar hypoventilation, correlates well with nocturnal hypoxemia. Serial vital capacity measurements give more details on the progression of the ventilatory failure. Vital capacity measurement in the upright and supine positions provides information on respiratory muscle strength and lung function. The drop in vital capacity from the upright to the supine position closely indicates diaphragm weakness. Division of vital capacity into its two components, inspiratory capacity and expiratory reserve volume, provides information on both inspiratory and expiratory muscle strength. Expiratory reserve volume is usually decreased in neuromuscular disorders, indicating weak expiratory muscles. This is of crucial importance, since coughing and clearance of bronchial secretions may be compromised. Forced expiratory volume in 1s in relation to vital capacity provides information on accompanying air-flow limitation contributing to the reduction of vital capacity and worsening respiratory function. Serial estimation of maximal inspiratory and expiratory pressures may also be useful in indicating the progression of inspiratory and expiratory muscular weakness. Control sleep studies give more details on nocturnal breathing pattern and are essential for detecting intermittent upper airway obstruction and nocturnal hypoxemia.

In chronic ventilatory failure due to muscular weakness early intermittent ventilatory support is recommended. Mechanical ventilation should be instituted if vital capacity falls below 13–15 ml/kg body weight, daytime blood gas tensions worsen

($PaCO_2 > 45\,mmHg$), and maximal inspiratory pressure is less than 30 mmHg. During the initial period of mechanical ventilation, arterial oxygen saturation and carbon dioxide tension (transcutaneous or end-tidal) should be closely monitored to guarantee adequate ventilation and rapid response to any complications. The ideal type of ventilatory assistance depends on the underlying disease. In neuromuscular disorders intermittent positive-pressure ventilation through a custom-made nasal mask seems to be the treatment of choice. This noninvasive approach allows early support in chronic ventilatory failure, is well accepted, and is a suitable method for home care. Intermittent negative-pressure ventilation using cuirass or jackets is also utilized in many countries. In contrast to nasal positive-pressure ventilation, this mode may be complicated by upper airway obstruction during REM sleep and higher frequency of aspiration and bronchopulmonary infections. Patients with any loss of reflex airway control should be ventilated through a tracheostomy. If uncuffed tracheostomy tubes are used, inadequate ventilation may occur during sleep due to increased leakage around the tracheal cannula. This may be avoided by cuffed tracheal cannula or by pressure-control ventilation which compensates for air leaks. If these patients are designated for at-home mechanical ventilation, close surveillance and back-up equipment have to be provided by home care organizations.

Neurogenic Pulmonary Edema

Pathophysiology

Neurogenic pulmonary edema (NPE) is a clinical entity that follows serious central nervous system insults, such as head trauma, subarachnoid or intracerebral hemorrhage, lesions of the hypothalamus and the medulla, or other causes of increased intracranial pressure. NPE may also account for sudden unexpected death in persons with epilepsy, as a single cause or combined with cardiac arrhythmia. Patients who require massive doses of narcotics may also develop NPE. The precise pathogenetic mechanism of NPE is still a matter of controversy. In animal models injuries of the central nervous system, particularly lesions of the medulla, the mesencephalon, and increased intracranial pressure, result in pulmonary edema, whereas sectioning of the cervical cord prevents it. A combination of a high-pressure and capillary leak edema may be responsible for the development of NPE. The pronounced autonomic sympathetic activity following central nervous injuries dramatically increases pulmonary hydrostatic microvascular pressure transients, thereby increasing fluid filtration and protein permeability. Depending on the capacity of the lymphatic flow, extravascular lung water increases, leading finally to alveolar edema. With large increases of pulmonary vascular pressures, focal endothelial injury may occur, increasing the protein permeability ("blast effect").

Recent experimental and clinical data suggest that a neurogenic increase in permeability may be the pivotal step in the development of NPE. Increased permeability is presumably induced by the release of vasoactive peptides from the nerve endings. Serial quantification of bronchoalveolar protein content and extravascular lung water in NPE revealed that increased permeability persists even in the absence of hydrostatic vascular disorders.

Diagnosis and Treatment

The incidence of NPE is probably much higher than reported. The diagnosis is a matter of awareness and exclusion. NPE may be present in patients with a history of cerebral insult and initial radiographic findings of pulmonary edema of any type. Differential diagnosis includes cardiogenic pulmonary edema, pulmonary edema due to systemic inflammatory response syndrome, and direct lung injury such as aspiration and toxic inhalation.

The initial therapeutic approach includes mechanical ventilation with controlled hyperventilation ($PaCO_2$ 30–35 mmHg) and low positive end-expiratory pressure (5 cm H_2O). The inspiratory oxygen fraction should be adjusted to maintain adequate oxygenation (PaO_2 90–100 mmHg). Pulmonary artery catheterization should be performed with the therapeutic goal of minimizing hydrostatic pulmonary vascular pressures. This will be achieved by decreasing pulmonary and peripheral vascular resistance, inotropic support, and mild reduction of the circulating blood volume. Dobutamine and furosemide are the drugs of choice.

Summary

In ventilatory failure, airway integrity is lost and secretions pool. Further weakness causes loss of ventilatory strength and, finally, abnormalities of central ventilatory drive. Patients who meet criteria for ventilatory failure are transferred to our critical care unit, intubated, and mechanically ventilated. In weaning we first try to optimize drive and the recovery of muscular strength by paying meticulous attention to nutrition, sedation, parenchymal disease, and electrolytes. Muscular retraining is encouraged by a gradual withdrawal of ventilatory support (and exercise in appropriate cases), while avoiding fatigue. Appropriate mechanical ventilation is established and withdrawn as respiratory muscle function improves. Finally, airway support is withdrawn as airway integrity improves and secretions are managed.

Suggested Reading

Ampel L, Hott KA, Sielaff GW, Sloan TB (1988) An approach to airway management in the acutely head-injured. J Emerg Med 6:1–7

Borel CO, Tilford C, Nichols DG, Hanley DF, Traystman RJ (1991) Diaphragmatic performance during recovery from acute ventilatory failure in Guillain-Barré syndrome and myasthenia gravis. Chest 99:444–451

Ell SR (1992) Neurogenic pulmonary edema. A review of the literature and a perspective. Invest Radiol 26:499–506

Ferguson IT, Murphy RP, Lascelles RG (1982) Ventilatory failure in myasthenia gravis. J Neurol Neurosurg Psychiatry 45:217–222

Ferguson R, Wright D, Willey R, Crompton GK, Grant I (1981) Suxamethonium is dangerous in polyneuropathy. Br Med J 282:298–389

Gibson G, Pride N, Davis J, Loh L (1977) Pulmonary mechanics in patients with respiratory muscle weakness. Am Rev Respir Dis 115(3):389–395

Goldberg AI (1990) Mechanical ventilation and respiratory care in the home in the 1990s: some personal observations. Respir Care 35:247–259

Gracey DR, McMichan JC, Divertie MB, Howard FMJ (1982) Respiratory failure in Guillain-Barré syndrome: a 6-year experience. Mayo Clin Proc 57:742–746

Gracey DR, Divertie MB, Howard FMJ (1983) Mechanical ventilation for respiratory failure in myasthenia gravis. Two-year experience with 22 patients. Mayo Clin Proc 58:597–602

Leger P, Jennequin J, Gerard M, Robert D (1989) Home positive-pressure ventilation via nasal mask for patients with neuromuscular weakness or restrictive lung or chest-wall disease. Respir Care 34:73–79

MacIntyre N (1986) Respiratory function during pressure support ventilation. Chest 89:677–683

Marini JJ (1990) Lung mechanics determinations at the bedside: instrumentation and clinical application. Respir Care 35:669–696

Marini JJ, Roussos CS, Tobin MJ, MacIntyre NR, Belman MJ, Moxham J (1988) Weaning from mechanical ventilation. Am Rev Respir Dis 138:1043–1046

McCool FD, Mayewski RF, Shayne DS (1986) Intermittent positive-pressure breathing in patients with respiratory muscle weakness. Chest 90:546–552

Mier Jedrzejowicz A, Brophy C, Moxham J, Green M (1988) Assessment of diaphragm weakness. Am Rev Respir Dis 137:877–883

Miller RD, Savarese JJ (1990) Pharmacology of muscle relaxants and their antagonists. In: Miller RD (ed) Anesthesia, 3rd edn. Churchill Livingstone, New York, p 389

Montgomery AB, Holle ROH, Neagley SR, Pierson DJ, Schoene RB (1987) Prediction of successful ventilation weaning using airway occlusion pressure and hypercapnic challenge. Chest 91:498–499

Moxham J (1984) Respiratory muscle fatigue – aspects of detection and treatment. Bull Eur Physiopathol Respir 20:437–444

Newsome DJ, Goldman M, Loh L, Casson M (1976) Diaphragm function and alveolar hypoventilation. Q J Med 177:87–100

Plummer AL, Gracey DR (1989) Consensus conference on artificial airways in patients receiving mechanical ventilation. Chest 96:178–180

Rochester DF, Arora NS (1983) Respiratory muscle failure. Med Clin North Am 67:573–597

Sahn S, Lakshminarayan S (1973) Bedside criteria for discontinuation of mechanical ventilation. Chest 63:1002–1005

Sassoon CS, Te TT, Mahutte CK, Light RW (1987) Airway occlusion pressure. An important indicator for successful weaning in patients with chronic obstructive pulmonary disease. Am Rev Respir Dis 135:107–113

Sassoon CSH, Mahutte K, Light RW (1990) Ventilator modes: old and new. Crit Care Clin 6:605–634

Shneerson J (1988) Disorders of ventilation. Backwell Scientific, Boston

Sporn PH, Morganroth ML (1988) Discontinuation of mechanical ventilation. Clin Chest Med 9:113–126

Torres A, Serra-Batlles J, Ros E et al. (1992) Pulmonary aspiration of gastric contents in patients receiving mechanical ventilation: the effect of body position. Ann Intern Med 116:540–543

Unertl K, Ruckdeschel G, Selbmann HK et al. (1987) Prevention of colonization and respiratory infections in long-term ventilated patients by local antimicrobial prophylaxis. Intensive Care Med 13:106–113

Vaz Fragoso CA, Kacmarek RM, Systrom DM (1992) Improvement in exercise capacity after nocturnal positive-pressure ventilation and tracheostomy in a postpoliomyelitis patient. Chest 101:254–257

Yang KL, Tobin MJ (1991) A prospective study of indexes predicting the outcome of trials of weaning from mechanical ventilation. N Engl J Med 324:1445–1450

Chapter 13

Swallowing Disturbances

Manfred Hörmann

Anatomy and Physiology of Feeding and Swallowing

Voluntary aspects of feeding (mastication and swallow initiation) are controlled by centers in the cerebral cortex. Corticobulbar tracts descend bilaterally to the pons and medulla with bilateral centers that control the muscles of swallowing. These centers consist of well-known cranial nerve nuclei (e.g., the nucleus ambiguus) as well as ill-defined groups of neurons nearby that are essential for the regulation of swallowing. The input from each cerebral hemisphere to the brainstem nuclei is distributed bilaterally so that the brain-stem centers continue to work after unilateral cortex or corticobulbar tract destruction.

There is also a sensory output from the brain-stem centers to the cortex regarding bolus characteristics, head position, and muscle activity and tension, essential for normal control of the swallowing process.

The brain stem can initiate swallowing without cortical input, and it

governs then the *involuntary* phase of swallowing. The muscles on each side of the tongue, palate, pharynx, and larynx are controlled by cranial nerves from the ipsilateral motor nuclei. The bolus then is normally propelled from the oral cavity, through the pharynx, into the esophagus without penetration into the nasopharynx or pharynx. The esophagus has an intrinsic neural network, regulating peristalsis automatically.

Swallowing entails three phases: (a) an oral voluntary phase influenced by the cortex and brain stem, (b) a pharyngeal involuntary phase controlled by the brain stem, and (c) an esophageal phase mediated by the brain-stem and intrinsic esophageal neurons.

Swallowing Disturbances in Neurologic Diseases

Neurologic diseases cause dysphagia by disturbing the oral and pharyngeal phases of swallowing. Dysphagia can result from diseases of (a) the cerebral cortex/brain stem, (b) the cranial

Section Editor: Daniel F. Hanley

nerves, (c) the neuromuscular junction, and (d) the muscles (of swallowing).

Cerebral Cortex

Stroke is the most frequent neurologic cause of dysphagia. If only one hemisphere is affected, brain-stem nuclei receive input from the other hemisphere, but there may still be swallowing apraxia or contralateral face and tongue weakness, with resulting poor bolus control. Serious dysphagia may occur after bilateral supratentorial lesions (pseudobulbar palsy). Multiple lacunar strokes may affect corticobulbar pathways in the deep white matter bilaterally, causing pseudo bulbar palsy. Brain-stem stroke can also result in pseudobulbar (upper brain stem with corticobulbar tracts) or bulbar (lower brain stem with the nuclei) palsy. Along with dysphagia, the patients present with different syndromes depending on the location of the disease in the brain stem. In patients with intracranial hemorrhage the occurrence of dysphagia depends on the location, extent of injury, and presence of secondary mass effect. Many patients with dysphagia after stroke have a good outcome after swallowing rehabilitation, although swallowing disturbances sometimes remain impediments to rehabilitation and sometimes require tracheotomy and gastrostomy.

Parkinson's disease may include dysphagia as an additional feature. The improvement of this symptom corresponds with relief of other motor disturbances, especially in the upper, extremities. Various neurodegenerative diseases also may cause dysphagia, such as spinocerebellar degeneration, progressive supranuclear palsy, or olivoponto-cerebellar atrophy, as may metabolic diseases and enzyme deficiencies in children. Progressive feeding impairment requires gastrostomy. Dystonia and dyskinesia, characterized by involuntary localized muscle contractions, can also prevent feeding.

In motor neurodiseases symptoms of dysphagia and dysarthria are found very often, especially in the elderly. Gastrostomy and sometimes tracheotomy may become necessary to avoid dehydration, aspiration, and asphyxia.

CNS-depressant drugs can reversibly impair swallowing, especially in the patient with opercular cortical lesions.

Cranial Nerves

Intrinsic brain-stem neoplasms and extrinsic tumors such as acoustic neuromas can compromise brain-stem swallowing centers and nuclei. Only some of these lesions are treatable by surgery, radiotherapy, or chemotherapy. Developmental abnormalities of posterior fossa structures are often associated with serious brain-stem dysfunction, including dysphagia. They may be treatable by surgical intervention.

Head trauma often includes brain-stem concussion or brain-stem hemorrhage. Where corticobulbar pathways are affected bilaterally, or lower brain-stem centers and/or nuclei only unilaterally, dysphagia may occur. Outcome of dysphagia in traumatically brain damaged people depends also on consciousness, memory, and learning abilities.

Neuromuscular Junction

Paired nerves innervate the muscles of mastication and swallowing: Nerves V (jaw), VII (face), IX/X (palate, pharynx, and larynx), and XII (tongue) are included in this process. They may be interrupted in their course from the brain stem through the skull base to the target muscle. Neoplasms can infiltrate and damage the nerves (leukemia, lymphoma, metastases); meningiomas, chordomas, or nasopharyngeal carcinomas may compress the nerves as they pass through the skull. Infections can be intense in the subarachnoid space, or they can cause neuropathic-mediated dysphagias.

Inflammatory or immune-mediated disorders such as sarcoid meningitis may infiltrate the nerves or induce demyelinating processes such as in Guillain-Barré syndrome.

In myasthenia gravis dysphagia occurs frequently. The Eaton-Lambert syndrome often occurs in the setting of malignancy or in immune-mediated processes. Dysphagia is then improved by treating the underlying malignancy or modulating the immune system. Botulinum toxin impairs release of acetylcholine from nerve terminals and frequently leads to swallowing disturbances.

Muscular Dysphagia

Myotonic dystrophy, with its delayed relaxion of muscles after contraction, may cause swallowing problems, which occasionally require tube feeding. Duchenne's dystrophy is less likely to be connected with dysphagia, but in oculopharyngeal dystrophy dysphagia is an essential symptom. In mitochon-drial myopathy dysphagia may result from pharyngeal myopathy and disordered brain-stem control. Dysthyroid myopathies are often associated with myasthenia gravis. Dysphagia in polymyositis, dermatomyositis, and sarcoid myopathies responds well to corticosteroids and immunosuppressants.

Esophageal Dysphagia

Esophageal dysphagia is caused by peptic and other inflammatory strictures, esophageal rings (Schatzki), neoplastic strictures, motility disorders (achalasia), and diffuse esophageal spasm. Diffuse esophageal spasm can be induced by inflammatory diseases or reflux esophagitis.

Diagnostic Procedure

History taking is important for the efficient use of more numerous and more complex diagnostic tests. Are there problems with swallowing liquids or a dry bolus, is the transport of the bolus impaired, or is swallowing painful? Have there been recurrent pneumonias or increased coughing?

The neurologic examination includes examination of the cranial nerves V (jaw), VII (face), IX/X (palate, pharynx, and larynx), and XII (tongue). Special attention is given to the separate examination of voluntary and involuntary movements, and reflex actions of these muscles.

Function of the larynx is best examined by the otolaryngologist. The ENT specialist also can answer the question of relaxation behavior of the upper esophageal sphincter by means of simultaneous manometry and electromyography.

Cineradiography is used to document the swallowing process. Since deglutition takes only 0.7 s after tiggering of the swallowing reflex, and since there is a very complex interaction of 5 cranial nerves and 26 cervical muscle groups, a recording system of high temporal (50 frames/s) and special resolution is needed. Various motor events during the short period of the pharyngeal swallowing process can be recognized. Differentiation between the pre-, intra-, and postdeglutitory aspiration is of crucial therapeutic importance. An individual surgical and/ or conservative program of rehabilitation is usually suggested. Additionally the risk of aspiration is usually assessed.

Therapy

Facilitative and compensatory strategies are used in the therapy of dysphagia. They involve therapeutic use of food or liquids as well as exercises to improve motor control or techniques to stimulate, inhibit, or improve oropharyngeal control. The methods prevent secondary atrophy, they may improve frequency of eating and drinking, and they use the muscles for their intended function, swallowing.

Facilitative strategies include swallowing of small volumes per swallow in severe dysfunction, the use of a straw in impaired oral transit of liquids, the use of a syringe or plunger-type spoon in impaired solid bolus formation by the tongue or in isolated problems with opening of the proximal esophageal segment.

Other methods (indirect therapies) include preparing exercises for facilitation and stabilization of orofacial and laryngeal voluntary movements, if the pre- and intradeglutitory phases of swallowing are disturbed. Techniques of facilitation (thermal stimulation, brushing, stretching, tapping, vibration, pressure, resistance) and voluntary movement exercises can be used, and the patient can be taught to exercise independently.

Compensatory strategies include neck flexion prior to swallow in poor laryngeal protection with glottic penetration, neck rotation to the weak side of the pharynx in unilateral pharyngeal retention or weakness, supraglottic swallow in laryngeal protection problems, and the "Mendelsohn maneuver" in impaired laryngeal elevation.

Medical treatment strategies have been used in esophageal disorders with hyper- or dysmotility. The use of calcium channel antagonists can be beneficial, at least in some patients with esophageal spasm at the level of entrance of the esophagus.

Operative Methods

Complete lack of sufficient opening of the P-E segment may necessitate myotomy of the upper sphincter of the esophagus. Unilateral weakness of the pharynx may necessitate operative diminution of the pharynx.

Gastrostomy and tube feeding can become necessary if serious impairments of swallowing and feeding remain. Gastrostomy seems to be better, because a nasogastric tube may inhibit movements of the larynx additionally.

In cases of continuous aspiration, tracheotomy may become necessary. New devices which allow both tracheal occlusion and speech are being developed and may enter clinical practice soon.

| # Prophylaxis of Deep Venous Thrombosis

MICHAEL A. DE GEORGIA, RAINER ZIMMERMANN, and
GREGORY J. DEL ZOPPO

Introduction

Nearly every patient entering a critical care unit is at risk for acute deep venous thrombosis (DVT) and its most devastating sequela, pulmonary embolism (PE). Although the exact incidence is unknown, PE is one of the leading causes of mortality in hospitalized patients, causing more than 50 000 deaths each year. Several methods of DVT prophylaxis have been proven safe and effective in other high-risk patients (Table 1); however, there is little consensus on the best method of prophylaxis for patients with neurological diseases (acute stroke, Guillain-Barré syndrome, and other neuromuscular diseases) and those undergoing neurosurgical procedures. The following is a brief review of the mechanisms, risk factors, and methods of DVT prophylaxis as they pertain to these patients.

Mechanisms and Risk Factors

The conditions that predispose to the development of venous thrombosis are well known and include stasis, vessel wall injury, and hypercoagulability (Virchow's triad). At least two of these elements are required for venous thrombosis to occur. A thrombus forms when a small nidus of fibrin deposition occurs on the vessel wall. In contrast to arterial thrombi, platelets contribute relatively little to the composition of venous thrombi, in which formation and propagation primarily involves the coagulation cascade. Venous stasis contributes to thrombus formation by causing vessel wall dilatation, promoting endothelial injury, and retaining coagulation factors. Local activation of coagulation and further fibrin deposition begins a cyclic process resulting in thormbus growth and propagation. Although most thrombi begin in the venous sinuses of the soleus and gastrocnemius muscles, approximately 20% proceed into the popliteal, femoral, and iliac veins, where the risk of embolization to the pulmonary circulation is greatly increased.

Section Editor: Thomas P. Bleck

Table 1. Recommendations for DVT prophylaxis for high-risk medical and surgical patients

Type of patient	Therapy
Undergoing elective general or gynecologic surgery, immobilized more than 48 h	Low-dose heparin (5000 IU s.c. every 12 h) or intermittent pneumatic compression
Undergoing elective urologic or major knee surgery	Intermittent pneumatic compression
Undergoing elective hip surgery	Adjusted-dose heparin to keep the aPTT in the high-normal range Moderate-dose warfarin to prolong the PT to an INR of 2.0–3.0 (corresponding approximately to a PT ratio of 1.2–1.5 times control)
Patients with hip fracture	Moderate-dose warfarin to prolong the PT to an INR of 2.0–3.0 (corresponding approximately to a PT ratio of 1.2–1.5 times control)

Table 2. Factors predisposing to venous thrombosis

- Surgery
- Malignancy/myeloproliferative diseases
- Immobilization
- Trauma
- Acute stroke
- Acute myocardial infarction
- Previous deep venous thrombosis
- Pregnancy and estrogen use
- Deficiencies of antithrombin III, protein C, protein S
- Nephrotic syndrome
- Congestive heart failure
- Obesity
- Age > 40 years
- Disseminated intravascular coagulation
- Anticardiolipin antibody, lupus anticoaglant
- Dysfibrinogenemia
- Venulitis (thromboangiitis obliterans, Behçet's disease)

A number of different conditions are associated with an increased risk of venous thrombosis; the patient entering a neurocritical care unit often has multiple risk factors (Table 2). Venous stasis is a common theme, and immobilization is probably the most important setting in which venous thrombosis occurs. Without prophylaxis, 60–75% of patients with severe hemiplegia after acute stroke develop a DVT in the paralyzed limb. Among patients undergoing neurosurgical procedures, 29–43% develop a DVT, and the risk doubles for operations lasting longer

than 4 h. Stasis from anesthesia induction contributes to the postsurgical risk of DVT. Hypercoagulability is also known to predispose to venous thrombosis in patients with inherited deficiencies of antithrombin III, protein C, and protein S and may also play a part in patients with acute stroke in whom impaired fibrinolysis has been reported. Direct cranial trauma and the resulting intravascular coagulopathy increase the risk of deep venous thrombosis and other thrombotic complications.

Methods of Prophylaxis

Mechanical Methods

Flexion and extension exercises of the lower extremities and early ambulation have often been recommended as simple and safe ways of preventing DVT. These measures have not been proven effective, however, and usually are not feasible for patients in a critical care setting. The use of properly fitted graduated elastic compression stockings has been shown to be effective in reducing the incidence of DVT, although it is more effective when combined with other methods, especially when multiple risk factors are present. Intermittent pneumatic compression (IPC) has been shown to help decrease the incidence of DVT (through activating the fibrinolytic system in addition to decreasing venous stasis), although no study has documented a clear reduction in the incidence of PE. The combination of graduated elastic compression and IPC (with the stockings worn underneath) has been shown to be better than IPC alone. IPC has not been associated with any adverse effects and should be used in patients who are at substantial risk from anticoagulation (e.g., patients with large intracranial hemorhages, selected neurosurgical patients).

Pharmacological Methods

Heparin. Heparin and warfarin are potent anticoagulants used in clinically evident thrombotic disease. The anticoagulant action of heparin results from its ability to bind and accelerate antithrombin III inhibition of thrombin and coagulation factors IXa, Xa, XIa, and XIIa. Heparin is the most widely used and extensively evaluated method of DVT prophylaxis, and a typical regimen involves 5000 IU given every 8 or 12 h by subcutaneous injection (low-dose heparin). Otherwise, the dosage is adjusted to keep the activated partial thromboplastin time (aPTT) in the high-normal range. A multitude of

controlled randomized trials have shown low-dose heparin to be safe and effective in other high-risk patients; however, there is widespread reluctance to use this method in patients with neurological diseases and those undergoing neurosurgical procedures for fear of intracranial hemorrhage. In patients with acute stroke, three randomized placebo-controlled trials have demonstrated a significant reduction in the incidence of DVT with low-dose heparin and, although none of the studies had a large patient sample, the incidence of hemorrhagic complications was not increased in patients receiving prophylaxis. Other studies have found no increase in intracranial bleeding when low-dose heparin was given to most patients undergoing neurosurgery.

Therefore, we recommend DVT prophylaxis with low-dose heparin 5000 IU every 12 h for patients with acute stroke and patients undergoing elective neurosurgical procedures (particularly those over the age of 40 and those with multiple risk factors). Controlled trials have not evaluated low-dose heparin in patients with cranial or spinal trauma, and these patients should preferably receive IPC. Although the combination of dihydroergotamine (DHE) and low-dose heparin has been shown to be more effective than low-dose heparin alone in reducing the incidence of DVT, we do not recommend it because the vasoconstrictor effect of DHE may cause worsening ischemia in patients with ischemic cerebrovascular disease.

Heparin is a polydisperse collection of glycosaminoglycans with anticoagulant activity, and molecular-weight-dependent prothrombotic features. Low-molecular-weight heparin fractions (LMWH, <9 kD) have lower prothrombotic activity than higher molecular-weight fractions, but anti-thrombotic activity can be adjusted by factor Xa assay to levels equivalent to those of unfractionated heparin preparations. Whether LMWH use may be associated with a decreased risk of hemorrhage is under study. Clinical trials, mainly from the surgical literature, have shown conflicting results. A recent meta-analysis of over 70 trials directly comparing LMWH with standard heparin in patients undergoing general and orthopedic surgery showed an equivalent reduction in the incidence of DVT, but no reduction in the incidence of hemorrhagic events. For patients with acute stroke, studies have shown equivalent or better efficacy in reducing the incidence of DVT, but again no significant reduction in the incidence of hemorrhagic complications. Low-molecular-weight heparin, not generally available at this time, may play an important role in DVT prophylaxis in the future.

Warfarin. Thrombocytopenia, arterial or venous thrombosis, or both may complicate the use of heparin for DVT presenting diagnostic and mangement difficulties in the critical care setting. Small amounts of heparin, including those contained in arterial flushes, may be enough to induce thrombocytopenia or thrombosis. An alternate approach is the use of warfarin, a vitamin-K antagonist which inhibits terminal alpha-carboxylation of coagulation factors II, VII, IX, and X by the hepatocyte. Warfarin causes a loss of functional factors VII, IX, X, and II in sequence which is dependent upon their half-lives and is maximal at 72 h. Adjustment of warfarin anticoagu-

lation according to the prothrombin time (PT) has been studied for DVT in several settings (Table 1). Dose adjustment should be according to the international normalized ratio (INR), although the relative PT prolongation from patient control is more often used clinically. Recommendations for warfarin dosage are given in Table 1.

Warfarin is routinely used for reatment of DVT (see Dalen and Hirsch 1986). Long-term treatment with warfarin is recommended for patients with a history of DVT or other vascular thrombosis and documented deficiencies of anti-thrombin III, protein C, or protein S, or evidence of an anticardiolipin antibody or lupus anticoagulant.

Table 3. Recommendations for DVT prophylaxis in the neurocritical care unit

1. All patients should be fitted with graduated elastic compression stockings.
2. Patients with acute stroke in whom intracranial hemorrhage has been excluded with computed tomography and patients undergoing elective neurosurgical procedures (particularly those over the age of 40 and those with multiple risk factors) should receive low-dose heparin 5000 IU subcutaneously every 12 h. In the surgical setting, prophylaxis should be started 2 h before surgery and should be continued postoperatively until the patient is ambulatory.
3. Patients with acute stroke in whom computed tomography reveals intracranial hemorrhage, selected neurosurgical patients (e.g., patients with cranial or spinal trauma), and patients at increased risk of bleeding (because of other medical or surgical reasons) should receive intermittent pneumatic compression. In the surgical setting, prophylaxis should be started before or during surgery and should be continued postoperatively until the patient is ambulatory.

Conclusion

The optimal prophylaxis of deep venous thrombosis for patients with neurological diseases and patients undergoing neurosurgical procedures has not been determined. General recommendations can be given based on the available literature (Table 3); however, it is emphasized that decisions regarding prophylaxis must be based upon a reasonable assessment of the risk/benefit ratio for each individual patient.

Suggested Reading

Barnett HG, Clifford JR, Llewellyn RC (1977) Safety of mini dose heparin administration for neurosurgical patients. J Neurosurg 47: 27–30

Black PM, Crowell RM, Abbott WM (1986) External pneumatic calf compression reduces deep venous thrombosis in patients with ruptured intracranial aneurysms. Neurosurgery 18:25–28

Cerrato D, Ariano C, Fiacchino F (1978) Deep vein thrombosis and low-dose heparin prohylaxis in neurosurgical patients. J Neurosurg 49:378–381

Consensus Conference (1986) Prevention of venous thrombosis and pulmonary embolism. JAMA 256:744–749

Dalen JE, Hirsch J (co-chairmen) (1986) American College of Chest Physicians and the NHIBI National conference on antithrombotic therapy. Chest 89[Suppl]:1s

Feinberg WM, Bruck DC, Ring ME, Corrigan JJ (1989) Hemostatic markers in acute stroke. Stroke 20:592–597

Fisher M, Francis R (1990) Altered coagulation in cerebral ischemia. Arch Neurol 47: 1075–1079

Joffe SN (1975) Incidence of postoperative deep vein thrombosis in neurosurgical patients. J Neurosurg 42:201–203

Kakkar VV, Howe CT, Flanc C et al. (1975) Natural history of postoperative deep vein thrombosis. Lancet 2:45–51

McCarthy ST, Turner JJ, Robertson D, Hawkey CJ, Macey DJ (1977) Low-dose heparin as a prophylaxis against deep-vein thrombosis after acute stroke. Lancet 2:800–801

McCarthy ST, Turner J (1986) Low-dose subcutaneous heparin in the prevention of deep-vein thrombosis and pulmonary emboli following acute stroke. Age Ageing 15:84–88

Nicolaides AN, Kakkar VV, Fields ES et al. (1971) The origin of deep vein thrombosis: a venographic study. Br J Radiol 44: 653–663

Nurmohamed MT, Rosendaal FR, Büller HR, Dekker E, Hommes DW, Vandenbroucke JP, Briet E (1992) Low-molecular weight heparin versus standard heparin in general and orthopedic surgery: a meta-analysis 340:152–156

Powers SK, Edwards MSB (1982) Prophylaxis of thromboembolism in the neurosurgical patient: a review. Neurosurgery 10:509–513

Prins M, Grelsema R, Sing AK, van Heerde LR, den Ottolander GJ (1989) Prophylaxis of deep venous thrombosis with a low-molecular weight heparin (Kabi 2165/Fragmin) in stroke patients. Haemostasis 19:245–250

Turpie AGG, Gent M, Cote R, Levine M, Ginsberg J, Powers P, Leclerc J, Gerts W, Jay R, Neemeh J, Klimek M, Hirsch J (1992) A low-molecular weight heparinoid compared with unfractionated heparin in the prevention of deep vein thrombosis in patients with acute ischemic stroke. Ann Int Med 117:353–357

Turpie AGG, Levine MN, Hirsh J, Carter CJ, Jay RM, Powers PJ et al. (1987) Double-blind randomized trial of ORG 10172 low-molecular weight heparinoid in prevention of deep venous thrombosis in thrombotic stroke. Lancet 1:523–526

Valldres JB, Hankinson J (1980) Incidence of lower extremity deep vein thrombosis in neurosurgical patients. Neurosurgery 6: 138–141

Warlow C, Ogston D, Douglas AS (1972) Venous thrombosis following strokes. Lancet 1:1305–1306

Chapter 15

Principles of Immunomodulatory Therapy

DAVID R. CORNBLATH and REINHARD HOHLFELD

Introduction

This chapter concerns the principles of immunomodulatory therapy for use in the neurologic intensive care unit (ICU). These principles, which are derived from those generally used for patients receiving immunomodulatory therapy, are particularly important in the ICU. This is because the side effects of the drugs used are considerable and will be compounded by the concurrent illnesses of patients in the ICU. However, there are differences between the use of these agents in the ICU setting and their use in the general clinical setting. For most intensive care patients the ICU stay is relatively short, and thus the long-term responsibility for immunomodulatory therapy will rest with other physicians. In many cases, patients in the ICU are sicker than others receiving immunomodulatory therapy, and the temptation is to use greater degrees of immunosuppression than would be used in the outpatient setting, in the belief that the potential benefit outweighs the ad-

Section Editor: Thomas P. Bleck

ditional risk. In selected cases this is justified, but this premise should be examined for each patient. As mentioned above, the complications and side effects of the individual agents should be borne in mind, as these will be exacerbated by the patient's coexisting illnesses.

Basic Principles

The basic principles for the use of immunomodulatory therapy in neurologic disease in the ICU are listed in Table 1. First, one should establish the diagnosis unequivocally, so that the appropriate drugs can be given for the correct indication. In ICU patients, most of the neurologic diseases requiring immunomodulatory therapy can be diagnosed over a 1–2 day period. The combination of history, clinical examination, selected laboratory tests, and electrophysiologic studies will usually establish the diagnosis. In some cases, a tentative diagnosis must be made pending further laboratory studies, such as the anti-acetylcholine receptor antibody titer.

Table 1. Principles of immunomodulatory therapy

---

1. Establish the diagnosis unequivocally.
2. Evaluate the patient comprehensively.
3. Define objective parameters of the disease.
4. Establish the goal(s) of therapy.
5. Understand the agents to be used.
6. Measure the risk : benefit ratio of treatment.

This first principle can not be emphasized too strongly. If the original diagnosis is incorrect, then therapy may be continued incorrectly with resultant complications.

Second, it is important to evaluate the patient comprehensively for evidence of other disease(s) than that primarily present. Several autoimmune diseases may occur in the same patient, and failure to treat all of them may make treatment of the primary disease difficult or impossible. For example, in patients with myasthenia gravis, treating associated hypo- or hyperthyroidism makes treatment of the primary disease more successful. In other instances, an infectious disease may accompany another disease, which would necessitate modifying therapy. For example, the Guillain-Barré syndrome may be seen in individuals with human immunodeficiency virus infection, and knowledge of the co-existence of these two disorders plays an important role in decisions concerning therapy. In the ICU, co-existing disorders such as hypertension, diabetes, or pulmonary tuberculosis, may also influence the choice of therapy.

Third, one should define objective parameters of the disease to measure. In the ICU setting this is usually easy, as patients are quite sick, severely neurologically affected, and frequently artificially ventilated. All of these can be quantified serially, so as to determine the changes with therapy. As decisions are made later about the effectiveness of specific therapies or lack thereof, it is helpful to have quantitative predictors to support such decisions.

Fourth, the primary treating physician should establish the goal(s) of therapy. In many instances in the ICU, this is straightforward such as the patient ventilating adequately. In other cases the goal of therapy is not as clear. In any case, establishing a goal of therapy and a time frame for the reaching of that goal is useful. Fifth, the treating physician should have an excellent understanding of the disease in question and the agents to be used. In some cases, this knowledge will reside with the ICU physicians, but in other cases neuromuscular or other consultative assistance will be required. Since these are the individuals likely to be following the patient over the long term, consultation should involve the appropriate people at the earliest point of therapy. The treating physician should be well aware of the expected benefits and risks of the drugs to be used. For example, with long-term corticosteroid treatment the risk of osteoporosis is significant, especially in postmenopausal women, and therapeutic strategies are available to prevent this, particularly if instituted early.

Sixth and last, the risk/benefit ratio of treatment should be clearly understood by the patient and his or her family. This is the basis of an informed decision regarding therapy.

Specific Agents

Adrenocorticosteroids. Steroids, usually prednisone or prednisolone, are the immunomodulatory agents commonly used in neurologic practice. In the ICU setting, intravenous preparations such as methylprednisolone and dexamethasone are used more commonly and generally in extremely high doses. Steroids have immunomodulatory effects on both the cell- and the antibody-mediated arms of the immune system.

The potential side effects of adrenocorticosteroids are well known. In the ICU setting, intravenous methylprednisolone is associated with electrolyte imbalance, hyperglycemia, and elevation of the white blood cell count, all of which are transient. However, the electrolyte imbalance may lead to cardiac arrhythmias, and there are reports of sudden death from the intravenous infusion of methylprednisolone. All corticosteroids have other known side effects that need to be monitored continuously. Most of these side effects can be managed when patients are followed closely. In general, intravenous preparations are delivered several times during the day, while oral preparations are given daily. Over the long term, alternate-day oral corticosteroid therapy is safer and usually as effective as daily therapy for many, but not all, immunologic conditions.

Plasmapheresis. Plasmapheresis has been used in an extraordinary number of disorders, mostly without clear benefit. In the ICU setting, plasmapheresis is useful in patients with acute myasthenic crisis, Lambert-Eaton syndrome, and Guillain-Barré syndrome. Regarding the latter disorder, several controlled clinical trials have shown a clear benefit (see Chap. 67). While most authors state that plasmapheresis works through the depletion of pathogenic antibodies, other immunomodulatory effects occur during plasmapheresis, for example, removal of cytokines and other inflammatory mediators. Plasmapheresis is a temporary therapy, and if long-term immunosuppression is desired other agents must be used. The main difficulty with plasmapheresis is adequate vascular access, which occasionally requires the insertion of central venous catheters.

Azathioprine. Azathioprine is a purine analog that is metabolized to 6-mercaptopurine and two other cytotoxic derivatives. It acts on proliferating cells. However, it is useful in antibody-mediated disorders that are T-cell dependent such as myasthenia gravis. Azathioprine usually takes weeks to months to have an effect on the immune system. For this reason, it has limited value in the ICU setting.

Cyclosporine. Cyclosporine is a fungal peptide with potent immunosuppressive activity. It appears to have a preferential effect upon early activation of helper/inducer T lymphocytes, sparing suppressor T-cell responses. Cyclosporine has been used predominantly in the transplant population, but also in patients with myasthenia. Rarely, it is used in other presumed autoimmune disorders. Like azathioprine, the immunomodulatory effects of cyclosporine may take weeks to months to become manifest, and thus its use in the ICU is limited. The main toxicities, hypertension and nephrotoxicity, can be managed with the frequent use of trough blood level determinations.

Human Immune Globulin. Human immune globulin is manufactured from large pools of human plasma in which the immunoglobulin contents are removed under sterile conditions and reconcentrated, providing a "pool" of human immunoglobulin. The mechanism of action in autoimmune disorders is unknown, and a large number of possible mechanisms have been postulated such as anti-idiotypic interactions or blockage of Fc receptors. Human immune globulin has recently received considerable attention because of its ease of administration. Peripheral venous access is required, and current preparations are quite safe, with little in the way of serious toxicity. Thus, human immune globulin, like plasmapheresis, has been used in an extraordinary number of diseases but is of proven benefit in few. A recent study by van der Meché and colleagues suggests that human immune globulin was as good as, or better than, plasmapheresis in the treatment of Guillain-Barré syndrome. This single study requires confirmation.

Cyclophosphamide. Cyclophosphamide, an alkylating agent, has been used in myasthenia gravis. It is much more toxic than azathioprine and should be reserved for patients in whom azathioprine or cyclosporine is ineffective or contraindicated. The immunosuppressive action is secondary to the cytotoxic effect on hematopoietic cells, particularly lymphocytes and monocytes/macrophages. Cyclophosphamide may have serious side effects. The major and often limiting side ef-

fect is bone marrow suppression, which affects leukocytes more than erythrocytes and platelets. The active metabolites are concentrated in the urine, resulting in damage to the epithelium of the bladder (hemorrhagic cystitis or malignant transformation). This toxicity can be reduced by appropriate fluid supply and by the simultaneous administration of a uroprotective agent. Nausea and vomiting, once a major problem, can now be effectively reduced with ondansetron. During prolonged therapy serious side effects may develop.

Illustrative Case

A 19-year-old, right-handed college student was transferred to the Johns Hopkins Neurosciences Intensive Care Unit in December, 1991, for further evaluation of progressive dyspnea and dysarthria. In the year before admission, she had had episodic double vision lasting seconds to minutes. Six months before admission, she had had an episode of right ptosis, which resolved spontaneously. Over the previous 6 months, her voice would become nasal with prolonged speech, but this always resolved completely. Over the week before admission, she had become generally fatigued and had noted difficulty in swallowing, with resultant mild weight loss. Two days before admission, the volume of her voice dropped, and she became dyspneic. She was admitted to a local hospital, where she was found to have ophthalmoparesis, bulbar dysfunction, and a forced vital capacity of 0.91. She was transferred to Johns Hopkins for further evaluation and treatment.

The past history revealed an episode of Hashimoto's thyroiditis, treated with synthroid. Thyroid disease had also been present in her mother. On initial examination, she was dyspneic with a respiratory rate of 30/min. The cranial nerves were remarkable for their inability to elevate the palate, and there were nasal speech and neck-flexor and tongue weakness. The remainder of the examination was normal. The forced vital capacity on admission was 1.2l, and the negative inspiratory force was $-21\,cm/H_2O$. Over the first night of admission, the vital capacity declined, and she was intubated the following morning. A tensilon test resulted in an increase of both vital capacity and negative inspiratory force. A tentative diagnosis of myasthenia was made, and plasmapheresis was instituted; this was done 5 times while the patient was in hospital. After the second plasmapheresis her vital capacity improved, and she was extubated 6 days after initial intubation. At the same time as plasmapheresis was begun, the search for associated autoimmune diseases was undertaken, and none were found. A chest CT scan failed to reveal evidence of a thymoma. She was started on oral corticosteroids while in hospital, in an effort to provide long-term immunosuppression. The AChR antibody titer drawn at the local hospital was positive and reported on the tenth hospital day.

This case illustrates the appropriate and successful use of immunomodulatory therapy in the Neurological ICU. Initially, the diagnosis of myasthenia gravis was based on the history, physical examination, and positive tensilon test. Plasmapheresis therapy was begun while the AChR antibody titer was pending. Because of the past

history of thyroid disease and the known association of other autoimmune diseases in myasthenics, the patient was evaluated for those other disorders. In this case, it was easy to define objective parameters of her disease, specifically the respiratory parameters. The goal of initial plasmapheresis therapy was straightforward, i.e., the return to independent ventilation. The long-term goal was to return her to normal functioning. Neuromuscular consultation was involved early in this case, as those physicians became her primary caregivers.

Suggested Reading

Baxter JD (1990) Minimizing the side-effects of glucocorticoid therapy. Adv Intern Med 35:173–194

Baylink DJ (1983) Glucocorticoid-induced osteoporosis. N Engl J Med 309:306–309

Consensus Conference (1986) The utility of therapeutic plasmapheresis for neurological disorders. JAMA 256:1333–1337

Cornblath DR, McArthur JC, Kennedy PGE, Witte AS, Griffin JW (1987) Inflammatory demyelinating peripheral neuropathies associated with human T-cell lymphotropic virus type III infection. Ann Neurol 21: 32–40

Dau PC (ed) (1979) Plasmapheresis and the immunobiology of myasthenia gravis. Houghton Mifflin, Boston

Drachman DB (1962) Myasthenia gravis and the thyroid gland. N Engl J Med 266:330–333

Drachman DB, McIntosh KR, DeSilva SD, Kuncl RW, Kahn C (1988) Strategies for the treatment of myasthenia gravis. Ann N Y Acad Sci 540:176–186

Dwyer JM (1992) Drug therapy: manipulating the immune system with immune globulin. N Engl J Med 326:107–116

French Cooperative Group on Plasma Exchange and Guillain-Barré Syndrome (1987) Efficacy of plasma exchange in Guillain-Barré syndrome: role of replacement fluids. Ann Neurol 22:753–761

Guillain-Barré Study Group (1985) Plasma-pheresis and acute Guillain-Barré syndrome. Neurology 35:1096–1104

Hohlfeld R, Toyka KV, Besinger VA, Gerhold B, Heininger K (1985) Myasthenia gravis: reactivation of clinical disease and of autoimmune factors after discontinuation of long-term azathioprine. Ann Neurol 17: 238–242

Kehrl JH, Fauci AS (1983) The clinical uses of glucocorticoids. Ann Allergy 50:2–8

Newsom-Davis J, Ward CD, Wilson SJ, Pinching AJ, Vincent A (1979) Plasmapheresis: short- and long-term benefits? In: Dau PC (ed) Plasmapheresis and the immunobiology of myasthenia gravis. Houghton Mifflin, Boston, pp 199–208

Osterman PO, Lundemo G, Pirskanen R, Fagius J, Pihlstedt P, Siden A (1984) Beneficial effects of plasma exchange in acute inflammatory polyradiculoneuropathy. Lancet 2:1296–1298

Shumak KH, Rock GA (1984) Therapeutic plasma exchange. N Engl J Med 310: 762–771

Thorn GW (1966) Clinical considerations in the use of corticosteroids. N Engl J Med 274: 775–781

Tindall RSA, Rollins JA, Phillips T, Greenlee RG, Wells L, Belendiuk G (1987) Preliminary results of a double-blind, randomized, placebo-controlled trial of cyclosporine in myasthenia gravis. N Engl J Med 316: 719–724

van der Meché FGA, Schmitz PIM, Dutch Guillain-Barré Study Group (1992) A randomized trial comparing intravenous immune globulin and plasma exchange in Guillain-Barré syndrome. N Engl J Med 326:1123–1129

Warmolts JR, Engel WK (1972) Benefits from alternate-day prednisone in myasthenia gravis. N Engl J Med 286:17–20

Wekerle H, Hohlfeld R (1992) Principles of therapeutic approaches to autoimmunity. In: Rose NR, Mackay I (eds) The autoimmune diseases. II. Academic, San Diego, pp 387–408

Witte AS, Cornblath DR, Parry GJ, Lisak RP, Schatz NJ (1984) Azathioprine in the treatment of myasthenia gravis. Ann Neurol 15:602–605

Chapter 16

General Management of Immunosuppressed Patients

MATTHIAS BLUMENSTEIN and KARL M. EINHÄUPL

Introduction

Advances in the therapy and management of malignancies and immunologic diseases, together with improved survival of patients with various transplanted organs, have added to the number of patients with profound derangements of the immune system. For the same reasons the number of immunocompromised patients with medical, surgical, or neurologic conditions requiring the expertise and facilities of intensive care treatment has increased within recent years. This group of patients is particularly susceptible to an adverse outcome in case of serious illness. Thus, a thorough understanding of any host defense impairment, diagnostic dilemmas, therapeutic approaches, and possible preventive strategies is essential for an effective treatment. Impairment of the immune system either by a predisposing disease state or by chemotherapy may change the typical clinical pattern of a disease. For example, patients with neutropenia and infec-

tion exhibit less fever and less striking physical findings of infection (e.g., local heat, swelling, adenopathy, exudate) than are ordinarily encountered in non-immunosuppressed patients with similar disorders. Furthermore, standard diagnostic tools, such as laboratory and serologic studies, often give inadequate results in such patients; this which may complicate differential diagnostic possibilities and therapeutic strategies. In addition, in transplanted patients or those with autoimmune diseases, the medical or surgical treatment of the condition requiring intensive care treatment may conflict with cytotoxic chemotherapy or other immunosuppressive therapeutic regimens of the primary disease. In the same patients immunosuppressive drugs often interfere with those commonly used in intensive care treatment, causing side effects and complications. Overall, although substantial progress has been made in our understanding of the mechanisms causing a derangement of the host's immune response, the treatment of such patients remains an intensive care challenge with a high death rate. Detailed discussion of each prob-

Section Editor: Thomas P. Bleck

Table 1. The major elements of host defense mechanisms

Exterior defenses	Skin, mucous membranes
	Sebaceous gland secretions
	Cilia lining organs (e.g., trachea)
	Gastric acidity
	Endogenous microbial flora
Soluble factors	Lysozymes
	Acute-phase proteins
	Complement
	Cytokines
	Immunoglobulins
Cellular components	Phagocytes
	Natural killer cells
	T/B lymphocytes

lem is beyond the scope of this chapter. The goal here is to supply information on those problems commonly encountered in the treatment of immuncompromised patients in the intensive care unit.

A functioning immune system depends on a variety of mechanisms. The exterior of the body and an intact intestinal mucosal wall present an effective biochemical and physical barrier to most pathogenic organisms. In addition, immunocompetent cells and soluble molecules distributed throughout the body are involved in host defense mechanisms. All the different systems interact to maintain the integrity of the body and to limit the spread of tissue damage, whether it is caused by physical damage or by infectious agents (Table 1).

Impairment of the immune system might be caused by defects related to malignancies, chronic infections, and metabolic diseases, or it might be due to medical treatment. Typical conditions associated with immunocompromised states include leukemia, lymphoma, solid tumors, or the ac-

quired immune deficiency syndrome. Furthermore, impaired response to infectious agents is a prominent feature of metabolic disease such as chronic kidney failure or diabetes. Malnutrition has been shown to have multiple effects on the human defense system, and this common problem in hospitalized patients may add to the high risk of infection. On the other hand, modification of immune function by pharmacological agents for organ transplantation and the treatment of certain autoimmune diseases is emerging as a major area of therapeutics.

Infections in Immunocompromised Patients

Infection remains the leading cause of death among immunocompromised patients. In ICU treatment the risk for infection is even more increased by the need for invasive procedures. Several studies have concluded that among intensive care patients, those with the highest risk of nosocomial pneumonia are individuals treated with mechanical ventilation. The routine placement of intravascular cannulae and urinary catheters may add to the risk of the compromised host.

Preventive strategies are aimed at reducing the incidence of infectious complications in the critical care unit. As a general rule, invasive procedures should be minimized in such patients. Special care should be taken to prevent microbial contamination of central catheters, tubing lines, and ventilation equipment. In the febrile patient such material should always be examined and suspected as a causative factor in bacteremia and septicemia. Clinical

Table 2. Common etiologic agents of infection in compromised patients

Bacteria	Gram-negative	*Escherichia coli*, *Klebsiella* species, *Pseudomonas aeruginosa*, *Haemophilus*, *Legionella pneumophila*
	Gram-positive	*Staphylococcus aureus*, *Streptococcus pneumoniae*
	Other	Mycobacteria, *Nocardia* species
Fungi		*Candida* species, *Aspergillus* species, *Cryptococcus*, *Mucor* species
Protozoa		*Pneumocystis carinii*, *Toxoplasma gondii*
Viruses		Cytomegalovirus, varicella-zoster virus, herpes-simplex virus, measles

infection mandates removal of the artificial device and institution of antibiotics. In intubated patients gram-negative pneumonia may result from retrograde colonization of the pharynx from the stomach. Numerous studies have shown that this complication may be more likely when gastric pH levels are elevated by antacids or H_2-receptor antagonists (e.g., cimetidine, ranitidine). Therefore, the use of a prophylactic agent against gastrointestinal bleeding that preserves the natural gastric acid barrier against bacterial overgrowth, such as sucralfate, may be preferable to antacids and H_2-blockers. In the same patients prevention of lower airway colonization and infection by the use of locally administered antibiotics has been shown to reduce the incidence of nosocomial lung infection significantly. While in general, the prophylactic use of antibiotics in intensive care treatment for prevention of bacterial infection is not recommended, in ventilated patients with known preexisting host defense impairment gut sterilization has proven useful as a temporary measure. Protocols commonly used for such prophylactic treatment include nonabsorbable antibiotics such as polymyxin, gentamycin, and amphotericin B. As a rule any microbial organism is able to cause

serious illness in a patient with a derangement of the immune system (Table 2). However, by far the most predominant microbials are gram-negative bacilli, followed by gram-positive cocci such as *Staphylococcus aureus*, coagulase-negative staphylococci, and streptococci.

The determination of the specific underlying immunologic defect is of clinical relevance, since the patterns of disease as well as the therapeutic consequences may differ depending on the mechanism of immunosuppression. For example, derangement of phagocytic function increases the risk of infection by bacteria and fungi, while a defect in cell-mediated immunity is significantly more often associated with infections due to viruses and protozoa.

Clinical and Diagnostic Approach

Common sites of infection include the lungs, the skin, and the gastrointestinal and urinary tracts. Among these, pneumonia developed in the hosptial is the infection most likely to causally contribute to death of patients. Patients with central intravascular catheters are

Table 3. Laboratory studies in the febrile compromised host

Routine laboratory testing	White blood count and differential, electrolytes, liver chemistry, creatinine
Chest roentgenography	
Culture	Blood, urine, sputum, swabs from suspected lesions: Direct microscopic examination Detection of microbial antigen, by-products, and genomes Detection of specific antibodies
Specific techniques in case of CNS involvement Pneumonia Odynophagia	 Lumbar puncture, biopsy Brochoscopy, open lung biopsy Endoscopy

threatened by systemic manifestations of bacteremia, septicemia, and metastatic infection.

As already mentioned, immunocompromised patients may have altered presentation of infection, making detection of the infection site and the invading microbial organism difficult. Fever alone may be the only indicator of infection. Fundamental goals are to establish the identification of the invading micro-organism as quickly as possible and to detect possible visceral involvement with disseminated infection. Historical, physical, and laboratory findings are helpful in determining if infection is present, and if so, which etiologic agent is responsible and what kind of therapy should be instituted. A thorough physical examination with particular attention to organ sites of high risk is critical for the early diagnosis. Besides routine laboratory testing, invasive diagnostic culture techniques such as endoscopy, bronchoscopy, or histologic examination of the infected organ site should be considered early in any event of refractory fever (Table 3).

Therapy

Due to the early development of septic complications any infection may become a life-threatening event in the compromised host. Despite the fact that the infectious agent often cannot be identified, the immediate start of broad-spectrum antibiotic therapy is indicated for the prevention of fatal complications. This has been proven to reduce morbidity and mortality in patients with a defective immune response.

The primary goal of treatment is to select antibiotic coverage for microorganisms that are most likely to be involved. Optimization of antimicrobial chemotherapy in immunocompromised patients has been addressed in numerous clinical studies. However, the results reported remain controversial. The primary selection is still based on the physician's empiricism, which should reflect the signs and symptoms of the various infectious diseases, an understanding of the antibiotic spectrum of available drugs, and knowledge of sensitivity patterns of the hospital in which the patients are treated.

The simultaneous use of two or more antimicrobial agents that are synergistic against infecting bacteria as initial empiric therapy is employed in most institutions. Examples of such combinations are vancomycin, ticarcillin, and amikacin, or ceftazidime and amikacin. If the patient remains febrile on antibiotics the addition of an antifungal agent is mandatory. In addition, viral infection and infection with protozoa should be considered in any patient who does not respond to the initial therapy.

Drug Interaction and Toxicity

The widespread use of immunosuppressive drugs, like steroids, cyclosporine, or azathioprine, is not only associated with a higher incidence of infections, but also increases the risk of drug interactions and clinical toxicity. This is especially true in intensive care medicine in which the physician frequently encounters patients who exhibit extreme changes in physiology and pharmacokinetic parameters. Furthermore, critically ill patients require aggressive therapy, and multiple-drug therapy is the norm to obtain a desired therapeutic objective or to treat coexisting diseases. Numerous clinically significant interactions between immunosuppressants and other drugs have been described. By far the majority of these involve interference with the metabolism of the immunosuppressive drug, either by causing rejection of the transplanted organ due to reduced blood concentrations, or by increasing the risk of toxicity by interference with clearance mechanisms. Therefore, with the use of immunosuppressive agents, knowledge of known drug interactions and careful monitoring of serum concentrations (if a sensitive and specific analytic procedure is available) are important to minimize the risk of overtreatment and adverse reactions.

Withdrawal of immunosuppression in patients with infectious complications is often of major concern in intensive care medical treatment. The risk of life-threatening complications due to excessive immunosuppression on the one side and rejection of a transplanted organ on the other outline the therapeutic conflict. Unfortunately, general guidelines for the management of immunosuppression, e.g., when to reduce, withdraw, or restart therapy in a given patient with infectious disease, are not available. Thus, the decision is based on the physician's judgement.

Suggested Reading

Bach JF (1989) The risk/benefit ratio in immunointervention for autoimmune diseases. In: Bach JF (ed) Immunointervention in autoimmune diseases. Academic, London, pp 215–224

Craven DE, Steger KA, Barber TW (1991) Preventing nosocomial pneumonia: state of the art and perspectives for the 1990s. Am J Med 91:44S–53S

Davies DM (1985) Textbok of adverse drug reactions, 3rd edn. Oxford University Press, New York

Nossal GJV (1987) Current concepts: immunology: the basic components of the immune system. N Engl J Med 316:1320

Rubin RH, Young LS (1988) The clinical approach to infection in the immunocompromised host, 2nd edn. Plenum, New York

Simmons BP, Wong ES (1982) Guideline for prevention of intravascular infections. Infect Control 3:61–72

Washington JA (1990) Bacteria, fungi and parasites, the clinician and microbiology laboratory. In: Mandell GL (ed) Principles and practice of infectious diseases, 3rd edn. Wiley, New York

Chapter 17

Infection Control in Neurocritical Care

Volker Schuchardt and Heinrich K. Geiss

Introduction

Nosocomial infections (NI) may involve not only patients but anyone else in contact with the hospital environment: staff members, technical services, visitors. NI significantly contribute to hospital morbidity and mortality, causing prolonged hospital stays and an excessive economic burden. The highest infection rates are found in specialized care units and they exceed infection rates for routine inpatients five- to tenfold. Sixteen to 36% of patients treated in intensive care units (ICU) suffer from NI. For the high incidence of infection there are several causes, including severity of the acute illness, age, multiple comorbid diseases, immunocompromised host, invasive procedures, mechanical ventilation, artificial nutrition, inadequate asepsis in emergency situations, and clustering of susceptible and infective individuals.

More than half of nosocomial infections are endogenous in origin; that

is, they are derived from pathogens with which the ICU patient is already colonized. The rest are exogenous and are caused by transmission of infective agents. The most important source of micro-organisms causing exogenous infections are the hands of staff members. In medical and surgical ICUs, pneumonias and urinary tract infections are the most frequently reported NI, followed by bacteremia, sepsis, and wound infections. Information on the infection rate in neurologic ICUs is sparse. In a retrospective Austrian study including 337 consecutive patients, the authors describe NI in 20% of their neurologic ICU patients and colonization without infection in another 15%. In our own prospective study of 99 patients, we found NI in 17 and colonization in another nine. An additional 13 patients entered the ICU with pre-exsisting infections (Tables 1–3). None of these 99 patients died of NI, nor did they experience sequelae from NI. Considering the extremely long ICU stays with a high incidence and long duration of artifical ventilation, this infection rate seems surprisingly low. This may be because neurologic ICU patients in general

Section Editor: Thomas P. Bleck

Table 1. Infection status in 99 neurologic ICU patients

No infection	60
Admitted to the ICU with infection	13
Microbial colonization without infection	9
Nosocomial infection acquired on ICU	17

tend to be younger and suffer less frequently from severe co-morbid diseases than patients of medical units. Additionally, most invasive procedures are performed within the first days after ICU admission, with the frequency of NI declining to zero after 4 weeks of treatment. Patients may reach a steady state between non-specific and specific host-defense mechanisms and the infective environment. We cannot, however, rely on this "auto defense". From the point of view of hygiene, prophylaxis in the neurologic ICU must focus on three points: (a) protection of the patient

Table 2. Distribution of clinically manifest infections in 30 neurologic ICU patients

	Nosocomial	Preexisting
Tracheobronchitis	8	1
Bacterial pneumonia	9	10
Fungal pneumonia	1	
Urinary tract infection	2	1
Skin infection (tracheostomy)	1	
Catheter-related infection	2	
Systemic candidiasis		1
Total	17	13

Table 3. Distribution of positive cultures in neurologic ICU patients ($n = 28$)

Organisms isolated	Trachea	Urine	Wound	Catheter tip
Coagulase-negative staphylococci	14	10		3
Nonhemolytic streptococci	12	2	1	
Staphylococcus aureus	10	1	1	
Enterococcus faecalis		7		1
Streptococcus pneumoniae	2			
Corynebacterium spp.	2	1		
Neisseria spp.	3			
Escherichia coli	2	6	1	2
Pseudomonas aeruginosa	2			
Serratia marcescens	1			
Candida spp.	10			
Aspergillus fumigatus	1			
Total number of patients affected	24	16	2	5

The total number of patients surveyed was 99. In 28 patients positive microbiological cultures were found with or without evident infections; 71 patients did not show microbial colonization at any culture site.

against exogenous infections, (b) protection of the patient against his own flora, and (c) protection of hospital staff, visitors and fellow patients.

General Measures

Personnel

Health care workers (HCW) in the neurologic ICU, including nurses, doctors, technicians, and assistants, must understand their responsibility for preventing nosocomial infections (NI). Continuous appreciation of the hygienic situation, ongoing education, and skilled training are essential. Preventive and control measures are primarily the responsibility of the ICU nursing supervisor. Written regulations ("hygienic guidelines") are helpful and facilitate decisions in daily practice.

ICU workers' hands are the most crucial factor in transmitting microorganisms, as mentioned above. Therefore, hand antisepsis is recognized as the most important single measure for infection control (the term "hand antisepsis" is used instead of the misleading term "hand washing"). The method used involves the application of alcohol solution (isopropanol 70%) for 30 s. This will reduce the transient flora by 99.999%. It is recommended that one disinfects hands when entering the unit, before and after patient manipulation, and after contact with potentially contaminated items. When dealing with blood or secretions, gloves are to be worn. Hand washing with soap and water may be restricted to the beginning of the work shift and to the case

of visually soiled hands. When hands are soiled with potentially infective material to avoid accidental contamination of the environment, hand washing should be preceded by hand disinfection. Skin care with hand creams or lotions is a self-evident part of individual hygiene and occupational health. Intact and smooth skin withstands colonization far better than rough and cracked skin. Bracelets, rings, and wristwatches are not allowed in high-risk areas as, firstly, they may serve as a contamination source and, secondly, they pose the risk of injury when nursing immobilized and unconscious patients.

The ICU staff wears special clothing that is restricted to the ward and that must be changed at least daily or in case of soiling. To avoid contamination of these uniforms, protective gowns or aprons are used during close patient contact (e.g., washing the patient). Protective equipment like goggles or face masks are restricted to situations discussed below. Consulting physicians and visitors without direct patient contact should similarly wear gowns that are changed daily and in case of soiling.

Acutely ill staff members, suffering, for example, from gastroenteritis, influenza, or infectious skin diseases, should be excluded from direct nursing contact with patients (Table 4). Currently, there is a worldwide debate about to whether HIV-positive health care workers pose a risk of transmission for patients. In general, seropositivity with HIV, HBV, or other bloodborne pathogens is not an argument for barring affected persons from any active care of patients. Seropositive health care workers should be counseled to avoid procedures that have

Table 4. Recommendations and work restrictions for health care workers (HCW) with infectious diseases

Disease/problem	Relieve from direct patient contact	Partial work restriction	Duration
Infectious conjunctivitis	YES		Until discharge ceases
Diarrhea			
Acute stage	YES		Until symptoms resolve
Salmonella carriers or other enteric pathogens	NO	HCW should not take care of high-risk patients	Until stool is free of the infecting agent
Enteroviral infections	NO	HCW should not take care of infants or newborns	Until symptoms resolve
Group-A streptococcal disease	YES		Until 24 h after onset of adequate treatment
Hepatitis A	YES		Until 7 days after onset of jaundice
Hepatitis B and C Acute disease and chronic antigenemia	NO	HCW must wear gloves for procedures that involve trauma to tissues or contact with mucous membranes or nonintact skin	Until antigenemia resolves
Herpes simplex			
Whitlow	YES		Until lesions heal
Orofacial	NO	HCW should not take care of high-risk patients	Until lesions heal
HIV positive	NO	Same as acute hepatitis B	Period of infectivity has not been determined
Staphylococcus aureus skin lesions	YES		Until lesions heal
Upper respiratory tract infections	NO	HCW should not take care of high-risk patients	Until acute symptoms resolve
Varicella	YES		Until lesions dry and crust
Zoster	NO	HCW should not take care of high-risk patients	Until lesions dry and crust

been epidemiologically linked to the transmission of HIV, HBV, or other blood-borne infections. Most patient contacts, including the majority of invasive procedures, can safely be carried out by health care workers infected with HIV or other blood-borne pathogens, provided they are familiar with and adhere to proper infection control. Those invasive procedures, however, that involve manipulations of pointed or sharp objects by feel within body cavities might pose a greater risk of accidental injury and inadvertent transmission of blood-borne pathogens and should therefore be voluntarily avoided.

ICU Environment

Although micro-organisms on walls and floors play an insignificant role in causing human diseases, the following recommendations are of importance. They are based on recognition of what reductions in microbial content can be consistently achieved with moderate effort rather than what levels are required to prevent infections.

Patient rooms should be cleaned twice daily with a disinfectant-detergent and, in the case of visible contamination (soiled floor, wall, or bed, etc.) should be disinfected immediately with an aldehyde-based disinfectant. A thorough cleaning of the patient's room should be performed at discharge and at least once a month.

Although soiled linen is heavily contaminated with human pathogens, the infection risk from it seems to be very low. It is prudent, nevertheless, to handle soiled linen cautiously and to dispose of it immediately into a laundry bag in the patient's room. Laundry from patients with highly contagious diseases must be collected separately in special water-tight bags. Excretions from patients (urine, stool, drainage fluids, or sputum) may contain large amounts of infective agents, and adequate and contamination-free disposal is therefore essential. In communities with modern and adequate sewage disposal systems, excretions including feces from patients suffering from salmonella gastroenteritidis, shigellosis, hepatitis A, etc. can be discharged directly into the sewers without preliminary disinfection. Exceptions are epidemics and some rare diseases such as cholera or Lassa fever. Used instruments are disposed or returned for decontamination and reprocessing immediately.

Invasive Procedures

Invasive procedures with perforation of the intact skin and introduction of prosthetic devices bypass host defenses and so are correlated with an increased risk of NI. Therefore, asepsis is most important with ICU patients. Invasive procedures should be performed in separate procedure rooms. If such a room is not available, invasive procedures may be done in the patient's room. The treated patient must be protected against infections from his roommate, from potentially infective material in the room, and from assistant personnel – no spectators!

Patients' risk of acquiring NI is one problem, potential transmission of serious infections to health care workers is another. AIDS has heightened the awareness of occupational risks, and methods to reduce bloodborne infections have become increasingly important. To avoid hazards by needle-stick and sharp injuries, all sharp items must be discarded promptly after use into impermeable disposal collection containers. Recapping of needles is strictly prohibited. Operations and other invasive procedures, at least in HIV- or HBV-positive patients, should be performed with protection by double gloves, waterproof garments, and face shields.

Intravenous and Intra-arterial Catheters

The insertion of intravenous and intra-arterial cannulas, as well as punctures of the ventricular system or the pleural space, must be performed under meticulous asepsis. Critical evaluation of the indication for any invasive procedure is crucial, as the potential for producing nosocomial septicemia is largely underappreciated. It is estimated that one third of all nosocomial bacteremias originate from infusion therapy in some form.

The following basic guidelines for intravascular cannulas and punctures should be adhered to:

1. Wearing of sterile gown, face mask, and cover
2. Disinfection of the insertion site with alcohol or iodine solution for 1 min
3. Hand disinfection with alcohol solution for at least 30 sec
4. Sterile gloves
5. Sterile draping of the insertion site
6. Atraumatic puncture
7. Fixing and covering of the cannula with a sterile gauze
8. No local antiseptics or antibiotics
9. Documentation of insertion and care on the covering

Peripheral cannulas and venous catheters should usually be changed every 72 h, whereas the duration of central venous catheters is restricted only by mechanical problems and infectious complications. However, in case of suspected catheter-related infection, the line must be removed as soon as possible. Antibiotic therapy alone is ineffective. Care of intravascular catheters includes visual control of the wound dressing every 12 h and changing of it every 48 h, in case of soiling immediately. After removal of the dressing, the insertion site is cleaned with sterile water or a disinfectant, dried, and again covered with a sterile gauze. Reentering of dislocated catheters is strictly forbidden. Prior to all manipulations of the delivery system

including stopcocks, side-ports, and "piggybacks", the nurse must perform hand disinfection with an alcohol solution. Delivery systems should be changed every 48 h. If inline infusion filters are used, this interval may be extended to 96 h. Maximal asepsis is needed when compounding parenteral admixtures to prevent infusate contamination. Admixtures should be prepared immediately before infusion.

Urinary Tract Catheters

Most urinary tract infections are caused by transurethral catheters, which therefore should be placed with caution and only if indicated. Insertion is done under strictly aseptic conditions and catheters must be removed as soon as possible. The catheter material influences the infection risk: Latex catheters are restricted to 1 week of use, whereas for catheterization of longer duration silicone catheters are recommended. To minimize infection hazards, intermittent straight catheterization (ISC) is recommended, especially in paraplegic patients. The lowest infection risk is correlated with the suprapubic catheter. It is always indicated for long-term catheterization and is beneficial for training sphincter function. For the placement of transurethral and suprapubic catheters, the aseptic technique is adapted from that for intravascular catheters (see above).

Intubation and Artificial Ventilation

Endotracheal intubation is necessary for unconscious patients, for those with pareses of oropharyngeal muscles, and for patients needing artificial ventilation. There are advantages and disadvantages of orotracheal versus nasotracheal intubation; both methods have an inherent risk of infection. Due to the high percentage of patients requiring long-term artificial ventilation, tracheostomy is a frequent procedure in the neurologic ICU. With tracheostomy, there is an additional risk of wound infection but the care of the oropharynx is easier. The risk factors of intubation-related NI are the following:

1. Translocation of oro-/nasopharyngeal flora into the trachea
2. Obstruction of sinuses with nasotracheal tubes
3. Risk of parotitis with orotracheal intubation
4. Impossible voluntary expectoration
5. Decreased function of ciliated epithelium
6. Microbial contamination during endotracheal suctioning
7. Silent aspiration of oropharyngeal and gastric secretions

With impaired respiratory muscle function, especially in patients with oropharyngeal pareses, when there is an important risk of aspiration, intubation must be done very early, even if blood gases are still normal. To prevent hazards of intubation and mechanical ventilation, some points are of importance:

(a) early intubation; (b) meticulous physiotherapy; (c) medical secretolysis; (d) endotracheal suctioning only when needed, at least every 4 h; (e) suction catheters introduced only once, not reintroduced; (f) ventilation tubes replaced every 48–72 h, up to 1 week with humidifying filters; (g) tracheostomy tubes changed every 10–14 days, daily if local infection is present; (h) restricted use of H_2 selective blockers and early introduction of enteral feeding; and (i) possibly gut decontamination.

Antimicrobial Prophylaxis

In immunocompetent patients, general antibiotic, antimycotic, or antiviral prophylaxis is not recommended. Any kind of antimicrobial treatment should be based on sound clinical suspicion (calculated therapy) or introduced after proper microbiological diagnosis. However, prophylactic intratracheal use of aminoglycosides in artificially ventilated persons is still under discussion. Calculated antimicrobiological therapy is based on resistance patterns, which should be discussed regularly together with the microbiological laboratory. With knowledge of resistance patterns, it is usually possible to reduce the number of antibiotics used on the ward to about ten. On this basis, it is easier for all physicians in charge to choose an appropiate initial antimicrobial therapy.

Prevention and Control of Transmission of Infections

Infections can be transmitted within hospitals from patients to personnel, from personnel to patients, among patients and employees themselves, and finally from patients and personnel to visitors or other community contacts. The most frequent mode of

Table 5. Recommendations for isolation procedures

Disease	Private room	Kind of isolation	Duration/remarks
Creutzfeld-Jakob disease	NO	Body fluid	Duration of disease; no cases of nosocomial transmission known
Enteroviral infections	NO	Enteric	Until symptoms resolve
Meningoencephalitis	NO	Enteric	Until enteroviral origin is excluded
Tuberculosis			
– pulmonary	YES	Respiratory	About 2 weeks after initiation of adequate tuberculostatic therapy
– extrapulmonary	NO	Body fluid	Same as pulmonary tuberculosis
Meningococcal diseases	YES	Respiratory	24 h after initiation of adequate therapy
Hepatitis A	NO	Enteric	Until 7 days after onset of jaundice
Hepatitis B	NO	Body fluid	Until antigenemia resolves
Hepatitis C	NO	Body fluid	Until antigenemia resolves
AIDS	NO	Body fluid	Private room necessary if patient cannot comply with basic hygiene rules. In USA, AIDS patients with cough should be isolated in a negative-pressure room until multi drug-resistant tuberculosis is excluded.
Zoster generalisatus	YES	Respiratory	Until lesions dry and crust
Nosocomial pneumonia	NO	Respiratory	

transmitting infective agents is direct spread via hands and, to a far lesser degree, via fomites. Therefore, it is indisputable that health care workers can decrease the risk of acquiring and transmitting infections by meticulous hand antisepsis after touching a source that is likely to be contaminated and after taking care of patients with transmissible diseases. Besides the widespread legislative regulations and standards, each hospital should have a written comprehensive plan for management of hospital personnel exposed to communicable diseases. This plan should include at least:

(a) management of each of the common infectious diseases (e.g., isolation precautions, disinfection, and sterilization), (b) protocols for immunization of hospital personnel, and (c) protocols for management after exposure to infectious agents.

Isolation

Isolation may be designed to protect personnel, immunocompetent patients, and visitors (source isolation: enteric, respiratory, body fluid precautions) or to protect the immunocompromised patient from exogenous infections (protective isolation). The aim of all these measures is to inhibit the spread of micro-organisms by: (a) spatial separation, (b) protective measures, and (c) control of supply and waste management.

Different methods of isolation depend on the kind of disease and the way specific infecting agents are trans-

Table 6. Recommendations for immunization of health care workers (HCW)

Disease	Active immunization	Additional remarks
Hepatitis A	HCW in substantial risk areas (Newborn nurseries, ICU, transplantation units).	Testing sera for pre-existing AB before passive immunization is probably not cost-effective.
Hepatitis B	All hospital personnel	After completing a 3-dose series, serologic testing for anti-HBs, because up to 5% of vaccine recipients will not develop protective levels of anti-HBs even after revaccination with additional doses of vaccine. In case of proven exposure nonresponders should be treated immediately with hepatitis B immune globulin.
Influenza	Strongly recommended annually for all HCW	
Measles	Recommended for all hospital personnel unless they have a record of physician-diagnosed measles, or laboratory evidence of immunity.	Because of the theoretical risk to the fetus, live virus vaccines generally are not given to pregnant women or to those who are likely to become pregnant within 3 months.
Rubella	All – male and female – HCW who might transmit rubella to pregnant patients or to other HCW	Routine serologic tests for female HCW to ensure immunity are advisible.
Poliomyelitis	HCW with increased risk of exposure	In HCW working in high-risk areas (transplantation unit, ICU) enhanced-potency inactivated polio vaccine is preferred because virus can be shed after oral vaccination.

mitted. It is beyond the scope of this chapter to describe isolation procedures in detail. General recommendations regarding isolation procedures in neurologic ICUs for some of the more frequent infections may be found in Table 5.

Immunization of Personnel

With the increasing availability of vaccines the risk of acquiring hospital-related infections can be reduced to almost zero in health care workers. Table 6 summarizes the recommended

immunizations for hospital personnel. Health care workers are not at a higher risk of acquiring diphtheria, pneumococcal disease, mumps, pertussis, or tetanus than the general adult population and therefore need no special immunization for these diseases.

Prophylaxis after Exposure

Hospitals should establish an exposure control plan that includes reporting and investigating procedures to be followed after accidental exposures. The postexposure evaluation must docu-

Table 7. Recommendations for postexposure prophylaxis (adapted from Williams)

Disease	Recommendation
Hepatitis A	Nonimmunized personnel who have had direct fecal-oral exposure to excretions from a patient incubating hepatitis A should be given IG (0.02 ml/kg).
Hepatitis B	Immune status of exposed person is unknown or immunization is not complete: HBsAg testing. If HBsAg is negative: HBIG (0.06 ml/kg) IM plus hepatitis B vaccine series; if HBsAg is positive: no prophylaxis.
Hepatitis C	After needle-stick exposure involving patients with known hepatitis C IG (0.06 ml/kg) IM should be given, although the effectivity of IG is not proven.
HIV	After needle-stick exposure involving patients with proven HIV treatment with AZT (zidovudine) should be considered. Treatment must be started within 30 min with 250 mg p.o. or 200 mg i.v. (starting later then 6 h after exposure seems to be ineffective) followed by 5 × 250 mg p.o. daily for 2 weeks.
Meningococcal disease	There are very few cases of proven nosocomial transmission of *Neisseria meningitidis* to hospital personnel taking care of patients with meningococcemia and meningococcal meningitis. Therefore, antimicrobial prophylaxis (2 × 600 mg rifampin for 2 days) should be offered to HCW only if intimate exposure to nasopharyngeal secretions occurs (e.g., unprotected mouth-to-mouth resuscitation).
Tuberculosis	If personnel are exposed to an infective patient and proper precautions were not used, it is important to skin-test these personnel immediately for baseline testing and a second time 10 weeks later. If a conversion occurs, further diagnostic steps (chest X-ray, bacteriology) must be initiated and INH therapy should be considered. BCG vaccination is not recommended generally; however, in areas with a high incidence it should be considered.
Varicella-zoster	HCW not known to be immune to varicella should receive VZIG (15–25 units/kg) within 96 h after exposure.

ment the route and circumstances of exposure and the identity of the person whose body fluid was involved in the exposure, unless such identification is not feasible or is illegal. Blood from the source individual must be tested as soon as possible for HIV and HBV status unless the patient is already known to be positive (OSHA Blood-borne Hazard Standard). Serologic testing of the exposed health care worker should be done immediately and after 1, 2, 3, and 6 months. When postexposure prophylatic treatment is deemed necessary and is offered, personnel must be informed of alternative means of prophylaxis, risk of infection if treatment is not accepted, degree of protection provided by the prophylactic therapy, and potential side effects (Table 7).

Suggested Reading

ACP Task Force on Adult Immunization (1989) Guide for adult immunization, 2nd edn. American College of Physicians, Philadelphia, PA

Benenson AS (ed) (1985) Control of communicable diseases in man, 14th edn. American Public Health Association, Washington, DC

Decker MD (1992) The OSHA bloodborne hazard standard. Infect Control Hosp Epidemiol 13:407–417

Fedson DS (1987) Immunization for health care workers and patients in hospitals. In: Wenzel RP (ed) Prevention and control of nosocomial infections. Williams and Wilkens, Baltimore, pp 116–173

Kappstein I, Daschner F (1988) Hygienic and organizational precautions to prevent transmission of selected viral infections in hospital. Immun Infekt 16:192–196

Klein JO (1981) Management of infections in hospital employees. Am J Med 70:919–923

Kretzschmar HA, Dahme E (1990) BSE – Die spongiformen Enzephalopathien und die Prionhypothese. Dtsch Arztebl 87:C1681–1686

Polder JA, Tablan OC, Williams WW (1992) Personnel health services. In: Bennett JV, Brachman PS (eds) Hospital infections, 3rd edn. Little Brown, Boston, pp 31–62

Ravilochan K, Tyler KL (1992) Human transmissible neurodegenerative diseases. Semin Neurol 12:178–192

Riegler R, Schmutzhard E, Skladal D, Stronegger W (1990) Nosokomiale Infektionen bei neurologischen Intensivpatienten. Eine retrospektive klinische und epidemiologische Analyse. Antibiot Monitor (Austria) 6:93–95

Williams WW (1983) CDC guidelines for infection control in hospital personnel. Infect Control 4[Suppl]:326–332

World Health Organisation (1992) Inactivated hepatitis A vaccine. Weekly Epidemiol Rec 67:261–263

Chapter 18

Organizing Nursing Care in a Neurocritical Care Unit

JUDITH SKI LOWER and BERTHILDE GANZ

Introduction

The organization of nursing and nursing care in a neurocritical care unit should be driven by a specific vision that becomes both the foundation and the driving force behind the organization of the nurses and their work processes. Organized correctly, the outcome will be quality, cost-efficient, holistic care produced by competent, satisfied nurses well served by each other and their unit.

Getting started is as simple as deciding what the nurses need to *do* and what they need to *know* every day in the "ideal unit." To achieve this, there are five critical factors that must be addressed: (1) daily and weekly processes, (2) clinical knowledge and skills, (3) patient care delivery system, (4) professional development, and (5) an environment that supports and maximizes the nurses' ability to do their job.

Organizing Daily and Weekly Processes

Establishing Clinical Standards

First, clinical expectations must be established that: (1) allow safe, acceptable practice regardless of patient acuity during a shift or the experience of the caregiver, (2) clearly distinguish nursing responsibility from that of the physician, (3) provide nurses with the autonomy to act independently and interdependently to initiate appropriate interventions, and (4) optimize outcomes.

These clinical standards may be designed around a medical diagnosis, nursing diagnosis, psychosocial state, or a body system. They must clearly identify what is expected of the nurse in terms of assessment, intervention, documentation, and reportable conditions. Examples of clinical standards are protocols, procedures, standardized plans of care, and standing orders. In order to have firsthand knowledge of these standards that guide their daily practice, the staff nurses should be involved in their de-

Section Editor: Michael N. Diringer

velopment, have mandatory review sessions at least twice a year, and review/revise them annually. These standards should then be critically assessed and approved by the medical director of the unit, both to provide validation and to support the nurses in their practice.

Establishing Operational Standards

Secondly, the operational expectations or standards must be addressed. These include, but are not limited to: (1) the chain of command to be used for clinical and administrative issues, (2) the method to be used to insure qualified neurocritical care nurses are always available to care for the patients, and (3) a communication system that allows issues to be addressed in a timely, productive manner while fostering teamwork.

A chain of command is essential in the NCCU. Nurses must clearly understand who is to be notified and in what order for clinical issues/events. An algorithm called "the nurse is concerned" is useful in defining what is expected (Fig. 1). A copy may be placed in each bedside chart for ready reference. The focus is safe management of the patient. It is important that nurses be supported in their use of this algorithm, even when they are inaccurate in their assessment, so that they will always be willing to act as a patient advocate.

The ability to notice subtle, clinical changes, and to understand the implications of those changes, is essential in caring for a critically ill neurological patient. When high acuity necessitates an increase in staffing, it is imperative that skilled neurocritical care nurses be available. There are several ways to organize a staff to achieve this goal. One is to salary the staff so that they may be flexed up, or down, to meet the demands of the current patient population. An on-call system, compensated with pay-back of time worked, is a cost-effective way of matching patient care demands with the supply of staff. Nurses may work extra when the demand is high, and be able to go/stay home when the census drops while still receiving a full pay check. An alternative used in Heidleberg is to mobilize additional nurses when needed by calling them on a rotational basis on their time off to request assistance.

Several strategies allow organization of a communication system to ensure the timely and productive attendance to issues. A senior staff nurse can be assigned each week to keep his/her eyes and ears open and "antennae UP". The role, in addition to his/her regular duties, is to literally monitor the environment, the relationships, teamwork, acuity, patient care issues, clinical practice, adequacy of support services, and the effectiveness of daily processes. Having a formalized process to review how each week has gone is essential to determine what facilitates or hinders ideal practice, to develop action plans, and to implement them immediately. This is accomplished during a weekly meeting with the senior nurse, the nurse manager, and the physician in charge.

It is helpful to establish a formal mechanism for identifying problematic issues or events that insures a critical retrospective review to determine what could have been done differently. If the issue needs to be followed up, the formal mechanism must include a

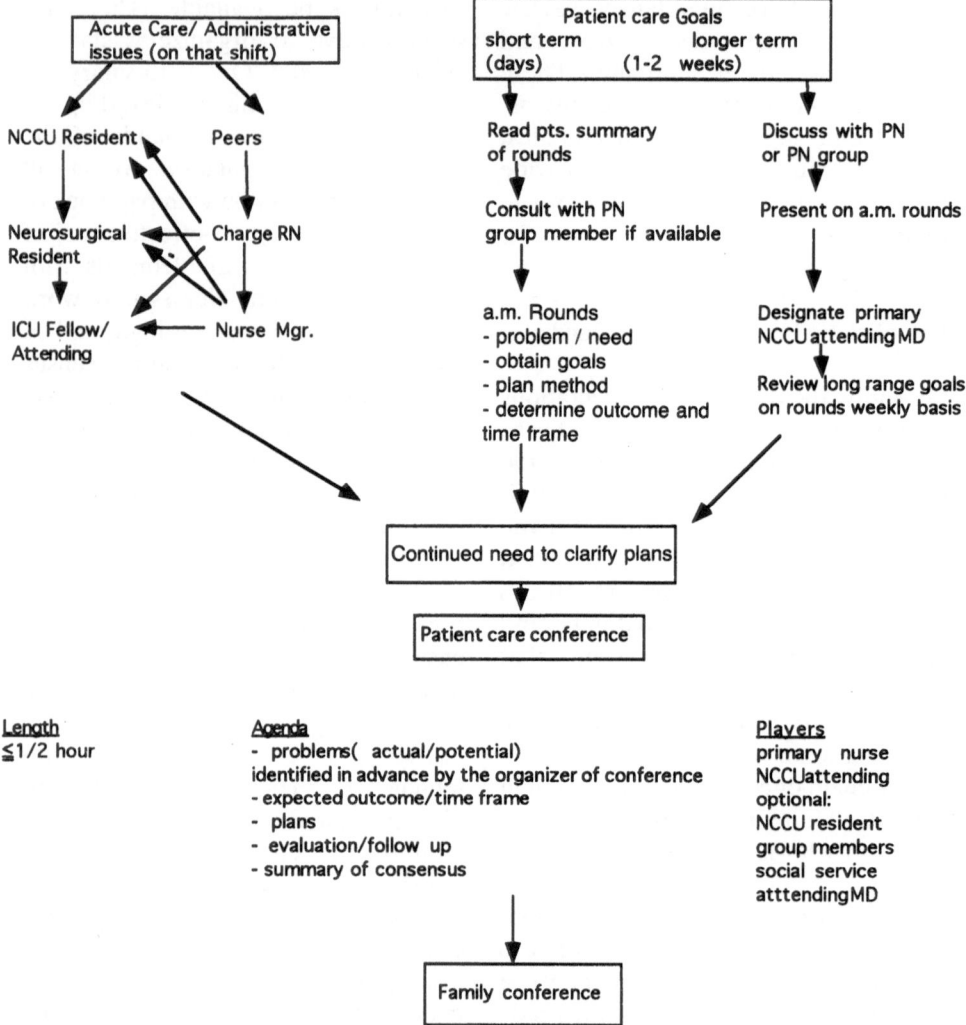

Fig. 1. The nurse is concerned algorithm

means of doing this. A Problem Identification Sheet is used to initiate this process and is shown in Fig. 2.

The Role of Nursing in a Multidisciplinary Team

Multidisciplinary rounds are an excellent way to maximize and accentuate the contribution of nursing to the team. Because the nurse is the care giver most often at the bedside, the nurse caring for a particular patient can present the raw patient data for the past 24h to the rest of the team utilizing a systems approach (see Fig. 3). The nurse benefits from participating in discussions about trends, academic questions, formulating plans, and evaluating the results from a mul-

Problem Identification Sheet NCCU

Date _____	If a patient is involved:
Time of Problem _____	Name _____
Reported by: _____	History: _____
Department Involved _____	Confidential? No Yes
Name of Person involved _____	

Type of Problem: (circle) Equip/supplies, MD/Rx Plan, Support Service, other _____

Problem Describe nature/circumstances. State time sequence. Be specific

What was done at that time to solve the problem?

In retrospect, is there something that you could have done to minimize, prevent, or solve the problem?

Outcome:

Fig. 2. Problem identification sheet for the neurocritical care unit

tidisciplinary perspective. At the end of each patient discussion, plans are verbally summarized, orders written, and then read out loud to all participants to ensure concensus. All are now focused on the same outcome for the patient and family for the next 24 h. The nurse participating in rounds summarizes the plans, rationale, desired outcome, etc. on a communication sheet for ready reference for nurses who follow her, or who have been off for a few days and want to catch up.

Our nursing colleagues in Germany also participate in daily morning rounds, which include a short discussion of each patient's problems with all the physicians involved in that patient's care. They are proud of the fact that the work is shared between the nurses and doctors without a strict line between what each should do. The focus is on working as a team, which improves both patient care and the overall working environment.

Clinical Knowledge and Skills

Empowering nurses with the knowledge base needed to perform competently and confidently is the second critical factor in organizing a nursing staff.

Envisioning what the nurse's fund of knowledge should include in order to handle *any* clinical situation is the starting point. This ideal nurse is usually one who has been in an NCCU for at least 3 years. In order not to overwhelm the new nurse and yet insure adequate knowledge of the essential *basics* of neurological, cardiac, and respiratory knowledge, what the nurse needs to know to be *safe*, confident, and able to handle routine patients and common emergencies is pulled from that large, ideal fund of knowledge. This list becomes what is taught first. The fund of knowledge may be divided into multiple levels

Dx/Operation
Day shift

		rounds	evenings	nights

```
N  ICU Day_____  Post-OP_____
E  GCS_____  Pupils_____  CN_____
U  Motor_____  RUE_____  LUE_____
R  _____  RLE_____  LLE _____
O  ICP_____  Rx: HVL_____
   Steroids_____
   DPH_____  Level_____
   Psych_____
   Sleep_____
   Pain MGMT_____
   Other_____
   _____

C  BP_____  Goal_____
A  Rx BP_____
R  Hr_____  Rhythm/ectopy_____
D  Hemodynamics:              Rx
I  CO/CI_____
A  Preload_____
C  Afterload_____
   Contractility_____
   _____

   Fluid status: ____
   TF/hr__  24 hr. balance_____
   Wt_____  UO_____  SpGr_____
   IV's_____
   _____

   Labs_____
   _____
```

Fig. 3. Systems approach

and taught on an annual, progressive basis (e.g., Year One, Year Two, Year Three) or in relation to a career ladder requirement (e.g., clinical nurse, master nurse, expert nurse). This progressive program allows an already established forum to teach new information or procedures.

Each level must have specific objectives, standardized class content, audiovisual aids to enhance learning, and a method of testing the learning. An example is given in Table 1. The education should be on a predetermined schedule which continuously builds on previously learned information and moves the nurse to a higher level of "critical thinking" capability. To move to one level, the nurse must pass a written competency examination based on the previous level's material.

The written competency exam: (1) provides staff with an opportunity to demonstrate their academic learning, (2) allows management to objectively assess their staff's level of knowledge, and (3) promotes planned reviewing and updating of material based on trends in test results.

Much of the neurological content of the classes is taken from the American Association of Neuroscience Nurses Core Curriculum and the cardiac and respiratory content is taken from the American Association of Critical Care Nurses Core Curriculum. Thus the nurses are simul-

		rounds	evenings	nights
R	day shift			
E	Mode___ Resp Rate_____			
S	FIO2_____ PEEP/CPAP_____			
P	PS___ Vt___ Ex VOL_____			
I	SaO2_____ EndTidal CO2_____			
R	ABG_____			
	Wean_____			
	NHO_____			
	CXR_____ Breath sounds_____			
	Secretions_____ Sx_____			
	CPT_____ IS_____			
	Other_____			
	_____			
	Diet_____			
	Rate_____ Residuals____			
G	GI Meds_____			
I	Stools_____			
	Rx_____			
	Glu_____ Ca_____ Phos_____			
	Supplements_____			
	Dexi_____			
	Other_____			
	_____			
	T max_____ WBC_____			
I	Antibiotics: Day/dose_____			
D	_____			
	Cultures_____			
	Line Status_____			
	Wound Status_____			
	_____			
	Spokesperson_____			
	FM Issues_____			
	_____			
	Physical care given_____			
	_____			

Fig. 3

taneously being prepared to take their national certification examinations in both neuroscience nursing (CNRN) and critical care (CCRN).

As to the teaching, a clinical nurse specialist or a clinical instructor may be employed to develop and teach all the classes. An alternative successful strategy is to give staff the opportunity to select different levels and be responsible for teaching them to their peers. The benefits of this alternative method are several: (1) peer staff nurses are available on all shifts to serve as sources of information in clinical questions, (2) it is an excellent developmental strategy, (3) the teaching nurse's confidence and competence are both increased. Unit teachers are carefully mentored in the beginning by a seasoned lecturer to insure adequate ability and a pleasing style.

Skills that are essential to the safe care of the neuroscience patient must be validated annually. The focus should be high-volume, high-risk skills as well as low-volume, high-risk skills or procedures which have changed in

Table 1. NCCU educational levels

Level 1	Level 2	Level 3	Level 4
Neuro A & P	Spinal cord injury	12-Lead ECGs	Brain resuscitation
Neuroassessment	(incomplete lesions,	Infarct patterns	Oxygen delivery
Increased ICP	autonomic dysreflexia)	Electrical activity	Oxygen consumption
ICP monitoring	Hypoxemias	of the heart	Jugular bulbs
Head injury	V/Q mismatch	Oxygen content	Clinical application of
Spinal cord injury	Pulmonary emboli	Infections (basic	AVDO$_2$
Hydrocephalus	DVT	principles,	Vasoactive substances
Cerebral circulation	ARDS	antimicrobial	(arachodonic acid
CVA	Advanced hemodynamics	therapy)	cascade, leukotrienes,
AVM	Pharmocology II	WBC and	prostaglandins, and
SAH	CPK curves	differential	thromboxane A)
Brain death	Ventilation	AaDO$_2$	Sepsis (clinical
Myasthenia	Pneumothorax		application of
Guillain Barré	Visual pathways		vasoactive substances)
Seizures	Cerebellar s/s		DIC
Brain tumors	UMN/LMN		Renal tubular physiology
Encephalitis	S/S r/t vessel		
Respiratory	Pacemakers		
Dysrhythmias	Junctional rhythms		
Pharmacology I			
Cardiac Output			
Hemodynamics I			
Shock			
Monitors			

A & P, anatomy & physiology; ICP, intracranial pressure; CVA, cerebrovascular accident; AVM, arteriovenous malformation; SAH, Subarachnoidal hemorrhage; DVT, deep vein thrombosis; ARDS, acute respiratory distress syndrome; CPK, creatine phosphokinase; UMN/LMN, upper and lower motor neuron; WBC, white blood cell; DIC, disseminated intravascular coagulation.

the past year. The review should be planned to be fun as well as educational. One way of organizing a skills review is to hold it annually or semiannually and conduct it with multiple stations that each participant must pass through. Each station has objectives, content, and a post test (usually a return demonstration).

The instructors should be members of the unit staff so they know the real issues and problems associated with this skill, can field any question relative to that unit's practice, and be available as resources in the future.

The annual review is a good opportunity to upgrade skills, demonstrate continued competency, and clarify practice or procedures.

Nurses in Germany approach clinical knowledge in quite a different way. All nurses train for 3 years to gain a registered nurse certificate; however, in order to qualify as an advanced nurse, which earns a degree as an qualified intensive care unit (ICU) nurse, one must continue for 2 more years. That additional 2-year program consists of academic and clinical training and is divided into two main areas. One is oriented to internal medicine (general internal medicine, cardiology, gastroenterology, nephrology with dialysis and neurology) and the other has a surgical focus (general surgery, neurosurgery, cardiac and vascular surgery, and organ transplantation). The nurse must obtain experience on all types of ICUs involved in this program. The neurologic ICU in Heidelberg is utilized for the internal medicine focus. Training in different ICUs is accomplished by teaching sessions, on-the-job training with a qualified ICU nurse, periodic written tests, and an overall examination at the end of the 2-year period. Specific areas of training during the first 6 weeks in the Heidelberg neurological ICU include: observation of respiratory, cardiac, and renal function; recognition of pathologic patterns and dysfunctions; care of the artifically ventilated patient and the patient with increased intracranial pressure; and care of long-term neurologic patients (stroke, meningitis and Guillain-Barré syndrome).

In Germany, as well as most European countries, it remains difficult to hire and retain ICU nurses, despite modernization of the ICUs, the provision of the newest technologies, the utilization of more flexible schedules, and more satisfactory working conditions.

Patient Care Delivery System

There are several patient care delivery systems available. Whichever one is utilized, (1) its demands and practice must be known by all nurses in the unit and (2) it must make adequate provision for the three A's (autonomy, authority, and accountability) in clinical practice.

Primary nursing is an ideal system for a neurologic unit because it provides for *consistency* in care. Neurologic changes are often subtle and noted only by those most familiar with the patient. Inherent in this concept is the need to provide support for the Primary Nurse. A method for accomplishing this is by use of Primary Nursing Groups. The goals of this approach are to: (1) provide support and accountability to the Primary Nurse, (2) provide 24-h consistency in caregivers, (3) capitalize on the talents/abilities of each member of the group, and (4) provide mentorship in the process to insure growth in both critical thinking and bedside skills.

How does one organize a staff to do this? See Fig. 4. Each group should contain nurses on different shifts, with a variety of different skills (cardiac, psychosocial, neurologic research, etc.) and a range of experience. Recognizing that a two-patient assignment is typical (or maximal) in an intensive care unit, each group will carry a two-patient primary load. Each group self-schedules, as a group, to provide the best 24-h coverage they can for their patients. Daily assignments are made to match: e.g., a group three patient with a group three nurse. Although one nurse (the primary nurse) remains accountable for the outcome of the patient, the entire group is there to support him/her in this effort. Care planning is a group effort, as is bringing in educational articles dealing with the patient's diagnosis, medications, etc., and seeking out additional resources to assist the patient and or family.

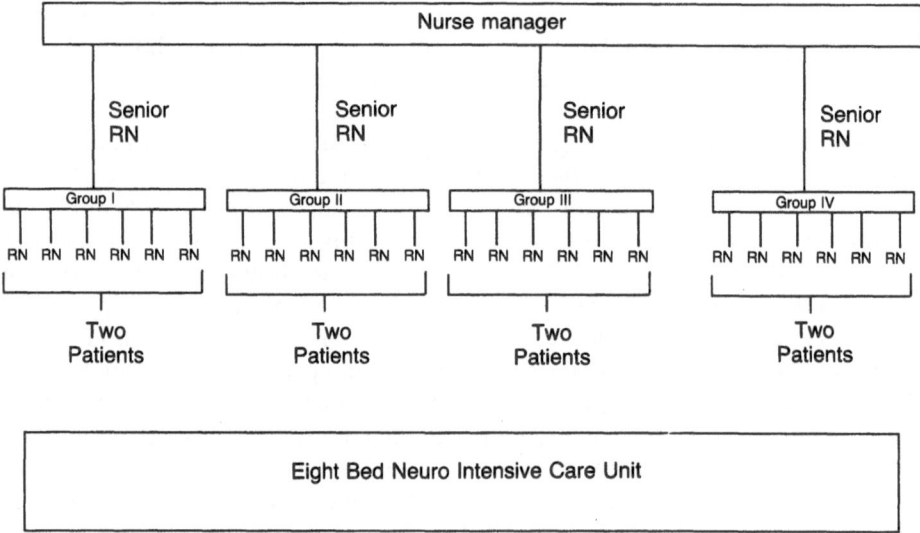

Fig. 4. Organizing primary nursing group (in the USA only). *RN*, registered nurse

Functioning as a group allows increased risk taking in creative approaches to care, less "burn out" in regard to long-term patients, a care plan that is the result of five or six nurses' input based on their experience with this patient and family as well as with the disease, and reduced time spent in reporting because all members are so familiar with the patient.

The quality of care given to these two patients is often *directly* related to the ability of the group to function as a cohesive team with clear patient/family goals. To insure that they do work as a team, there is a Senior Nurse who heads each group, carefully mentored and supervised by the Nurse Manager. This group leader is responsible for the growth and development of each nurse, for monitoring the daily process of the group (clinically as well as interpersonally), and for being a role model to other staff. The group meets for 4 h every six weeks, outside the unit and on unit time, to get to know each other better, to review audits done on their patients during the last 6 weeks, to critically review the care and outcomes of their patients, to pursue a formal educational program for their own development, and to provide support/encouragement to each other.

In order to insure adequate knowledge of the patient care delivery system, a series of classes staged over a minimum of 2 years is helpful. These classes may include the definition and source of the three A's, group structure/process, care planning, auditing, group dynamics, patients' developmental needs, families in crisis, etc. (Table 2).

Professional Development

The unit and institution in which nurses work have a responsibility to ensure

Table 2. Four-phase primary nursing classes

	Phase I (0–3 months)	Phase II (6 months)	Phase III (1 year)	Phase IV (18–24 months)
Concept autonomy, authority, account-ability	Definition Historical perspective Team nursing vs, primary nursing	Definition of the three A's M. Manthey's 5 principles Accountability to patient/fm	Source of three A's Utilization of the 3 A's in daily practice Accountability to peers	Impact of todays healthcare environment on the tenets of the PN concept Accountability to physicians
Care planning	Patient profile Nursing diagnosis Use of the care plans to organize care	Assessment, problem identification, goals, interventions, evaluation Use of protocols	Monitoring of PN paperwork via process and outcomes audits	Theorist (nursing and others) Orem, Maslow, Erickson, etc.
Family and crisis	Initial interview Immediate needs Teaching Spokesperson for the family	Family conference: timing, goal, content, participants	Acute crisis: Phases, approach influencing factors, needs Genograms	Chronic crisis Complex genograms
Rounds	Times, format, goals and participants	Taking a strong patient advocate stand Facilitating long term planning on rounds	Critiquing peer adherence to the established format of rounds	
PN groups	Purpose and structure PN Meetings	Function of the group in R/T: pt/ fm, peers, and NCCU ID mechanisms for group PN patient pickup.	Utilizing audit tools to evaluate group process in PN goals	

PN, primary nursing; R/T, related to; pt/fm, patient/family; NCCU, neurocritical care unit; ID, identification.

on-going opportunities that allow each nurse's talents to be nurtured and developed, maximize interpersonal relationships so energies are focused where they should be, and allow the staff to both be "stretched" and to feel good about their professional development.

Unit-Based Committees

Nurses need opportunity, experience, and responsibility in managing their own unit beyond hands-on patient care. Unit-based committees afford this opportunity. The number and type of committees depends on unit needs. Examples of committees might be:

primary nursing, education, scheduling, code, social, helicopter, equipment, budget, quality assurance/improvement, peer review, and recruitment. Unit time should be provided to do the work for these committees in predetermined amounts. Annual goals and outcomes should be communicated to the entire staff on a quarterly basis. Bulletin boards, staff meetings, or a unit-based newsletter offer excellent media for such communication. Minutes from each meeting are reviewed by the Nurse Manager to keep her informed, to utilize her ideas and suggestions for resources, and to prevent duplication or confusion between multiple committees addressing similar issues.

Interpersonal Relationships

Often ignored, but perhaps the most critical area if there is a problem, is that of fostering supportive, open peer relationships. Nurses should be educated in how to give feedback to peers, to negotiate (not give way), to reach concensus, and to resolve conflict. Mechanisms should be established to handle situations where one-to-one feedback is not effective. They can include assistance from a Senior Nurse, the Nurse Manager, or a Peer Review Committee.

Essential to the tone of each shift is the role of the Charge Nurse and the ability of that nurse to manage routine as well as crisis occurrences. The preparation for this role must be equal to its level of importance. Topics for an all-day preparatory class for this role are shown in Table 3. The nurse new to the role must be mentored for at least a month before assuming the role

Table 3. Content for "charge nurse" class

Purpose/expectations of role
Making assignments
Giving report
Assigning jobs
Conflicts with assignments
Routine admissions
Routine transfers
Bed reservations
Hold bed
Triage rounds: MD and RN
Emergencies:
  Codes
  Fires
  Disasters
  Helicopter admission
  Deteriorating patient on the floor
Administrative issues:
  Sick calls
  Lateness
  Holidays
  Vacation
  Decreased census
  Increased acuity
  When to call the nurse manager
  Calls from the police
  Calls from the media
Requests for nursing consults from other units
Borrowing/lending equipment
Needle sticks and on the job injuries
Change in patient status
When to call the medical director
Questioning a residents plan
Handling angry patient/family/physican
Handling controlled substances
Support services:
  Housekeeping
  Pharmacy
  Escort
  Dietary
  Lab medicine
  Social services
  Pastoral services
  Clinical engineering
Patient valuables
Medications brought from home
Isolations procedure review
Visitor faints/is injured
Peer conflicts:
  Inappropriate behavior
  Can't handle assignment
  "Super Nurse"
Triage decisions
Use of students, assistants
Pediatric cases

independently. Back-up advisors (even if only by telephone) should always be available to guide or support the Charge Nurse in decision making should the need arise.

Nurse Managers must always be alert for opportunities to stretch the capabilities of their more talented staff with expanded roles. One approach is to divide the role of the Nurse Manager into administrative, staffing/scheduling, education, budget, and clinical practice areas (primary nursing and quality improvement). Senior staff may be rotated through each section for a 4-month rotation, carefully mentored by the Nurse Manager. The goal is to educate and empower the staff nurses to make decisions and manage these areas in ways that best meet the needs of the unit. Scheduled time is provided to accomplish these tasks. The result is not only professional growth for the staff, but a unit with extremely knowledgable nurses who can make decisions from a globally informed position even in the absence of the Manager. Advanced levels on a career ladder can be easily reached through this system.

The nursing organizational structure in Germany is quite different and reflects the fact that their existing system does not provide for a true "career" for nurses. This situation is currently being addressed. There are three types of nurses: those who do routine nursing jobs, those who have qualified to be shift leaders (which requires an additional 3 months of on-the-job training), and the Managing Nurse. The Managing Nurse is usually assigned to one department and has a truly administrative focus. The Nurse Manager has a very powerful and important position, being on the same political level as the Director of the department.

Quality Assurance/Quality Improvement

Ideal, successful units view this topic as a shared opportunity to improve care rather than as a punitive task carried out by some outsider. Professional nurses need to understand the process of moving from a problem focus (quality assurance) or an ideal focus (quality improvement) to a focus on outcome. Properly focused, this process can improve patient outcomes, make the nurses' job easier, and be fun to do. In the Neurocritical Care Unit at Johns Hopkins Hospital, it is a requirement that *all* nurses do both a quality assurance and a quality improvement project each year to insure their understanding of the process and to improve practice in many small ways. Their peers on the Quality Assurance/Quality Improvement Committee are the ones that mentor them through this exercise.

Creating an Environment that Supports and Maximizes Nurses' Ability to Do Their Jobs

Everyday hassle factors found on the job will, over time, undermine even the most cohesive, productive staff. These factors must be continuously sought out, addressed by whoever owns the problem, and put to rest. Staff need to have consistent avenues of communication to express their feelings about these factors without fear of reprisal.

Staff meetings, held at least quarterly, whose only function is to identify current unresolved hassle factors are helpful. Surveys conducted at least annually on a variety of topics provide staff with a forum to communicate how well the environment is working for them. Surveys around the subjects of job satisfaction, relationships with the medical team or Nurse Manager, adequacy of support services, educational opportunities, etc., provide the Nurse Manager with the necessary information to make changes in the unit's practice and/or processes. Frequently seemingly unresolvable issues that the staff have given up on, e.g., less than adequate service from the Pharmacy Department, can be resolved in time, freeing up the staff's energies to do their real jobs.

Neurocritical care units in both the USA and Germany are increasing their utilization of non-nursing personnel to provide for transportation of supplies, medications, and patients and to assist with care and tasks. This is an effort to allow nurses more time and opportunity to devote to performing truly nursing-oriented tasks.

Summary

The bottom line in organizing a nursing staff is to remember that *THE MOST VALUABLE COMMODITY* any unit has is its nursing staff, each and every one of them. We must learn to respect and treasure their individuality and diversity. We must also remember that, treated with respect, made to feel like valuable members of a team, given opportunities to be challenged and grow professionally, they are an invaluable asset in creating an excellent neurocritical care unit.

| # Early Rehabilitation

VOLKER HÖMBERG and JAMES N. DAVIS

Introduction

The improvement in neurocritical care, extensively reviewed in this volume, has magnificently increased the number of patients surviving major brain injury and prolonged states of coma. This development has raised the question of when to begin the rehabilitation process. We must confess that we know only very little about the proper techniques to be used in this "early" rehabilitation. The goal of this chapter is to discuss some of the aims and rationales of rehabilitation in the early stages, when the patient is still in coma or in a confused state.

Early Rehabilitation: Attempt at a Definition

We want to define early rehabilitation as an integrated multiprofessional approach combining pharmacological and training techniques, which should start as soon as the patient is out of immediate life-threatening distress but still needs monitoring. There is general agreement that such a systematic early rehabilitation approach can start as soon as the patient no longer needs artificial ventilation and his or her other vital functions, including intracranial pressure, are sufficiently stabilized. The aim of early rehabilitation is to facilitate spontaneous recovery and to improve the disease state as far as possible, in order to prevent permanent disability and handicap. In this sense early rehabilitation is the beginning of an ongoing chain of rehabilitation programs leading to optimal return of the patient to his previous social and vocational environment.

The most frequent target groups for early rehabilitation in neurology and neurosurgery are patients with head injuries, severe stroke, or brain operations and those with severe afflictions of the peripheral nervous system such as acute polyradiculitis, giving rise to a severe paralysis.

Section Editor: Michael N. Diringer

Goals of Early Rehabilitation

A simple, easily understandable goal of early rehabilitation measures is the prevention of further damage to the central or peripheral nervous system, mostly by using appropriate pharmacological treatment for brain edema or neuroprotective agents. Another goal is to prevent possible sequelae of immobilization such as bed sores, contractures, or muscle ossification by intensive physiotherapy. Furthermore, early rehabilitation techniques should be aimed at facilitating the process of spontaneous recovery after brain injury, e.g., by introducing systematic challenges to the inborn plasticity of the central nervous system. An example of such a strategy is coma stimulation, to improve the state of consciousness, or language facilitation, to improve the communicative abilities of the patient.

The Therapeutic Team

At present the organization of early rehabilitation units is highly variable between hospitals and between different countries. Early rehabilitation units can be attached to emergency hospitals where the primary neurological or neurosurgical interventions take place. This has the advantage that the patient is close to all the necessary facilities for immediate intervention in case of complications. The disadvantage of this location is that in emergency hospitals the knowledge and expertise in rehabilitative techniques is relatively low, and hence it may be difficult to install an appropriate therapeutic team in such an environment. Therefore, it is often preferable to set up such a unit in a rehabilitation hospital with existing professional knowledge of rehabilitative techniques where a therapeutic team specialized in aspects of early rehabilitation can more easily be created. The optimal size of an early rehabilitation unit is between ten and 15 patients. Smaller units usually cannot work in a cost-effective way; on the other hand, it is difficult to manage team interactions in larger units.

Of key importance for the efficacy of an early rehabilitation unit is the construction of a multidisciplinary team of physicians, nurses, and therapists. The team should be directed by a neurologist or neurosurgeon with special training in neurological rehabilitation and a solid background in the neurobiology of brain plasticity. This physician has to decide about the necessary qualifications of the staff, and is also responsible for in-house training of staff and for the organization of academic activities in the unit, e.g., the organization of therapeutic trials.

The nursing staff must combine qualifications in acute critical care of patients with those in activation nursing, i.e., the use of facilitation techniques to improve the patient's state. This encompasses special skills in mobilizing the patient, positioning the patient in bed, neurourological interventions such as bladder training, and handling communication problems, as well as skills concerning the re-teaching of activities of daily living.

The physical therapist's primary tasks in an early rehabilitation unit are to improve the motor and sensory state of the patient, to avoid sequelae such as bed sores or contractures, to decrease possible symptoms such as spasticity or involuntary movement, and to facilitate residual motor abilities of the patient.

The occupational therapists should be able to handle stimulation techniques together with the nurses and to perform cognitive training procedures to improve perception and motor abilities of the patients, including orofacial movements such as swallowing and vocalization.

The speech pathologists must have experience in early facilitation of communication as well as experience in the application of orofacial training.

Psychologists should also be part of the early rehabilitation unit. Generally, it is not possible to use the standard neuropsychological evaluation techniques with patients at this very early stage. Therefore, the psychologists must know about cognitive assessment methods in confused states as well as about possible learning mechanisms in these states (see below). They should further be able to design learning procedures for the patients according to their present cognitive states. Finally, it is of great importance for the functioning of a rehabilitation team working permanently with patients in critical conditions to stabilize the psychological balance between the patient, the team, and – not least – the relatives. Relatives usually are overwhelmed by the condition of the patient, who appears to them as a strange and altered person. This generates much psychological distress both in families and in the team. Therefore, the psychologist in early rehabilitation should be sufficiently trained in psychotherapeutic techniques to deal both with the relatives and with the team, in order to cope with such an emotionally stressful situation.

Hence, a large number of therapeutic professionals participate in such an early rehabilitation team. Nevertheless, it is extremely important that these experts from various disciplines act as a homogeneous team with well-structured communication. There must be clearly defined responsibilities but also clearly defined overlap between responsibilities.

So far, there is no gold standard concerning the optimal environmental setup for an early rehabilitation unit. On the one hand, there are requirements such as technical monitoring equipment, which has to be present around the patient. On the other hand, there is good evidence that a friendly and somewhat "enriched" environment is preferable to clean and sterile hospital surroundings. It has been shown that just the chance to look out of a window may improve the status of patients after surgery (Ulrich 1984). Details about including the possible risk of overstimulation of patients are discussed below in the section on coma stimulation. Apart from this, an early rehabilitation unit should provide a friendly, psychologically stable atmosphere with various means of audiovisual stimulation as well as the possibility of rooming-in relatives.

Rationales for Neurorehabilitation Treatments

Table 1 gives a hierarchically organized list of possible intervention strategies to improve a particular behavior after a permanent lesion has occurred in the central nervous system.

Table 1. Hierarchy of intervention strategies

- Restoration of impaired structure
- Unmasking of alternative structures
- Teaching behavioral bypass strategies
- Using technical aid devices
- Adapting the environment

By far the most desirable would be the restoration of impaired structure. There have been numerous attempts in this direction, e.g., by means of implantation of autogeneic or heterogenic nervous tissue into the brains of patients suffering from degenerative disorders affecting major wide-projecting neurotransmitter systems, such as in Parkinson's disease. However, these methods today are restricted to simple neurotransmitter systems, and the evidence is far from complete that these attempts work in the long term. Nevertheless, advances in molecular biology and neurogenetics make it likely that this avenue will become more and more feasible.

The next possible rationale is to unmask or "wake up" possible alternative structures, which have escaped central nervous system damage, to take over the task of the damaged tissue, thus exploiting the redundancy and plasticity of the system. There is ample evidence from animal studies that changes in peripheral sensory inputs either in terms of reduction of the input, e.g., caused by limb amputation, or by additional sensory input, e.g., by stimulation of particular limb segments, gives rise to structural changes in the cortical projection areas of experimental monkeys. Furthermore, following circumscribed lesions in somatosensory or motor cortical areas in primates, functional reorganization in the intact cortical tissue neighboring the site of the lesion has been shown (for a review see Jenkins et al. 1992). These studies elegantly demonstrated that changes in ongoing information lead to reorganizational changes in the brain.

In addition, it has been shown that such "plastic" cerebral changes can be facilitated by certain pharmacological agents and may be inhibited by others. Especially in early rehabilitation the exploitation of this strategy is a useful approach. The problem is that up to now very little work has been directed at sorting out which particular environmental challenges are able to provoke both pace and extent of functional brain reorganization.

If the unmasking of alternative structures is not possible, hierarchically, the next possible rationale for neurological rehabilitation is to teach the patient systematic bypass strategies to achieve a particular goal by a behavior which is not critically dependent on the lesioned tissue, but uses unimpaired brain structures for its control and completion. Especially in later stages of rehabilitation this approach certainly is the most frequently used. A simple example of such an approach is mnemonic strategies for memory retraining, such as using diaries or first-letter priming. For rehabilitation in the early stages possible applications of bypass strategy learning can be derived from the concept of implicit or procedural learning, which is distinct from explicit or declarative learning. Explicit learning is characterized by the formation of new associations, which is an attention-requiring process linked with conscious recollection of the learned information. In contrast, the implicit learning mechanism is characterized by the strengthening of already existing associations, and is a non-attention-requiring "automatic" process, which can be demonstrated experimentally by more effective processing when information is repeated at a later time. This process of implicit learning is one example of the ability of the central nervous system to process information without awareness. Other examples include the so-called blindsight phenomenon, i.e., the nonconscious identification of objects in "blind" parts of the visual field after infarction of primary visual cortex, or the preservation of motor skills (motor memory) in patients who otherwise have severe impairment in declarative or episodic memory. By comparison between patient groups (for a review see Soliveri et al. 1992) it has been demonstrated that these two distinct memory subsystems also have different neuroanatomical substrates, with the explicit memory system being primarily dependent on the intactness of the midtemporal thalamic and cortical connections, in contrast to the implicit memory system, in which the basal ganglia and the cerebellum appear to be involved. Also on an ontogenetic basis these two memory systems can be separated. Furthermore, it has been demonstrated that using such implicit memory mechanisms, events occurring under general anesthesia can be remembered, and learning of certain motor activities can be achieved even in deep coma. The exploitation of processing without awareness is one of the most challenging neurobiological principles of neurological rehabilitation, especially in the very early stages.

If the teaching of behavioral bypass strategies is not possible, the next step down in the hierarchy of rehabilitation rationales is to use technical aid devices designed to take over particular functions completely. These can be, for example, highly computerized tools for communication and environmental control in a patient with tetraplegia. A critical review of the possibilities of aid devices is given in the chapter by Mauritz (Chap. 20).

Finally, especially in those patients who have lost the ability to learn either behavioral bypass strategies or the use of external aid devices, the only possible means remaining for rehabilitation is to adapt the environment to the patient. This rationale is of particular importance in geriatric populations with vascular or degenerative dementia. However, in early stages of rehabilitation this rationale plays only a minor role and may even be counterproductive, as it does not offer challenges to the system in reorganization.

Pharmacological Approaches

The impact of pharmacological agents for the neuroprotective prevention of further damage after an acute lesion has been discussed in an earlier chapter (Ch. 9). When it comes to problems of early rehabilitation, this aspect of pharmacological enhancement of recovery is important. Much of this work has originated from the laboratory of Feeney and his colleagues (for a review see Feeney and Sutton 1987). In particular, amphetamines have been proven to enhance the recovery of motor impairment in rats after brain injury using the beam-walking paradigm. In contrast, the use of dopamine receptor blockers such as haloperidol proved to delay recovery. Up to now, only a few studies have looked at the impact of recovery-enhancing drugs in man. In a recent study, Crisostomo et al. (1988) demonstrated that the combined use of amphetamines and physical therapy promoted recovery of motor function in patients with stable hemiparesis after an acute stroke with CT-proven lesions restricted to motor cortex: 10 mg of amphetamine in fruit juice administered to four patients resulted in superior improvement in a functional score compared with a matched group of four patients receiving fruit juice alone. Unfortunately, these results have not been replicated so far, although they seem to be promising. Of probably even greater importance is the fact that certain drugs (see Table 2) may be detrimental to rehabilitative outcome. These unfortunately include substances frequently used for the control of high blood pressure, seizures, or psychomotor agitation in patients in the early phase after brain injury. It has to be stated that, for the time being, a recommendation of pos-

sibly useful drugs facilitating recovery cannot be made on firm grounds, whereas the avoidance of certain drugs appears to be more straightforward.

Coma Stimulation

Following the above-mentioned animal experimental data on changes in synaptic connectivity following sensory stimulation, in appears feasible to use sensory stimulation in various modalities to enhance the level of consciousness in coma patients. Much of the enthusiasm for "coma stimulation" was generated by an article published in 1978 in *The Lancet* by Le Winn and Dimanescu. These authors discussed the impact of an "enriched" environment on synaptic reinnervation as a possible means of recovery after brain damage, making the point that an "enrichment" of the environment around the patient is apt to improve recovery. This follows the simple model that the interruption of afferent input to central nervous system networks causes deprivation and lowering of arousal. The concept follows the work of Galbraith et al. (1978) comparing synaptic reinnervation in rats with the rate of recovery after head injury in man.

Since then the idea of stimulating patients in coma by enrichment of the environment has become a feasible issue. The question remains, however, as to which particular pattern, dosage, and modality mixture of sensory stimulation is the most helpful in achieving this goal in patients with a particular pathology. It must be noted that up to now we do not definitely know which doses and which patterns

Table 2. List of drugs and their classification in the study of the effect of drugs on recovery of function (From Goldstein et al. 1990)

Detrimental drugs
- Clonidine
- Prazosin
- Phenytoin
- Benzodiazepines
- Dopamine receptor antagonists

Neutral drugs
- Other antihypertensives
- Other anticonvulsants

of stimulation are useful or not. Although it appears, at first glance, reasonable to deliver as much sensory stimulation to a coma patient as possible, it cannot be excluded that overstimulation may have even counterproductive effects on recovery in the central nervous system due to habituation effects. Many of these problems have recently been reviewed by Wood (1991). It is certainly necessary in the future for coma stimulation techniques to be based on clearly defined clinical trials. Coma stimulation appears to bear a promising potential for reorganization of consciousness using the above-mentioned modes of processing without awareness.

Suggested Reading

Bach-y-Rita P (1991) Applications of principles of brain plasticity and training to restore function. In: Young RR, Delwaide PJ (eds) Principles of restorative neurology. Butterworth, London

Corkin S (1968) Acquisition of motor skill after bilateral medical temporal lobe excision. Neuropsychologogia 6:155-265

Crisostomo EA, Duncan PW, Propst MA, Dawson DB, Davis JN (1988) Evidence that amphetamine with physical therapy promotes recovery of motor function in stroke patients. Ann Neurol 23:94-97

Feeney DM, Sutton RL (1987) Pharmacotherapy for recovery of function after brain injury. Crit Rev Neurobiol 3:135-197

Galbraith S, Jennett B, Raismang B (1978) Recovery from coma and reinnervation rate. Lancet 1:710

Goldstein LB, Matchar DB, Morgenlander JC, Davis JN (1990) Drugs influence the recovery of function after stroke. Stroke 21:179

Hömberg V, Bickmann U, Müller K (1993) Ontogeny is different for explicit and implicit memory in humans. Neurosci Lett 150:187-190

Jenkins WM, Merzenich MM, Ochs MT, Allard T, Guic-Robies E (1990) Functional reorganization of primary somatosensory cortex in adult owl monkeys after behaviourally controlled tactile stimulation. J Neurophysiol 63:82-104

LeVere TE, Brugler T, Sandin M, Gray-Silva S (1989) Recovery of function after brain damage: facilitation by the calcium entry blocker nimodipine. Behav Neurosci 103:561-565

Le Winn EB, Dimanescu MD (1978) Environmental deprivation and enrichment in coma. Lancet 2:156-157

Merzenich MM, Nelson RJ, Stryker MP, Cynader MS, Schoppmann A, Zook JM (1984) Somatosensory cortical map changes following digit amputation in adult monkeys. J Comp Neurol 224:591-605

Merzenich MM, Recanzone G, Jenkins WM, Allard TT, Nudo RJ (1988) Cortical representational plasticity. In: Rakic P, Singer W (eds) Neurobiology of neocortex. Wiley, New York, pp 41-67

Rader MA, Alston JB, Ellis DW (1989) Sensory stimulation of severely brain-injured patients. Brain Inj 3:141-147

Roorda-Hrdlickov V, Wolters G, Bonke B, Phaf RH (1990) Unconscious perception during general anaesthesia, demonstrated by an implicit memory task. In: Bonke B, Fitch W, Milar K (eds) Memory and awareness in anaesthesia. Swets and Zeitlinger, Vienna, pp 150-155

Shacter DC (1987) Implicit memory: history and current status. J Exp Psychol [Learn Mem Cogn] 13:501-518

Soliveri P, Brown RG, Jahanshahi M, Marsden CD (1992) Procedural memory and neurological disease. Eur J Cogn Psychol (in press)

Ulrich R (1984) View through a window may influence recovery from surgery. Science 224:420-421

Watson MJ, Shiel AM, Wilson BA, Horn SA, Mc Lellan DL (1922) Learning during coma: a preliminary study. J Clin Exp Neuropsychol 14:385

Weiskrantz L (1986) Blindsight. Oxford University Press, New York

Wood RL (1991) Critical analysis of the concept of sensory stimulation for patients in vegetative states. Brain Inj 4:401-409

Chapter 20

Communication Aids for Paralytic Patients

KARL-HEINZ MAURITZ and PETRA DENZLER

Patients with impairments of motor abilities and speech functions are no longer able to communicate with their environment in a sufficient way, since alternative strategies (writing, sign language, gestures) are not available to them either. With improved methods of intensive care in neurology the number of patients who are severely handicapped and nonvocal has increased enormously. Among them are patients suffering from locked-in syndrome, patients with lesions in the caudally located brainnerve nuclei, as in amyotrophic lateral sclerosis, or patients under mechanical ventilation suffering from Guillain-Barré syndrome or high cervical spinal lesions. Most of these patients are mentally alert and feel the need to be in contact with their human surroundings, to express their thoughts and ideas, their basic needs, and their feelings. Communication aids for them are not only used to convey facts but they also have an important psychosocial integration function.

One of the oldest methods of communication for a nonvocal person is described by Dumas in his novel: *The Count of Monte Cristo*. In that novel a typical locked-in patient is described. The patient indicates "yes" or "no" by blinking with his eyes once or twice. The relatives use a dictionary to leaf through the alphabet and by that he can testify his last will.

With the advances in microelectronic technology new methods for augmentative or prosthetic communication are available today for nonspeaking patients. However, before selecting a communication aid a thorough analysis of motor, sensory, cognitive, and social abilities of the patient is required. There are three different applications of communication aids in nonvocal severely handicapped patients. Depending on the severity of the physical disabilities, communication aids are used either as a primary communication system (replacing the lost speech functions) or as a means to improve communication ability (in case of problems with formulation or understanding) or to make communication easier (in patients

Section Editor: Michael N. Diringer

whose speech cannot be sufficiently understood).

Communication aids have to meet several criteria. They should

– Be adapted to the individual requirements and abilities of a patient
– Be accepted by the user and his social environment
– Allow a certain communication speed (communication speed during normal conversation is 180 words/min; simple communication aids allow rates of 2–3 words/min)
– Include the possibility to correct and modify messages
– Be battery driven and portable
– Have printer options or other features to store communication contents

Moreover, the training should be easy and the usage has to be possible without external help.

The expected duration of the communication problem must also be taken into consideration. In case of short-term, transient speech impairments a rather simple communication aid without a personal computer (PC) may be appropriate. Intensive care patients who are under sedatives and analgesics often do not meet the requirements of alertness and intact mental abilities necessary for handling a sophisticated communication aid. A PC is not advisable in persons with permanent memory deficits who cannot concentrate or work consistently over a prolonged period of time either. However, in nonverbal patients with preserved cognitive functions even expensive and elaborate systems seem warranted.

Input Devices and Control Elements

Input switches and control elements as interfaces between the patient and the communication aid have to take into account the physical functions that are still intact, and they have to offer different modes of activation (see Table 1). Therefore it has to be determined which voluntary actions the user can reliably perform. These actions should not cause undue fatigue, nor should they compromise good muscle tone or cause pain to vulnerable joints.

Speech and Phonation

If a patient with severe motor impairment can make a noise above a certain volume he can control technical aids and scanning devices by that input. Portable intercoms between rooms and portable buzzers activated by the sound of a voice enable patients to be left unattended. Speech recognition devices are an adequate means to control electronic aids. They analyze spoken words or sounds and compare them to speech patterns of the user

Table 1. Various input devices

Speech-input, speech-recognition devices
Written-word recognition devices
(Adapted) keyboards
Joystick, computer mouse
Light pen
Game paddles
Touch tablet
Touch screen
Light pointer and pointer system
Optical systems
Ability switches: pneumatic (sip and puff), proximity, pressure, bioelectric etc.

that have been stored. If the spoken word and the stored speech pattern are congruent, a previously defined function is performed.

Finger Activation

For persons with intact handwriting, a graphic tablet can be used as an input device for the computer (written word recognition device). A patient with

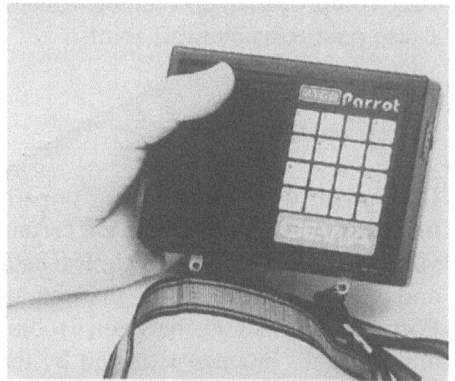

a

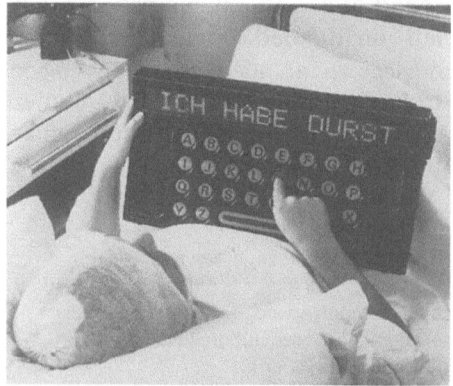

b

Fig. 1. a Portable communication aids (Zygo and Epitech): "Zygo Parrot" (up to 16 individual messages in natural speech). **b** Electronic communication aid with large LED display. The macro keys are recessed, allowing the user to stabilize the hand. Storage of over 2000 letters possible. Very useful for intensive care units (Boehringer Ingelheim)

residual motor functions is often able to press buttons of a portable aid or to to use an adapted keyboard. Simple messages can be written (Fig. 1b; "I am thirsty") or prestored messages can be selected (Fig. 1a). In these cases, macro or "elefant keyboards" or keyboards for single-hand use are advisable. For patients with limited hand or finger dexterity a finger positioning grid (keyguard) covers the keyboard and prevents unintentional activation of more than one key at a time (Fig. 2). Moreover, different key types can be used, ranging from simple pressure buttons to infrared light barriers with variable reaction time and repetition rate. An electronic communication aid with a macro keyboard and an illuminated LED display of large, moving letters has been described by Metz et al. (1984). In this case, a modest pressure (below 10 g) and medium motor ability are sufficient to activate stored messages. At the Institute of Rehabilitation Medicine of the University of Gothenburg, Sweden, a similar system has been developed

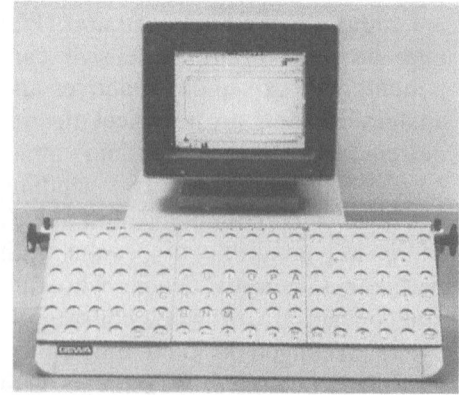

Fig. 2. Communication aid with macro keyboard, keyguard, and personal computer (Epitech)

(Lindberg and Höök 1974) which uses a perforated plate over the keyboard; the text is projected electronically on two display screens, one directed to the writer and one towards the "audience."

If the patient is not able to use a commercially available keyboard, the software can be adjusted to make the system more user friendly by a keyboard emulator.

Other computer input devices activated by hand and finger movements available are the joystick, the computer mouse, game paddles, touch tablets, light pens as well as the touch screen, whereby in the latter case complex movements should be possible (albeit within a limited scope).

Head Movements

If the patient is able to move his head, simple head pointers (Fig. 3) or light pointers are used, by means of which specific fields of communication can be indicated on an individually adjusted table. Sophisticated pointer systems (camera systems) are based on the same principle.

Eye Movements

If the head cannot be kept in a stable position and is not sufficiently mobile, optical systems can be chosen which are able to analyze the eye movements or blinking (Fig. 4) of the patient (cornea reflection method, and especially the photoelectric eye measuring

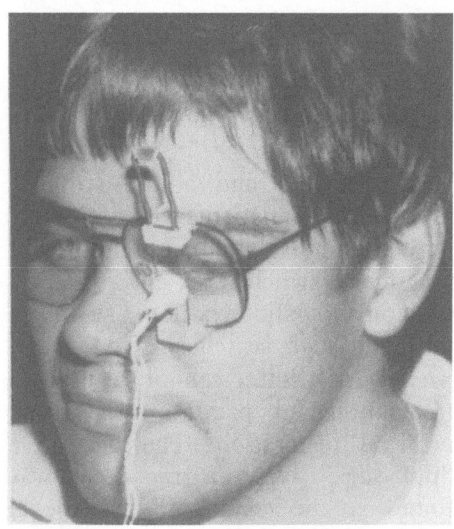

Fig. 4. Optical switch with infrared sensor mounted to an eyeglasses frame and activated by eye blinking

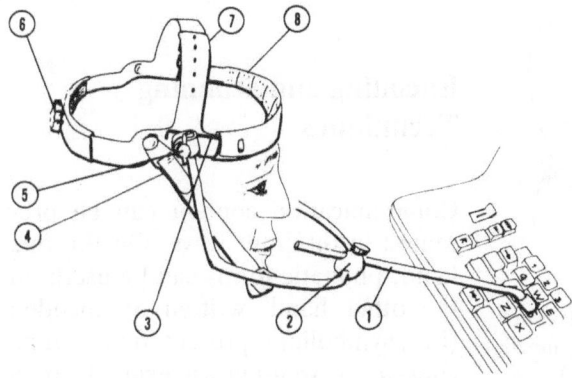

Fig. 3. Head pointer for use as input device. Useful for paralytic patients with sufficient control of head movements. The head stick (*1*) is fastend by a head band. The *numbers 2–8* indicate specific technical details (Epitech)

method and the infrared limbus pupil reflection method). By means of these systems, for example, by using sensor glasses, a high rate of communication of more than a hundred letters per minute can be achieved by alert and well-trained patients (ten Kate et al. 1980, 1989). All optical systems, however, have the disadvantage that extensive mechanical procedures are necessary and the transmission of contents normally has to remain limited.

Other Minimal Movements

Touch devices and ability switches may be used in patients with extremely limited motor abilities. There are pneumatic switches as, for example, cushion and balloon switches as well as puff and suck switches (see Fig. 5), whereby the latter cannot be used in tracheotomized patients undergoing artificial respiration. The use of a "puff-suck" type of transducer was found to be useful for high-level quadriplegic individuals who are mentally alert and have good neuromuscular control of the head and neck (Lywood and Vasa 1974; Vasa and Lywood 1976). In conductivity and

tongue sensors the contact with conducting parts poses a problem.

Proximity switches work without touch and do not require accurate movements. Moreover, magnetic switches can be fastened on the body of the patient, as well as movement, tilt and acceleration switches, which respond to changes in several directions.

Bioelectric Switches

For the most severe forms of impairment, bioelectric switches may be recommended. They use electrical signals from muscles (emg), eye movements (eog) or from the brain (eeg or contingent negative variation CNV: "neurocybernetic man-machine communication link"). The switch function is triggered when an adjustable threshold has been passed. Trials in normal individuals using computer systems via "brain power" ("brain-guided typewriter"), however, demonstrate the currently limited possibilities of use: the writing velocity of this next system amounts to about 2.3 signs per minute. In general a considerably high number of training hours is required to achieve very simple effects so that the use of biotechnologically developed devices is still very remote for the patient.

Encoding and Scanning Techniques

Communication content can be presented in different ways. On the one hand, phonetic forms can be used; on the other hand, written or encoded (i.e., symbolic) representations can be chosen. A well-known example of a

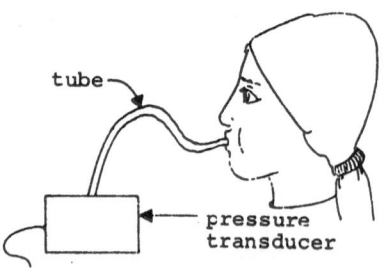

Fig. 5. Mode of action of a suck and puff switch. (The switch is operated by very small, mouth-controlled pressure changes in the tube)

language based on symbols is BLISS (see Fig. 6; Frey 1987), which was initially developed only for children with cerebral motor disturbances. BLISS comprises 26 basic symbols and can be used to produce any type of text even with abstract contents (Rossdeutscher et al. 1989). In the meantime, a programmable BLISS communication aid is on the market. The communication by symbols, in contrast to strings of letters, enables the patient to communicate at a higher speed.

As an alternative to BLISS there are purely pictorial representations without the strict rules of a symbolic language (see Fairhurst and Stephanidis 1985, 1989). Both in the "Touch-Talker" and the "Light-Talker" messages are stored by means of pictures and recalled when these pictures are activated by touch, light sensor, or a control switch. The messages are then translated into synthesized speech.

Combinations of different forms of representation (symbols, pictures, letters) offer a high degree of flexibility for the user. The LOGOS system, for example, offers the user complete freedom of choice in the combination of pictograms, text, and vocal utterances (Fairhurst and Hasan 1990).

Communication elements can be chosen directly or by scanning proce-dures. A direct selection requires the user to perform precise movements (pointing, indicating). The advantages of this method are the high rate of communication as well as the fact that it can be learned easily.

Scanning procedures present individual elements one after the other which can be selected by the handicapped person by means of a defined voluntary action. Especially communication boards with a matrix-like display and different overlays or light diodes using the scanning procedure (Kugele 1984: Börsig-communication board) can easily be produced, at a low price, and they offer certain advantages over more complex displays (see Sprague and Sprague 1983). Yeongchi and Voda (1985) presented a user-friendly communication board, the display of which is comprised of 36 squares in a 6 × 6 matrix. The alphabet is arranged according to the normal sequence, each row beginning with a vowel; letters are selected by naming the vowels vertically, then the consonants horizontally (listener-controlled system). This arrangement allows a functional use for the patient, attendant, and staff also during dressing, bathing, or traveling outside. A direct computer-based scanning procedure is the basis of several commercially available word processing methods for handicapped persons: A cursor moves automatically over a matrix of letters (autoscan). A letter is selected by activating various sensors. However, the time-consuming, strenuous transmission of more complex content is a disadvantage of these methods. This might be improved by a so-called "predictive scanning," which is a computer-aided scanning technique that anticipates the next letter based

Fig. 6. Bliss symbol language. Although the Bliss language follows simple rules, even very complex messages can be represented

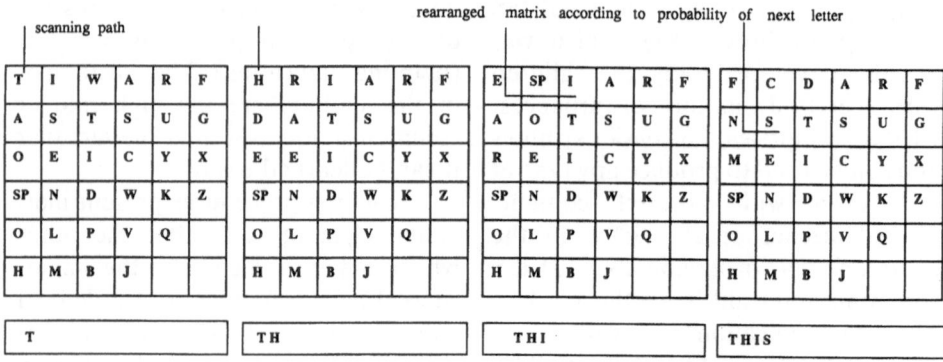

Fig. 7. Predictive scanning. The cursor starts in the left upper corner of the matrix. The matrix is rearranged according to the probability of the next letter so that the scanning pathway is short and communication speed is increased

upon probability. For instance, if the last two letters were "t" and "h" the aid would know that the following letter would most probably be "e" or "a" or "i" to form the word "the," "that" or "this" (see Fig. 7).

High cognitive abilities are required by encoding procedures, which offer rapid access to a large number of elements (for example, a specific number code represents an entire term). A combination of different scanning techniques is offered by "Hawkings communication system," the "Equalizer" by Word+ Inc., a portable, battery-operated, computer-aided system with speech synthesizer and printer.

Rossdeutscher and Boenick (1985) presented a system by means of which the handicapped person with very limited motor functions (eye movements and movement of a finger) can call up the letters of the alphabet (also in the sequence of their most frequent occurrence) as well as numbers and signs, whole words (for example, stored names of relatives, the doctor, etc.), parts of sentences as well as whole sentences (in each case with storage function). A help function has

been installed, which, in the simplest form, can trigger an alarm signal for the nurse.

Output Devices

Visual output devices are most commonly used. They are the most flexible and fastest displays. Computer monitors, printers, LED displays are among them. When selecting appropriate output devices, it should be taken into consideration that the processing for acoustic (speech output, signal sounds) and tactile displays (for example, Braille lines via relief printer) is more time consuming. Therefore a combined display should be chosen if possible, i.e., using several display units, including optical devices.

Suggested Reading

Evans AL, Gowdie RA, Keating D, Smith DC, Wyper DJ, Cunningham E (1985) A versatile speech output communication aid. J Med Eng Technol 9:180–182

Fairhurst MC, Hasan MQ (1990) Characteristics of user interaction with a communication system for the non-vocal using a hierarchically structured interface. J Biomed Comput 26:53–61

Fairhurst MC, Stephanidis C (1985) An interactive aid for expressive communication with pictographic symbols. Int J Biomed Comput 17:177–184

Fairhurst MC, Stephanidis C (1989) A model-based approach to the specification of computer-based communication aids. J Med Eng Technol 13:13–17

Frey H (1987) Die Bliss-Symbol-Kommunikationsmethode. Eine Einführung. Julius Groos, Heidelberg

Kate JH ten, Hepp B (1989) Optical and eye-controlled communication aids. J Med Eng Technol 13:63–67

Kate JH ten, Frietman EEE, Stoel FJML, Willems W (1980) Eye controlled communication aids. Med Progr Technol 8:1–21

Kugele L (1984) Kommunikation mit äußerungsbehinderten Patienten. Dtsch Krankenpflege Z 6:344–346

Linberg B, Höök O (1974) Communication aid for patients with anarthria. Scand J Rehab Med 6:102–103

Lywood DW, Vasa JJ (1974) Computer-terminal operating and communication aid for the severely handicapped. Med Biomed Eng 693–697

Metz G, Horst D, Krüger H (1984) Elektronische Kommunikationshilfe mit Makrotastatur für Beatmungspatienten auf Intensivstation. Anästhes Intensivtherap Notfallmed 19:204–205

Rossdeutscher W, Boenick U (1985) Ein Kommunikationssystem für Patienten mit Sprachausfall als Folge hochgradig zentraler Lähmung. Orthopädie-Technik 7:124–129

Rossdeutscher W, Rüssing K, Pischke M (1989) Elektronische Kommunikationshilfen für motorisch Behinderte. Krankengymnastik 41:116–120

Sprague L, Sprague C (1983) Equipment-free communication. Commun Outlook 4: 6–7

Vasa JJ, Lywood DW (1976) High-speed communication aid for quadriplegics. Med Biol Eng 1:445–450

Walsh MJ, Westphal LC (1986) A prototype portable electronic speaking aid for the nonvocal handicapped. Trans Biomed Eng 33:985–988

Yeongchi W, Voda JA (1985) User-friendly communication board for nonverbal, severely physically disabled individuals. Arch Phys Med Rehab 66:827–828

Appendix: Addresses of Producers

Boehringer Ingelheim
Medizintechnik
Postfach
55218 Ingelheim am Rhein
Germany

Canon Inc.
Audio & Visual Aids Center
7-1 Nishi- Shinjuku 2-chome,
Shinjuku-ku,
Tokyo 163
Japan

Epitech GmbH
Pivitstr. 13
32120 Hiddenhausen
Germany

Fondation Suisse pour les Téléthèses
Crêt-Taconnet 32
Case postale 1755
2002 Neuchâtel, Switzerland

Medicom
MATAM Advanced Technology
Center
31905 Haifa
Israel

Prentke Romich Company (PRC)
1022 Heyl Road
Wooster, OH 44691
USA

tash Inc.
Technical Aids & Systems for the
Handicapped Inc.
70 Gibson Drive, Unit 1
Markham, Ontario L3R 2Z3
Canada

Chapter 21

Diagnosis of Brain Death

MICHAEL N. DIRINGER, THORSTEN STEINER, and HEINZ ANGSTWURM

Introduction

Until recently, death was defined only as irreversible cardiopulmonary arrest. However, advances in medical technology, such as pulmonary ventilation, advanced cardiac resuscitation, and pharmaceutics, have created the ability to maintain cardiopulmonary function artificially, even in patients who do not recover any brain function. This situation has led to the concept of brain death as a new definition of death. Additionally, the concept allows the transplantation of viable organs.

Over the past 25 years medicine has struggled with the ethical, legal, and practical aspects of these issues. In order to understand these issues it is necessary to develop a concept of brain death, to define criteria which can reliably identify brain death, and to understand the legal constraints on medical decisions.

The Concept of Brain Death

Development of criteria for the definition of brain death can be approached philosophically or operationally. We have to differentiate clearly between the determination of brain death, which is based on assessment of clinical signs, and the concept of brain death, which must be approached philosophically.

Numerous definitions of brain death have been offered. Plum and Posner stated that "brain death occurs when irreversible brain damage is so extensive that the organ enjoys no potential for recovery and can no longer maintain the body's internal homeostasis." The ad hoc Committee of the Harvard Medical School to examine the definition of brain death suggested that brain death should be declared when the brain "no longer functions and has no possibility of functioning again." The NIH collaborative study called it "total destruction of the brain," while the Conference of Royal Colleges and Faculties of the United Kingdom "agreed that permanent functional death of the brain stem constitutes brain death."

Section Editor: Michael N. Diringer

These definitions point to the lack of conceptual clarity about death in brain-injured patients. Thus, while irreversible loss of brain function is widely accepted as a prerequisite for declaring brain death, there is little consensus on the concept of why brain-dead patients are dead. Health care workers, even those involved in organ procurement for transplantation, often do not consistently apply a coherent concept of death. This lack of clarity has resulted in differing criteria for the diagnosis of brain death, inconsistencies in the use of "confirmatory" tests, discomfort in managing such patients, and interference with donation of organs for transplantation.

The initial premise in conceptually defining death on a neurologic basis is that a patient who has irreversible loss of all brain function is dead, irrespective of cardiac function. This premise evolved out of the need to procure organs for transplantation and is based on the facts that these patients never regain any brain function and eventually suffer cardiac arrest. Therefore, it became necessary to define what constitutes irreversible loss of all brain function. One philosophical concept of brain death is the higher-brain concept. It defines life and death based on consciousness, cognition, and responsiveness to environmental stimuli, functions primarily attributed to the cortex. The lower-brain concept argues that the capacity for consciousness resides in the brain stem (reticular activating system) and is essential for cortical function. Thus irreversible loss of brain-stem function would define death. Finally, the whole-brain concept requires loss of function of both the brain stem and cortex.

The operational approach to defining brain death also lacks uniformity. One approach is to delineate a state of brain unresponsiveness from which survival of bodily function has never been seen and to use that state to define brain death. Another is to define a state which will reliably predict widespread severe brain necrosis. A third is to define the diagnosis based on the demonstration of an isoelectric electroencephalogram (EEG) or the absence of cerebral blood flow. These varying philosophical and operational approaches have resulted in the development of numerous criteria for the determination of brain death and persistent uneasiness in their application.

Criteria for the Diagnosis of Brain Death

Historical Aspects

In 1968 the Harvard Medical School Ad Hoc Committee to Examine the Definition of Brain Death (see Appendix) set out to "define irreversible coma as a new criterion for death." The clinical diagnosis required: (a) unreceptivity and unresponsiveness, (b) no movements of breathing, and (c) absence of brainstem reflexes. An isoelectric EEG was considered "of great confirmatory value," and it was recommended that it be used when available. They indicated that, in order to determine irreversibility, all of these tests should be repeated in 24 h. While it was not necessary to determine the etiology of the coma, the exam had to be performed in the absence of hypothermia or sedative drugs. Once the determination had been made, the report indicated that the family should be informed, death was to be declared, and then the respirator turned off. It was suggested that the physician in charge of the patient consult with one or more other physicians "so that the responsibility is shared over a wide range of medical opinion." The Committee recommended that the decision to withdraw ventilation not be made by those physicians involved in organ or tissue transplantation. This report served as the basis for the development of brain death criteria by many institutions and was the basis for including the requirement for an isoelectric EEG.

The Conference of the Royal Colleges and Faculties of the United Kingdom published the *Diagnosis of Brain Death* in 1976 (see Appendix), in which they defined brain death as brain-stem death. Brain-stem death may not be applied as a synonym for brain death and must therefore be used with caution: It should be considered that isolated brain-stem death is rare and derives from infratentorial processes such as ischemic hemorrhage which produce loss of brain-stem function – an infratentorial function. EEG activity might then occur despite brainstem death with apnea. It is difficult to judge the meaning of remaining EEG activity in definite brain-stem-dead individuals. In many cases this remaining EEG activity in isolated brain-stem deaths will cease within 24–36 h. The Conference of the Royal Colleges and Faculties of the United Kingdom did not require an EEG, angiography, or cerebral blood flow studies. However, the Conference did require that the condition which led to brain death be fully established. The search for

potential factors which could mimic brain death or worsen a patient's neurologic condition was emphasized; depressant drugs, neuromuscular blocking agents, respiratory depressants, and metabolic or endocrine disturbances had to be excluded. A flexible period of observation was recommended, such that prolonged observation was needed in cases of hypoxic or ischemic injury, whereas only a few hours might be needed following severe head injury or intracerebral hemorrhage. Finally, the technique for apnea testing was refined to include preoxygenation, continued oxygen administration during apnea, administration of 5% CO_2 to raise arterial CO_2 to at least 50 torr, and careful investigation in patients with chronic respiratory insufficiency (Table 1).

The United States Collaborative Study of Cerebral Death was an NIH multicenter, prospective study which assessed criteria for brain death in the USA. An operational definition was used to determine failure of the brain to return to any function: death within

Table 1. Performance of apnea testing

1. Hypoventilation for 20 min with 100% O_2, then
2. Blood-gas control: $PaCO_2 < 40$ mmHg
3. If no, repeat 1; if yes, disconnect from the ventilator
4. 6 l O_2 (100%) via tracheal tube
5. After 5–10 min (depending on the starting $PaCO_2$): blood-gas control
   a) If $PaCO_2 > 60$ mmHg: apnea proved
   b) If $PaCO_2 < 60$ mmHg and if $PaO_2 > 150$ mmHg, continue apnea testing
   c) If $PaCO_2 < 60$ mmHg and if $PaO_2 < 150$ mmHg, short ventilation with 100% O_2 (hypoventilation), then continuation of apnea testing

3 months despite all therapy. The project sought to determine which criteria would establish brain death by requiring that they predict bodily death within 3 months despite all therapy. To be included, patients had to demonstrate cerebral unresponsiveness and apnea. Of the 503 patients who met these criteria, 87% died within 3 months. When the Harvard criteria were applied, only 19 of the 503 patients met them, but all 19 died. Thus the Harvard criteria were completely accurate but not very sensitive. Therefore, a third set of criteria was applied: cerebral unresponsiveness, apnea, one isoelectric EEG. Of the 189 patients who met these criteria, 187 died; the other two were cases of drug intoxication. The final recommended criteria required one examination at least 6 h (unlike the 24 h required by the Harvard criteria) after the onset of coma and apnea. The exam should demonstrate cerebral unresponsiveness, apnea, dilated pupils, absent brain-stem reflexes, and isoelectric EEG. Apnea was defined as the need for controlled ventilation for at least 15 min; that is, the patient made no effort to override the ventilator but was not disconnected from it. Although it was recognized that not all brain-dead patients had dilated pupils, the requirement was included to avoid incorrect diagnosis in cases of drug intoxication. It was noted that spinal reflexes are poor indicators of brain death and were present in approximately one third of the patients who died. They also recommended an additional "confirmatory" test demonstrating absence of cerebral blood flow when an early diagnosis is desired, particularly when brain-stem reflexes are untestable or when sedatives have been administered. Finally, the report recognized that the criteria overlapped and preferred the added assurance so that errors would not occur.

The German Scientific Advisory Board of the Federal Physicians Organization (*Wissenschaftliche Beirat der Bundesärztekammer*) published two comments on "the criteria of brain death" in 1982 and 1986. The recommendations for diagnosis and documentation include a clinical examination by two independent physicians; one must be specially experienced in intensive care medicine. The criteria for determination of brain death include demonstration of unreceptivity, unresponsiveness, absent brain-stem reflexes, and apnea. The protocol currently used in Germany will be described below (Fig. 1).

In the USA, the Report of the Medical Consultant on the Diagnosis of Death to the President's Commission, published in 1981, included guidelines which represented a distillation of the current practice at that time. They attempted to develop criteria that: (a) eliminate error in classifying a living individual as dead; (b) allow as few errors as possible in classifying a dead body as alive; (c) allow determinations to be made without unreasonable delay and to be adaptable; and (d) are explicit and accessible to verification. The guidelines addressed only commonly available and verified tests, were deemed advisory, and recommended consultation with other physicians. Brain death was defined as the "irreversible cessation of all [clinically ascertainable] functions of the entire brain including the brain stem." This was to be demonstrated by unreceptivity, unre-

---

Protokoll zur Feststellung des Hirntodes*)

Klinik: _____

Patient: _____ Vorname: _____ geb.: _____ Alter: _____

Protokoll-Nr.: _____

Voraussetzungen:

1.1 Diagnose _____

   Primäre supra-tentorielle ☐ infra-tentorielle ☐ Hirnschädigung

   Zeitpunkt des Unfalls/Krankheitsbeginns: _____

   Untersuchungsdatum: _____ Uhrzeit: _____

   Feststellungen und Befunde beantworten mit ja oder nein:**)

		1. Untersucher	2. Untersucher
1.2 Intoxikation	ausgeschlossen	_____	_____
Relaxation	ausgeschlossen	_____	_____
Primäre Hypothermie	ausgeschlossen	_____	_____
Hypovolämischer Schock	ausgeschlossen	_____	_____
Metab. od. Endokr. Koma	ausgeschlossen	_____	_____
Blutdruck, mmHg syst.		_____	_____

Maßgebliche Symptome des Ausfalls der Hirnfunktion:

2.1 Koma   _____   _____

2.2 Ausfall der Spontanatmung   _____   _____

2.3 Pupillen mittelweit/weit
    Pupillen-Licht-Reflex fehlt beidseits   _____   _____

2.4 Oculo-zephaler Reflex fehlt
    (Puppenkopfphänomen)   _____   _____

2.5 Corneal-Reflex erloschen beidseits   _____   _____

2.6 Trigeminus-Schmerzreaktion erloschen   _____   _____

2.7 Pharyngeal-/Tracheal-Reflex erloschen   _____   _____

                    Untersuchende Ärzte (Druckbuchstaben)   _____   _____
                                       (Unterschrift)   _____   _____

Gegebenenfalls ergänzende Untersuchungen:

3.1 Isoelektrisches (Null-Linien) EEG 30 Min. abgeleitet _____ Uhr _____
                                                    Arzt _____

3.2 Frühe akustisch evozierte Hirnstammpotentiale Welle III–V beiderseits erloschen   ja ☐   nein ☐
    Datum _____ Uhr _____ Arzt _____
    Medianus-SEP beiderseits erloschen   ja ☐   nein ☐
    Datum _____ Uhr _____ Arzt _____

3.3 Zerebrale Angiographie: Zirkulationsstillstand beiderseits festgestellt:
    Datum _____ Uhr _____ Arzt _____

Gegebenenfalls Beobachtungszeit:

4. Zum Zeitpunkt der hier protokollierten Untersuchungen besteht das eindeutige
   Hirntod-Syndrom seit _____ Stunden.
   Weitere Beobachtung erforderlich (Lebensalter!)   ja ☐   nein ☐
   Zusammen mit den Befunden in den Protokollbogen Nr. _____ wird der
   Hirntod und somit der Tod des Patienten diagnostiziert am _____ um _____ Uhr
       Ärzte 1. _____ 2. _____ (Druckbuchstaben)
             _____ _____ (Unterschrift)

---

*) für die geforderte 2malige Untersuchung ist je ein Protokollformular auszufüllen
**) Befundkatalog aus: »Kriterien des Hirntodes«; gem. Stellungnahme der Arbeitsgruppe d. Wiss. Beirates d.
    BÄK u. Arbeitsgem. d. Wiss. Med. Fachges., DÄB 79, H. 14/82, S. 45 – Überarbeitete Fassung 1986

Fig. 1. German brain-death protocol form

sponsiveness, absent brain-stem reflexes, and apnea. Apnea testing was described in detail to include preoxygenation, passive flow of oxygen during apnea, and hypercarbia of at least 60 torr confirmed by arterial blood-gas sampling. The report specifically indicated that true decerebrate or decorticate posturing or seizures are inconsistent with the diagnosis of brain death. Irreversibility was recognized by: (a) establishing the cause of coma, (b) excluding the possibility of recovery of any brain function (exclusion of reversible conditions), and (c) a period of observation. This report was the first to include shock as a reversible condition. The period of observation was considered a matter of clinical judgement; 6 h was appropriate in uncomplicated cases with a confirmatory EEG or test of cerebral blood flow, 12 h with a well-established irreversible cause of coma without a confirmatory test, and 24 h for anoxic damage. Finally, the observation period could be reduced if tests showed isoelectric EEG or absent cerebral blood flow for 10 min in an adult without drug intoxication, hypothermia, or shock.

Legal Considerations in the United States

For most of the legal history of the United States, the determination of death was simply a matter of observing that a patient's heart had ceased to beat. Thus the time of death was a question of fact which was established by medical expertise. While the concept of neurologically defined death was introduced into the legal system in the later 1970s, it was the advent of organ transplantation that was the driving force in the evolution of the legal definition of brain death. Shortly after the publication of the Harvard criteria, statutes were enacted which permitted the determination of death based on cessation of brain function. These laws were developed to protect physicians against civil and criminal liability. Early statutes permitted the use of "ordinary standards of medical practice" to determine the moment of death based on the absence of either brain or cardiopulmonary function.

In 1972, Capron and Kass proposed a model statute:

A person will be considered dead if in the announced opinion of a physician, based on ordinary standards of medical practice, he (or she) has experienced an irreversible cessation of respiratory and circulatory functions, or, in the event that artificial means of support precludes a determination that these functions have ceased, he (or she) has experienced an irreversible cessation of total brain function. Death will have occurred at the time when the relevant functions ceased.

It must be kept in mind that it is not possible to determine clinically the exact time of the individual death. Death has probably occurred prior to the time of clinical determination. Thus what is clinically determined as time of death is a legal concept and does not reflect cessation of the individual's vital functions.

The Uniform Determination of Death Act is the most widely accepted model for determination-of-death statutes. It was developed through a joint effort involving the American Bar Association, The American Medical Association, the National Conference of Commissioners on Uniform State Laws, and the President's Commission for the Study of Ethical Problems in Medicine and Biomedical and Behavioral Research. The act reads:

An individual who has sustained either (1) irreversible cessation of circulatory and respiratory functions, or (2) irreversible cessation of all functions of the entire brain, including the brain stem, is dead. A determination of death must be made in accordance with accepted medical standards.

The American Medical Association issued a model which recapitulated the Uniform Determination of Death Act but also added sections which were designed to provide protection from civil and criminal liability. The American Bar Association proposed a model which defined exclusively brain death.

At the present time, all 50 states and the District of Columbia have determination-of-death statutes. The majority conform to the Uniform Determination of Death Act. Some include the requirement that the determination be made by two physicians, and one requires the hospital to attempt to notify next of kin and establish a policy for reasonable accommodation of religious or moral objections to the determination. Others dictate that death be pronounced prior to termination of artificial means of support.

Almost all statutes make the determination of brain death based on "accepted medical standards." Therefore, what compromises these standards is a question of law, determined by the trial court based on expert testimony regarding care and treatment given by physicians within the same speciality of medicine, practicing under like and similar circumstances.

Legal Considerations in Germany

In Germany, brain death is defined as complete and irreversible cessation of the whole brain function, while cardiopulmonary function is artificially maintained. The period of observation to prove irreversibility is 12 h in primary (for patients over age 3 years) and 72 h in secondary brain lesions. Additional observation periods and ancillary tests are required in children up to the 4th week and until the 2nd year. Apnea is proven if pCO_2 levels rise to 60 mmHg.

Relevance of Ancillary Testing in Germany

An EEG recording fulfilling the criteria set by the German EEG Society may be used to shorten the observation period in a patient fulfilling the clinical criteria for brain death. This EEG must be artifact free and isoelectric. Standardized EEG is obligatory only in primary infratentorial lesions. If there is an isoelectric EEG in a primary infratentorial lesion no further observation is necessary (see Table 1). Brain-stem acoustic evoked potentials (BAEP), supraspinal somatosensory evoked potentials (SEP), and transcranial Doppler ultrasound (TCD) are approved for ancillary testing. Angiographic demonstration of absent intracranial circulation is also a valid indicator of brain death and may shorten the observation period. However, for legal reasons angiography may not be performed in order to prove brain death, because of the theoretical possibility of causing cessation of some preserved perfusion. If angiography is performed to determine the cause of the underlying disease, e.g., search for an aneurysm in a grade-V SAH patient, and cessation of intracranial circulation is found while doing this study, angiography is accepted as an ancillary test.

uVL T/DIV
0,25

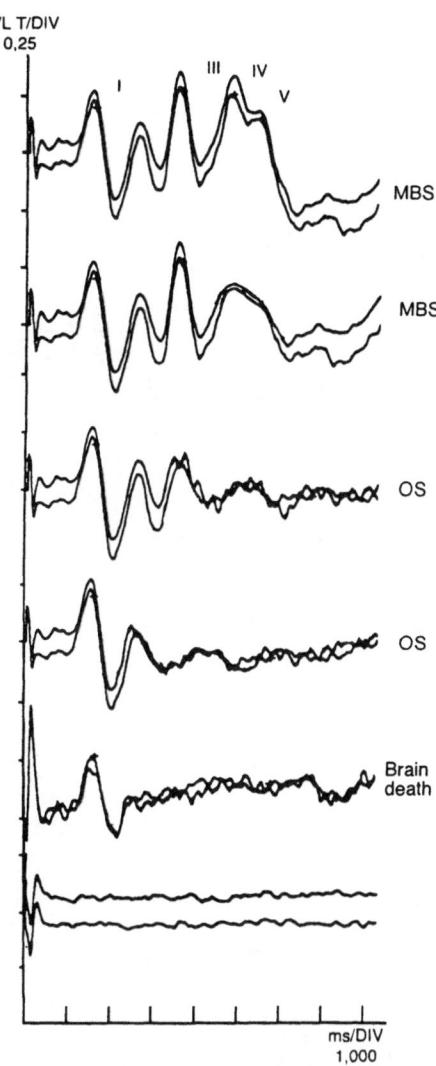

Fig. 2. Course of acoustic-evoked brain-stem potentials in brain-stem compression. *MBS*, Mid-brain syndrome; *OS*, oblongata syndrome (from Hacke W, 1988, with permission)

Table 2. Recommendation of the German EEG Society for EEG monitoring in brain death

- 30 min monitoring without artifacts
- time constant 1.0, upper limiting frequency 70 c/s
- beside amplification (7 mm/50 μV), intermediate higher amplification with 12–14 and 20 mm/50 μV
- distance between electrodes less than 10 and more than 8 cm
- all resistances of electrodes less than 10 k Ohm
- parallel ECG monitoring
- registration of EMG of the orbicular oris muscle

Legal Considerations in Other European Countries

Legal considerations regarding brain death in other European countries differ mainly in period of observation, time of EEG application, and acknowl-

edgment of ancillary tests. While irreversibility in the UK is dependent on the clinical situation after primary brain damage, and proven after 24-h observation in secondary brain damage, the period of observation in Switzerland (patient older than 6 years) has to be 6 h after primary and 48 h after secondary lesions. In Austria a 6-h observation after primary brain lesions and 24-h observation after secondary brain lesions is required, together with one isoelectric EEG. Other ancillary tests are acknowledged only in Germany. The pCO_2 peak level after 5–10 min hypoventilation with 100% O_2 is 50 mmHg in Switzerland and 60 mmHg in the UK. A comparison of brain-death criteria in selected European countries and the USA is given in Table 3.

In Japan, there are still major difficulties with the concept of brain death. Currently, brain death is not accepted as death in Japan. This causes (a) major problems with transplantation (in fact, no transplantation programs with the exception of kidney and liver transplantation from living donors are possible), and (b) the need to continue critical care therapy in

Table 3. International brain death criteria

	Germany	USA	UK	Swiss	France	Greece	Sweden	Italy	Finn-land	Netherlands
I. Preconditions										
– diagnosis	+	+	+	+	+	+	+	+	+	+
– no hypothermia	+	+	+	+	<35°C	+	+	?	<35°C	+
– no shock	+	+	+	+	+	+	+	?	+	+
– no sedative drugs	+	+	+	+	+	+	+	?	+	+
– no neuromuscular blocking agents	+	+	+	+	+	+	+	?	+	+
– no severe electrolyte disturbances	+	+	+	+	+	+	+	?	+	+
– endocrine disturbances	+	+	+	+	+	+	+	?	+	+
– no fluid imbalance	+	+	+	+	+	+	+	?	+	
II. Clinical determination										
– number of physicians	2	1 (most states)	2	1	?	2	?	3	?	1
– number of clinical examinations	2	2	2	2	4?	2	2	12	2	
– coma	+	+	+	+	+	+	+	+		+
– apnea testing	+	+	+	+	+	+	?	no spontaneous respiration for at least 2 min		+

Table (rotated; criteria as rows, 11 columns):

Criterion	1	2	3	4	5	6	7	8	9	10	11
pCO_2 mmHg	>60	>60 (>20 Torr)	>50	>50		>60					>50
– no brain-stem reflexes			+	+	+	+	+	+	+	+	
– no pupillary response to light	+	+	+	+	+	+	+	+	+	+	+
– no vestibulo-ocular reflex	+	+	+	+	+	+	+	+	+	+	+
– no corneal reflex	+	+	+	+	+	+	+	+	+	+	+
– no gag reflex	+	+	+	+	+	+	+	+	+	+	+
– no cough reflex	+	+	+	+	+	+	+	+	+	+	+
III. Period of observation											
– in primary brain damage	12	6–12	6	6	12	?	12	≥2	12	6	no differentiation
– in secondary brain damage	72	24	12	48	?	?	12	?		72	
IV. Ancillary tests										only if brain death remains in doubt	
– isoelectric EEG	1	2	−	−	2x: 2nd after 24h	2x: 2nd after 6h[a]	−	occasional	4	+	2x: 2nd after 24h
– duration of recording	30 min[a]	6 h/30 min	−	−					30 min		
– TCD	(+)	+	−	−	−	−	−	−	(+)	−	−
– loss of BAEP	(+)	−	−	−	−	−	−	−		−	−
– cessation of circulatory function	angiography	radioisotope CBF	angiography			angiography in case of intoxication	−	2x: arch angiography; 2nd after 30 min		2x: arch angiography; 2nd after 25 min	
– ICP above systolic BP	−	−	+	−	−	−	−	−	−	−	−

[a] See Table 1.

patients with brain-death syndrome. In those cases, therapy cannot be terminated upon diagnosis of brain death.

Diagnosis

There are four elements in the diagnosis of brain death which are common to all published criteria: irreversibility, absence of neurologic function, apnea, and additional tests. Each of these elements must be considered when evaluating a patient.

Irreversible brain damage can be demonstrated by radiographic studies indicating a clear etiology and/or severe anatomical damage. Lacking such evidence, it is necessary to employ a longer period of observation or, alternatively, to demonstrate absent cerebral blood flow or electrical activity. In addition, determination of irreversibility requires that no reversible factors which could contribute to the clinical picture may be present. In every clinical evaluation the following conditions should be considered: hypothermia, shock, sedative drugs, neuromuscular blocking agents, severe electrolyte or endocrine disturbances, hepatic or renal encephalopathy and infratentorial disease, brain-stem stroke, encephalitis, or tumor. There is no consensus regarding the severity of these conditions which would preclude the diagnosis of brain death. For instance, some clinicians consider that a serum level of barbiturates in the normal anticonvulsant range does not preclude the declaration of brain death. Others do not declare brain death until sedative drugs are no longer detectable. Similarly, there is no consensus on the degree of metabolic disturbance (hyponatremia, renal or hepatic insufficiency) which would preclude the diagnosis of brain death. The lack of definitive data makes the decision a matter of clinical judgement.

There are not enough data to show the correlation between clinical, neurophysiological, and angiographic results of brain death and certain drug levels. Experience with anesthesia and intoxication in subjects with normal brain function revealed that thiopental levels below $5 \mu g$ and methohexital levels below $2 \mu g$ do allow awakening. These levels may be taken into consideration during assessment of patients with absent brain function. The effects of low-dose barbiturates are not altered by pre-existing brain lesions. Serum drug levels should, if possible, be collected from an arterial line, since these may correlate better with brain tissue drug levels.

The neurologic examination is the primary determinate of neurologic function. It should include unresponsiveness to all environmental stimuli and absence of brain-stem reflexes. Testing of reflexes should employ potent stimuli. Brain-stem reflexes tested should include the pupillary response to light, vestibulo-occular, corneal, gag, and cough reflexes. While spinal reflexes, including deep tendon reflexes, and a triple flexion response to plantar stimulation may be present, posturing or seizures are incompatible with a diagnosis of brain death. When these criteria are not, met further testing is not warranted.

While respiratory drive can be considered a brain-stem reflex, the clinical implications of its absence have given this function a special role in diagnosing brain death. In apnea testing preoxygenation as well as passive oxygen flow during apnea are important to prevent cardiovascular instability. The patient should be pre-oxygenated with 100% oxygen for 5–10 min prior to beginning the test. Passive oxygenation should be continued during apnea by inserting a catheter into the endotracheal tube down to the carina and maintaining an oxygen flow of 2–6 l/min. The test should always begin at normal arterial CO_2 and pH and persist until CO_2 rises to 20 torr and significant acidosis develops.

Ancillary Tests

The need for additional tests such as an EEG or cerebral blood flow studies is controversial. When the etiology and severity of damage are clearly demonstrated and the clinical exam has persisted for a 24-h period, further testing is probably unnecessary. These tests may be useful when the etiology is unclear, or the period of observation is short. They are often useful when other conditions, such as the use of sedative drugs or metabolic disturbances, are present. However, use of these tests can be problematic.

The most widely used test to confirm brain death is the EEG. A properly performed isoelectric EEG is widely accepted as "confirmation" of brain death. However, the ICU environment makes it difficult to meet the published technical criteria for the determination of electrocerebral silence. In addition, EEG conveys little information about brain-stem function. The EEG cannot be used in all cases, as several factors may produce an isoelectric EEG when there is potential for recovery. Isoelectric

EEGs with subsequent recovery have been reported with sedative drug overdose, after anoxia, during hypothermia, and following head injury.

Evoked Potential

EEG monitoring in the ICU might sometimes be limited by insuperable methodical difficulties. This does not apply for acoustic and somatosensory evoked potentials (BAEP, SEP). To prove loss of brain function the Scientific Advisory Board of the Federal Physicians Organization in Germany requires the total loss of BAEP after they have been proven normal at the beginning of the observation period. Interestingly, waves I and II may be present in brain-dead patients because they are generated outside the brain stem. Phenytoin intoxication and hypothermia can suppress BAEP.

Loss of initially normal SEP can also demonstrate absence of brain function. There is no cortical response in brain death, while spinal SEP above T_7 will be normal. However, double-sided hemispheric lesions will also lead to total loss of cortical SEP. In single cases the T_2 amplitude might be lowered, whereas the T_7 response is normal. This constellation suggests damage of the posterior fascicles in the medulla and might thus support the diagnosis of brain death.

Angiography

Determination of cerebral blood flow is frequently used to "confirm" brain death. Arteriography was the imaging technique first used to demonstrate absence of intracranial blood flow. Various procedures have been employed to demonstrate the absence of cerebral blood flow, including selective internal carotid and vertebral angiography and aortic arch injections using conventional and digital techniques. The absence of angiographic vessel opacification in brain death is thought to be due to intracranial pressure elevation or impedance of cerebral venous outflow. While the lower limit of blood flow detectable by angiography and the best technique have not been rigorously defined, failure of injected contrast medium to reach the intracranial circulation is widely accepted as "confirmatory" of brain death. Radioisotopic studies of cerebral blood flow using technetium have also been used to confirm brain death. However, theoretical uncertainty may arise from persistent filling of venous sinuses, and because the posterior fossa circulation is not visualized. In addition, it is not valid when cerebral blood flow is low.

However, in Germany angiography is not allowed if performed to prove brain death because of the possibility that the *dye* could cause the final cessation of blood flow in a few remaining vessels.

Recently, single photon-emission computer tomography has been employed to demonstrate absence of cerebral blood flow in brain death. It offers advantages over technetium, since it has higher resolution and visualizes the posterior fossa; however, its lower limit of blood flow detectability is not known. Xenon-enhanced computer tomography has been used less extensively to confirm brain death. Xenon has anesthetic effects which could potentially interfere with the clinical appearance of patients and has a 10–15% error in measuring cerebral

blood flow. Disadvantages inherent in these techniques include the need to transport critically ill patients to and from the ICU, cumbersome equipment, lengthy duration, and interference with patient care. Transcranial Doppler (TCD) ultrasound is a simple, noninvasive, inexpensive test which is useful in determining the absence of cerebral blood flow.

Doppler Ultrasound

Several patterns of linear blood flow velocities (LBFV) determined by TCD have been described as intracranial pressure rises leading to brain death. These include an oscillating pattern of LBFV and reversal of intracranial diastolic blood flow. TCD findings suggesting brain death have been confirmed by 4-vessel angiography and technetium radionuclide scanning.

Five patterns of TCD profile changes have been identified which occur as intracranial hypertension progresses to brain death:

1. Low diastolic LBFV: There is a rapid, sharp peak of the TCD waveform during systole, followed by a rapid decline of diastolic LBFV to near zero. Anterograde flow is present throughout the entire cardiac cycle and there is no evidence of retrograde flow. This pattern may be reversible. Low diastolic velocity corresponds to the diminished cerebral perfusion pressure gradient as intracranial pressure approaches diastolic blood pressure.
2. Systolic peaks: Only systolic LBFV is detected. A sharp peak in the waveform, which may last through the entire cardiac cycle, is seen.

There is no diastolic blood flow. This may be reversible.

3. Oscillating blood flow: Anterograde short systolic spikes (see 4 below) alternate with brief, sharply contoured, retrograde diastolic blood flow. With careful measurement of LBFV in both directions, a net zero velocity may be calculated. This also may be reversible. The typical angiographic findings which correlate with this pattern are a delayed, tapered filling of the basal cerebral arteries.

4. Short systolic spikes: The only detectable signals are brief anterograde spikes in the wave-form which last for only a brief portion of the cardiac cycle (as opposed to systolic peaks, which are longer). These are associated with angiographic absence of blood flow.

5. Absence of TCD signal: There is no detectable intracranial TCD signal. Extracranial internal carotid flow may be detectable with submandibular insonation. This pattern has been associated with extracranial angiographic arrest of flow in all vessels. Absence of TCD signal to confirm intracranial circulatory arrest should be restricted to patients who have had previously demonstrable TCD waveforms. Otherwise, the absence of signal could be the result of a thickened skull and inadequate cranial "windows".

The use of TCD to confirm brain death in comatose patients has been found to be highly specific (100%) and sensitive (91.3%), but false-positive test results may occur. To reduce the chance of false-positive results, the entire intracranial circulation must be surveyed, with evaluation of both the anterior circulation and the vertebrobasilar system. False-positive confirmation of brain death by TCD may also occur if one fails to study arteries from each hemisphere in the anterior circulation. Undetectable TCD flow in the internal carotid artery and middle cerebral artery in one hemisphere has been seen in the presence of normal TCD waveforms in the other hemisphere.

Since the comment of the German Scientific Advisory Board of the Federal Physicians' Organization from 1991, TCD is an acknowledged ancillary test in Germany; it proves cessation of cerebral perfusion if certain standardized conditions are fulfilled.

Communication with Family

The declaration of brain death is a process which requires not only precise clinical assessment but also effective and humane communication with the patient's family. While each case is unique, some general guidelines may be offered. When brain death is suspected it may be helpful for the physician to tactfully inform the family of the suspected diagnosis and that it is currently being evaluated. This provides an opportunity for the family to prepare for the outcome and to later raise the possibility of organ donation. Following the determination of brain death, the patient is pronounced dead and the family should be informed in an unambiguous manner that the patient has died. Opportunity should be provided for visits from family and clergy. The request for organ donation is best made in a separate discussion with the family. Often it is useful to enlist the aid of a third-party clergyman, social worker, or member of the organ procurement team to facilitate the discussion. Following the declaration of death, either the patient is taken to the operating room for organ harvest or ventilation is discontinued. Since the patient is medically and legally dead, the family's permission is not needed to remove the ventilator. It is usually preferable that the family not be present during the discontinuation of ventilation because of the possible occurrence of spinally mediated reflexive movements. Privacy, as well as emotional support from physicians, nurses, social workers, or clergy, should be available for the family.

When to Diagnose Brain Death

Circumstances where it is appropriate to pursue the diagnosis of brain death are limited. It is currently necessary in order to harvest organs for transplantation. Otherwise the diagnosis will allow for the removal of life support, including ventilation, from a dead body. Current medical practice, however, allows withdrawal of life-sustaining therapies when they are considered futile (see Chap. 9). Thus, in patients who are not candidates for organ donation, a formal diagnosis of brain death is no longer necessary before support can be withdrawn.

Suggested Reading

Ad Hoc Committee of the Harvard Medical School to Examine the Definition of Brain Death (1968) A definition of irreversible coma. JAMA 205:337–340
Capron JM, Kass A (1972) Legal definition of death. Ann NY Acad Sci 315:349
Conference of Royal Colleges and Faculties of the United Kingdom (1976) Diagnosis of brain death. Lancet I:1069–1070
Editorial (1983) Brain death criteria (in Dutch). Ned Tijdschr Geneeskd 127:2293
Frowein RA, Richard KE, Hamel E (1985) In: Gänshirt H, Berlit B, Haack G (eds) Verhandlungen der deutschen Gesellschaft für Neurologie, vol 3. Springer, Berlin Heidelberg New York, pp 543–533
Hacke W, Ringelstein EB, Buchner H, Ferbert A (1985) Neurophysiologische und neurosonologische Verlaufsunter suchungen beim drohenden Hirntod. In: Gänshirt H, Berlit B, Haack G (eds) Verhandlungen der deutschen Gesellschaft für Neurolgie, vol 3. Springer, Berlin Heidelberg New York
Kaste M, Palo J (1981) Criteria of brain death and removal of cadaveric organs. Ann Clin Res 13:313–317
Le Ministre Delegue charge de la Sante (1990) Decret n° 90-844 du 24 septembre 1990. Le Ministre Delegue charge de la Sante, France
Marku K, Matti H, Jorma P (1979) Diagnosis and management of brain death. Br Med J 1:525–527
NIH Collaborative Study (1977) An appraisal of the criteria of cerebral death. A summary statement. JAMA 237:982–986
Ogata J, Imakita M, Yutani C, Miyamoto S, Kikuchi H (1988) Primary brainstem death: a clinico-pathological study J Neurol Neurosurg Psychiatr 51:646–650
Pallis C (1984) Brainstem death: the evolution of a concept. In: Morris PJ (ed) Kidney transplantation 2nd edn. Grune and Stratton, New York, pp 101–127
Plum F, Posner JB (1982) Brain death. In: Plum F, Posner JM (eds) The diagnosis of stupor and coma, 3rd edn. Davis, Philadelphia, p 313
Pohlmann-Eden B (1991) Zur Problematik der Hirntod-Diagnose. Dtsch Med Wochenschr 116:1523–1530
President's Commission for the Study of Ethical Problems in Medicine and Biomedical and Behavioral Research (1981) Guidelines for the determination of brain death. JAMA 246:246–149
Takeuchi K, Takeshita H, Takakura K (1987) Evolution of criteria for determination of brain death in Japan. Acta Neurochir 87:93–98
Wissenschaftlicher Beirat der Bundesärztekammer (1982) Stellungnahme zur Frage der Kriterien des Hirntodes. Dtsch Artzebl Mitteilg 79:45–55
Wissenschaftlicher Beirat der Bundesärztekammer, "Kriterien des Hirntodes" (1986)

Fortschreibung der Stellungnahme des
Wissenschaftlichen Beirates "Kriterien
des Hirntodes". Dtsch Artzebl Mitteilg
83:2904–2946
Wissenschaftlicher Beirat der Bundesärzte-
kammer, "Kriterien des Hirntodes" (1991)
Kriterien des Hirntodes. Dtsch Artzebl
Mitteilg 87:2855–2860

Appendix. Criteria established for brain death by various authorities

Harvard criteria (1968)

1. Unresponsive coma
2. Apnea
3. Absence of cephalic reflexes
4. Absence of spinal reflexes
5. Isoelectric EEG
6. Persistence of condition for at least 24 h
7. Absence of drug intoxication or hypothermia

Swedish criteria (1972)

1. Unresponsive coma
2. Apnea
3. Absent brain-stem reflex
4. Isoelectric EEG
5. Nonfilling of cerebral vessels on two aortocranial injections of contrast media 25 min apart

British criteria (1976)

Conditions:

1. Patient deeply comatose
   a) No depressant drugs
   b) No hypothermia
   c) No remediable metabolic or endocrine disturbance as cause

2. Spontaneous ventilation inadequate or absent
   a) Relaxants and other depressant drugs excluded

3. Cause established; condition due to irremediable structural brain damage

Diagnostic tests:

1. Pupils fixed and nonreactive to light
2. No corneal reflex
3. Vestibulo-ocular reflexes absent
4. Stimulation anywhere elicits no motor responses mediated via cranial nerves
5. No gag or tracheal suction reflex
6. No respiratory movements when ventilator removed and $PaCO_2$ rises above threshold

U.S. Collaborative Study Criteria (1977)

1. Basic prerequisite – completion of all appropriate and therapeutic procedures
2. Unresponsive coma
3. Apnea
4. Absent cephalic reflexes with dilated, fixed pupils
5. Isoelectric EEG
6. Persistence of the above for 30 min to 1 h, and 6 h after onset of coma and apnea
7. Optional confirmatory test indicating absence of cerebral circulation

President's Commission

1. Unreceptive and unresponsive coma
2. Absent brain-stem function: absent pupillary, corneal, oculocephalic, oculovestibular, oropharyngeal reflexes
3. Apnea with $PaCO_2$ greater than 60 torr
4. Absence of posturing or seizures
5. Irreversibility demonstrated by establishing cause and excluding

reversible conditions (sedation, hypothermia, shock, and neuromuscular blockade)

6. Period of observation determined by clinical judgement

7. Use of cerebral blood flow test when brain-stem reflexes are not testable, inability to establish sufficient cause, to shorten period of observation

Chapter 22

Organ-Preserving Therapy After Brain Death

WILLIAM A. BAUMGARTNER, HUBERT BÖHRER, and
EIKE MARTIN

Introduction

Appropriate management of the brain-dead patient who is considered for multiple organ donation can be a challenging but rewarding experience. With the increasing success of all solid organ transplants, the number of potential recipients who would benefit has increased exponentially. In order to maximize the number of suitable organs, knowledgeable and careful management of the potential donor is imperative. This chapter will attempt to define the role of the caregiver, review the general management strategies, and emphasize the factors, specific to each different organ as they relate to care of the donor patient.

Identification of Donors

Although approximately 90% of all organ donors originate from intensive care units, 25% are not recognized as potential donors for 48 h or more or until the time of death. As the inci-

dence of complications increases progressively with time, 20% of potential donors die within 6 h of admission and 50% die within 24 h if not appropriately supported. Although early identification of the donor and subsequent communication with the family remains a difficult proposition for many physicians, it remains the single most effective method to obtain consent for organ donation. Legislative efforts of various kinds cannot replace the communication between the primary care physician and the family of the brain-dead patient. The suggestion of organ donation gives the family a chance to make their own decision and may result in some feeling of satisfaction in an otherwise tragic situation.

General exclusionary criteria for organ donation include:

– Malignancy (except primary brain tumor)
– Untreated septicemia
– Acquired immunodeficiency syndrome
– Viral hepatitis and encephalitis
– Intravenous drug abuse
– Significant history of drug abuse or homosexuality

Section Editor: Michael N. Diringer

In the past several years, the arbitrary age limit for using specific organs for transplantation has increased. At the present time, the majority of transplant centers would consider any donor up to 60 years of age for heart, lung, liver, and pancreas donation. Kidney donation would be considered up to the age of 70 years.

Evaluation of Donors

Evaluation of the potential donor consists of a thorough history taking and physical examination. In many institutions this evaluation is reviewed by a donor organ coordinator, thereby not inconveniencing the attending physician. Previously held donor exclusionary criteria, including cardiac arrest, chest and abdominal trauma, and requirement for high-dose inotropes, no longer immediately exclude donors. Further work-up and evaluation often result in successful procurement and subsequent function of these organs after transplantation.

Some particular organs have unique characteristics which are important in the evaluation process. A fixed serum creatinine value >2 mg/dl (177μmol/l) is the limit at which donors are excluded for kidney donation. If, however, the creatinine value decreases with aggressive resuscitation, kidneys can be used for transplantation in the majority of cases. Similarly, decreasing serum transaminase levels will usually result in the liver being used for transplantation.

In evaluating a patient as a potential heart donor, the primary electrocardiographic abnormality precluding use of the organ is the presence of pathological Q-waves. Chest trauma, high levels of inotropes (e.g., dopa-

mine), and cardiac arrest do not necessarily preclude the use of the heart for transplantation. Echocardiography prior to procurement and physical examination both prior to and during the organ procurement procedure determine the extent of myocardial injury. In general, most donor hearts with a normal echocardiogram and no significant abnormalities observed by palpation at the time of cardiectomy function well following transplantation. Older donors (males > 40 yrs and females > 45 yrs), especially with associated risk factors, will often require coronary angiography.

Patients being considered as lung donors should have an arterial $PO_2 > 350$ mmHg determined at an inspired oxygen concentration of 100%. Peak airway pressure should be <30 cmH$_2$O and the chest X-ray should show no evidence of major pulmonary contusion, atelectasis, or infiltration. Often these X-ray abnormalities are responsive to various lung expansion procedures. Bronchoscopy is the standard method to assess the trachea and bronchi as well as to obtain aspirates for Gram stain, culture, and sensitivity.

There are no contraindications to the use of the pancreas for transplantation except a history of diabetes. Approximately 40% of pancreas donors exhibit hyperamylasemia.

Medical Management of the Multiorgan Donor

Prior to the actual declaration of death, the medical management of neurologically injured patients consists of methods which lower intracerebral pressure. Patients are generally hypovolemic during this phase. Once death is imminent or declared, the overall goals of management change. Since brain death is often associated with marked hemodynamic changes, recognition and intervention to maintain hemodynamic stability is of primary importance. In addition, these patients often need hydration to provide adequate perfusion pressure for those organs which might potentially be transplanted.

Hemodynamic management is often the single most difficult issue that confronts a physician and/or coordinator taking care of these patients. Monitoring lines facilitate fluid management and titration of various medications including antidiuretics and vasopressors. A patient should have an arterial line for continuous recording of the arterial pressure. In addition, a central venous pressure catheter is also important to adjust fluids appropriately. A Foley catheter and temperature probe are also indicated for purposes of monitoring urine output and core temperature, respectively.

Several problems associated with patients that undergo brain death include:

- Hemodynamic variations
- Respiratory problems
- Fluid and electrolyte abnormalities
- Temperature variations
- Diabetes insipidus
- General care

Hemodynamic Variations

Immediately prior to brain death, the donor may exhibit a hypertensive response to progressive increase in intracranial pressure. This is also associated with increased sympathetic activity and circulating catecholamines. All of these effects contribute to the development of microinfarcts of the heart, seen both clinically and experimentally, which subsequently result in impaired graft function following transplantation. When recognized, this hypertensive response can be treated with either nitroprusside or esmolol (β-blocker), both of which have short half-lives making them ideal agents in the management of unstable patients. On occasion, bradycardia may be observed. Since atropine has no particular effect in patients undergoing brain death, a chronotropic drug such as isoproterenol can be used effectively to treat these transient bradyarrhythmias.

Following brain herniation and irreparable damage to the medullary and pontine vasomotor areas, hypotension often results. The cause of this frequently observed hemodynamic perturbation may be a lack of sympathetic vasomotor control, fluid loss from the concomitant occurrence of diabetes insipidus, and/or the overall hypovolemia observed in these patients at the time of brain death.

Hypotension resulting in decreased perfusion pressure is harmful to all organs considered for transplantation. Optimal organ function following procurement and transplantation is associated with a systolic blood pressure maintained above 90 mmHg for the majority of time prior to procurement. Adequate blood pressure is maintained by both fluid resuscitation and/or vasopressor medications.

Respiratory Management

Since all brain-dead patients are on controlled mechanical ventilation, ventilator adjustments can be employed to maintain a normal pH of 7.4. Metabolic acidosis, however, should be treated with sodium bicarbonate. Avoidance of higher minute ventilation volume will result in lower intrathoracic pressures avoiding any compromise in cardiac output. Oxygenation is considered adequate if the arterial oxygen saturation is above 95%. The majority of these patients are placed on positive end-expiratory pressure (PEEP) (5 cmH$_2$O). Excessive use of PEEP is discouraged in order to maintain adequate venous return and cardiac output. Patients being considered for lung transplantation are maintained disregard on the lowest inspired oxygen concentration resulting in adequate oxygenation (PaO_2 > 70 mmHg) to reduce the potential for atelectasis associated with hyperoxia. In all other brain-dead donors, PaO_2 should be maintained above 100 mmHg.

Fluid and Electrolytes

Following the declaration of brain death, clinical assessment of the potential donor will often reveal a state of hypovolemia. Administration of 1–2 l Ringer's lactate solution is often needed to maintain the blood pressure. The central venous pressure should be kept between 5 and 10 mmHg. General guidelines for the management of organ donors are listed in Table 1. Elevating the central venous pressure above 10 mmHg can be associated with cardiac dilatation and pulmonary edema, which could preclude successful transplantation of the heart and lungs. If significant blood loss has occurred, blood should be administered to maintain a hematocrit of more than 30%. Although Ringer's lactate is used as the primary replacement fluid,

Table 1. General Guidelines for the Management of the Potential Multi-Organ Donor

1. Review the history and conduct a physical examination.
2. Assess height and weight.
3. Assess the monitoring lines. The patient should have an arterial line, a central venous pressure line, a Foley catheter and temperature probe. If the patient is hypotensive, administer 1–2 l Ringer's lactate over 30–60 min. Subsequent fluid management should be based upon urine output and maintaining central venous pressure between 5 and 10 mmHg.
4. Maintain intravenous fluids at 100 ml hourly plus the previous hour's urine output. If hypernatremia is observed, switch replacement fluid to 5% dextrose in water.
5. Monitor potassium, sodium, glucose levels, and arterial blood gases every 2–4 h. At the initial evaluation, measure hematocrit, magnesium, blood urea nitrogen, creatinine, calcium, liver function, urine analysis, prothrombin and partial thromboplastin times, and phosphate levels.
6. If hematocrit is below 30%, transfuse cross-matched blood.
7. If systolic pressure remains below 90 mmHg after adequate volume replacement, begin dopamine infusion to maintain systolic pressure above 90 mmHg. If dopamine is inadequate, maintain dopamine and start dobutamine infusion.
8. Apply a warming blanket to maintain temperature above 35°C.
9. If the patient develops diabetes insipidus with urine output exceeding 250 ml/h for 2 h, start a vasopressin infusion. Titrate infusion to maintain urine output at 100–200 ml/h. Initial suggested dose would be 0.5–1.0 U/h for adult patients.
10. Send tracheal aspirate, urine, and blood for routine and fungal culture.
11. Send blood for ABO typing, HLA tissue typing, and serum titers for human immunodeficiency virus, cytomegalovirus, hepatitis B and C virus and toxoplasmosis.
12. Continue general care of the patient with nasogastric aspiration and frequent and sterile endotracheal suctioning. After cultures have been obtained, start a broad-spectrum non-nephrotoxic agent.
13. Obtain chest X-ray, electrocardiogram, and echocardiogram.

the serum sodium concentration increases occasionally. This necessitates changing the resuscitation fluid to 5% dextrose and water until the serum sodium concentration returns to the normal range. Some centers also suggest the use of colloid (e.g., hydroxyethyl starch) solutions in addition to crystalloid fluids, on the premise that hemodynamic stability is achieved with a smaller infused volume.

Temperature Variations

The majority of patients who undergo brain death will become hypothermic. Since this may cause severe cardiovascular problems, patients will require warming blankets to maintain a temperature above 35°C. In addition to a warming blanket, heat lamps and warming the intravenous fluids and inspired air can be advantageous in maintaining body temperature.

Following adequate volume expansion, assessed by clinical examination and central venous pressure monitoring (urine output may be influenced by diabetes insipidus), inotropic medication should be started if hypotension persists. In intensive care units where the insertion of a pulmonary artery catheter is routine, this additional monitoring line may be of benefit in further assessing the volume status of the patient. Excessive catecholamines, occurring either endogenously or administered as inotropes, increase myocardial oxygen consumption and can result in postoperative kidney and myocardial dysfunction. For these reasons every effort should be made to limit these medications. The primary inotropic agent used in the management of organ donors is dopamine. It is generally believed that doses in excess of 15–20 µg/kg per minute are associated with decreased myocardial function following transplantation. If an additional inotrope is needed, dobutamine is generally recommended.

Diabetes Insipidus

Diabetes insipidus occurs during brain death in the majority of patients. Diabetes insipidus is the result of the decrease in circulating antidiuretic hormone caused by injury to the hypothalamic-pituitary regions of the brain. Two vasopressant preparations are presently used. Desmopressin, a synthetic analogue of arginine vasopressin, is given intravenously at a dose of 0.5–2.0 µg every 8–12 h. Its potential advantage over aqueous vasopressin is the longer duration of action and low pressor/antidiuretic ratio. The pressor activity seen with all of these compounds has been associated with decreased kidney and liver function following transplantation. Vasopressin is generally administered in a continuous intravenous infusion at a rate of 0.5–1.0 U/h. These drugs are titrated to maintain urine output at the rate of 100–200 ml/h.

On occasion the potential organ donor will exhibit oliguria. Decreased urine output leads to postoperative acute tubular necrosis in renal allografts. Build-up of fluid in the donor is also detrimental to potential liver, heart, and lung transplantation. Mannitol or furosemide administration will usually result in a brisk diuresis in the majority of cases.

Associated with these fluid fluxes are occasional electrolyte imbalances. The serum potassium and sodium concentrations should be checked frequently (see Table 1). In addition to potassium and sodium, magnesium and phosphate should also be determined and corrected if the levels are low. Serum glucose should also be examined since hyperglycemia will lead to osmotic diuresis.

General Care

Patients considered for potential organ donors should continue to have standard care. This includes lubrication of the eyes, frequent airway suctioning, and intermittent manual lung inflation to prevent atelectasis. Nasogastric suction is used to reduce the risk of aspiration. All invasive catheters should be dressed and maintained sterilely. The majority of centers also employ routine broad spectrum (nonnephrotoxic) antibiotics.

Hormonal Therapy

Both experimental and human studies have documented a reduction in circulating hormones following brain death. Since a reduction in hormones has been shown to result in organ injury experimentally, the concept of hormonal therapy in potential organ donors was developed. The administration of triiodothyronine, cortisol, and insulin has shown conflicting results. At the present time, randomized controlled trials are necessary to adequately evaluate the potential beneficial effect of hormonal therapy.

Conclusion

The availability of organs is a limiting factor in transplantation. The successful management of the potential donor following declaration of death and consent is crucial. The commitment to maintaining such potential patients following declaration of death will lead to an increasing number of recipients who will benefit from well-preserved organs.

Suggested Reading

Baumgartner WA (1990) Evaluation and management of the heart donor. In: Baumgartner WA, Reitz BA, Achuff SC (eds) Heart and heart-lung transplantation. Saunders, Philadelphia, pp 86–102

Bodenham A, Park GR (1989) Care of the multiple organ donor. Intensive Care Med 15:340–348

Darby JM, Stein K, Grenvik A, Stuart SA (1989) Approach to management of the heartbeating 'brain dead' organ donor. JAMA 261:2222–2228

Soifer BE, Gelb AW (1989) The multiple organ donor: identification and management. Ann Intern Med 110:814–823

Timmins AC, Hinds CJ (1991) Management of the multiple-organ donor. Curr Opin Anaesthesiol 4:287–292

Part II
Differential Diagnosis of Symptoms and Signs

Chapter 23

The Comatose Patient

Erich Schmutzhard, Allan H. Ropper, and Werner Hacke

Definition

Impairment of consciousness and coma are important problems in neurocritical care. The ascending reticular activating system (ARAS) exerts the most influence on consciousness and any damage to this system, either directly or indirectly, impairs consciousness. Consciousness is defined as the state of awareness of one's self and the environment. Coma is the opposite of consciousness and is the total absence of awareness of one's self and the environment, even when externally stimulated.

Gradation of Coma

Although the commonly used coma scales, such as the Glasgow Coma Scale or Innsbruck Coma Scale, do not actually reflect "depth" of coma, they are useful prognostically, especially in patients with trauma. The introduction of terms such as "midbrain syndromes" and "bulbar brain syndrome" reflects

---

Section Editor: Allan H. Ropper

an attempt to stage coma after cranial trauma. This classification allows better documentation of disease progression and resolution. The use of neurological scoring systems allows reliability and objectivity in assessing comatose patients. Most coma scales were developed for evaluation of supratentorial brain injuries. However, neither infratentorial structural disturbances nor diffuse cortical or subcortical dysfunction from hypoxic, metabolic, or toxic causes fit into this classification. In addition, the abundance of descriptive terms employed (such as "clouding of consciousness," "lethargy," "delirium," "obtundation," and so on) has made it difficult to assess patients objectively. This also applies, though to a much lesser extent, to the terms used to describe "depth of disturbance of consciousness": (1) somnolence, (2) sopor (continental Europe) or stupor (North America), and (3) coma. Unless stimulated, somnolent patients are sleepy and apathetic. They often have difficulty cooperating with the examination and may have bouts of motor restlessness. Soporous or stuporous patients can be aroused only by strong external stimuli. Patients may respond verbally during these short periods of arousal. Comatose patients cannot be aroused even by strong, painful stimuli. The eyes remain closed and no communication is possible. The depth or grade of coma (I–IV) can be assessed by the presence or absence of spontaneous movements, brainstem reflexes, abnormal posturing, normal or abnormal muscle tone, and the ability to breathe spontaneously.

Pathogenesis

The existence of the ARAS was first postulated in 1949 by Moruzzi and Magoun, and although revisions have been made since then, the fundamental concept of the physiology underlying arousal and consciousness is still based on this pioneering work. The ARAS is a poorly defined group of neurons located in the center of the upper brainstem (extending from the midbrain into the thalamus). This system transmits the effects of external stimuli to the cerebral cortex. Stimulation of the thalamic nuclei from cortical activity and sensory projections to the limbic system are important modulators of alertness. The ARAS receives many collaterals from all major somatic and sensory pathways.

The anatomy and physiology of the ARAS is not fully understood, but at least three main projections have been identified: (1) via the thalamic reticular nucleus to the cerebral cortex, (2) via the hypothalamus to the limbic system and forebrain structures, and (3) from the midbrain raphe and locus ceruleus to the neocortex via widespread and diffuse projections. Coma can result from large, particularly bilateral, hemispheric lesions that disrupt the ARAS projections. More often, the projections are disrupted indirectly by secondary impairment, such as increased intracranial pressure or a mass. Coma can result from any lesion to this complex system, including structural damage to the upper brainstem or both hemispheres, metabolic, hypoxic, or toxic causes, or severe disturbances of the endocrine system.

The following is a review of the clincal features, diagnostic workup, treatment, and prognosis of comatose patients. Each of the different causes of coma will be discussed separately. In addition, conditions that mimic coma, such as the locked-in syndrome, akinetic mutism, and persistant vegetative state (or apallic syndrome) will also be reviewed.

Clinical Features

A complete past medical history and details about the onset of coma are essential for diagnosis and early treatment. Table 1 summarizes important parts of the initial evaluation of comatose patients.

Primary and Secondary Structural Damage to the Brainstem

Secondary damage to the brainstem and impairment of consciousness and coma can result from any expanding supratentorial disease that causes increased intracranial pressure and downward transtentorial herniation or any unilateral mass that causes uncal and transtentorial herniation. Deter-

Table 1. Emergency assessment of a comatose patient

1. Data from medical history, if available, including previous drug treatment

Neurological:	Other:
seizures	arterial hypertension
cerebrovascular disease	cardiac disease
alcohol or drug use or abuse	pulmonary disease
	psychiatric disorder, including suicide attempts
	diabetes
	any other major disease:
	cancer
	immunosuppressive/autoimmune disorder

2. Earlier factors probably related to the present condition:
   headache
   vomiting
   recent trauma to head and neck
   fever, infection, or sepsis
   earlier focal neurological signs such as
       hemiparesis
       aphasia
       hemianopia
       diplopia
       vertigo
       etc.
   type of onset:
       progressive
       abrupt
       fluctuating
3. General examination:
   pattern of respiration
   signs and symptoms of pulmonary dysfunction
   cardiac evaluation
       arrhythmia
       blood pressure
       shock
   body temperature
   fits: focal/generalized
   myoclonus
   concomitant injuries
   tongue bite
   incontinence
   fomites: content
   skin
       color
       petechiae
   anuria/polyuria
   signs of dehydration

mining the level of brainstem damage on the basis of clinical signs, such as pupillary reflexes, oculocephalic reflexes, posture, muscle tone, and breathing patterns, was introduced by Gerstenbrand and Lücking and by Plum and Posner. In general, although this clinical classification is applicable to selected patients with cranial trauma, it is not applicable to most other patients in coma (for example, those with coma secondary to metabolic or toxic disorders or those with infratentorial lesions). Moreover, it has recently become clear that coma from supratentorial lesions is not simply the result of downward herniation since most patients have signs of brainstem dysfunction before they develop coma.

Rapidly expanding, space-occupying supratentorial diseases include trauma, spontaneous intracerebral hemorrhage, abscesses, tumors, focal ischemia, sinus venous thrombosis, purulent meningitis, subarachnoid hemorrhage, diffuse vasculitis (in patients with autoimmune disease), cerebral malaria, air embolism, and brain edema following eclampsia.

Metabolic Disorders

In patients with metabolic encephalopathy, patients progress from mild changes in mentation, and particularly in attention, to an acute confusional state, to coma. Patients may develop decorticate and decerebrate posturing similar to those with coma after structural damage. The progressive signs of brainstem dysfunction are almost always bilateral and may worsen acutely. Important features in patients with severe metabolic encephalopathy include respiratory abnormalities, such as changes in frequency, rhythm, or depth of breathing. Certain respiratory changes are almost diagnostic for some conditions. For example, *hyperventilation* is frequently seen in patients with metabolic acidosis (as in those with diabetes mellitus, uremia, lactic acidosis, or ingestion of acids). Other patients, such as those with hepatic failure, pulmonary disease, sepsis, and psychiatric illness, may have hyperventilation associated with respiratory alkalosis. Mixed metabolic acidosis and respiratory alkalosis may occur in patients with hepatic coma and salicylate intoxication. *Hypoventilation* often results in respiratory acidosis and may occur in patients with damage to the respiratory center (located in the lower brainstem), neuromuscular disorders, or primary pulmonary disease. Hypoventilation can also occur as a compensatory response to metabolic alkalosis. Structural damage to the brainstem results in irregular, shallow, or ataxic breathing whereas neuromuscular disorders and primary pulmonary diseases result in tachypnea.

Normal pupillary reaction to light in a comatose patient with other signs of midbrain dysfunction is strongly suggestive of a metabolic cause of coma rather than a structural cause. In patients with metabolic coma, the eyes are in the forward position, although in those with rapidly developing metabolic disorders any eye position or eye movement can be transiently observed. Sustained conjugate deviation and dysconjugate positioning (including skew deviation) suggests structural damage. Oculomotor reflex responses are usually conjugate in patients with metabolic disorders.

Any type of changes in muscle tone or reflexes as well as focal or generalized seizures may occur throughout the course of metabolic brain disease. Frequently, patients have tremor, asterixis, and myoclonus. Because tremor and asterixis are present only in noncomatose patients, the clinician must depend on the description of others involved in the patient's care earlier in the course of the disease. Myoclonus is frequently multifocal and may consist of irregular, nonpatterned gross twitching of various muscle groups. Myoclonus is often prominent in proximal muscles. It may be triggered by external stimuli and is most commonly seen after anoxia. Pronounced unilateral weakness is rare in metabolic disorders and usually occurs with hypoglycemia or after seizures. Preexisting compensated focal motor deficits, however, may result in severe weakness in the presence of almost any metabolic disorders.

Table 2 lists possible causes of metabolic coma, specific neurological signs, and diagnostic steps. Laboratory values that accompany severe impairment of consciousness are listed separately. In general, rapid changes are more likely to cause severe symptoms rather than particular absolute values. In many instances, a detailed history and physical examination will allow one to choose the correct diagnostic test. In general, blood samples should be

Table 2. Metabolic coma

Etiology	Specific neurologic signs	Diagnostic steps
Hypoxia	Flaccid muscle tone, myoclonus	Preceding cardiac disease, polytrauma, resuscitation, attempted suicide
Hyperosmolar diabetic coma	Frequently: coma, seizures (20%–25%), focal signs	Blood glucose >1100 mg%, high serum osmolarity
Diabetic ketoacidosis	Clouding of consciousness but rarely coma	Ketonuria, blood glucose >400 mg%
Hypoglycemia	High variability, incl. coma, seizures, focal signs	Blood glucose <30 mg%
Hepatic encephalopathy	Tremor, asterixis (wing beating); final stage: severe clouding of consciousness	Ammonia
Uremia	Delirium, seizures, myoclonus, asterixis; final stage: clouding of consciousness	Serum creatinine, urea, potassium
Dysequilibrium syndrome	Muscle cramps, seizures, coma	Postdialysis, urea, sodium, osmolarity
Hyponatremia	Clouding of consciousness; seizures and coma only in case of rapid change of serum sodium level	Serum sodium <126 mmol
Hypernatremia	Delirium, "muscle weakness"; coma only in case of rapid change	Serum sodium >156 mmol, reduced urinary sodium excretion
Hypercalcemia	Delirium, headache, "muscle weakness"	Calcium and phosphate in serum and urine, parathormone
Hypocalcemia	Tetanic syndrome, delirium, pseudopsychotic behavior, seizures	Calcium and phosphate in serum and urine, parathormone
Thiamine deficiency	Wernicke encephalopathy; very rarely coma	Vitamin B1 level, 100 mg vitamin B1 i.v.

obtained for analysis of blood gases, serum glucose, electrolytes, transaminases, blood urea nitrogen (BUN), and creatinine. In the emergency department, a disturbance in glucose metabolism, which can be diagnosed and treated quickly, is the most frequent cause of metabolic coma. Patients with coma from hepatic failure or renal failure frequently have triphasic waves on EEG.

Endocrinological Disorders

Impairment of cognitive functions (mentation and awareness) and even acute confusional states, such as delirium, occur frequently in patients with diseases of the endocrine system. Coma is a rare complication and is seen most often in patients with thyreotoxicosis (thyroid storm) and adrenal insufficiency. The onset is usually slow. A sudden onset of coma may be seen in patients with acute dysfunction of the anterior pituitary gland or infarction of the pituitary gland (these patients usually have preceding ophthalmoplegia, amaurosis fugax, and severe headache).

Hypoxia

Global, sustained hypoxic damage may be the result of a cardiac arrest, submersion injury, respiratory failure or arrest (from pulmonary or extrapulmonary causes), systemic vascular disease, vasculitis, hypertensive encephalopathy, cerebral malaria, air embolism, or poisoning (e.g., carbon monoxide or cyanide poisoning). Hypoxia leads to glial swelling, secondary neuronal ischemia, and diffuse brain edema. Hypoxia is suggested as the cause of coma in patients without focal signs, decerebrate or decorticate posturing, myoclonus, decreased PO_2, increased PCO_2, metabolic acidosis, and a markedly abnormal EEG with generalized slowing.

Drug Overdose

Drug overdose – accidental or intended – may result in coma of varying degrees. Table 3 summarizes important aspects of the most common types of drug overdose (for a detailed review see Schuster 1983).

Seizures

Patients presenting in the postictal period after a seizure may be comatose. Often the seizure itself is not observed. High doses of antiseizure medications, such as benzodiazepines or barbiturates, given in the emergency department are frequently the reason for prolonged recovery after a single seizure. Occasionally, such overzealous treatment is complicated by aspiration pneumonia or shock. Sometimes generalized or focal seizures occur in the setting of severe intracranial disease, such as subarachnoid hemorrhage, encephalitis, sinus thrombosis, or hemorrhage into a tumor.

Status epilepticus (continuous seizures or failure to regain consciousness between seizures) also may be accompanied by hypoxia. Petit mal (absence) status and partial complex status are confirmed by EEG and should not be confused with coma. In most patients, neurocritical care monitoring and management are needed for a few hours or days. Structural, meta-

Table 3. Clinical features and diagnostic steps in patients in coma after a drug overdose[a]

Drug	Main clinical features[b]	Main diagnostic steps
Alcohol (ethanol)	Hypothermia, average to wide pupil size, tachycardia, vomiting, typical smell	Blood level of alcohol
Antidepressants (tricyclic)	Myoclonus, epileptic seizures	Urine level of drug ECG: sinus tachycardia arrhythmia conduction defects
Atropine-scopolamine	Raised body temperature, flush, dry skin, dilated pupils	ECG: tachycardia
Arsenic	Diarrhea, seizures, hemolysis	Arsenic at hair roots ECG: arrhythmia
Barbiturates	Flaccidity, apnea, blisters, hypothermia, hypotension	EEG: burst-suppression Urine/serum level of drug
Benzodiazepines	Usually stupor, no severe cardiac or respiratory alteration	Urine/serum level of drug
Bioiogical toxins:		
plants containing atropine	See atropine-scopolamine	Investigate for ingestion of plants
poisonous mussels (containing domoic acid)	Within 1.5–48 h after ingestion: myoclonus, seizures	Investigate for exposure to or ingestion of contaminated seafood, domoic acid levels in feces
mushrooms, e.g, *Amanita* spp.	Nausea, vomiting, diarrhea, jaundice, seizures	Investigate for ingestion of mushrooms
Carbon monoxide	See hypoxia (Table 2)	CO Hemoglobin CT scan: hypodensities in basal ganglia
Cocaine	Seizures, cerebrovascular ischemia	Serum level of drug
Cyclosporine	S.p. kidney transplantation, flaccid tetraparesis, seizures	CT (MRI) scan: white matter changes Serum level of drug
Ethanol	See alcohol	
Glycol	myocloni	Renal failure (oxalate in urine), acidosis CT scan: hypodensities in basal ganglia
Heroin (opiates)	Seizures, pulmonary edema, rhabdomyolysis, needle marks, extreme miosis	Opiate in urine creatine kinase, myoglobin in urine
Lead	Seizures, anemia, neuropathy, lead line in gingiva	Anemia, basophilic stippling, lead levels in blood and tissue
Lithium	Preceding abdominal pains, vomiting, exsiccosis, myocloni, seizures	Renal failure Lithium levels in serum
Methanol	Blindness	Blood level of methanol, acidosis
Opiates: see heroin		
Pesticides (or ganophosphates)	Agricultural background, abdominal pains, profuse sweating, miosis, paraparesis, seizures	Low cholinesterase in serum, tachycardia, tachyarrhythmia

Table 3. *Continued*

Drug	Main clinical features[b]	Main diagnostic steps
Phenytoin	Nystagmus	Serum level of phenytoin
Salicylate	Seizures, hyperventilation, hyperthermia	Acidosis, CT scan: brain swelling salicylate level
Tricyclic antidepressants	See antidepressants	
Thallium	Neuralgia, seizures, loss of hair, constipation	Coagulation disturbance, thallium at hair roots Raised blood pressure

CT, Computed tomography; ECG, electrocardiography; EEG, electroencephalography; MRI, magnetic resonance imaging.
[a] Adapted from Plum and Posner 1982, Einhäupl et al. 1990, Klein et al. 1970, and Teitelbaum et al. 1990.
[b] In addition to coma.

bolic, and toxic causes must be excluded by neuroimaging studies, cerebrospinal fluid analysis, and laboratory tests.

Diagnostic Workup

The immediate care of comatose patients depends on the history and results of examination (including the evolution of neurological symptoms and signs), and accompanying non-neurological problems. A stepwise approach is essential. Clinicians must be alert to subtle changes in neurological findings. Other clinical features (extracerebral and extracranial) may support the neurological diagnosis. Table 4 lists primary diagnostic steps to be taken at the site of the emergency. Table 5 lists diagnostic steps to be taken in the emergency department or neurocritical care unit (see Chap. 3).

Differential Diagnosis

This section reviews conditions that resemble coma. These "pseudoco-

Table 4. Primary diagnostic steps in a comatose patient at the site of emergency

1. Brief neurological assessment
2. Assessment of vital signs: blood pressure, heart rate, body temperature, blood sugar
3. Clearance of any airway obstruction
4. Orotracheal intubation, artificial ventilation, if appropriate
5. Insertion of a (central) venous catheter, intravenous fluid; blood samples for drug testing
6. Inspection of the patient's surroundings
7. History taking; if possible, ask relatives or witnesses
8. Immediate supervised transport to emergency or intensive care facility

matose conditions" include: (1) locked-in syndrome, (2) akinetic mutism, (3) apallic syndrome or persistent vegetative state, (4) extensive, generalized peripheral nerve disease, and (5) hypersomnia.

Locked-In Syndrome

The locked-in syndrome is defined as paralysis of all four extremities and almost all motor cranial nerves with the exception of those controlling verti-

Table 5. Diagnostic steps to be taken in the emergency room or intensive care unit

1. Reassessment and repetition of the steps in Table 4, if appropriate
2. Monitoring of blood pressure, pulse rate, ECG, body temperature, blood gas analysis
3. Central venous and arterial catheter; urinary catheter
4. Laboratory tests: red blood cell count, white blood cell count, thrombocytes, coagulation parameters, glucose, electrolytes, serum creatinine, creatinine phosphokinase including isoenzymes, transaminases
5. Neuroradiologic assessment:
   CT, MRI, angiography
6. If appropriate, call specialist consultants
7. Doppler ultrasound – extracranial blood vessels
8. Cerebrospinal fluid:
   cells
   glucose
   albumin and immunoglobulins
   Keep some fluid for further studies
9. Electroencephalogram
10. Blood, urine, and possibly gastric contents: toxicologic screening including alcohol, drugs, and other chemical compounds
11. Pregnancy test

cal eye movements, blinking, and respiratory function; patients are fully aware of their environment, that is, they are conscious. The syndrome results from bilateral destruction of the ventral part of the pons, leading to supranuclear motor deefferentiation. Most locked-in syndromes are caused by basilar artery thrombosis or, infrequently, pontine hemorrhage, primary brainstem contusion, brainstem encephalitis, tumor, or pontine myelinolysis. Most patients require assisted ventilation initially, though eventually spontaneous respiration may recur. Brainstem reflexes, such as the oculocephalic, oculovestibular, and, particularly, corneal reflexes are absent. Patients are unable to swallow, speak, or even phonate. Sensation is intact, including pain sensation. Sleep is frequently preserved. The EEG is abnormal and shows generalized slowing. Visual evoked potentials are preserved. The prognosis is variable depending on the exact cause and extent of the lesion. Patients with ischemia or hemorrhage never functionally recover; up to two-thirds die in the acute setting. Patients who survive are fully alert but can only communicate through a code of voluntary eye movements. They require life-long total care.

Akinetic Mutism

Patients with akinetic mutism are immobile, appear awake and alert, and have preserved cognition. The motor system is intact, both peripherally and centrally. Most patients have large bilateral frontal lobe lesions, frequently extending to and involving the cingulate gyri and the limbic system. There have been many case reports demonstrating lesions in various parts of the brain. Hydrocephalus and space-occupying lesions of the pineal gland have also been reported in patients with akinetic mutism. Briefly, the clinical features of akinetic mutism are most likely the result of lesions interfering with reticulocortical pathways or limbic-cortical integration (sparing corticospinal pathways). The condition is often reversible, even after months of apparent standstill. Prognosis depends on the primary disease and its evolution and the degree of destruction.

Apallic Syndrome or Persistent Vegetative State

Apallic syndrome (the term used in Germany) or persistent vegetative state (the term used in North America) is a subacute or chronic condition that can evolve after any severe brain disease. Other terms include "coma vigile" or "neocortical death." It is defined as a state of awakeness with apparent lack of cognition. Thus, patients keep their eyes open but do not fixate on the examiner. Patients neither obey commands nor show signs of emotional appropriateness. The motor activity of the extremities is extremely limited and may consist only of very slow, aimless motion. Muscle tone is usually increased. Patients are mute and show frequent oral automatisms, such as licking, sucking, and chewing. Even bruxism may exist. Reflexive oral gripping may emerge. Brainstem functions are either intact or become normal throughout the course of the disease. The EEG shows severe diffuse pathological changes such as severe slowing with no response to auditory or noxious stimuli.

The prognosis, in terms of rehabilitation and resocialization, depends primarily on the underlying lesion. Age is also a prognostic factor, as children have a much better chance of rehabilitation than elderly patients. Patients generally have a poor prognosis when they have been in a persistent vegetative state for more than 2–4 weeks after a cardiac arrest, diffuse cerebral hypoxia, and coma for 48–96 h. In patients with trauma or inflammatory diseases, however, substantial improvement in motor and cognitive functions can occur even after several months. The same is true for younger patients with subarachnoid hemorrhage or intracerebral bleeding. In patients with Jacob-Creutzfeldt disease and other diffuse progressive brain disease, the onset of persistent vegetative state usually heralds imminent death, which is frequently caused by pneumonia or other nosocomial infections.

Extensive Generalized Peripheral Nerve Disease

Patients with inflammatory polyradiculoneuropathies (for example, Guillain-Barré syndrome), paralytic poliomyelitis, severe hypokalemia, and myasthenia gravis may develop quadriplegia and cranial nerve involvement that resembles locked-in syndrome or coma. Even the pupils can be dilated and the pupillary reflexes can be lost. Nevertheless, characteristics of the primary disease and its evolution (including involvement of the respiratory muscles and acute respiratory failure) almost always allow differentiation of this condition.

Hypersomonia

Hypersomonia is defined as a condition of intense and permanent sleep. Patients can be aroused throughout the course of the disease, but frequently for only brief periods of time. This condition occurs in patients with bilateral paramedian thalamic lesions, tegmento-mesencephalic lesions, or both (either from ischemia or tumors). The caudal cranial nerves are never affected; swallowing is preserved and even phonation may be possible. Patients do not have decorticate or decerebrate posturing, two features that distinguish hypersomnia from locked-in syndrome and coma.

Prognosis

In general, prognosis depends on many factors including the underlying disease, the initial depth of coma, and complications such as infections, decubitus ulcers, contractions, and cachexia. Initial low scores on coma scales are almost always associated with a poor prognosis. For example, of more than 400 consecutive patients with brain trauma, none of the patients with a score of 0 to 1 on the Innsbruck Coma Scale survived. Similarly, of those with scores of 3 on the Glasgow Coma Scale, only 10% survived. The rapidity of the development of coma and early signs of resolution are also important prognostically. The location and extent of structural damage and the degree and duration of increased intracranial pressure are also crucial. Patients with very large lesions of major parts of the hemispheres almost never have a good outcome. Patient age and the presence of concurrent diseases strongly influence prognosis.

Early loss of somatosensory evoked potentials may also be helpful in predicting outcome. Prognostic scores (e.g., from APACHE III and the Levy-Boston-Corona algorithm) are also helpful. It is essential for patients in coma to be continually and regularly reevaluated. Decisions regarding the aggressiveness of therapy and life support (that is, "code status") need to be based on ethical considerations for each individual patient and not only on the probabilities derived from scoring systems (see Chap. 5).

Suggested Reading

Ashwal ST, Bale JF, Coulter DL, Eiben R, Carg BP, Hill A, Myer EC, Nordgren RE, Shewmon DA, Sunder TR, Walker RW (1992) The persistent vegetative state in children; report of the Child Neurology Society Ethics Committee. Ann Neurol 32:570–576

Becker DP, Gudeman SK (1989) Textbook of head injury. Saunders, Philadelphia

Benzer A, Mitterschiffthaler G, Marosi M, Luef G, Reindl H, Pühringer F, de la Renotiere K, Schmutzhard E (1991) Innsbruck Coma Scale–early prediction of non-survival in severe head-trauma. A 10 year experience. Lancet 11:977–978

Berek K, Luef G, Kiechl S, Schmutzhard E (1992) Neurologische Symptome im Rahmen endokriner Noträlle. Wien Klin Wochenschr 104:613–619

Berkovic SF, Bladen PF (1982) Absence status in adults. Clin Exp Neurol 19:198–207

Cairns H, Oldfield RC, Pennybacker JB (1941) Akinetic mutism with an epidermoid cyst of the 3rd ventricle. Brain 64:273–290

Critchley EMR (1988) Neurological emergencies. Saunders, London (Major problems in neurology, vol 17)

Dalle Ore G, Gerstenbrand F, Lücking CH, Peters G, Peters UH (1977) The apallic syndrome. Springer, Berlin Heidelberg New York

Gerstenbrand F, Lücking HC (1970) Die akuten traumatischen Hirnstammschäden. Arch Psychiatr Nervenkr 213:346–381

Gerstenbrand F, Hackl JM, Mitterschiffthaler G, Poewe W, Prugger M, Rumpl E (1984) Die Innsbrucker Koma-Skala: klinisches Koma-Monitoring. Methodik und Ergebnisse bei 102 Patienten einer neuro-

logischen Intensivpflegestation. Intensivbehandlung 9:133–144

Hacke W (1988) Neurologische Intensivmedizin,
2nd edn. Perimed, Eriangen

Haig AJ, Katz RT, Saghal V (1987) Mortality and
complications of the locked in-syndrome.
Arch Phys Med Rehabil 68:24–27

Jennett WB, Plum FC (1972) Persistent vegetative state after brain damage. Lancet 1:
734–737

Jones EG, Powell TPS (1970) An anatomical
study of converging sensory pathways
within the cerebral cortex of the monkey.
Brain 93:793–820

Jones JG, Vucevic M (1992) Not awake, not
asleep, not dead. Intensive Care Med 18:
67–68

Klein M, Namer R, Harpur E, Corbin R (1970)
Earthenware containers as a source of
fatal lead poisoning: case study and public
health considerations. N Engl J Med 283:
669–672

Kotagai S, Archer CR, Walsh JK, Gomez C
(1985) Hypersomnia, thalamic lesions and
altered sleep architecture in Kearns-Sayre
syndrome. Neurology 35:574–577

Marshall SB, Marshall LF, Vos HR, Chesnut
RM (1990) Neuroscience critical care.
Pathophysiology and patient management.
Saunders, Philadelphia

Moruzzi G, Magoun HW (1949) Brainstem reticular formation and activation of the EEG.
Electroencephalogr Clin Neurophysiol 1:
455–473

Mullie A, Buylaert W, Michem N, Verbruggen
H, Corne L, de Cock R, Mennes J, Quets
A, Verstringe P, Houbrechts H, Delooz
H, van den Broeck L, Lauwaert D,
Weeghmanns M, Bossaert L, Lewi P (1988)
Predictive value of Glasgow Coma Score
for awakening after out-of-hospital cardiac
arrest. Lancet 1:137–140

Plum F, Posner JB (1982) The diagnosis of stupor
and coma, 3rd edn. Davis, Philadelphia

Ropper AH (1989) Neurological intensive care.
In: Toole JF, Vincken PJ, Bruyn CW,
Klawans HL (eds) Handbook of clinical
neurology (revised series). Elsevier,
Amsterdam

Ropper AH (1993) Neurological and neurosurgical intensive care. 3rd edn. Raven,
New York

Rumpl E, Gerstenbrand F (1985) Verlaufsformen
schwerer Schädelhirntraumen. Intensivbehandlung 10:92–99

Schuster HP (1983) Soforttherapie bei
Vergiftungen. Perimed, Erlangen

Shwemon DA, de Giurgio CM (1989) Early
prognosis in anoxic coma. Neurol Clin 7:
823–843

Stöhr M, Brandt T, Einhäupl ICM (1990)
Neurologische Syndrome in der Intensivmedizin. Kohlhammer, Stuttgart

Teasdale G, Jennett B (1974) Assessment of
coma and impaired consciousness. Lancet
ii:81–84

Teitelbaum JS, Catorre RJ, Carpenter S,
Gendron D, Evans AC, Gjedde A,
Cashman NR (1990) Neurologic sequelae
of domoic acid intoxication due to the in-
gestion of contaminated mussels. N Engl J
Med 322:1781–1787

Tunkel AR, Wispelwey B, Scheld WM (1990)
Bacterial meningitis. Recent advances in
pathophysiology and treatment. Ann Intern
Med 112:610–623

Virgile RS (1984) Locked in syndrome. Clin
Neurol Neurosurg 86:275–279

Chapter 24

Acute Hemiparesis

Stefan Schwab, Thomas Brott, and Rüdiger von Kummer

Definition

Acute hemiparesis is often the leading symptom of patients admitted to the neurocritical care unit. The accompanying symptoms and the medical history give the first indication of the location of the patient's lesion and help to expedite treatment. Clinically, many of these patients present with a pronounced brachiofacial contralateral hemiparesis or -plegia with ipsilateral eye deviation, contralateral sensory loss, and extensor plantar reflexes.

In many cases the clinical history alone indicates the cause and location of the patient's lesion. First, the time-course of patient's symptoms is important. Did the hemiparesis occur suddenly or over hours or days? Vascular, hypoglycemic, postparoxysmal, or psychogenic hemipareses generally occur suddenly, whereas neoplastic and inflammatory or traumatic causes lead to a more subacute onset of symptoms. Other accompanying symptoms including headache, fever, nausea, vomiting, and vegetative dysfunction

should be elicited from the medical history, and information about the patient's family history, especially regarding migraine or epileptic disorders, is equally important. Finally, the presence of vascular risk factors including hypertension, diabetes, coronary heart disease, smoking, and hyperlipidemia should be determined.

Topography

General and specific guidelines for inference of lesion location are described below. The sensitivity and specificity of the guidelines have been addressed peviously in clinical-pathologic and clinical-radiographic case series, usually informally. The anatomic sensitivity and specificity of the guidelines have yet to be carefully tested during the first hours after onset of acute hemiparesis.

Pure Hemiparesis

Hemiparesis may be caused by a lesion anywhere between cerebral cortex and

---

Section Editor: Werner Hacke

cervical motor neurons. For further differentiation, additional symptoms have to be reviewed for anatomic localization and appropriate diagnosis.

Hemiparesis with Additional Hemispheric Symptoms

The human speech center, located in the dominant (usually left) hemisphere, requires the coordination of several different pathways. Cortical and subcortical lesions therefore lead to different grades and types of aphasia. In the acute setting, differentiation between Broca's and Wernicke's aphasia is impossible. Patients with acute hemiparesis usually present with global or nonfluent aphasia.

Unilateral neglect is the tendency of patients not to respond to stimuli contalateral to their lesion. Localization cannot be confined to one single area, although neglect usually occurs in patients with right posterior lesions.

Apraxia is often hard to demonstrate in patients who are critically ill, but when identified it can be of some relevance. Apraxia of the ideomotor type is frequently associated with global aphasia but occurs most commonly in the absence of aphasia in patients with right-hemispheric lesions. Other impairments including acalculia and agraphia, ideatoric apraxia, or anosognosia do not play a significant role in the acute assessment of the neurocritical care patient but may become relevant once early rehabilitation starts.

In most cases of acute hemiparesis a concomitant sensory impairment can be observed. This is most commonly due to lesions that involve the spinothalamic and thalamocortical fibers to the precentral gyrus.

Hemiparesis with Lesions in the Internal Capsule

Because fibers of the corticospinal and corticobulbar tracts are close together within the internal capsule, symptoms of internal capsule lesions include contralateral hemiparesis with facial palsy, sensory deficit, and dysarthria or dysphagia. The tongue may deviate to the paretic side and the soft palatine and throat muscles may show asymmetry.

Hemiparesis with Conjugate Deviation of the Eyes

In principle, conjugate deviation of the eyes can occur as a result of either an extended cortical or a small pontine lesion. In cortical lesions (between the frontal eye fields and the contralateral paramedian pontine reticular formations) the deviation is directed to the side of the lesion, usually ipsilateral, although an irritative lesion such as epilepsy may result in contralateral deviation. The opposite is seen with lesions or irritation of the paramedian pontine reticular formation. Eye deviation from lesions at this site may be disconjugate because other nearby fibers are often affected. Internuclear ophthalmoplegia (INO), vertical gaze palsy, or one-and-a-half syndrome may also be seen. Patients often present with head deviation and a horizontal gaze palsy which might be partial or total.

Hemiparesis Associated with Thalamic Lesions

The classic (single-sided) thalamic syndrome (occurring, for example, in a lesion of the ventroposterolateral nucleus) contains the following symptoms: contralateral sensorimotor deficit, hemiatxia and intention tremor, and pain that may be sponatneous or evoked by any form of stimulation. Eye movement abnormalities are not uncommon, particulary with thalamic hemorrhage. The eyes may be deviated to the side of lesion, downward, on the contralateral side. Upgaze is frequently abnormal.

Hemiparesis in Brain-stem Lesions

The cardinal manifestations of brainstem lesions are involvement of the long tracts of the brain stem combined with deficits of the cranial nerve nuclei. Oculomotor disturbances suggest a lesion in the midbrain as do INO and vertical gaze palsy (dorsal midbrain). Crossed brain-stem syndromes result from concomitant cranial nerve and long tract damages. Lesions of the medial medulla usually lead to contralateral weakness and dysarthria, although those of the lateral medulla (Wallenberg syndrome) do not result in hemiparesis. Brain-stem lesions almost always result in disturbances of consciousness and breathing, regardless of the specific location. Table 1 lists the possible causes and locations of specific hemiparetic syndromes.

Hemiparesis in High Cervical Lesions

When hemiparesis appears without facial involvement, a paresis of the eleventh cranial nerve may be present. Because of the extension of the fifth nerve nuclei down to the C-2 segment a dissociated sensory deficit of the face is sometimes found.

Etiology of Hemiparesis

Congenital Hemiparesis

Congenital hemiparesis may result from a number of different prenatal infections, such as congenital syphilis, toxoplasmosis, and viral encephalitis due to CMV or HIV infections. Other infections such as bacterial meningitis, Coxsackie B, and varicella may cause hemiplegia in the infant. Hemiplegia can also result from arterial or venous infarction or bleeding in high-risk and breech deliveries. Often, these patients are admitted to neurology because of hydrocephalus, which sometimes can lead to focal seizures or subdural hematoma. Following the acute phase, these patients tend to have a prolonged rehabilitation phase or other neurologic symptoms.

Vascular Hemiparesis

Vascular syndromes are subdivided into those occurring in the anterior and the posterior circulation (carotid arteries and basilar and vertebral arteries, respectively). Anatomic, and particularly etiologic, classification may be difficult and at times arbitrary. In one large series of very carefully studied cases of acute cerebral infarction, the etiology could not be established in 40% (508 of 1213).

Carotid Circulation

The majority of hemispheric infarcts are within the territory of the middle cerebral artery (MCA). Infarctions of posterior cerebral arteries rarely cause isolated hemiparesis. Acute infarctions of the anterior cerebral arteries (ACA)

Table 1. Topography of acute hemiparesis

Hemiparesis with . . .	Localization of the lesion	Cause with respect to the clinical history	Technical methods
Disturbance of consciousness	– extended hemispheric lesion – brain stem	– 1. acute: ischemia, bleeding, encephalitis, hypoglycemia – 2. subacute: neoplasm, sinus vein thrombosis, migraine, (esp. basilar migraine)	CCT (or MRI), ultrasound, angiography, CSF EEG
Aphasia	– on dominant hemisphere cortical or subcortical in the mid cerebral artery territory	– 1. acute: ischemia, bleeding, encephalitis, hypoglycemia – 2. subacute: neoplasm, sinus vein thrombosis	CCT (or MRI), ultrasound, angiography, CSF EEG
Neglect	– mostly right parietal lobe	See above	See above
Apraxia	– nondominant hemisphere	– in patients on an ICU, normally of anamnestic interest with hint to the nondominant hemispheric	CCT (or MRI), ultrasound, angiography, CSF EEG
Eye deviation	1. ipsilateral without brain-stem symptoms: cortical lesion 2. contralateral without brain-stem symptoms: cortical irritation or thalamic lesion 3. ipsilateral with brain-stem symptoms: ipsilateral pontine lesion 4. contralateral with brain-stem symptoms: contralateral pontine irritation	ad 1. and 2. acute: cortical ischemia, bleeding subacute: subdural or epidural hematoma ad 3. and 4. acute: Thrombosis of the basilar artery, brainstem bleeding, basilar migraine, trauma	CCT (or MRI), ultrasound, angiography, CSF EEG BAEP, SSEP
Motorsensory deficit Facial palsy Dysarthria Dysphagia	contralateral lesion of the internal capsule	acute: ischemia, bleeding, trauma subacute: encephalitis, neoplasm	CCT (or MRI), ultrasound, angiography, CSF EEG
Hemiataxia Intention tremor Spontaneous or evoked pain on any form of stimulation	contralateral thalamic lesion	acute: bleeding, ischemia subacute: neoplasm	CCT (or MRI), angiography, ultrasound, CSF EEG

Table 1. *Continued*

Hemiparesis with . . .	Localization of the lesion	Cause with respect to the clinical history	Technical methods
With symptoms of the brain stem:			
1. oculomotor symptoms:	mesodiencephalic	acute: bleeding, ischemia	CCT (or MRI), angiography,
– disconjugate gaze palsy (INO, horizontal and vertical gaze paresis)	– lesion of PPRF (parapontine reticular formation) und MLF (medial longitudinal fasciculus)		ultrasound, CSF BAEP EEG
2. pupillomotor dysfunction	– affection at side of Edinger's nucleus or parasymphathetic	mesencephalon	
– wide pupils not reacting to light	efferent fibers (third nerve)	– sign of herniation	
3. impaired or no corneal reflex	– fifth nerve nuclear lesion or central or peripheral lesion of sixth nerve		
4. Horner's Syndrome	– lesion of sympathetic trunk	– dissection of vertebral artery	
– with neck pain and/or twelfth nerve palsy		– dissection of internal carotid artery	
Crossed brain stem (with contalateral hemiparesis)		mostly cardioembolic infarction, bleeding	CCT (or MRI), angiography, ultrasound,
1. Weber	– base of the midbrain		CSF
+ ipsilateral third nerve paresis			BAEP EEG
2. Millard-Gubler	– caudal pontine lesion		
– ipsilateral nuclear seventh nerve paresis			
3. Brissaud			
+ ipsilateral seventh nerve spasm			
4. Foville	– inferior medial pontine	infarction in the posterial inferior cerebellar artery territory	
+ ipsilateral hemiataxia,			
+ Horner's syndrome			
+ contralateral numbness			
5. Wallenberg (with hemiparesis in extended lesions):	– dorsolateral medulla	– infarction in the posterior inferior cerebellar artery and vertebral artery territory	
– ipsilateral Horner's syndrome,			
– hemiataxia,			
– nystagmus			

Table 1. *Continued*

Hemiparesis with . . .	Localization of the lesion	Cause with respect to the clinical history	Technical methods
– nuclear fifth nerve palsy – ninth nerve palsy – tenth nerve palsy – contralateral loss of pain and temperature sensation			
Brown-Séquard: – ipsilateral, spastic hemiparesis – at height of lesion: floppy paresis, paresthesia, radicular pain, – ipsilateral, below the lesion: first floppy, then spastic hemiparesis, vasomotoric disturbances, contralateral loss of pain and temperature sensation	– high cervical	acute: stick and shooting wounds, neoplasms	MRI, myelography, ultrasound, CSF, SSEP

are infrequent. They are caused by emboli, vasospasm following SAH, vasculitis, local atherosclerotic disease (particularly in blacks), and other rare conditions. Clinically, the leg is more involved than the arm or the hand; the face is spared.

Ischemic infarction of the MCA is usually apoplectic in onset. The syndrome characterically consists of a severe contralateral brachiofacial accentuated hemiparesis with ipsilateral conjugated eye deviaton, facial palsy, and global aphasia or contralateral neglect (depending on whether the lesion is in the dominant or nondominant hemisphere, respectively). Severe dysarthria is frequently ob-

served, mimicking infarction of the brain stem, and, depending on the degree of cerebral edema, altered consciousness and coma may occur.

Thromboembolism into the MCA is the most common cause of acute ischemia in the MCA territory. Atheromatous occlusion of the internal carotid artery as well as dissection tend to launch additional (supraocclusive) emboli into the MCA. Events marked by sudden onset and maximal severity suggest an embolic cause, either cardiac embolic or artery-to-artery embolic. The patient's medical history might include arrhythmia, atrial fibrillation, or internal carotid artery stenosis. Multiple or single ischemic attacks may occur after internal arterial dissection, especially after an even seemingly trivial trauma. Dissections can occur spontaneously, however. Neck pain is common in the setting of carotid dissection, and ipsilateral Horner's syndrome and a history of pulsatile tinnitus may also be detected. High-grade, hemodynamically induced watershed infarctions usually are found in the subcortical white matter. They may be subacute in onset and fluctuating, and the proximal arm and leg may be more involved. A past history of TIAs suggests a thrombotic cause, and auscultation might reveal a murmur that indicates stenosis of neck vessels. In younger patients with severe hemiparesis other causes such as fibromuscular dyplasia and paradoxical embolism should be considered. In MCA infarcts it is sometimes possible to correlate the site of occlusion to the clinical presentation. In occlusion of the MCA proximal to the lenticulostriate branches extensive deep hemispheric and cortical infarction will occur. The deficit with therefore include a dense hemiplegia, hemisensory disturbances, and hemianopia. Often these patients tend to become comatose, with forced eye deviation and signs of increased intracranial pressure. Occlusion distal to the lenticulostriate branches results in an infarct with variable extent to the frontal, parietal, and temporal cortex. A brachiofacial hemiparesis of varying severity can be seen. Diagnosis can be made with cerebral angiography or, in many patients, with transcranial Doppler ultrasonography.

Although rare, acute occlusions of the MCA can occur secondary to vasculitis, and one may find a history of fever, weight loss, and involvement of

Table 2. Autoimmune vasculitis causing cerebral ischemia

Wegener's granulomatosis
Takayasu's disease
Systemic lupus erythematosus
Scleroderma
Polyarteritis nodosa
Isolated central nervous system angiitis
Giant cell arteritis
Churg-Strauss angiitis

other organs in these patients. The cause of vasculitis may be infectious, autoimmune, or toxic (Table 2).

Certain drugs including heroin, cocaine, and LSD may cause intracerebral bleeding or ischemia. In addition to the clinical history, the physical examination will usually reveal signs of intoxication such as tachycardia, hypertension, disturbances of pupillary function, and altered consciousness.

Posterior Circulation

Twenty percent of the macroangiopathic disturbances of the cerebral blood supply involve the posterior circulation. Clinical signs of posterior circulation disease are almost always complex and include acute limb and gait ataxia, oculomotor abnormalities, dysarthria, dysphagia, perioral numbness, and hemi- or tetraparesis. Other symptoms may be tempory loss of vision and double vision.

The typical signs of basilar artery thrombosis consist of oculomotor abnormalities, tetraparesis, and an extensor plantar reflex. Isolated hemiparesis previously was thought to be an extremely rare symptom in posterior circulation stroke. Now, with MRI, small pontine infarctions may be detected in association with isolated hemiparesis. Such patients do not require ICU treatment if no evidence is found for significant vertebral or basilar artery disease.

Occlusions of the paramedian branches of the basilar artery or vertebral artery can lead to hemiparesis combined with other brain-stem symptoms. Depending on the location of the lesion, classical brain-stem syndromes can be found (Table 1). However, paramedian pontine infarction sometimes leads to pure hemiparesis/hemiplegia.

Infarction within the posterior circulation may be caused by emboli, local atherosclerosis, or small-vessel disease. The diagnostic approach is principally the same as described for infarctions of the anterior circulation. Dissection and inflammatory causes must be excluded.

Lacunar Infarction

Lacunar infarctions are small, deep infarcts which result from thrombosis of or emboli to small penetrating arteries or arterioles in the thalamus (aa. thalamoperforantes), basal ganglia (aa. lenticulostriatae), and brain stem (Rr.ad pontem). Patients with lacunar infarction often present with pure motor hemiplegia or pure sensory stroke. Hypertension is the major risk factor, and diabetes is frequent. These patients are not often candidates for critical care treatment. Indeed, many small, deep lacunar infarctions are clinically asymptomatic.

Metabolic Causes of Acute Hemiparesis

Although the main cause of hemiparesis is a vessel occlusion, other causes should also be considered. Hypoglycemia (with serum glucose levels below 60 mg/dl) can cause an acute hemiparesis. It may be accompanied by headache, confusion, and a generalized tonic-clonic seizure.

Nonatherosclerotic Vasculopathies Causing Cerebral Ischemia

Acute hemiparesis can also stem from migraine, as in basilar migraine, complicated migraine, and familial hemiplegic migraine. Patients with migraine-related hemiparesis are usually younger (between ages 20 and 40), may have a history of headache, and may have a positive family history. If hemiparesis occurs with symptoms of classic migraine (i.e., severe headache, visual disturbances, photophobia, and prodromal signs) the diagnosis is highly probable. Patients with basilar migraine, however, may present with symptoms mimicking brain-stem or cerebellar infarction. These patients may present with severe occipital headache, confusion, bilateral visual symptoms, and numbness of hands and lips. EEG and cerebral angiography are often necessary to make the correct diagnosis. Attacks of complicated migraine usually start with a motor aura with mono- or hemiparesis, followed by headache. Familiar hemiplegic migraine is a subtype of migraine.

Hemiparesis following focal seizures lasting less than 24 h is called Todd's paresis. In the rare cases in which paresis lasts longer, focal damage is likely and differentiation from hemiparesis of vascular origin is difficult. The patient's clinical history and EEG findings are helpful in detecting this cause of hemiparesis. Sneddon syndrome, moyamoya disease, and mitochondrial myopathy may cause

Table 3. Nonatherosclerotic vasculopathies causing cerebral ischemia

Sneddon syndrome
Moyamoya disease
Mitochondrial myopathy, encephalopathy, lactic acidosis, stroke-like episodes (MELAS)
Migraine
Drug abuse
Cervicocephalic arterial dissection
Arterial trauma

hemiparesis in a very few cases (Table 3).

Spontaneous Intracerebral Hemorrhage

Clinically, ischemic infarction cannot reliably be differentiated from intracerebral hemorrhage (ICH). CT or MRI is essential for diagnosis. ICH occurs in descending incidence in the basal ganglia, thalamus, central white matter, and posterior fossa. Usually, the initial symptom is headache, followed by altered consciousness. However, depending on the localization of the bleeding, hemiparesis may be the leading symptom. Although a number of neurologic diseases may cause intracerebral bleeding, arterial hypertension and advancing age are the main risk factors of parenchymal cerebral hematoma.

The most common site of bleeding is the putamen. Patients present with contralateral hemiparesis, extensor plantar reflexes, and sensory deficit. Depending on the size of the hematoma, other clinical signs such as altered consciousness or even coma may occur. In thalamic hemorrhage, prognosis depends on hematoma size and presence of intraventricular blood. The classic "thalamic syndrome" is seldom seen in the acute phase. Hypertension is the most common risk factor of lobar hemorrhage. However, other causes include arteriovenous malformations, anticoagulation, or cerebral amyloid angiopathy in the elderly. Patients with lobar hemorrhage have less dramatic initial symptoms than those with basal ganglia hemorrhage, but mortality is only slightly lower.

Cerebellar, mesencephalic and medullary hemorrhage cause mainly altered consciousness and rarely hemiparesis as a leading symptom.

Vascular Malformation

Aneurysms, arteriovenous malformation (AVM), and angioma may cause hemiparesis either directly or by acute parenchymal bleeding. Typical symptoms of acute subarachnoid hemorrhage (SAH) are sudden headache, photophobia, and meningismus. Loss of consciousness and nausea are also frequently seen. The range of symptoms (the Hunt and Hess classification) depends on the site and amount of bleeding, subsequent onset of vasospasm, and degree of cerebral edema.

Bleeding from aneurysms must be distinguished from bleeding from an AVM. Symptoms such as relapsing migraine-like headache, seizures, and signs of local ischemia point toward an AVM. These patients are usually younger than those with aneurysmal bleeding. It is important to note that patients with an angioma may also present with SAH. Vasospasm following SAH is frequent cause of delayed hemiparesis, particularly in the setting of a ruptured aneurysm.

Venous Sinus Thrombosis

Up to 1% of cerebral infarctions are caused by thrombosis of the cerebral veins and sinuses. Thrombosis may arise from a hypercoagulability (pregnancy, malignancy, paraneoplastic) or from penetrating, nearby inflammatory processes (otitis media, paranasal sinusitis). The course may be slow or subacute, in most cases beginning with headaches, followed by seizures, focal signs, and decreased alertness. Papilledema and meningeal signs are frequently present. Hemiparesis is usually mild to moderate and may show atypical patterns of paresis distribution.

Infections

The mechanisms that lead to hemiparesis in patients with cerebral infection involve the infection itself (e.g., herpes encephalitis or abscess) or an associated inflammatory vasculitis (e.g., bacterial meningitis). Intracerebral abscesses, spread hematogenously as microemboli, are often multiple and located between the gray and white matter (where small vessels are located). Patients should be examined for the presence of endocarditis and penetrating local inflammations. Organisms causing abscesses in immunocompromised patients include various Fungi, *Toxoplasma*, and *Listeria*. Fever, headache, meningismus, seizures, and decreased alertness may occur in patients with abscesses, as well as hemiparesis with aphasia or cranial nerve abnormalities, depending on the localization of the abscess. Cerebrospinal fluid analysis can be normal in these patients, and lumbar puncture should be deferred unless a mass effect is excluded by brain imaging.

Theoretically, a variety of bacterial infections can lead to hemiparesis. In most cases, however, the hemiparesis will not be the leading symptom except in paretic neurosyphilis. Usually, hemiparesis occurs in addition to fever, confusion, and seizures. Meningococcal meningitis may be distinguished from pneumococcal meningitis by the presence of petechial bleeding. In the exudative phase, neurosyphilis may present like cerebral tuberculosis with vasculitis-related infarction or, less commonly, as a space-occupying granuloma.

An infectious focus often occurs in herpes simplex encephalitis, which is characterized by a bilateral, asymmetric inflammation of the anterior temporal lobes and limbic system. Physical examination reveals focal signs with or without hemiparesis, aphasia, and seizures. Almost all viral infections of the CNS may present with focal signs, although seizures, drowsiness, and an organic brain syndrome are more prominent. Examination of CSF and an EEG are important in patients suspected of having viral encephalitis. A parasitic infection should be considered when there is a combination of eosinophilia with a history of foreign travel.

Neoplasm

Bleeding into an intracranial tumor can result in acute hemiparesis. This is more common in patients with glioblastoma ("apoplectic glioma") and metastases from malignant melanoma, kidney, thyroid, testicular, or ovarian carcinoma. The patient's history of a malignancy or accompanying symptoms such as weight loss, cachexia, hormonal disorders, or pain will point to the diagnosis. Clinically, it is difficult to differentiate the neurologic symptoms of bleeding into an intracranial tumor from those of intracerebral bleeding. Primary cerebral lymphomas may present with acute hemiparesis.

Trauma

Trauma may cause subdural, epidural, or concussion bleeding, which may then lead to a hemiparesis. An intracranial hemorrhage must be excluded in every case of hemiparesis with a history of trauma. An epidural hematoma results frequently from rupture of the middle meningeal artery or from bleeding of perforated veins as a result of trauma. A subdural hematoma results from rupture of small arteries or veins close to the surface of the gray matter. Diagnosis is made by CT scan.

Demyelinating Diseases

Multiple sclerosis can occasionally cause acute, severe hemiparesis. The hemiparesis is often combined with other signs of multifocal CNS involvement such as optic nerve dysfunction, oculomotor disturbances with or without sensory loss, and coordination deficits. Acute disseminated encephalomyelitis characteristically occurs after active or passive vaccinations or acute viral infections. Patients usually present with seizures, brain-stem symptoms, and altered consciousness.

Spinal Lesions

Rarely, a high spinal lesion can result in acute hemiparesis. In neoplasms the diagnosis will not cause difficulties be-

cause the hemiparesis develops slowly. Specific trauma (e.g., gunshot or stab wounds) is a common cause of the Brown-Séquard syndrome.

Psychogenic Hemiparesis

Floppy paresis of one arm or leg, of one side of the body without facial involvement, or with sensory disturbances restricted to one side of the body (without crossing the midline) are suspicious of a psychogenic disorder. However, all other organic causes of hemiparesis have to be ruled out before this diagnosis is confirmed.

Ancillary Tests

Computed Tomography

Emergency CT is still the first diagnostic step after physical examination in patients with acute hemiparesis. The head scan can be performed within 5 min. Even the comatose, artifically ventilated patient can be easily monitored throughout the procedure. In acute hemiparesis, CT may be normal or may reveal brain hemorrhage or another type of lesion. Under these circumstances, a normal early CT does not rule out focal ischemia, encephalitis, migraine, hypoglycemia, Todd's paresis, or psychogenesis. Severe and extended hemispheric ischemia can be detected as early as 2 h post-ictus (Fig. 1a–c). Small and infratentorial ischemic areas are more difficult to detect. If the CT scan shows a lesion, one must determine whether the lesion is appropriate to the history

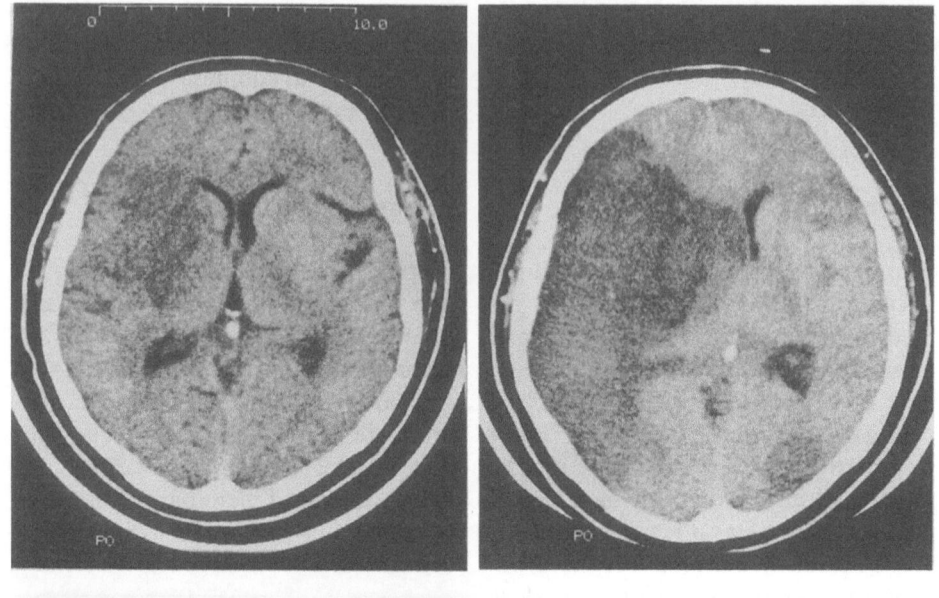

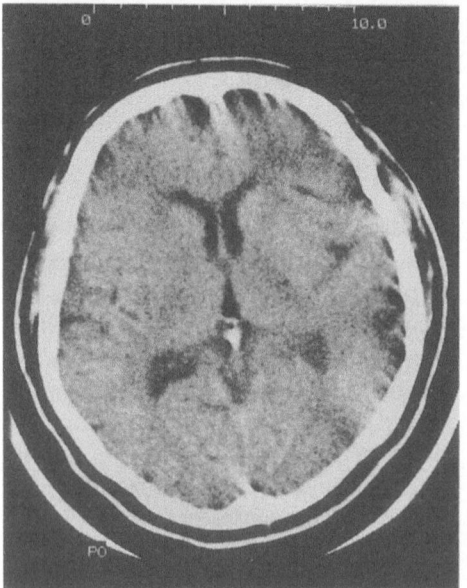

Fig. 1a–c. Cranial CT series in a 71-year-old man after sudden left-sided hemiparesis: **a** 90 min after symptom onset a slight hypo-density of the right lentiform nucleus is seen; **b** 24 h after symptom onset the area of hypo-density has increased. There is slight com-pression of the right ventricle; **c** 4 days after symptom onset there is complete hypodensity of the total MCA territory with considerable mass effect with contralateral shift of midline structures. There is additional hypodensity of the occipital lobe of the left hemisphere

and the neurologic findings. In selected patients with acute MCA occlusion, the CT may be positive immediately. Acute thrombus results in intraluminal increased attenuation, visible as a snake-like hyperintensity (i.e., the hyperdense MCA sign) (Fig. 2).

Magnetic Resonance Imaging

CT is usually preferable to MRI in acute hemiparesis, as the latter is more time consuming. In the environment of MRI, patient observation is difficult; MRI is less sensitive for acute brain

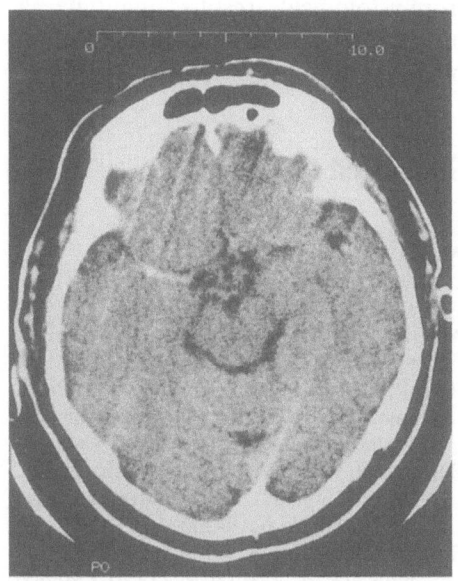

Fig. 2. Dense middle cerebral artery sign in accite right hemispheric stroke

hemorrhage than CT, particularly in subarachnoid hemorrhage. Small and infratentorial ischemic lesions are easier to detect by MRI (Fig. 3). MRI in combination with MR angiography can give important additional infor-

mation when arterial or venous blood flow disturbances are suspected.

Cerebral Angiography

Cerebral angiography using the transfemoral approach and digital subtraction technique is now a procedure of low risk in experienced hands. In acute hemiparesis, angiography is indicated with a view to therapeutic consequences only, e.g., thrombolysis of major intracranial arterial occlusions, anticoagulation in venous thrombosis, surgery for gross hemorrhage from an AVM.

Extra-/Intracranial Doppler Sonography (ECD, TCD)

Doppler ultrasonography is a noninvasive, fast, and informative examination of the cerebral vessels. In cases of normal CT or MRI it may reveal evidence of stenosis or occlusion and indicate the need for cerebral angiography. Transcranial Doppler (TCD)

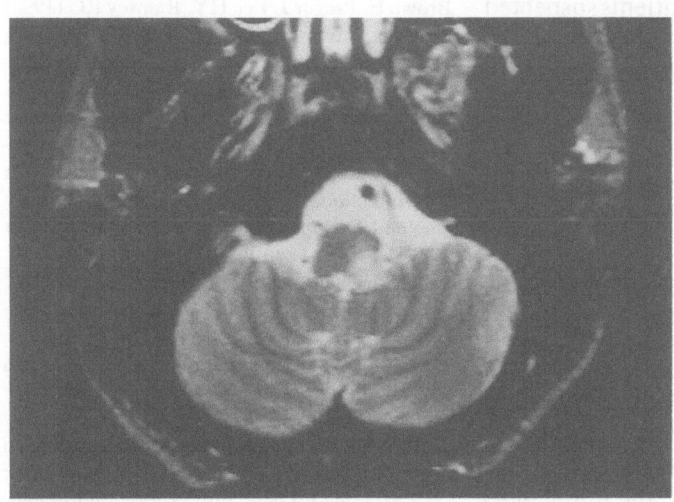

Fig. 3. T2-weighted spin-echo sequence of MRI in a 30-year-old man with left sided Wallenberg syndrome shows an increased signal of the dorsolateral medulla oblongata

may be most useful in the setting of aneurysmal subarachnoid hemorrhage. Intracranial arterial blood flow velocities may be followed serially to detect and follow delayed arterial vasospasm.

Electroencephalography (EEG)

The EEG still has value in the assessment of acute hemiparesis. The EEG may show a focus in cases of postseizure paresis, encephalitis, or migraine. In migrainous hemiparesis, delta wave focus may be present for hours and days after the clinical symptoms have cleared. In herpes simplex encephalitis typical periodic lateralized epileptiform discharges are usually found in advanced stages of the disease. Early EEG changes may be only minor focal changes and a slight slowing of frequency.

Cerebrospinal Fluid (CSF)

The examination of CSF is the essential diagnostic tool in CNS infections. In autoimmune processes it may show oligoclonal bands. In patients suspected of having SAH but with normal CT scans, blood in the CSF may establish the diagnosis.

Evoked Potentials

With the help of brain-stem acoustic evoked potentials (BAEP) and somatosensory evoked potentials (SSEP) it is possible to determine the extent of a brain-stem lesion. Although neither examination is usually indicated in the acute setting and these tests are best reserved for follow-up, the initial elec-trophysiological results may be a prognostic paremeter and helpful in planning therapy.

Suggested Reading

Adams HP, Butler MJ, Biller J (1986) Non-hemorrhagic cerebral infarction in young adults. Arch Neurol 43:793–796

Ameri A, Bousser MG (1992) Cerebral venous thrombosis. Neurol Clin 10:87–111

Berlit P, Endemann B, Vetter P (1991) Zerebrale Ischämien bei jungen Erwachsenen. Fortschr Neurol Psychiatr 59:322–327

Bernsen HJ, van de Vlasakker C, Verhagen WI, Prick MJ (1990) Basilar artery migraine stroke. Headache 30:142–144

Bitoh S, Hasegawa H, Ohtsuki H, Obashi J, Fujiwara M, Sakurai M (1984) Cerebral neoplasms initially presenting with massive intracerebral hemorrhage. Surg Neurol 22:57–62

Broderick JP, Brott T, Tomsick T, Huster G, Miller R (1992) The risk of subarachnoid and intracerebral hemorrhages in blacks as compared with whites. N Engl J Med 326: 733–736

Brott T, Broderick JP (1993) Intracerebral hemorrhage. Heart Dis Stroke 2:59–63

Brott T, Thalinger K, Hertzberg V (1986) Hypertension as a risk factor for spontaneous intracerebral hemorrhage. Stroke 17:1078–1083

Brown E, Prager J, Lee HY, Ramsey RG (1992) CNS complications of cocaine abuse: prevalence, pathophysiology, and neuroradiology. AJR 159:137–147

Caekebeke JF, Peters AC, Vandvik B, Brouwer OF, de Bakker HM (1990) Cerebral vasculopathy associated with primary varicella infection. Arch Neurol 47:1033–1035

Caplan LR (1991) Migraine and vertebrobasilar ischemia. Neurology 41:55–61

Chambers BR, Norris JW, Shurwell BL, Hachinski V (1987) Prognosis in acute stroke. Neurology 37:221

Del Zoppo GJ (1988) Thrombolytic therapy in cerebrovascular disease. Stroke 19: 1174–1179

Del Zoppo GJ, Ferbert A, Otis S, Brückmann H, Hacke W, Zyroff J, Harker L, Zeumer H (1988) Local intra-arterial fibrinolytic therapy in acute carotid artery territory stroke. A pilot study. Stroke 19:307–313

DiNubile MJ (1988) Septic thrombosis of the cavernous sinuses. Arch Neurol 45:567–572

Einhaupl KM, Villringer A, Meister W, Mehraein S, Garner C, Pellkofer M, Haberl RL, Pfister HW, Schmiedek P (1991) Heparin treatment in sinus venous thrombosis. Lancet 338:597–600

Fisher CM (1982) Lacunar strokes and infarcts: a review. Neurology 32:871–876

Foster JW, Hart RG (1987) Hypoglycemic hemiplegia: two cases and a clinical review. Stroke 18:944–946

Green RM, Kelly KM, Gabrielsen T, Levine SR, Vanderzant C (1990) Multiple intracerebral hemorrhages after smoking "crack" cocaine. Stroke 21:957–62

Hacke W, Zeumer H, Ferbert A, Brückmann H, del Zoppo GJ (1988) Intra-arterial fibrinolytic therapy improves outcome in patient with acute vertebrobasilar occlusive disease. Stroke 19:1216–1222

Heistinger M, Rumpl E, Illiasch H, Turck H, Kyrle PA, Lechner K, Pabinger I (1992) Cerebral sinus thrombosis in a patient with hereditary protein-S deficiency: case report and review of the literature. Ann Hematol 64:105–109

Kelly MA, Gorelick PB, Mirza D (1992) The role of drugs in the etiology of stroke. Clin Neuropharmacol 15:249–275

Krieger D, Adams HP, Rieke K, Schwarz S, Forsting M, Hacke W (1993) Prospective evorluation of the prognostic significance of evoked potentials in acute basilar occlusion. Crit Care Med 21:1169–1174

Levine SR, Twyman RE, Gilman S (1988) The role of anticoagulation in cavernous sinus thrombosis. Neurology 38:517–522

Malouf R, Brust CM (1985) Hypoglycemia: causes, neurological manifestations, and outcome. Ann Neurol 17:421–430

May EF, Jabbari B (1990) Stroke in neuroborreliosis. Stroke 21:1232–1235

Milandre L, Perot S, Salamon G, Khalil R (1989) Spontaneous dissection of both extracranial internal carotid arteries. Neuroradiology 31:435–439

Mokri B, Schievink WI, Olsen KD, Piepgras DG (1992) Spontaneous dissection of the cervical internal carotid artery. Presentation with lower cranial nerve palsies. Arch Otolaryngol Head Neck Surg 118:431–435

Mori E, Tabuchi M, Yoshida T, Yamadori A (1988) Intracarotid urokinase with thromboembolic occlusion of the middle cerebral artery. Stroke 19:802–812

Mullges W, Ringelstein EB, Weiller C, Leibold M, Bruckmann H (1991) Dissektionen der A. carotis interna – neue diagnostische und pathogenetische Aspekte. Fortschr Neurol Psychiatr 59:12–24

Pfister HW, Borasio GD, Dirnagl U, Bauer M, Einhaupl KM (1992) Cerebrovascular complications of bacterial meningitis in adults. Neurology 42:1497–1504

Roos KL, Scheld WM (1988) The management of fulminant meningitis in the intensive care unit. Crit Care Clin 4:375–392

Rother J, Schreiner A, Wentz KU, Hennerici M (1992) Hypoglycemia presenting as basilar artery thrombosis. Stroke 23:112–113

Ruggieri PM, Masaryk TJ, Ross JS, Modic MT (1992) Intracranial magnetic resonance angiography. Cardiovasc Intervent Radiol 15:71–81

Sacco RL, Ellenberg JH, Mohr JP, Tatemichi TK, Hier DB, Price TR, Wolf PA (1989) Infarcts of undetermined cause: the NINCDS stroke data bank. Ann Neurol 25:382–390

Schlake HP, Grotemeyer KH, Hofferberth B, Husstedt IW, Wiesner S (1990) Brain-stem auditory evoked potentials in migraine – evidence of increased side differences during the pain-free interval. Headache 30:129–132

Tinuper P, Aguglia U, Laudadido S, Gestaut H (1987) Prolonged ictal paralysis: electrencephalographic confirmation of its epileptic nature. Clin Electroencephalogr 18:12–14

Trenkwalder P, Trenkwalder C, Feiden W, Vogl TJ, Einhaupl KM, Lydtin H (1992) Toxoplasmosis with early intracerebral hemorrhage in a patient with the acquired immunodeficiency syndrome. Neurology 42:436–438

Von Kummer R, Hacke W (1992) Safety and efficacy of intravenous tissue plasminogen activator and heparin in acute middle cerebral artery stroke. Stroke 23:646–652

Chapter 25

Confusion, Psychosis, and Neuropsychological Symptoms

KLAUS POECK

Introduction

The phenomena described in this chapter are assessed exclusively on the basis of observing the patient's spontaneous behavior, talking to him and listening to him. Ancillary examinations are of little help. This is a field intermediate between neurology and psychiatry. Doctors who are uncertain about terminology and classification should take great care to describe in as much detail as possible what they have observed personally and what they have learned about the patient's behavior from nurses and relatives. A correct and vivid description will eventually permit the diagnosis.

Delusion and Hallucination

Patients presenting with acute delusion will be admitted to the intensive care ward mainly if the condition has an organic basis. Possible causes are acute or chronic intoxication, withdrawal

syndromes, epileptic states, metabolic psychoses, and dehydration in the elderly.

Patients may be excited or even agitated, or they may be apathetic. Frequently, they are tense and intimidated. Often patients do not spontaneously report their delusions and hallucinations. It is important to observe their suspicious or anxious gaze, aimless looking around, or attraction to a nonexisting target. In many cases it requires a good deal of experience to make the patient talk. Frightening or threatening experiences are rarely reported freely. The flow of thought will often be incoherent, speech may be slurred and the voice low-keyed.

Often the pupils are abnormal, that is, dilated or miotic. Sweating and tremor may be present. Usually patients are too tense to permit an orderly neurological examination. The EEG electrodes or the CT machine may be interpreted as damaging tools.

Extensive laboratory and toxicological investigations are necessary to diagnose the underlying disease state. In most cases, emergency therapy must be applied before the final diagnosis is made.

Section Editor: Werner Hacke

Rarely, a patient presents with a profound emotional alteration, usually with anxiety, suspicion, and sometimes even panic attacks. The condition may be purely psychic in nature or it may be the result of delusion or hallucination. "Pure ictal fear" has been described in patients with temporal lobe epilepsy.

Delirious State

The delirious state is similar to that of delusion and hallucination as described in the preceding paragraphs, but it is more dangerous because the underlying causes may be life-threatening disease states. There are psychiatric and somatic signs and symptoms, and the latter deserve the utmost attention.

Virtually all patients are conspicuous by alteration of their mood and affect. Anxiety is the prominent feature, the cause of which is difficult or impossible to recognize. There may be outbreaks of aggressiveness directed against any person, even members of the family.

Patients are uncooperative, will pull out catheters or tubes and will need to be restrained by handcuffs. This, in turn, will make them more aggressive and will necessitate sedation. Given the severe medical condition, the required dose of sedative drugs may produce sleepiness or even coma.

The patient's attention is easily distracted by objectively irrelevant stimuli which are perceived in a delusional way. The nurse may be interpreted as a life-threatening person and the air conditioning as the source of poisonous gas or dangerous irradiation.

There may also be hallucinations; these are usually visual, often moving. Acoustic hallucinations are rare, but when they are experienced, patients hear unpleasant or threatening voices talking to them and sometimes about them. The logical sequence of thought as can be judged from verbal expression is disrupted. Speech is a fluent monologue without turn-taking. Articulation is slurred. It is necessary to repeat questions and commands, and answers are mostly random, or they consist of rude and abrupt comments.

A very characteristic feature of delirium is the fluctuation of behavior that makes it advisable to rely on the description given by nurses who observe the patient for long periods. This is especially important because there may be reversal of sleeping and waking periods, the patient being particularly active at night, while profoundly sleepy or even comatose during the day. Medical findings include tachycardia, elevated blood pressure, and sweating.

Amnesia

In patients requiring neurocritical care, amnesia is most frequently observed as global amnesia, that is, the inability to record and store, i.e., to learn any new items, associated with the inability to retrieve items experienced (and recorded) prior to the onset of the disease state.

The most common variant is *transient global amnesia*. The condition has an abrupt onset without a recognizable cause. All of a sudden, patients have lost awareness of where they are, how they got there, and what they had intended to do. They appear perplexed and keep asking the same questions about their current situation. They forget the answers immediately, which has an alarming effect on their surroundings. They are awake and have no paresis, ataxia, or hemianopia.

The striking feature is that, in contrast to their inability to report on themselves and their situation, their behavior, other than that they continuously ask the same questions, is quite normal. Patients who do not "know" how and why they went to a certain place will nonetheless behave according to the requirements of the situation, which they will not be able to report verbally immediately afterwards. Thus they do not "know" that they are in hospital, yet they will obediently and correctly place their arm in the position for an intravenous injection. When asked afterwards whether they have received an injection they will say that they do not know.

Neurological signs are unremarkable, and the results of ancillary examinations do not give a clue to the etiology of the condition. The course is benign. The global amnesia clears up gradually over a period of hours, with or without any treatment, hence the term "transient". If amnesia lasts longer than 24 h the diagnosis should be questioned.

The cause of transient global amnesia is not known. It is most likely not caused by ischemia and does not herald a stroke. Epilepsy, as well as migraine, has been incriminated, but the evidence is circumstantial. The condition may recur, but this does not alter its basically benign nature.

Long-lasting or *persistent amnesia* is an important consequence of anoxic brain damage. Most frequently, the underlying cause is cardiac arrest. In young patients this may remain unexplained in spite of extensive evaluation. In elderly patients bilateral thalamic infarcts, usually from multiple emboli, may be seen on CT. A short period of coma is followed by global amnesia, as described above. In the critical care unit, these patients are lucid, and usually they do not present with neurological deficits of any sort. They are quiet, often show decreased spontaneity, and are usually friendly. Their affect is remarkably flat. When addressed nonverbally they are well behaved. They will eat and drink and cooperate with nursing care. It is clear, however, that they are not aware of being in the hospital and that they forget any event, be it the doctor's visit, the care of the nurse, or even a visit by the family. Patients recognize familiar faces but do not remember persons' names, and they do not learn to recognize unfamiliar faces, such that doctors and nurses must introduce themselves time and again. The patients are not able to give a verbal report on past events. The main feature, again, is the contrast between the lack of awareness of place and time and their behavior, which is appropriate to the situation.

Ancillary studies usually are not diagnostic. Every experienced neurologist has seen a number of these patients with normal EEG, CT scan, and MRI.

The syndrome may clear up over a period of some days or a week. If it lasts longer, it becomes likely that global amnesia will be permanent. At a later stage it is recognized by others that in these patients procedural memory is preserved to a remarkable extent in the presence of severely disrupted declarative memory. For instance, a patient may be able to drive a car to his home without being able to name the streets.

Aphasia and Apraxia

Language and speech are frequently impaired in patients requiring neuro-critical care. Typical disease states are stroke, traumatic contusion of the brain, and inflammatory brain disease. Some of these disease states lead to a central language disorder by affecting the language area of the brain which, in most people, is located in the left frontotemporoparietal area. Others interfere only with the motor functions of speech, which are articulatory movements, phonation, and breathing. In the first instance there is aphasia and in the second there is dysarthria or, as specialists prefer to say, dysarthrophonia. The conditions may coexist.

The neurologist is used to considering aphasia in terms of the traditional syndromes, e.g., Broca's, Wernicke's, amnestic, or global aphasia. These syndromes are frequently found in patients with a stable condition of vascular origin, at least 4–6 weeks following stroke. They should not be expected in acute disease; neither are they found in acute cerebral disease of nonvascular etiology.

In most instances, the patient admitted to the intensive care unit does not speak at all. His expression will be blank, and he does not react to verbal or other stimuli. He will be unable to swallow and might not be able to open his mouth on request. It is not easy to realize that the lack of communication stems from a disruption of language functions and not from stupor or psychosis. Of course, if there is right hemiplegia, it is sound to assume that the patient is aphasic. The behavioral distinction, however, is next to impossible if no vocal reaction whatsoever can be elicited.

Some patients develop fluent paraphasic speech and even unintelligible jargon in the very acute stage of disease. This is particularly true in those with herpes simplex virus encephalitis. Again, the distinction between aphasia and psychosis is difficult to make, even more so, because these patients, like those with acute stroke in the territory of the posterior temporal artery, may not present with hemiplegia.

A strong indicator of aphasia is the presence of apraxia, which usually can be recognized on the second day after onset. The diagnosis of apraxia cannot be made when the patient simply does not execute oral or gestural movements required on verbal command, or by requesting imitation. It is necessary that the patient perform movements other than those requested. This type of movement is termed parapraxic. Two examples are: The patient is asked to stick out his tongue and he opens and closes his mouth instead, or he is requested to show his fist in a threatening gesture, and the response is a movement like waving good-bye. A very important phenomenon in apraxia is perseveration. This is the inappropriate repetition of a movement or part of a movement that had been correctly or incorrectly performed before. If the patient does react in the examination for apraxia and he performs parapractic movements, then it is highly unlikely that his failure to speak is due to psychosis or stupor.

When the patient had been mute for a day or two, the first sign of communication is the utterance of sounds which eventually can be identified as Yes or No, even though these might be spoken in a random way. Also, nodding and head shaking might not reflect the appropriate or supposed meaning.

Examining patients with acute aphasia in the setting of an intensive care ward cannot been done by means of the well-known aphasia tests developed for the detailed description and quantitative assessment of the language deficit in patients with stable conditions 4–6 weeks after stroke. Short versions of these tests are psychometrically not valid. There exist some tests specifically developed for the examination of acute impairment of language and speech. For the English language there are the Frenchay Aphasia Screening Test, which requires 3–10 min, and the Acute Aphasia Screening Protocol, requiring about 10 min. For the German language the Aachen Aphasia Bedside Test has been developed, which includes standardized stimulation procedures. These are particularly relevant in aphasic patients with acute severe illness who are frequently impaired, not only in language and speech but also in motivation, drive, and attention. Application of this test requires 15–40 min.

Acute dysarthria has been studied mainly in cases of acute traumatic brain damage. In a study of 110 patients, Ziegler and von Cramon (1987) found aphasia to be present in 19%, in contrast to dysarthria, which was present in 52%. Signs and symptoms of dysarthria varied depending on the localization of traumatic brain damage. The most severe form was observed in patients with damage to the upper brain stem. In the initial phase, after re-

gaining consciousness these patients do not produce any vocal utterance even though they may follow commands requesting nonverbal reactions. While the vocal cords cannot be activated voluntarily, reflex activity is present, though without any sound. Articulatory movements are absent, and this is true also for nonspeech movements of the oral musculature. This stage may last for several months, until the first whispered utterances are produced.

Neglect and Anosognosia

Following the acute onset of hemiplegia, hemianopia, or even blindness (see below) the patient may behave as though these signs and symptoms were not present. Usually the patients are elderly and bedridden. When addressed, they do not complain of a motor or sensory defect.

Visual Neglect. It is easily noted that the patients turn their head and gaze only towards one side, usually to the right. When the examiner approaches the bed from the left side they will answer towards the right, and they may give a confabulatory answer when pressed to describe the appearance of the examiner.

Motor Neglect. When asked to move the paralyzed left-sided limbs the patients will move their right arm or leg. When the examiner particularly requests that they move the left arm they will lift the right arm and insist it is the left one, or they lift the left arm with the help of the right one.

Sensory Tactile Neglect. On tactile sensory stimulation the patients will report only on right-sided stimuli. In milder forms of neglect, they report on both sides when this particular side is stimulated, but on bilateral simultaneous stimulation they report only on the right side of the body.

It may be difficult to distinguish neglect from hemiparesis or hemisensory loss. Frequently, it helps to observe the spontaneous behavior of patients who do move the arm that remained flat on the bedcover when they were asked to move it. Transcranial magnetic stimulation will help to distinguish paralysis from severe motor neglect.

Anosognosia. In the most striking forms, neglect is expressed as anosognosia. The term is derived from the Greek words "nosos", meaning illness, and "gnosis", meaning recognition. A-noso-gnosia thus means nonrecognition of a disease state or denial of illness. The patients will strictly deny any neurological deficit. In the presence of hemiplegia they will try to stand up just to demonstrate that they are not paralyzed. Some patients strongly deny being ill at all, and they will not admit to staying in the hospital. When pressed, they will give evasive answers or produce some delusional elaboration to explain why they are staying in bed and do not immediately get up, which they say they are perfectly able to do.

Cortical Blindness. An important instance of anosognosia is cortical blindness. It is observed only in acute visual loss of cortical origin. These patients are obviously blind. They do not look at silently moving visual stimuli. When they look at the examiner who talks to them, their gaze is slightly off-target. Yet they do not complain of visual loss and, when asked to describe what they see, they produce an intelligent guess or give a purely confabulatory answer. Pupillary light reactions are normal, which makes the distinction from psychogenic blindness difficult. In the latter condition the patients do complain of visual loss, and optokinetic nystagmus can usually be elicited. I have seen a patient with psychogenic blindness, however, who did not fixate and therefore had no optokinetic nystagmus. In case of doubt, alpha-blocking during EEG recording is very helpful, the phenomenon being absent in cortical, but not in psychogenic blindness.

The most frequent cause of cortical blindness is top of the basilar artery embolus, and it is very urgent to demonstrate both the embolic occlusion at the top of the basilar artery and its cause. Recurrence is likely and may be fatal.

With hemineglect and anosognosia, other than with blindness, there usually is extensive damage to the right parietal lobe, and the origin is either vascular or neoplastic.

Acute Alexia

There are patients who discover, after being admitted to the hospital, that they have acutely lost the ability to read. This may be true for sentences, words, or even letters. Aphasia need not be present, and usually there is no hemiplegia. In the classical situation the patient has complete or partial right-sided hemianopia. Even though reading is severely impaired, the patient will be able to single out a Cyrillic letter or a number mistakingly included in an English word. It is very curious that some patients who cannot correctly read a word are nevertheless able to recognize its semantic field. For "czar" they will read "Russia", for "sympathy", "orchestra" (two errors in one answer), and one of my patients reacted to visual stimulus by a photograph of the late president Kennedy by saying: "Poor man, he was murdered."

Most of the patients are able to write, but they cannot read what they have written. They will identify the same letters they could not read on visual presentation when they are "written" on their skin without visual control. Color naming is frequently impaired also, and sometimes even questions of the type, "What color is a banana?" are answered at random. This is a typical posterior disconnection syndrome, and the cause usually is infarction in the territory of the left posterior cerebral artery. The explanation is that visual stimuli can no longer be processed in the ischemic left, but only in the right visual area. Interruption of posterior callosal fibers prevents the relay of visual stimuli to the language area.

For the same reason, some patients are unable to name visually presented objects. This is a visual naming deficit and not object agnosia. The patients will promptly identify and name objects they are permitted to palpate when visual perception is excluded. The condition is not only of theoretical but also of medical interest, because acute occlusion of the posterior cerebral artery may be embolic in origin, and recurrence of the event may lead to life-threatening embolism into the basilar artery.

Suggested Reading

Biniek R, Huber W, Willmes K, Glindemann R, Brand H, Fiedler M, Annen C (1991) Ein Test zur Erfassung von Sprach- und Sprechstörungen in der Akutphase nach Schlaganfällen. Nervenarzt 62:108–115

Crary MA, Haak MY, Malinsky AE (1989) Preliminary psychometric evaluation of an acute aphasia screening protocol. Aphasiology 3:611–618

Enderby PM, Wood VA, Wade DT, Langton Hewer R (1987) The Frenchay Aphasia Screening Test: a short simple test for aphasia appropriate for non-specialists. Int J Rehabil Med 8:166–170

Geschwind N (1965) Disconnexion syndromes in animals and man. Brain 237–294, 385–644

Poeck K (1985) Clues to the nature of disruption of limb praxis. In: Roy EA (ed) Neuropschological studies of apraxia and related disorders. North Holland, Amsterdam, pp 99–109

Ziegler W, von Cramon D (1987) Differentialdiagnostik der traumatisch bedingten Dysarthrophonien. In: Springer L, Kattenbeck G (eds) Aktuelle Beiträge zur Dysarthrophonie. Tuduv, Munich

Chapter 26

Seizures

Hermann Stefan and Ronald B. Lesser

Basic Mechanisms of Intra- and Extracellular Epileptic Activity

Epilepsy does not occur due to one disturbing mechanism or one disease, but is to be considered as a multifactorial polyetiological phenomenon. Clinically, the epileptic syndrome is characterized by an episodic functional disturbance. It occurs due to excessive neuronal discharges as a consequence of increased irritability or decreased inhibitory functions. There is no uniform explanation of all epileptic phenomena, even though the understanding of cellular mechanisms leading to epileptic activity has increased considerably in recent years. In the development of epilepsies a genetic dispostion may be the cause as well as realization factors, for instance, perinatal or postnatal brain disturbances in early childhood, infections of the brain, brain tumors, cerebral disturbances of blood flow, deformations, and disturbance of metabolism.

There is a wide pathogenetic spectrum between the poles of genetic disposition and the acquired trigger mechanisms, in which the different epileptic syndromes are to be classified. Therefore, the epileptic syndromes occur as a result of innate genetic as well as acquired realization factors. An increased neuronal irritability develops by means of molecular-biological-biochemical mediation, finally leading to the epileptic process (Fig. 1). The latter process explains the spontaneous, recurring, chronic epileptic seizures. The permanent imbalance of excitatory and inhibitory mechanisms in the brain may finally lead to status epilepticus.

International Classification of Epileptic Seizures

An international terminology for the classification of epileptic seizures was introduced for better international communication. In focal epileptic seizures the symptoms and the beginning of seizure activity in the EEG point to an initial activation of a circumscribed neuronal system of one brain hemisphere. As the onset of epi-

Section Editor: Werner Hacke

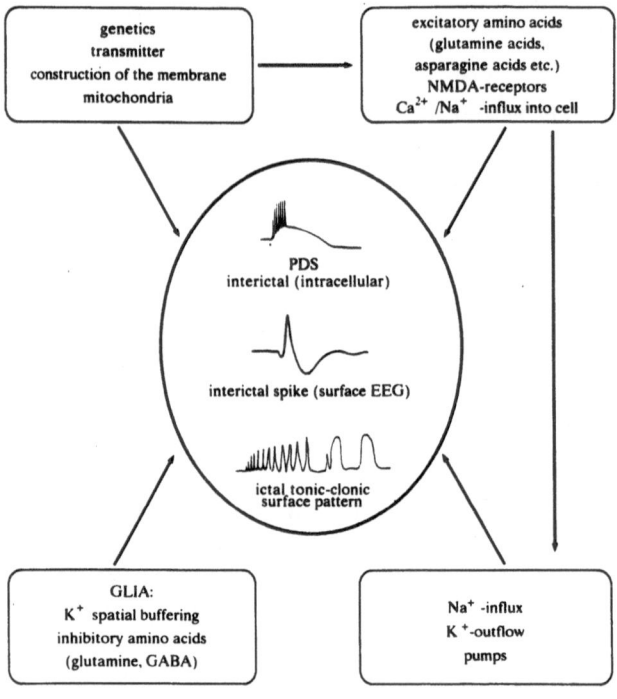

Fig. 1. The electrophysiological intracellular elementary epileptic phenomenon is called paroxysmal depolarization shift (PDS). Several factors are responsible for the excessive neuronal excitation. Aminoacids (e.g., glutamate) and NMDA receptors mediate a massive calcium influx into the neuron. This may lead to prolonged epileptic activity (e.g., series of seizures or status) and cell damage

leptic activity concerns only one part of a hemisphere, focal seizures are internationally classified as "partial" seizures. Simple- and complex-partial seizures are differentiated according to the international classification of epileptic seizures: Simple-partial seizures show no impairment of consciousness, while in complex-partial seizures "consciousness" is impaired. Impairment of consciousness was defined pragmatically in these cases by disturbances in consciousness as well as an impaired capacity to contact and report during a seizure (amnesia) and an impaired capacity to react to a call or certain tasks. Complex-partial seizures can start with an impairment of consciousness in the sense defined above or can follow simple-partial seizures (Table 1). Simple-partial and complex-partial seizure symptoms can develop into secondary generalized seizures with tonic-clonic convulsions. In the list of generalized seizures, absences are defined as well as myoclonic, clonic, tonic, tonic-clonic, and atonic seizures.

Differential Diagnosis

Syncopes

Syncopes of short duration and weak accentuation can easily be mistaken for a complex-partial seizure. In experiencing a short syncope the patient notices only a feeling of emptiness in the head, vertigo, tinnitus, or dark vision. Longer duration can be accompanied by a "pale" fainting fit.

Syncopes lasting more than 10 s can be accompanied by motoric symptoms (convulsive syncopes). In this case the bulbi are turned upwards or

Table 1. International classification of epileptic seizures (From Commission on Classification and Terminology of the International League Against Epilepsy 1985)

I. Partial (focal, local) seizures
Partial seizures are those in which, in general, the first clinical and electroencephalgraphic changes indicate initial activation of a system of neurons limited to part of one cerebral hemisphere. A partial seizure is classified primarily on the basis of whether or not consciousness is impaired during the attack. When consciousness is not impaired, the seizure is classified as a simple partial seizure. When consciousness is impaired, the seizure is classified as a complex partial seizure. Impairment of consciousness may be the first clinical sign, or simple partial seizures may evolve into complex partial seizures. In patients with impaired consciousness, aberrations of behavior (automatisms) may occur. A partial seizure may not terminate, but instead progress to a generalized motor seizure. Impaired consciousness is defined as the inability to respond normally to exogenous stimuli by virtue of altered awareness and/or responsiveness.

There is considerable evidence that simple partial seizures usually have unilateral hemispheric involvement and only rarely have bilateral hemispheric irrvolvement: complex partial seizures, however, frequently have bilateral hemispheric involvement.

Partial seizures can be classified into one of the following three fundamental groups:
A. Simple partial seizures
B. Complex partial seizures
  1. With impairment of consciousness at onset
  2. Simple partial onset followed by impairment of consciousness
C. Partial seizures evolving to generalized tonic-clonic convulsions (GTC)
  1. Simple evolving to GTC
  2. Complex evolving to GTC (including those with simple partial onset)

Clinical seizure type	EEG seizure type	EEG interictal expression
A. Simple partial seizures (consciousness not impaired)	Local contralateral discharge starting over the corresponding area of cortical representation (not always recorded on the scalp)	Local contralateral discharge

  1. With motor signs
    (a) Focal motor without march
    (b) Focal motor with march (Jacksonian)
    (c) Versive
    (d) Postural
    (e) Phonatory (vocalization or arrest of speech)
  2. With somatosensory or special-sensory symptoms (simple hallucinations, e.g., tingling, light flashes, buzzing)
    (a) Somatosensory
    (b) Visual
    (c) Auditory
    (d) Olfactory
    (e) Gustatory
    (f) Vertiginous
  3. With autonomic symptoms or signs (including epigastric sensation, pallor, sweating, flushing, piloerection and pupillary dilatation)
  4. With psychic symptoms (disturbance of higher cerebral function). These symptoms rarely occur without impairment of consciousness and are much more commonly experienced as complex partial seizures
    (a) Dysphasic
    (b) Dysmnesic (e.g., deja-vu)
    (c) Cognitive (e.g., dreamy states, distortions of time sense)

Table 1. *Continued*

    (d) Affective (fear, anger, etc.)
    (e) Illusions (e.g., macropsia)
    (f) Structured hallucinations (e.g., music, scenes)

B. Complex partial seizures (with impairment of con- sciousness: may sometimes begin with simple symptomatology)	Unilateral or frequently bilateral discharge, diffuse or focal in temporal or frontotemporal regions	Unilateral or bilateral generally asynchronous focus: usually in the temporal or frontal regions

    1. Simple partial onset followed by impairment of consciousness
        (a) With simple partial features (A1–A4) followed by impaired consciousness
        (b) With automatisms
    2. With impairment of consciousness at onset
        (a) With impairment of consciousness only
        (b) With automatisms

C. Partial seizures evolving to secondarily generalized seiures (This may be generalized tonic-clonic, tonic, or clonic)	Above discharges become secondarily and rapidly generalized	

    1. Simple partial seizures (A) evolving to generalized seizures
    2. Complex partial seizures (B) evolving to generalized seizures
    3. Simple partial seizures evolving to complex partial seizures evolving to generalized seizures

II. Generalized seizures (convulsive or nonconvulsive)

Generalized seizures are those in which the first clinical changes indicate initial involvement of both hemispheres. Consciousness may be impaired and this impairment may be the initial manifestation. Motor manifestations are bilateral. The ictal electroencephalographic patterns initially are bilateral, and presurnably reflect neuronal discharge which is widespread in both hemispheres.

Clinical seizure type	EEG seizure type	EEG interictal expression
A. 1. Absence seizures	Usually regular and symmetrical 3 Hz but may be 2–4 Hz spike-and-slow-wave complexes and may have multiple spike-and-slow-wave complexes. Abnormalities are bilateral	Background activity usually normal although paroxysmal activity (such as spikes or spike-and-slow-wave complexes) may occur. This activity is usually regular and symmertical

        (a) Impairment of consciousness only
        (b) With mild clonic components
        (c) With atonic components
        (d) With tonic components
        (e) With automatisms
        (f) With autonomic components (b through f may be used alone or in combination)

2. Atypical absence	EEG more heterogeneous: may include irregular spike-and-slow-wave complexes, fast activity or other paroxysmal activity. Abnormalities are bilateral but often irregular and asymmetrical	Background usually abnormal; paroxysmal activity (such as spikes or spike-and-slow-wave complexes) frequently irregular and asymmetrical

Table 1. *Continued*

May have:
(a) Changes in tone that are more pronounced than in A1
(b) Onset and/or cessation that is not abrupt

B. Myoclonic seizures		
Myoclonic jerks (single or multiple)	Polyspike and wave, or sometimes spike and wave or sharp and slow waves	Sames as ictal
C. Clonic seizures	Fast activity (10 c/sec or more) and slow waves; occasional spike-and-wave patterns	Spike-and-wave or polyspike-and-wave discharges
D. Tonic seizures	Low voltage, fast activity or a fast rhythm of 9–10 c/sec or more decreasing in frequency and increasing in amplitude	More or less rhythmic discharges of sharp and show waves, sometimes asymmetrical. Background is often abnormal for age
E. Tonic clonic seizures	Rhythm at 10 or more c/sec decreasing in frequency and increasing in amplitude during tonic phase, interrupted by slow waves during clonic phase	Polyspike and waves or spike and wave, or, sometimes, sharp and slow wave discharges
F. Atontric seizures (astatic seizures) (combinations of the above may occur, e.g., B and F, B and D)	Polyspikes and wave or flattening or low-voltage fast activity	Polyspikes and slow wave

III. Unclassified epileptic seizures
Includes all seizures that cannot be classified because of inadequate or incomplete data and some that defy classification in hitherto described categories. This includes some neonatal seizures, e.g., rhythmic eye movements, chewing, and swimming movements.

IV. Addendum
Repeated epileptic seizures occur under a variety of circumstances:
(1) As fortuitous attacks, coming unexpectedly and without any apparent provocation; (2) as cyclic attacks, at more or less regular intervals (e.g., in relation to the menstrual cycle, or the sleep-waking cycle); (3) as attacks provoked by: (a) nonsensory factors (fatigue, alcohol, emotion, etc.), or (b) sensory factors, sometimes referred to as "reflex seizures".
Prolonged or repetitive seizures (status epilepticus). The term status epilepticus is used whenever a seizure persists for a sufficient length of time or is repeated frequently enough that recovery between attacks does not occur. Status epilepticus may be divided into partial (e.g., Jacksonian), or generalized (e.g., absence status or tonic-clonic status). When very localized motor status occurs, it is referred to as epilepsia partialis continua.

extremities are stretched tonically. Tonic symptoms can be accompanied by mydriasis, nystagmus, salivation, and incontinence; more rarely, even a bite on the tongue can occur or aura-like symptoms with nausea. The EEG shows generalized slowing during the syncope. Subsequently, flattenting in the EEG during temporary loss of muscle tonus can occur, followed by a convulsive tonic muscle pattern. The simultaneous registration of ECG during EEG or even video-controlled EEG recordings are important for the proof of tachycardia, bradycardia, or asystolias. A syncope is proved by the record of bradycardia (40 beats/min), tachycardia (150 beats/min), asystolia lasting longer than 4 s, or systolic blood pressure of more than 70 mmHg. Reflex syncopes, however, occur most frequently. Twenty to 30% of syncopes are either diagnostically not correctly classified or mistaken for epileptic seizures. In tentative diagnosis of syncopes additional long-term ECG recordings and activation measures are necessary, as for instance examination of bulbus pressure, vasal maneuver, and perhaps also examination of carotid pressure. The differentiation of a "temporal syncope" as a consequence of a complex-partial seizure in temporal lobe epilepsy and syncopal fainting (for instance, induced psychovagally) can be particularly difficult, as in both cases symptoms can be similar (aura, change of consciousness, automatisms).

Absences

To enable acurate treatment, the typology of complex-partial seizures has to be distinguished meticulously from that of other epileptic seizures. In generalized spike-wave epilepsies and complex-partial seizures with seizure onset in the temporal lobe differentiation of absences is of utmost importance. In both cases the main clinical symptom consists in a disturbance of consciousness. The patient is absentminded and shows a stare gaze. Simultaneous video-EEG registration with the proof of 3-cps spike-wave complex in generalized spike-wave epilepsy with absence and of focal EEG pattern of a complex-partial seizure is

decisive for a correct diagnostic characterization. Differentiation of both types on the basis of seizure symptoms is aggravated, as not only the main symptom can be similar but also automatisms can occur in both seizure types. Oral automatisms are frequent in absences as well as in complex-partial seizures. In generalized 3-cps spike-wave epilepsy, absences often are accompanied by mild rhythmical myoclonia of the eyelid in the frequency of spike-wave complexes. The median duration of these absences is 7–10 s, whereas complex-partial seizures frequently last more than a few minutes.

Onset and end of change of consciousness cannot be clearly differentiated. The aura has to be classified in the case of a complex-partial seizure, as it is missing in generalized absences with 3-cps spike-wave complexes.

Ictus Emeticus

Autonomous and visceral phenomena frequently occur during epileptic seizures. These are acute symptoms, and they are generally accompanied by a change of behavior as well as by changes of consciousness during the seizure. Repeated ictal vomiting is present in patients with complex-partial seizures and interictal focus in the temporal brain region. Epileptic activity is predominantly in the medial and frontal temporal brain region. Before vomiting, feelings of nausea occur as well as salivation. This is followed by contractions of the abdominal musculature, and finally vomiting results as a consequence of vagus activation. Frequently the patient does not remember vomiting. In differential diagnosis for migraine these clinical characteristics are important, as are other cyclic or repeated conditions of vomiting without any conceivable internal basic affliction.

Transient Global Amnesia (TGA)

Episodes with a sudden incapacity to follow new thoughts while consciousness and other cognitive functions are intact are the main symptoms of transient, global amnesia. Functional disturbances of hippocampal or diencephalic structures seem to be the pathophysiological cause of this. The duration of the TGA ranges between 2 and 12 h (median 6 h). In anamesis exhaustion, diseases of coronary circulation, and migraine are frequently found. In these cases there are normally no pathological findings in the EEG and no potentials typical for epilepsy. In case of hippocampal epileptic focal seizure, status difficulties can occur if the leading symptom consists in a transient amnesia with changes of consciousness being more or less pronounced. It is not imperative that changes in the surface EEG show potentials typical for epilepsy in this circumscribed focal status. These can be identified only by means of special electrodes (e.g., sphenoidal, foramen ovale). An indication of epileptic seizure activity can be obtained by serum-prolactin recordings as in complex-partial seizures an excessive rise in prolactive can occur postictally. Whereas Single Photon Emission Computed Tomography (SPECT) in TGA, as a consequence of inadequate circulation, can show a temporal hypoperfusion, frequently a regional hyperperfusion occurs temporally in ictal SPECT in temporal lobe epilepsy.

Hysteric Seizures

In the past several decades a change of symptoms of hysteric seizures was seen; hysteric seizures formerly occurred predominantly as large seizures with "Arc de Cercle". Psychically induced seizures of the conscious as well as the remotely conscious type can be accompanied by discrete symptoms as in complex-partial seizures; 12–37% of patients with conscious or remotely conscious pseudoepileptic seizures simultaneously show paroxysmal interictal EEG changes. In this situation it is recommended that further diagnosis include video-controlled long-term EEG recordings and postictal serum-prolactin analysis under standardized conditions (one must beware of pseudohysteric seizure symptoms in frontal lobe epilepsy; here there is often no increase in prolactin). Hysteric seizures may also mimic tonic or tonic-clonic grand-mal status. In case of therapy-resistant status one should re-examine the diagnosis.

Hypovigilance in Dyssomnia

Conditions of hypovigilance can occur during the day in connection with the narcoleptic syndrome. Diagnostically, they are to be differentiated from the eppileptic twilight state. In this case a special sleep-polygraphic diagnosis is necessary, which might be supplemented by the analysis of the human leukocyte antigen (HLA-DR2). The proof of HLA-DR2 is mostly successful in patients with narcolepsy. However, HLA-DR2 is also found in healthy persons without narcolepsy. Status narcolepticus with loss of muscle tone and hallucination may mimic status epilepticus or schizophrenic psychosis.

Suggested Reading

Bauer J, Stefan H, Huk WJ, Feistel H, Hilz MJ, Brinkmann HG, Druschky KF, Neundörfer B (1989) CT, MRT and SPECT neuroimaging in status epilepticus with simple partial and complex partial seizures: case report. J Neurol 236:296–299

Commission on Classification and Terminology of the International League Against Epilepsy (1985) Proposal for classification of epilepsies and epileptic syndromes. Raven, New York, pp 268–278 (Epilepsia, vol 26, 3.)

Dasheiff RM, La Vera J, Dickinson RN (1986) Sudden unexpected death of epileptic patients due to cardiac arrhythmia after seizure. Arch Neurol 43:194–196

Gastaut H (1974) Syncopes: generalized anoxic cerebral seizures. In: Vinken PJ, Bruyn GW (eds) The epilepsies. Elsevier/North Holland, Amsterdam, pp 815–835 (Handbook of clinical neurology, vol 15.)

King DW, Gallagher B, Murvin AJ et al. (1982) Pseudoseizures: diagnostic evaluation. Neurology (NY) 32:18

Kramer RE, Lüders H, Lesser RP et al. (1988) Ictus emeticus: an electroclinical analysis. Neurology 38:1048–1052

Miller JW, Yanagihara T, Petersen RC, Klass DW (1987) Transient global amnesia and epilepsy. Arch Neurol 44:629–633

Penry JK, Porter RJ, Dreifuss FE (1975) Simultaneous recording of absence seizures with video tape and electroencephalography: a study of 374 seizures in 48 patients. Brain 98:427

Chapter 27

Neck Stiffness and Headache

BRIGITTE WILDEMANN and GERALD DAL PAN

Introduction

Neck stiffness and headache are important features of various disorders presenting as neurological or neurosurgical emergencies. Their simultaneous appearance usually reflects meningeal irritation and together with accompanying signs and symptoms is of significant diagnostic value.

Neck stiffness is felt as resistance to passive flexion of the neck. It may be accompanied by additional signs such as Brudzinski's and Kernig's sign. In severe cases hyperextension of the neck (opisthotonus) may be present. Usually head rotation is not limited. Neck rigidity and related phenomena tend to disappear in deepening coma and often fail to be elicited in infants and in the elderly. Neck stiffness is thought to arise from reflex tonic innervation of cervical muscles as a mechanism to minimize tension on irritated meninges and spinal nerve roots. The associated head pain is nonspecific and its characteristic features vary with the type and evolution of the

etiological process. It is caused by stimulation of pain-susceptible meningeal nerve fibers; depending on the underlying pathology, additional mechanisms such as displacement or distension of other pain-sensitive structures may contribute to its emergence. In the intracranial compartment these include basal and dural arteries, venous sinuses, and sensory fibers of cranial nerves V, VII, IX, X and of the upper cervical nerves.

Differential Diagnosis

Neck stiffness accompanied by headache most characteristically results from meningeal disorders such as subarachnoid hemorrhage, intracranial infection, and meningeal malignant infiltration. It may also occur secondary to raised intracranial pressure, in particular if obstruction of cerebrospinal fluid (CSF) pathways and impending tonsillar herniation are present. Rarely it may be a feature of arteritis.

Nuchal rigidity may be a symptom of various other conditions; in these processes any type of head movement

---

Section Editor: Werner Hacke

may be compromised and headache is not invariably present. Thus, it may appear with disorders of the cervical spine including cervical spondylosis, disk herniation, trauma, and metastases. It may develop secondary to osteoarthritis such as occurs in rheumatoid arthritis of the atlantoaxial joint, or result from structural cervical spine abnormalities including basilar impression, atlas and axis malformations, and Klippel-Feil syndrome. It also may be a feature of tumors in the vicinity of the foramen magnum or of posterior fossa deformities, including the Dandy-Walker and Arnold-Chiari syndromes. Neck rigidity in the context of more generalized increase in muscle tone occurs in extrapyramidal disorders such as Parkinson's disease, the malignant neuroleptic syndrome, malignant hyperthermia, and catatonia. Among muscular causes, tetanus and focal or more widespread myositis may induce resistance to neck flexion. Head retraction and neck stiffness are also features of paratonic rigidity or "gegenhalten" resulting from diffuse forebrain dysfunction. This appears with metabolic encephalopathy, cerebral atrophy, and hypertensive vascular disease, or

it may reflect a diencephalic disturbance in progressive tentorial herniation. Unlike extrapyramidal rigidity, paratonia disappears with slow and careful passive movements (Table 1).

Clinical Presentation

In patients presenting with severe headache and neck stiffness, a detailed history and physical examination are essential components of the clinical approach. Important features are the length of the illness, the mode of onset and nature of headaches, associated symptoms, presence of focal or diffuse neurologic impairment, and clinical or laboratory evidence of disease outside the nervous system. The patient should also be questioned about previous trauma.

Subarachnoid Hemorrhage

Key features of subarachnoid hemorrhage are headache and neck stiffness of acute or fulminating onset in a previously healthy patient. The headache

Table 1. Differential diagnosis of nonmeningeal neck stiffness

Cervical spine disorders	Extrapyramidal disorders
Spondylosis	Parkinson's disease
Disk herniation	Malignant neuroleptic syndrome
Trauma/fracture	Malignant hyperthermia
Metastases	Catatonia
Osteoarthritis	
Structural abnormalities	
Tumors	
Muscle disorders	Paratonia
Myositis	Metabolic encephalopathy
Tetanus	Cerebral atrophy
Whiplash injury	Hypertensive vascular disease
	Transtentorial herniation

is excruciating and neck or back pain may be additionally present. Vomiting is a frequent feature and alteration of consciousness and coma may rapidly occur. Focal neurologic signs may be found if intraparenchymal bleeding has also occurred. Spontaneous subarachnoid hemorrhage most often results from rupture of an intracranial aneurysm or arteriovenous malformation and these conditions should be considered first. Less commonly, a spinal or dural-based arteriovenous malformation may rupture, leading to neck stiffness and back pain with little or no headache.

An indistinguishable clinical presentation may arise with secondary access of blood to the subarachnoid space. This occurs as a complication of hypertensive cerebral hemorrhage or bleeding into a primary or metastatic intracranial neoplasm. However, in these conditions focal neurologic signs are more frequently observed. Occasionally subarachnoid hemorrhage may result from spontaneous intracranial carotid artery dissection. It rarely develops secondary to vasculopathies predisposing to aneurysm formation and arterial dissection such as fibromuscular dysplasia, moyamoya disease, and Marfan's syndrome. Other causes include rupture of mycotic aneurysms in infective endocarditis and hematologic disorders including leukemia, thrombocytopenia, and coagulopathies. In these conditions clinical and laboratory evidence of systemic disease are helpful.

Intracranial Infections

Headache and nuchal rigidity of inflammatory origin are of variable intensity, but usually have typical accompanying symptoms. Severe headache and neck rigidity followed by serious neurological deterioration and coma within a few hours may result from fulminant purulent meningitis. Associated findings at onset are fever, chills, photo- and phonophobia, vomiting, irritability, and altered sensorium. The presence of a purpuric or petechial skin rash is highly suggestive of meningococcal meningitis. Pneumococci, streptococci, staphylococci, or *Haemophilus influenzae* are more likely to be the causative organism if there is a history of preceding otitis media, sinusitis, head trauma, or neurosurgical intervention.

Moderate head pain and nuchal rigidity in the context of fever, mental status changes, seizures, and significant diffuse or focal central nervous system involvement are classical manifestations of infectious or parainfectious encephalitis. With most encephalopathies of viral origin, evolution of symptoms takes place gradually over a few days. However, a fulminant clinical course is not unusual and is particularly frequent in herpes simplex encephalitis. In this condition signs of temporal lobe dysfunction are highly suggestive diagnostic features. Subacute or chronic encephalitis and meningitis syndromes with duration of symptoms for weeks to months are more likely to be caused by other pathogens. The differential diagnosis includes mycobacterial or spirochetal disease and, in patients with severe immunodeficiency, a fungal or parasitic origin. A similar clinical presentation may occur with subacute bacterial endocarditis and in this disorder results from single or repeated septic cardiogenic embolization. In addition, septic emboli may cause the formation of mycotic aneurysms and their rupture may provoke dramatic clinical deterioration with features of acute subarachnoid hemorrhage.

Meningeal Malignant Infiltration

Headache and nuchal rigidity may be symptoms of leukemic or carcinomatous spread to the meninges. Signs of cranial or spinal nerve involvement are usually present. Intensive care management is usually not necessary but may be required if rapid alteration of consciousness occurs and an aggressive therapeutic approach has been decided on.

Raised Intracranial Pressure

Headache and neck stiffness may reflect raised intracranial pressure and may arise with both supra- and infratentorial expanding lesions. Most frequently, acute or rapidly growing infratentorial space-occupying processes leading to hydrocephalus and incipient tonsillar herniation are associated with their appearance. Examples include cerebellar hematomas or large cerebellar ischemic infarction as well as posterior fossa tumors. A dramatic presentation with headache of acute onset, vomiting, mental obtundation, and nuchal rigidity may be due to sudden obstruction of CSF pathways, such as ensues from colloid cysts of the III ventricle or from other mobile tumors growing within the ventricular system.

Vasculitis

Vasculitic involvement of the meninges and central nervous system may be accompanied by headache and neck stiffness. Associated abnormalities include encephalopathic clinical syndromes and seizures or focal and multifocal neurological deficits of either ischemic or hemorrhagic origin. Central nervous system arteritis may be a feature of systemic necrotizing vasculitides and collagen vascular disorders or may evolve in relation to drug abuse or malignancy. In these conditions extracerebral vasculitic involvement and/or alterations of laboratory-tested variables will be found in the majority of cases. Isolated central nervous system vasculitis may complicate meningitis and meningoencephalitis of nearly any origin. A rare cause is isolated granulomatous angiitis of the central nervous system.

Principles of Diagnosis

Neuroimaging

The management of a patient presenting with headache and neck stiffness requires prompt recognition of the underlying (potentially serious) neurological disease and rapid institution of therapy. The most important tests in the emergency situation are imaging procedures such as computed tomography (CT), magnetic resonance imaging (MRI), and angiography, as well as cerebrospinal fluid (CSF) studies and (occasionally) Doppler ultrasonography and electroencephalography. Laboratory studies may provide helpful information in inflammatory conditions.

Table 2 summarizes principal diagnostic features of some important causes of neck stiffness.

Table 2. Diagnostic features of some important causes of neck stiffness

Condition	Imaging study	CSF analysis[a]	Other diagnostic tests
Subarachnoid Hemorrhage	Subarachnoid blood visible on cranial CT in >85% of cases. Intracranial hematoma may be present	Bloody CSF with xanthochromia	Angiography necessary to evaluate for intracerebral aneurysm and vascular malformation
Posterior fossa mass lesion	Posterior fossa lesion, with or without obstructive hydrocephalus	Generally not performed	Cranial MRI generally more informative than CT in defining the lesion
Spinal arteriovenous malformation	Cranial study may be normal	Bloody CSF with xanthochromia	Spinal MRI and/or myelography necessary to define the lesion. Angiography may also be needed
Neck trauma/ fracture	Cranial study normal if no concomitant head trauma	Generally not performed	Conventional radiography and CT of the spine necessary to establish diagnosis of fracture. Spinal MRI helpful in assessing damage to cord
Meningeal infection	Unenhanced images may be normal; gadolinium-enhanced MRI may reveal meningeal enhancement	Mononuclear or polymorphonuclear pleocytosis, elevated protein content, and variable glucose content	CSF and blood cultures/serology necessary to establish diagnosis. Emergency CSF Gram stain also helpful
Carcinomatous or leukemic meningitis	Unenhanced images may be normal if no concomitant intracerebral lesion. Gadolinium-enhanced MRI may reveal meningeal enhancement	Malignant pleocytosis, generally with elevated protein content	CSF cytologic examination necessary to establish diagnosis

[a] When any of these conditions is suspected, CSF analysis should be performed only after a cranial imaging study has been performed and shows no indication of mass effect.
CT, Computed tomography;
MRI, magnetic resonance imaging;
CSF, cerebrospinal fluid.

In most instances an immediate CT scan is the diagnostic procedure of choice. It will help to decide whether further management is primarily neuro-logical or neurosurgical. CT will almost always reveal recent subarachnoid hemorrhage (generally up to 4–5 days), and helps rapidly to distinguish

290   B. Wildemann and G.D. Pan

hematoma from other focal lesions. Areas of ischemic infarction may not yet be demarcated, but early signs of ischemia may be apparent. It also allows evaluation for the presence and degree of brain edema and hydrocephalus. In intracranial infections CT is of significant value, although not specifically diagnostic. CT should be carried out before lumbar puncture to exclude significant brain swelling and impending transtentorial herniation, particularly in stuporous or comatose patients. CT reveals complications such as communicating hydrocephalus, subdural empyema, ventriculitis, and brain abscess. It may suggest sinus venous thrombosis, but definite diagnosis of cerebral venous thrombosis requires additional tests in most cases. In bacterial meningitis or brain abscess visualization of adjacent structures may identify the potential source of infection such as nasal sinusitis or mastoiditis. The presence of multiple ischemic areas together with CSF pleocytosis and laboratory evidence of infection may be compatible with septic embolization from infective endocarditis.

While CT remains the primary imaging modality in the clinical situation mentioned above – particularly if acute subarachnoid hemorrhage is suspected – MRI may be also necessary to exclude other pathologies. MRI plays a major role in the assessment of additional structural changes such as leptomeningeal enhancement in meningitis, subtle changes of the brain tissue adjacent to inflamed structures, and secondary ischemic changes due to vasculitic complications of meningitis. MRI is the method of choice if a cervical cause of neck stiffness is suspected.

CSF Examination

CSF examination must be performed in any patient suspected to suffer from acute meningitis or meningoencephalitis and, whenever possible, should be undertaken before antibiotic treatment is started. In the emergency situation, cell count, cytology and the search for bacteria in a Gram-stained smear are the most important diagnostic procedures. Purulent intracranial infections can be distinguished from nonpurulent infections with relative certainty. Protein content as well as glucose and lactate estimations will provide additional information. In acute bacterial meningitis CSF contains more than 3000 cells/μl and polymorphonuclear leukocytes are the main cell type; however, moderate pleocytosis or absence of cells does not exclude a bacterial etiology. Extra- or intracellular organisms can be identified microscopically in Gram-stained smears in the majority of cases, but may be absent in patients treated with antibiotics prior to lumbar puncture. Protein content and lactate are significantly increased, CSF glucose is low. CSF abnormalities in viral meningitis or meningoencephalitis include a moderately increased cell count (100–3000/μl) and protein content. Cytology may show granulocytes in the very acute stage, but typically lymphocytes and monocytes are predominant. A mixed polymorphonuclear and mononuclear pleocytosis is often found with granulomatous infections or may occur with brain abscesses or septic embolization from endocarditis. Slightly increased lactate and normal glucose is found in viral infections. Glucose is typically decreased in granulomatous processes such as tuberculous or fungal meningitis. Laboratory studies including blood count and erythrocyte sedimentation rate may support a presumptive diagnosis of bacterial meningitis or infective endocarditis.

In patients with suspected subarachnoid hemorrhage who are admitted a few days after the onset of clinical symptoms a spinal tap may be of considerable diagnostic value. In these cases the CT scan is often negative, but the presence of xanthochromia and the cytologic appearance of phagocytes containing red blood cells and/or hemosiderin are of pathognomonic significance.

Angiography

Angiography is required in subarachnoid hemorrhage for definitive demonstration of an intracranial aneurysm or arteriovenous malformation. It should be performed as an emergency procedure if early neurosurgical intervention is intended. Angiography may be necessary to evaluate large parenchymal hematomas prior to surgical evacuation, particularly if their distribution is not consistent with chronic hypertension. In suspected sinus venous thrombosis or arterial dissection angiography is the diagnostic procedure of choice unless emergency MRI is available.

Doppler Ultrasonography

Transcranial Doppler ultrasonography is important to identify and monitor the presence of vasospasm following subarachnoid hemorrhage or secondary to vasculitis in acute intracranial infections.

Electroencephalography

Electroencephalography is required as an emergency diagnostic test to record seizure activity in unresponsive patients suspected to suffer from persistent focal or generalized convulsions. Temporal abnormalities may reflect the earliest localizing alterations in presumed herpes simplex encephalitis.

Suggested Reading

Blau JN (1986) Headache: history, examination, differential diagnosis and special investigations. In: Vinken PJ, Bruyn GW, Klawans HL (eds) Handbook of clinical neurology, vol 48. Elsevier, New York, pp 43–58

Campbell JK, Caselli RJ (1991) Headache and other craniofacial pain. In: Bradley WG, Daroff RB, Fenichel GM, Marsden CD (eds) Neurology in clinical practice. The neurological disorders, vol 2. Butterworth-Heinemann, Boston, pp 1507–1548

Headache Classification Committee of the International Headache Society (1988) Classification and diagnostic criteria for headache disorders, cranial neuralgias and facial pain. Cephalalgia 8 [Suppl 7]:1–96

Moore PM, Cupps TR (1983) Neurological complications of vasculitis. Ann Neurol 14: 155–167

Ray BS, Wolff HG (1940) Experimental studies on headache: pain sensitive structures of the head and their significance in headache. Arch Surg 41:813–856

Simpson JF (1969) Meningeal signs and symptoms. In: Vinken PJ, Bruyn GW (eds) Handbook of clinical neurology, vol 1. Wiley Interscience Division, New York, pp 536–549

Swanson JW (1991) Cranial and facial pain. In: Bradley WG, Daroff RB, Fenichel GM, Marsden CD (eds) Neurology in clinical practice. The neurological disorders, vol 1. Butterworth-Heinemann, Boston, pp 231–237

| # Tetraplegia and Paraplegia

ROMAN HABERL and DENNIS G. VOLLMER

Introduction

Tetraplegia and paraplegia are syndromes which may have a traumatic, inflammatory, degenerative, or neoplastic etiology. The clinical signs differ depending on the causative process and the level of the lesion. Diseases at all levels of the neuraxis, from cerebral cortex to muscle, may cause the clinical syndromes of para- and tetraplegia (Table 1).

The patient's history may give the first clue to the etiology of the syndrome. Trauma usually is obvious, but occasionally neurological deficits occur in delayed fashion, where the inciting trauma may not be apparent. Fever is indicative of an inflammatory cause, and preceding systemic neoplasia should raise suspicion of metastatic spinal cord compression. The acuteness of onset is of special diagnostic relevance; Table 2 summarizes typical temporal courses for some causes of para- and tetraplegia.

Section Editor: Werner Hacke

Clinical Findings

Clinical signs useful for differentiating central and peripheral causes of paraplegia include the presence of exaggerated tendon reflexes, with increased muslce tone (spasticity), pathological reflexes (e.g., Babinski's sign, Gordon's sign), the segmental versus nonsegmental distribution of sensory deficits, and the presence of cranial nerve palsies. Peripheral – radicular or neurogenic – diseases produce loss of tendon reflexes and a flaccid para-/tetraparesis, whereas central lesions may cause either flaccidity with loss of muscle reflexes (particularly in the acute stage) or spasticity. The reduction of muscle tone and muscle reflexes with acute spinal lesions, especially of traumatic origin, is called "spinal shock", which may last up to 6 weeks before spastic signs develop.

One goal of the primary neurological examination of a patient with para- or tetraplegia is to decide on the level of the causal process. Figure 1 lists typical neurological signs related to the level of the lesion. Lesions above the spinal level produce additional symptoms such as cranial nerve palsies,

Table 1. Differential diagnosis of para- and tetraplegia as related to the level of the lesion

Level	Frequent causes	Clinical characteristics	Best diagnostic technique
Parasagittal cortex	Tumor	Flaccid paraparesis, no sensory deficit, Jackson seizures	Cranial CT scan
Bilateral white matter, bilateral internal capsule	Infarcts	Spastic tetraparesis	Cranial CT scan
Bilateral brain stem	Infarcts, encephalitis, multiple sclerosis, tumor, central pontine myelinolysis	Spastic tetraparesis, cranial nerve palsies	Cranial MRI
Pyramidal decussation	Trauma, tumor	Flaccid tetraparesis	Cranial MRI
Upper cervical spinal cord (C1–4)	Trauma	Spastic tetraparesis, diaphragmatic paresis	Craniocervical MRI
Central cervical medulla	Intramedullary tumor, syrinx, contusion	Brachial paraparesis, sensory level at neck, bladder dysfunction	Cervical MRI
Lower cervical spinal cord (C5–8)	Disk prolapse, spinal stenosis, tumor	Spastic paraparesis, nuclear arm palsies	Myelography, cervical MRI, CT scan
Thoracic spinal cord	Tumor, anterior spinal artery syndrome, multiple sclerosis	Spastic paraparesis, sensory level, paresis of abdominal wall muscles	Myelography, spinal MRI
Thoracolumbar spinal cord ("epiconus", L4–S2)	Occlusion of the artery of Adamkiewicz, tumor	Incontinence, spastic paraparesis except hip flexors, sensory level at L4	Myelography, MRI
Conus (S3–C)	Tumor, disk prolapse	Incontinence, saddle anesthesia, loss of anal reflex, impotence	Myelography, MRI
Cauda equina	Medial disk prolapse	Sensory loss from L4, saddle anesthesia, nuclear leg palsies, incontinence, impotence	Myelography, MRI
Multiple nerve roots	Polyradiculitis (GBS, CIDP), porphyria	Areflexia, flaccid para- or tetraparesis	CSF, electrophysiology
Peripheral nerves	Acute polyneuropathy (e.g., intensive care polyneuropathy)	Areflexia, flaccid para- or tetraparesis	Electrophysiology
Muscle	Myasthenia gravis, botulism, dyskalemic palsies		Electrophysiology, laboratory parameters

Table 2. Differential diagnosis in para- and tetraplegia – acuteness of onset

Acute (seconds to minutes)	Subactue (30 min to several hours)	Chronic (days to weeks)
Trauma	Transverse myelitis	Tumor
Anterior spinal artery syndrome	Guillain-Barré syndrome	Myasthenia gravis
Dyskalemic palsies	Decompression illness	Tuberculous spondylitis, epidural abscess
Epidural/subdural spinal hemorrhage	Cervical disk prolapse	Multiple sclerosis
Electrical injury		Guillain-Barré syndrome
		Syringomyelia
		Poliomyelitis

epileptic seizures, or neuropsychological alterations. When the neurological syndrome is incomplete, localization of the spinal level may be difficult or misleading. In this situation, the entire spinal axis, extending to include the foramen magnum, must be evaluated.

Situations with acute or incomplete subacute para-/tetraplegia are emergencies. The diagnostic evaluation must be completed within hours, because motor and vegetative symptoms due to spinal cord compression are less likely to be reversible with delayed treatment. Figure 2 shows the sequence of diagnostic steps. Plain radiographs of the spine are recommended before myelography or magnetic resonance imaging (MRI) because fractures or osteodestruction may be obscured by contrast within the spinal canal and may be missed on MRI. In addition, the observation of bony changes may allow tailoring of the appropriate radiological studies.

Ancillary Tests

The relative roles of myelography, spinal computed tomography (CT) and MRI are evolving. When the level of involvement is unclear or multifocal, CT may be less useful; MRI and panmyelography are better suited to studying long segments of the spinal axis. Bony detail is best appreciated on CT, whereas evaluations of intramedullary processes are best done with MRI. Myelography, possibly coupled with postmyelogram CT scanning, is still the most widely available and generally the most rapid method of screening for spinal cord compression. In addition, critically ill patients, as well as those with certain metallia implants, are better evaluated with myelography. When a spinal mass lesion has been excluded, inflammatory causes, vascular causes, supraspinal diseases, or a psychogenic syndrome should be considered.

Etiologies

Vascular Causes

There are both cerebral and spinal causes of para- and tetraplegia (Table 3). Multifocal lacunar lesions in the white matter or bilateral infarction in the internal capsule may, on rare occasions, produce tetraparesis. More

Level	Clinical symptoms
C1–C8:	
Tract for vibratory and position sense	Ipsilateral hypesthesia for posture/vibration
Pyramidal tract, leg and arm	Spastic tetraparesis/paraparesis
Tract for pain and temperature	Contralateral hypalgesia
Sympathetic tract for the whole body: temperature and vessel tone regulation, tone of internal bladder sphincter	Ipsilateral anhidrosis, hyperthermia, Horner syndrome, orthostatic hypotension/paroxysmal hypertension
Motor neurons for diaphragma (C4) and arm (C5–C8)	Diaphragmatic palsy, segmental flaccid and atrophic arm paresis
Tract for touch, pressure	Sensory level
Th 1–L2:	
Tract for vibratory and position sense	Ipsilat. hypesthesia for posture at legs
Pyramidal tract, leg	Spastic paraparesis
Tract for pain and temperature	Contralateral level for pain, temperature
Segmental sympathetic innervation, sympathetic nuclei for bladder (Th 12–L2)	Level with anhidrosis below, urine incontinence
Motor neurons for thoracic and abdominal wall muscles	Ipsilat. abdominal wall palsy, abdominal wall reflex lost
Tract for touch, pressure	Sensory level, loss of cremaster reflex
L3–S1:	
Tract for vibratory and position sense at legs	Ipsilateral hypesthesia for posture at legs
Pyramidal tract, leg	Spastic paraparesis
Tract for leg pain and temp.	Contralateral hypalgesia
Motor neurons for leg muscles	Segmental flaccid, atrophic leg palsy
Tract for touch, pressure	Sensory level
S2–S4:	
Parasympathetic nuclei for bladder, sexual organs, descending colon	Autonomic bladder with high urine volume, impotence
Motor neurons for spincter ani, external urethral sphincter	Stool and urine incontinence
Sensory tract for "saddle region"	Saddle anesthesia

Fig. 1. Clinical symptoms related to the level of the spinal cord injury

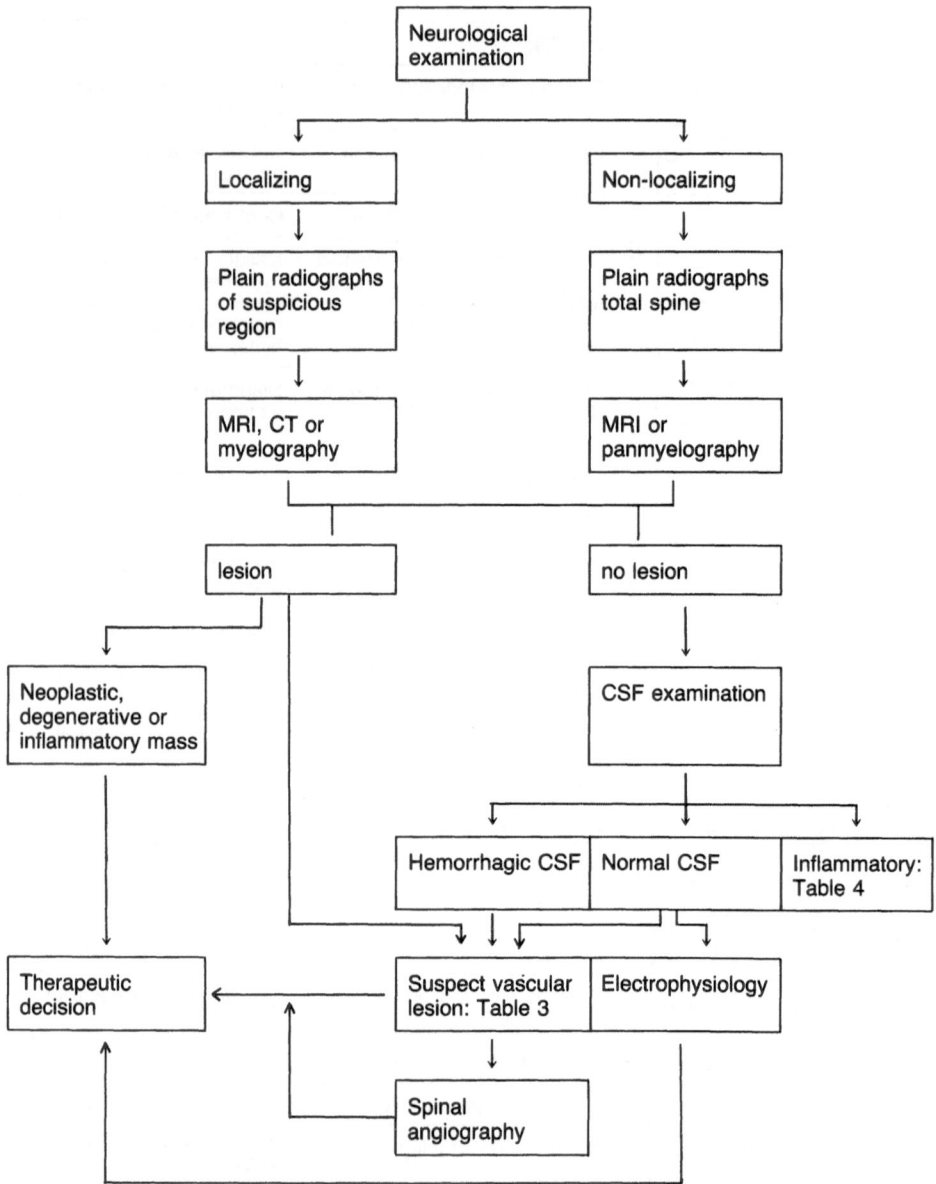

Fig. 2. Diagnostic process in para- and tetraplegia

frequently, tetraparesis develops after brain-stem infarction due to occlusion of the basilar artery. Both brain-stem infarction and spinal ischemia may have a staggering or binodal onset rather than an acute beginning. This opens a window for preventive anticoagulation therapy with early diagnosis.

Spinal ischemia is usually due to occlusion of the anterior spinal artery or the artery of Adamkiewicz with the characteristic clinical syndrome of

Table 3. Vascular causes of tetra- and paraplegia

Cause	Vessel	Onset	Characteristic features	Etiology
Brain stem infarction	Basilary artery	Acute or spasmodic, minutes to hours	Cranial nerve palsies, vertigo	Thrombosis or embolism, vertebral artery dissection
Vasculitis (panarteritis, allergic vasculitis, Wegener, Churg-Strauss, lamphomatoid granulomatosis, Behçet's disease (Moore and Cupps 1983)	Brain-stem vessels, spinal arteries, multifocal cerebral arteritis	acute	ANAs or ANCAs in serum positive, systemic or visual system involvement, eosinophilia	
Spinal infarction (Brosch et al. 1990; Hands et al. 1991; Riggle and Oddi 1989; Waring and Karunas 1991; Zull and Cydulka 1988)	Anterior spinal artery	Acute or spasmodic, bitemporal	Umbelliform acute pain, dissociated pain/temperature sensory deficit, spastic para-/tetraparesis	Aortic dissection DeBakey I–III, aortic surgery, cardiogenic embolism, intra-aortic balloon insertion, thrombotic
	Central spinal artery (A. sulcocomissuralis)	Acute or spasmodic	Brown-Sequard syndrome	Atherosclerosis, disk prolapse, embolism
	Artery of Adamkiewicz	Acute or spasmodic	Complete motor and sensory loss at thoracolumbar level	Atherosclerosis, infrarenal aortic dissection, embolism, tumors, abdominal surgery, during profound hypotension

Table 3. *Continued*

Cause	Vessel	Onset	Characteristic features	Etiology
Spinal arteriovenous malformation	Intradural and extradural vascular malformations, dural fistulas	Chronic, fluctuating over weeks, acute deterioration with hematomyelia	Fluctuating symptoms with segmental pain, spastic paraplegia, bladder dysfunction	Spinal compression, spinal ischemia
Intramedullary hemorrhage (hematomyelia)	Intraparenchymal vascular malformation	Chronic fluctuating or acute deterioration with hematomyelia	Fluctuating symptoms, characteristic intramedullary lesion on MRI	
Spinal subarachnoid, epidural or subdural hemorrhage	Vertebral artery, spinal arteries	Acute within seconds	Acute neck pain, progressive symptoms, blood stained CSF	Spinal berry aneurysm, vertebral dissecting aneurysm, dural fistula
Spinal microvascular compression (claudicatio spinalis, vascular myelopathy)	Branches of the spinal anterior art. and the spinal posterior arteries, artery of Adamkiewicz	Subacute or chronically progressive	Progressive paraparesis, bladder dysfunction	Spinal stenosis, spinal vascular malformation, secondary to spinal trauma or tumor, venous stop

beltlike pain, paraparesis, and loss of sensation for pain and temperature below this level. The cause of the occlusion may be cardiogenic embolism, spinal compression, aortic dissection, or iatrogenic. Radiographic examination is required to detect spinal vascular malformations (myelography, spinal angiography), spinal epidural or subdural bleeding (myelography, CT, MRI), and to exclude nonvascular causes of paraparesis. The finding of blood-stained CSF on lumbar puncture may be consistent with the diagnosis of spinal subarachnoid or subdural hemorrhage. Intraspinal microvascular compression may result from degenerative spondylosis (e.g., cervical spondylotic myelopathy), posttraumatic spinal swelling, and spinal compression by space occupying lesions. In the setting of spondylotic cauda equina compression, there is an increase in back pain and occasionally paraparesis with exercise ("claudication spinalis").

Inflammatory Causes

Inflammatory diseases of the spinal cord include viral, bacterial, and parasitological infections, granulomatous inflammations, and demyelinating immunological disease (Table 4). Bacterial involvement includes osteomyelitis and/or disk space infection, epidural abscess, subdural empyema, and meningitis. Intramedullary abscess is rare at present. The hallmark of vertebral osteomyelitis or subdural abscess is localized spinal pain and tenderness. These findings would tend to differentiate epidural abscess or osteomyelitis from the other infections noted above. Systemic signs of infection are frequently, but not always observed. Although *Staphylococcus aureus* is still the most common etiologic agent, gram-negative organisms and opportunistic agents are increasingly reported. Tuberculous involvement, an important consideration in underdeveloped countries, is becoming more prevalent in developed countries as well.

Tetraparesis can be a presenting symptom of brain-stem encephalitis. Listeriosis and tick-borne encephalitis are the most frequent causes. Polyradiculitis should be included in the differential diagnosis of patients with areflexia, flaccid paraparesis, lack of sensory level, and a normal myelogram.

Since many inflammatory conditions produce spinal cord compression, radiological examination with myelography or spinal MRI is mandatory. MRI may also reveal focal intramedullary spinal cord lesions (hyperintense on the T2 sequence and gadolinium enhancing when acute) in multiple sclerosis and transverse myelitis. Radiological signs may suggest an etiology, such as massive prevertebral swelling and kyphosis in vertebral tuberculosis and osteolysis of ribs in vertebral hydatidosis (Table 4).

Cerebrospinal fluid examination aids in the diagnosis of inflammatory conditions. The diagnosis may be made by cell count, protein level, glucose level, cell differential, evaluation of CSF-specific oligoclonal proteins by isoelectric focusing, comparison of albumin and immunoglobulin G levels in CSF and serum, and comparison of specific antibody titers in CSF and serum. Of particular interest for early diagnosis is the identification of pathogens by polymerase chain reaction (PCR) in CSF.

Table 4. Inflammatory causes of para- and tetraplegia

Cause/literature	Typical localization	Onset	Diagnostic features	CSF	MRI	Diagnosis by
Listeriosis (Simpson 1971)	Brain stem	Subacute, cheese consumption days before	Fever, cranial nerve palsies	Up to 1000/μl cells, high protein (1200 mg/100 ml)	Hyperintense focal brain-stem lesions on T2	PCR in CSF
Toxoplasmosis	Multifocal cerebral involvement	Subacute	HIV infection	IgM titers and increasing IgG titers	Multifocal enhancing lesions	Improvement during therapy
FSME	Brain stem	Subacute, tick bite weeks before	Fever, cranial nerve palsies	50–150/μl cells, lymphocytic, moderate protein elevation	Diffuse brain-stem swelling	Specific IgM antibodies in serum
Vertebral tuberculosis (Pott's disease) (Moula et al. 1981)	Mid-thoracic (Th 4-9)	Chronic	Urinary incontinence, kyphosis and prevertebral swelling on X-ray/CT scan	Up to 1000/μl cells, high protein, low glucose	Meningeal contrast enhancement	Ziehl-Neelsen staining and PCR in CSF
Lyme (Steere 1989)	Myelitis (stage 2, rare) or multifocal demyelination (stage 3)	Chronic	Spastic paraparesis, ataxic gait	CSF-specific oligoclonal protein	Focal hyperintensities on the T2-sequence	Intrathecal antibody production
Varicella zoster	Radiculomyelitis, cauda	Subacute	Radicular pain, skin eruptions, incontinence	Low cell count (up to 30/μl), protein elevation		PCR, specific antibodies in CSF
Transverse myelitis[a]	Thoracic segments	Acute	Fever (50%), progressive motor and sensory signs, beltlike hyperpathy	30–150/μl cells, 50–200 mg/100 ml protein	Segmental hyperintensity on the T2 sequence	

Disease	Location	Time course	Clinical symptoms	CSF	Imaging	Diagnosis/remarks
Vertebral hydatidosis (Kaoutzanis et al. 1989; Karray et al. 1990)	Thoracic, lumbar spine	Subacute to chronic	Backache, bone destruction (also ribs) with disk preservation		Paravertebral cysts and spinal cysts	MRI, antibodies against *Echinococcus granulosus*
Epidural abscess (Dei-Ahang et al. 1990)		Subacute	Backache, fever, meningism, numbness	Increase in cell count and protein, aspiration of pus	Enhancing space-occupying lesion in the epidural space	Previous paravertebral puncture, risk factors like Crohn's disease, diabetes mell. [1,10]
Tropical spastic paraparesis (Roman 1988; Roman and Roman 1988)		Subacute to chronic	Asymmetrical spastic paraparesis, backache, dysesthesias of feet, bladder dysfunction	Normal		Endemic for tropical islands, anti-HTL V-I serum antibodies
HIV myelopathy (Fisher and Enzensberger 1987)	Thoracic segments	Chronic (late stages of HIV infection)	Spastic paraparesis, spinal ataxia, incont.			
Multiple sclerosis (Ringelstein et al. 1987)	Cervical and thoracic	Subacute to chronic	Disseminated motor, cerebellar and brain-stem symptoms	Normal cell count and protein level, oligoclonal protein/IgG in CSF	Hyperintensity on T2, gadolinium enhancement	MRI, CSF, evoked potentials
Polyradiculitis (GBS., CIDP) (Ropper 1992)		Subacute, infection 2–4 weeks before	Symmetrical flaccid weakness, areflexia	Increased protein, normal cell count	Normal	Electrophysiology (delayed F-waves)

a Described with viral infections (smallpox, varicella, measles, rubella, mumps, influenza, echovirus, herpes simpex 6, EBV), postvaccinial (rabies, smallpox) and bacterial infections (streptococcus, pertussis, mycoplasma, pneumococcus).

Tumors

A variety of intraspinal tumors may produce para- and tetraplegia (Table 5). These may be localized to the vertebrae, epidural space, intradural ex- tramedullary space, intramedullary space, or a combination of the above.

Vertebral and epidural involvement are most common with metastatic lesions, myeloma, and primary tumors of the bone. Intradural extramedullary

Table 5. Tumors causing paraplegia or tetraplegia

Tumor (frequency)	Typical localization	Typical clinical signs
Primary intraspinal tumors (Helseth and Mork 1989):		
meningioma (47%)	Intradural extramedullary – thoracic	Slowly progressive paraparesis, older women, high CSF protein
neurinoma (11%)	Intradural extramedullary – all regions	radicular symptoms at onset, 30–60 years, high CSF protein
angioma (4%)	Intradural extramedullary	Fluctuating paraparesis, segmental pain
glioma (5%)	Intradural intramedullary – cervical	Back pain, slowly progressive paraparesis, central medullar syndrome, <30 years
ependymoma (19%)	Intradural intramedullary – cervicothoracic (epithelial type) or conus/cauda (papillary type)	Lumbar pain
Metastatic tumors (Waring and Karunas 1991):	Extradural (98%) or rarely intradural intramedullary (1–2%)	Sixth decade
lung. (appr. 20%)	Upper thoracic segments	
breast (appr. 14%)	Lower thoracic segments	
prostate (appr. 20%)		
kidney (appr. 10%)	Lower thoracic segments	
lymphoma (8%)		
myeloma (4%)		
melanoma (3%)		
rectum, colon (4%)		
Meningeal carcinomatosis		Meningism, radicular pain, paraparesis, tumor cells in CSF, high CSF protein
Vertebral tumors (Hamel et al. 1984):	Extradural	Adolescents and young adults
hemangioma, osteoblastoma, lipoma, histiocytosis X (Gandolf: 1983), chordoma, aneurysmal bone cysts, lipoma		
Dermoid cysts	Extradural, conus	

[a] Of all intraspinal tumors.
[b] Of all spinal metastases.

Table 6. Other and rare causes of para- and tetraparesis

Cause (literature)	Onset	Clinical features	Diagnosis by	Clinical situation
Degenerative myelopathy	Chronic	Exercise-dependent back pain, spastic para- or tetraparesis, radicular symptoms	Myelography, CT scan	
Syringomyelia	Chronic	Pain, segmental sensory deficit for pain and temp., radicular symp., trophic lesions	MRI	Post-traumatic, craniocervical dysplasia, impairment of CSF passage
Hypokalemic paralysis	Acute, for hours to 3 days	Pure flaccid tetraplegia	Low serum potassium	Familial, induced by glucose, cold
Rare:				
Cervical radiation myelopathy (Berlit et al. 1987; Berlit and Schwechheimer 1987)	Subacute to chronic	Spastic paraparesis, dissociated sensory loss for pain/temperature	Exclusion of other causes	1–1.5 years after radiation, total dose > 40 Gy
Intrathecal methotrexate (Werner 1988)	Subacute	Transient, rarely permanent paraparesis	Elevated protein and myelin basic protein in CSF	5–20 days after injection
Epidural lipomatosis (Kaplan et al. 1989)	Gradually progressive	Back pain, radiculopathy, paraparesis, thoracic/lumbar sensory level	Hyperintesity on T1 and T2 MRI, myelography, posterolat. fat on CT scan	Long-term high-dose steroid therapy (>4 months)
Chronic fluoride intoxication (Fisher et al. 1989)	Chronic	Radiculopathy, spastic paraparesis	Osteosclerosis sparing the skull (DD: Paget's disease)	High fluoride conc. (>3 mg/l) in drinking water
Brown tumor (Yokota et al. 1989)	Chronic	Back pain, paraparesis		Hyperparathyroidism
"Spinal coning" (Wong et al. 1992)	Acute to subacute (0.5–4 h)	Paraparesis, sensory level	MRI	Lumbar puncture in the presence of spinal block

tumors are frequently benign, such as schwannoma, meningioma, and, at the level of the cauda equina, myxopapillary ependymoma. Common intramedullary tumors include ependymoma and astrocytoma, with other lesions such as hemangioblastoma, oligodendroglioma, and metastatic disease being less common.

Although the specific location dictates the clinical syndrome, considerable overlap in presentation exists. Generally, the first symptom with vertebral and epidural tumors is pain (70%), initially radicular in nature, which may be present for days to weeks before other symptoms develop. Paraparesis, seen in 60% of patients, generally follows. Urinary retention and leg numbness are less common – 35% and 30% respectively. Spinal cord involvement is reported to occur in 5% of all cancer patients, with higher incidence in special types of cancer (Table 5).

The clinical features of intradural intra- or extramedullary tumors are often indistinguishable. Pain, though often seen, is generally less severe than with epidural involvement. Nocturnal pain is a symptom which is particularly indicative of neoplastic spinal involvement. Sensorimotor signs are more often asymmetrical with extramedullary lesions and are related to the location of spinal cord compression. Intramedullary tumors occasionally present with a syringomyelic syndrome of suspended sensory loss, segmental muscle atrophy, and long tract signs.

Persistent radicular symptoms, especially in the thoracic region, should prompt evaluation for neoplastic involvement by spinal MRI or myelography. Since spinal cord symptoms may acutely deteriorate following myelography, the possibility for neurosurgical intervention should be readily available. A reversal of symptoms after surgical decompression becomes unlikely when complete paraplegia or urinary retention lasts for more than 24 h. Meningeal carcinomatosis may produce paraparesis without an obvious spinal cord compression. Repeated CSF examination is diagnostic in 80–90%. The rare association of a spastic paraparesis or lower extremity monoparesis with intracranial meningioma in a parasagittal location should be recognized.

Other Causes and Rare Reasons

There are a number of other causes of para- and tetraplegia. The list includes motor neuron diseases (amyotrophic lateral sclerosis, familial spastic paraplegia), disturbances of neuromuscular transmission (myasthenia gravis, Lambert-Eaton syndrome, botulism), and metabolic derangements of the muscle (dyskalemic paralysis, mitochondrial myopathy). In addition, many rare causes of the syndrome have been reported (Table 6).

Suggested Reading

Aitken RJ, Wright JP, Bok A, Elliot MS (1986) Crohn's disease precipitating a spinal extradural abscess and paraplegia. Br J Surg 73:1004–1005

Bach F, Larsen BH, Rohde K, Borgesen SE, Gjerris F, Boge-Rasmussen T, Agerlin N, Rasmusson B, Stjernholm P, Sorensen PS (1990) Metastatic spinal cord compression. Occurrence, symptoms, clinical presentations and prognosis in 398 patients with spinal cord compression. Acta Neurochir (Wien) 107:37–43

Berlit P, Schwechheimer K (1987) Neuropathological findings in radiation myelopathy of the lumbosacral cord. Eur Neurol 27:29–34

Berlit P, Harle M, Johann A (1987) Cervical radiation myelopathy with spastic paraparesis of the arms. Case report and a review of the literature. Nervenarzt 58: 40–46

Boustany RM, Fleischnick E, Alper CA, Marazita ML, Spence MA, Martin JB, Kolodny EH (1987) The autosomal dominant form of "pure" familial spastic paraplegia: clinical findings and linkage analysis of a large pedigree. Neurology 37: 910–915

Britton CB, Mesa-Tejada R, Fenoglio CM, Hays AP, Garvey GG, Miller JR (1985) A new complication of AIDS: thoracic myelitis caused by herpes simplex virus. Neurology 35:1071–1074

Brosch T, Kolmel HW, Christe W (1990) Acute spinal ischemia in diseases of the aorta. Nervenarzt 61:231–234

Copeman MC (1988) Presenting symptoms of neoplastic spinal cord compression. J Surg Oncol 37:24–25

Dei-Anang K, Hase U, Schurmann K (1990) Epidural spinal abscesses. Neurosurg Rev ' 13:285–288 .

Femminineo AF, LaBan MM (1988) Paraparesis in a patient with Crohn disease resulting from septic arthritis of the hip and psoas abscess. Arch Phys Med Rehabil 69:223–225

Fischer PA, Enzensberger W (1987) Neurological complications in AIDS. J Neurol 234:269–279

Fisher RL, Medcalf TW, Henderson MC (1989) Endemic fluorosis with spinal cord compression. A case report and review. Arch Intern Med 149:697–700

Gandolfi A (1983) Vertebral histiocytosis-X causing spinal cord compression. Surg Neurol 19:369–372

Hamel E, Frowein RA, Karimi-Nejad A, Muller W (1984) Tumors of the cervical spine. Nervenarzt 55:285–292

Hands LJ, Collin J, Lamont P (1991) Observed incidence of paraplegia after infrarenal aortic aneurysm repair. Br J Surg 78:999–1000

Helseth A, Mork SJ (1989) Primary intraspinal neoplasms in Norway, 1955 to 1986. A

population-based survey of 467 patients. J Neurosurg 71:842–845

Kaoutzanis M, Anagnostopoulos D, Apostolou A (1989) Hydatid disease affecting the vertebrae. Acta Neurochir (Wien) 98: 60–65

Kaplan JG, Barasch E, Hirschfeld A, Ross L, Einberg K, Gordon M (1989) Spinal epidural lipomatosis: a serious complication of iatrogenic Cushing's syndrome. Neurology 39:1031–1034

Karray S, Zlitni M, Fowles JV, Zouari O, Slimane N, Kassab MT, Rosset P (1990) Vertebral hydatidosis and paraplegia. J Bone Joint Surg [Br] 72:84–88

Moore PM, Cupps TR (1983) Neurological complications of vasculitis. Ann Neurol 14: 155–167

Moula T, Fowles JV, Kassab MT, Sliman N (1981) Pott's paraplegia. A clinical review of operative and conservative treatment in 63 adults and children. Int Orthop 5:23–29

Riggle KP, Oddi MA (1989) Spinal cord necrosis and paraplegia as complications of the intra-aortic balloon. Crit Care Med 17: 475–476

Ringelstein EB, Krieger D, Hunermann B (1987) Evaluation by MRI of paraparesis and tetraparesis of undiagnosed aetiology. J Neurol 234:401–407

Roman GC (1988) The neuroepidemiology of tropical spastic paraparesis. Ann Neurol 23 [Suppl]:S113–S120

Roman GC, Roman LN (1988) Tropical spastic paraparesis. A clinical study of 50 patients from Tumaco (Colombia) and review of the worldwide features of the syndrome. J Neurol Sci 87:121–138

Ropper AH (1992) The Guillain-Barré syndrome. N Engl J Med 326:1130–1136

Simpson JF (1971) Listeria monocytogenes meningitis: an opportunistic infection. J Neurol Neurosurg Psychiatry 34:657–663

Steere AC (1989) Lyme disease. N Engl J Med 321:586–596

Waring WP, Karunas RS (1991) Acute spinal cord injuries and the incidence of clinically occurring thromboembolic disease. Paraplegia 29:8–16

Werner RA (1988) Paraplegia and quadriplegia after intrathecal chemotherapy. Arch Phys Med Rehabil 69:1054–1056

Wong MC, Krol G, Rosenblum MK (1992) Occult epidural chloroma complicated by acute paraplegia following lumbar puncture. Ann Neurol 31:110–112

Yokota N, Kuribayashi T, Nagamine M, Tanaka M, Matsukura S, Wakisaka S (1988) Paraplegia caused by brown tumor in primary hyperparathyroidism. Case report. J Neurosurg 71:446–448

Zull DN, Cydulka R (1988) Acute paraplegia: a presenting manifestation of aortic dissection. Am J Med 84:765–770

Chapter 29 | # Acute Muscular Weakness

Wolfgang Müllges, Klaus V. Toyka, and
Hans-Peter Hartung

Introduction

The differential diagnosis of diseases
presenting with muscle weakness is
broad. It includes disorders of the
motor neuron, of the neuromuscular
junction, and of muscle, and systemic
conditions affecting the motor system
diffusely, such as metabolic, toxic, and
endocrine disorders. Severe generalized muscle weakness once had a
poor prognosis due to respiratory impairment and pulmonary infections.
Today, modern intensive care has
greatly changed this dim prognosis.
Early recognition of potentially life-
threatening conditions and expectant
management are required to institute
effective therapy.

In this chapter we provide a diagnostic framework for approaching
patients with severe weakness. For a
more detailed description of individual
disorders, the reader is referred to the
appropriate specific chapter.

Weakness results from impairment of the strength of contraction
and power of movement. Loss of en-

durance, i.e., the ability to perform a
motor act repeatedly over a period of
time, may be an early manifestation of
weakness. Weakness manifests itself
not only by loss of power but also by
fatigability and variation in strength on
repeated effort.

Muscle strength should be examined immediately by assessing
sustained contractions such as head
and limb elevation time, grip strength,
loudness of voice, and swallowing, and
by measuring vital capacity and forced
expiration.

Selection of Patients with
Weakness for Intensive Care
Monitoring and Treatment

As outlined in Fig. 1, patients with
primary weakness should immediately
be evaluated as to organic or nonorganic causes of this symptom. *Nonorganic* weakness is almost invariably
dramatic. Early diagnosis will save expensive and potentially harmful medical intervention. Clues to identify
hysterical weakness are given in Table
1. Only if this diagnosis is not readily

Section Editor: Daniel F. Hanley

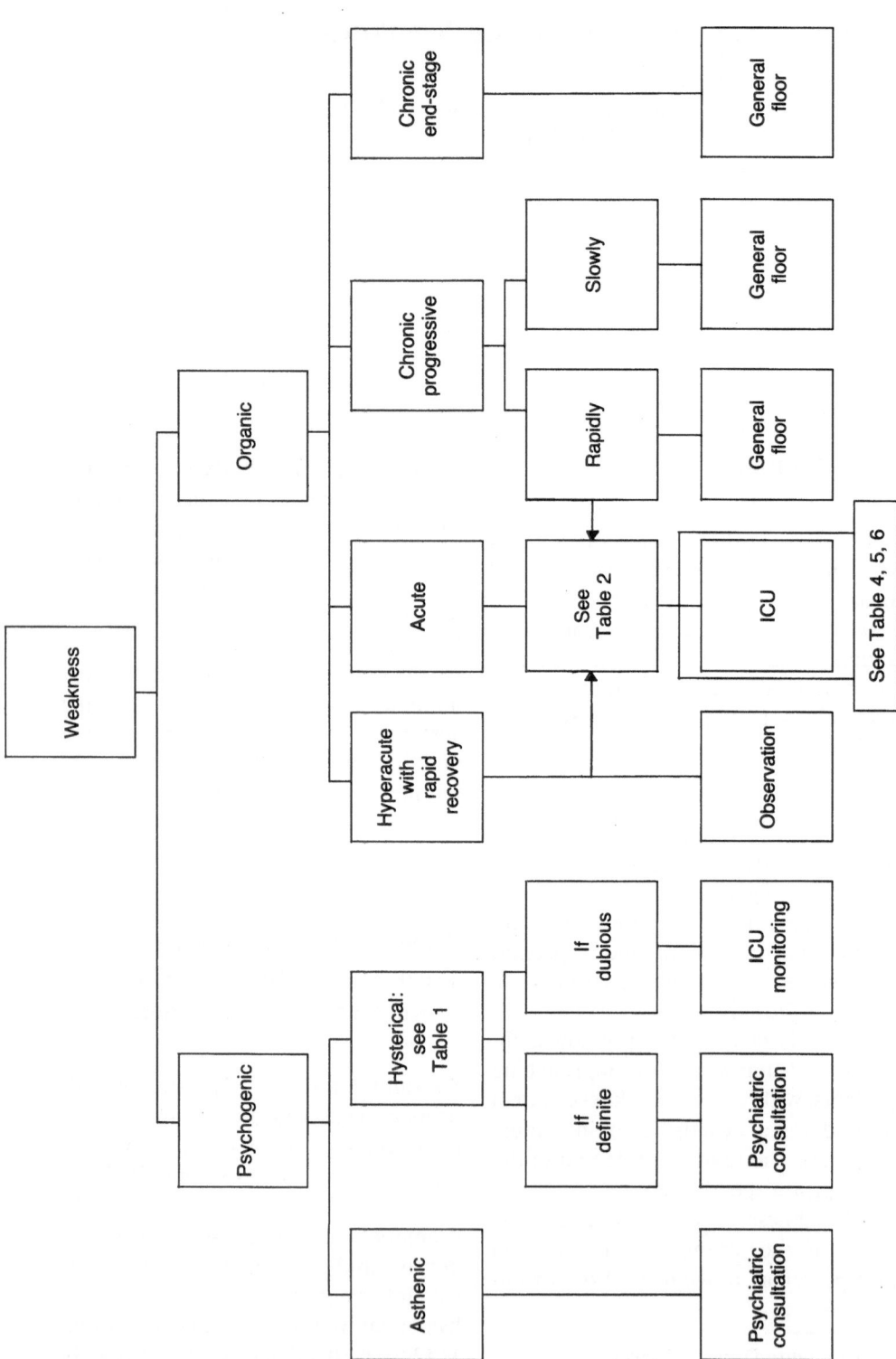

Fig. 1. Operational diagram for admission of patients with complaint of weakness to ICU

Table 1. Clues to diagnosing hysterical weakness (DSM III: 300.11, 300.81. ICD 9: 306)

History:
- Medically unexplained symptoms
- Multiple hospital emergency admissions without clear diagnosis
- Multiple surgical operations (e.g., von Münchhausen's syndrome)
- Previous episodes of severe unexplained weakness (except for dyskalemia and porphyria!)
- Abuse of psychotropic drugs
- (Self-) admittance directly to ICU with announcements fitting the patient's dramatic life-style

General examination:
- Sudden onset of paresis without signs of general disease, malaise, or pain (healthy-looking patient)
- Apparently dramatic weakness in an awake patient
- Normal cranial nerve function
- Anatomic pattern of involvement incompatible with organic disorders
- Normal or brisk reflexes with apparently flaccid weakness
- No impairment of breathing or swallowing with severe flaccid tetraparesis
- Rapid fluctuations of paresis without obvious cause
- Active resistance to examiner's movements[a]
- Absent or rapidly changing reaction to painful stimuli and tickling in an awake patient[a]
- General or sharply limited anesthesia; loss of hearing, smell, and vision[a]
- Small but jerky movements in the affected limbs
- Lack of rebound if resistance is suddenly withdrawn

Special testing:
- Hoover's sign: simultaneous and intermittent activation of agonists and antagonists[a]
- Babinski's trunk-thigh test: lack of involuntary leg raising when sitting up from recumbent position
- Apparent gaze palsy with normal optokinetic response[a]

Note that only a pattern of several abnormal findings proves nonorganic weakness. None of these exclude an underlying organic disorder.
[a] Signs with a high diagnostic value.

apparent should patients be monitored carefully because a superposition of nonorganic and organic weakness is possible. In patients with *organic* weakness classification according to the time in which muscle weakness evolves is most helpful for establishing the diagnosis and judging imminent deterioration.

Diseases with *sudden* loss of muscle tone and recovery within seconds to minutes are almost never due to primary neuromuscular dysfunction. In neuromuscular disorders weakness may develop rapidly over hours to days in a previously healthy person, or may run a chronic course with ultimate failure of mucle function. In *end-stage* dis-

orders such as amyotrophic lateral sclerosis or muscular dystrophy admission to the ICU is usually discouraged, but this remains a difficult ethical and medical decision in the individual case. End-stage disease is suggested by generalized muscle wasting, fasciculation, and cachexia and this should prompt a careful history of the patient's previous complaints. The primary care physician should be consulted before unnecessary intubation and supportive measures are undertaken. As long as the diagnosis is in doubt we do not withhold intensive care treatment (see Table 2).

Optional indications in *advanced chronic* disorders are the expressed

Table 2. Criteria for admission to the ICU

1. Acute crisis with respiratory failure:
   severe weakness of accessory respiratory
   muscles (shoulder girdle), orthopnea,
   cyanosis, oxygen saturation below 90%
   without oxygen breathing and after suction
2. [a] Inability to swallow, anarthria/dysarthria
3. Rapidly progressive weakness occurring in an
   observational environment, e.g., hospital
   ward
4. High-grade tetraparesis of unknown origin
5. Myoglobinuria

[a] May occur as a conversional symptom (cf.
Table 1; ICD 9: 306).

wish of the patient for long-term home ventilation where this is appropriate, and potentially reversible secondary disorders such as pneumonia. Apart from these, we usually do not admit terminally ill patients to the ICU since the patient's expected deterioration may prompt intubation by the staff, producing serious ethical conflicts. Admission should therefore be confined to the *rapidly progressive* disorders as defined in Table 2. Depending on the local setting, admittance to the ICU may be preferable to management in the emergency room since diagnosis and therapeutic procedures can be performed more rapidly. Some routine laboratory tests should be carried out immediately, while others should be ordered only when a specific diagnosis is being considered (Table 3).

General Considerations for ICU Management

In each case close monitoring is obligatory (Table 4). Patients are seriously endangered by respiratory failure due either to muscle weakness or to aspiration, both of which may arise within a few minutes. Delaying intubation in a progressively weak patient can result in serious complications. In our experience, small doses of fentanyl and haloperidol often suffice for quick and painless intubation that gives the patient sudden relief from respiratory distress. With local administration of an anesthetic ointment, intubation can be done even transnasally; this is often a prerequisite for the patient to tolerate the tube without sedation. If inability to swallow necessitates intubation, artificial ventilation with assisted-mode techniques is preferable. Cardiac and renal function should be carefully monitored. One should routinely check for signs of deep venous thrombosis and developing decubital ulcers. Having stabilized vital functions, one should then proceed with the differential diagnostic approach to the cause of weakness.

Differential Diagnostic Approach to Patients with Acute Tetraparesis

If a patient is admitted already intubated and sedated, a detailed neuromuscular examination is not possible, and the course of the examination will follow that carried out in patients with coma of undetermined cause. In more cooperative patients the level of motor system disturbance must be delineated. Severe generalized weakness may be accompanied by sensory symptoms or deficits, signs of CNS disturbance, and lower cranial nerve involvement. The rapidity of symptom evolution provides

Table 3. Laboratory tests

Immediately on admission
– blood pressure, body temperature, ECG
– blood-gas analysis
– hemoglobin
– urinary hemostix: if positive → RIA for myoglobin
– serum electrolytes
– muscle enzymes

Special laboratory tests
(maintain appropriate quantity of body fluids)
Blood:
– thyroid hormones (thyroid dysfunction may mimic or exacerbate other neuromuscular disease)
– liver function (alcoholic myopathy)
– autoantibodies (myasthenia gravis, Lambert-Eaton syndrome)
– toxic screen (see Table 9)
– calcium and phosphate; parathyroid hormone
Urine:
– porphyrins
CSF:
– inflammatory cells (transverse myelitis, infectious myelitis, poliomyelitis)
– protein elevation (AIDP, diphtheria, spinal trauma/tumor)
– IgG Index (myelitis)

Additional technical investigations
– Spinal cord disease:
  neuroimaging by myelography, MRI (if ventilation is stable), or CT
  magnetic and sensory evoked potentials
– Neuropathy:
  nerve conduction studies including F-waves[a],
  electromyography
  sural nerve biopsy
– Myopathy
  electromyography[a]
  (muscle biopsy)
– Neuromuscular junction disorder
  repetitive nerve stimulation

---

[a] If complete nerve conduction studies are not immediately available a short electrical stimulus by an electrophysiologic stimulator to the ulnar and peroneal nerves gives information about nerve and muscle excitability. Only in hypokalemia or magnesium intoxication is the response to electrical stimulation absent in all affected muscles early in the disease.

the most helpful clues for the final diagnosis (Fig. 2).

Tetraparesis with Sensory Signs

Patients with predominant motor disturbance often also have sensory findings. The paresis may be flaccid, with diminished reflexes, or spastic, with signs of upper motor neuron involvement. In acute *spinal cord* disease, pyramidal signs may be absent initially due to spinal shock (cf. Table 9). In spinal lesions sphincter disturbances are frequent, whereas they are uncommon in lower motor neuron disorders.

Table 4. General management of neuromuscular diseases in the ICU

1. Continuous monitoring
   Oxygen saturation (percutaneous measurement) give 2 l oxygen/min if below 95%
   ECG; if heart rate variability is abnormal consider pacemaker
2. Assessment of muscle strength
   Measurement of vital capacity
   Hand grip strength (dynamometer)
   Arm abduction time
   Head lifting time
   Loudness of voice
   Ability to swallow secretions
   Use of accessory muscles of ventilation
3. Management of inability to swallow
   Frequent suction (possibility of sudden death by bolus aspiration!)
   Head positioning to allow outflow of secretions
   Wendel or Guedel tube
4. Others
   Assessment of cardiac output (e.g., in myositis) and arrythmias (e.g., autonomic fiber
      involvement in GBS)
   Heparinization for prevention of deep venous thrombosis
   Measures against skin lesions and decubital ulcers
   In case of myoglobinuria:
      – monitor electrolytes frequently
      – initiate forced diuresis with monitoring of pulmonary arterial pressure (or at least central
        venous pressure)
      – consider dialysis
5. Indications for intubation and artificial ventilation
   Oxygen saturation below 90% (<85% if more chronic)
   Exhaustive respiratory work
   Forced vital capacity falling below 15 ml/kg
   Recurrent minor aspiration
6. Intubation technique
   In awake patients explain procedure.
   Do it quickly with minimal help of drugs (see p. 310).
   Avoid muscle relaxants.
   Transnasal approach preferred after local anesthetic spray
7. Artificial ventilation
   Use assisted ventilation with IMV mode.
   Low PEEP setting of 3 cm H_2O (except in pneumonia atelectasis)
   Use as few sedatives as possible to monitor neurologic findings
   Try to communicate verbally; check for dyspnea, pain, and anxiety.

Pyramidal tract lesions may evolve with or without pain. If *pain* is *present* (Table 5), trauma, other mechanical causes, or inflammation are likely. Concerning trauma, there may not always be an obvious history, e.g., in rheumatoid arthritis with dislocation of the odontoid process.

If *pain* is *absent* (Table 6) knowledge of the time course is of paramount importance: if weakness is hyperacute, vascular accidents are the most likely cause. The only exception to this general rule is necrotizing myelitis, which is a very rare condition. If supraspinal diseases are suspected ap-

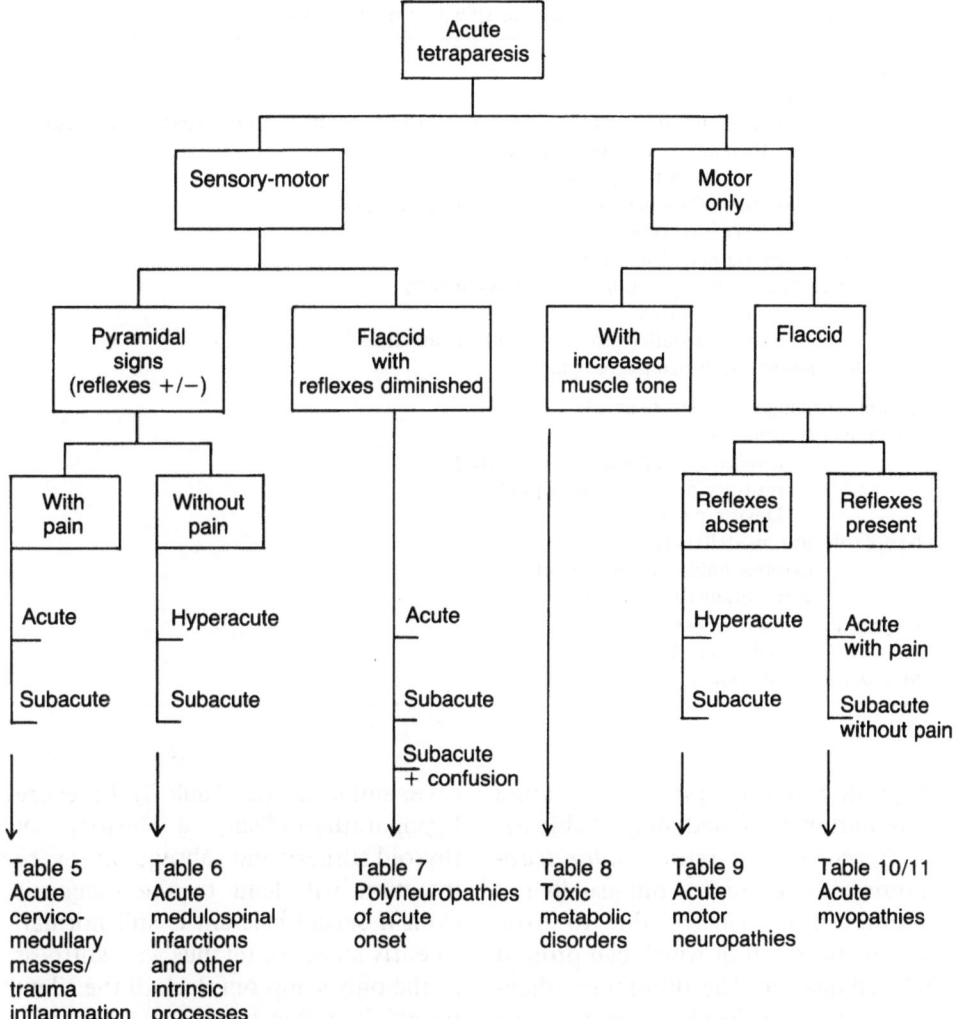

Fig. 2. Differential diagnostic approach to patients with severe acute tetraparesis rubricated according to general findings

Table 5. Differential diagnosis of spinal cord lesions with pain

Acute (evolving over minutes to hours)
- traumatic: spinal contusion, fracture with dislocation of the cervical spine
- mechanical: cervical disk protrusion, dislocation of the odontoid process with compression of C-1 and C-2 spinal cord segments

Subacute (evolving over hours to days)
- inflammatory: meningomyelitis, abscess

Table 6. Differential diagnosis of sensorimotor spinal cord lesions without pain

---

Hyperacute (evolving over minutes to hours)
  With cranial nerve involvement:
    – ischemic: bilateral infarction of the medullary pyramids due to vertebral artery occlusion or of
                their anterior spinal branches
                basilar artery thrombosis
                pseudobulbar palsy (history of multiple strokes)
  Without cranial nerve involvement:
    – ischemic: arterial spinal artery syndrome
    – hemorrhagic (warfarin or anticoagulant treatment!)
              hematomyelia
              intramedullary/epi- or subdural hemorrhage
    – inflammatory: necrotizing myelopathy

Subacute (evolving over hours to days)
  Inflammatory: poliomyelitis
                myelitis (granulomatous, post viral)
                postvaccinal (rabies, smallpox)
                Devic syndrome
  Neoplastic: intramedullary (glioma)
              extramedullary (meningioma)
              extradurally (metastasis)
  Degenerative: cervical spondylosis
               syringomyelia
  Metabolic: B_{12} deficiency

---

propriate diagnostic procedures should be undertaken immediately (Table 3).

Severe flaccid sensorimotor tetraparesis with diminished but usually not absent reflexes can be due to toxic neuropathies, all of which can prompt ICU admission. The differential diagnosis given in Table 7 focuses on the more common disorders, which may take a severe and rapid course. Often the CNS and other organs are also affected in these critically ill patients.

Tetraparesis Without Sensory Signs

Rarely, patients with severe tetraparesis of rapid onset have accompanying *stiffness* (increase in motor tone) as a major finding on neurological examination (cf. Table 8). In severe hypoparathyroidism, a history of thyroid surgery and subsequent severe infection will lead to the diagnosis even if serum calcium is still normal. In early stages of tetanus with stiffness as the only symptom, lack of the silent period in reflex testing is diagnostic. The black widow spider's venom initially causes cramps and spasms, which are followed by generalized paralysis for about 48 h.

If tetraparesis is *flaccid*, neuropathies, myopathies, or defects of neuromuscular transmission are likely. Electrodiagnosis is of great importance in differentiating these disorders rapidly. As a rule of thumb, weakness will be pronounced in the legs and distally in neuropathic diseases, while in myopathies weakness is most pro-

Table 7. Differential diagnosis of severe sensorimotor flaccid tetraparesis with diminished reflexes

Acute
   Diphtheria (rare; Landry-type palsy preceded by bulbar and accommodation disturbance 5–8
      weeks earlier; high CSF protein; cardiomyopathy)
   Porphyria (colicky pain; confusion; tachycardia; truncal dysesthesia)
   TOCP (endemic; preceded by a cholinergic phase 1–4 days earlier)
   GBS (see Table 9)

Subacute with confusion
   TOCP
   Heavy metals: lead, mercury, thallium, arsenic, lithium, gold
   Industrial: methyl-*n*-butyl-ketone, *n*-hexane, methyl-bromide, ethylene oxide, acrylamide,
      ethylene glycol (coolant)

Subacute without confusion
   Drug induced: amphetamine, chloramphenicol, clioquinol, dapsone, disulfiram, ethionamide,
      hydralazine, isoniazid, nitrofurantoin, phenytoin, vincristine, others
   Metabolic: beriberi (vitamin B_1 deficiency), pellagra, vitamin B_{12} deficiency
   Uremic

TOCP, triorthocresylphosphate; GBS, Guillain-Barré syndromé.

Table 8. Differential diagnosis of rapid-onset tetraparesis with increased muscle tone

Tetany (spasms never generalized)
Hypoparathyroid crisis (generalized spasms)
Tetanus (spasms triggered by unspecific external stimuli)
Hypothyroid crisis (slow DTRs; myoedema on percussion testing)
Addisonian crisis
Black widow spider bite (early)

minent in proximal muscles or in fastest-acting muscles. Furthermore, deep tendon reflexes are preserved.

If *deep tendon reflexes* (DTRs) are *absent* (cf. Table 9) and weakness evolved *hyperacutely*, hypokalemia is probable but spinal shock should still be considered. Hyperkalemic episodic paralyses are shorter in duration and only occasionally severe enough to necessitate artificial ventilation. Serum potassium is helpful in hypokalemia but less so in hyperkalemia to establish the diagnosis. With severe electrolyte dysfunction other systemic changes have to be looked at, such as endocrine dysregulation. More frequently, *subacute* flaccid tetraparesis with diminished or absent DTRs evolves in an ascending distribution and is related to the Guillain-Barré syndrome or other acute polyneuropathies which may be associated with minor sensory symptoms and signs (see Chap. 67). Facial diplegia and, less frequently, lower cranial nerve palsies may occur early in the course. Monitoring as described in Table 5 is important. Poliomyelitis, although now rare in industrial countries, may occasionally mimic GBS.

If *DTRs* are *preserved* this may be accompanied by *muscle pain*. Overt pain may indicate rhabdomyolysis, which is exceedingly important to look for because of impending renal failure and cardiac arrhythmias caused by secondary hyperkalemia and hypophosphatemia. Dark discoloration of the urine is seen only in very severe

Table 9. Differential diagnosis of rapid-onset flaccid tetraparesis with loss of deep tendon reflexes

Hyperacute
  Rule out spinal shock! (see Tables 5 and 6)
  Hypokalemic familial periodic paralysis (may be seemingly sporadic; appears overnight after
    heavy work or excessive meal)
  Severe hypokalemia: hyperinsulinism, hyperaldosteronism, hyperthyroidism, addisonian crisis,
    renal failure, chronic dialysis treatment, chronic ingestion of thiazides or laxatives, barium
  Hyperkalemic episodic paralysis (rare)

Subacute
  Global
    – Severe electrolyte imbalance (potassium, sodium, calcium, magnesium metabolism)
  Ascending
    – Guillain-Barrè syndrome with minor sensory involvement (high CSF protein; prolonged
      F-waves; nerve conduction block)
    – Paraneoplastic polyneuropathy
    – Polyneuritis associated with connective-tissue disease (lupus, panarteritis)
    – Poliomyelitis (preceding illness; CSF pleocytosis)

Table 10. Differential diagnosis of acute flaccid tetraparesis with deep tendon reflexes usually preserved and muscle pain/myoglobinuria

Drug induced/toxic: alcohol, amphotericin B, barbiturates, chloroquine, clofibrate, epsilon
  aminocaproic acid, fenfluramin, lovastatin, heroin, phenylcyclidine, cocaine, amphetamine,
  licorice, tetanus toxin, snake venoms
Infectious: influenza, *Legionella* pneumonia, pneumococcal pneumonia, severe sepsis
Malignant hyperthermia, malignant neuroleptic syndrome (high fever; rigidity; lethargy)
Fulminant poly-/dermatomyositis
Traumatic: crush injury, widespread surgical procedures; electric shock
Ischemic: proximal arterial occlusion
Postexertional: forced march, catatonic stupor, status epilepticus

cases. A positive test for hemoglobin in the absence of red blood cells suggests myoglobinuria until disproved otherwise. All conditions associated with myoglobinuria may produce acute illness with muscle pain, swelling of extremities, headache, vomiting, and even loss of consciousness. Most frequently, this is encountered in alcoholics at the height of a drinking bout, but a number of other underlying causes should be excluded (Table 10).

If *pain* is *absent*, myopathies or disorders of neuromuscular transmission are likely (Table 11). Elevation of the serum creatine kinase (CK) points to a myopathy. It is normal in myasthenic syndromes and myasthenia gravis, with the exception of a few toxic causes. Characteristically, in myopathies serum enzyme activities decrease in the following order: CK > aldolase > LDH > AST > ALT. Early EMG examination is important. If this reveals spontaneous activity, poly-/dermatomyositis is a likely cause. Endocrine myopathies are chronic disorders but may occasionally deteriorate rapidly, especially in a stress situation due to surgical intervention or severe infection.

Table 11. Differential diagnosis of painless acute flaccid tetraparesis with deep tendon reflexes usually preserved

---

Muscular:
  Poly-/dermatomyositis: idiopathic, associated with connective-tissue disease, paraneoplastic, drug induced (penicillamine)
  Infectious myositis: trichinosis (facial, bulbar, diaphragmal muscles severely affected; myocardium), Coxsackie B (arthralgia)
  Alcoholic myopathy
  Endocrine myopathies: thyroid, hyperinsulinism, aldosteronism, hyperparathyroidism

Neuromuscular transmission defects
  Myasthenia gravis (aquired autoimmune, rarely congenital)
  Myasthenic syndromes:
  – Lambert-Eaton syndrome (look for neoplasm)
  – Drug-induced[a]: aminoglycosides, some tetracyclines, neomycin, kanamycin, colistin, polymyxin, sulfonamides, phenytoin, carbamazepine, trimethadione, quinine, quinidine, all local anesthetics, verapamil, propanolol, all muscle relaxants[b], D-penicillamine[c], chloroquine, resochine, barbiturates, lithium, chlorpromazine, diazepam, opioids, cortisone, thyroid hormones, magnesium salts
  Botulism (accommodation paralysis; dry mouth)
  Inadvertent overdose of botulinum toxin for treatment of movement disorders
  Organophosphate poisoning (confusion; coma; mydriasis, red face, profuse diarrhea and sweating)

---

[a] Only in toxic doses or with underlying transmission disorder.
[b] In therapeutic doses.
[c] May cause a subtype of autoimmune myasthenia.

If the EMG does not reveal spontaneous activity a disturbance of neuromuscular transmission is probable and repetitive nerve stimulation and edrophonium testing are warranted. The most common of these disorders is myasthenia gravis. While myasthenia usually develops insidiously, severe infections or precipitation by drugs interfering with neuromuscular transmission may lead to a dramatic presentation.

Suggested Reading

American Psychiatric Association (1987) Diagnostic and statistical manual of mental disorders, 3rd edn. Washington DC, 300.18, 300.81

Cassem NH, Barsky AJ (1990) Functional somatic symptoms and somatoform disorders. In: Cassem NH (ed) Massachusetts General Hospital handbook of General Hospital psychiatry. Mosby, St Louis, pp 131–157

Haerer AF (1992) De Jong's The neurologic examination. Examination in cases of suspected hysteria and malingering, 5th edn. Lippincott, Philadelphia, pp 733–751

Koffler A, Friedler RM, Massry SG (1976) Acute renal failure due to non-traumatic rhabdomyolysis. Ann Intern Med 85:23–28

Koppel C (1989) Clinical features, pathogenesis, and management of drug-induced rhabdomyolysis. Med Toxicol Adverse Drug Exp 4:108–112

Landy HJ, Tucci KA (1992) Nonpenetrating spinal cord injury. In: Weiner WJ (ed) Urgent and emergent neurology. JB Lippincott, Philadelphia, pp 261–276

Layzer RB (1985) Neuromuscular manifestations of systemic disease. Davis, Philadelphia, pp 268–279

London SF, Ringel SP (1992) Neuromuscular emergencies. In: Weiner WJ (ed) Urgent and emergent neurology. Lippincott, Philadelphia, pp 59–78

Mandell GL, Douglas RG Jr, Bennett JE (eds) (1990) Principles and practice of infectious disease, 3rd edn. Churchill Livingstone, New York

May HL (ed) (1992) Emergency medicine. Little and Brown, Boston

Ringel SP, Carrol JE (1980) Respiratory complications of neuromuscular disease. In: Weiner WJ (ed) Respiratory dysfunction in neurologic disease. Futura, New York, pp 113–119

Sheehan MF, Sheehan DV (1992) Psychiatric diagnosis in neurological emergencies. In: Weiner WJ (ed) Urgent and emergent neurology. Lippincott, Philadelphia, pp 559–599

Further references for specific diagnoses are given in the specific chapters of this book.

Chapter 30

Brain-Stem Syndromes

DERK KRIEGER, MICHAEL S. PESSIN, and ANDREAS FERBERT

Introduction

No other region of the CNS compares with the brain stem in being as densely packed with vital structures. Crowded into the small space of the brain stem are the nuclear groups and nerve fibers of the cranial nerves, sensory tracts ascending from the spinal cord of cochlea to the thalamus and cortex, and the motor pathways descending from the cortex and the subcortical nuclei to the brain stem and spinal cord. In addition, the brain stem contains the reticular formation, with autonomic centers that control respiration, blood pressure, and gastrointestinal functions, as well as centers that mediate arousal and wakefulness. Finally, the brain stem is surrounded by a narrow passage for the circulation of cerebrospinal fluid. For both clinical and therapeutic purposes it is critical to determine whether a lesion lies within or outside the brain stem. Thus, depending on the acuteness of the disease process, brain-stem syndromes require immediate neurological eval-

uation. Acute lesions within the brain stem frequently cause coma, either by directly invading and destroying the central core of the brain stem or by impairing its blood supply with subsequent ischemia, necrosis, or hemorrhage. The most common pathologic process that causes primary destruction of the brain stem is cerebrovascular occlusive disease; however, hemorrhage, demyelinating disorders, and encephalitis may produce similar effects. Acute posterior fossa lesions lying adjacent to but outside the brain stem likewise cause brain-stem disturbance in three different ways: (a) direct exertion of pressure on the tegmentum of the pons and midbrain, (b) upward herniation of the superior vermis of the cerebellum through the tentorial notch and, (c) downward herniation of the cerebellar tonsils through the foramen magnum.

Since a comprehensive review of all brain-stem syndromes would be far beyond the scope of this chapter, we focus on circumstances that are predominantly relevant to neurocritical care. The etiology of brain-stem syndromes is judged by accompanying features, such as known underlying

Section Editor: Daniel F. Hanley

diseases or results of laboratory tests during further evaluation. Treatment considerations depend on establishing a diagnosis, which in turn dictates the urgency and specificity of therapeutic measures for conditions as diverse as acute vascular occlusive disease, cerebellar mass lesions, Wernicke's disease, or central pontine myelinolysis. Atypical conditions, such as brain-stem encephalitis, are often diagnosed only on retrospective grounds or by exclusion and generally require symptomatic rather than immediate specific treatment. However, in all patients with presumed brain-stem encephalitis, CSF examination should rule out bacterial causes, in particular *Listeria monocytogenes*, requiring immediate antibiotic coverage.

Clinical Signs and Symptoms

Intrinsic Lesions of the Brain Stem

Patients with acute intrinsic lesions of the brain stem often present with unconsciousness; however, medullary lesions as well as anterior pontine lesions may spare consciousness. The most common cause for acute intrinsic brain-stem lesions is vertebrobasilar occlusive disease.

Intracranial Vertebral Occlusive Disease. Occlusive disease of the intracranial vertebral artery is associated with several clinical pictures depending on the individual anatomy of the vertebrobasilar system. Wallenberg's syndrome (lateral medullary infarction) is somewhat variable but usually involves a wedge of the lateral medulla containing a portion of the olive ventrally and

a section of the corpus restiforme dorsally. It may also be accompanied by cerebellar infarction. The clinical symptoms are explained by the distinctive anatomy of the lesion. Vertigo or more indecisive dizziness is the leading symptom, often in combination with moderate to severe posterior headache. Facial pain and reduced ipsilateral sensation is related to involvement of the descending spinal tract of the 5th cranial nerve; occipital pain radiating to the neck reflects the acute vascular distension and collateral blood flow produced by the acute vertebral occlusion. Intensive posterior neck pain associated with clinical symptoms and signs of brain-stem ischemia is often seen in vertebral dissection. Alteration of vision is another common complaint and may be described as diplopia or sometimes as the illusion of oscillating objects. In rare cases even upside-down vision has been described. The usual symptoms probably reflect skew deviation and nystagmus due to the sudden alterations in the vestibulo-ocular system. Nausea and vomiting are also due to acute vestibular dysfunction or to involvement of the dorsal tegmentùm in the floor of the 4th ventricle. Ataxia is another important feature; almost all patients with lateral medullary infarcts have difficulty in walking with veering to the side, leaning, or stumbling. In addition, many patients describe ipsilateral limb clumsiness. Hiccups are frequent and can be very annoying, interfering with food intake and respiration. The origin is uncertain, but it is most likely related to involvement of the 10th nerve fibers or disintegration of the respiratory controls. Patients often have difficulties swallowing. Food or secretions may penetrate into the air passages producing aspiration. Hoarseness is also common but may be absent in the ventral or more superficial lesions. Some patients mention numbness, burning, or painful sensations in the contralateral limbs or trunk caused by alteration of the spinothalamic tract. The principal clinical signs accompanying lateral medullary infarction include (a) diminished sensation in the ipsilateral face, (b) diminished pain and temperature sensation on the contralateral body, (c) ipsilateral Horner syndrome, (d) gait ataxia and ipsilateral limb ataxia, (e) horizontal or frequently rotatory nystagmus toward the side of the lesion, (f) paralysis of the ipsilateral vocal cord and weakness of the ipsilateral palate, and (g) slight ipsilateral facial weakness.

In some instances ischemia extends beyond the lateral medullary territory and also affects the inferior lateral pons or the medial medulla, thus explaining associated pyramidal tract involvement and additional signs of the 5th, 6th, and 7th cranial nerves. The resulting hemiparesis is usually crossed, that is, contralateral to the infarct and on the same side of the body as the limb pain and temperature loss. In other instances bilateral symptoms and signs occur from bilateral vertebral occlusions. Depending on the collateralization, dislodgement of embolic material, and thrombus propagation into the caudal and mid-basilar, the clinical syndrome becomes indistinguishable from basilar artery occlusion.

Occlusion of the Mid-basilar Artery (for review see Kubic and Adams 1946; Ferbert et al. 1990). The onset is frequently sudden with partial or progressively severe brain-stem signs, but it can also begin with transient symp-

toms. Particularily in embolic basilar occlusions, a severe brain-stem disturbance may be preceded by bilateral or even unilateral transient symptoms reflecting temporal occlusions at different sites of the vertebrobasilar vasculature caused by the migrating clot. Premonitoring symptoms (TIAs) are common, as in internal carotid occlusive disease, and reflect perfusion insufficiency due to the occlusive disease. The first symptoms are often headache, difficulty in speaking, dizziness, confusion, or coma. The core clinical findings are usually pupillary abnormalities, disorders of ocular movement, facial palsy, and hemiplegia (or quadriplegia) with bilateral extensor plantar reflexes. There is no unifying clinical syndrome and, depending on the extent of the brain-stem ischemia, the following clinical phenomena are often recognized: (a) Internuclear ophthalmoplegia (INO) involves paralysis of the adducting eye during voluntary horizontal gaze in combination with a nystagmus of the abducting eye. Adduction may be preserved during convergence and on labyrinthine stimulation. In MRI studies of patients with INO medial tegmental lesions involve the ipsilateral medial longitudinal fasciculus. Vertical nystagmus and skew deviation are frequent concomitant findings. (b) Conjugate horizontal gaze palsies involve lesions of the fibers from the frontal eye fields crossing near the level of the abducens nucleus. This region is usually referred to as the paramedian pontine reticular formation (PPRF). Lesions which include the abducens nucleus probably produce an ipsilateral voluntary gaze palsy including caloric or vestibulo-ocular reflexes. If the 6th nerve nucleus is spared, reflex movements of the ipsilateral eye are preserved. Bilateral lesions of the pontine tegmentum involving the abducens nucleus and the PPRF produce paralysis of all horizontal eye movements, sparing vertical gaze, since this is mediated at a further rostral level. A unilateral pontine lesion involving the PPRF and the MLF causes the combination of INO and horizontal gaze palsy, referred to as the one-and-a-half syndrome. These patients move only a single eye in abduction to one side, thus lacking one and one half of the components of normal horizontal gaze. (c) Ocular bobbing (see Fisher 1964) refers to unusual eye movements where both eyeballs intermittently dip briskly downward and then return to the primary position. Depending on the actual extent of the pontine lesion, ocular bobbing can be unilateral and exaggerated by labyrinthine stimulation. The proposed mechanism of this abnormality relates the bobbing to roving eye movements in patients with coma due to widespread bilateral supratentorial lesions. In pontine lesions, since horizontal gaze is lost and vertical gaze preserved, the vertical vector of gaze is accentuated so that the eyes bob down. Ocular bobbing usually indicates severe intrinsic pontine dysfunction, but can also be seen with extrinsic and toxic or metabolic dysfunction. (d) Ptosis in pontine lesions is attributed to involvement of descending sympathetic fibers in the lateral pontine tegmentum. It can be modified by concomitant involvement of the 7th nerve nucleus or hemiplegia. (e) Pontine pupils are frequently pinpoint and must be distinguished from morphine-induced miotic pupils. In pure pontine lesions, light reactions are preserved; however, with co-

existing midbrain lesions they may be poorly reactive. Since pupillary constriction is more severe with pontine infarction than with peripheral Horner syndrome, it has been postulated that the lesion involves both parasympathetic irritation and sympathetic destruction of the central autonomic pathways. (f) Nystagmus is a frequent finding without clear-cut localizing value, since it is dependent upon the site of lesion and the degree of paresis of eye movements. (g) Skew deviation is of diagnostic localizing value in combination with INO, but in isolation it can be found with a wide spectrum of lesions in the region of the vestibular nuclei, brachium pontis, cerebellum, and rostral midbrain. (h) Palatal myoclonus is a rhythmic involuntary jerking movement of the soft palate and pharyngopalatine arch, often involving the diaphragm and laryngeal muscles. It appears some time after the acute brain-stem process and is thought to be generated by a lesion involving the triangle of Mollaret, which refers to a circuit between the ipsilateral nucleus dentatus of the cerebellum and the contralateral inferior olive of the medulla and the red nucleus of the midbrain. (i) Coma is often encountered in patients with bilateral pontine destruction; however, it has to be carefully distinguished from "locked-in" states that may mimic coma and are found with extensive lesions of the pontine base. Usually, but not always, the "locked-in" patient can communicate by way of vertical eye movements or blinking and can demonstrate full comprehension of his situation and environment. Because of the importance of distinguishing "locked-in" states from diminished consciousness in patients with pontine infarction, we recommend bedside evaluation of evoked potentials to gain further information on the disintegration of brain-stem function in these patients. (j) Paresis almost always accompanies acute basilar occlusion. Due to variations in the extent of ischemia, different degrees of quadriplegia are often observed. Initial motor weakness may even be quite lateralized ("herald hemiparesis" of basilar occlusion), initially confusing the diagnosis before bilateral signs emerge. (k) Respiratory abnormalities are frequent but difficult to characterize because of the extent of the brain-stem ischemia and interfering general medical factors, such as aspiration and neurogenic pulmonary edema. The traditional clinicoanatomic concept derived from idealized cross sections at different levels of the brain stem that defined discrete inspiratory and expiratory centers has to be questioned, based on recent findings (see Chap. 34, Autonomic Instability). (l) Ataxia of the limbs is common but frequently hidden by weakness. (m) Dysarthria, dysphagia, and uncontrolled laughing and crying (tearing) probably reflect pseudobulbar paralysis, apparent to some degree in most patients. Sensory findings are quite variable and difficult to assess, due to stupor or altered communication.

Top-of-the Basilar Syndrome (for review see Caplan 1980). Occlusive lesions of the rostral tip of the basilar artery (usually embolic in origin) lead to variable bilateral infarction of midbrain, thalamic, and occipital and medial temporal lobe structures. The clinical picture is somewhat variable, but the following major clinical syndromes are frequently observed: (a) Pupillary reactivity is usually abnormal, because the afferent limb of the pupillary reflex arc is interrupted in the vicinity of the Edinger-Westphal nucleus. If the Edinger-Westphal nucleus is affected, pupils are generally fixed and dilated. However, if additional rostral lesions alter the descending sympathetic pathways, the deficit includes a midposition, fixed pupil. Thalamic involvement results in small, poorly reactive pupils. (b) Ocular convergence abnormalities arise probably within the medial midbrain. Rostral brain-stem lesions may cause convergence nystagmus, convergence movements during voluntary horizontal gaze (pseudo sixth), and lid retraction (Collier's sign). (c) Voluntary vertical gaze impairment is generated by simultaneous bilateral activation of the frontal and parietal occipital conjugate "gaze centers". The descending pathways converge on the periaqueductal region near the interstitial nucleus of Cajal and the posterior commissure. Clinically, a clear disparity between voluntary upgaze and well-preserved reflex-induced vertical eye movements (Bell's phenomenon, doll's eyes maneuver) suggest a central vertical gaze paresis, although the anatomic basis for the disparity is not established. Most commonly, up- and downgaze palsies occur together, although lesions of the pretectum in the vicinity of the posterior commissure produce isolated upward-gaze paralysis (Parinaud syndrome). Selective paralysis of downward gaze is rare, and lesions have been found to be more caudal and ventral in the vicinity of the red nucleus. (d) Abnormal sleeping patterns in combination with 3rd nerve palsies have been described following infarcts in the territory of the paramedian mesencephalic artery and following survival from transtentorial herniation syndromes. Vivid visual hallucinations have been attributed to rostral brain-stem lesions from infarcts and Wernicke's encephalopathy. Similar hallucinations may occur in sleep-deprived individuals and in drug intoxication and are most likely related to dysfunction of the reticular activating system. Confabulations may occur, possibly due to the anatomic relationship to neuronal circuits related to memory function. (e) Behavioral abnormalities in bilateral thalamic ischemia include general cognitive abnormalities, such as lack of initiation and spontaneity, also referred to as abulia. Clinically, they can be indistinguishable from frontal lobe disease and thus probably indicate broad loss of function of corticothalamic projections from the anterior thalamus. Disorientation and severe amnestic syndromes are often associated with hypersomnolence in these patients. (f) Cortical blindness may accompany top-of-the-basilar occlusions in patients with extended bilateral infarcts in the posterior cerebral artery distribution.

Pontine Hemorrhage. Hemorrhage into the pons, usually due to chronic hypertension, arises from the paramedian arterioles, begins at the base of the tegmentum, and variably dissects in all directions in a symmetrical fashion. It is usually restricted to the pons, but in some instances rupture into the 4th ventricle occurs. The clinical signs accompanying large medial pontine hematomas are coma, quadriparesis, often with limb stiffness and rigidity, absent horizontal eye movements, pontine pupils, and respiratory rhythm abnormalities. Headache and vomiting occasionally occur in the premonitory phase. Usually the onset of clinical

signs is rapid; however, some pontine hemorrhages develop gradually, and early findings may be asymmetrical. Thus deafness, dysarthria, facial numbness, and dizziness may sometimes precede the onset of coma. Since the hemorrhage can be confined to the basis pontis, "locked-in" states may occur. Vertical reflex eye movements are usually present, and some patients demonstrate ocular bobbing. Nearly all patients with pontine hemorrhages who survive more than a few hours develop body temperatures above 40°C, not attributable to infectious complications. Hemorrhages confined to rupture of the short lateral circumferential arteries or posterior penetrators may result in lateral tegmental hemorrhages and carry a better prognosis. Depending on the clinical status of the patient and the CT or MRI appearance of the hemorrhage, the diagnostic workup should include angiography to rule out AV malformations.

Basilar Migraine (for review Bickerstaff 1961; Fisher 1979; Caplan 1991). Altered states of consciousness in combination with symptoms attributed to the posterior circulation impairment, including blurred vision, vertigo, dysarthria and numbness, and tingling of the limbs and face may be attributed to migraine attacks in some patients. In many instances, but not all, symptoms clear with the onset of headache. Current data suggest that this syndrome has a female predominance and is almost always correlated with a family history of migraine. Basilar migraine deficits are sometimes indistinguishable from brain-stem ischemia due to occlusive vertebrobasilar disease. However, in migraine, deficits develop over a period of time and are most often preceded by scintillations or brightness that gradually spread within the visual sphere. These "positive" symptoms are followed by defective "negative" phenomena that also spread and clear subsequently. Depending on the timing of angiography, vasoconstriction of the basilar artery may be seen.

Central Pontine Myelinolysis. Central pontine myelinosis (CPM) has to be considered whenever a patient gravely ill with a general medical disease develops quadriplegia, pseudobulbar palsy, and progressive mental dullness over a period of several days. The name describes the locus and essential features of the pathological process. CPM occurs sporadically, with no hint of genetic disposition. The outstanding clinical characteristic of CPM is its invariable association with some other serious, often life-threatening disease. In many cases CPM appears in the late stages of chronic alcoholism, often in association with Wernicke's disease and polyneuropathy. Other medical conditions and diseases associated with CPM are chronic renal or hepatic failure, advanced neoplastic disease, dehydration, and electrolyte disturbances (particularily in burn victims). In the majority of cases of CPM seen at autopsy, there were no signs related to a pontine lesion, presumably because lesions can be small, located in the median raphe, and involve only a few corticopontine fibers. In other cases CPM is obscured by coma from a metabolic or other associated condition. In rare cases CPM can be recognized on clinical grounds.

Wernicke's Disease. Wernicke's disease (WD) is described by the triad of clinical features including ophthalmoplegia, ataxia, and mental disturbance or decreased consciousness. Often the disease begins with ataxia, followed by mental confusion over a period of days or even weeks. WD has to be considered in the presence of the following ocular signs: (a) vertical and horizontal nystagmus, (b) weakness or paralysis of the external rectus muscles, and (c) weakness or paralysis of the conjugate gaze. Pupils are usually spared but may become miotic or nonreacting in advanced states. The ataxia involves primarily the stance and gait and is therefore more likely to be brought out by heel-to-knee than by finger-to-nose testing. Mental disturbances include hallucination, confusion, and agitation, or progressive states of decreased consciousness. Patients who die of WD demonstrate symmetrical lesions in the paraventricular regions of the thalamus and hypothalamus, in the mammillary bodies, in the periaqueductal gray, in the floor of the 4th ventricle and in the superior vermis. Clinical-pathologic correlation indicates that the ocular muscle and gaze palsies are attributable to lesions of the 6th and 3rd nerve nuclei and adjacent tegmentum, and the nystagmus to lesions in the regions of the vestibular nuclei. The lack of significant destruction of nerve cells in these lesions accounts for the rapid recovery after initiation of the appropriate therapy.

Extrinsic Lesions of the Brain Stem
(for review see Sypert and Alvord 1975; Heros 1982; Amarenco 1991; Rieke et al. 1993)

Extrinsic brain-stem lesions produce their effects via compression of the brain stem or aqueduct of Sylvius. Large basilar artery aneurysms may compress the basis pontis or cerebral peduncles, cause obstructive hydrocephalus, or present as a cerebellopontine angle mass. Also, benign or malignant tumors within the posterior fossa may compromise brain-stem function. In general, these conditions only rarely present as neurologic emergencies. More commonly, *acute cerebellar vascular events* lead to subacute brain-stem compression and subsequent obstructive hydrocephalus. Often cerebellar vascular conditions, either infarction or hemorrhage, present with clinical symptoms, sometimes misdiagnosed as labyrinthine or peripheral vestibular disease. Small lateral cerebellar hemorrhages and infarcts present with unilateral clumsiness and limb and gait ataxia. Since most cerebellar infarcts are caused by vertebral artery occlusions, about one fifth of the cases present with signs of lateral medullary dysfunction. The most common symptom at onset is an inability to stand or walk or a sudden fall. Headache, vomiting, dizziness, and dysarthria are also common features. In general, there is a period of 6–12 h of stability; however, in some cases there is progressive neurologic deterioration within a time period varying between a few hours to several days. Uncommonly, there have been subacute courses simulating posterior fossa tumors with days or weeks of headache and dizziness followed by gradual onset of ataxia and clouding of consciousness.

The pathophysiology of acute cerebellar mass lesions is currently not well understood. Pupils are usually small but reactive, and the pupil ipsilateral to the cerebellar lesion may be smaller. The crucial diagnostic findings involve the oculomotor system. The eyes may be conjugately deviated to the contralateral side, with course

nystagmus or a gaze paresis to the side of the infarct. The gaze paresis is often dysconjugate, with more severe weakness of the abducting eye (6th nerve palsy). This phenomenon can be explained by ascent of the vermis toward the transtentorial notch. Large infarcts often cause drowsiness, confusion, and decreased spontaneity of activity and verbal communication. The head can be tilted toward the lesion and patients frequently resist head movements. Depending on the amount of dorsofrontal shift, the brain stem can be distorted, usually leading to bilateral hyper-reflexia and extensor plantar responses. Sometimes nerve structures within the cerebellopontine angle are compressed by swollen cerebellar tissue, giving rise to a reduced corneal reflex (5th nerve) and an ipsilateral facial nerve paralysis (7th nerve). Due to the acuteness of the pathologic process, papilledema is only rarely present. A relatively small proportion of large cerebellar infarcts (more than a third of a cerebellar hemisphere) produce progressive deterioration. Once significant swelling has developed, the process becomes self-perpetuating. Compression of the rostral orifice of the 4th ventricle causes obstructive hydrocephalus. Cerebellar tonsils are forced into the foramen magnum and the lower brain-stem tegmentum is compressed directly. The clinical picture becomes indistinguishable from that of acute intrinsic brain-stem lesions caused by basilar artery occlusion. Additionally, ascending vermal tissue herniates through the tentorial notch, thus leading to midbrain compression with oculomotor nucleus destruction, responsible for the ipsilateral pupillary dilatation in the later stages of the disease.

Conditions Mimicking Brain-Stem Syndromes

Miller-Fisher Syndrome. (for review see Ropper et al. 1991) The essentials of this syndrome, originally described by Fisher in 1956, include areflexia with ophthalmoplegia and ataxia. Approximately two thirds of the patients have diplopia as the presenting symptom; the remainder are divided between ataxia first and both symptoms appearing simultaneously. Some patients complain of dizziness, but only rarely does vertigo or vomiting precede the acute disease. Ataxia is usually noticed as a gait disorder rather than as limb clumsiness. The syndrome is now widely accepted as a variant of Guillain-Barré syndrome, thus explaining a number of diverse signs now viewed as Miller-Fisher syndrome variants. The controversy over the pathologic site of the Miller-Fisher syndrome, whether the brain stem or a combined central and peripheral pathology, remains unsettled. The central nervous system proposition is appealing because of the truly cerebellar appearance of ataxia and the eye signs. Supranuclear eye signs include an internuclear ophthalmoplegia, conjugate recovery of vertical before horizontal eye movements, Parinaud's syndrome, Bell's phenomenon despite voluntary paralysis of upgaze, ptosis in the presence of severe ophthalmoplegia, dissociated horizontal nystagmus suggesting an internuclear ophthalmoplegia, upper lid jerks, rebound nystagmus, abnormal vertical vestibulo-ocular responses, and convergence spasm. However, each of these signs can be mimicked by myasthenia gravis and thus the origin of these signs may be misinterpreted because of the greater frequency of central disorders with ocular manifestations in clinical practice.

Guillain-Barré Syndrome Variants. Initial symptoms are proximal arm weakness and difficulty in swallowing, almost always with ptosis and usually with incomplete ocular paresis. The reflexes are diminished and eventually lost in the arms and may be diminished in the legs, but leg power is unaltered and patients usually can walk. Most patients require tracheostomy because of the duration of the oropharyngeal paralysis. A few individuals may present with blurred vision from accommodation paralysis, thus closely imitating botulism, making it advisable to administer botulism antitoxin if the diagnosis is not clear.

Myasthenia Gravis. Ocular palsies can present more or less exclusively as diplopia, ptosis, or strabismus, sometimes in association with exophthalmus but rarely with pupillary change. As a rule, primary diseases of muscle do not involve the pupil, and in most instances their involvement is bilateral. The differential diagnosis has to include exophthalmic ophthalmoplegia of thyroid disease.

Intoxication. Botulism is a rare form of food-borne illness, caused by the exotoxin of *Clostridium boltulinum*. Outbreaks are due more often to home-preserved than to commercially canned products, and vegetables are implicated in most instances. Symptoms usually appear within 12–36 h following ingestion and include blurred vision and diplopia as the initial neurologic features. In many cases of botulism the pupils are dilated and unreactive.

Other symptoms of bulbar involvement follow in quick succession, including vertigo, deafness, nasality or hoarseness of the voice, dysarthria, and dysphagia. Diphtheria, an acute infectious disease caused by *Corynebacterium diphtheriae*, can also mimic acute brain-stem disease. It usually begins locally, with palatal paralysis between the 5th and 12th days of illness. In addition other cranial nerves (5th, 17th, 10th, and 12th) can be affected. Ciliary paralysis with loss of accommodation and blurring of vision is the main clinical sign that distinguishes diphtheria from intrinsic brain-stem disease.

Other Conditions. Acute hypoglycemia or global hypoxia may resemble clinical syndromes found in acute vascular accidents of the posterior circulation. Decreased levels of consciousness associated with focal neurologic deficits have been decribed in acute hypoglycemia following inadequate doses of insulin. Coma and midbrain signs, such as dilated pupils with only mild degrees of quadriparesis, resembling top-of-the-basilar occlusion, are sometimes encountered after cardiac arrest. Similar syndromes are sometimes encountered in hospitalized patients who have received repetitive high doses of narcotics or sedatives for various reasons. In particular, if there is no conclusive history available, metabolic derangements, cumulative effects of sedative drugs or narcotics, and global hypoxic states have to be considered.

Suggested Reading

Amarenco P (1991) The spectrum of cerebellar infarctions. Neurology 41:973–979

Bickerstaff E (1961) Basilar artery migraine. Lancet 1:15

Caplan LR (1980) "Top of the basilar" syndrome: selected clinical aspects. Neurology 30:72

Caplan LR (1991) Migraine and vertebrobasilar ischemia. Neurology 41:55

Ferbert A, Brückmann H, Drummen R (1990) Clinical features of proven basilar artery occlusion. Stroke 21:1135–1142

Fisher CM (1964) Ocular bobbing. Arch Neurol 11:543–545

Fisher CM (1979) Transient migrainous accompaniments of late onset. Stroke 10:96

Heros RC (1982) Cerebellar hemorrhage and infarction. Stroke 13:106–110

Kubic CS, Adams RD (1946) Occlusion of the basilar artery. A clinical and pathological study. Brain 69:73–121

Rieke K, Krieger D, Adams H-P, Aschoff A, Meyding-Lamadé U, Hacke W (1993) Management of acute cerebellar stroke. Cerebrovasc Dis 3:45–55

Ropper AH, Wijdicks EFM, Truax BT (1991) Guillain-Barré syndrome. Davies, Philadelphia

Sypert GW, Alvord EC (1975) Cerebellar inarction: a clinicopathological study. Arch Neurol 32:357–363

Chapter 31

Ocular Motor Disturbances

Marianne Dieterich and Ronald J. Tusa

Introduction

In this chapter the characteristics of spontaneous and evoked eye movements in severely ill patients are described. Eye movements provide valuable information on lesion location and on the grade and prognosis of coma. While voluntary eye movements such as saccades, smooth pursuit, vergence, and optokinetic nystagmus (OKN) can be examined in the cooperative patient, spontaneous eye position and movement and the vestibulo-ocular reflex (VOR) can be evaluated only in patients with stupor and coma. The following sections provide a guideline for the differentiation and assessment of various eye movement disorders in both alert and comatose patients.

Pathophysiology of Ocular Motor Subsystems

In order to move the eyes conjugately in the orbits, three pairs of eye muscles

are employed on three major planes; the horizontal, vertical, and torsional or roll plane. These planes correspond to those of the three semicircular canals of the vestibular end organs. Several different ocular motor subsystems exist. Saccades act by bringing images of the seen world to the fovea. Smooth pursuit, OKN, VOR, and vergence eye movements function to stabilize visual images on the retina.

Saccades and Quick Phases of Nystagmus

Saccades and quick phases of nystagmus are conjugate rapid eye movements. Saccades have peak velocities as high as 500–700°/s and are used to redirect the line of sight. Quick phases have peak velocities up to 500°/s and reset the position of the eyes during vestibular and optokinetic nystagmus. Horizontal saccades and quick phases are generated by burst cells in the parapontine reticular formation (PPRF), which project to the sixth nerve nucleus. Vertical saccades and quick phases are generated by burst cells in the rostral interstitial nucleus

Section Editor: Daniel F. Hanley

of the medial longitudinal fasciculus (RiMLF) in the midbrain, which project to the third and fourth nerve nuclei. The PPRF and RiMLF receive input from the superior colliculus, a structure crucial for converting the motor error signal for saccades and quick phases into a temporal signal that can be used by the burst cells. The trigger for quick phases of nystagmus during VOR and OKN probably comes from the secondary neurons within the vestibular nucleus.

Disorders of saccades and quick phases consist of abnormalities of initiation, accuracy, and velocity. Spontaneous and quick phases of nystagmus can still be initiated following unilateral ablation of cerebral cortex and basal ganglia (hemispherectomy), whereas volitional (visual and goal-guided) gaze cannot be initiated contralateral to the side of the lesion for several weeks. Dysmetria (hypermetria and hypometria) occurs primarily following lesions involving the cerebellar vermis, fastigial nucleus, or cerebellar peduncles. Slow saccades and quick phases are due to a decreased number of functioning burst cells in the PPRF and RiMLF.

Smooth Pursuit

Smooth pursuit eye movements are voluntary, conjugate slow eye movements (peak eye velocity = 100°/s) which stabilize images of moving objects on the fovea for continuous clear vision. During normal pursuit, the gain (eye velocity/target velocity) = 0.8–1.0, and the eye stays on target nearly exactly. Pursuit is triggered by retinal slip (target motion minus eye motion) of selected targets. Retinal slip is me-

diated by a pathway involving the dorsal-lateral geniculate, striate cortex, and occipitotemporal cortex. Two cortical efferent pathways are responsible for bringing this information to the ocular motor nuclei. These include occipitotemporal and frontal eye field projections to the pons, which in turn project to the cerebellar flocculus and vermis, then to the medial vestibular nucleus, and finally to the sixth and third nerve nuclei.

Dysfunction of the smooth pursuit system causes decreased pursuit gain, which forces patients to use saccades to keep up with the target (saccadic pursuit). Unilateral lesions of the cerebral hemisphere, pons, and cerebellum all cause decreased pursuit gain in the ipsilateral direction. Bilateral lesions cause decreased pursuit gain horizontally and vertically.

Optokinetic Nystagmus

OKN consists of conjugate visual-following responses (slow phases), interrupted by resetting quick phases. The optokinetic system can be stimulated either by rotating a large pattern around a stationary subject or by sustained self-rotation in a lit stationary background. The slow phases in OKN are mediated by two subsystems, an *immediate tracking system*, that may overlap the smooth pursuit system, and a *velocity-storage system*, which is a more sluggish system that involves visual input into the vestibular system. Unilateral lesions of the cerebral hemisphere, pons, and cerebellum all cause decreased OKN gain in the ipsilateral direction, which at the bedside appears as a reduced frequency of nystagmus.

Vestibulo-ocular Reflex (VOR)

The VOR helps to stabilize images of the visual surround on the retina during head movements. Angular head accelerations are sensed by three pairs of semicircular canals, and linear head accelerations are sensed by two pairs of otoliths. These sensors induce compensatory eye movements (slow phases) in the opposite direction of head acceleration by a three-neuron arc (vestibular afferents-vestibular nucleus-ocular motor nuclei). Sensorimotor transformation occurs from canal planes to the planes of eye movements, such that the neurons always contact their two respective extraocular eye muscles. Static head tilt causes ocular counter-rolling (torsional eye movements) about the line of sight and a slight hypertropia (elevation of eye on side of head tilt), which is mediated primarily by the otoliths. This counter-rolling and hypertropia in response to lateral head tilt only partly compensate for the degree of head tilt but help maintain binocular vision along the earth horizontal plane.

Horizontal VOR can be stimulated either by thrusting the head in one direction (causes contralateral slow phase) or by caloric irrigation. Warm water produces a nystagmus with quick phases to the ipsilateral side, and cold water (30°C or ice water) causes nystagmus to the contralateral side. Vertical VOR can be stimulated by vertical head thrust and occasionally by simultaneous caloric irrigation (bilateral ice-water irrigation induces a conjugate, upbeat nystagmus, whereas bilateral warm water irrigation produces a conjugate downbeat nystagmus). In comatose patients, 100–200 ml ice water is slowly infused into the external auditory meatus. Caloric irrigation is performed with the head of the supine subject tilted upwards by 30° in order to place the horizontal canals in a vertical plane. In awake patients, only a few milliliters of ice water are used and the head is first tilted such that the external auditory meatus of one ear is pointing up to allow the ice water to sit in the ear for 30 s. After 30 s, the head is rotated with the nose pointed up, and fixation is blocked by a Ganzfeld or Frenzel lens. Caloric stimulation should not be performed in patients with lesions of the tympanic membrane or fractures of the middle ear; head thrust should not be performed in patients with possible lesions of the cervical spine.

In conscious patients and patients with psychogenic disorders of consciousness, unilateral caloric irrigation induces caloric nystagmus with both slow and quick phases of nystagmus. Rapid head thrusts elicit a compensatory, rapid, conjugate deviation of both eyes to the opposite side. If both stimuli (warm and cold) in one ear cause decreased nystagmus, this usually indicates a peripheral vestibular disorder.

Cervico-ocular Reflex

Rotation of the head on the trunk, or of the trunk under a fixed head, stimulates proprioceptive afferents of the cervical spine and induces the cervico-ocular reflex. In normal subjects the gain of this response is very low (<0.1). In patients with chronic loss of peripheral vestibular function (e.g., previous ototoxicity) there is usually a much larger response.

Vergence and Ocular Alignment

Vergence eye movements are discon-jugate, with both slow and fast components that carry the eyes in opposite directions to enable binocular foveation of near objects. They are mediated by vergence neurons in the vicinity of the third nerve nuclei. Abnormalities of vergence occur in mesencephalic lesions, which are often accompanied by vertical gaze palsies.

Ocular misalignment can occur horizontally (eso- or exodeviation) and vertically (hypo- and hypertropia). It is due either to a paralytic lesion of the third, fourth, or fifth nerve or to a central lesion (nonparalytic strabismus). It can be detected by the different positions of the light reflex on each pupil or the correcting movements in the alternating cover test. (Each eye is covered alternately with an occluder held obliquely to permit simultaneous observation of both eyes. The position of the covered eye is compared with that of the fixating eye.)

Neural Integrator

Whenever the eyes are moved to an eccentric position in the orbit, the soft tissue around the eyes normally forces the eyes back to the center of the orbit within 1 s. To counteract this force, all oculomotor subsystems use a common "position-neural integrator", which adds an appropriate increase in neural firing to the oculomotor nuclei during an eccentric eye movement. The neural integrator for horizontal eye movements is mediated by neurons at the junction of the medial vestibular nucleus and prepositus hypoglossi nucleus (MVN/NPH) in the dorsal medulla, and the vertical neural integrator is mediated by the interstitial nucleus of Cajal (INC) in the dorsal midbrain. The function of both integrators is improved by the cerebellar flocculus.

Impairment of the neural integrators (leaky neural integrator) causes the eyes to drift to center of gaze during eccentric gaze, which impairs eccentric fixation. When the subject is asked to hold eccentric fixation, outward corrective saccades must be made repeatedly to refixate the target (gaze-position nystagmus). The neural integrator also is impaired during sleep and by a variety of GABA-enhancing drugs, including benzodiazepines and certain anticonvulsants.

Ocular Motor Abnormalities with Topographic Relevance

The diagnostic value of single ocular-motor abnormalities is variable because some have a high topographic specificity (e.g., convergence retraction nystagmus, downbeat nystagmus, upbeat nystagmus) whereas others are induced by lesions along the whole length of the brain stem (e.g., skew deviation, ocular tilt reaction). In Table 1, abnormalities are summarized according to different brain regions.

Eye Movement Disorders in Stupor and Coma

During drowsiness, saccade number and velocity are decreased; smooth pursuit, OKN, and VOR slow-phase

Table 1. Ocular motor abnormalities

Description	L: Site of the lesion A: Etiology
Hemispheres Horizontal deviation	Ipsilateral conjugate deviation L: parietal lobe, rarely frontal lobe A: trauma, hemorrhage, infarction, tumor, encephalitis, rarely focal seizures Contralateral conjugate deviation L: parietal or frontal lobe A: seizures
Ocular motor apraxia	Disturbance of voluntary eye movements (and pursuit), weakness of convergence, VOR eye movements relatively normal L: acute bilateral frontal or frontoparietal lesions A: infarctions, multiple sclerosis, hemorrhage
Diencephalon Seesaw nystagmus	Synchronous, alternating elevation and intorsion of one eye and depression and extorsion of the other eye L: interstitial nucleus of Cajal (INC), zona incerta A: chiasmal/parasellar tumor (i.e., pituitary adenoma), hydrocephalus, trauma, infarction, hemorrhage
Skew deviation	Supranuclear vertical divergence of both eyes in primary position and different positions of gaze, contraversive (contralateral eye undermost); at times alternating (higher eye reverses on gaze to either side) L: contralateral INC, often involved in paramedian thalamic lesions A: infarction, hemorrhage, tumor parasellar/chiasmal, hydrocephalus, trauma
Ocular tilt reaction	Tonic or paroxysmal triad of head tilt, skew deviation, and ocular torsion towards the undermost eye, contraversive L: contralateral INC (RiMLF), often involved in paramedian thalamic lesions A: infarction, hemorrhage, tumor parasellar/chiasmal, trauma, inflammatory
Midbrain Vertical gaze palsy	Vertical gaze deficit for all types of eye movements, though VOR often spared (Parinaud syndrome) L: upward gaze abnormalities from involvement of the posterior commissure or nuclei; downward gaze abnormalities from involvement of portions of the RiMLF A: tumor, vascular, hydrocephalus, degenerative, metabolic, encephalitis, trauma
Convergence retraction	Convergent jerks combined with jerks backward into the orbit, spontaneous or nystagmus elicited by upward saccades or quick phases (elicited by OKN drum); often associated with vertical gaze palsy, lid retraction and pupillary abnormalities (i.e., dorsal midbrain syndrome, Koerber-Salus-Elschnig syndrome) L: dorsal midbrain (RiMLF), posterior commissure A: tumors of the pineal gland and the third ventricle, hydrocephalus, vascular, trauma, encephalitis

Table 1. *Continued*

Description	L: Site of the lesion A: Etiology
Acquired pendular	Small amplitude, high frequency (2–7 Hz), often dissociated or monocular, in the horizontal, vertical or torsional planes; often associated with palatal myoclonus L: Central tegmental tract in brain stem A: multiple sclerosis (70%), infarctions, rarely in Kearns-Sayre syndrome and with monocular or binocular visual loss, toxic
Upbeat nystagmus	Upbeating nystagmus in the primary position of gaze (not suppressed by fixation), maybe modulated by static head tilt; INO occasionally present L: pontomesencephalic (brachium conjunctivum), dorsal medulla (ventral tegmental tract) A: brain stem tumor, infarction, hemorrhage, multiple sclerosis, encephalitis, degeneration, drugs
Ocular tilt reaction	(see above), contraversive and skew deviation L: contralateral INC and MLF A: unilateral infarction, hemorrhage, tumor, multiple sclerosis
Pons Internuclear ophthalmoplegia	Monocular adduction paresis with lateral gaze on the side of the lesion and dissociated abducting nystagmus on the contralateral side; convergence mostly intact; associated gaze evoked nystagmus on upward gaze, vertical smooth pursuit deficits, sometimes skew (ipsilateral eye uppermost) L: ipsilateral MLF A: multiple sclerosis (~80%), infarction, hemorrhage, tumor, encephalitis, toxic, metabolic, cerebellar ectopia
One-and-a-half syndrome	Ipsilateral horizontal gaze paresis and ipsilateral adduction paresis (INO) (i.e., paralytic pontine exotropia) resulting in exotropia and, with lateral gaze, abduction of the contralateral eye only; associated ocular bobbing in coma L: ipsilateral paramedian pontine reticular formation (PPRF) and ipsilateral A: brain-stem infarction, multiple sclerosis, hemorrhage, tumor
Downbeat nystagmus	Downbeating nystagmus in the primary position of gaze (no fixation suppression), increasing on lateral gaze and head extension L: craniocervical junction (flocculus); floor of the 4th ventricle A: cerebellar ectopia (≈25%), cerebellar degeneration (≈20%), multiple sclerosis, drugs, tumor, infarction, vitamin B_{12} deficiency, magnesium depletion
Ocular bobbing	Paroxysmal, usually conjugate, rapid downward deviation followed by slower returning upward drift, often combined with a pause in between; variants are reverse bobbing (rapid upward deviation, slow downward return), ocular dipping (slow downward drift, rapid return), reverse dipping (slow upward drift, rapid return); often associated paresis of horizontal VOR; intact pupillary light reactions L: acute bilateral pontine lesion, directly or by compression of the pontomedullary brain stem A: infarction, hemorrhage, tumor, concussion, encephalitis, hypoxic, metabolic, multiple sclerosis

Table 1. *Continued*

Description	L: Site of the lesion A: Etiology
Ocular tilt reaction	(see above), ipsi- or contraversive and skew deviation L: contralateral in the upper pons, ipsilateral vestibular nuclei in the pontomedullary region A: unilateral infarction, hemorrhage, multiple sclerosis, tumor, brain stem encephalitis
Periodic alternating	Horizontal spontaneous nystagmus with periodic changing of direction nystagmus (mean duration of a period 100–200 s). increases on lateral gaze, inhibited during sleep L: pontomedullary brain stem, archicerebellum (?) A: infratentorial tumor, cerebellar ectopia, multiple sclerosis, degenerative, toxic, vascular, congenital
Upbeat nystagmus	(see above)
Ocular tilt reaction	(see above), ipsiversive, disconjugate or monocular torsion with predominance of the ipsilateral eye L: ipsilateral vestibular nuclei (medial and superior)
Cerebellum Opsoclonus	Rapid, conjugate, mainly horizontal with different amplitudes without intersaccadic interval (6–12 Hz), spontaneously or induced by eye movements (vertical), activated by lid closure, persisting during sleep; associated ataxia, dysarthria, myoclonus of the limbs L: Purkinje cells in the cerebellum, rarely brain stem (pons, midbrain, thalamus) A: in children: paraneoplastic syndrome in neuroblastoma, encephalitis, hydrocephalus, thallium intoxication; in adults: encephalitis, paraneoplastic syndrome (carcinoma of breast, lung, uterus), pontine or thalamic hemorrhage or infarction, hydrocephalus, multiple sclerosis, glioma, trauma, toxic (amitriptyline, haloperidol, lithium, thallium, chlordecone, DDT)
Periodic alternating nystagmus	(see above)
Flocculus Downbeat nystagmus	(see above)

eye velocity are decreased; and the neural integrator becomes leaky. During light sleep and stupor, even with the eyes open all voluntary as well as spontaneous eye movements are absent. Irregular, mainly horizontal, periodic deviations of the eyes may occur, caused by insufficient fixation. These roving eye movements cannot be produced voluntarily, and their presence is useful to discriminate organic from psychogenic disorders of consciousness. In coma, there is usually complete loss of quick phases of nystagmus due to dysfunction of the reticular formation (encompassing the PPRF and RiMLF), and the VOR elicits only a deviation of the eyes. In addition, spontaneous eye deviations (conjugate and disconjugate) and spontaneous eye movements frequently occur in coma.

Spontaneous Eye Deviations

Conjugate Eye Deviations

Horizontal. Deviations towards the side of the lesion may occasionally occur from seizures involving the cortical pursuit eye fields, but they usually occur from ablative lesions of structures involved with visual spatial attention (posterior parietal cortex, pulvinar, superior colliculus, and their interconnections). These deviations usually can be overcome (eyes cross the midline) by a passive head thrust (VOR) but may require a combination of caloric irrigation and head rotation.

Deviations away from the side of the lesion may be due either to seizures involving cortical saccade eye fields or to ablative lesions involving either the PPRF or sixth nerve nucleus on one side. In the latter case, the deviation is accompanied by a defect in the ability to generate quick phases or saccadic eye movements towards the side of the lesion, and the deviation cannot be overcome with VOR or caloric irrigation.

Vertical. Downward deviation of the eyes is caused by a dorsal midbrain lesion involving the posterior commissure, RiMLF, or INC (e.g., thalamic hemorrhage, hydrocephalus) or may be due to drugs. Upward deviation of the eyes is rarely observed in coma but occasionally occurs in hypoxic brain damage after cardiac arrest. It is associated with a bad prognosis. Periodic tonic elevation of both eyes combined with lid elevation and neck hyperextension is seen in oculogyric crisis, an extrapyramidal disorder due to postencephalic parkinsonism, or as dystonic side effects of drugs (e.g., phenothiazines).

Disconjugate Eye Deviation

Disconjugate eye deviations are a frequent sign of altered consciousness due to loss of the voluntary control of eye movements and fixation. When the deviation is severe, ocular motor defects should be looked for, including oculomotor nerve palsies (third, fourth, and sixth), skew deviation, internuclear ophthalmoplegia, and one-and-a-half syndromes (see Table 1).

Oculomotor nerve palsies in comatose patients may be difficult to identify because one has to rely on observation of abnormal spontaneous eye position and VOR. A third nerve palsy is the most common, frequently associated with unilateral pupil dilation (the earliest sign of uncal herniation) and ptosis. The most vulnerable part of the nerve is the area along the peripheral course via the base of the skull and the cavernous sinus to the orbit, whereby it passes over the petroclinoid ligament lateral to the posterior clinoid process. Causes of a third nerve palsy other than the uncal herniation are midbrain lesions (hemorrhage or infarction) and nerve trauma. Unilateral or bilateral sixth nerve palsies (deviation of the eye in adduction) are frequent in patients with increased intracranial pressure due to direct damage of the nerve along the clivus through stretching during herniation. The fourth nerve is rarely susceptible to herniation (protected by the tentorium) but very susceptible to head trauma.

Spontaneous Eye Movements

Horizontal

Spontaneous Nystagmus. Spontaneous nystagmus is uncommon in coma, since the quick phases are no longer generated because of diminished activity of brain stem burst neurons in the PPRF and RiMLF. Peripheral vestibular lesions in comatose patients induce ipsilateral conjugate tonic deviation of the eyes. Monocular or disconjugate pendular nystagmus in the two eyes is found in pontine lesions involving the central tegmental tract.

Roving Eye Movements. Similar to the slow eye movements of light sleep in healthy persons, the eyes in a light (diencephalic) comatose stage show conjugate or disconjugate, usually horizontal, slow random deviations. They represent a benign prognostic value by indicating an intact ocular-motor function of the brain stem. These movements are slower than the conjugate rapid eye movements (REM) during sleep.

Periodic Alternating or "Ping-pong" Gaze. Periodic alternating, slow, conjugate, horizontal deviations of the eyes in stupor or coma are referred to as ping-pong gaze. These episodic rhythmic deviations of the eyes with a pause of 2–3 s at lateral gaze occur every few seconds for a period of hours. Ping-pong gaze has been observed in bilateral hemispheric infarctions or lesions of the cerebral peduncles.

Vertical

Ocular Bobbing and Dipping. These are paroxysmal, usually conjugate vertical eye movements that move the eyes eccentrically and then back to center of gaze. Frequently, there is a pause of up to 10 s after each recentering eye movement. Although the pathophysiological mechanism is unknown, the different phenomena seem to represent a varying imbalance of vertical gaze. *Ocular bobbing* consists of an intermittent, rapid downward deviation of the eyes, followed by a returning slower upward drift. Typically, the spontaneous and VOR eye movements are absent, indicating a deleterious prognosis. *Reverse ocular bobbing* is a rapid upward deviation of the eyes with a slower downward return to the midposition, which can develop from ocular bobbing. *Ocular dipping, i.e., inverse ocular bobbing*, is characterized by the rare combination of a slow downward deviation with a rapid return to the primary position, whereas *reverse dipping (i.e., converse bobbing)* is a slow upward drift followed by a rapid return. Although ocular bobbing (and perhaps its rare variants) is usually observed in intrinsic pontine lesions such as infarctions, hemorrhages, and tumors, it has also been reported in toxic, anoxic, and metabolic disorders. Ocular dipping has no localizing value. Variants of ocular bobbing in association with divergence or convergence indicate a dorsal midbrain dysfunction.

Acute Ocular Myoclonus. Large pendular eye movements in the vertical direction have been observed in acute brain stem infarctions.

Locked-in Syndrome. Patients with a locked-in syndrome (i.e., supranuclear motor de-efferentation with quadriplegia and aphonia mostly due to a bilateral, ventral pontine lesion) are often awake and communicate by use of vertical eye movements and blinking. In the acute phase, the locked-in syndrome can be misinterpreted as coma or a vegetative state; therefore, it always must be considered in the differential diagnosis.

Evoked Eye Movements

In coma, the cerebral control of eye movements is lost and only the VOR can be evoked. If unilateral caloric irrigation or a horizontal head thrust fails to induce any horizontal eye movement, an ipsilateral pontomedullary junction lesion (vestibular nuclei) or a contralateral dorsal pontine lesion (sixth nerve nucleus) is likely, provided that a peripheral vestibular lesion is excluded.

Disconjugate VOR may occur with a number of different lesions. Intact abduction of one eye and reduced or abolished adduction of the other eye is due to a lesion of the MLF in the pontine brain stem (internuclear ophthalmoplegia) or to involvement of the medial rectus portion of the third nerve nucleus. The eye with the abolished adduction indicates the side of the lesion. Disconjugate VOR may also occur in peripheral nerve palsies or with involvement of the nerve fascicles within the brain stem; destruction of the ocular motor nerves or nuclei prevents all responses of the ipsilateral eye except that mediated by the lateral rectus muscle, and destruction of the sixth nerve fascicle or nerve will impair abduction of the ipsilateral eye but spare movements of the other eye.

Loss of vertical VOR with intact horizontal VOR indicates a midbrain lesion involving the ocular motor nuclei or nerves bilaterally.

Brain Stem Herniation

In comatose patients, the level of brain stem injury can often be determined by the VOR and other eye movements. With total loss of the VOR the likelihood of a lethal outcome is high (92%), and it becomes even higher in combination with the loss of pupillary reflexes (100%), providing pre-existing vestibular disorders or ototoxic drugs and vestibular sedatives are not present (Table 2). Corresponding to the altered state of consciousness (with rostral-caudal deterioration), the following phenomena can be observed: In light supratentorial coma (early diencephalic stage) due to lesions of the hemispheres the impairment of

Table 2. Conditions and agents that may lead to a misinterpretation of eye movements in coma

Peripheral vestibular lesions including ototoxic agents (e.g., aminoglycoside antibiotics, loop diuretics, high-dose salicylate, alkylating chemotherapeutic anticancer agents)
Drugs suppressing the vestibular system: sedatives (benzodiazepines, barbiturates), antiepileptic drugs (phenytoin, carbamazepine), tricyclic antidepressants, alcohol, vestibular sedatives
Infranuclear/supranuclear ocular motor disorders with external ophthalmoplegia (e.g., endocrine myopathy, Fisher's syndrome)
Toxic agents causing various ocular motor disturbances by acting within the brain stem or cerebellum (e.g., opsoclonus by amitriptyline, haloperidol, lithium, thallium, toluene, chlordecone, DDT; internuclear ophthalmoplegia by opiates, bromides; vertical gaze palsy by barbiturates/primidone)
Neuromuscular blockers (e.g., succinylcholine)
Metabolic coma (e.g., hepatic coma induces INO, ocular bobbing, skew deviation)

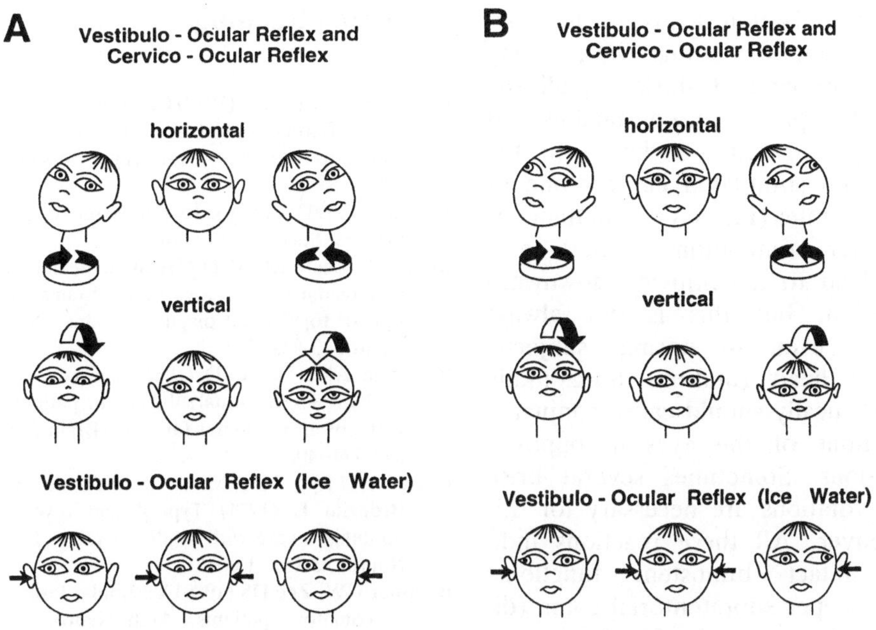

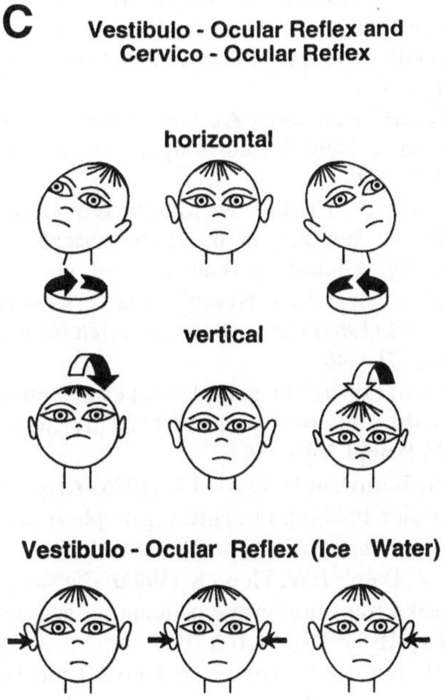

A Vestibulo - Ocular Reflex and
Cervico - Ocular Reflex

horizontal

vertical

Vestibulo - Ocular Reflex (Ice Water)

B Vestibulo - Ocular Reflex and
Cervico - Ocular Reflex

horizontal

vertical

Vestibulo - Ocular Reflex (Ice Water)

C Vestibulo - Ocular Reflex and
Cervico - Ocular Reflex

horizontal

vertical

Vestibulo - Ocular Reflex (Ice Water)

Fig. 1A–C. VOR in comatose patients. Passive head rotations (horizontal and vertical) with high frequency or ice water (unilateral and bilateral) stimulates the VOR. Passive head rotation also can induce a cervico-ocular reflex in patients who had previous loss of the VOR (e.g., ototoxicity). **A** In light supratentorial coma (diencephalic stage) with intact brain-stem function passive head rotations about the Y- and Z-axis (*top* and *middle*) cause compensatory, conjugate deviations of the eyes in opposite horizontal and vertical directions. Caloric stimulation by ice water (*bottom*) produces a conjugate, tonic deviation to the ipsilateral stimulated ear with unilateral maneuver and a conjugate downward deviation with bilateral maneuver. **B** In deeper comatose states (midbrain-upper pons stage) or with pontine lesions of the medial longitudinal fascicle (MLF) the horizontal VOR movements become disconjugate, i.e., intact abduction of one eye and reduced or abolished adduction of the other eye. Vertical VOR is usually absent due to involvement of the midbrain. **C** Loss of all VOR indicates a deep coma (pontomedullary stage) with a bad prognosis (provided that the coma is not metabolic and an infranuclear ophthalmoplegia can be excluded) gaze stabilization leads to horizontal periodic deviations, i.e., roving eye movements. Caloric stimuli (by ice water) produce no nystagmus, but a conjugate tonic deviation to the ipsilateral stimulated ear for one or a few minutes (Fig. 1A). Simultaneous ice-water stimulation of both ears may lead to a conjugate downward deviation, but this is not always elicited even in normal subjects. Passive head rotations horizontally and vertically should cause conjugate deviations of the eyes in opposite directions. Sometimes several brisk head rotations are necessary for this maneuver. All these reactions indicate intact brainstem functions. With deeper supratentorial coma (diencephalic stage) the VOR becomes more lively, so that one single head rotation is enough to provoke compensatory eye deviation.

In deeper comatose states, the midbrain-upper pons stage, the normal conjugation of both eyes during spontaneous and reflex eye movements disappears; disconjugate eye positions and movements occur (Fig. 1B). VOR eye movements become more and more difficult to induce. Repeated head rotation maneuvers are necessary to produce impaired and sometimes disconjugate deviations, which are also seen with ice-water stimulation.

As coma deepens (ponto-medullary stage) the eyes become immobile, and all spontaneous and VOR eye movements are abolished (Fig. 1C). This is a sign of bad prognosis if the lesion is not metabolic.

The medullary stage is characterized by a loss of reflex eye movements as well as of all brain stem reflexes. Death is inevitable.

Suggested Reading

Barnes GR, Forbat LN (1979) Cervical and vestibular afferent control of ocular motor response in man. Acta Otolaryngol (Stockh) 88:79–87

Brandt T (1991) Vertigo. Its multisensory syndromes. Springer, London

Brandt T, Dieterich M (1993) Skew deviation with ocular torsion, a vestibular brainstem sign of topological diagnostic value. Ann Neurol 33:528–534

Bronstein AM, Hood JD (1986) The cervico-ocular reflex in normal subjects and patients with absent vestibular function. Brain Res 373:399–408

Brusa A, Firpo MP, Massa S, Piccardo A, Bronzini E (1984) Typical and reverse bobbing: a case with localizing value. Eur Neurol 23:151–155

Buettner UW, Zee DS (1989) Vestibular testing in comatose patients. Arch Neurol 46:561–563

Cannon SC, Zee DS (1988) The neural integrator of the oculomotor system. In: Lessel S, van Dalen JTW (eds) Current neuro-ophthalmology. Mosby, St. Louis, pp 123–138

Daroff RB, Waldmann AL (1965) Ocular bobbing. J Neurol Neurosurg Psychiatry 28:375–377

Drake ME Jr, Erwin CW, Massey EW (1982) Ocular bobbing in metabolic encephalopathy: clinical, pathologic, and electrophysiologic study. Neurology 32:1029–1031

Fisher CM (1964) Ocular bobbing. Arch Neurol 11:543–546

Fisher CM (1969) The neurological examination of the comatose patient. Acta Neurol Scand 45 [Suppl 36]:1–56

Hata S, Bernstein E, Davis LE (1986) Atypical ocular bobbing in acute organophosphate poisoning. Arch Neurol 43:185–186

Henn V, Baloh RW, Hepp K (1984) The sleep-wake transition in the oculomotor system. Exp Brain Res 54:166–176

Katz B, Hoyt WF, Townsend J (1982) Ocular bobbing and unilateral pontine hemorrhage. J Clin Neuro Ophthalmol 2:193–195

Keane JR (1985) Pretectal pseudobobbing. Five patients with "V"-pattern convergence nystagmus. Arch Neurol 42:592–594

Keane JK (1986) Acute vertical myoclonus. Neurology 36:86–89

Larmande P, Dongmo L, Limodin J, Ruchoux M (1987) Periodic alternating gaze: a case without any hemispheric lesion. Neurosurgery 20:481–483

Leigh RJ, Zee DS (1991) The neurology of eye movements, 2nd edn. Davis, Philadelphia

Mueller-Jensen A, Neunzig H-P, Emskoetter T (1987) Outcome prediction in comatose patients: significance of reflex eye movement analysis. J Neurol Neurosurg Psychiatry 50:389–392

Nakada T, Kwee IL, Lee H (1984) Sustained upgaze in coma. J Clinical Neuro Ophthalmol 4:35–37

Noda S, Ide K, Umezaki H, Itoh H, Yamamota K (1987) Repetitive divergence. Ann Neurol 21:109–110

Plum F, Posner JB (1980) The diagnosis of stupor and coma, 3rd edn. Davis, Philadelphia

Ropper AH (1981) Ocular dipping in anoxic coma. Arch Neurol 38:297–299

Rosenberg ML, Calvert PC (1986) Ocular bobbing in association with other signs of midbrain dysfunction. Arch Neurol 43:314

Senelick R (1976) "Ping-pong" gaze. Periodic alternating gaze deviation. Neurology 26: 532–535

Simon RP (1978) Forced downward ocular deviation. Occurrence during oculovestibular testing in sedative drug-induced coma. Arch Neurol 35:456–458

Stewart JD, Kirkham TH, Mathieson G (1979) Periodic alternating gaze. Neurology 29: 222–224

Susac JO, Hoyt WF, Daroff RB, Lawrence W (1970) Clinical spectrum of ocular bobbing. J Neurol Neurosurg Psychiatry 33:771–775

Tusa RJ, Zee DS, Herdman SJ (1986) Effect of unilateral cerebral cortical lesions on ocular motor behavior in monkeys: saccades and quick phases. J Neurophysiol 56:1590–1625

Tusa RJ, Ungerleider LG (1988) Fiber pathways of cortical areas mediating smooth pursuit eye movements in monkeys. Ann Neurol 23:174–183

Tusa RJ, Kaplan PW, Hain TC, Naidu S (1990) Ipsiversive eye deviation and epileptic nystagmus. Neurology 40:662–665

Tusa RJ (1989) Saccadic eye movements. Supranuclear control. Bull Soc Belge Ophthalmol 237:67–111

Walsh FB, Hoyt WF (1988) Clinical neuro-ophthalmology, 4th edn. Williams and Wilkins, Baltimore

Chapter 32

Acute Visual Loss Due to Retrochiasmatic Lesions

MARIANNE DIETERICH

Acute visual disturbances in unilateral retrochiasmatic lesions of the optic tract result in homonymous visual field defects or local scotoma, depending on the size of the lesion, caused by (a) lesions of the lateral geniculate nucleus (LGN), (b) lesions of parts of the visual radiation near the lateral geniculate nucleus, (c) complete lesions of the visual radiation white matter below the visual cortex, or (d) a unilateral destruction of the primary visual cortex (area 17, V1).

The accompanying visual field defects do not demonstrate perfect congruency in both eyes because of the spatial arrangement of the axons in the optic tract or in the visual radiation. In retrochiasmatic disorders the corresponding visual field defects are always homonymous; however, shape and extension vary according to the site of the lesion. In LGN lesions and those in the surrounding area the defect marks a contralateral upper quadrant anopia; in complete visual radiation lesions and complete primary visual cortex lesions the defect marks

a contralateral homonymous hemianopia with macular sparing. Lesions of the minor, most occipital, supracalcarine part of the visual cortex induce wedge-shaped homonymous field defects in a contralateral quadrant (upper or lower). Homonymous visual field defects occur in posterior cerebral artery infarctions, chronic cerebral hypoxia, intracerebral hemorrhages, and severe head trauma. Traumatic brain damage affecting the visual radiation is the chief cause (in 52%) of persisting visual field defects.

Bilateral damage of the LGN, the visual radiation, and the primary visual cortex results in loss of all conscious vision, in cortical blindness. It may appear suddenly as a transient or chronic symptom, but it can also develop from bilateral hemianopia when the blindness in the two hemifields does not occur simultaneously. Acute cortical blindness is a result of subarachnoid hemorrhage, transient cardiac arrest, extended occipital tumors (e.g., glioblastomas) with acute decompensation, and carbon monoxide or mercury poisoning. The most common etiology in cortical blindness, however, is a cerebrovas-

Section Editor: Daniel F. Hanley

cular disease with bilateral posterior cerebral artery infarctions or a basilar artery occlusion. In patients in an intensive care unit, bilateral occipital lobe infarctions are often due to increased intracranial pressure, inducing a transtentorial herniation and compressing the posterior cerebral arteries. In recent years the occurrence of cortical blindness with invasive procedures such as cerebral angiography and open heart surgery has further increased. Occipital lobe infarctions in the latter case indicate a poor prognosis. In rare cases, cortical blindness may occur as an ictal or postictal symptom. Patients recovering from cortical blindness may experience a limited visual field, especially in the region of the fovea, i.e., tunnel vision, or a transient state of cerebral asthenopia, with blurred vision or visual fatigue, and visual agnosia. Cortical blindness is associated with anosognosia in cases where the cortical defect of the occipital lobes extends beyond area V1.

Suggested Reading

Aguilar MJ, Gerbode F, Hill JD (1971) Neuropathological complications of cardiac surgery. J Thorac Cardiovasc Surg 61: 676–685

Aldrich MS, Vanderzant C, Abou-Khalil B et al. (1985) Cortical blindness as an ictal manifestation. Electroencephalogr Clin Neurophysiol 61:37P

Aldrich MS, Alessi AG, Beck RW, Gilmann S (1987) Cortical blindness: etiology, diagnosis, and prognosis. Ann Neurol 21:149–158

Gloning I, Tschabitscher H (1969) Rückbildung einer corticalen Blindheit. Wien Z Nervenheilkd 11:406–407

Gloning I, Gloning K, Tschabitscher H (1962) Die occipitale Blindheit auf vaskulärer Basis. Graefes Arch Ophthalmol 165: 138–177

Grüsser O-J, Landis T (1991) Visual agnosias and other disturbances of visual perception and cognition, vol 12. Macmillan, London, pp 144–148

Sadeh M, Goldhammer Y, Kuritsky A (1983) Postictal blindness in adults. J Neurol Neurosurg Psychiatry 46:566–569

Smith JL, Cross SA (1983) Occipital lobe infarction after open heart surgery. J Clin Neuro Ophthalmol 3:23–30

Wilbrand H, Saenger A (1917) Die homonyme Hemianopsie nebst ihren Beziehungen zu den anderen cerebralen Herderscheinungen. In: Wilbrand H, Saenger A (eds) Die Neurologie des Auges. Ein Handbuch für Nerven- und Augenärzte, vol 7. Bergmann, Wiesbaden

Zihl J, von Cramon D (1986) Zerebrale Sehstörungen. Kohlhammer, Stuttgart

Chapter 33

Acute Visual Loss – Monocular Blindness

Detlef Kömpf and Werner Hacke

Introduction

Acute monocular blindness is usually caused by vascular disease or trauma. Less common causes include space-occupying lesions, vascular malformations, or inflammatory processes. These can be differentiated mainly by the different time course of the visual loss (Fig. 1).

Binocular visual loss is rare (except after trauma). Cerebral (cortical or geniculocalcarine) blindness refers to subnormal visual acuity as a result of bilateral retrogeniculate lesions, usually from bilateral infarctions in the territories supplied by the posterior cerebral arteries. The bilateral lesions need not develop simultaneously or be anatomically symmetrical. For example, a patient may have a left hemianopia from a right hemispheric stroke and then develop cortical blindness when a second infarct occurs on the contralateral side. There may be no other clinical signs of nervous system disease (that is, pupillary light reactions may be brisk and fundi may be normal), but various degrees of dementia and memory loss are often present. A curious phenomenon often encountered in patients with cerebral blindness is denial of blindness (Anton's syndrome). Patients behave as if they are blind but deny that they cannot see, often giving rather bizarre excuses for their abnormal behavior. These patients do not call attention to their deficit. Cerebral blindness can easily be confused with factitious or functional blindness, two syndromes that present with a similar clinical picture with preserved light reactions, clear media, and normal fundi (see below).

Approach to Acute Monocular Blindness

The key step in the approach to acute visual loss is a meticulous history of the onset and progression of visual symptoms. The evaluation of the clinical circumstances and accompanying neurological deficits often allows early diagnosis. Patients should be questioned about trauma, infection, pre-

Section Editor: Daniel F. Hanley

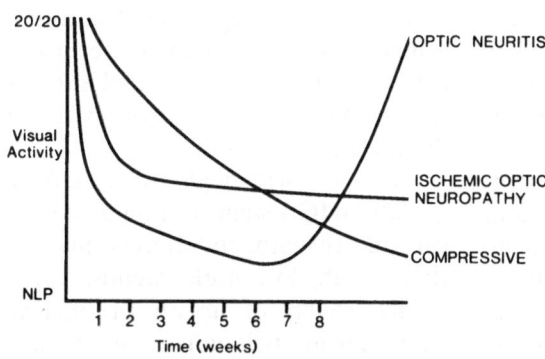

20/20

Visual
Activity

NLP

OPTIC NEURITIS

ISCHEMIC OPTIC
NEUROPATHY

COMPRESSIVE

1 2 3 4 5 6 7 8
Time (weeks)

Fig. 1. Time course of visual loss in optic neuritis, anterior ischemic optic neuropathy (AION), and compressive optic neuropathy. *NLP*, No light perception

ceding stroke, myocardial infarction, and cardiac arrhythmias.

Three different patterns of monocular visual loss often disclose the underlying etiology:

1. Transient (seconds, minutes)
   – Obscurations, amaurosis fugax
2. Abrupt and persistent
   – Ocular stroke, trauma, or functional
3. Acute or subacute (hours, days, weeks)
   – Vasculitic, inflammatory, compressive, infiltrative, or degenerative

Neurological examination with special emphasis on the cranial nerves and the ocular, cranial, and cervical vascular systems adds important information. The visual impairment must be thoroughly assessed immediately, including:

1. Corrected visual acuity, stereopsis
2. Visual fields and color vision
3. Examination of eye and orbit
4. Examination of the fundus
5. Amsler grid for metamorphopsia

The pupils can be pharmacologically dilated for funduscopy in patients without signs of major neurological disease or impaired consciousness.

Special emphasis should be placed on the shape and color of the optic disk, presence of retinal emboli, microinfarcts, or venous stasis. Additional changes, such as diabetic or hypertensive retinopathy, should also be assessed.

Additional studies include computerized tomography (CT) of the orbits, base of the skull, and brain. Vascular examination using extracranial and transcranial Doppler ultrasound, as well as B-mode techniques and ophthalmodynamometry, should be done in those with a presumed ischemic cause of monocular blindness.

Ischemic Visual Loss

Amaurosis fugax (AF) – Transient Visual Loss

Transient ocular ischemia is characterized by an attack of partial or complete transient monocular blindness (TMB) lasting seconds to minutes with complete recovery thereafter. Frequently, AF begins abruptly and shows a moving pattern of visual loss developing like a falling curtain. AF may recur frequently if the underlying cause is not treated. Most attacks are due to embolism of fresh thrombus in the ophthalmic circulation from an atheromatous carotid plaque. Patients frequently have bright yellowish Hollenhorst plaques on funduscopic examination (Fig. 2). Cardiac lesions associated with thromboembolism include myocardial infarction (producing mural thrombus), mitral stenosis with or without atrial fibrillation, and vegetative valvular lesions.

AF may precede both cerebral stroke and retinal infarction. Although the risk of permanent visual loss is relatively low (3% per year), patients have an above-average risk of stroke (about 10% per year). Furthermore, AF is a marker for generalized arteriosclerotic vascular disease. Many patients have significant coronary artery disease and are at greater risk of early death. Their decreased survival is due more often to coronary artery disease than to stroke.

Patients with high-grade (≥70%) ipsilateral ICA stenosis should undergo carotid thromboendarterectomy. In those with low-grade stenosis or a cardiac source of emboli, prophylaxis with aspirin, ticlopidine, or warfarin should be considered.

Other infrequent causes of an AF include:

1. Retinal vascular insufficiency in patients with extensive extracranial arterial occlusive disease. Low-pressure retinopathy is characteristic. Another pattern of amaurosis

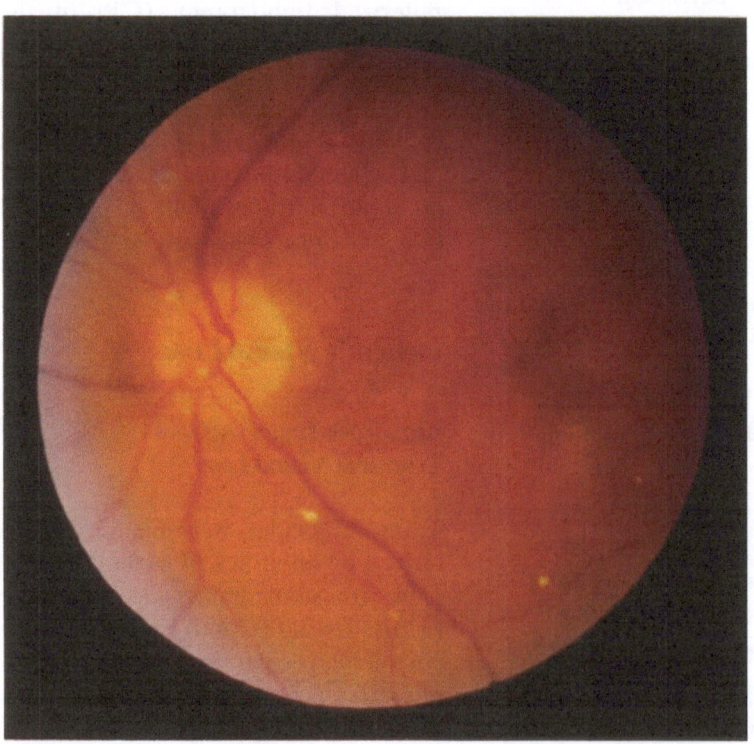

Fig. 2. Yellowish cholesterol Hollenhorst plaques in amaurosis fugax. Source: Prof. Hacke

can occur in which the attacks are less rapid in onset and longer in duration (from several minutes up to 2 h). Factors that predispose to these attacks are systemic hypotension, venous hypertension, and extracerebral steal.

2. Angiospasm of the ophthalmic or retinal arteries, or the choroidociliary circulation. Patients may present with flickering optical sensations and may have a history of migraine headaches.

Central Retinal Artery and Branch Retinal Artery Occlusion – Persistent Visual Loss

The major symptom of central retinal artery occlusion (CRAO) is sudden, unilateral blindness that is persistent. Blindness is confirmed by failure of the pupil to react to direct light. If the fundus is examined early (within minutes), a striking finding is the presence of segmentation of blood columns because of slow flow within the retinal veins. After an hour or more, the ischemic retina appears white and the normal red color of the choroid at the fovea accentuates the central cherry-red spot of the macula (Fig. 3). After days, optic atrophy develops.

The most important principal cause of CRAO is, again, an embolic obstruction. AF as a premonitory symptom suggests an embolus (cardiac or carotid) or, uncommon but important, temporal arteritis.

In acute embolic CRAO, treatment strategies differ widely. Recently,

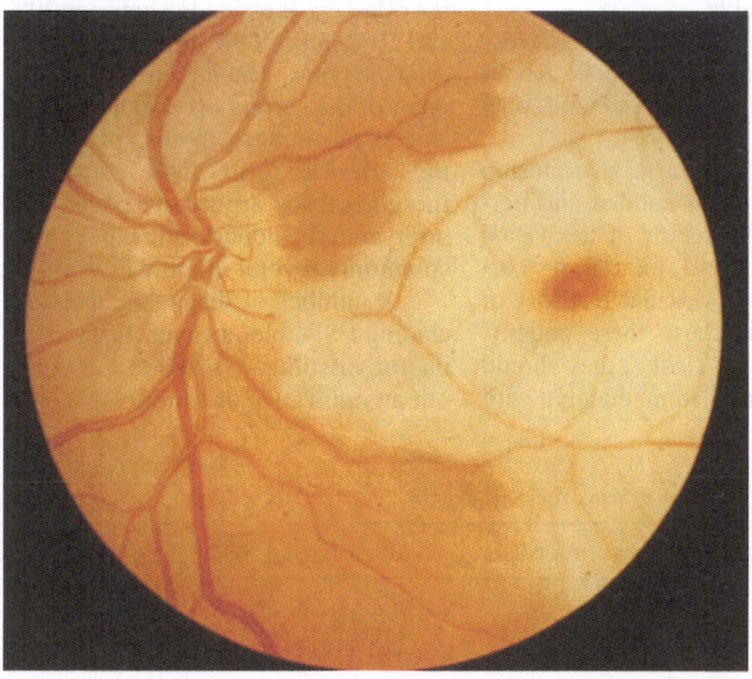

Fig. 3. Cherry-red spot at the macula in central retinal artery occlusion (CRAO). Source: Prof. Kömpf

superselective intra-arterial thrombolysis of acutely occluded ophthalmic vessels using urokinase or rt-PA has been reported. As in the treatment of acute stroke, anticoagulation with heparin is widely used but not of proven value. One reasonable treatment, proposed by Sfytche et al. (1974), is firm ocular massage (with the patient supine) to decrease the intraocular pressure and help dislodge the embolus into the peripheral arterial circulation. Breathing into a paper bag to increase the pCO_2 concentration and giving Diamox 500 mg intravenously have also been advocated. Anterior chamber paracentesis may be of benefit only in the very early stage when there is no flow in the arterial and venous retinal circulation and the cherry-red spot has not yet developed. There is currently no controlled validation of these strategies available.

The prognosis for visual recovery in CRAO is extremely poor. About 58% of eyes remain blind and only 21% retain useful vision.

Branch retinal artery occlusion (BRAO) presents as sudden and permanent loss of a sector of the visual field from retinal infarction corresponding to the vascular territory of the arteriole. Because these patients are also at risk for stroke, they should also be examined immediately, with

emphasis on the cerebrovascular and cardiovascular systems.

Anterior Ischemic Optic Neuropathy

Patients with anterior ischemic optic neuropathy (AION) present with sudden persistent visual failure due to acute infarction of the optic nerve head. Patients typically have an altitudinal field defect and pallor and swelling of the optic disk on examination. There are two types of AION (Table 1): the nonarteritic type in patients past middle age with diabetes mellitus and hypertension, and the arteritic type in those with giant cell arteritis. Embolism is not thought to be a major factor in the pathogenesis of AION.

The risk of AION developing in the other eye is estimated between 30% and 50% in both the arteritic and nonarteritic types. The interval of involvement of the second eye can be as short as several minutes, hours, or days in the arteritic form. This constitutes the emergency aspect of AION. The interval in the nonarteritic type is most commonly several months to years.

A number of diagnostic tests, including ESR, blood chemistry, screening for vasculitis, CT and MRI (to rule out an infiltrative or compressive optic

Table 1. Two types of acute ischemic optic neuropathy

	Nonarteritic AION	Arteritic cranial arteritis
Age peak (years)	60–65	70–80
Visual dysfunction	Minimal-severe	Severe
Second eye involvement	40%	75%
Systemic	Hypertension, diabetes	Weight loss, fever, headache
ESR (mm/h)	Normal	High (50–120)
Response to steroids	None	Systemic symptoms + return of vision −/(+)

neuropathy), and carotid noninvasive studies, should be performed when AION is suspected. Temporal artery biopsy is indicated when there is a high index of clinical suspicion of temporal arteritis (anorexia, malaise, proximal arthralgia, myalgia, headache, increased ESR). It is important to note that temporal arteritis may spare certain areas of the temporal artery. Thus, the biopsy should be large enough (at least 2 cm in length) for histological examination.

There is no effective treatment for nonarteritic AION. Optic nerve sheath decompression is highly controversial. The treatment of choice in the arteritic type is urgent high-dose corticosteroids pending temporal artery biopsy. Prebiopsy corticosteroid treatment does not affect the results of the biopsy; inflammatory changes may be seen as late as 2 weeks after beginning treatment with corticosteroids. Therefore, if AION is suspected for any reason, corticosteroid treatment should be started immediately and a temporal artery biopsy should be done. Prompt diagnosis of temporal arteritis and treatment with high-dose corticosteroids usually prevents involvement of the second eye.

The prognosis for recovery of vision in arteritic AION is extremely poor. In the nonarteritic type, improvement has been noted in 33% of patients. The prognosis of patients suffering from a vasculitic cause of AION is comparable.

Traumatic Optic Neuropathy

The diagnosis of traumatic optic neuropathy is usually suggested by the history. The most common form of injury to the optic nerve is direct injury by orbital penetrating wounds. Indirect injuries occur as a result of orbitofacial or cranial trauma. Sudden blindness results from optic nerve contusion, usually within the optic canal. Frontal impact deformation of the skull concentrates forces at the orbital apex (orbital opening of the optic canal), where blood vessels may be sheared and nerve tissue may be compressed. Secondary edema may play a role in worsening visual outcome. Hemorrhage within the nerve substance or sheaths can often be seen on CT scan. Radiological studies for orbitocranial fractures and orbital foreign bodies should be done, though the severity of visual loss does not correlate well with the presence of craniofacial or optic canal fractures or with the level of consciousness. Even blunt trauma to the eye and adnexa can result in severe visual loss not accounted for by visible injury to the globe.

Treatment of traumatic optic neuropathy is controversial, though corticosteroid pulse therapy and surgical decompression have been recomended. Indications for transethmoidal decompression in indirect optic nerve trauma include:

1. Complete visual loss immediately after injury
2. Vision is present but is impaired or fails to improve to 20/40 or better after 3 weeks of treatment with corticosteroids (dexamethasone 1 mg/kg/day).

Optic Neuritis

Optic neuritis (ON) includes the inflammatory and demyelinative optic neuropathies. Pain is present at the time of visual failure in two thirds of patients, aggravated characteristically by moving or touching the eye. Vision typically worsens over several days (Table 2). The disk is normal ("retro-bulbar neuritis"), edematous ("papillitis"), or atrophic (in the late course). The risk of developing multiple sclerosis after an attack of apparently idiopathic ON is quite high: about two thirds of patients will develop multiple sclerosis within 15 years. Other possible causes of ON are listed in Table 3.

Papilledema

Optic disk swelling, due to an increase of the intracranial spinal fluid pressure, is a dynamic process. The severity varies with the chronicity and the cause. Diagnosis of papilledema represents a major neurological emerg-

Table 3. Causes of optic neuritis

Multiple sclerosis
Unknown etiology
Viral infections of childhood (measles, mumps, chickenpox)
Viral encephalitides
Post-, paraviral infections
Herpes zoster
Contiguous inflammation
Granulomatous inflammations (syphilis, tuberculosis, cryptococcosis, sarcoidosis)

ency. As a general rule, visual acuity is normal, at least in the early stages. Although visual symptoms (always bilateral) are rare, typically transient visual obscurations occur. Brief symptoms of amaurosis fugax, lasting only 10–30 s and described as a "veil" over the eye, may occur.

Compressive/Infiltrative Optic Neuropathy

The signature of compressive optic neuropathy (CON) is slow progressive painless loss of vision in one eye.

Table 2. Clinical characteristics of optic neuritis, papilledema, and ischemic optic neuropathy

Symptoms	Optic neuritis	Papilledema	AION (nonarteritic)
visual	rapidly progressive loss of central vision	no visual loss, transient obscurations	acute field defect commonly altitudinal
other	tender globe, pain on motion	headache, nausea, focal neurological signs	none
Bilateral	rare	almost always	typically unilateral
Pupil LR	diminished LR no anisocoria	normal LR no anisocoria	diminished no anisocoria
Acuity	diminished	normal	variable
Fundus	normal	disc swelling	pallid segmental disk edema

Because vision declines slowly over weeks and months, CON does not play an important role in the differential diagnosis of acute visual loss. The visual disturbance can, however, be a confounding neurological deficit if it is discovered by chance at the time of an emergency.

Patients usually notice visual loss when the central visual field is affected (central scotoma), producing loss of visual acuity. Subjectively, decreased color saturation is common, though patients often do not report this spontaneously. The optic disk is normal, atrophic, or even edematous.

Causes of CON can be grouped as follows:

1. neoplastic
   - pituitary adenoma/apoplexy
   - craniopharyngeoma
   - lymphoma
   - primary optic nerve tumors
2. non-neoplastic
   - carotid aneurysm
   - sarcoidosis, tuberculosis
   - fungal, parasitic infections (AIDS)

Although there may be a number of other symptoms that suggest regional or generalized disease, the visual symptom is frequently the only indication that a lesion is present.

Functional Visual Loss

The possibility of a functional origin of visual loss should always be considered in patients with isolated findings and an otherwise normal neurological examination. Functional visual loss can occur in children and adults, in the elderly and the adolescent. Some patients have obvious psychiatric disorders, while others appear emotionally healthy.

The diagnosis of functional visual loss should particularly be considered

- Whenever there is a mismatch between subjective complaints and objective findings
- When there is no relative afferent pupil defect
- When the fundus is normal months after the onset of visual loss
- When there is inconsistency in the acuity fraction when the patient is tested at various distances from the eye chart
- When the visual field is tubular or spiral
- When the visual evoked responses are normal

Suggested Reading

Bernstein EF (1988) Amaurosis fugax. Springer, Berlin Heidelberg New York

Boghen DR, Glaser JS (1975) Ischemic optic neuropathy. The clinical profile and natural history. Brain 98:689

Glaser JS (1990) Neuro-ophthalmology. Lippincott, Philadelphia

Gmeiner H-J, Kömpf D, Ruprecht K-W (1989) Ischämisch bedingte Augenerkrankungen und extrakranielle Carotisstenose/-verschluss. In: Fischer P-A, Baas H, Enzensberger W (eds) Gerontoneurologie, Enzephalitiden, Neurogenetik. Springer, Berlin Heidelberg New York, pp 1063–1066 (Verhandlungen der Deutschen Gesellschaft für Neurologie 5)

Hayreh SS (1975) Anterior ischemic optic neuropathy. Springer, Berlin Heidelberg New York

Hollenhorst RW (1961) Significance of bright plaques in the retinal arterioles. JAMA 178:123–129

Lessel S (1989) Indirect optic nerve trauma. Arch Ophthalmol 107:382

Miller NR (1985) Walsh and Hoyt's clinical neuro-ophthalmology, 4th edn, vol 2. Williams and Wilkins, Baltimore

Müller M, Wessel K, Mehdorn E, Kömpf D, Kessler C (1993) Carotid artery disease in vascular ocular syndromes. J Clin Neuro-ophthalmol 13:175–180

Miller NR (1990) The management of traumatic optic neuropathy. Arch Ophthalmol 108: 430–435

Rizzo JF, Lessell S (1988) Risk of developing multiple sclerosis after uncomplicated optic neuritis. Neurology 38:185

Ruprecht KW, Kömpf D (1987) Amaurosis fugax. In: Lund O-E, Waubke TN (eds) Okuläre Symptome. Strategien der Untersuchung. Enke, Stuttgart, pp 35–46

Savino PJ, Glaser JS, Cassady J (1977) Retinal stroke: Is the patient at risk? Arch Ophthalmol 95:1185–1189

Savino PJ (1988) Risk of cerebrovascular disease in patients with anterior ischemic optic neuropathy. In: Bernstein EF (ed) Amaurosis fugax. Springer, Berlin Heidelberg New York

Sfytche TJ, Bulpitt CJ, Kohner EM (1974) Effect of changes in intraocular pressure on the retinal microcirculation. Br J Ophthalmol 58:514–522

Unsöld R, Seeger W (1989) Compressive optic nerve lesions at the optic canal. Springer, Berlin Heidelberg New York

Wray SH (1988) Visual aspects of extracranial carotid artery disease. In: Bernstein EF (ed) Amaurosis fugax. Springer, Berlin Heidelberg New York, pp 72–80

Wray SH (1988) Occlusion of the central retinal artery. In: Bernstein EF (ed) Amaurosis fugax. Springer, Berlin Heidelberg New York, pp 81–89

Wray SH (1991) Neuro-ophthalmologic diseases. In: Rosenberg RN (ed) Comprehensive neurology. Raven, New York, pp 659–698

Zeumer H, Freytay HJ, Knospe U (1992) Intravascular thrombolysis in central nervous system cerebrovascular disease. Neuroimag Clin North Am 2:359–369

Chapter 34

Acute Autonomic Instability

DERK KRIEGER and SHREYAS V. PATEL

Introduction

This chapter concerns acute autonomic instability in neurologic diseases
affecting the anatomic integrity of central and peripheral autonomic control
loops. In particular, cardiovascular
and respiratory dysfunction may act as
life-threatening complications during
neurocritical care treatment and
deserve further discussion. The autonomic nervous system orchestrates a
wide range of vegetative functions via
either the sympathetic nervous system
or the parasympathetic system, or
both. Furthermore, there is evidence
for diffuse interaction between the
autonomic and endocrine systems.
Thus cardiovascular and pulmonary
function, electrolyte-fluid balance, and
adaptation to variable demands contribute to the integrity of autonomic
control mechanisms. Responses of
peripheral end-organs are determined
by transmitter release; catecholamines
at the sympathetic nerve ending,
acetylcholine at the parasympathetic
neuron effector junction, and addi-

tional humoral contribution of circulating epinephrine and norepinephrine
from the adrenal medulla. Overactivity of the sympathetic limb of the
autonomic system is thought to be
the phenomenon that links cardiac and
pulmonary pathology found in acute
central nervous accidents. Profound
effects on the heart and the lungs may
contribute to the death rates of many
primary neurologic conditions such
as subarachnoid hemorrhage, stroke,
status epilepticus, and head trauma.
The cardiovascular system plays a
pivotal role in homeostasis by adjusting the blood supply to various vascular beds in proportion to their level
of activity. The maintenance of arterial
pressure and the regulation of cardiac
output in the face of different behavioral demands can be achieved by
integration of peripheral reflex inputs
and central drives at the level of the
brain stem. Additionally, the autonomic nervous system affects cardiovascular function through influences
on electrolyte and fluid balance and
hormonal mechanisms. Cardiorespiratory interactions involve a complex and still unresolved integration at
different sites of the nervous system;

Section Editor: Daniel F. Hanley

however, they may play a crucial role in explaining respiratory arrest or fatal cardiac arrhythmia in neurologic disease.

Circulatory Reflex Control

Several groups of peripheral receptors contribute to the reflex control of circulation, the role and characteristics of the baroreceptor reflex being defined in most detail. The nucleus of the tractus solitarius (NTS) seems to be the primary site of integration of most cardiovascular afferents within the central nervous system, as it receives extensive afferents from arterial baro- and chemoreceptors, other vagal afferents, and input from diverse regions of the CNS. Neurophysiologic studies in animals using extra- and intracellular recordings from NTS neurons were performed to elucidate synaptic pathways of baroreceptor inputs. This approach revealed a significant convergence of excitatory and inhibitory carotid sinus and aortic depressor nerve inputs on NTS neurons; however, the detailed synaptic organization of the NTS remains unresolved. Regarding NTS output, there are numerous pathways discovered by neuroanatomic tracing studies, which include projections to the ventrolateral medulla, nucleus ambiguus (NA), nucleus parabrachialis, other midbrain regions, spinal cord, hypothalamus, and the amygdala nuclei. Among these different interactions, the most important for baroreceptor control of heart rate appears to be the link between NTS and NA.

Regarding sympathetic output, evidence suggests that preganglionic activity is controlled by several pathways originating in the rostral ventrolateral medulla and terminating on neurons in the intermediolateral cell column (IML) of the thoracic spinal cord. Baroreceptor activity inhibits sympathetic efferent discharge, probably by a direct connection from the NTS to the rostral ventrolateral medulla. Current opinion, however, regards regulation of IML activity to be complex and mediated by numerous bulbospinal pathways, suggesting integrative processes for the control of preganglionic neuron activity within the spinal cord. Further modulation of spinal preganglionic sympathetic activity is achieved by various transmitters which serve the multiple inputs of the IML.

Serotonergic pathways arise from the rapheal nuclei and the ventral medulla. Adrenergic efferents appear to arise from neuronal clusters in the lateral medulla. Noradrenergic efferents arise from the lateral pons. Neural pathways using oxytonin appear to arise from the paraventricular nucleus and synapse in the IML. Other neuropeptides such as angiotensin II, substance P, and thyrotropin-releasing hormone are found in the IML, but their sites of origin are yet undetermined. Thus, the regulation of sympathetic preganglionic activity involves a complex interplay of excitatory and inhibitory inputs at the level of the IML.

Cardiorespiratory Interactions

Neurons collectively known as respiratory neurons are found at many different sites in the CNS and share the common attribute of having their discharge patterns modulated by respiration. Neurons with inspiratory and expiratory discharge patterns are located in the pons and medulla. As with cardiovascular control, respiratory neurons seem to be integrated at different CNS levels. However, the exact anatomy and neurobiology of the respiratory controller remain speculative. Currently, experimental evidence locates the site of the respiratory rhythm pacemaker to be in the vicinity of the Bötzinger complex rostral to the ventral respiratory group. Neurons in a very limited region of the ventrolateral medulla, called the pre-Bötzinger complex, are capable of generating respiratory rhythm through communications with interneurons and premotoneurons that transmit oscillatory drive to spinal respiratory motoneurons. Sensory inputs to the respiratory controller include numerous peripheral chemo- and mechanoreceptors and central chemoreceptors found at the ventral surface of the medulla at the exit of the 9th and 10th nerves.

Hypercapnia stimulates a progressive increase in respiration and arterial pressure. It is well recognized that the respiratory response to hypercapnia emanates primarily from the central chemoreceptors. These same chemoreceptors also mediate the circulatory response. Hence, it is postulated that coordination of the respiratory and cardiovascular systems is achieved by the parallel output of the respiratory rhythm generator to the respiratory and cardiovascular control networks. However, respiration must exceed a certain threshold before respiratory-related discharge of sympathetic activity becomes manifest, suggesting that the rhythm generator predominantly

serves the respiratory neurons. If central respiratory drive exceeds a given level, as in hypercapnia, the rhythm is "shared" with the sympathetic control neurons, thus coupling both vital systems.

An example of cardiorespiratory interaction occurs in the moment-to-moment variation of sinus rhythm known as sinus arrhythmia. This is the consequence of respiratory control of the vagal output to the heart and involves two factors: (a) vagal cardiomotor neurons suppressed by activity of the respiratory generator during inspiration and (b) inhibitory peripheral vagal afferents stimulated by lung inflation. The firing pattern of inhibitory cardiac vagal efferents closely mirrors the output of postinspiratory neurons in the medulla that discharge in phase with the phrenic nerve and continues after inspiratory discharge has ceased. Like the postinspiratory neurons, cardioinhibitory neurons are particularly sensitive to inputs from irritant receptors in the airways or to electrical stimulation of the superior laryngeal nerve in animal models. Such stimuli evoke a prolonged respiratory pause with continuing phrenic nerve avtivity (resembling apneusis) and vagal bradycardia.

Neuroendocrine Interactions in Autonomic Control

It is becoming increasingly evident that attempts to separate endocrine from neural factors in autonomic regulation force an artificial division upon an integrated neuroendocrine system. Hormones such as angiotensin II and vasopressin act as important cardiovascular effectors in the CNS and peripherally in vascular tissues. Several other peptides may be involved in central blood-pressure control. The NTS has been shown to contain endogenous opioids, substance P, and somatostatin.

Endogenous opioids have been shown to attenuate baroreceptor-reflex function, which can be reversed by naloxone in animal models. Adrenal steroids are known to act both pre- and postsynaptically by influencing neurotransmitter uptake and release and even to alter the synthesis of neuronal proteins. Important CNS effector sites for blood pressure regulation by catecholamines are the NTS, dorsal vagal nucleus, and nucleus reticularis lateralis. The content of noradrenergic and adrenergic neurons has slight regional variation and the transmitters bind to a_1, a_2 and b-receptors. The a_2 receptor seems to be most important, since a_2-receptor agonists such as clonidine lower bood pressure in normotensive and hypertensive subjects. The fall in blood pressure is associated with a fall in plasma norepinephrine secondary to a central inhibition of sympathetic tone.

The distinction between peripheral peptide hormones and neuropeptides is now meaningless, as almost all the classical peptide hormones have been discovered in the brain. It appears that neuropeptides exert their neuromodulatory effects by processes other than synaptic transmission, and that CNS peptidergic neurons may act quite similar to their glandular counterparts in the periphery. Brain monoamines, however, function primarily by means of synaptic transmission.

Clinical Relevance and Management

Neurogenic Heart Disease

Cardiographic abnormalities in patients with neurologic disease can be divided in two major categories: cardiac arrhythmias and repolarization abnormalities. Most often, the changes are seen best in the anterolateral and inferolateral leads with large inverted T waves, large U waves, and prolonged QT intervals. Numerous cases of neurogenic electrocardiographic changes have been reported; however, little is known about the mechanism of these changes. Their similarity to those produced by either intravenous or intracoronary catecholamine infusion has been noted. Likewise, in patients with subarachnoid hemorrhage ECG abnormalities were consistent with myocardial infarction but in autopsied cases infarction was not demonstrated. Acute autonomic dysregulation involving the orbital-frontal cortex and hypothalamus was postulated. Currently, it is felt that disinhibition of hypothalamic or other autonomic regulatory centers in these individuals results in elevated catecholamine levels and concomitant ECG changes. Raised norepinephrine levels have been found after cerebral infarction and subarachnoid hemorrhage, lending some support to this hypothesis. Furthermore, stress-induced myocardial lesions can be prevented by sympathetic blockade, using antiadrenergic agents (mecamylamine) and catecholamine – depleting agents (reserpine). Cardiac enzymes are also elevated in many, but not all patients with presumed neurogenic electrocardiographic changes. The isoenzyme creatine kinase myocardial band (CK MB) was found elevated in these patients, supporting the presumption that there is a myocardial cell injury. Autopsy studies in patients who experienced sudden death due to neurogenic cardiac complications revealed myofibrillar degeneration. Myofibrillar degeneration is also known as coagulative myocytolysis with contraction band necrosis and is easily distinguishable from coagulation necrosis, the major lesion in myocardial infarction. In coagulation necrosis muscle cells die in a relaxed state, whereas in myofibrillar degeneration cells die in a hypercontracted state with prominent contraction bands. Furthermore, calcification occurs almost immediately in myofibrillar degeneration, but only late in coagulation necrosis. Myofibrillar degeneration with immediate calcification is also known in cardiac surgery as the "stone heart", a complication that occurred at reperfusion following cardiopulmonary bypass prior to the use of adequate cardioplegic solutions. Since myofibrillar degeneration is predominantly subendocardial, it may involve the cardiac-conducting system, giving rise to cardiac arrhythmias.

The phenomenon of electrocardiographic abnormalities in neurologic disease is not rare: in a large series of consecutive stroke patients, 90% showed transient abnormalities on the ECG, compared with only 50% of a control population. Despite the fact that stroke and coronary artery disease often co-exist and that it is difficult to distinguish between cause and effect, there are obviously a fair number of stroke patients presenting with authentic neurogenic electrocardio-graphic changes. The rapid appearance and disappearance of electrocardiographic changes with perturbations of the nervous system strongly suggests that effects are due more likely to neural than to humoral factors. Thus, from another perspective neurogenic cardiac complications can be explained by nervous system stimulation. It has been established that stimulation of the lateral hypothalamus produces hypertension and electrocardiographic changes similar to those detected in patients with central nervous system damage. Spinal section at the C-2 level and stellate block, but not vagotomy, prevent this. In contrast, stimulation of the anterior hypothalamus causes bradycardia, prevented by vagotomy. Bilateral hypothalamic stimulation consistently produces the typical histologic features of myofibrillar degeneration. There have been reports of cardiac dysrhythmogenesis arising from the insular cortex, presumably due to profuse interconnections with the limbic system, the hypothalamus, and other regions of autonomic control. Animal experiments further suggest that lesions in specific regions of the insular cortex cause isolated cardiac dysrhythmias without alterations in blood pressure or respiration.

Neurogenic Pulmonary Edema

Neurogenic pulmonary edema (NPE) is a rapidly developing, protein-rich alveolar pulmonary edema that occurs in a variety of neurologic diseases, such as head injury, epileptic seizure, brainstem and supratentorial lesions, subarachnoid hemorrhage, dysautonomia, and intoxications. The underlying mechanisms involve autonomic dysregulation disturbing the pulmonary capillary-tissue-lymphatic system, mediated mainly by sympathetic limb overactivity and, to a lesser extent, by release of catecholamines from the adrenal glands. Medullary neuronal populations in the region of the nuclei reticularis gigantocellularis and parvicellularis probably mediate the arterial hypertension and pulmonary edema associated with acute supratentorial mass lesions. This condition, also referred to as the Cushing response, is characterized by an acute increase of cardiac output, blood pressure elevation, tachycardia, and augmented oxygen utilization. Currently, ICP-induced arterial hypertension is thought to result from central mediated vasoconstriction, increased cardiac output, or a combination of both mechanisms.

Additionally, the abovementioned medullary centers are thought to be inhibited by NTS neurons, since bilateral NTS lesions are known to produce NPE. Finally, ablation and stimulation experiments of the caudal hypothalamus and lateral preoptic region in animal models have produced similar symptoms. Both mechanisms producing NPE and systemic hypertension may be prevented by either cervial cord trans-section or sympathetic blockade at different levels of the effector system, but not by vagotomy and parasympathatic agents.

At the pulmonary capillary level, transcapillary fluid migration is governed by the hydrostatic pressure and the interstitial tissue colloid osmotic pressure. Both favor water moving out, and the plasma colloid osmotic pressure and the interstitial hydrostatic pressure draw water into the capillary. Plasma colloid osmotic pressure is maintained by tight interendothelial junctions of the capillary wall. Plasma hydrostatic pressure is regulated by the smooth muscle tone of the precapillary arterioles and the postcapillary venules. Thus, enhanced transcapillary fluid migration occurs in the presence of mismatch of these four Starling components. Small amounts of extra fluid in the interstitium can be cleared by the lymphatic outflow; however, when the amount of fluid exceeds lymphatic drainage capacities, alveolar pulmonary edema develops.

Pulmonary vessels have both a sympathetic and a parasympathetic nerve supply. Parasympathic fibers arise from the trunk of the vagus nerve, and stimulation results in pulmonary vasodilation with a drop in capillary hydrostatic pressure of unclear significance. Sympathetic innervation probably arises at multiple thoracic levels and reaches the pulmonary vessels via segmental ganglia. Alpha-receptor activation seems to cause vasoconstriction, while beta-receptor activation induces vasodilation. Additionally, there is evidence that alpha-receptor activation has pronounced effects on the venous side of the pulmonary circulation. In conclusion, NPE results from a massive centrally mediated alpha-adrenergic discharge producing generalized vasoconstriction with high systemic and pulmonary vascular pressures and redistribution of blood volume.

Several factors are putatively related to the genesis of NPE. Left atrial pressure elevation induced by associated acute systemic hypertension may cause a sudden rise in capillary hydrostatic pressure with subsequent pulmonary edema. In a few NPE patients studied with Swan-Ganz catheters, left atrial pressure was elevated, but not severely enough to explain pulmonary edema. Pulmonary outflow constriction at the site of the pulmonary venules may contribute to hydrostatic pressure elevation independent of the left atrial pressure. In addition, arteriovenous shunting augments hydrostatic pressure and may further explain the severely decreased O_2 saturation often encountered in these patients. Furthermore, sympathetic stimulation affects capillary permeability by direct influence on contractile elements of endothelial cells, thus explaining the high protein content in NPE.

To summarize, excluding pulmonary edema secondary to cardiac factors, NPE appears to be modulated by the sympathetic arm of the autonomic nervous system via a combination of hemodynamic and endothelial factors.

Clinical Situations in Neurocritical Care

Cerebral Lesions

Focal and diffuse cerebral lesions, particularly associated with elevated ICP or brain stem disease, may cause autonomic complications involving the cardiovascular, pulmonary, and gastrointestinal systems. Autonomic instability has been most extensively studied in head-injured patients, but it may also occur in association with cerebral infarction and intracerebral and subarachnoid hemorrhage. In clinical practice, the severity of autonomic dysfunction may vary greatly between minor and central importance. Careful monitoring of basic parameters, such as heart rate, rhythm variability, breathing pattern, and blood pressure, is indicated, and depending on the severity of the autonomic dysfunction, further invasive monitoring precedures, such as blood gas analysis, pulmonary wedge pressure, and cardiac output determination may be necessary to recognize and treat these conditions. Besides cardiopulmonary deterioration, patients presenting with acute cerebral lesions are at risk for gastrointestinal complications, in particular hemorrhage. In head-injured patients a hyperdynamic state characterized by increased cardiac output, blood pressure, heart rate, and oxygen utilization that responds to beta-blockade (propranolol) is seen and results from increased sympathetic activity. The Cushing reflex, hypertension secondary to raised ICP, is due to centrally mediated vasoconstriction or increased cardiac output. Cardiac arrhythmias and myofibrillar degeneration have also been described in head injury. Neurogenic pulmonary edema is a potentially fatal source of hypoxemia and has to be distinguished from disseminated intravascular coagulation, pneumonia, and pulmonary embolism. All three conditions might eventually progress to ARDS, which has a particularly high mortality. In severely traumatized individuals pulmonary fat embolism may appear within 24–48 h and causes hypoxemia, tachypnoea, tachcardia, fever, bronchospasm, and ECG abnormalities. Pulmonary embolism from deep-vein thrombosis is a major threat to immobilized or comatose patients and tends to occur at a later stage of the disease. Gastrointestinal bleeding is relatively frequent in severely head injured patients and may result from steroids and sympathetic overactivity. However, the exact mechanisms and importance of gastric secretion, hydrogen ion concentration, and ischemia remain unclear. In practice, the most frequent lesion is erosive gastritis in the presence of hyperacidity. Approximately 40% of gastrointestinal bleeding begins within 48 h and only 20% after 1 week. As a consequence, antacids or H_2-blockers should be routinely administered to these patients.

Subarachnoid hemorrhage in particular is associated with ECG changes. The exact figure is unknown. Sudden death in subarachnoid hemorrhage is frequently due to serious arrhythmias and may account for the high number of patients who die before reaching the hospital. Experience in most stroke units indicates that cardiac arrhythmias are frequent but rarely serious or fatal in ischemic stroke.

Electroconvulsive therapy (ECT) is an interesting model for the study of systemic effects of seizures. In ECT-treated patients cardiovascular complications are rare, but severe hypertension and pulmonary edema are the leading causes of death. In animal experiments, it has been shown that autonomic instability is attenuated by beta-adrenergic blockade or adrenalectomy. Clinical studies have revealed an abrupt increase in sympathetic activity and circulating catecholamine levels in patients undergoing ECT. Further attention has to be directed towards ECG abnormalities, since T-wave changes frequently occur and an initial parasympathetic discharge may cause asystole.

Neuroleptic malignant syndrome caused by administration of neuroleptics to psychotic patients and catatonic states of schizophrenia are often associated with autonomic instability. The core syndrome of muscle stiffness and rigidity in combination with hyperthermia has been successfully treated with dantrolene and dopaminergic agents intravenously. Hypertension and tachycardia may be early signs of the syndrome or may represent a forme fruste in some patients.

Spinal Lesions

In acute, severely disabling spinal lesions, dysautonomia causes several problems that merit discussion. In high cervical cord injuries worsening of the respiratory status frequently develops during the first few days. This is attributed to cord expansion with edema, exceptionally ascending to the medulla. Particularly pertinent to critical care is a syndrome of hypoventilation and, in its extreme form, sleep apnea in patients with high cervical injuries. It may be exaggerated by mechanical factors such as immobilization and constitutional factors such as diminished oropharyngeal space and is currently attributed to decreased sensitivity of the central ventilatory drive to carbon dioxide. Clinically, a vague subjective sensation of air hunger may progress to a confusional state with sighing respirations. In later stages patients may progressively hypoventilate and eventually cease to breathe, especially during sleep. Oxygen should be administered with care, as these patients are often dependent on hypoxic drive and may require mechanical ventilation at night. Besides respiratory problems with high cervical injuries, there can be significant variations in blood pressure and heart rate following tracheal suctioning or position changes. Gastrointestinal atony may persist for several days, and patients with thoracolumbar fractures can have a reflex ileus for up to 2 weeks. Autonomic dysfunction, in particular "cholinergic crises" with reflex bradycardia and even cardiac arrest, profuse sweating, pilomotor erection, and headaches, can occur after recovery from spinal shock. These crises can be precipitated by bladder fullness, tracheal suctioning, and other painful stimuli below the level of trans-section. They can be treated with anticholinergic drugs, but these drugs exacerbate bladder and bowel atony and careful use is mandatory. Spontaneous temperature fluctuations due to dysautonomia are common and may complicate the recognition and adequate management of serious infectious disease.

Peripheral Lesions

Dysautonomia in peripheral lesions requiring neurocritical care is almost exclusively described in Guillain-Barré syndrome (GBS). Autonomic dysfunction is a relatively common but somewhat overestimated clinical problem in GBS. Cardiovascular abnormalities include absence of sinus arrhythmia, fixed or paroxysmal arrhythmias, orthostatic hypotension, and sustained or paroxysmal hypertension. Complete heart block with GBS requiring pacemaker implantation is dangerous but rare. Morphological ECG changes such as ST-T-segment and T-wave ab-

nomalities may occur in some patients and may raise the question of associated myocarditis. Intermittent or persistent hypertension is an issue in GBS and should be treated at higher levels. As in high cervical spine lesions, tracheal suction procedures or position changes may cause considerable blood pressure and heart rate changes. Other features of dysautonomia in peripheral lesions include potentially dangerous ileus and bladder dysfunction, in particular urinary retention. The most profound abnormalities occur in patients with severe weakness and respiratory failure. Episodes of acute and severe hypotension seen in GBS appear to be due to a vasodepressor sesponse with an accompanying drop in the systemic vascular resistance. Pulse rate is usually unchanged or only slightly slowed, within a range of 70–90 bpm. In some patients vasodepressor episodes alternate with extreme hypertension. The mechanism of GBS dysautonomic vasodepressor episodes is unknown, whereas hypertension may be due to the loss of the baroreflex buffering capacity caused by an afferent neuropathy.

The syndrome of inappropriate ADH secretion (SIADH) has been attributed to dysautonomia in Guillain-Barré patients. Afferent inputs from cardiovascular receptors, including atrial, aortic, and carotid receptors, inhibit ADH release, so autonomic afferent demyelination in GBS could result in SIADH. In other cases, however, ADH secretion is triggered by reduced venous return in positive end-expiratory airway pressure breathing.

Generalized tetanus produces increased muscle tone and spasms. An accompanying hyperactive sympathetic state includes labile or sustained hypertension, profuse diaphoresis, and fever, associated with increased circulating catecholamine levels. Tetanus toxin is thought to have a direct effect on the autonomic system, because adrenergic overactivity persists when muscle activity is eliminated by curare.

In botulism an anticholinergic state is characteristic, with blurred vision and dry mouth. Blood pressure and heart rate control are impaired due to the absence of parasympathetic baroreflex modulation. For the management of patients with botulism it is important to consider that the autonomic component of the illness may recover more slowly than the neuromuscular blockade.

Suggested Reading

Agar JM (1966) The medical complication of the early management of head injury in the adolescent. Med J Aust 78:1182–1183

Appenzeller O, Marshall J (1963) Vasomotor disturbance in Landry-Guillain-Barré syndrome. Arch Neurol 9:368–372

Barger AC, Liebowitz MR, Herd JA (1961) Chronic catheterization of the coronary artery: infusion of autonomic drugs in the unanesthetized dog. Fed Proc 20:107

Barman SM, Gebber GL (1985) Axonal projection patterns of ventrolateral medullospinal sympathoexcitatory neurons. J Neurophysiol 53:1551–1566

Baroldi G (1975) Different morphological types of myocardial cell death in man. In: Fleckenstein A, Rona G (eds) Recent advances in studies of cardiac structure and metabolism, vol 6. Pathophysiology and morphology of myocardial cell alteration. University Park Press, Baltimore, pp 385–397

Bredin DP (1977) Guillain-Barré syndrome: the unresolved cardiac problems. Ir J Med Sci 146:273–279

Buisseret P (1982) Acute pulmonary oedema following grand mal epilepsy and as a complication of electric shock therapy. Br J Dis Chest 76:194–195

Burch GE, Myers R, Abildskov JA (1954) A new electrocardiographic pattern observed in cerebrovascular accidents. Circulation 9:719–726

Carlson RW, Shaeffer RC, Michaels SG, Weil MH (1979) Pulmonary edema following intracranial hemorrhage. Chest 3:319–325

Clifton GL, Robertson CS, Kyper K et al. (1983) Cardiovascular response to head trauma. J Neurosurgery 59:447–454

Cropp CF, Manning GF (1960) Electrocardiographic change simulating myocardial ischemia and infarction associated with spontaneous intracranial hemorrhage. Circulation 22:24–27

Cruickshank JM, Neil-Dwyer G, Stott A (1974) The possible role of catecholamines, corticosteroids and potassium in the production of ECG changes associated with subarachnoid hemorrhage. Br Heart J 36:697–706

Cushing HC (1932) Peptic ulcers and the interbrain. Surg Gynecol Obstet 55:1–34

Dampney RAL, Kumada M, Reis DJ (1979) Central neural mechanisms of the cerebral ischemic response. Circ Res 44:48–62

Darragh TM, Simon RP (1985) Nucleus tractus solitarius lesions elevate pulmonary arterial pressure and lymph flow. Ann Neurol 17:565–569

Dimant J, Grob D (1977) Electrocardiographic changes and myocardial damage in patients with acute cerebrovascular accidents. Stroke 8:448–455

Donoghue S, Felder RB, Gilbey MP, Jordan D, Spyer KM (1985) Postsynaptic activity evoked in the nucleus tractus solitarius by carotid and aortic nerve afferents in the cat. J Physiol (Lond) 360:261–273

Ducker TB, Simmons RL (1968) Increased intracranial pressure and pulmonary edema, part II: the hemodynamic response of dogs and monkeys to increased ICP. J Neurosurgery 28:118–123

Estanol BV, Marin OS (1975) Cardiac arrhythmias and sudden death in subarachnoid hemorrhage. Stroke 6:382–386

Faulhauer K, Hermann H, Harbauer G (1971) Cardiovascular response to slowly increased ICP. Acta Neurochir (Wien) 24:63–70

Fitts CT, Cathcaut RS, Artz CP et al. (1971) Acute GI tract ulceration: Cushing's ulcer, steroid ulcer, Curling's ulcer and stress ulcer. Am J Surg 37:218–223

Hammer WJ, Leussenhop AJ, Weintraub AM (1975) Observations on the electrocardiographic changes associated with subarachnoid hemorrhage with special reference to their genesis. Am J Med 59: 427–433

Hawkins WE, Clower BR (1971) Myocardial damage after head trauma and simulated intracranial hemorrhage in mice: the role of the autonomic nervous system. Cardiovasc Res 5:524–529

Hersch G (1961) Electrocardiographic changes in head injuries. Circulation 28:853–860

Hodson AK, Hurwitz BJ, Albrecht R (1984) Dysautonomia in Guillain-Barré syndrome with dorsal root ganglion neuropathy, Wallerian degeneration, and fatal myocarditis. Ann Neurol 15:88–95

Hugenholtz PG (1962) Electrocardiographic abnormalities in cerebral disorders: report of six cases and review of the literature. Am Heart J 63:451–461

Iversen IL (1983) Nonopioid neuropeptides in mammalian CNS. Annu Rev Pharmacol Toxicol 23:1–27

Jordan D, Spyer KM (1986) Brainstem integration of cardiovascular and pulmonary afferent activity. In: Cervero F, Morrison JFB (eds) Progress in brain research, vol 67. Elsevier Science, Amsterdam, pp 295–314

Kamada T, Fusamoto H, Kawano S et al. (1977a) Acute gastrointestinal bleeding following head injury. Am J Gastroenterol 68:249–253

Kamada T, Fusamoto H, Kawano S et al. (1977b) Gastrointestinal bleeding following head injury: a clinical study of 433 cases. J Trauma 17:44–47

Kolin A, Kvasnicka J (1963) Pseudoinfarction pattern of the QRS complex in experimental cardiac hypoxia induced by noradrenaline. Cardiologia 43:362–370

Krull F, Schuchardt V, Haupt WF, Meves J (1988) Prognosis of acute polyneuritis requiring artificial ventilation. Intensive Care Med 14:388–392

Li C, Gefter WB (1992) Acute pulmonary edema induced by overdosage of phenothiazines. Chest 101:102–104

Lichtenfield P (1971) Autonomic dysfunction in the Guillain-Barré syndrome. Am J Med 50:772–780

Loewy AD, Neil JJ (1981) The role of descending monoaminergic systems in central control of blood pressure. Fed Proc 40:2278–2285

Lopes OU, Palmer JF (1976) Proposed respiratory "gating" mechanisms for cardiac slowing. Nature 264:454–456

Maire FW, Patton HD (1956) Neural structures involved in the genesis of preoptic pulmonary edema, gastric erosions and behavior changes. Am J Physiol 184:345–350

Malik AB (1985) Mechanisms of neurogenic pulmonary edema. Circ Res 57:1–18

Maron MB, Dawson CA (1980) Pulmonary venoconstriction caused by elevated cerebrospinal fluid pressure in the dog. J Appl Physiol 49:73–78

McAllen RM, Spyer KM (1976) The location of cardiac vagal preganglionic motoneurones in the medulla of the cat. J Physiol (Lond) 258:187–204

McAllen RM, Spyer KM (1978a) Two types of vagal preganglionic motoneurones projecting to the heart and lungs. J Physiol (Lond) 282:353–364

McAllen RM, Spyer KM (1978b) The baroreceptor input to cardiac vagal motoneurones. J Physiol (Lond) 282:365–374

Mc Ewen BS, Davis PG, Parsons B, Pfaff DW (1979) The brain as a target for steroid hormone action. Annu Rev Neurosci 2: 65–112

Melville KI, Blum B, Shister HE et al. (1963) Cardiac ischemic changes and arrhythmias induced by hypothalamic stimulation. Am J Cardiot 12:781–791

Mesulam M-M, Mufson EJ (1982) Insula of the old world monkey, III: efferent cortical output and comments on function. J Comp Neurol 212:38–52

Mifflin SW, Spyer KM, Withington-Wray DJ (1986a) Hypothalamic inhibition of baroreceptor inputs in the nucleus of the tractus solitarius of the cat. J Physiol (Lond) 373: 58P

Mifflin SW, Spyer KM, Withington-Wray DJ (1986b) Lack of respiratory modulation of baroreceptor inputs in the nucleus of the tractus solitarius of the cat. J Physiol 376:33P

Millhorn DE (1986) Neural respiratory and circulatory interaction during chemoreceptor stimulation and cooling of the ventral medulla in cats. J Physiol (Lond) 370: 217–231

Moore RY, Bloom FE (1979) Central catecholamine neuron systems: anatomy and physiology of the norepinephrine and epinephrine systems. Annu Rev Neurosci 2:113–168

Myers M, Norris J, Hachinski VC (1981) Plasma norepinephrine in stroke. Stroke 12: 200–204

Nandiwada P, Hyman AL, Kadowitz PJ (1983) Pulmonary vasodilatory response to vagal stimulation and acetylcholine in the cat. Circ Res 53:86–95

Nathan MA, Reis DJ (1975) Fulminating arterial hypertension with pulmonary edema from release of adrenomedullary catecholamines after lesion of the anterior hypothalamus in the rat. Circ Res 37:226–235

Norris JW, Hachinski VC (1976) Intensive care management of stroke patients. Stroke 7: 573–577

Norris JW, Hachinski VC, Myers MG et al. (1979) Serum cardiac enzymes in stroke. Stroke 10:548–553

Norton L, Green J, Eiseman B (1970) Gastric secretory response to head injury. Arch Surg 101:200–204

Oppenheimer SM, Hachinski VC, Cechetto DF (1989) Cardiac chronotropic organization of the rat insular cortex. Soc Neurosci Abstr 15:595

Oppenheimer SM, Cechetto DF, Hachinski VC (1990) Cerebrogenic cardiac arrhythmias. Cerebral electrocardiographic influences and their role in sudden death. Arch Neurol 47:513–519

Pace NL (1976) Cardiac monitoring and demand pacemaker in Gullain-Barré syndrome. Arch Neurol 33:374

Petty MA, Reid JL (1981) Opiate analogs, substance P, and baroreceptor reflexes in the rabbit. Hypertension 3 [Suppl 1]:142–147

Raab W, Stark E, MacMillan WH et al. (1961) Sympathogenic origin and anti-adrenergic prevention of stress-induced myocardial lesions. Am J Cardiol 8:203–211

Reid JL (1981) The clinical pharmacology of clonidine and related central antihypertensive agents. Br J Clin Pharmacol 12:295–302

Reynolds RW (1963) Pulmonary edema as a consequence of hypothalamic lesion in rats. Science 141:930–932

Richter DW (1982) Generation and maintenance of the respiratory rhythm. J Exp Biol 100:93–107

Robertson CS, Clifton GL, Grossman RG (1984) Oxygen utilization and cardiovascular function in head-injured patients. Neurosurgery 15:307–314

Ropper AH, Wijdicks EFM, Truax BT (1991) Guillain-Barré syndrome. Davies, Phiadelphia, pp 102–105

Rosell S (1980) Neuronal control of microvessels. Annu Rev Physiol 42:359–371

Ross CA, Ruggiero DA, Reis DJ (1985) Projections from the nucleus tractus solitarii to the rostral ventrolateral medulla. J Comp Neurol 242:511–534

Ruggiero DA, Mraovitch S, Granata AR, Anwar M, Reis DJ (1987) A role of insular cortex in cardiovascular function. J Comp Neurol 257:189–207

Sarnoff SJ, Sarnoff LC (1952) Neurohemodynamics of pulmonary edema. I. Autonomic influence of pulmonary vascular pressures and acute pulmonary edema state. Dis Chest 22:685–696

Scharrer B (1977) Peptides in neurobiology: historical introduction. In: Gainer H (ed) Peptides in neurobiology. Plenum, New York, pp 1–8

Simon RP, Gean-Marton AD, Sander JE (1991) Medullary lesion inducing pulmonary edema: a magnetic imaging study. Ann Neurol 30:727–730

Smith MK, Ray CT (1972) Cardiac arrhythmias, increased intracranial pressure, and the autonomic nervous system. Chest 61: 125–133

Smith JC, Ellenberger HH, Ballanyi K, Richter DW, Feldman JL (1991) Pre-Bötzinger complex: a brainstem region that may generate respiratory rhythm in mammals. Science 254:726–729

Sun M-K, Guyenet PG (1985) GABA-mediated baroreceptor inhibition of reticulospinal neurons. Am J Physiol 249:R672–R680

Swann KW, Black PM (1984) Deep vein thrombosis and pulmonary embolism in neurosurgical patients. A review. J Neurosurg 61:1055–1062

Swank RL, Dugger GS (1954) Fat embolism: a clinical and experimental study of mechanisms involved. Surg Gynecol Obstet 98: 641–652

Touho H, Karasawa J, Shishido H, Yamada K, Yamazaki Y (1989) Neurogenic pulmonary edema in the acute stage of hemorrhagic cerebrovascular disease. Neurosurgery 25: 762–768

Weir BK (1978) Pulmonary edema following fatal aneurysm rupture. J Neurosurg 49: 502–507

Yashon D (1978) Spinal injury. Appleton-Century-Crofts, New York

| # Abnormal Breathing Patterns

JEFFREY I. FRANK

Introduction

Normal respiratory function depends on the harmonious balance of numerous factors. The most important sensors of respiratory needs are the central and peripheral chemoreceptors and airway receptors. This information is communicated to various levels of the central nervous system (CNS) which, in turn, modulates the effector organs of respiration, including the lungs, upper airways, and respiratory musculature.

The brain stem is the primary site of automatic respiratory control, and the cerebral cortex governs voluntary respiration. Integration of the output of these anatomically and functionally separate respiratory control systems occurs primarily at the spinal cord level. The final common pathways of neural effector control are the inspiratory and expiratory spinal motor-neurons innervating respiratory musculature.

While this simplistic overview of the various neuroanatomical sites in-volved with respiratory feedback and control diminishes its complexity, it emphasizes the fact that neurological processes affecting any of these regions may cause respiratory dysfunction, manifest as abnormal breathing patterns. While respiratory pattern abnormalities are commonly associated with neurological insults, central and peripheral, they often go unrecognized. This chapter reviews some of the more important respiratory pattern abnormalities encountered in patients with neurological dysfunction, emphasizing their clinical significance and diagnostic and therapeutic implications.

Peripheral Disorders of Breathing

Myopathies, neuromuscular junction disorders, polyneuropathies, and motor neuronopathies all can cause respiratory dysfunction by impairing the function of respiratory effectors. Progressive respiratory musculature dysfunction, diaphragmatic and accessory, is the common denominator of all of these illnesses. Early in their

Section Editor: Daniel F. Hanley

course, the respiratory dysfunction is not readily apparent. It is not reflected in respiratory rate or appearance. However, diminished inspiratory pressures generated by the diaphragm progressively compromise lung capacity, sigh mechanisms, and cough. Atelectasis ensues, leading to perfusion of collapsed (nonventilated) alveoli, resulting in hypoxemia.

An increase in respiratory rate may be associated with the peripheral etiologies of respiratory dysfunction when peripheral and central sensors continue to drive breathing in response to the declining lung volumes and compromised oxygenation. Respiratory alkalosis can occur in some of these cases, but, more often, the minute volume of ventilation is unchanged since the increased respiratory rate is only to compensate for diminished tidal volumes.

The increase in respiratory rate which can occur with these patients further challenges respiratory musculature function. This can lead to a variety of abnormal breathing patterns that are common to non-neurological etiologies of breathing failure. Use of accessory musculature becomes exaggerated and, ultimately, grossly apparent (e.g., intercostal retraction, inspiratory scalene and abdominal muscular contractions).

A "paradoxical" breathing pattern would be common in the extreme. Whereas the abdomen usually becomes protuberant during inspiration due to inferior displacement of the diaphragm, abdominal musculature augmentation of inspiration causes the opposite to occur. This disparity in the surface contour of the abdomen during breathing is referred to as "paradoxical breathing." Similarly, with

progressive respiratory muscle dysfunction, there can be alternation between diaphragmatic breathing and accessory muscle breathing. This abnormal respiratory pattern is referred to as "respiratory alternans" and, like paradoxical breathing, conveys compromise in the effectors of respiratory function. Hypoventilation with carbon dioxide retention is a late phenomenon.

Complete aventilation is rare with peripheral etiologies of respiratory failure, but it certainly can occur. Most often, it occurs after passing through other patterns reflecting progressive ventilatory insufficiency. However, when complete aventilation is recognized in patients without an identified cause of respiratory failure or evidence of CNS dysfunction, peripheral neurological etiologies should be suspect. A common setting for this issue to arise is in the evaluation of patients who have unexpected difficulties in being "weaned" from mechanical ventilatory support.

Anatomy of CNS Respiratory Control Centers

Most of our insights into brain-stem control of automatic respiration come from animal lesioning experiments. The results of these studies provide a framework to understand the various levels of respiratory organization; we must accept that human respiratory control will deviate from that of experimental animals.

The brain stem is the seat of automatic respiratory control. However, the neural network in the brain stem controlling breathing is highly complex. From lesioning experiments in animals, it was discovered that characteristic respiratory patterns can be consistently induced. The clinical corollary of these observations is that recognition of certain characteristic breathing pattern abnormalities can provide useful information to enhance the neuroanatomical localization process. While the human control mechanisms for breathing vary from the more commonly studied animals (cats) in the classical lesioning experiments, there remain many practical similarities which allow insight into human control mechanisms.

Lumsden's classic lesioning studies proposed several levels for the automatic control of breathing by the brain stem. He proposed a pneumotaxic center (PNC) laying bilaterally in the rostral pons. The PNC probably has an auxilliary role in respiratory regulation, coordinating a variety of influences to affect balanced function. More inferiorly, in the pontine reticular formation, there is an apneustic center (APC). Recent studies suggest that the APC may be the location of the normal inspiratory cut-off switch, since it is the site of termination of various afferent inputs that can arrest an inspiration (e.g., intercostal afferents). In its absence, the normal inspiratory cut-off mechanisms are inactivated.

The medulla contains dorsal and ventral respiratory "groups." The dorsal respiratory group (DRG) is within the ventrolateral nucleus tractus solitarius (NTS). These are inspiratory neurons which project to the spinal cord, providing the principal rhythmic respiratory drive to phrenic motorneurons. In addition, the strategic location of the DRG in the NTS, the site of afferent projections from the glossopharyngeal and vagus nerves, supports its function as a center which integrates afferent information to affect a respiratory response.

The ventral respiratory group (VRG) is a subpopulation of inspiratory and expiratory neurons in the nucleus ambiguus and nucleus retroambiguus (NRA) of the medulla. Inspiratory neurons of the VRG are concentrated in the rostral NRA, in contrast to the more caudal location of expiratory neurons. The respiratory rhythmicity of the VRG output is derived from interneurons from the DRG.

The descending expiratory neurons of the VRG project predominantly to the contralateral thoracolumbar spinal cord, driving intercostal and abdominal respiratory motorneurons. The inspiratory neurons project to the contralateral spinal cord, 25% with phrenic motor nucleus branching and the remaining projecting to intercostal motorneurons.

Lesions above the PNC do not cause respiratory pattern abnormalities, but, in combination with vagotomy, a slow deep-breathing pattern results due to the loss of important afferent modulatory information conveyed through the vagus nerves. Lesions isolating the PNC from lower brain-stem centers (without vagotomy) lead to slow deep breathing, and apneusis (sustained inspiration) or apneustic breathing (rhythmic respiration with profound increase in inspiratory time) ensues when it is combined with vagotomy.

Lesions below the APC, isolating the medullary centers from higher modulatory regions, lead to a regular gasping respiratory pattern. When medullary lesions affect the DRG, there can be an arrhythmic or "ataxic" breathing pattern. Cervicomedullary junction lesions cause arrest of all respiration.

The descending cortical tracts which control voluntary (nonautomatic) respiration travel separately from the brain-stem control centers. While their specific origin in human beings has not been fully elucidated, both animal studies and human reports suggest that the lateral corticospinal or corticorubral tracts have an important role in carrying the descending cortical influences on voluntary respiration.

The spinal cord regions affecting the phrenic, intercostal, and abdominal respiratory motorneurons integrate the diverse supraspinal inputs mentioned above, ascending spinal pathways, and important local spinal reflexes. While the integratory role of the spinal cord is vital to normal respiratory functioning, it is highly complex and beyond the scope of this discussion.

Abnormal Breathing Patterns With CNS Lesions

Central Neurogenic Hyperventilation

Central neurogenic hyperventilation (CNH) is a rare condition and most confidently diagnosed by demonstration of an elevated PaO_2, a lowered $PaCO_2$, and an acutely elevated arterial pH which persists during sleep and occurs in the absence of respiratory stimulants (e.g., salicylates) or a parenchymal pulmonary process. While some classic autopsy case descriptions identified patients with sustained, rapid, and deep hyperventilation to have lower midbrain or upper pons lesions involving the paramedian reticular formation, the occurrence of such a syndrome has not been well verified by animal lesioning experiments. Since many patients may have concurrent parenchymal lung changes which can stimulate breathing (e.g., neurogenic pulmonary edema), skepticism has grown with regard to the actual significance of the syndrome of CNH.

More recently, however, numerous case reports have described CNH in patients with diverse brain-stem lesions, albeit with ambiguous localizations due to the nature of the pathology. It has even been described in fully awake patients. We have observed the syndrome in some patients with supratentorial mass lesions and horizontal brain tissue shifts distorting the upper brain stem, but it is difficult to clarify the anatomical implication of such cases.

Interestingly, there is a preponderance of descriptions of CNH in patients with CNS lymphoma. Those with postmortem examinations have not always had lesions involving the brain stem, suggesting that the syndrome of primary CNH should lend suspicion to underlying CNS lymphoma in the undiagnosed patient more than anatomical suspicion of high brain-stem dysfunction.

Clearly, the diagnosis of CNH is complex and of questionable localizing, diagnostic, or prognostic significance. Most importantly, it should remain a diagnosis of exclusion to ensure that significant metabolic acid-base disturbances or parenchymal pulmonary processes which can cause hyperventilation are identified and promptly treated. Therapeutically, the respiratory alkalosis induced by CNH can cause cardiovascular dysfunction and electrolyte disturbances (e.g., hypokalemia). Some have found morphine sulfate beneficial for attenuating the severity of hyperventilation, but these remain anecdotal reports.

Cheyne-Stokes Respiration

Cheyne-Stokes respiration (CSR) is a periodic breathing pattern characterized by a progressive increase and then decrease in the depth of breathing with a subsequent brief period of apnea. This crescendo-decrescendo pattern of periodic breathing effectively results in "hyperventilation" and diminished arterial carbon dioxide levels, in spite of the accompanying apneic periods. However, it does not qualify as CNH, since depressed arterial oxygen is usually the rule in these patients.

The pathophysiology of CSR is an increase in the ventilatory response to carbon dioxide, causing hyperpnea, and the posthyperventilatory apnea is due to impaired function of the forebrain respiratory stimulatory centers. It occurs with bilateral deep brain abnormalities including the upper brain stem, but the wide variability of pathology and lesion locations reported to be associated with CSR preclude its use as a specific localizer of brain abnormalities. While it can be observed in some normal patients during sleep, it generally reflects significant bilateral brain dysfunction. It can commonly be observed in patients with severe metabolic encephalopathy in addition to structural lesions affecting both hemispheres or the upper brain stem.

Apneustic Breathing

Apneustic breathing is characterized by sustained deep inspiration lasting several seconds followed by rapid exhalation and a brief postexpiratory pause. Its presence reflects a loss of the normal inspiratory cut-off mechanism, localizing dysfunction to the apneustic center in the inferior medial pontine region. It is an extremely useful localizing sign when observed. However, these patients are often acutely placed on mechanical ventilation, which masks the abnormal breathing pattern. When present, brief, closely monitored withdrawal of mechanical ventilation allows recognition of an apneustic breathing pattern, which, in turn, enhances the bedside neurodiagnostic process.

Gasping

Gasping is an abnormal breathing pattern most often characterized by an attenuated inspiratory period followed by a disproportionately long period of expiration. It can be a regular rhythmic breathing pattern, but often there is some simultaneous irregularity. We have observed numerous variations of gasping respirations, including an unusual "reversed" pattern with a normal inspiratory period and a markedly diminished expiratory period. Occasionally there can be abnormal head and neck movements with this respiratory pattern, including hyperextension of the head and platysma contraction during inspiration, as we once observed in a hanging victim without tracheal injury.

Gasping breathing patterns are most commonly due to lesions involving the medulla, but the variability in the manifestations reflects its multiple anatomical etiologies. Normal arterial blood gases are often seen with this respiratory pattern, since the minute volume of ventilation is not necessarily impaired. However, the disorders often causing such severe medullary dysfunction are progressive, thereby reflecting risk for impending ventilatory collapse.

Ataxic Breathing

As already mentioned, rhythmicity of breathing is predominantly controlled by the DRG neurons in the NTS in the medulla. Abnormalities of this brainstem region can lead to irregular rate and depth of breathing with interspersed apneic periods. Like gasping, ataxic breathing localizes a lesion to the medulla, but it can be caused by numerous pathological processes. Similar irregular breathing patterns have been described in some degenerative nervous system disorders including the Shy-Drager syndrome.

Aventilation/Hypoventilation

Complete aventilation can occur with medullary and/or high spinal cord lesions, in addition to the peripheral etiologies already discussed. Interestingly, it has been described in patients with unilateral brain-stem infarction. The complete apnea is usually not of much additional localizing value compared with the rest of patient's exam, which should be consistent with lower brain-stem or high spinal cord dysfunction. Obviously, all surviving patients are in-tubated and artificially ventilated. However, it should be noted that the time delay before respiratory resuscitation can be responsible for concomitant anoxic brain dysfunction. The prognosis for recovery to normal spontaneous breathing in patients with CNS etiologies of aventilation is variable, but it is certainly worse than that for the acute peripheral etiologies (e.g., Guillain-Barré syndrome, poliomyelitis) and better than that for chronic etiologies (e.g., amyotrophic lateral sclerosis).

In the absence of upper airway obstruction causing sleep apnea, complete aventilation during asleep with normal ventilation during wakefulness ("Ondine's curse") occurs when there is an interruption of the brain-stem respiratory generators or their spinal projections but maintained integrity of corticospinal pathways which control the more "voluntary" aspect of respiratory control. Clearly, this is a potential cause of death or anoxic damage. Anticipating its occurrence in patients with lower brain-stem abnormalities helps to plan appropriate patient care (e.g., continuous pulse oximetry, apnea monitor) to avoid the associated morbidity and mortality.

Idiopathic primary alveolar hypoventilation refers to a depressed respiratory drive during sleep in patients with brain-stem disorders. While it nonspecifically reflects brain-stem dysfunction, it has less localizing value than the extreme syndrome of aventilation mentioned above.

Spinal cord abnormalities can also cause hypoventilation, particularly during sleep, and damage to ascending spinoreticular fibers may be a more important etiology in some cases than disrupted descending respiratory motor pathways. This syndrome can be seen after anterior cervical spinal operations, bilateral cordotomies, etc.

Hiccups

Frequent hiccups usually have non-neurological causes such as intoxications or thoracoabdominal disorders causing diaphragmatic irritability. The neuroanatomy of hiccups is poorly understood. When associated with neurological disorders. hiccups usually reflect lower brain-stem (medullary) pathology. While recognition of the association of hiccups with brain-stem pathology may explain the phenomenon in certain patients, other etiologies should be systematically excluded, such as lower lobe pneumonia, pleural effusion, pulmonary infarction, myocardial infarction, perforated intestine, gastrointestinal ulcers, and hepatic and splenic abscess. It has been observed that diminished arterial carbon dioxide can accentuate hiccups, and elevated arterial carbon dioxide can attenuate them. Consequently, approaches to allow higher carbon dioxide levels can be helpful when hiccups are causing discomfort or complicating the care of patients with neurological etiologies, balancing the potential deleterious effects of elevated carbon dioxide on intracranial processes which increase intracranial pressure.

Suggested Reading

Aminoff MJ, Sears TA (1971) Spinal integration of segmental, cortical and breathing inputs to thoracic respiratory motorneurones. J Physiol (Lond) 215:557–575

Bateman DE, Gibson GJ, Hudgson P, Tomlinson BE (1985) Central neurogenic hyperventilation in a conscious patient with a primary cerebral lymphoma. Ann Neurol 17:402–405

Berger AJ, Mitchell RA, Herbert DA (1976) Properties of apneustic respiration. Fed Proc 35:633

Berger AJ, Mitchell RA, Severinghaus JW (1977a) Regulation of respiration (first of three parts). N Engl J Med 297:92–97

Berger AJ, Mitchell RA, Severinghaus JW (1977b) Regulation of respiration (second of three parts). N Engl J Med 297:138–143

Berger AJ, Mitchell RA, Severinghaus JW (1977c) Regulation of respiration (third of three parts). N Engl J Med 297:194–201

Bogousslavsky J, Khurana R, Deruaz JP, Hornung JP, Regli F, Janzer R, Perret C (1990) Respiratory failure and unilateral caudal brainstem infarction. Ann Neurol 28:668–673

Caplan LR (1983) Bilateral distal vertebral artery occlusion. Neurology 33:552–558

Cherniack NS, von Euler C, Homma I (1979) Experimentally induced Cheyne-Stokes breathing. Respir Physiol 37:185–200

Cohen MI, Piercey MF, Gootman PM (1974) Synaptic connections between medullary inspiratory neurons and phrenic motorneurons as revealed by cross-correlation. Brain Res 81:319–324

Devereaux MW, Keane JR, Davis RL (1973) Automatic respiratory failure associated with infarction of the medulla. Arch Neurol 29:46–52

Dubaybo BA, Afridi I, Hussain M (1991) Central neurogenic hyperventilation in invasive laryngeal carcinoma. Chest 99:767–769

Frank JI, Biller J (1993) Prognosis of respiratory failure with cervicomedullary infarctions. Neurology 43:A325 (abstract)

Gautier H, Bertrand F (1975) Respiratory effects of pneumotaxic center lesions and subsequent vagotomy in chronic cats. Respir Physiol 23:71–85

Gottlieb D, Michowitz SD, Steiner I, Wald U (1987) Central neurogenic hyperventilation in a patient with medulloblastoma. Eur Neurol 27:51–54

Hugelin A, Bertrand F (1973) Organization of the pneumotaxic oscillator in the cat. Acta Neurobiol Exp (Warsz) 33:91–107

Kahn N, Wang SC (1967) Electrophysiologic basis for pontine apneustic center and its role in integration of the Hering-Breuer reflex. J Neurophysiol 10:301–318

Krieger AJ, Rosomoff HL (1974) Sleep-induced apnea. I. A respiratory and autonomic dysfunction syndrome following bilateral and percutaneous cervial cordotomy. J Neurosurg 40:168–180

Krieger AJ, Rosomoff HL (1974) Sleep-induced apnea. II. Respiratory failure after anterior spinal surgery. J Neurosurg 40:181–185

Levin BE, Margolis G (1977) Acute failure of automatic respirations secondary to unilateral brainstem infarction. Ann Neurol 1:583–586

Lumsden T (1923) The regulation of respiration. I. J Physiol (Lond) 58:81–91

Lumsden T (1923) Observations on the respiratory centers in the cat. J Physiol (Lond) 57:153–160

Lumsden T (1923) Observations on the respiratory centers. J Physiol (Lond) 57:354–367

Merril EG (1970) The lateral respiratory neurons of the medulla: their associations with nucleus ambiguus, nucleus retroambiguus, the spinal accessory nucleus and the spinal cord. Brain Res 24:11–28

Newsome Davis J (1970) An experimental study of hiccup. Brain 93:851–872

Newsome Davis J, Plum F (1972) Separation of descending spinal pathways to respiratory motorneurons. Exp Neurol 34:78–94

North JB, Jennett S (1974) Abnormal breathing patterns associated with acute brain damage. Arch Neurol 31:338–344

Pauzner R, Mouallem M, Sadeh M, Tadmor R, Farfel Z (1989) High incidence of primary cerebral lymphoma in tumor-induced central neurogenic hyperventilation. Arch Neurol 46:510–512

Plum F, Alvord EC Jr (1964) Apneustic breathing in man. Arch Neurol 10:101–112

Plum F (1970) Neurological integration of behavioural and metabolic control of breathing. In: Porter R (ed) Breathing: Hering-Breuer centenary symposium. Churchill, London, pp 159–175

Remmers JE, Marttila I (1975) Action of intercostal muscle afferents on the respiratory rhythm of anesthetized cats. Respir Physiol 24:31–41

Remmers JE, Tsiaras WG (1973) Effect of lateral cervical cord lesions on the respiratory rhythm of anesthetized, decerebrate cats after vagotomy. J Physiol (Lond) 233:63–74

Rodriquez M, Baele PL, Marsh HM, Okazaki H (1982) Central neurogenic hyperventilation in an awake patient with brainstem astrocytoma. Ann Neurol 11:625–628

Salmoiraghi GC (1963) Functional organization of brain stem respiratory neurons. Ann NY Acad Sci 109:571–585

Salvesen R (1989) Pontine tumor with central neurogenic hyperventilation. J Neurol Neurosurgy Psychiatry 52:1441–1442

Severinghaus JW, Mitcheall RA (1962) Ondine's curse – failure of respiratory automaticity while awake. Clin Res 10:122

Shibata Y, Meguro K, Narushima K, Shibuya F, Doi M, Kikuchi (1992) Malignant lymphoma of the central nervous system presenting with central neurogenic hyperventilation. J Neurosurg 76:696–700

Sunderrajan EV, Passamonte PM (1984) Lymphomatoid granulomatosis presenting as central neurogenic hyperventilation. Chest 86:634–636

Part III
Neurocritical Care for Defined Diseases

Inflammatory Diseases: Bacterial Infections

Chapter 36

Bacterial Meningitis

HANS-WALTER PFISTER and KAREN L. ROOS

Introduction

The earliest clinical and pathological description of meningococcal meningitis appeared in 1806 in a medical and agricultural journal. The remarkable features of the pathological process were recognized and described, including the purulent exudate between the dura and pia mater over the cerebrum and cerebellum, and the turgidity of the blood in the veins and sinuses of the brain.

The recognition of the characteristic pathological process of this infection – the production of a purulent exudate in the subarachnoid space (SAS) – resulted in the earliest form of therapy, which was the removal or "washing out" of the cerebrospinal fluid. The advent of antimicrobial therapy altered the management of this infection, focusing the therapeutic process on the eradication of the micro-organisms in the SAS. With increasing understanding of the pathopysiology of this infection, management is again directed toward altering the primary pathological process, i.e., inflammatory exudation in the SAS, and managing the complications that arise as a result.

The incidence of bacterial meningitis is estimated at five to ten cases per 100 000 persons per year. There are approximately 25 000 cases of bacterial meningitis annually in the United States, 80% of which occur in children under the age of 10. This disease is much more common in developing countries and in specific geographic areas, such as the meningitis belt of Africa, where there is an estimated incidence of 70 cases per 100 000 persons per year.

Before the advent of antimicrobial agents, bacterial meningitis was almost exclusively a fatal disease with a case fatality rate of 95–100% for pneumococcal meningitis, 90% for *Haemophilus influenzae* meningitis, and 70–90% for meningococcal meningitis. However, despite further progress in antimicrobial therapy the fatality rate of meningitis due to pneumococcus, which is the organism most often responsible for bacterial meningitis in adults, has remained unchanged (20–30%) during the past

Section Editor: Thomas P. Bleck

several decades. The incidence of neurological sequelae, including sensorineural hearing loss, focal neurological deficits, and seizure disorders, remains high. The chance to improve the outcome of bacterial meningitis lies in a better management of the complications arising during the acute phase of the disease.

Definition

The diagnosis of bacterial meningitis is based on the presence of symptoms and signs of meningitis and detection of the bacterial micro-organisms in the cerebrospinal fluid (CSF). The symptoms of bacterial meningitis are stiff neck, headache, fever, photophobia, vomiting, and lethargy or an altered level of consciousness. The classic sign of meningeal irritation is nuchal rigidity. The neck resists flexion but can be passively rotated from side to side. There may be a history of a recent upper respiratory tract infection or an acute or chronic otitis media. Focal or generalized seizures, signs of increased intracranial pressure, and cranial nerve palsies are also common at the time of presentation. The laboratory diagnosis of bacterial meningitis is made by at least one or both of the following: (a) detection of the bacterial micro-organism in the CSF by microscopic examination of a Gram-stained smear, culture for bacterial pathogens, or detection of bacterial antigen using the latex agglutination method; or (b) CSF pleocytosis >1000 white blood cells per microliter with >60% polymorphonuclear leukocytes, a low CSF glucose concentration, and exclusion of other causes of meningitis.

Pathophysiology

Most of the knowledge on pathophysiological mechanisms of bacterial meningitis has been derived from rabbit and rat models. These experimental studies have shown that components of bacterial cell walls initiate the local production of cytokines, including tumor necrosis factor alpha and interleukin-1β, within the CSF that subsequently elicit inflammatory changes in CSF. Cerebral edema formation, alterations in cerebral blood flow, increased intracranial pressure (ICP), and obstruction to CSF outflow and resorption have been demonstrated in animal models of bacterial meningitis. An increase of regional cerebral blood flow (rCBF) occurs early in experimental bacterial meningitis, while in advanced stages of the disease, rCBF was reduced. Morphological alterations of the blood-brain barrier result in increased blood-brain barrier permeability. The complex pathophysiological mechanisms of the major intracranial complications, i.e., cerebrovascular complications, brain edema, and increased ICP, are not completely understood; however, a number of phenomena have been observed during experimental bacterial meningitis which may contribute to the ultimate brain injury. These factors include leukocytes and their products, endothelial adhesion of leukocytes, cytokines, reactive oxygen intermediates, cyclo-oxygenase metabolites, and platelet-activating factor.

Clinical Features

The spectrum of meningeal pathogens is dependent on a patient's age, concomitant or underlying diseases, or clinically predisposing factors. Such factors include a parameningeal infectious source (e.g., otitis, sinusitis, mastoiditis, brain abscess, subdural empyema), recent intracranial surgery, a history of head trauma with or without a dural sinus fistula, a distant infectious focus (e.g., pneumonia, endocarditis), immunodeficiency, or malignancy.

The three major etiologic agents causing bacterial meningitis are *Haemophilus influenzae* (30–40% of all bacterial meningitis cases), *Neisseria meningitidis* (20–30%), and *Streptococcus pneumoniae* (15–20%). *Listeria monocytogenes* is emerging as a frequent pathogen as well. Gram-negative bacilli are responsible for 10% of cases of bacterial meningitis overall; however, they are responsible for 60–70% of all cases of meningitis in postneurosurgery patients and are a common cause of meningitis in the elderly adult and in adults debilitated by chronic illness. The meningeal pathogen cannot be detected in approximately 10–30% of patients with purulent meningitis.

The presence of a purpuric or petechial rash is suggestive of meningococcal infection or, more rarely, *Staphylococcus aureus* infection. Ten percent of meningococcal infections have an overwhelming course with development of the Waterhouse-Friderichsen syndrome. This syndrome is characterized clinically by fever, large petechial hemorrhages in the skin and mucous membranes, cardiovascular insufficiency, and disseminated intravascular coagulation.

The clinical presentation of bacterial meningitis is usually rapidly progressive over several hours; however, bacterial meningitis may also have a more subacute presentation evolving over 24–72 h. Because of the characteristic clinical presentation of this infection, antibiotic therapy is started within the first 48 h of the disease in approximately 50% of patients. With adequate therapy, clinical symptoms usually improve within several days. If the patient's clinical condition does not improve, a change of antibiotics may be considered; however, the possibility of a persistent infectious focus or complications of bacterial meningitis should be investigated.

Approximately 10% of patients with bacterial meningitis develop focal cerebral signs, e.g., hemi- or tetraparesis, ataxia, aphasia, and hemianopia. Seizures occur in 30–40% of patients. Approximately 10% of the patients develop cranial nerve palsies, usually of the third, sixth, seventh, or eighth cranial nerve. Sensorineural hearing loss develops in 10–30% of patients with bacterial meningitis.

Predictors for an unfavorable course of the disease are: apurulent bacterial meningitis, i.e., high bacterial density in the CSF combined with a low cell count; age over 40 years; underlying or concomitant disease, e.g., splenectomy or endocarditis; type of bacterial pathogen (e.g., gram-negative bacteria or pneumococci); and a long time between onset of neurological symptoms and initiation of therapy.

Differential Diagnosis

The differential diagnosis in the acute phase of bacterial meningitis includes: (a) viral meningitis or meningoencephalitis, (b) rickettsial infection, (c) Lyme disease, (d) subarachnoid hemorrhage, (e) fungal meningitis, (f) focal infectious mass lesions, and (g) neuroleptic malignant syndrome.

The clinical presentation of viral meningitis is headache, fever, nuchal rigidity, and lethargy. Patients with viral meningitis are typically awake and alert, although they complain of incapacitating, throbbing headache. On examination the cerebrospinal fluid is clear, and the opening pressure is either normal or only slightly elevated. The CSF cell count ranges from 50 to 2000 white blood cells per cubic millimeter with a predominance of lymphocytes. CSF protein concentration is only mildly elevated, and the glucose concentration is usually normal.

The term meningoencephalitis is used when there are signs of brain parenchymal inflammation by the infectious process. When this occurs, the clinical presentation is characterized by focal neurological deficits, such as hemiparesis, an altered level of consciousness, and focal or generalized seizure activity.

In herpes simplex virus type-I (HSV-1) encephalitis, initial symptoms are fever, hemicranial headache, confusion, or a change in behavior. The headache may be present for several days prior to the onset of the confusional state. As the infection progresses, focal neurological deficits and seizure activity develop. HSV-1 has a predilection for the temporal and orbitofrontal areas; as such, the ab-

normalities on neurological examination suggest infection in these localized areas of the brain. The following abnormalities are typical of HSV-1 meningoencephalitis on examination of the CSF: (a) elevated opening pressure, (b) white blood cell counts ranging from 50 to 500 cells per μl, with a lymphocytic predominance, (c) red blood cells and/or xanthochromia, (d) elevated protein concentration (averaging approximately 200 mg/dl), and (e) normal or moderately low glucose concentration. Electroencephalographic (EEG) abnormalities are very specific for this infection and often very useful, in addition to the abnormalities on CSF examination, in making the diagnosis. The characteristic EEG abnormalities in HSV-1 encephalitis are periodic sharp wave complexes that arise from one or both temporal regions and recur every 1–5 s.

Rocky Mountain spotted fever (RMSF) may present like bacterial meningitis. The initial symptoms of RMSF are fever, headache, myalgias, and gastrointestinal disturbances. The neurologic manifestations of RMSF include focal deficits, stupor, delirium, coma, and seizure activity. The rash of RMSF is maculopapular and/or purpuric, typically diffuse, and involves the palms and soles; it may be difficult to distinguish clinically from the rash of meningococcemia. The rash of RMSF usually does not involve the mucous membranes, while the rash of meningococcemia may appear on them. The diagnosis of RMSF may be made by biopsy of the skin lesions. Examination of the CSF can also distinguish RMSF from bacterial meningitis. In RMSF, the white blood cell count in the CSF is typically less than

100/mm³ (cells may be absent), the protein concentration is mildly to moderately elevated, and the glucose concentration is normal.

A clinical presentation typical of viral meningitis may also be a manifestation of CNS involvement by *Borrelia burgdorferi*, the etiologic organism of Lyme disease. The CSF inflammatory changes are much less pronounced in Lyme disease than in bacterial meningitis, and the clinical presentation is more typically subacute. There is a mild CSF mononuclear pleocytosis, a mild elevation in protein concentration, and a normal glucose concentration. In the majority of cases, intrathecal production of anti-*B. burgdorferi* antibodies can be detected in CSF.

The typical presentation of a subarachnoid hemorrhage is a severe, explosive headache with vomiting or a sudden transient loss of consciousness followed by a severe headache. Nuchal rigidity is usually present within a few hours of onset. Subarachnoid hemorrhage may be visualized on computerized tomographic (CT) scan; however, in 5–10% of cases the CT scan is negative, and the diagnosis is made by finding red blood cells or xanthochromia in the CSF.

Fungal meningitides may resemble bacterial meningitis; however, fungal meningitides tend to have a more insidious onset of fever, headache, and increasing confusion over several days or weeks. The CSF usually shows a mononuclear pleocytosis, an elevated protein concentration, and a low glucose concentration. India ink examination of CSF is positive in approximately 50% of cryptococcal meningitis cases; this percentage increases in the setting of HIV infection.

The diagnosis of fungal meningitis is established by a positive culture, although fungal cultures are typically slow growing. When coccidioidal meningitis is suspected, culture of CSF obtained from a cisternal, rather than a lumbar, puncture is recommended. The detection of fungal antigen in serum and CSF and complement-fixing antibodies are useful in the diagnosis of fungal meningitis.

Brain abscess and subdural empyema may have a clinical presentation similar to that of bacterial meningitis. The presentation of either of these mass lesions is dominated by hemicranial headache that becomes increasingly more severe and generalized, focal neurological deficits, and seizure activity. Either of these lesions can be readily visualized by CT or magnetic resonance (MR) scan. The similarity between the initial presentation of these mass lesions and that of bacterial meningitis has prompted the use of neuroimaging prior to lumbar puncture in patients with fever and headache; however, careful neurological examination can often distinguish a focal mass lesion from meningitis.

The diagnostic criteria of neuroleptic malignant syndrome are fever, generalized lead-pipe rigidity, fluctuating level of consciousness, autonomic instability, and a marked elevation in the serum creatine kinase concentration.

Complications

Major determinants of the prognosis of bacterial meningitis are based on the occurrence of the following complications: (a) central nervous system complications including cerebral arterial or venous ischemia or infarction, cerebral edema, hydrocephalus, brain abscess, subdural empyema, or subdural effusion (noted in 15–45% of cases of bacterial meningitis in infants <18 months of age), and, rarely, central diabetes insipidus, or the syndrome of inappropriate secretion of antidiuretic hormone, and spinal vasculitis; (b) systemic complications including septic shock, disseminated intravascular coagulation (DIC), adult respiratory distress syndrome (ARDS), septic or reactive arthritis and rhabdomyolysis; and (c) typical complications arising during intensive care therapy including pneumonia, deep venous thrombosis, pulmonary embolism, pharmacogenic or alcoholic withdrawal syndrome, electrolyte disturbances (e.g., central diabetes insipidus or the syndrome of inappropriate secretion of antidiuretic hormone), and adverse effects of drug or surgical therapy.

Cerebral arterial or venous complications should be investigated in patients with bacterial meningitis who have focal neurological deficits or persistent unexplained coma despite 3 days of adequate antibiotic therapy. Such vascular involvement became evident from (a) autopsy studies showing arteritis and thrombophlebitis; (b) angiographic evidence of vasculitis (Fig. 1) or thrombosis of the superior sagittal sinus and cortical veins; (c) observations of altered cerebral blood flow and blood velocity; and (d) CT studies revealing cerebral infarctions.

Vascular complications may raise ICP by different mechanisms, including: (a) vasogenic brain edema from endothelial damage, (b) cytotoxic brain edema from brain infarction, and (c) failure of autoregulation. There is a risk of cortical necrosis when the cerebral perfusion pressure decreases as a result of increased ICP.

In Pfister and colleagues' prospective study of 86 adult patients with

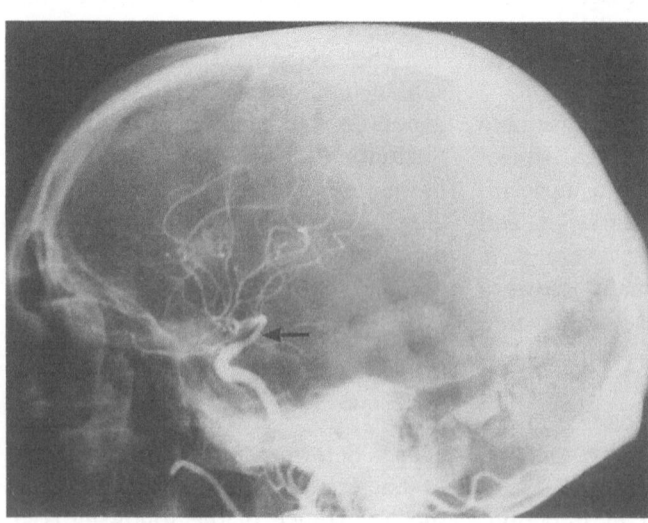

Fig. 1. Right carotid angiography (lateral view from a common internal carotid artery injection) in a 66-year-old patient with pneumococcal meningitis revealed marked narrowing in the supraclinoid portion of the right internal carotid artery (*arrow*)

bacterial meningitis, 43 developed complications. The major CNS complications were vascular involvement (15.1% of the patients), cerebral edema (14.0%), and hydrocephalus (11.6%). The systemic complications were dominated by septic shock (11.6%), ARDS (3.5%), and DIC (8.1%). Seven patients had cerebral herniation, three with a fatal outcome. Likewise, in a retrospective study of children with bacterial meningitis performed by Horwitz et al., 18/302 children (6.0%) had cerebral herniation during the acute phase of the disease, three died, and four had severe disability.

An autopsy study done by Dodge and Swartz revealed that ten of 30 patients who died during the acute phase of bacterial meningitis had diffuse brain edema. Because of the efficiency of the pia as a barrier, brain abscess is a very rare complication of bacterial meningitis.

Ancillary Tests

After admission of the patient and clinical examination, a cranial CT should be performed to identify the following:

1. Parameningeal infectious foci via the bone window technique, e.g., sinusitis, mastoiditis (Fig. 2)
2. Intracranial free air due to a dural leak (Fig. 3)
3. Brain abscess or subdural empyema (Fig. 4)
4. Early complications of bacterial meningitis, e.g., venous sinus thrombosis, hydrocephalus, or infarction

MR is superior to CT for detecting parenchymal ischemic changes. Vascular involvement can be detected by cerebral angiography, transcranial Doppler sonography, and SPECT investigation. Transcranial Doppler sonography may be useful in diag-

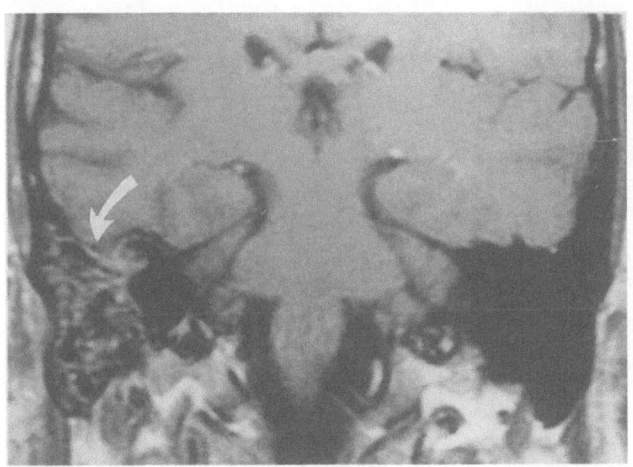

Fig. 2. Acute mastoiditis with dural involvement in a 53-year-old man. T1-weighted coronal MR image obtained after IV administration of paramagnetic contrast agent shows abnormal enhancement of both thickened mucosa of right mastoid air cell system and dura above tegmen tympani (*arrow*). (Courtesy of Klaus Sartor and Marius Hartmann, Heidelberg)

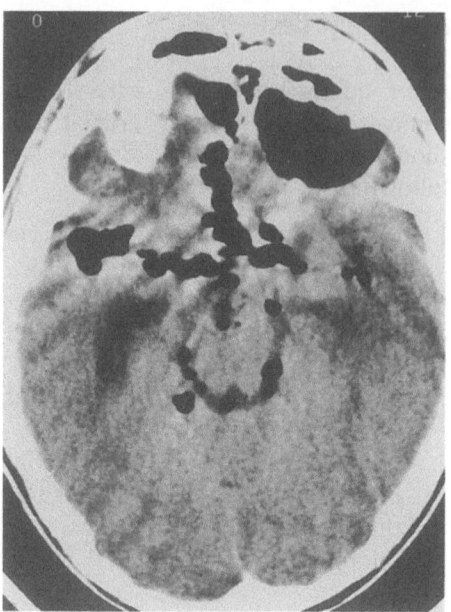

Fig. 3. Pneumocephalus in a 33-year-old man which was due to a craniocerebral injury caused by a shooting device used to kill cattle (suicide attempt). Axial CT scan shows multiple smaller and larger collections of air, most of which are located extra-axially, which have entered the intracranial cavity through leaks in the frontobasal dura. (Courtesy of Klaus Sartor and Marius Hartmann, Heidelberg)

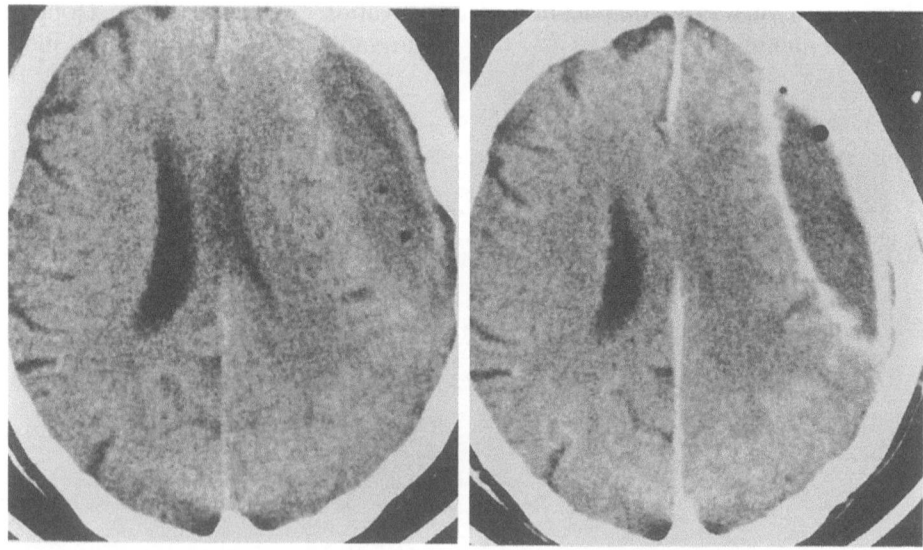

a   b

Fig. 4a,b. Subdural empyema in a 70-year-old man with a changed mental status occurring 4 weeks after drainage of a chronic subdural hematoma through a burr hole. Axial CT scans obtained before (a) and after (b) IV administration of iodinated contrast material reveal extraaxial mass lesion of low density compared with normal brain parenchyma that is biconvex and enhances peripherally, with short extensions of the enhancement into several sulci. The ipsilateral ventricle is largely compressed due to the mass effect. (Courtesy of Klaus Sartor and Marius Hartmann, Heidelberg) nosing involvement of great arteries at the base of the brain. However, vasculitis or thrombosis of small vessels, major sinuses, and cortical veins cannot be detected by this technique. Cerebral angiography may be considered if at least one of the following criteria is fulfilled: the development of focal neurological deficits or focal seizure activity; evidence of a focal lesion on cranial CT or MR (e.g., infarction, focal brain edema); or no improvement in coma (Glasgow Coma Scale score less than eight) after 3 days of adequate antibiotic therapy, provided that other causes for coma, e.g., metabolic or pharmacologic causes, hydrocephalus or brain abscess, have been excluded. In addition, MR angiography can diagnose sinus thrombosis.

Cerebrospinal fluid typically shows a pleocytosis with more than 1000 cells/μl. There is a predominance of polymorphonuclear leukocytes (PMNs); 80–90% of patients with bacterial meningitis have more than 80% PMNs in their CSF. A cell count below 1000 cells/μl may be found in the following conditions:

– Very early stage of bacterial meningitis
– Partially treated bacterial meningitis
– Overwhelming bacterial meningeal infection usually due to pneumococci (so-called apurulent bacterial meningitis), characterized by a very low cellular response but a high density of bacteria in the CSF
– Leukopenic or immunosuppressed patients

Certain bacterial pathogens such as Listeria monocytogenes may not induce a purulent CSF.

The protein concentration in the CSF usually exceeds 120 mg/dl, and the glucose concentration is normally below 30 mg/dl. The CSF/serum glucose ratio is typically less than 0.31. Gram's stain discloses bacteria in approximately 80–90% of patients with a positive CSF culture. The likelihood of a positive culture of Gram's stain result decreases to 5–40% in patients treated with antibiotics prior to examination of the CSF. An elevated CSF lactate concentration or C-reactive protein may be useful in differentiating bacterial from viral meningitis, especially in patients who have been partially treated with antibiotics prior to examination of the CSF.

Management

General Aspects

Clinical suspicion of bacterial meningitis (high fever, headache, stiff neck, impairment of consciousness) should prompt a cranial CT, including the bone window technique, and examination of the CSF. Only clinical signs of cerebral herniation or a focal mass lesion constitute a clear contraindication to lumbar puncture. In the case of suspected raised ICP, hyperosmolar agents (e.g., 0.25 g/kg body wt. of mannitol) may be infused intravenously, just before lumbar puncture. CSF should be immediately examined for cell count with differential, protein, and glucose concentration, Gram's stain, and bacterial antigen detection by latex agglutination; in addition, agar plates should be inoculated for routine culture for bacteria. Thereafter, intravenous antibiotic therapy should be started. If CT scan is delayed, antibiotic therapy should be initiated and CT scan and CSF examination obtained as soon as possible. The goal should be to limit the period from examination of the patient to the initiation of antibiotic therapy to less than 1 h. The possibility of an extracranial infectious focus should be investigated. Surgical intervention for parameningeal infections, such as otitis or mastoiditis, should be performed as soon as possible when indicated. CSF leaks are surgically corrected once the meningeal infection is under control, not during the acute phase of bacterial meningitis.

If the meningeal pathogen is known, an antibiotic is chosen with bactericidal activity against the pathogen, good blood-CSF barrier penetration, and effective concentrations in the CSF, with a relatively low incidence of adverse effects (Table 1). Experimental studies have demonstrated that the best response is achived with CSF antibiotic concentrations that exceed the minimal bactericidal concentration (MBC) of the infecting organism by 10- to 20-fold. If the meningeal pathogen is unknown, empiric therapy is started based on the age of the patient, predisposing factors, and the most likely meningeal pathogen (Table 2). The total daily dosages of the most frequently used antibiotics in bacterial meningitis are listed in Table 3. The susceptibility of the identified meningeal pathogen to several antibiotics should be determined. The CSF cultures usually become sterile within 24–48 h after starting therapy; however, enteric gram-negative rods and

Pseudomonas aeruginosa may remain culturable for 2–3 days after the initiation of antibiotic therapy. If the CSF is not sterile within 3 days, a change in the antibiotic regimen should be considered; in addition, a persistent source of infection should be investigated. Within 24 h of the onset of antibiotic therapy, almost 50% of samples of CSF from patients with bacterial meningitis have an increase in cell count in the CSF. This has no prognostic significance.

Antibiotics Most Often Used in the Therapy of Bacterial Meningitis

Penicillin G is very effective against gram-positive and gram-negative cocci and anaerobic bacilli, with the exception of penicillinase-producing staphylococci, enterococci, and *Bacteroides fragilis*. Penicillin G is insufficiently effective against *Haemophilus influenzae*, gram-negative Enterobacteriaceae, and *Pseudomonas aeruginosa*. The blood-CSF penetration is adequate in inflamed meninges but very poor in intact blood-CSF barrier (<1%).

Ampicillin is less effective than penicillin against streptococci and pneumococci, equally effective against meningococci, and more effective against *L. monocytogenes*, *H. influenzae*, and enterococci. Ampicillin is insufficiently effective against gram-negative Enterobacteriaceae and *P. aeruginosa*.

The broad-spectrum penicillins such as piperacillin, azlocillin, and mezlocillin are mainly effective against *P. aeruginosa*, Enterobacteriaceae, and enterococci, but they are inferior to cefotaxime against enteric gram-

Table 1. Recommended treatment of bacterial meningitis

Meningeal pathogen	Antibiotic	Alternatives
N. meningitidis	Penicillin G *or* ampicillin	Third-generation cephalosporin[a]
S. pneumoniae	Penicillin G *or* third-generation cephalosporin[a]	Ampicillin
H. influenzae type b	Third-generation cephalosporin[a]	Ampicillin plus chloramphenicol
Streptococci (group B)	Penicillin G *or* third-generation cephalosporin[a]	Ampicillin
Enterobacteriaceae	Third-generation cephalosporin[a]	Broad-spectrum penicillin[c] plus aminoglycoside[b]
Pseudomonas aeruginosa	Ceftazidime plus aminoglycoside[b]	Piperacillin plus aminoglycoside[b]
S. aureus (methicillin sensitive)	Oxacillin	Nafcillin *or* vancomycin *or* fosfomycin
S. aureus (methicillin resistant)	Vancomycin	
Coagulase-negative staphylococci	Vancomycin	
L. monocytogenes	Ampicillin (plus aminoglycoside[b])	Trimethoprim-sulfamethoxazole

[a] Cefotaxime or ceftriaxone
[b] Gentamicin or tobramycin
[c] Piperacillin or mezlocillin

negative rods. Since the CSF concentrations usually do not exceed the minimal bactericidal concentration for *P. aeruginosa*, a combination with an aminoglycoside is recommended because of the synergistic effect. The penicillinase-resistant oxacillins exhibit a high binding to plasma proteins (97%) and a moderate blood-CSF penetration in inflamed meninges. They are used in the treatment of staphylococcal meningitis.

The first-generation cephalosporins such as cefalotin and most second-generation cephalosporins such as cefamandol and cefoxitin have been shown to provide relatively poor CSF penetration with achieved CSF concentrations below the minimal bactericidal concentration of most meningeal pathogens, and are therefore inappropriate for the treatment of bacterial meningitis. A marked advancement in the therapy of bacterial meningitis was achieved with the development of the third-generation cephalosporins, such as cefotaxime, latamoxef, ceftizoxime, ceftriaxone, ceftazidime, and cefsulodine. The most frequently employed and best studied antibiotics in this group are cefotaxime and ceftriaxone.

Cefotaxime has a sufficient CSF penetration rate and has been used successfully in the therapy of pneumococcal, meningococcal, and *H. influenzae* meningitis and meningitis due to enteric gram-negative rods (reaching CSF concentrations of 10–500 times the minimal inhibitory concentration of *Escherichia coli* and *Klebsiella*). However, cefotaxime is only minimally effective or not ef-

Table 2. Initial empiric antibiotic therapy of bacterial meningitis

Age-groups	Frequent etiologic agents	Recommended antibiotic regimen
Neonates (≤2 months old)	Enteric gram-negative rods Group-B streptococci *Listeria monocytogenes*	Cefotaxime plus ampicillin
Infants and children (>2 months old)	*Haemophilus influenzae* *Streptococcus pneumoniae* *Neisseria meningitidis*	3rd-generation cephalosporin[a]
Adults		
• healthy, immunocompetent, community-acquired	*Streptococcus pneumoniae* *Neisseria meningitidis*	3rd-generation cephalosporin or penicillin G or ampicillin
• nosocomial (e.g., postneurosurgical) or recent head injury	*Staphylococcus aureus* *Staphylococcus epidermidis* Enteric gram-negative rods *Streptococcus pneumoniae*	3rd-generation cephalosporin plus oxacillin[b] plus aminoglycoside[c]
• immunocompromised	*Streptococcus pneumoniae* *Listeria monocytogenes* Enteric gram-negative rods	3rd-generation cephalosporin plus ampicillin
• shunt-related meningitis	*Staphylococcus epidermidis* *Staphylococcus aureus* Enteric gram-negative rods	3rd-generation cephalosporin plus vancomycin plus aminoglycoside

[a] Cefotaxime or ceftriaxone
[b] Alternatives: nafcillin or vancomycin
[c] Gentamicin or tobramycin

fective against *L. monocytogenes*, *P. aeruginosa*, enterococci, *S. aureus*, *Acinetobacter*, and *Clostridium difficile*.

Ceftriaxone has an activity comparable to that of cefotaxime and the advantage of a long serum half-life of about 8 h; therefore, ceftriaxone can be administered in a once- or twice-daily dose. In childhood bacterial meningitis, ceftriaxone has been proven to be superior to cefuroxime.

Ceftazidime is very effective against *P. aeruginosa* and is superior in vitro to cefsulodine and piperacillin. However, ceftazidime is less effective against gram-positive bacteria than cefotaxime. Ceftazidime's level of beta lactamase stability is high, and its CSF penetration rate is comparable to that of cefotaxime.

Latamoxef is not recommended for initial therapy of bacterial meningitis because it is insufficiently effective against gram-positive cocci; however, it has been used successfully in combination with ampicillin in the treatment of meningitis due to these organisms. The use of latamoxef is limited because of the potential adverse effects of hypoprothrombinemia, thrombopathy, and thrombocytopenia associated with this agent.

The aminoglycosides such as gentamicin, tobramycin, netilmicin, and amikacin are especially effective against gram-negative bacteria (enteric

Table 3. Recommended antibiotics in bacterial meningitis[a]

Antibiotic	Total daily dose (dosage interval)				Serum half-life (h)	CSF/serum ratio (%)[b]
	Adults	Infants	Neonates 1–4 weeks	<1 week		
Penicillin G	24–30 mega U/day (every 4 h)	250 000–400 000 U/kg/day (every 4 h)	150 000–200 000 U/kg/day (every 6 h)	50 000–150 000 U/kg/day (every 8 h)	0.6–1	3–5
Ampicillin	12 g/day (every 4 h)	150–200 mg/kg/day (every 4 h)	100–200 mg/kg/day (every 6 h)	50–100 mg/kg/day (every 12 h)	0.5–1	5–10
Cefotaxime	6 g/day (every 8 h)	200 mg/kg/day (every 6 h)	150 mg/kg/day (every 8 h)	100 mg/kg/day (every 12 h)	~1	6–16
Ceftriaxone	2(–4) g/day (every 24 h)	100 mg/kg/day (every 24 h)	–	–	6–8	4–9
Ceftazidime	6 g/day (every 8 h)	150 mg/kg/day (every 8 h)	100–150 mg/kg/day (every 8 h)	60 mg/kg/day (every 12 h)	1.8	~20
Gentamicin/tobramycin	240–360 mg/day (every 8 h)	5 mg/kg/day (every 8 h)	7.5 mg/kg/day (every 8 h)	5 mg/kg/day (every 8 h)	2–3	<10
Trimethoprim-sulfamethoxazol	10 mg/kg/day[c] (every 8 h)	10 mg/kg/day (every 8 h)	10 mg/kg/day (every 8 h)	10 mg/kg/day (every 8 h)	11	30–50
Chloramphenicol	4 g/day (every 6 h)	100 mg/kg/day (every 6 h)	50 mg/kg/day (every 12 h)	25 mg/kg/day (every 12 h)	1.5–3.5	40–90
Vancomycin	2 g/day (every 6 h)	40 mg/kg/day (every 6 h)	40 mg/kg/day (every 6 h)	20–30 mg/kg/day (every 12 h)	6	10–30
Oxacillin	9–12 g/day (every 4 h)	200 mg/kg/day (every 6 h)	100–200 mg/kg/day (every 6 h)	50–100 mg/kg/day (every 8 h)	0.7	<10
Piperacillin	12 g/day (every 8 h)	200–300 mg/kg/day (every 8 h)	200–300 mg/kg/day (every 8 h)	200–300 mg/kg/day (every 8 h)	1.3–1.5	~15
Fosfomycin	15 g/day (every 8 h)	200–300 mg/kg/day (every 8 h)	100 mg/kg/day (every 12 h)	100 mg/kg/day (every 12 h)	2	20–30

[a] Reduction of dosage of all antibiotics except ceftriaxone is necessary in renal failure.
[b] With inflamed meninges.
[c] Based on trimethoprim.

gram-negative rods and *P. aeruginosa*) and staphylococci. They are not effective or only insufficiently effective against meningococci, pneumococci, streptococci, enterococci, *L. monocytogenes*, *H. influenzae*, and anaerobic bacteria. The serum concentrations of the aminoglycosides should be monitored regularly (e.g., gentamicin concentration $<10\,\mu$g/ml). The CSF concentrations of the aminoglycosides, whose activity is decreased in acid milieu, usually do not attain the minimal bactericidal concentrations for most gram-negative bacteria because of their poor and variable CSF penetration, even in inflamed meninges. Therefore, especially during the 1970s, intraventricular administration of the aminoglycosides was recommended. However, with the advent of sufficient CSF-penetrating third-generation cephalosporins, this strategy has increasingly receded into the background. Currently, the intraventricular administration of gentamicin (dosage 5–10 mg/day in adults, 1–2 mg/day in children) is indicated only if gram-negative meningitis is unquestionable, the clinical picture is severe (coma), and clinical or bacteriological improvement does not occur during intravenous antibiotic therapy.

Once-daily Aminoglycoside Therapy

All aminoglycosides can potentially cause reversible and irreversible vestibular, cochlear, and renal toxicity, and, because of the narrow therapeutic range and wide pharmacokinetic variability among patients, optimal dosage regimens are often difficult to attain. In general, low serum trough levels of aminoglycosides are associated with decreased antibiotic accumulation in the renal cortex and endolymph and perilymph of the inner ear, and high serum peak levels correlate with increased bactericidal effect. Recently, it has been reported that toxicity can be reduced and efficacy can be improved when aminoglycosides are given only once daily compared with the conventional regimen of multiple times daily (that is, a single total dose of aminoglycosides results in higher peak levels and lower trough levels). Aminoglycosides should always be given intravenously because of the variable rate of absorption after intramuscular injection.

Fosfomycin has an effective CSF penetration and may be useful in staphylococcal meningitis; however, staphylococci may become resistant to this antibiotic during therapy. In addition, it is active against *H. influenzae*, meningococci, and gram-negative enterobacteria (*E. coli*, *Citrobacter*, *Serratia*). It is less effective against pneumococci, *Enterobacter*, *Klebsiella*, and *Proteus* and ineffective against *Bacteroides* species.

Vancomycin is an alternative antibiotic for bacterial meningitis due to oxacillin- or fosfomycin-resistant staphylococci. Vancomycin is often required in shunt infections or ventriculitis. In addition, vancomycin is effective against streptococci, including enterococci and pneumococci.

Trimethoprim-sulfamethoxazol (TMP-SMZ) has good CSF penetration and is used as an alternative antibiotic in the therapy of *Listeria* meningitis in cases of allergy to ampicillin. Furthermore, TMP-SMZ has been successful in the therapy of bacterial meningitis due to *Enterobacter*, *Acinetobacter*, and *Serratia*.

Metronidazole adequately penetrates into the CSF and is employed in the therapy of brain abscess and the very rare condition of anaerobic meningitis (e.g., meningitis caused by *Bacteroides fragilis*, *Fusobacterium*, *Peptococcus*, *Veillonella*, and *Peptostreptococcus*).

Chloramphenicol is not a first-choice antibiotic because of its possible side effects. It has a good degree of CSF penetration, even in intact meninges, and is very effective against meningococci, pneumococci, and *H. influenzae*. Chloramphenicol has a high failure rate in gram-negative meningitis because in this condition it reaches only bacteriostatic concentrations in the CSF. The serum concentrations of chloramphenicol have to be monitored regularly, and the maximum levels should not exceed 15–20 μg/ml.

Empiric Antibiotic Recommendations

The most common bacterial pathogens causing neonatal meningitis are enteric gram-negative rods, group-B streptococci, and *Listeria monocytogenes*. Therefore, a combination of ampicillin and cefotaxime or of ampicillin and an aminoglycoside is recommended (Table 2). A third-generation cephalosporin is recommended for initial empiric antibiotic therapy in infants and children (over 2 months of age). In controlled studies, cefotaxime or ceftriaxone were as effective as ampicillin and chloramphenicol. Moreover, an increasing number of strains of *Haemophilus influenzae*, the most frequent bacterial

pathogen of meningitis in infants and children, have been identified in recent years that are resistant to ampicillin and chloramphenicol.

The most frequent agents of bacterial meningitis in previously healthy adults are meningococci and pneumococci. Initial treatment with a third-generation cephalosporin (e.g., cefotaxime or ceftriaxone) is recommended before the meningeal pathogen is identified. Penicillin G or ampicillin may be substituted in cases of meningococcal infection as demonstrated by Gram's stain. CSF isolates of pneumococci and meningococci should be tested for penicillin and ampicillin susceptibility. A third-generation cephalosporin can be used for penicillin-resistant meningococci or relatively penicillin-resistant pneumococci, and vancomycin is recommended for highly penicillin-resistant pneumococci.

Initial therapy of bacterial meningitis associated with recent head trauma or a neurosurgical procedure should include a combination of a third-generation cephalosporin, such as cefotaxime or ceftriaxone, oxacillin (alternatively fosfomycin), and an aminoglycoside to treat staphylococci and enteric gram-negative rods. Ventriculitis associated with an external intraventricular drainage device should be treated with a combination of a third-generation cephalosporin, vancomycin (alternatively oxacillin or fosfomycin), and an aminoglycoside. When meningitis develops in association with a ventriculoperitoneal shunt, the shunt should be removed and a temporary external ventricular drainage device inserted. The latter will control hydrocephalus while the infection is being treated. Some clinicians have attempted antibiotic treatment without shunt removal, with limited success. Antibiotic therapy should include a combination of a third-generation cephalosporin, vancomycin (alternatively flucloxacillin or fosfomycin), and an aminoglycoside. If the shunt infection is caused by enteric gram-negative rods, which are susceptible to aminoglycosides, then gentamicin should be given intravenously and intraventricularly (dosage in infants and children 1–2 mg/day, in adults 5–10 mg/day). If there is a known underlying immunocompromised state or malignancy, the initial antibiotic therapy should be directed against a broad spectrum of bacterial pathogens, including *L. monocytogenes*; therefore, a combination of a third-generation cephalosporin and ampicillin is recommended.

Treatment Duration

The treatment duration of bacterial meningitis depends on the response to therapy and the type of bacterial pathogen. In meningitis caused by meningococci, pneumococci, *H. influenzae* and group-B streptococci, a 10–14 day course of antibiotic therapy is recommended. Alternatively, antibiotics should be continued for 7 days after the patient's fever has disappeared. Meningitis due to *L. monocytogenes* and enteric gram-negative rods is usually treated for 3–4 weeks.

Isolation

Patients with meningococcal meningitis should be isolated for the first 24 h after the onset of antibiotic therapy.

Chemoprophylaxis

The risk of secondary disease for close contacts of patients with *H. influenzae* type b or meningococcal meningitis is approximately 200–1000 times the risk for the general population. Chemoprophylaxis for eradication of the bacteria from the nasopharynx is recommended for family and household members, persons who have had close contact with the index case for more than 4 h daily during the week prior to the onset of the disease, and hospital staff members who have had potential contact with secretory products of the respiratory tract of the index case prior to the onset of antibiotic therapy. In contrast to meningococcal meningitis, the risk of infection in *H. influenzae* meningitis seems to exist only for children younger than 6 years of age. Since the bacterial pathogens are usually not eradicated from the upper respiratory tract in a patient with *H. influenzae* meningitis or meningococcal meningitis despite successful systemic antibiotic therapy, the patient is a potential carrier. Therefore, it is recommended that the index patient also receives chemoprophylaxis before discharge from the hospital. The recommended antibiotic for chemoprophylaxis is rifampicin (Table 4). Rifampicin usually has no toxic effects when administered for a short period of time; however, it should not be prescribed to pregnant women.

Up to 70% of meningococci were resistant to sulfadiazine in reported series in the 1970s; therefore, sul-

Table 4. Chemoprophylaxis of bacterial meningitis

Etiologic agent	Total daily dosage of rifampicin		
	Adults	Infants and children (>1 month)	Neonates (<1 month)
Haemophilus influenzae	600 mg/day orally over 4 days	20 mg/kg/day orally (maximum 600 mg/day) over 4 days	10 mg/kg/day orally over 4 days
Neisseria meningitidis	2 × 600 mg/day orally over 2 days	2 × 10 mg/kg/day orally over 2 days	2 × 5 mg/kg/day orally over 2 days

fadiazine is not recommended for chemoprophylaxis of meningococcal disease. Rifampicin is currently the recommended agent. An alternative to rifampicin, ciprofloxacin, has been given successfully as chemoprophylaxis in meningococcal infection (500 or 750 mg in a single oral dose).

Immunophrophylaxis (Vaccination)

The efficacy of the 23-valent preparation of pneumococcal vaccine against pneumococcal meningitis has not been proven. However, this preparation is usually recommended for high-risk patients over 2 years of age. The dose of the vaccine is 0.5 ml, intramuscularly, which is usually well tolerated. Booster injections should be given every 5 years. There is no effective vaccine against meningococci of the serogroup B, which accounts for the most frequent cases of meningococcal infection. A tetravalent meningococcal vaccine (serogroups A,C,Y, and W 135) is currently recommended for high-risk patients, including patients with terminal complement component deficiency or

dysfunction, asplenic patients, and travelers to areas with hyperendemic or epidemic meningococcal disease (e.g., Nigeria, Cameroon). *H. influenzae* type b conjugate vaccine is recommended for all infants at the age of 2, 4, and 6 months.

Management of Special Problems and Complications

Experimental studies on the pathophysiological mechanisms of pneumococcal meningitis have shown that the cell wall of the pneumococcus elicits an inflammatory response in the subarachnoid space. Since bacterial lysis by antibiotics releases cell-wall components, which in turn initiate the inflammatory cascade, adjunctive therapy to alter the inflammatory cascade may be more promising than further development of lytic antibiotics.

Two placebo-controlled doubleblind studies performend by Lebel et al. and Odio et al. in children with bacterial meningitis showed a beneficial effect of *dexamethasone* on hearing loss and neurological sequelae. These results may not be applicable to newborns but are most likely applicable to adults with bacterial meningitis. Dexamethasone reduced mortality in adults with pneumococcal meningitis in an open randomized study performed in Egypt. Dexamethasone may also have a beneficial effect in patients with cerebral edema, cerebral arterial complications, or apurulent bacterial meningitis. Recent studies to evaluate the effect of corticosteroids in septic shock do not, however, support the use of high-dose steroids in septic shock. The recommended dose of dexamethasone in children with bacterial meningitis is 0.15 mg/kg every 6 h intravenously for 4 days. The first dose of dexamethasone should be given before the first dose of antibiotic. The concomitant use of an intravenous H_2-receptor antagonist is recommended. For cerebral arterial complications there is no proven therapy. Vasospasm of the large arteries at the base of the brain, with a high risk of cerebral infarction, resembles vasospasm in subarachnoid hemorrhage after aneurysmal bleeding. In these patients, *hypervolemic hypertensive therapy* could be considered to prevent irreversible brain damage, but this has not yet been investigated in bacterial meningitis.

Anticoagulation of septic venous sinus thrombosis in bacterial meningitis is a subject of controversy. Recently, the beneficial effect of dose-adjusted intravenous heparin was reported in patients with aseptic venous sinus thrombosis. Although prospective controlled studies on the treatment of septic venous sinus thrombosis have not been performed, anticoagulation with intravenous heparin seems justified, since the outcome with antibiotic therapy alone is unsatisfactory, with mortality still between 50% and 78%.

Immediate treatment of hydrocephalus by ventricular drainage is easy and very effective. Subdural effusion (sterile) usually spontaneously resolves and does not require surgical therapy. Only in cases of clinical deterioration due to subdural empyema should *stereotactic aspiration* be performed.

Treatment of increased ICP is discussed in Chap. 9.

New Developments

Free-radical scavengers and non-steroidal anti-inflammatory agents such as indomethacin have had beneficial effects in experimental animal studies of bacterial meningitis, but so far they have not been investigated clinically. Further studies are needed to determine whether some of the approaches recently considered, such as application of monoclonal antibodies directed against leukocyte endothelial adhesion molecules, endotoxin, or cytokines (tumor necrosis factor alpha or interleukin 1β), may be applied in clinical practice.

Prognosis and Conclusions

Despite the improvement in antimicrobial therapy during the past few decades, the mortality and number of sequelae due to bacterial meningitis remain high. The unfavorable clinical outcome is often due to intracranial complications such as cerebral edema, hydrocephalus, and cerebrovascular complications during the acute phase of the disease. The availability of the third-generation cephalosporins has led to a decrease in mortality of gram-negative meningitis from 40–80% to 10–20%; however, the mortality of bacterial meningitis due to pneumococcus, which is the most frequent pathogen in adult bacterial meningitis, is still as high as 20–30%. The overall incidence of sensorineural hearing loss in children with bacterial meningitis is 10–30%. The antibiotics most often used for the treatment of bacterial meningitis are known to induce autolysis, which results in the release of inflammatory cell wall components. Further improvement of antibiotics so that they retain killing without lysis may substantially improve the prognosis of the disease. Likewise, it may also be helpful to identify agents capable of intervening with mediators which are believed to be of major importance in producing secondary brain damage. Thus, in clinical practice, early detection and better management of the complications may be important factors in decreasing mortality and improving prognosis of bacterial meningitis.

Suggested Reading

Arevalo CE, Barnes PF, Duda M, Leedom JM (1989) Cerebrospinal fluid cell counts and chemistries in bacterial meningitis. South Med J 82:1122–1127

Bone RC, Fisher CJ, Clemmer TB et al. (1987) A controlled trial of high-dose methyl-prednisolone in the treatment of severe sepsis and septic shock. N Engl J Med 317:563–568

Cabral DA, Flodmark O, Farrell K, Speert DP (1987) Prospective study of computed tomography in acute bacterial meningitis. J Pediatr 111:201–205

Cohen J, Glauser MP (1991) Septic shock: treatment. Lancet 338:736–739

DiNubile MJ, Boom WH, Southwick FS (1990) Septic cortical thrombophlebitis. J Infect Dis 161:1216–1220

Dodge PR, Swartz MN (1965) Bacterial meningitis – a review of selected aspects. II. Special neurologic problems, postmeningitic complications and clinicopathologic correlations. N Engl J Med 272:954–960

Dodge PR, Davis H, Feigin RD, Holmes SJ, Kaplan SL, Jubelirer DP, Stechenberg BW, Hirsh SK (1984) Prospective evaluation of hearing impairment as a sequela of acute bacterial meningitis. N Engl J Med 311:869–874

Durand ML, Calderwood SB, Weber DJ et al. (1993) Acute bacterial meningitis in adults. N Engl J Med 328:21–28

Einhäupl KM, Villringer A, Meister W et al. (1991) Heparin treatment in sinus venous thrombosis. Lancet 338:597–600

Felgenhauer K, Kober D (1985) Apurulent bacterial meningitis (compartmental leucopenia in purulent meningitis). J Neurol 232:157–161

Geiseler PJ, Nelson KE, Levin S, Reddi KT, Moses VK (1980) Community-acquired purulent meningitis: a review of 11 316 cases during the antibiotic era, 1954–1976. Rev Infect Dis 2:725–745

Gilbert DN (1991) Minireview: once-daily aminoglycoside therapy. J Antimicrob Chemother 35:399–405

Girgis NI, Farid Z, Mikhail IA, Farrag I, Sultan Y, Kilpatrick ME (1989) Dexamethasone treatment for bacterial meningitis in children and adults. Pediatr Infect Dis J 8:848–851

Haring HP, Rötzer HK, Reindl H, Berek K, Kampfl A, Pfausler B, Schmutzhard E (1993) Time course of cerebral blood flow velocity in central nervous system infections. A transcranial Doppler sonography study. Arch Neurol 50:98–101

Horwitz SJ, Boxerbaum B, O'Bell J (1980) Cerebral herniation in bacterial meningitis in childhood. Ann Neurol 7:524–528

Igarashi M, Gilmartin RC, Gerald B, Wilburn F, Jabbour JT (1984) Cerebral arteritis and bacterial meningitis. Arch Neurol 41:531–535

Kaplan SL, Fishman MA (1988) Update on bacterial meningitis. J Child Neurol 3: 82–93

Mustafa MM, Lebel MH, Ramilo O, Olsen KD, Reisch JS, Beutler B, McCracken GH (1989) Correlation of interleukin-1β and cachectin concentrations in cerebrospinal fluid and outcome from bacterial meningitis. J Pediatr 115:208–213

Odio CM, Faingezicht I, Paris M et al. (1991) The beneficial effects of early dexamethasone administration in infants and children with bacterial meningitis. N Engl J Med 324:1525–1531

Paulson OB, Brodersen P, Hansen EL, Kristensen HS (1974) Regional cerebral blood flow, cerebral metabolic rate of oxygen, and cerebrospinal fluid acid-base variables in patients with acute meningitis and with encephalitis. Acta Med Scand 196:191–198

Peltola H, Anttila M, Renkonen OV and the Finnish study group (1989) Randomised comparison of chloramphenicol, ampiciliin, cefotaxime, and ceftriaxone for childhood bacterial meningitis. Lancet 1:1281–1286

Peukonen OV, Sivonen A, Visakorpi R (1987) Effect of ciprofloxacin on carrier rate of Neisseria meningitidis in army recruits in Finland. Antimicrob Agents Chemother 31:962–963

Pfister HW, Koedel U, Haberl R, Dirnagl U, Feiden W, Ruckdeschel G, Einhäupl KM (1990) Microvascular changes during the early phase of experimental pneumococcal meningitis. J Cereb Blood Flow Metab 10:914–922

Pfister HW, Borasio GD, Dirnagl U, Bauer M, Einhäupl KM (1992a) Cerebrovascular complications of bacterial meningitis in adults. Neurology 42:1497–1504

Pfister HW, Koedel U, Lorenzl S, Tomasz A (1992b) Antioxidants attenuate microvascular changes in the early phase of experimental pneumococcal meningitis in rats. Stroke 23:1798–1804

Pfister HW, Feiden W, Einhäupl KM (1993) The spectrum of complications during bacterial meningitis in adults: results of a prospective clinical study. Arch Neurol 50: 575–581

Pugsley MP, Dworzack DL, Horowitz EA et al. (1987) Efficacy of ciprofloxacin in the treatment of nasopharyngeal carriers of Neisseria meningitidis. J Infect Dis 156: 211–213

Quagliarello V, Scheld WM (1992) Mechanisms of disease: bacterial meningitis: pathogenesis, pathophysiology, and progress. N Engl J Med 327:864–872

Raimondi AJ, DiRocca C (1979) The physiopathologic basis for the angiographic diagnosis of bacterial infections of the brain and its covering in children. Childs Brain 5:1–13

Roos KL, Tunkel AR, Scheld WM (1991) Acute bacterial meningitis in children and adults. In: Scheld WM, Whitley RJ, Durack DT (eds) Infections of the central nervous system. Raven, New York, pp 335–410

Saez-Llorens X, Ramilo O, Mustafa MM, Mertsola J, McCracken GH (1990) Molecular pathophysiology of bacterial meningitis: current concepts and therapeutic implications. J Pediatr 116:671–684

Sagar SM, McGuire D (1991) Infectious diseases. In: Samuels MA (ed) Manual of neurology. Diagnosis and therapy, 4th edn. Little, Brown, Boston, pp 127–182

Saukkonen K, Sande S, Cioffe C, Wolpe S, Sherry B, Cerami A, Tuomanen E (1990) The role of cytokines in the generation of inflammation and tissue damage in experimental gram-positive meningitis. J Exp Med 171:439–448

Schaad UB, Suter S, Gianella-Boradori A, Pfenninger J, Auckthaler R, Bernath O, Cheseaux JJ, Wedgwood J (1990) Comparison of ceftriaxone and cefuroxime for the treatment of bacterial meningitis in children. N Engl J Med 322:141–147

Scheld WM (1989) Drug delivery to the central nervous system: general principles and relevance to therapy for infections of the central nervous system. Rev Infect Dis 11 [Suppl 7]:1669–1690

Schmutzhard E, Aichner F, Berek K et al. (1989) Akute Komplikationen der Pneumokokken-Meningoenzephalitis. Intensivbehandlung 14:91–95

Smith AL (1988) Neurologic sequelae of meningitis. N Engl J Med 319:1012–1014

Southwick FS, Richardson EP jr, Swartz MN (1986) Septic thrombosis of the dural venous sinuses. Medicine (Baltimore) 65: 82–106

Sprung CL, Caralis PV, Marcial EH et al. (1984) The effects of high-dose corticosteroids in patients with septic shock. A prospective, controlled study. N Engl J Med 311: 1137–1143

Swartz MN (1984) Bacterial meningitis: more involved than just the meninges. N Engl J Med 311:912–914

Tuomanen E, Liu H, Hengstler B, Zak O, Tomasz A (1985) The induction of meningeal inflammation by components of the pneumococcal cell wall. J Infect Dis 151: 858–868

Tuomanen EI, Saukkonen K, Sande S, Cioffe C, Wright SD (1989) Reduction of inflammation, tissue damage, and mortality in bacterial meningitis in rabbits treated with monoclonal antibodies against adhesion-promoting receptors of leucocytes. J Exp Med 170:959–969

Tunkel AR, Wispelwey B, Scheld WM (1990) Bacterial meningitis: recent advances in pathophysiology and treatment. Ann Intern Med 112:610–623

Tureen JH, Dworkin RJ, Kennedy SL, Sachdeva M, Sande MA (1990) Loss of cerebrovascular autoregulation in experimental meningitis in rabbits. J Clin Invest 85:577–581

Veterans Administration Systemic Sepsis Cooperative Study Group (1987) Effect of high-dose glucocorticoid therapy on mortality in patients with clinical signs of systemic sepsis. N Engl J Med 317:659–665

Chapter 37

Tuberculous Meningitis and Central Nervous System Tuberculosis

ERICH SCHMUTZHARD and ULRICH ROELCKE

Definition and Epidemiology

Tuberculosis can affect almost any organ system in the body. It is caused by *Mycobacterium tuberculosis* and *M. bovis* and is characterized histologically by granuloma formation. Tuberculosis remains a major health problem and affects half the world's population, with an estimated 10 million new cases per year. In industrialized countries, tuberculosis occurs mainly among the poor, such as in drug addicts and in immigrants from developing countries. Although there was a steady decrease in the incidence of tuberculosis over the past century, the number of reported cases has dramatically increased in the past decade, most likely because of the acquired immune deficiency syndrome. The incidence of multiple-drug-resistant *M. tuberculosis* infection is also increasing.

Patients may present with tuberculous meningitis, tuberculous encephalopathy, intracranial tuberculomas, and rarely, tuberculous

---

Section Editor. Thomas P. Bleck

brain abscesses. Patients with tuberculous meningitis (basilar) may require neurocritical care for treatment of obstructive hydrocephalus or vasculitis-related cerebral infarction. Those with tuberculomas and tuberculous abscesses may present with symptoms and signs of space-occupying lesions (increased pressure on vital structures, such as the brain stem). Patients may also have seizures. Tuberculous spinal osteomyelitis, necrotizing myelopathy, and tuberculosis of the skull usually do not result in life-threatening complications.

Pathogenesis

M. tuberculosis is a nonmotile rod that measures $0.5 \times 4.0 \mu m$. It is acid fast with the Ziehl-Neelson stain and grows on egg-enriched media but may require up to 8 weeks for growth. Central nervous system tuberculosis occurs in about 10% of all patients with tuberculosis and spreads secondarily from a focus elsewhere in the body. The primary infection is usually in the lung, or rarely in the gastrointestinal tract. Sometimes the primary infection is not obvious. Miliary tuberculosis is found in about two thirds of patients. In 1933, Rich and Mc-Cordoch postulated that ruptured meningeal tuberculous foci ("Rich's focus") can spread mycobacteria through the CSF.

Clinical Features and Differential Diagnosis

Chronic meningitis can have many infectious and noninfectious causes. The differential diagnosis is listed in Table 1.

Tuberculous Meningitis

Tuberculous meningitis begins with a prodromal phase which lasts for several weeks; patients may become anorexic, apathetic, or irritable. Mental status changes, including abnormal behavior; confusion, and depression may occur. Patients have headache, photophobia, and neck stiffness. Fever may or may not be present. Patients with basilar meningitis present with the triad of cranial nerve palsy, arteritis of the basilar vessels, and hydrocephalus. If untreated, increased intracranial pressure leads to coma, decerebrate posturing, hypothalamic disturbances, and death within weeks. Rarely, the course is more chronic. Occasionally, the onset may be fulminant, similar to that of acute bacterial meningitis. Infrequently, patients can present with stroke resulting in acute focal neurological deficits. Seizures can occur at any stage of the disease.

Table 1. Differential diagnosis of chronic meningitis

Infectious causes
  cryptococcosis
  histoplasmosis
  candidiasis
  coccidioidomycosis
  other rare fungal diseases
  partially treated bacterial meningitis
  epidural and subdural empyema, brain abscess
  spirochetal infections:
    syphilis
    borreliosis
  brucellosis
  nocardiosis
  actinomycosis
  toxoplasmosis
  cysticercosis
  trypanosomiasis
  viral meningoencephalitis

Noninfectious causes
  carcinomatous and leukemic meningitis
  sarcoidosis
  Vogt-Koyanagyi-Harada syndrome
  granulomatous angiitis
  Behçet's disease
  systemic lupus erythematosus
  multiple emboli (e.g. septic emboli)

Tuberculous Encephalopathy

Tuberculous encephalopathy occurs almost exclusively in children and may occur even without meningitis. It is thought to be caused by an immune response and is characterized by diffuse edema of the white matter. Patients typically present with acute onset of seizures, coma, and decerebrate posturing.

Intracranial Tuberculomas

Single or multiple tuberculomas can occur anywhere in the brain, with or without meningitis. Most patients present with symptoms and signs of space-occupying, expanding lesions, such as seizures, hemiparesis, or other focal deficits. Patients with posterior fossa tuberculomas may have cerebellar or brain-stem syndromes and obstructive hydrocephalus. It is not possible to clinically distinguish patients with tuberculomas from those with tumors. Even during antituberculous treatment, tuberculomas can continue to expand. In some patients, tuberculomas may merely accompany tuberculous meningitis and not cause symptoms directly.

Table 2. Diagnostic workup of CNS tuberculosis

- detailed history and neurological examination
- examination of the retina for papilledema and retinal tubercles
- analysis of CSF for microbiolgy
- *leukocyte count, erythrocyte sedimentation rate
- *intradermal skin test
- *chest X-ray
- CCT scan (with contrast)
- MRI
- Transcranial Doppler sonography
- Cerebral angiography
- Biopsy of meninges or tuberculoma

* of minor importance but not invasive or hazardous to patients

Tuberculous Brain Abscesses

Patients with tuberculous brain abscesses clinically resemble those with bacterial abscesses and have increased intracranial pressure, focal deficits, and seizures. Tuberculous abscesses do not have granulomatous changes in their walls.

Diagnosis

If clinical features are suggestive of central nervous system tuberculosis, a stepwise approach of diagnostic steps is recommended (see Table 2). The following is a review of ancillary tests that may help to confirm the diagnosis.

Cerebrospinal Fluid, Microbiology, and Other Laboratory Tests

Results of CSF analysis in tuberculous meningitis are usually abnormal (except in patients with isolated intracranial tuberculomas). The CSF is usually clear or slightly opaque and the opening pressure is usually increased. The glucose concentration is decreased, but often not as much as in bacterial meningitis (blood: CSF ratio 2:1). It may be normal early in the course. Most patients have a mononuclear or lymphocytic pleocytosis (cell count between 100 and 1000/ml. Rarely, patients present with a neutrophilic pleocytosis.) When CSF circulation is impaired, the protein concentration may be markedly increased and the fluid may appear xanthochromic.

Detection of acid-fast bacilli (AFB) in the CSF is the most definitive way of diagnosing tuberculous meningitis and CNS tuberculosis; however, this is possible in fewer than 30% of patients. *M. tuberculosis* can be cultured in up to 75% of patients with tuberculous meningitis but, because of the slow growth, cultures are less important clinically. Concentration of tuberculostearic acid has been reported to be both a sensitive (100%) and a specific (92%) marker for CNS tuberculosis (positive predictive value of 78% and negative predictive value of 100%). These results have been difficult to reproduce. Various immunological methods, such as dot-immunobinding assays and enzyme-linked immunosorbent assays (ELISA), have been used to detect *M. tuberculosis* antigen 5 and antimycobacterial antibodies in the CSF. These methods are not widely available. Polymerase chain reaction (PCR) is probably the most sensitive technique, if cross-contamination can be kept to a minimum, to confirm tuberculous meningitis in culture-negative patients. Determination of CSF adenosine deaminase has been reported to be helpful in distinguishing CNS tuberculosis from bacterial meningitis. A recent controlled study, however, revealed no statistically significant difference in the concentrations in these two groups of patients.

The leukocyte count may be normal or decreased, though a relative lymphocytosis may be present. The erythrocyte sedimentation rate may be normal or increased (often greater than 100 mm/h). Intradermal skin tests are useful when positive; however, they may be falsely negative in about 20–40% of patients, even when there is no other evidence of immunosuppression. The tuberculin skin test may become positive during treatment. The radiographic findings, which frequently are nonspecific early in the disease, include hilar adenopathy, infiltrates, and cavities in the superior segment of the lower lobe, and pleural scarring or pleural effusions. The chest X-ray may be normal in about 50% of patients. Thoracocentesis or pleural biopsy should be done if pleural scarring or pleural effusions are present. Gastric secretions, sputum, and urine should be stained for AFB.

Neuroimaging and Ancillary Tests

Patients with CNS tuberculosis have characteristic, but not pathognomonic, findings on CT scan. Communicating or obstructive hydrocephalus is found in up to 80% of patients. Administration of contrast medium results in basal meningeal enhancement. Ischemic infarction may also be seen. Co-existing contrast-enhancing tuberculomas are occasionally found and may become calcified later. It may be impossible on CT scan to distinguish tuberculomas from tumors (for example, meningiomas) or other infectious diseases causing space-occupying lesions or to distinguish tuberculous abscesses from bacterial abscesses. Because tuberculous meningitis usually occurs at the base of the brain, MRI allows better visualization of granulomatous changes within the basal cisterns. MRI can show thickened basal meninges with enhancement, hydrocephalus, and ischemic cerebral infarction (Fig. 1). MRI can also visualize obstruction of the CSF circulation, enabling the clinician to closely monitor the effect of treatment. On angiography, findings are nonspecific and tuberculomas may simulate gliomas, metastases, and especially meningiomas. Vascular stenosis or occlusion can be visualized in some patients with tuberculous meningitis.

Other ancillary tests, including EEG, motor, and sensory-evoked potentials, and early auditory-evoked potentials, are usually not helpful in confirming the diagnosis of CNS tuber-

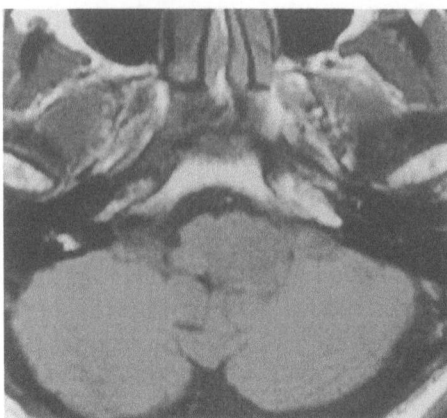
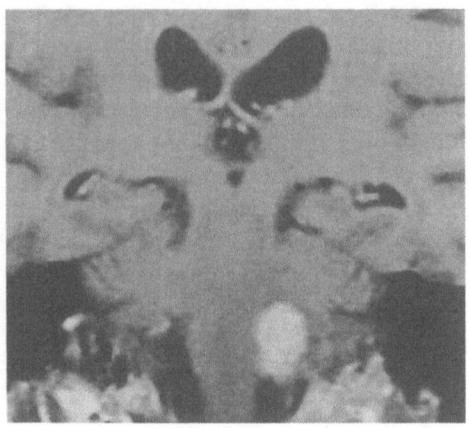

a   b

Fig. 1a,b. Tuberculous meningitis in a 47-year-old man with impaired oculomotor functions, signs of increased intracranial pressure, and abnormal CSF. T1-weighted MR images obtained before (**a**, axial view) and after (**b**, coronal view) IV administration of paramagnetic contrast agent show soft tissue mass next to swollen medulla oblongata that enhances markedly and homogeneously. Medullary enlargement likely reflects reactive edema or edema due to local vasculitis. (Courtesy of Klaus Sartor and Marius Hartmann, Heidelberg)

culosis. Focal or generalized seizure activity may occasionally be seen in patients with tuberculomas. Auditory-evoked potentials may be used to monitor side effects of antituberculosis treatment. Transcranial Doppler sonography may be helpful by detecting vasculitis in the basal intracranial arteries and in monitoring the course of disease.

Biopsy

Rarely, biopsy is performed for histological, microbiological, and immunological studies. It should be considered in immunocompromised patients, in whom the diagnosis of tuberculous meningitis is difficult to make and in whom delay of treatment may be harmful. It should also be considered in the rare cases where intracranial tuberculomas present without accompanying tuberculous meningitis.

Treatment

Specific Chemotherapy

Most patients with CNS tuberculosis can be treated on the regular ward. Table 3 lists criteria for neurocritical care. In general, there is no consensus on how and for how long CNS tuberculosis should be treated. Large controlled trials comparing various treatment regimens are under way, but definitive results are still lacking. Several antituberculous drugs are available, though there are differences in CSF penetration, drug-resistance patterns, and side effects. The mycobacterial strain and sensitivity to drugs should be ascertained as early as possible.

Table 4 lists the drugs currently recommended for the treatment of CNS tuberculosis, including dosages for adults, degree of CNS penetration, and major side effects. Usually, a

Table 3. Indications for neurocritical care in patients with CNS tuberculosis

---

- Reduced level of consciousness due to raised intracranial pressure (requiring ICP monitoring)
- Hydrocephalus (both occlusive and aresorptive)
- Tuberculomas in the posterior fossa
- Peri- or postoperative period (e.g. shunt procedure)
- Localizing brainstem and cerebellar signs and symptoms
- Multiple focal neurological deficits
- Tuberculomas precipitating status epilepticus
- Transient focal neurological deficit with evidence of severe vasculitis (by means of angiography or transcranial doppler-sonography)

---

three-drug combination of isoniazid (INH), rifampin, and ethambutol is recommended for the initial 3–4 months, followed by isoniazid and rifampin for 9–21 months. Sometimes a four-drug combination is used (adding pyrazinamide). This, or even a five-drug combination, may be necessary when treating patients with tuberculomas. Enlargement of tuberculomas has been reported during three-drug combination therapy. Rifampin, isoniazid, pyrazinamide, and streptomycin are bactericidal, while ethambutol is bacteriostatic.

If major side effects occur, the doses of isoniazid and rifampin should be decreased or treatment with the drugs should be stopped until clearance has occurred. Dose-dependent neuropathies of the 2nd cranial nerve (ethambutol) and 8th cranial nerve (streptomycin) may occur. Because they are inexpensive, thiacetazone and para-aminosalicylic acid are still widely used in some developing countries, though they are not highly effective. The peripheral neuropathy of isoniazid can be prevented by giving pyridoxine (50 mg/d). Rarely, treatment with isoniazid can result in a Jarisch-Herxheimer-type reaction. In the past, streptomycin and rifampin have been given intrathecally; however, there are no data showing this route to be better than the intramuscular or the oral route.

Adjunctive Therapy

Corticosteroids have been given to patients with CNS tuberculosis in an attempt to reduce arachnoid adhesions; however, improvement in outcome has never been shown. Corticosteroids may be useful in patients who already have hydrocephalus or masses causing ICP elevation once antituberculosis treatment has begun. Recently, intraventricular and intrathecal hyaluronidase have been given to reduce persisting arachnoiditis. Routine use of antiseizure drugs should be avoided. The metabolism of phenytoin is blocked by isoniazid and phenytoin toxicity may occur. In patients with documented seizures (clinically or by EEG), however, treatment with benzodiazepines, carbamazepine, or even phenytoin should be considered.

Neurosurgical Intervention

Ventriculoatrial or ventriculoperitoneal shunts should be performed as early as possible in patients with hydrocephalus (several studies have shown that eary shunting is beneficial). Surgical decompression and biopsy may be necessary in patients with space-occupying tuber-

Table 4. Drug therapy in CNS tuberculosis (modified from Tandon et al. 1988; Wood and Anderson 1988)

Drug	Adult dose	Route	CNS penetration	Major side effects
Isoniazid	8–10 mg/kg/d once daily (max 600 mg)	oral	+++	– peripheral neuropathy (due to pyridoxine antagonism) – very rarely encephalopathy
Rifampin	10 mg/kg/d	IV oral	++	– transient increase in LFTs – severe or permanent liver damage is rare – gastroeneritis
Ethambutol	15–25 mg/kg/d in divided doses (max 1600 mg)	oral	++	– optic neuropathy
Pyrazinamide	30 mg/kg/d in divided doses (max 2000 mg)	oral	+++	– gastrointestinal – liver toxicity – arthralgias
Streptomycin	15–20 mg/kg/d once daily (max 1000 mg)	IM	+	– vestibular and cochlear damage – renal toxicity
Ethionamide	15 mg/kg/d in divided doses	oral IV	+++	– gastrointestinal – liver toxicity – hypoglycemia in diabetics
Thiacetazone[a]	3 mg/kg/d in divided doses (max 150 mg)	oral	++	–
Para-amino salicylic acid	0.2 g/kg/d in divided doses (max 12 g)	oral	+	– gastrointestinal
Cycloserine	10–15 mg/kg/d in divided doses (slow build up)	oral	+++	– gastrointestinal – seizures – neuropsychological symptoms

[a] Very cheap, but not highly effective.
+, poor; ++, sufficient – good if meninges are inflamed; +++, good.

culomas or obstructive hydrocephalus or in those in whom tumor is a possibility. Usually, tuberculomas can be treated conservatively and can be monitored with CT scanning.

Other General Measures

Protection of airways, ventilatory support, and careful fluid management should also be provided. Patients with tuberculous meningitis frequently develop the syndrome of inappropriate secretion of antidiuretic hormone (SIADH) and fluid restriction may be helpful. Depending on the clinical course and the initial CSF and CT findings, patients should be followed closely; CSF analysis and CT scanning should be done twice weekly, or more frequently, if the patient is not improving. The level of consciousness and the extent of focal neurological signs are crucial factors. Evoked potentials have been suggested to detect side effects of treatment as early as possible (for example, 2nd and 8th cranial neuropathies). Transcranial Doppler sonography can be used to assess the risk of stroke in patients with vasculitis. Patients with severe CNS involvement must be monitored closely during the first few weeks of treatment.

Prognosis

The overall mortality in patients treated for CNS tuberculosis ranges from 15% to 30%. Adequate chemotherapy must be started as soon as possible whenever the diagnosis is considered. Even with adequate treatment, some patients with tuberculous meningitis or tuberculomas may worsen. Patients may be left with multiple infarctions, hydrocephalus, and cranial nerve damage. Residual cranial nerve palsies, blindness, seizures, impairment of cognitive function, and hydrocephalus occur in up to 25% of patients. About 50% of patients will have at least some residual damage. The prognosis of those infected with atypical mycobacteria is poor, especially in the setting of HIV infection.

Suggested Reading

Anderson JM, MacMilian JJ (1975) Intracranial tuberculoma – an increasing problem in Britain. J Neurol Neurosurg Psychiatry 38: 194–201

Anonymous (1984) Immune reaction in tuberculosis. Lancet 2:204

Brennan RW, Deheja H, Kutt H, Kerebely K, Mc Dowell F (1970) Diphenylhydantoin intoxication attendant to slow activation of isoniazid. Neurology 20:687–693

Bullock MR (1982) Diagnostic and prognostic features of tuberculous meningitis on CT scanning. J Neurol Neurosurg Psychiatry 45:1098–1101

Bullock MR, van Dellen JR (1982) The role of cerebrospinal fluid shunting in tuberculous meningitis. Surg Neurol 18:274–277

Chambers ST, Hendrickse WA, Record A, Rudge P, Smith H (1984) Paradoxical expansion of intracranial tuberculoma during chemotherapy. Lancet 2:181–184

Chawla RK, Seth RK, Raj B, Saini AS (1991) Adenosine deaminase levels in cerebrospinal fluid in tuberculosis and bacterial meningitis. Tubercle 72:190–192

Collins FM (1982) The immunology of tuberculosis. Am Rev Respir Dis 125:42–49

Des Prez RM, Heim CR (1990) Mycobacterium tuberculosis. In: Mandell GL, Douglas RG, Bennett JE (eds) Principles and practice of infectious diseases, 3rd edn. Churchill Livingstone, New York, pp 1877–1906

Fallon RJ, Kennedy DH (1981) Treatment and prognosis in tuberculous meningitis. J Infection 3 [Suppl]:39–44

Fitzsimons JM (1963) Tuberculous meningitis: a follow-up study on 198 cases. Tubercle 44: 87–102

French GL, Chan CY, Cheng SW, Teoh R, Humphries MJ, O'Mahony G (1987) Diagnosis of tuberculous meningitis by detection of tuberculostearic acid in cerebrospinal fluid. Lancet 2:117–119

Klein NC, Damskr B, Hirschmann SZ (1985) Mycobacterial meningitis: retrospective analysis 1970 to 1983. Am J Med 79:29–34

Kocen RS (1977) Tuberculous meningitis. Br J Hosp Med 18:436–444

Kocen RS, Parsons M (1970) The neurological complications of tuberculosis: some unusual manifestations. Q J Med 34:17–31

Lebas J, Malkin JE, Cognin Y, Modai J (1986) Cerebral tuberculomas developing during treatment of tuberculous meningitis. Lancet 2:84

Luef G, Allerberger F, Cheng A, Chang C, Berek K, Pfausler B, Schmutzhard E (1992) Diagnosis of tuberculous meningitis by detection of tuberculostearic acid in cerebrospinal fluid. Wien Klin Wochenschr 104:322–324

Molouvi A, Le Fock JL (1985) Tuberculous meningitis. Med Clin North Am 69: 315–331

Offenbacher H, Fazekas F, Schmidt R, Kleinert R, Payer F, Kleinert G, Lechner H (1991) MR in tuberculous meningoencephalitis: report of four cases and review of the neuroimaging literature. J Neurol 238: 340–344

O'Mahoney M, Sister C, Lawrence A, Wong P (1976) Tuberculous meningitis. Br Med J 402

Parsons M (1988) Tuberculous meningitis, tuberculomas and spinal tuberculosis. A handbook for clinicians, 2nd edn. Oxford University Press, Oxford

Radhakrishnan VV, Mathai A (1991) A dot-immunobinding assay for the laboratory diagnosis of tuberculous meningitis and its comparison with enzyme-linked immunosorbent assay. J Appl Bacteriol 71: 428–433

Rich AR, McCordock HA (1933) The pathogenesis of tuberculous meningitis. Bull Johns Hopkins Hosp 52:5–38

Rieder HJ, Cauthen GM, Block AB (1988) Tuberculosis and acquired immunodeficiency syndrome – Florida. Arch Intern Med 149:1268–1273

Riggs HE, Rupp C, Ray H (1956) Clinicopathologic study of tuberculous meningitis in adults. Am Rev Tubercul 74:830–834

Roetzer HK, Haring HP, Lehner H, Schmutzhard E (1991) Transcranial Doppler-sonography in infections of the central nervous system. Trop Med Parasitol 42:467 (abstract)

Schachter EH (1972) Tuberculin-negative tuberculosis. Am Rev Respir Dis 106:587–593

Schlossberg D (1990) Infections of the nervous system. (Clinical topics in infectious disease.) Springer, Berlin Heidelberg New York

Schoeman JF, Le Roux D, Bezuidenhout PB, Donald PR (1985) Intracranial pressure monitoring in tuberculous meningitis: clinical and computerized tomographic correlation. Dev Med Child Neurol 27:644–654

Schoeman J, Hewlett R, Donald P (1988) MR of childhood tuberculous meningitis. Neuroradiology 30:473–477

Selwyn PA, Hartel D, Lewis VA, Schoenbaum EE, Vermund SH, Klein RS, Walker AT, Friedland GH (1989) A prospective study of the risk of tuberculosis among intravenous drug abusers with immunodeficiency virus infection. N Engl J Med 320:545–550

Shankar P, Manjunath N, Mohan KK, Prasad K, Behari M, Ahiya GK (1991) Rapid diagnosis of tuberculous meningitis by polymerase chain reaction. Lancet 1:5–7

Tandon PN, Bhatia R, Bhargava S (1988) Tuberculous meningitis. In: Harris AA (ed) Microbial disease. Elsevier Science, Amsterdam, pp 195–226 (Handbook of clinical neurology, vol 8, 52)

Traub M, Colchester ACF, Kingsley DPE, Swash M (1984) Tuberculosis of the central nervous system. Q J Med 53:81–100

Van Scoy RE, Wilkowske CJ (1983) Antituberculous agents. Mayo Clinic Proc 58: 233–240

Wood M, Anderson M (1988) Neurological infections. Saunders, London (Major problems in neurology, vol 16)

Chapter 38 | **Brain Abscess and Empyema**

Philip A. Villanueva

Introduction

Although variable in their presentation, brain abscesses and empyema share a common tendency to produce a disappointing outcome. This may be due to a number of causes: (a) They may occur in cases where there has been a previous central nervous system (CNS) insult (e.g., trauma, infarct, surgery). (b) The immune response of the CNS has previously been impaired (e.g., trauma, underlying systemic disease). (c) The immune response of the CNS is relatively limited, even under normal circumstances. (d) By their nature, an abscess, especially in the cerebritic stage, and an empyema may create a significant vasculitic picture, both macro- and microscopically, which may in turn lead to further ischemic tissue damage. (e) Brain abscesses, either in the cerebritic or the "mature" phase, may act as mass lesions creating major intracranial pressure (ICP) problems.

As a result, these pyogenic conditions may lead to permanent tissue

damage in areas beyond their topographical extent. Therefore, the clinician must be concerned not only with treating the actual lesion itself, but also with minimizing the deleterious effects upon the surrounding tissues. The intensive care unit (ICU) management of this disease process is critical to limiting the amount of tissue lost or damaged. Likewise, as many patients with these entities are systemically ill, they may require intensive management for their extracranial problems.

On a pathophysiological basis, there may be a continuum between intracranial empyema and abscess. For organizational purposes, this chapter will treat the two entities separately. Each section will briefly discuss the major pathophysiological features of the disease process and therapy, emphasizing the ICU aspects.

Brain Abscess

Brain abscess remains a frustrating entity. The ease of diagnosis has improved significantly with the devel-

Section Editor: Thomas P. Bleck

opment of modern neuroimaging techniques such as CT and MRI; however, the causative organisms have apparently increased greatly both in number and in virulence. This may be due to increasing antibiotic resistance, as well as to the increasing number of potential patients with compromised immunity.

Bacterial abscesses generally develop in four stages. Following inoculation of the site, days 1–3 show a microscopic picture of an "early" or diffuse cerebritis. From day 4 to 9, the picture is that of a more organized, or "late" cerebritis. Early capsule formation is noted from day 10 to 13, and late capsule formation after 2 weeks. Generally, the single thick-walled abscesses are due to contiguous spread, while the thin-walled variety, especially if multiple, are associated with hematogenous spread.

The abscess almost always occurs at the point of inoculation. This may be via direct contiguity or blood-borne spread. In the cases of contiguous spread, several conditions may predispose the patient to infection. These are traumatic injury, surgery, and sinus infections. Overlying scalp and skin infections have also been included among these causes, but in actuality, spread is via the blood, presumably through emissary veins which traverse the skull.

Traumatic injury predisposes the patient to brain abscess in several ways. In the case of an open but not penetrating injury, there may be bone and dural violation overlying ischemic or necrotic brain. Retention of foreign bodies within the wound may increase the likelihood of abscess formation. If there has been penetrating trauma, the presence of retained foreign bodies or bone fragments surrounded by devitalized tissue may similarly increase the risk. The concomitant immune compromise associated with head trauma may also be a significant predisposing factor. Brain abscess development following operative intervention for nontraumatic causes is associated with CSF leakage, intraoperative wound contamination, and placement of surgical prostheses, including ICP-monitoring devices. Local areas of ischemia and necrosis provide further support for bacterial growth.

The development of brain abscess due to a contiguous sinusitis probably remains the most common cause of this disease entity. As would be expected, the location of the involved sinus will determine the portion of the brain affected. Therefore, frontal and ethmoidal sinus infections are associated with frontal lobe abscesses, infections in the maxillary sinuses with temporal lobe abscesses, and mastoid sinus disease with cerebellar, temporal, and occipital infections. Sinusitis of the ethmoid or sphenoid sinuses may be associated with temporal or frontal abscesses.

Brain abscesses which develop due to blood-borne bacteria are associated with several factors. Congenital right-to-left intracardiac shunting remains a cause, as does intrapulmonic shunting. The net result of both processes is to bypass the normal filtration process of the lung, with the resulting escape of bacteria into the systemic arterial circulation. Blood-borne abscess formation is also associated with immune compromise. This state is associated with several etiologies: the use of immunosuppressive drugs, as in cancer chemotherapy or organ transplantation; the acquired immune deficiency state (AIDS); and the immune suppression which occurs as a result of trauma. The first of these causes has long been known; the second has become associated with more "exotic" agents; the third cause, especially neurotrauma, has only recently been recognized as a major cause of immune suppression. Other disease states which are associated with brain abscess formation are endocarditis, diverticular disease, osteomyelitis, and oral/gingival infections. However, in a significant number of patients the source remains undetermined.

The most common bacteria associated with abscesses are streptococci (aerobic and beta-hemolytic), *Staphylococcus aureus*, *Pneumococcus*, and *Enterococcus*. Also found, depending upon the culturing technique, are *Bacteroides* species and anaerobic *Streptococcus*. These latter two may have a higher incidence than previously identified. Careful anaerobic technique is necessary to allow their growth from abscess tissue. Blood-borne infections have a tendency to follow the intracranial arterial paths with the greatest flow. Therefore, the incidence of abscess formation is greatest in the parietal lobes, due to the flow from the middle cerebral arteries, while bacterial "deposition" tends to occur where blood flow is slowest, that is, in the capillary level at the gray-white junction.

Clinical Presentation and Diagnosis

Several factors influence the clinical presentation of the patient with a brain abscess: size, location, nature of the infecting organism, and host response.

There is no clear-cut or universal picture seen in with abscesses. In general, there are four major clinical pictures.

The first pattern is that of the focal mass with rapid expansion. These lesions present with focal findings initially, but they progress rapidly to a diffuse picture with elevated ICP. The next pattern is that of a diffuse depression of cerebral function, with little or no focality but elevated ICP. The third clinical picture is that of a diffuse destructive lesion with multiple deficits. The ICP may well be less than initially expected. The final pattern is that of the small, discrete lesion with focal deficits and little or no elevation of ICP. These lesions tend to be more irritative and chronic in nature, and seizures may be the first sign.

There are several other findings which are noted in varying degrees with brain abscesses. These are: fever (usually low grade and seen in approximately 50% of cases), nausea and vomiting (which may be associated with ICP elevation), and a diffuse alteration in mental status which is seen to varying extent in approximately half the cases.

Ancillary Tests

Most laboratory tests are not conclusive in the diagnosis of a brain abscess. Peripheral white cell count may be only mildly elevated, but the erythrocyte sedimentation rate (ESR) may be elevated significantly. Lumbar puncture seldom yields useful information and, because of the risk of herniation, should be avoided.

410   P.A. Villanueva

Computerized tomography (CT) has provided the major advance in the diagnosis of brain abscesses (Fig. 1). The radiographic findings of brain abscesses in their various stages have been described elsewhere. CT has significantly decreased the time to diagnosis in these cases, enabling earlier definitive therapy to be started. It is also of value in determining the progress of medical therapy (e.g., antibiotics during the cerebritis stage) or the degree of surgical success in aspiration or excision. MRI allows for even better resolution and early identification of additional chanels such as subdural abscess or additional meningeal involvement (Fig. 2).

Surgical Management

Surgical therapy, which may range from drainage to excision, provides the opportunity to treat several aspects of the abscess picture. First, definitive identification of the organism(s) may be obtained via proper culture. Next, devitalized tissue and cavity fluid may be removed or reduced in volume. This, in turn, may reduce or relieve the elevated intracranial pressure.

The first technique, simple drainage, employs the insertion of a pliable tube, via a needle, into the abscess cavity. The tube is then withdrawn over days, allowing the abscess cavity both to drain as well as to shrink.

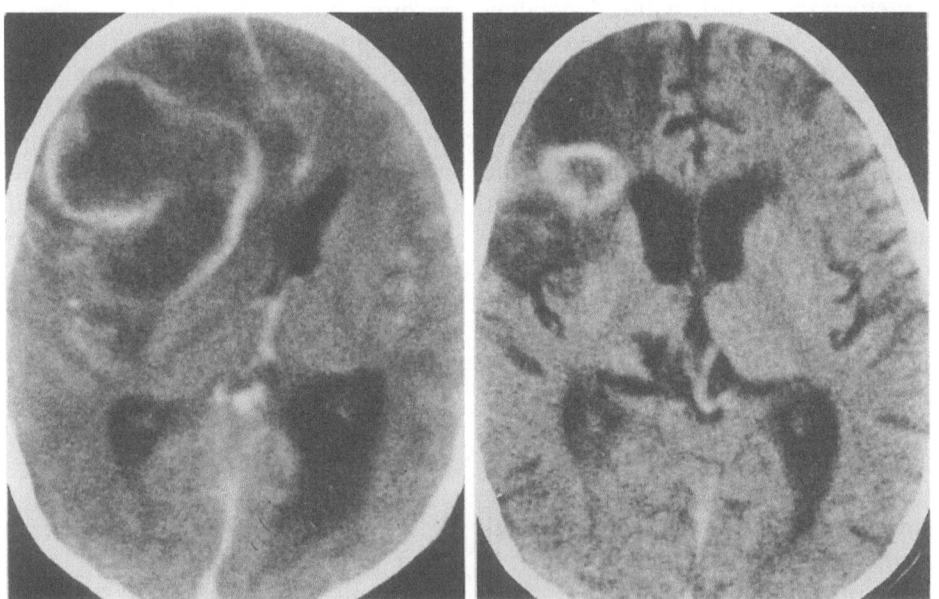

a   b

Fig. 1a,b. Cerebral abscess in a 2-year-old boy who, after aspiration of a peanut, first developed pneumonia and then signs of increased intracranial pressure. Initial CT scan obtained after IV administration of iodinated contrast material (**a**) demonstrate large, slighly lobulated and hypodense mass lesion with peripheral (ring) enhancement involving the frontotemporal region of the right cerebral hemisphere; there is severe mass effect. After surgical drainage and treatment with antibiotics the lesion became much smaller, with correspondingly reduced mass effect (**b**), but some, presumably permanent damage to the brain parenchyma remained. (Courtesy of Klaus Sartor and Marius Hartmann, Heidelberg)

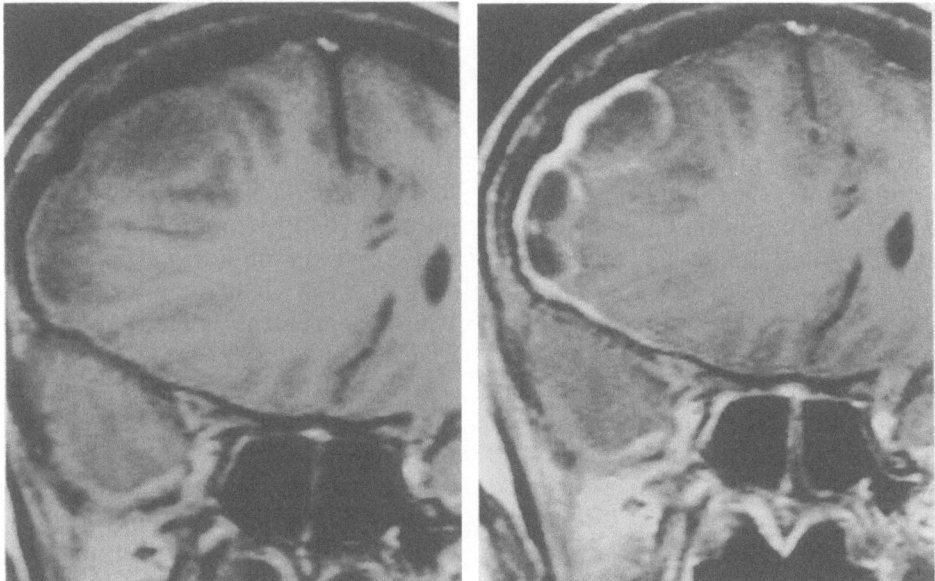

a   b

Fig. 2a,b. Subdural empyema in a 66-year-old woman with increasing headache but no fever or focal neurologic signs 6 weeks after a right mastoidectomy. T1-weighted coronal MR images obtained before (**a**) and after (**b**) IV administration of paramagnetic contrast agent demonstrates lobulated or partially septated extra-axial mass lesion of low signal intensity that exhibits marked peripheral enhancement. Note that there is additional enhancement of the frontobasal dura. (Courtesy of Klaus Sartor and Marius Hartmann, Heidelberg)

Improvements in perioperative management have meant that this approach is applied less frequently. Currently, the two techniques most applied are aspiration and excision. The factors which influence the choice between these two methods include size and age of the abscess, its location, the patient's neurological and systemic status, and the risk(s) of perioperative complications. Excision tends to be associated with a lower recurrence rate than does aspiration, but studies comparing the two techniques tend to include in the aspirated groups a higher percentage of multiple and or deeply situated abscesses in "sicker" patients. Aspiration may be performed via CT or other stereotactically guided techniques; the anesthetic risks are fewer, with less systemic stress to the patient, and it may be performed more than once, as in the case of the patient who remains unstable for a prolonged time period. When excision is opted for, certain operative principles are employed: wide exposure; accurate localization of the lesion(s) using intraoperative ultrasound; control of the cavity contents to prevent spillage; meticulous care in obtaining adequate anaerobic cultures; thorough irrigation using an antibiotic solution; and repeated use of ultrasound to ensure removal of all necrotic material. The bone flap is replaced unless there is gross spillage of the abscess contents. An ICP monitor is usually placed (if not inserted preoperatively) and kept in place for 5–7 days. Where abscesses occur in contiguity with extradural infections, the latter are treated at the same time to minimize re-infection. This may be done by the neurosurgeon, oral/maxillofacial surgeon, or otolaryngologist. Empiric antibiotic coverage is begun based upon Gram-stain results unless an etiology is already known; coverage usually includes ceftriaxone, vancomycin, and metronidazole. If *Listeria monocytogenes* is suspected, penicillin and/or sulfa-trimethoprim are added. The antibiotics are continued for 4–8 weeks with CT scans performed weekly or when needed as dictated by the patient's condition.

Nonsurgical Management

Nonsurgical therapy remains a somewhat controversial approach. In general, it is reserved for those patients who, for medical reasons, are not able to undergo aspiration or excision. In general, the lesions which best lend themselves to nonoperative therapy are smaller and thinner walled (preferably in the cerebritic stage). In many cases, the causative organism will have been determined via blood or aspirate culture. Antibiotic therapy is maintained for 6–8 weeks. Serial CT scans are performed to monitor the efficacy of therapy. This method of therapy appears effective when there are multiple, poorly accessible lesions or when the patient is considered a poor operative risk. An aspirate culture should be obtained from the most accessible lesion (in the case of more than one) to determine the appropriate antibiotic coverage.

Intensive Care Unit Management

ICU management of the patient with a brain abscess is directed toward maintenance of CNS homeostasis. This is done by the maintenance of ICP and acceptable cerebral perfusion pressure (CPP), conntrol of seizures, and provision of adequate systemic support. For ICP monitoring and ICP management please refer to Chaps. 8 and 9.

Corticosteroids are not used in the management of brain abscess in our institution. It is felt that whatever benefit may accrue in terms of brain swelling control is greatly outweighed by the further impairment of immune function. Others use them after appropriate antibiotic treatment has begun in patients with cerebral edema surrounding the abscess.

Several other neurological monitoring techniques may be utilized in ICU management of the brain abscess, including cerebral blood flow, jugular venous bulb O_2 saturation ($SJVO_2$), and evoked potential monitoring. These techniques may provide an effective indication of the functional status of the brain. At this time, they are not a suitable alternative for ICP monitoring, but may be used in conjunction with it. Jugular bulb saturation monitoring has been an especially helpful technique, with saturations below 50% alerting the clinician to potential intracranial ischemia. A regional/focal cerebral blood flow (CBF) monitoring device may be placed at the time of operation in the surgical field so as to follow CBF postoperatively. This technique, though limited to a single gyrus, can provide valuable information regarding CBF in the affected area. The CBF may be monitored globally using xenon-133 or N_2O via inhalation methods. The global rate of cerebral oxygen utilization ($CMRO_2$) may be determined if CBF and $SJVO_2$ are known. As $CMRO_2$ is probably the most accurate indicator of CNS function, the clinician has access to real-time data regarding the status of the brain. PET scanning can reveal local changes in $CMRO_2$ or glucose utilization.

From a systemic standpoint, ICU management of the brain abscess patient is directed toward avoiding the systemic causes of secondary CNS insult and treating the infection, both at the CNS level and at its original source (if known). Airway control and ventilatory support may be required, depending upon the level of consciousness of the patient. If intubation beyond 7 days is expected, early tracheostomy should be considered. This has proven to be of value for several reasons: the effectiveness of pulmonary toilet is improved, ICP control may be facilitated, patient comfort is usually increased, and sinus drainage is enhanced. This latter point may be of considerable significance in the case of an infection which has extended from an infected sinus. Conversion of a naso- or endotracheal tube to a tracheostomy will allow reduction of mucosal swelling and improve drainage of the sinus contents. Muscle relaxation and sedation are used to prevent struggling and control agitation, two patient responses which may worsen brain swelling.

Nutritional support is provided in all cases. The enteral route is used as early as possible, but the parenteral route may be used in the early phase. Blood sugars and serum electrolytes are monitored closely to avoid hyperglycemia and electrolyte disturbance, especially hyponatremia. Prophylactic anticonvulsants are frequently used and continued for a minimum of 6 months postoperatively if no seizures have occurred; if seizures have been a part of the abscess picture, they are usually continued for at least 1 year. Initially, phenytoin and phenobarbital may be used, but other agents such as carbamazepine may be substituted or added as needed. Unless ongoing seizure activity is identified or suspected, electroencephalography (EEG) is of uncertain value in the acute phase. It is subsequently performed and is of value in following the patient who has had seizures.

The placement of a central venous access line with a port/reservoir for chronic drug administration is useful for patients whose therapy will require prolonged parenteral antibiotics. These systems allow antibiotic therapy during the rehabilitation and outpatient stages, since the patient need not remain attached to a constant intravenous infusion. Rehabilitation evaluation and therapy are initiated as soon as the patient is stable for the manipulation required.

Epidural Abscess

This entity is frequently associated with suppurative sinusitis, although it may also be associated with trauma or prior surgical intervention. *Streptococcus* species and *Staphylococcus aureus* are the most frequently encountered organisms. Concomitant findings reveal sinusitis and its attendant symptoms, osteomyelitis, and soft tissue scalp or facial swelling.

Diagnostic studies of value are plain skull radiography, radionuclide bone scanning, and CT or MR scanning. These latter two tests are the most valuable.

Surgical therapy, i.e., craniectomy, is the therapy indicated, although some authors advocate craniotomy if no osteomyelitis is present. Bone is removed until diploic bleeding is encountered. The dura is carefully debrided of the infected granulation tissue, which may be attached with variable tenacity. Attempts should be made, as previously described, to obtain accurate cultures of the purulent collection including culture for anaerobes. If the dura is intact, and the preoperative studies and clinical exam do not indicate parenchymal involvement, then the dura is usually not opened. Of course, if during the course of the operation the dura is opened, then the subdural space is irrigated with copious amounts of antibiotic solution. The otolaryngology or oral/maxillofacial surgery services may be required for surgical intervention in the sinuses if these are involved. An epidural, closed-suction drain is placed and kept in place for up to 72 h postoperatively. Antibiotic coverage is as described for brain abscesses, as is ICU management, if indicated.

If a craniectomy has been performed, the defect is not repaired for a minimum of 6 months. In the interim, skull radiography is performed, usually at 2- to 3-month intervals, to watch for osteomyelitis. Serial ESR may be followed, with an upward trend indicating a possible unresolved or recurrent osteomyelitis. Serial CT scanning is also of value to watch for the delayed development of intradural collections.

Subdural Empyema

There have been various descriptions and terms assigned to this entity. However, it is generally considered to apply to an exudative, spreading, purulent collection in the subdural space, not contained by a membrane. Occasionally loculated abscesses may be encountered in the subdural space, but these are clearly walled off.

The condition usually arises from an extracranial infection transmitted through an emissary vein. In these cases, the dura and overlying bone appear uninvolved. When the infection arises in a sinus, an epidural abscess may be encountered. In pediatric cases, the infection may develop from an infected subdural effusion. Three basic presentations are noted; acute, subacute, and the infantile form.

The acute presentation is one of rapid onset and progression. Headache, fever, nausea, vomiting, and neck stiffness are noted. There may be a history of sinusitis or prior otolaryngological intervention. However, the patient may present with progressive neurological deficit(s) or epilepsy. In the subacute form, there is usually a relatively long history of headache, fever, and a prior cranial procedure. There is usually some degree of membrane formation. The infantile form usually develops in a patient with a postmeningitic subdural effusion. The organism involved is frequently *Haemophilus influenzae*. Seizures are frequently a presenting sign, as well as fever, vomiting, progressively altered consciousness, and evidence of an intracranial expanding mass.

In all cases, the underlying pathophysiological process is that of inflammation, vasculitis, and infarction. Coalesced areas of infarction may be seen grossly at operation, along with obviously thrombosed vessels.

Diagnosis

CT scanning, including skull base scans in the bone window technique, is probably the best diagnostic tool for the acutely ill patient. Hypodense areas may be noted over the convexity, as well as in the interhemispheric fissure and above the tentorium. Secondary evidence of infection, e.g., osteomyelitic changes, sinusitis or abscess formation, may be seen. Brain edema with shift (often out of proportion to the size of the collection) is frequently noted. MR scanning may also be valuable.

The pertinent clinical findings, as noted previously, should provide the clinician with clues to the presence of this entity. The diagnosis of subdural empyema prompts a determination of the source of the infection, permitting simultaneous treatment and minimizing the risk of reinfection.

Therapy

The treatment is operative, ranging from burr holes and irrigation to large flaps (free or osteoplastic) with debridement. We routinely perform a craniotomy and replace the flap if

there is no evidence of extradural disease. However, if even the slightest suspicion exists, the bone flap is left open, to be replaced by a cranioplasty no sooner than 6 months later. The wide exposure afforded by this method allows adequate examination of the area affected, as well as other areas which may harbor infection not clearly visualized on the diagnostic study(ies). Cultures are obtained as described previously. The purulent material is carefully irrigated. No attempt is made to strip away adherent material. The dura is closed in a watertight manner.

We frequently place a subdural catheter/monitor to assist in the management of any ICP problems. This latter maneuver is not performed by all clinicians and may, in theory, complicate the healing process by including a foreign body, but, in our experience, this has not been the case.

ICU Management

The ICU phase of management is critical. The patient frequently presents in an obtunded state and is rarely improved immediately after surgery. Brain swelling is often marked, and the ICP may be elevated in spite of the craniectomy. ICP is controlled via the methods described previously, although care must be taken to avoid techniques which may worsen the underlying ischemia, e.g., overly aggressive hyperventilation or diuresis. Antibiotics will usually have been begun in surgery. Empiric antibiotic choices were described above. Definitive antibiotic coverage is maintained for a minimum of 4 weeks, with longer courses maintained under certain circumstances. Respiratory and nutritional support are of signal importance, given the patient's obtunded and frequently immunocompromised state.

Seizure control requires special attention. The cortical damage frequently results in a focus or foci for seizures. The resultant epilepsy may be especially difficult to control. In the early or ICU stage of management, the parenteral route should be used. Phenytoin and/or phenobarbital may therefore be the only agents available. Multiple-drug therapy may well be necessary. Continuous EEG monitoring may likewise be necessary, especially if the fits are difficult to control or if status epilepticus is suspected. The treatment of status epilepticus is discussed in Chap. 66. If the disease is treated successfully, then the antiepileptic drugs are continued for a minimum of 1 year post control, although frequently, these patients must remain under medication permanently.

CT scanning is performed usually within 24 h postoperatively and repeated at weekly intervals during the course of antibiotic therapy and, of course, if changes in the patient's condition indicate it.

Recurrent collections, in our experience, usually require a full reopening of the operative site. If the bone was originally replaced, it will be left out after the second operation. Even nowadays the mortality of subdural empyema remains high.

Conclusion

The suppurative or pyogenic intracranial infections remain, in spite of advances in antibiosis as well as diagnosis, extremely serious conditions. Even if survival is achieved, the potential for long-term morbidity in terms of neurological deficit or epilepsy remains high.

Suggested Reading

Bannister G, Williams B, Smith S (1981) Treatment of subdural empyema. J Neurosurg 55:82–88

Black KP, Gray G Jr, Charache P (1973) Penetration of brain abscesses by systemically administered antibiotics. J Neurosurg 38:705–709

Brand B, Caparosa RJ, Lubic L (1984) Otorhinologic brain abscess therapy – past and present. Laryngoscope 94:483–487

Britt RH (1985) Brain abscess. In: Wilkins RH, Rengachary SS (eds) Neurosurgery. McGraw-Hill, New York, pp 1928–1956

Britt RH, Enzmann DR (1983) Clinical stages of human brain abscesses on serial CT scans after contrast infusion: computed tomographic, neuropathological, and clinical correlation. J Neurosurg 59:972–989

Carter LP (1991) Surface monitoring of cerebral cortical blood flow. Cerebrovasc Brain Metab Rev 3:246–255

DeLouvois J (1978) The bacteriology and chemotherapy of brain abscess. J Antimicrob Chemother 4:395–413

Dobkin JF, Healton EB, Dickinson T et al. (1984) Nonspecificity of ring enhancement in "medically cured" brain abscesses. Neurology 34:139–144

Rosenblum ML, Levy RM, Bredesen DE (1988) Neurosurgical implications of the acquired immunodeficiency syndrome (AIDS). Clin Neurosurg 34:419–445

Fairbanks DV, Milmoe N (1985) The diagnosis and management of sinusitis in children: complications and sequelae. Pediatr Inf Dis 4:875–879

Garvey G (1983) Current concepts of bacterial infections of the central nervous system. Bacterial meningitis and bacterial brain abscess. J Neurosurg 59:735–744

Hockley AD, Williams B (1983) Surgical management of subdural empyema. Child Brain 10:294–300

Jooma OV, Pennybacker JB, Tutton GK (1951) Brain abscesses: aspiration, drainage or excision. J Neurol Neurosurg Psychiatry 14:308–313

Mosely IF, Kendall BE (1984) Radiology of intracranial empyema. Neuroradiology 26: 333–345

Obrist WD, Thompson HK, Wang HS et al. (1975) Regional cerebral blood flow estimated by xenon-133 inhalation. Stroke 6:245–249

Ohaegbulam SC, Saddegi NU (1980) Experience with brain abscesses treated by simple aspiration. Surg Neurol 13:289–291

Robertson CS, Narayan RK, Gokasian ZL (1989) Cerebral arteriovenous oxygen difference as an estimate of cerebral oxygen delivery in comatose patients. J Neurosurg 70:222–228

Rosenblum ML, Hoff JT, Norman DA et al. (1980) Nonoperative treatment of brain abscesses in selected high-risk patients. J Neurosurg 52:217–225

Rosenblum ML, Mampalam T, Pons V (1986) Controversies in the management of brain abscess. Clin Neurosurg 33:603–632

Rubin RH, Hooper DC (1985) Central nervous system infections in the compromised host. Med Clin North Am 69:281–296

Sable NS, Hengerer A, Powell KR (1981) Acute frontal sinusitis with intracranial complications. Pedriatr Inf Dis 3:58–61

Sharif HS, Ibrahim A (1982) Intracranial epidural abscess. Br J Radiol 55:81–84

Williams B (1982) Subdural empyema. Adv Tech Stand Neurosurg 9:133–170

Young B, Ott LG, Thompson JS et al. (1985) The cellular immune depression of the non-steroid-treated head injury patient. Neurosurgery 16:725

Chapter 39

Neurosyphilis

HILMAR W. PRANGE and THOMAS P. BLECK

Definition and Epidemiology

Patients suffering from one of the manifestations of neurosyphilis may be misdiagnosed and thus fail to receive adequate treatment for a long time. For this reason, the routine use of appropriate antisyphilitic antibody testing is advisable in all patients with unexplained neurologic diseases. Neurosyphilis should be suspected in any person with a positive antitreponemal antibody test and at least two of these three clinical and cerebrospinal fluid (CSF) features:

1. A progressive or relapsing-remitting course of CNS dysfunction for which other causes have been excluded
2. Pathologic CSF findings including a lymphocytic pleocytosis, elevated total protein, or intrathecal immunoglobulin synthesis
3. Improvement (either clinical or in the CSF) following appropriate antibiotic therapy

The diagnosis of neurosyphilis is proven by demonstration of the intrathecal synthesis of antitreponemal antibodies (ITpA index $\geq$ 2).

Traditionally, syphilitic CNS manifestations are classified according to their clinical phenomenology and the stage of infection in which they appear. CNS manifestations in the secondary stage or the early latent stage are usually less severe, and vary with respect to symptoms, signs, and acuity.

Typical CNS manifestations of late syphilis include general paresis (called progressive paralysis in Europe, and accounting for about 30% of cases), meningovascular neurosyphilis (about 25%), and tabes dorsalis (25%). In about 15% of cases the symptoms are less distinct and classification is difficult. When the disease does not progress as expected, the patient has often received antibiotic therapy for another bacterial infection which has been at least partially effective.

The epidemiology of neurosyphilis is closely correlated with the prevalence of *Treponema pallidum* infection in a given population. The incidence of syphilis varies greatly

---

Section Editor: Thomas P. Bleck

around the world. While running as high as 360 per 100 000 inhabitants in several African countries, the incidence of new syphilitic infection in the United States is about 15 per 100 000/year. In Germany, the number of cases ranges from 0.6 to 4.9 per 100 000/year: in 1990 the mean value was 1.4 per 100 000/year. A high infection risk exists in males aged 25–30 years. Men are afflicted more than twice as often as women. The most exposed social group are heterosexual drug addicts, whereas the incidence among homosexuals is declining.

Concurrent infection with *T. pallidum* and HIV is not uncommon, since the modes of transmission are similar and the risk groups overlap. Several authors have hypothesized that patients who contract this dual infection show a shortened latency of CNS involvement and increased acuity of the clinical symptoms.

Pathogenesis

To date it remains unclear why only about 35% of syphilitic patients develop symptomatic tertiary syphilis, and why one patient contracts cardiovascular disease, a second gummatous syphilis, and a third a CNS manifestation. Untreated, 9.4% of male and 5.0% of female syphilitic patients develop CNS manifestations. The penetration of *T. pallidum* into the CNS can occur in all phases of the disease. The life cycle of treponemes is characterized by parasitism. The organisms attach to cell surfaces to obtain the constituents of the host cell for their own metabolism. Several authors have concluded from in vitro

and in vivo experiments that host-associated treponemes lack the ability to synthesize N-acetyl-D-glucosamine. Attachment to host cells provides them with hyaluronic acid, a polymer of N-acetyl-D-glucosamine and D-glucuronic acid. As a consequence, the spirochete has a special affinity for tissues containing high amounts of mucopolysaccharides. These are, for example, cartilaginous structures, perivascular regions, and distinct constituents of neural tissues. Treponemes prefer to reside in these regions, which they reach using hyaluronidase as a "spreading factor."

In perivascular areas, multiplication of *T. pallidum* results in a resorption of the mucopolysaccharide support material surrounding arteries and capillaries, leading to deformation of the vessel wall and, consequently, to a severe inflammatory reaction. A pathomechanism like this may be applicable to meningovascular neurosyphilis and, to a certain extent, to general paresis. In tabes dorsalis, treponemes reach their target structures via CSF bulk flow. The inflammatory process occurs at dorsal root ganglia and the dorsal root entry zone of the spinal cord, preferentially damaging spinal ganglion cells. Consequently, the dorsal tracts (mainly the fasciculus gracilis) degenerate. Dorsal root fibers coming from the gut may also be affected.

A peculiar phenomenon of the different phases of treponemal infection is the changing host reactivity to the invading microorganisms. During the early stages the host's defense mechanisms seem impaired. Large numbers of treponemes appear within mucous and cutaneus structures without remarkable tissue damage, substantiating the assumption that *T. pallidum* is not provided with the potent toxins that some other bacteria possess. The inflammatory reaction of the host is minor because the mechanisms necessary to recognize the foreign organisms are altered. One explanation suggests that treponemes disguise themselves by coating themselves with host proteins and mucopolysaccharides. During the later stages of syphilis the immune reaction apparently overshoots against a small quantity of spirochetes located perivascularly or intraparenchymally. A massive cellular and humoral immune reaction is launched, resulting in the synthesis of excessive amounts of antibody. Autoaggressive defense mechanisms have been discussed, including an immunogenetic predisposition.

Clinical Features and Differential Diagnosis

During secondary syphilis, CNS involvement is present in about one-third of the patients; they complain of recurring headache, irritability, and affective instability; nausea and vomiting may occur at times. Neurologic examination may reveal slight nuchal rigidity, tremor, and, occasionally, lesions of one or more cranial nerves (preferentially cranial nerves VIII, VII, and III). Unilateral or bilateral papilledema may at times occur. CSF abnormalities include modest pleocytosis, increased total protein and, to a lesser extent, intrathecal synthesis of immunoglobulins. In most cases, hospital admission is necessary for a few days to initiate

antibiotic treatment, because of the risk of a Jarisch-Herxheimer reaction, which is not uncommon at this stage of the disease. Indications for intensive care at this stage are rare, and include (1) a pronounced meningitic syndrome resembling Lyme borreliosis, and (2) a syphilitic polyradiculopathy with a course similar to the Guillain-Barré syndrome. The most distinctive marker for differentiating these two syndromes is the pleocytosis (up to 100 cells/μl), which only occurs in syphilitic polyradiculitis. These patients present with bilateral leg pain and weakness, depressed tendon reflexes, and distally decreased sensation. The motor alterations may ascend, affecting the respiratory muscles and, later, swallowing. The electrodiagnostic examination reveals reduced motor conduction and prolonged or unrecordable F-wave responses; needle electromyography shows the characteristics of acute denervation. Patients developing this symptom complex need to be referred to an intensive care unit for monitoring of respiratory and autonomic functions, and to receive respiratory support as required.

Meningovascular neurosyphilis is a manifestation of the tertiary stage, and more frequently requires critical care management. One intriguing point is that the symptoms are nonspecific and vary considerably, justifying the term "the great imitator" for this syphilitic CNS manifestation. The vasculitic process, progressing with minor symptoms which are hardly noted by the patient for a long period, can result in an acute stroke due to brain infarction or intracerebral hemorrhage. The latter occurs predominantly in elderly patients who are also suffering from hypertension or diabetes as concurrent risk factors. In contrast, infarctions mainly arise in younger patients (age 35–50 years). The syphilitic origin of the condition becomes apparent when serologic tests are performed. Lumbar puncture should only be carried out following exclusion of massive brain edema by computed tomography (CT). CSF analysis generally yields modest pleocytosis, signs of a disturbed blood/CSF barrier, and oligoclonal IgG antibodies. The underlying vasculitic process may be demonstrated by cerebral angiography, which shows concentric narrowing of the larger intradural vessels, or occlusion of the proximal branches of the anterior and middle cerebral arteries (signified by smooth symmetrical tapering). This vasculitic pattern differs markedly from that of arteriosclerosis; in older syphilitic patients, both patterns can be encountered.

In some patients with meningovascular neurosyphilis, the basilar artery or one of its branches may be predominantly affected, resulting in an infarction of the occipital lobe or cerebellum. When compression of the mesencephalic aqueduct or fourth ventricle occurs, cerebellar infarctions may produce acute obstructive hydrocephalus. The patient presents with brain stem symptoms and reduced alertness. To avoid fulminant herniation, ventricular drainage (with a spillover pressure of at least 20 mmHg to avoid upward herniation) is necessary. Obstructive hydrocephalus may also arise due to a space-occupying gumma situated in the diencephalon or infratentorial cisterns. However, intracranial gummata are extremely rare today.

Even Merritt found only one cerebral gumma among several hundred patients with neurosyphilis. Intracranial gummatous masses are easily identified by CT or magnetic resonance imaging (MRI). They are preferentially located within basal cisterns or around the cranial nerves, and show modest contrast enhancement but only scanty perifocal edema. Other infrequent complications of meningovascular neurosyphilis that may require intensive care therapy are subdural hematoma (hemorrhagic pachymeningitis) and subarachnoid bleeding due to ruptured syphilitic aneurysms.

In contrast to meningovascular neurosyphilis, general paresis is characterized by progressive tetraparesis, chronic dementia, disturbances of speech and articulation, abnormal pupillary reactions (Argyll-Robertson pupils), and abnormal CSF (intrathecal IgG synthesis and pleocytosis up to 150 cell/μl). In severe cases, general paresis may follow a course similar to viral encephalitis and thus be erroneously diagnosed as herpes simplex encephalitis (HSE). In such cases, a useful distinction is provided by the IgG index, which is initially normal in HSE but always increased in general paresis. Such fulminant manifestations of general paresis call for continuous surveillance in order to recognize the Jarisch-Herxheimer reaction early on if it occurs. Frequent seizures or status epilepticus (see Chap. 66) may also mandate admission to an intensive care unit.

The signs and symptoms of tabes dorsalis are largely restricted to signs of dorsal column degeneration. These include ataxia, areflexia, paresthesiae, disturbances of micturition (from the deafferented bladder), impotence, lancinating pain, reduced vibratory and joint position sense, and abnormal pupils. Moreover, almost 50% of the patients show lesions of the optic nerve. The course of disease is chronically progressive; acute events seldom intervene. Nevertheless, acute gastric crises, quickly progressive parapareses, unbearable pain attacks, and spontaneous fractures of femur or other bones constitute unequivocal emergencies. Gastric crises associated with epigastric pain, severe nausea and vomiting, or permanent retching leading to hematemesis, may tempt the surgeon to perform a laparotomy until the pupillary or other tabetic findings are noted. The rapid development of flaccid paralysis of the legs should prompt emergency myelography or spinal MRI since tabetic changes of the lumbar spine (Charcot spine) can result in compression of the spinal cord or cauda equina.

In tabes dorsalis, the abovementioned conditions rarely require admission to the critical care unit unless secondary complications occur, such as pulmonary embolism or serious electrolyte imbalances. The only life-threatening event peculiar to the pre-ataxic stage of tabes is the so-called oblongata crisis. In 1913, Dusser de Barenne published a case report of a tabetic who suddenly died during inpatient treatment. Within a short time he had become pale and unconscious, and soon after stopped breathing and remained pulseless. Postmortem examination did not yield a specific cause of death. Later authors explained such events as acute irritation of the autonomic system possibly due to recurrent dorsal ganglionitis involving the sympathetic nerves. The symptomatology usually starts with recurring intense abdominal pain, then cyanosis and coma occur abruptly. Finally, apneic episodes, frequently accompanied by fits and sinus tachycardia, emerge. The actual trigger mechanisms remain unknown. Keeping this infrequent complication in mind, we recommend that respiration and heart rate be monitored in every patient suffering from the pre-ataxic stage of tabes in periods of severe recurrent gastric crises.

The rare spinal manifestations of neurosyphilis, such as cervical hyperplastic pachymeningitis, Erb's spastic spinal paralysis, and syphilitic amyotrophy are not conditions requiring intensive care. Terminal stages which require respiratory support have not been reported to date.

Ancillary Tests

The most important confirmatory tests are serologic assays and CSF analysis. Serologic tests can be classified into (1) specific antitreponemal tests (such as the MHA-TP, TPHA, and FTA-ABS), and (2) the non-treponemal reactions using cardiolipin as the antigen (such as the VDRL, RPR, and the cardiolipin complement fixation reaction). The non-treponemal tests are usually an adequate screening test for previous infection in otherwise healthy patients younger than 60 years of age; older patients, or those with impaired immunity, may lose reactivity to cardiolipin and should be tested with an antitreponemal procedure. In patients suspected of having neurosyphilis, quantitative antitreponemal antibody testing and CSF analysis are necessary to verify the diagnosis. The procedure of choice for CSF antibody studies remains debated. In the United States, many laboratories will not perform antitreponemal tests in the CSF because standardization is lacking, and because very small amounts of serum contaminating the CSF may produce a positive test. In Europe, the TPHA is used routinely in CSF. Further CSF studies include cell counts, determinations of total protein, albumin, and IgG concentrations, and electrophoretic analysis for oligoclonal antibodies. Albumin and IgG determination as well as oligoclonal antibody detection should be performed simultaneously in serum and CSF samples to obtain CSF/serum quotients. The IgG production index is a measure of intrathecal immunoglobulin synthesis, and is calculated from the albumin and IgG quotients as follows:

$$\text{IgG index} = \frac{\text{IgG}_{CSF} \times 10^3 / \text{IgG}_{serum}}{\text{albumin}_{CSF} \times 10^3 / \text{albumin}_{serum}}$$

The upper limit of the normal range is 0.69. Indices exceeding this limit indicate intrathecal IgG production due to a local humoral immune reaction within the CNS. To verify the syphilitic nature of the latter, local production of antitreponemal antibodies must be proven. For this purpose, the ITpA (intrathecally produced *T. pallidum* specific antibodies) index seems most suitable. It is calculated according to the formula:

$$\text{ITpA index} = \frac{\text{TPHA}_{CSF} / \text{Total IgG}_{CSF}}{\text{TPHA}_{serum} / \text{Total IgG}_{serum}}.$$

Since antibodies of the IgM type hardly cross the blood/CSF barrier, the titre of the TPHA test reflects the rate of antitreponemal IgG antibody production in each compartment. The upper limit of this index is 2.0. Higher values confirm the diagnosis of neurosyphilis. Since the ITpA index remains positive in many cases of tabes dorsalis and general paresis throughout the life of the patient, it cannot be regarded as a criterion of activity.

The activity of the syphilitic CNS process can be estimated from the CSF pleocytosis and from positive antitreponemal IgM in serum established by the 19S-(IgM)FTA-ABS test. However, about one-third of patients with untreated neurosyphilis do not have pleocytosis. Therefore, other markers of disease activity have been sought. A positive CSF-VDRL test, regardless of previous antibiotic therapy, and a positive polymerase chain reaction in CSF samples may be taken as evidence of disease activity. The IgG index is not a reliable criterion of activity but it is well suited for long-term monitoring of the therapeutic response, since it falls in a logarithmically linear fashion after effective therapy. Six to twelve months after antibiotic treatment the CSF cell count should be normal, the treponemal-specific IgM antibodies should have disappeared from the serum, and the CSF-VDRL test should be negative.

Other ancillary tests such as CT, MRI, electroencephalography, chest X-ray, ophthalmologic and otologic examination, cerebral and aortic angiography, as well as evoked potentials, may help to exclude other CSF diseases, discover serious complications, and reveal related findings (e.g., aortic aneurysms, syphilitic hearing loss, etc.), and establish the functional state of the CNS. Application of these techniques depends on the clinical presentation of the patient and will not be discussed in detail here. Conventional angiography and MR angiography are useful in patients with luetic vasculitis (Fig. 1a–c).

Treatment

Antibiotic therapy is essential in all cases of untreated active neurosyphilis. The treatment of choice is intravenous administration of aqueous crystalline penicillin G, at least 12 million IU/day for 10–14 days. We prefer short infusions of 5–10 million IU penicillin G four times daily for 14 days. In cases of penicillin allergy, some of the third-generation cephalosporins can be employed. Since the CSF concentrations of ceftriaxone attained by 2 g/day i.v. greatly exceeds the minimum immobilizing concentration for *T. pallidum*, this compound can be employed. Doxycycline (100 mg i.v. four times daily for 28 days) should be given in the infrequent cases of life-threatening β-lactam allergy (e.g., anaphylaxis).

In the first few days it is necessary to pay increased attention to potential complications of antibiotic therapy, e.g., anaphylactic reactions, hypernatremia, convulsions, and the Jarisch-Herxheimer reaction. The incidence of anaphylactic reactions after penicillin administration is reported to be 0.04%; less severe allergic reactions are encountered in 0.7–10% of patients. β-Lactam allergy, including allergic reactions to third-generation cephalosporins, is quite infrequent and rarely predictable even when skin tests are performed. Convulsions and hypernatremia are more common side effects of highdose penicillin therapy, especially in severely handicapped patients. The Jarisch-Herxheimer reaction, presumably an escape from immunotolerance following increased antigen release, commonly occurs during the first 24 h and presents with fever, arterial hypotension, tachycardia, hyperventilation, and worsening of the CNS findings. This may justify the administration of prednisolone. The incidence of this reaction is higher in the early stages of syphilis but low in cases of neurosyphilis. Steroid treatment may also be useful in cases of severe luetic vasculitis.

Other therapeutic measures in neurosyphilis are symptomatic. In cases of extensive hemispheric or cerebellar infarction brain edema and elevated ICP need to be treated as discussed in Chap. 9. Acute hydrocephalus may require drainage by means of ventriculostomy. Epileptic states can be treated according to the recommendations given in Chap. 66. Attacks of lancinating pain and gastric crises should be treated with potent analgesics. If tabetics with less pronounced symptoms have severe gastric crises, monitoring of the autonomic function is mandatory. In general paresis, massive agitation or excitation associated with psychotic episodes may require neuroleptics. Syphilitic polyradiculitis can be managed like the Guillain-Barré syndrome, including artificial ventilation

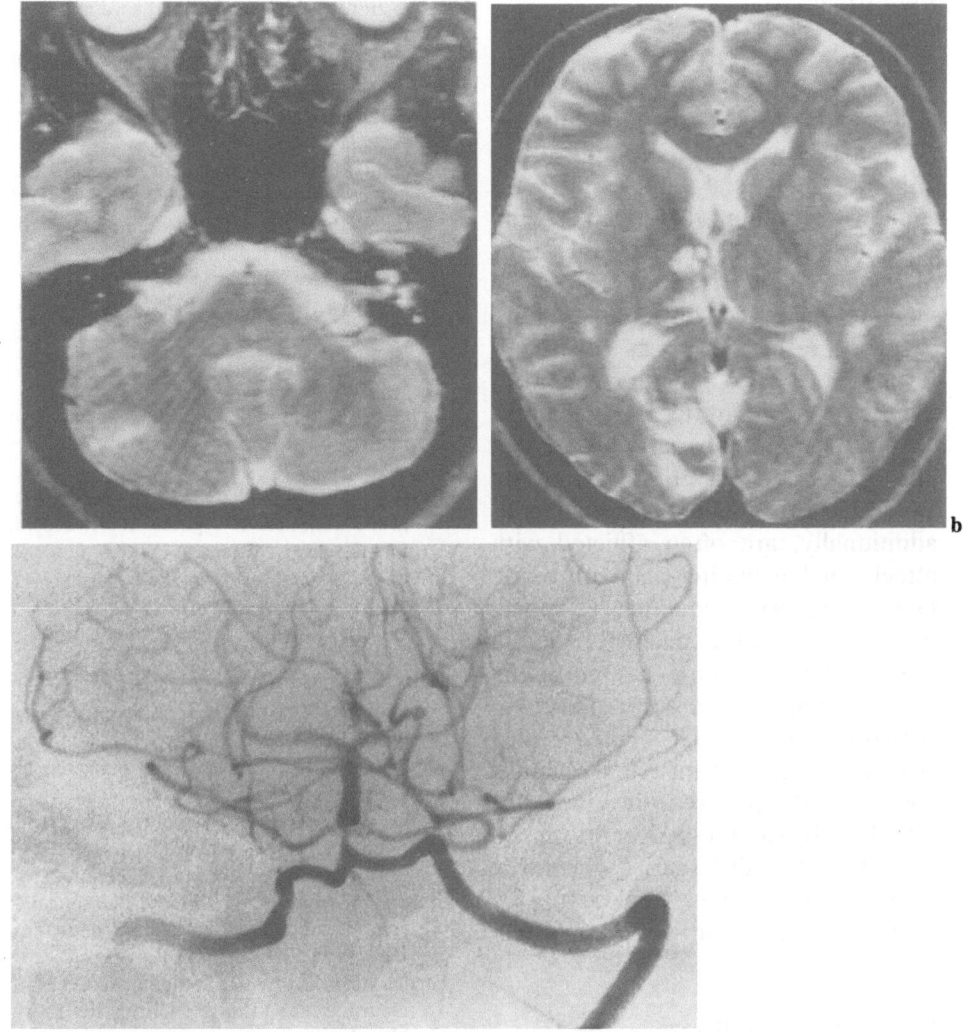

Fig. 1a–c. Neurosyphilis with vascular complications in a 44-year-old woman with subacute left hemiparesis, right homonymous hemianopsia and an 8-week history of headaches. T2-weighted axial MR images reveal multiple areas of abnormally increased signal intensity involving right cerebellar hemisphere (**a**) plus right medial occipital lobe, right medial thalamus, and bilateral paratrigonal white matter (**b**). Lesions have relatively sharp margins and are both morphologically and topographically consistent with ischemic infarcts. Frontal view of vertebral angiogram, arterial phase, shows severe circular stenosis of proximal basilar artery extending onto origins of both inferior anterior cerebral arteries (**c**). (Courtesy of Klaus Sartor and Marius Hartmann, Heidelberg)

if necessary. Acute meningitis during the secondary stage usually shows a less severe course than other bacterial meningitides, apart from the occasional occurrence of a Jarisch-Herxheimer reaction after the beginning of antibiotic therapy, which justifies admission to an intensive care unit.

Prognosis

The management of neurosyphilis requires intensive care only in exceptional cases. Severe complications are rare and fatal courses are extremely uncommon. Nevertheless, the outcome of the therapeutic measures discussed above is variable. Cases of early syphilis show, as a rule, excellent results, whereas the manifestations of meningovascular, tabetic, and paretic neurosyphilis generally end in only partial remission after therapy. Tabetics retain the signs of dorsal column lesions and, additionally, are often afflicted with attacks of lancinating pain for years. General paresis sometimes gradually progresses to a more distinct dementia after antibiotic therapy, and persisting spastic hemipareses are not unusual in patients with vascular neurosyphilis. In spite of earlier claims, neurosyphilis has not disappeared in the last decades. It should be therefore included in the differential diagnostic consideration in all cases of acute vascular or inflammatory CNS processes.

Suggested Reading

Brandon WR, Boulos LM, Morse A (1993) Determining the prevalence of neurosyphilis in a cohort co-infected with HIV. Int J AIDS 4:99–101

Burstain JM, Grimprel E, Lukehart SA et al. (1991) Sensitive detection of Treponema pallidum by using the polymerase chain reaction. J Clin Microbiol 29:62–69

Canale-Parola E (1977) Physiology and evolution of spirochetes. Bacteriol Rev 41:181–204

Clark EG, Danbolt N (1955) The Oslo study of the natural history of untreated syphilis. An epidemiologic investigation based of a restudy of the Boeck-Brunsgaard material. J Chronic Dis 2:311–344

Dusser de Barenne JG (1913) Über einen Fall von Tabesparalyse mit "Medulla-oblongata-Krisen". Z Ges Neurol Psychiatr 14:545–551

Fitzgerald TJ (1983) Attachment of treponemes to cell surface. In: Schell RF, Musher DM (eds) Pathogenesis and immunology of treponemal infection. Dekker, New York, pp 195–228

Goodman LJ, Karakusis PH (1988) Neurosyphilis. In: Harris AA (ed) Handbook of clinical neurology, vol 8. Elsevier, Amsterdam, pp 273–287

Hutchinson CM, Hook EW (1990) Syphilis in adults. Med Clin North Am 74:1389–1416

Idsoe O, Guthe T, Willcox RR (1972) Penicillin in the treatment of syphilis. World Health Organisation, Geneva (WHO Bulletin 47)

Jordan KG (1988) Modern neurosyphilis – a critical analysis. West J Med 149:47–57

Korting HC, Walther D, Riethmuller U, Meurer M (1986) Comparative in vitro susceptibility of Treponema pallidum to ceftizoxime, ceftriaxone and penicillin G. Chemotherapy 32:352–355

Lanska MJ, Lanska DJ, Schmidley JW (1988) Syphilitic polyradiculopathy in an HIV-positive man. Neurology 38:1297–1301

Libman LJ, Matthews JH (1976) "Oblongata" crises in tabes dorsalis. J Neurol Neurosurg Psychiatry 39:1240–1241

Merritt HH, Adams RD, Solomon HC (1946) Neurosyphilis. Oxford University Press, New York

Muller F (1981) Der 19S(IgM)-FTA-Abs-Test in der Serodiagnostik der Syphilis. Technik, Fehlermöglichkeiten und diagnostische Aussage. Immun Infekt 9:23–24

Nau R, Prange HW, Muth P et al. (1993) Passage of cefotaxime and ceftriaxone into cerebrospinal fluid in patients with uninflamed meninges. Antimicrob Agents Chemother 37:1518–1524

O'Neill P, Nicol CS (1972) IgM class antitreponemal antibody in treated and untreated syphilis. Br J Vener Dis 48:460–463

Prange HW, Moskophidis M, Schipper HI, Muller F (1983) Relationship between neurological features and intrathecal synthesis of IgG antibodies to Treponema pallidum in untreated and treated human neurosyphilis. J Neurol 230:241–252

Reiber H, Felgenhauer K (1987) Protein transfer at the blood cerebrospinal fluid barrier and the quantitation of the humoral immune response within the central nervous system. Clin Chim Acta 163:319–328

Vatz KA, Scheibel RL, Keiffer SA, Ansari KA (1974) Neurosyphilis and diffuse cerebral angiopathy: a case report. Neurology 25: 472–476

Wicher K, Wicher V (1983) Immunopathology of syphilis. In: Schell RF, Musher DM (eds) Pathogenesis and immunology of treponemal infection. Dekker, New York, pp 139–159

Chapter 40

Neuroborreliosis

WOLFGANG PANKL

Definition and Epidemiology

Lyme disease (neuroborreliosis) is a tick-borne infection caused by the spirochete *Borrelia burgdorferi*. It is initially characterized by a typical rash at the site of the tick bite (erythema migrans) and "flulike" or "meningitis-like" symptoms (stage I). This may be followed by frank meningitis, cranial or peripheral neuritis, carditis, and migratory musculoskeletal pain (stage II). Months to years later, intermittent or chronic arthritis or chronic neurological and dermatological abnormalities may develop (stage III).

Lyme disease has a world-wide distribution, corresponding to the distribution of the usual vector, the tick (*Ixodes dammini* and *I. pacificus* in the U.S., *I. ricinus* in Europe, and *I. persulcatus* in Asia). Ticks are not found in Australia and the vector there remains unknown. *B. burgdorferi* has also been isolated from horse flies and mosquitoes.

In Europe, strains of *B. burgdorferi* are more heterogeneous

than those in North America. This heterogeneity may be responsible for the variabilty in extraneurological clinical features. There is less variability, however, in the CNS manifestations of Lyme disease in Europe and in North America. Because of the high rate of seropositivity (10–30% of the general population) in endemic areas, strict clinical criteria should be used for diagnosis. It remains unclear what percentage of seropositive individuals develop symptoms.

Pathogenesis

After deposition of *B. burgdorferi* in the skin, local proliferation of the spirochete occurs, resulting in the characteristic erythema migrans rash. Within days to weeks, the spirochetes spread hematogenously throughout the body. The exact mechanism by which *B. burgdorferi* causes disease is unclear, but a direct inflammatory response and cross-reaction of anti-*B. burgdorferi* antibodies to human antigens may play an important role. In general, a cellular immune response to

Section Editor: Thomas P. Bleck

the spirochete precedes a humoral response, and specific antibodies are not found when erythema migrans is present. IgM antibody titers peak between the third and sixth week and then decline (although titers may remain high during late stages of the disease). IgG antibody titers rise slowly and often persist for years (even during clinical remission).

Clinical Features and Differential Diagnosis

CNS Manifestations

An overview of CNS manifestations is given in Table 1.

Stage I. Patients with early Lyme disease often present with headache and neck stiffness. Given the nonspecific nature of these symptoms, however, unless patients give a history of a tick bite or have erythema migrans on examination, it is difficult to diagnose Lyme disease early.

Stage II. Meningitis is the most common neurological feature of stage II and may be the presenting symptom of patients with Lyme disease. A history of erythema migrans is reported by

Table 1. CNS manifestations of Lyme disease

Stage I	Headache
	Neck stiffness without pleocytosis
Stage II	Lymphocytic meningitis
	Encephalitis
	Myelitis
	Meningopolyradiculitis
Stage III	Progressive encephalomyelitis

only 40% of patients. Patients have headache, neck stiffness, photophobia, nausea, and vomiting. Fever is usually low grade (37.5°–38.5°C) but occasionally may be higher. CNS involvement occurs in about half of patients and includes encephalitis, transverse myelitis, and meningopolyradiculitis (Bannwarth's syndrome). Patients with encephalitis have somnolence, emotional lability, memory impairment, ataxia, chorea, focal and generalized seizures, and hemiplegia (acute or subacute in onset). Transverse myelitis is usually incomplete, may be either acute or subacute in onset, and results in spastic paraparesis or quadriparesis with disturbances of gait and micturition. Sensory loss occurs less commonly. Patients with meningopolyradiculitis have intense, migrating, radicular pain and peripheral or cranial nerve palsies. Approximately 50% of patients in stage II present with cranial nerve palsies, usually facial palsy (bilateral in 30–70%).

Stage III. Progressive encephalomyelitis represents the chronic manifestation of Lyme disease, observed months to years after infection. Because of involvement of both the central and peripheral nervous systems, symptoms are diffuse and multifocal. Patients usually have gait disturbances, bladder dysfunction, sensory loss, and spastic paraparesis or quadriparesis. Cerebral involvement may lead to mood changes and impaired memory and concentration. Less commonly, patients may have severe dementia, delirium, somnolence, and seizures. The differential diagnosis of patients suspected of

Table 2. Differential diagnosis of CNS symptoms

Acute meningoencephalitis
Brain-stem encephalitis
Progressive encephalomyelitis
Cerebral demyelinization
Acute aseptic meningitis
Cerebral vasculitis
Dementia
Chronic lymphocytic meningitis
Transverse myelitis

---

having neuroborreliosis is listed in Table 2.

Peripheral Nervous System Manifestations

Some patients with Lyme disease may present with the Guillian-Barré syndrome (GBS). The clinical course of patients with GBS secondary to Lyme disease is identical to that of primary GBS.

Diagnosis

Lyme disease should be suspected in patients with a history of a tick bite, erythema migrans, peripheral or cranial neuropathy, and meningitis (especially when exposed to endemic regions).

Cerebrospinal Fluid and Other Laboratory Tests

Analysis of CSF shows a lymphocytic pleocytosis of about 100 cells/ml (may be up to 4000 cells), increased protein concentration, and normal or slightly decreased glucose concentration. Specific serum antibodies can be measured with hemagglutination tests, immunofluorescence (IFA), and enzyme-linked immunosorbent assay (ELISA). In stage I, 20–50% of patients have anti-*B. burgdorferi* antibodies (mainly IgM). In stage II, 70–90% show IgM antibodies, and later IgG antibodies. In stage III nearly all patients have IgG antibodies. Patients with syphilis or relapsing fever may also have high IgG titers and those with rheumatoid arthritis, Rocky Mountain spotted fever, infectious mononucleosis, tuberculous meningitis, and leptospirosis may have low IgM titers. Western blot analysis is highly sensitive and specific for Lyme disease. Patients should have western blot analysis if they are suspected to have Lyme disease but are seronegative by IFA or ELISA, or if they are suspected not to have Lyme disease but are seropositive (that is, false positivity is suspected). To demonstrate intrathecal antibody production, CSF and serum levels must be measured and the CSF:serum ratio must be calculated (a ratio greater than 2 is considered positive). The presence of specific oligoclonal bands is the most sensitive and specific indicator of intrathecal antibody production.

B. burgdorferi can also be detected with polymerase chain reaction (PCR), and the spirochete has been isolated successfully from the skin (from the erythema migrans rash), blood, joint fluid, and CSF. It can be cultured in Barbour-Stoenner-Kelly medium, but the technique is time consuming and difficult. Serology is currently the only practical laboratory aid.

Neuroimaging and Ancillary Tests

Radiologic changes are frequently absent in patients in stage I of the disease. CT scans of patients in stage II have shown enhancing and non-enhancing low-density lesions, midline shift due to mass effect, and focal demyelinization. In stage III, CT and MRI scans are abnormal in nearly all patients. Findings include white matter changes (both periventricular and subcortical) and infarcts of the internal capsule and thalamus. Cerebral angiography in patients with symptoms of progressive encephalomyelitis may demonstrate vasculitic changes.

Within several weeks after disease onset, about 8% of patients develop cardiac involvement. The most common abnormality is a fluctuating degree of atrioventricular block. Complete heart block, when it occurs, rarely persists for more than a week, and usually only temporary pacing is needed. Some patients have acute myopericarditis, mild left ventricular dysfunction, or – rarely – cardiomegaly. Only one case of fatal pancarditis has been reported (albeit in a patient with both Lyme disease and babesiosis). Less common manifestations of Lyme disease include generalized lymphadenopathy, splenomegaly, and recurrent hepatitis. Respiratory failure is rare.

Treatment

Based on available data from randomized trials, patients with neuroborreliosis should be treated with either ceftriaxone or cefotaxime (either is preferred over penicillin G). Both ceftriaxone and cefotaxime penetrate the blood-brain barrier well, but ceftriaxone has the advantage of requiring only once-daily dosing. Alternatively, doxycycline can be used (see Table 3). All patients with neuroborreliosis need intravenous treatment

Table 3. Treatment of Lyme disease

Stage I	Doxycycline[a]	2 × 100 mg/day p.o.	14–21 days
	Amoxicillin	3 × 500 mg/day p.o.	
	Penicillin V	3 × 1.2 million units/day p.o.	
	Erythromycin	3 × 500 mg/day p.o.	
Stage II	Neuroborreliosis:		
	Ceftriaxone	1 × 2 g/day i.v.	14–21 days
	Cefotaxime	3 × 2 g/day i.v.	
	Penicillin G	4 × 5 million units/day i.v.	
	other manifestations:		
	Doxycycline[a]	2 × 100 mg/day p.o.	
Stage III	Progressive encephalomyelitis		
	Ceftriaxone	1 × 2 g/day i.v.	14–28 days
	Cefotaxime	3 × 2 g/day i.v.	
	Penicillin G	4 × 5 million units/day i.v.	
	other manifestations:		
	Doxycycline[a]	2 × 100 mg/day p.o.	

[a] Children under the age of 8 years should not receive Doxycycline.

to maintain high serum and CSF antibiotic levels. Although there are no exact guidelines, patients should be treated for at least 2–3 weeks, depending on their clinical response. If there is no clinical response, if patients relapse after initial improvement, or if lymphocytic pleocytosis remains unchanged 6 months after treatment, then patients should be re-treated with a longer course (such as for 4 weeks). An alternative antibiotic can be considered.

The effect of corticosteroids on clinical course and outcome is not clear, but generally corticosteroids are not recommended. A Jarisch-Herxheimer reaction, with shaking chills and fever, occurs in about 10% of patients in the first 24 h after beginning treatment. Corticosteroids do not prevent this reaction.

Prognosis

In general, the earlier the treatment, the better the outcome. Patients treated while still in stages I and II have a good prognosis. Meningeal symptoms improve quickly; improvement of radicular pain and weakness follows days to weeks later. Patients with severe CNS involvement (especially those with spinal cord involvement) may be left with residual deficits. In stage III, recovery of patients takes months and is usually incomplete.

Suggested Reading

Ackermann R et al. (1988) Chronic neurologic manifestation of erythema migrans borreliosis. Ann NY Acad Sci 539:16–23

Burgdorfer W et al. (1982) Lyme disease – a tick-borne spirochetosis? Science 216: 1317–1319

Halperin JJ et al. (1989) Lyme neuroborreliosis: central nervous system manifestations. Neurology 39:753–759

Halperin JJ et al. (1991) Central nervous system abnormalities in Lyme neuroborreliosis. Neurology 41:1571–1582

Pachner AR et al. (1989) Central nervous system manifestations of Lyme disease. Arch Neurol 46:790–795

Pfister HW (1993) Lyme-Neuroborreliose (Bannwarth-Syndrom) In: Brandt T, Dichgans J, Diener HC (eds) Therapie und Verlauf neurologischer Erkrankungen. Kohlhammer, Stuttgart

Reik Louis Jr (1991) Lyme disease. In: Scheld WM, Withley RJ, Durack DT (eds) Infections of the central nervous system. Raven, New York

Rousseau JJ et al. (1986) Acute transverse myelitis as presenting neurological feature of Lyme disease. Lancet 2:1222–1223

Stanek G (1991) Laboratory diagnosis and seroepidemiology of Lyme borreliosis. Infection 19:263–367

Steere Allen C (1989) Medical progress – Lyme disease. N Engl J Med 321:586–594

Chapter 41

Tetanus and Botulism

THOMAS P. BLECK and KLAUS UNERTL

Definitions

Tetanus and botulism are toxin-mediated diseases of synaptic (including neuromuscular) transmission. The toxins producing these two conditions are very similar in size and sequence and are derived from members of the genus *Clostridia*, a group of anaerobic gram-positive rods. Both *C. tetani* and *C. botulinum* produce spores, which are the form of the organism transmitted. *C. tetani* spores are inoculated into the host and produce toxin in the body. *C. botulinum* spores usually contaminate food and produce their toxins prior to ingestion by the patient; production of toxins in the patient is less common. The major mechanism of action of both types of toxins is presynaptic inhibition of transmitter release. The different clinical manifestations of the toxins derive from (a) preferential binding of each toxin to different types of synapses, and (b) differences in the transport and dissemination of the toxins.

Section Editor: Thomas P. Bleck

Tetanus

Tetanus is a disease in which central inhibitory neurotransmission is disabled by tetanospasmin, a 150-kD toxin elaborated by *C. tetani*. The major clinical expression is in the upper motor neuron system, resulting in spasms and increased resting muscle tone. Some patients also manifest deficits in excitatory systems. Four clinical forms are recognized:

1. Generalized tetanus is the most commonly recognized form of the disease, but it usually represents a complication of unrecognized local tetanus. Its major symptoms include trismus ("lockjaw," an inability to open the mouth due to masseter spasm), risus sardonicus (an unusual, and often subtle, change in facial appearance resulting from straightening of the upper lip), and generalized spasms (episodes of tonic contraction of all muscle groups, producing opisthotonus, flexion of the arms, and extension of the legs. This posture resembles decorticate posturing, but the patient with

tetanus remains conscious. Spasms are typically elicited by sensory stimuli.).

2. *Local tetanus* produces fixed rigidity and hyper-reflexia in the muscles associated with the site of spore inoculation. Neuromuscular transmission may also be affected locally, superimposing a lower motor neuron lesion.

3. *Cephalic tetanus* is a special type of local tetanus which is confined to the head.

4. *Neonatal tetanus*, which is usually generalized, affects the newborn after contamination of the umbilical stump.

Botulism

Botulism is a disease in which peripheral cholinergic neurotransmission, both nicotinic and muscarinic, is predominantly disabled. At least eight immunologically distinct types of botulinum toxin have been reported; all are similar in size and peptide sequence to tetanospasmin. The major manifestations are motor paralysis, due to failure of neuromuscular transmission, and autonomic dysfunction. Four clinical forms are recognized:

1. Food-borne botulism follows germination of *C. botulinum* spores in food, which is then ingested without being heated adequately to denature the botulinum toxin.

2. Infant botulism occurs when ingested *C. botulinum* spores germinate in the gastrointestinal tract of an infant, resulting in local toxin production.

3. Wound botulism results from germination of *C. botulinum*

spores in the anaerobic environment of a wound, resulting in local toxin production.

4. Botulism of undetermined etiology is an uncommon condition diagnosed when the mechanism of infection cannot be determined.

Pathogenesis

Both tetanus and botulism result from inhibition of neurotransmitter release. In order for this to occur, the toxin must reach its target cells, bind to the presynaptic membrane, be internalized, and disrupt the coupling of depolarization to exocytosis.

Tetanus

In tetanus, the major cells affected are the glycinergic inhibitory neurons of the spinal cord and the descending GABAergic inhibitory neurons of the brain stem. The lower motor neuron dysfunction of local tetanus results from a similar failure of acetylcholine release by the alpha motor neuron. The toxin reaches these cells from the periphery by retrograde transport in motor neurons. It is released into the extracellular space, from which it appears to be bound preferentially by its target cells (although all neurons have tetanospasmin receptors). Once internalized, it prevents transmitter release at a step after calcium entry has occurred. The affected synapses are rendered inactive for weeks, perhaps permanently.

The autonomic nervous system is also affected by tetanospasmin. The clinical manifestation is usually that of a hypersympathetic state, resembling a pheochromocytoma, resulting from disinhibition of adrenal catecholamine release. Much less frequently, hyper-parasympathetic manifestations are noted.

Botulism

Botulinum toxins are disseminated via the bloodstream from the gastro-intestinal tract (primarily the stomach and small intestine) in food-borne and infant botulism, or from the site of injury in wound botulism. Although the steps of binding and internalization of botulinum toxins are similar to those of tetanospasmin, the different forms of botulinum toxin appear to differ in the modes by which they prevent acctylcholine release.

Clinical Features and Differential Diagnosis

Despite their similarities of mechanism, the differences in the types of neurons preferentially affected by the toxins result in very different clinical phenomena.

Tetanus

The major clinical sign of tetanus is increased muscle tone. This produces trismus and risus sardonicus when it affects the facial musculature and abdominal rigidity in the generalized form. Muscular hypertonia in the neck may mimic the nuchal rigidity of meningitis, but it is usually present in all directions of movement (rather than simply on flexion of the neck). In addition, the lack of inhibition of reflex arcs leads to generalized spasms. Local and facial tetanus have more confined symptoms, usually related to the portal of entry. In these states, a lower motor neuron lesion is often present near the site of inoculation, reflecting inhibition of acetylcholine release at the neuromuscular junction. Autonomic, usually hypersym-pathetic, symptoms occasionally develop toward the end of the first week of illness. These problems reflect failure to inhibit adrenal cate-cholamine release. On rare occasions, hypervagal syndromes are noted.

There is a very limited differential diagnosis for tetanus. Strychnine poisoning, which specifically blocks the glycine receptors responsible for spinal motor neuron inhibition, is the only true mimic of tetanus. Although strychnine poisoning is sometimes reported to lack tetanus's character-istic increase in muscle tone between generalized spasms, there is little evidence to support this contention. Dystonic reactions to phenothiazines and other dopamine-blocking agents are often characterized by increased muscle tone, but the patients suffering from such a reaction almost always have head deviation to one side, a phy-sical finding almost unheard of in tetanus. The abdominal rigidity of peritonitis can be distinguished by the presence of abdominal pain, vomiting, and rebound tenderness. Meningitis was discussed above.

There is no diagnostic laboratory test for tetanus. However, almost all patients who are adequately im-munized with tetanus toxoid will be immune to the disease. A few case reports of patients with severe tetanus who had antibody titers well in excess of the level commonly thought to be protective (0.01 IU/ml) call into question the value of determining the antitoxin titer as part of the diagnostic process. However, most tetanus patients lack any detectable anti-tetanus antibodies. Strychnine can be detected in blood and urine; since the initial treatment for tetanus and strychnine poisoning are the same, one should not delay emergency management while these studies are being performed. Drug screening for dopamine-blocking agents should be performed, and a diagnostic challenge with an anticholinergic agent (e.g., benztropine, 1–2 mg) is advisable to rapidly exclude this possibility.

Botulism

The major clinical manifestation of botulism is muscle weakness. This results from the presynaptic deficit in neuromuscular transmission induced by the toxin. Other peripheral cholinergic synapses are variably affected.

The three major forms of botulinum toxin affecting humans are A, B, and E. A and B are predominantly associated with improperly canned or prepared food; type E usually follows ingestion of fish or other marine life. There are some epidemiologically important differences in symptoms and signs among the toxin types, but these are of minimal clinical relevance since the antitoxin used is polyvalent.

The most frequent symptoms of botulism are dysphagia, dry mouth, diplopia, and dysarthria, followed by weakness of the extremities. Constipation is seen in about three fourths of patients, with nausea, vomiting, and abdominal cramping less frequently represented. A minority of patients may experience diarrhea early in their course. Ptosis, a diminished gag reflex, ophthalmoparesis, and facial weakness are common findings on examination. Fixed, dilated pupils are seen in only a minority of cases and are more common in type B than type A. Deep tendon reflexes are usually decreased or absent, but rare cases of hyperactive reflexes have been described. Altered consciousness has been reported in about 10% of botulism patients; the mechanism of this problem is unknown.

The actual incidence of autonomic dysfunction in botulism is uncertain. Quantitative evidence of this problem has been sought, and it appears to be very frequent. It is manifested as failure of both sympathetic and parasympathetic function.

Ancillary Tests

Both tetanus and botulism are diagnosed primarily by clinical means. Laboratory testing for the toxins (or antibodies to tetanospasmin) are important confirmatory tests but are usually not available quickly enough to influence treatment decisions.

Tetanus

Measurement of antitetanus antibodies is frequently performed in an attempt to retrospectively disprove the diagnosis of tetanus. However, several cases of severe tetanus have been described in patients with antibody concentrations exceeding the usually accepted level of 0.01 IU/ml. Based on current understanding, an antibody level of 0.5 IU/ml appears to be protective. The efficacy of different epitopes of antitetanus antibodies probably differs, partially explaining the lack of protection in some patients with supposedly protective antibody titers.

The major use of ancillary tests in tetanus is to exclude other diagnostic possibilities. Serum and urine testing for strychnine is the most important diagnostically; since the initial treatments of tetanus and strychnine poisoning are the same, therapy need not await the results of these studies. Dystonic reactions to neuroleptics and other dopamine-blocking agents are usually easily distinguished from tetanus, but assays for these drugs may be useful.

Botulism

The most important diagnostic test for botulism is electromyography with repetitive nerve stimulation. Patients with botulism will typically show either no change or a slight decrement in the motor response to repetitive nerve stimulation at low rates (about 5 Hz). At high rates (40 or 50 Hz), the diagnostic increment in motor response will appear. Studies of several different muscles may be necessary to prove the diagnosis. Nerve conduction studies are also useful in evaluating the possibility of the Miller Fisher variant of the Guillain-Barré syndrome.

Assays for botulinum toxin should be performed in the serum and stool of suspected patients. These assays will determine the type of toxin present, which is of epidemiologic value. The antitoxin treatment of suspected botulism cases should not be delayed while waiting for the results of this testing, however.

Management

The physician's major concern in both tetanus and botulism is the adequacy of ventilation. Tetanus patients occlude the upper airway during spasms and may have similar difficulties with diaphragmatic function. Botulism patients have hypotonic upper airways, difficulty with oropharyngeal secretions, and diaphragmatic weakness. In both clostridial conditions, autonomic dysfunction is common.

Tetanus

Patients with suspected tetanus should receive passive immunization with human tetanus immune globulin (HTIG), 500 U i.m. Intrathecal administration of HTIG does not appear to be superior to the systemic route. Intravenous pooled (i.e., not hyperimmune) immunoglobulin preparations have also been used but do not appear to confer an advantage. Since tetanus does not provoke an adequate immune response to confer protection, a regular tetanus toxoid series must also be administered (at a separate site from the HTIG for the first injection).

Benzodiazepines are the first-choice therapeutic agents for controlling the motor symptoms of tetanus. These drugs do not directly affect the loss of glycinergic inhibition of motor neurons, but rather enhance the GABA-mediated descending inhibitory influences on the motor system. Diazepam has been studied most extensively. When administered in adequate quantities, diazepam will relieve muscular rigidity and decrease the frequency and intensity of tetanic spasms. The diazepam doses required may be astronomical by other standards, sometimes exceeding 400 mg/day. When given intravenously in such doses, the propylene glycol vehicle of the diazepam may produce a lactic acidosis. For this reason, as well as nutrition, we advise early placement of a feeding tube after airway safety has been assured. Midazolam infusion is another alternative, since this water-soluble compound is not given with propylene glycol. The sedative and amnestic effects of these agents are an added benefit. While a variety of other drugs have been proposed for the rigidity and spasms of tetanus, none has emerged as a superior agent. Because they lack the GABA agonism of the benzodiazepines, and because of the theoretical epileptogenicity of tetanospasmin, phenothiazines should not be employed.

Most patients with severe tetanus require endotracheal intubation. Because pharyngeal manipulation is a potent stimulus of tetanic spasms, this procedure should usually be performed in the setting of neuromuscular junction blockade, following a dose of diazepam adequate to produce sedation. We employ either succinylcholine or vecuronium for this purpose. Some experts recommend immediate tracheostomy once the endotracheal tube has been placed,

since the tube itself may trigger spasms. This should be decided on an individual basis, but it is frequently advantageous. Once the airway is secure, the patient may receive sufficient doses of diazepam to control spasms and rigidity without fear of airway obstruction. Ventilatory support may be required. With adequate doses of benzodiazepines, long-term neuromuscular junction blockade (e.g., with pancuronium) is seldom necessary.

Sympathetic hyperactivity is now the leading cause of death in tetanus. This circumstance is initially manifested by tachycardia and hypertension (labile or sustained). The hypercatecholaminergic state producing this complication should be treated in a manner similar to a pheochromocytoma. We prefer intravenous labetolol; others have employed intravenous morphine, or epidural blockade of the renal nerves.

Botulism

Patients presenting with botulism are at imminent risk of respiratory failure and must be carefully observed for autonomic dysfunction as well. At the first sign of hypoventilation or difficulty with pharyngeal secretions, they should undergo endotracheal intubation and mechanical ventilation. Although their flaccid paralysis may make communication impossible, one must always remember that the patients are sentient and must therefore provide explanation, reassurance, analgesia, and sedation as indicated.

The efficacy of botulinum antitoxin, debated for several decades, now appears clear. This therapy will remove circulating botulinum toxin, but it does not appear to affect the toxin already in place at the neuro-muscular junction. Therefore, the clinician, the patient, and the family should anticipate at least 2 weeks of illness before recovery begins. The patient must first be tested for hyper-sensitivity to horse serum, and desensitized if necessary. The usual dose is one vial i.v. and one vial i.m., which can be repeated in 4 h if the symptoms progress. Antitoxin is not usually recommended in infant botulism because the prognosis is generally very good. In cases of sus-pected wound botulism, the wound should be widely debrided. Whether antitoxin should be injected in the vicinity of the wound has not been determined, but it seems reasonable. Care should be taken to inject it into viable, well-vascularized muscle, however.

The use of antibiotics for food-borne botulism does not appear justified. If intercurrent infection occurs, aminoglycosides should not be used for treatment since they worsen the defect in neuromuscular trans-mission. In cases of infant or wound botulism, penicillin or metronidazole should be given to eradicate the source of continuing toxin production.

Botulism patients who manifest hypotension as a sign of autonomic dysfunction should be treated with volume repletion first. If vasopressors are necessary, low initial doses should be used because of the possibility of receptor denervation hypersensitivity.

The rate of recovery from botulism also appears to differ among types, but this has not been controlled for toxin dose. Type A patients take an average of 2 months to recover, while type B patients take about half as much time.

Prognosis

Tetanus

The progonsis of tetanus patients de-pends upon the severity of the illness, the accessibility of intensive care services, the patient's underlying health, and the development of com-plications. Severity of illness in tetanus is rated as mild, moderate, severe, or very severe depending on the in-cubation period (time from presumed inoculation to the first symptom, usually neck stiffness), the period of onset (time from first symptom to first generalized spasm), the portal of entry (some carry worse prognoses), high

Table 1. Prognostic rating scale for tetanus

I. Score one point for each:
   A. Incubation period <7 days
   B. Period of onset <48 h
   C. High-risk portal of entry (burns, umbilical stumps, surgical procedures, compound fractures, septic abortions, intramuscular injections, illicit narcotic injections)
   D. Generalized tetanus
   E. Core temperature above 40°C
   F. Tachycardia (heart rate above 120/min in adults, or 150/min in neonates)

II. Severity and prognosis

Score	Severity	Mortality
0–1	Mild	<10%
2–3	Moderate	10–20%
4	Severe	20–40%
5–6	Very severe	>50%

III. Exceptions: cephalic tetanus is rated at least severe; neonatal tetanus is always rated very severe.

fever, and tachycardia. A prognostic rating scale is presented in Table 1.

Botulism

The death rate among patients with botulism varies with the type of toxin involved and, to some extent, with the epidemiologic aspects of the infection. The overall mortality in developed countries is about 7%. Mortality is higher among patients with type A toxin than with the other forms and increases with the age of the patient. Interestingly, the first patient in an outbreak incurs a higher mortality risk; the relative contributions of the toxin load and the more rapid recognition of other cases have not been dissected.

The prognosis of infant botulism is apparently better, with a reported mortality of about 4%. Wound botulism carries a mortality of about 15%.

Suggested Reading

Bleck TP (1989) Clinical aspects of tetanus. In: Simpson LL (ed) Botulinum neurotoxin and tetanus toxin. Academic, San Diego, pp 379–398

Bleck TP (1991) Tetanus. In: Scheld WM, Whitley RJ, Durack DT (eds) Infections of the central nervous system. Raven, New York, pp 603–624

Hughes JM, Blumenthal JR, Merson MH et al. (1981) Clinical features of type-A and type-B botulism in the U.S. Ann Intern Med 95:442–445

Tacket CO, Rogawski MA (1989) Botulism. In: Simpson LL (ed) Botulinum neurotoxin and tetanus toxin. Academic, San Diego, pp 351–378

Veronesi R, Foccacia R (1981) The clinical picture. In: Veronesi R (ed) Tetanus: important new concepts. Excerpta Medica, Amsterdam, pp 183–206

Vita G, Girland P, Puglisi RM et al. (1987) Cardiovascular-reflex testing and single-fiber electromyography in botulism. Arch Neurol 44:202–206

| # Other Bacterial Infections

HANS-WALTER PFISTER

Neurobrucellosis

Definition, Epidemiology, and Clinical Features

The most common etiologic agents of brucellosis (Malta fever), *Brucella melitensis* and *B. abortus* (Bang's bacillus), are ingested via raw milk or milk products as well as via direct contact with animals infected with *Brucella* species (sheep, goats, cattle, pigs, camels). Predisposed to this disease are agriculturists, butchers, veterinarians, dairy workers, and slaughterhouse workers. Brucellosis is endemic in Middle Eastern countries (in particular in Saudia Arabia and Kuwait) and in the Mediterranean region (e.g., Spain and Portugal) and therefore should be considered in visitors to these countries. The course of brucellosis is subclinical in about 50% of infected persons. After an incubation period of several weeks, fever periods of 1–2 weeks' duration may develop including chills, night sweat, nausea, fatigue, myalgia,

weight loss, arthralgia, hepatosplenomegaly, and lymphadenopathy, interrupted by afebrile asymptomatic periods lasting several days. In about 5–10% of treated patients symptoms reoccur during the following three months. Involvement of the central or peripheral nervous system occurs in 2–5% of patients.

Neurobrucellosis may present as (a) acute meningoencephalitis (rarely myelitis), (b) subacute or chronic meningitis, or (c) radiculoneuritis (cranial nerve involvement in 50% of patients, most often the sixth, seventh, and eighth nerves). Cerebral meningovascular involvement includes vasculitis, vasospasm, or mycotic aneurysm and may result in stroke, subarachnoid hemorrhage, or intracerebral bleeding. The infection is usually the result of a hematogenous spread of *Brucella*, and is rarely the consequence of extension of infection from a contiguous infectious focus (e.g., infective spondylitis). Neurological symptoms and signs may be the only clinical manifestation. The CSF reveals a lymphocytic pleocytosis (40–1400 cells/μl) and an elevated total protein content (82–510 mg/dl). The

Section Editor: Thomas P. Bleck

diagnosis is confirmed by the detection of elevated IgG antibody titers (agglutination titer for *Brucella* in serum of >1:160). CSF cultures are positive in about 50% of cases.

Management and Prognosis

Controlled clinical studies in neurobrucellosis have not been performed. For treatment of neurobrucellosis usually a combination of doxycycline (2 × 100 mg/day i.v. in adults) and trimethoprim-sulfamethoxazole (e.g., 10 mg/kg/day i.v. of trimethoprim) is recommended for a duration of 2–4 months. After 2 weeks of intravenous therapy the drugs can be administered orally. An alternative antibiotic is rifampin (10 mg/kg per day orally). Several authors even recommend a triple-drug therapy using doxycycline, trimethoprim-sulfamethoxazole, and rifampin. In addition, the administration of corticosteroids (e.g., dexamethasone 24 mg/day i.v.) is recommended during the acute phase of the disease. About 90% of treated patients show a complete recovery within 1 year. Mortality of untreated brucellosis is 2%. The most frequent cause of death is bacterial endocarditis with septic embolism.

Whipple's Disease

Definition, Epidemiology, and Clinical Features

Whipple's disease (intestinal lipodystrophy) is a rare disorder caused by the gram-positive "Whipple's bacillus". It usually affects middle-aged men. The clinical symptoms include recurrent arthralgias, diarrhea, weight loss, abdominal pain, attacks of fever, increased erythrocte-leukocyte sedimentation rate, and leukocytosis. In about 5–10% of patients neurological manifestations evolve including a granulomatous encephalitis with perivascular infiltrates, in particular in the diencephalon, brain stem and cerebellum, and ependymitis with possible development of an occlusive hydrocephalus. Rarely, aseptic meningitis, radiculoneuritis, or myositis may occur. The typical neurological syndrome is characterized by the triad of dementia, supranuclear ophthalmoplegia, and myoclonic jerks. In addition, hypothalamic dysfunction (polydipsia, hyponatremia, altered circadian rhythm) or cerebellar signs (in particular ataxia) may develop. Intestinal symptoms may be preceded for years by neurological manifestations.

The detection of abnormal macrophages plays a major diagnostic role. In affected tissues macrophages with a foamy cytoplasm full of periodic acid-Schiff (PAS)-positive, amylase-resistant bodies can be visualized. These bodies contain fragments of bacteria and intact bacilli. The abnormal macrophages are most frequently detected in the jejunal mucous membrane, the mesenteric lymph nodes, in the CSF, and in brain tissue. The bacillus has not yet been grown in culture media, but polymerase chain reaction techniques have shown that it resembles actinobacteria.

Cranial CT may show hypodense parenchymal areas and granulomas in or near the upper brain stem, or hydrocephalus. MRI may show the existing abnormalities in greater detail. Granulomas are generally enhanced by the administration of paramagnetic agents.

The CSF usually reveals a normal cell count and a normal protein content. Rarely, CSF cells may contain PAS-positive substances.

Management and Prognosis

The disease is chronic, progressive, and ultimately fatal when untreated. Preferred treatment is trimethoprim-sulfamethoxazole (e.g., 10 mg/kg per day trimethoprim i.v.) or doxycycline (2 × 100 mg/day i.v. in adults). With antibiotic therapy one third of the patients attain a clinical standstill or even improvement. The organisms remain intact within macrophages for a long period. Therefore, a treatment duration of 1–3 years is usually recommended, e.g., 360–480 mg/day trimethoprim orally or doxycycline 100 mg/day orally. In patients with hypothalamic-hypophysial dysfunction endocrine maintenance therapy may be necessary.

Legionellosis (Legionnaires' Disease)

Legionnaires' disease is an acute febrile illness associated with pneumonia, caused by the gram-negative bacillus *Legionella pneumophila*. *Legionella* may colonize water supplies and respiratory equipment. About 30% of the patients who suffer from legionellosis have neurological manifestations including (a) encephalopathy with disorientation, altered consciousness, headache, cerebellar or extrapyramidal signs, or rarely, seizures; (b) myelopathy (rare); or (c) axonal polyneuropathy (rare). The cause of the neurological disorder is thought to be *Legionella* toxins. The CSF exhibits a slightly increased cell count and total protein content in 20–25% of patients. Neurological symptoms and signs lasting several days may precede pneumonia. They usually completely resolve with adequate antibiotic therapy using erythromycin (4 × 500 mg/day i.v. for 10–14 days). An alternative antibiotic appears to be ciprofloxacin (2 × 200 mg/day i.v.), which is effective in vitro and in clinical reports.

Actinomycosis/Nocardiosis

The mycelium-forming bacteria *Actinomyces* and *Nocardiae* cause chronic purulent infections which may result in the formation of an abscess (pseudotumor), granuloma, and fistula. Neurological manifestations which occur in up to 10% of patients who suffer from *actinomycosis* include brain abscess and, rarely, intracranial epidural abscess or subdural empyema, meningitis, or spinal epidural abscess. They may develop by hematogenous spread from a primary infectious focus (thoracic, abdominal, pelvic, or disseminated actinomycosis) or by extension from a contiguous infectious focus. Cervicofacial actinomycotic infection, which most often follows dental infections or manipulations, may extend to the base of the skull and reach the meninges. Primary actinomycosis of the central nervous system has been reported anecdotally. The diagnosis is proven by the microscopic or cultural detection of actinomyces (most often *Actinomyces israelii*) in the abscess pus.

The therapy of choice for actinomycosis is intravenous penicillin G for 4–6 weeks (adults 20–24 megaunits/day, children 200 000–250 000 units/kg/day i.v.), followed by oral maintenance therapy for 6–12 months to prevent relapses (e.g., phenoxymethyl-penicillin 3 × 1.2 megaunits/day orally). In case of allergy to penicillin, erythromycin is administered (2–4 g/day i.v. in adults, 50 mg/kg/day i.v. in children).

Surgical intervention is required in a solitary brain abscess or spinal abscess. Despite adequate therapy, recurrences may occur over a period of several years.

Central nervous system *nocardiosis* is caused by hematogenous spread from a primary pulmonary infectious focus and occurs in 20–30% of patients with nocardiosis. Neurological manifestations include brain abscess, and rarely meningitis or spinal abscess. Diagnosis is made by the microscopic (gram-positive, partly acid fast) and cultural detection of *Nocardia* in the abscess pus. Nocardiosis is most often observed as an opportunistic infection in immunocompromised patients.

Therapy of choice in nocardiosis is trimethoprim-sulfamethoxazole (480–640 mg/day i.v. trimethoprim dose in adults, 15–20 mg/kg/day i.v. in children) for 6–8 weeks. To prevent relapses oral maintenance therapy is recommended for 6–12 months (e.g., 160 mg/day trimethoprim orally in adults). A single brain abscess is usually surgically excised. The mortality is approximately 50%, but it may reach 90% in patients with multiple, inoperable brain abscesses.

Suggested Reading

Al Deeb SM, Yaqub BA, Sharif HS, Phadke JG (1989) Neurobrucellosis: clinical characteristics, diagnosis, and outcome. Neurology 39:498–501

Bahemuka M, Shemena AR, Panayiotopoulos CP, Al-Aska AK, Obeid T, Daif AK (1988) Neurological syndromes of brucellosis. J Neurol Neurosurg Psychiatr 51:1017–1021

Barnicoat MJ, Wierzbicki AS, Norman PM (1989) Cerebral nocardiosis in immunosuppressed patients: five cases. Q J Med 268:689–698

Burden P (1989) Actinomycosis. J Infect 19:95–99

Donaldson RM Jr (1992) Whipple's disease – rare malady with uncommon potential. N Engl J Med 327:346–348

Finegold SM (1988) Legionnaires' disease – still with us. N Engl J Med 318:571–573

Fishman RA (1992) Cerebrospinal fluid in diseases of the nervous system, 2nd edn. Saunders Harcourt Brace Jovanovich, Philadelphia

Hall WH (1990) Modern chemotherapy for brucellosis in humans. Rev Infect Dis 12:1060–1099

Johnson JD, Raff MJ, Van Arsdall JA (1984) Neurological manifestations of legionnaires' disease. Medicine (Baltimore) 63:303–310

Keinath RD, Merrell DE, Vlietstra R, Dobbins WO (1985) Antibiotic treatment and relapse in Whipple's disease. Gastroenterology 88:1867–1873

McLean DR, Russell N, Khan MY (1992) Neurobrucellosis: clinical and therapeutic features. Clin Infect Dis 15:582–590

Mousa ARM, Elhag KM, Khogali M, Marafie AA (1988) The nature of human brucellosis in Kuwait: study of 379 cases. Rev Infect Dis 10:211–217

Relman DA, Schmidt TM, MacDermott RP, Falkow S (1992) Identification of the uncultured bacillus of Whipple's disease. N Engl J Med 327:293–301

Ryser RJ, Locksley RM, Eng SC, Dobbins WO, Schoenknecht FD, Rubin CE (1984) Reversal of dementia associated with Whipple's disease by trimethoprim-sulfamethoxazole, drugs that penetrate the blood-brain barrier. Gastroenterology 86: 745–752

Shakir RA, Al-Din ASN, Araj GF, Lulu AR, Mousa AR, Saadah MA (1987) Clinical categories of neurobrucellosis. A report on 19 cases. Brain 110:213–223

Smego RA (1987) Actinomycosis of the central nervous system. Rev Infect Dis 9:855–865

Unertl K, Lenhart FP, Forst H, Vogler G, Wilm V, Ehret W, Ruckdeschel G (1989) Brief report: Ciprofloxacin in the treatment of legionellosis in critically ill patients including those cases unresponsive to erythromycin. Am J Med 87 (Suppl 5A): 128S–131S

Wiethölter H, Dichgans J (1982) Diagnosis of cerebral Whipple's disease by cerebrospinal fluid cytology. Arch Psychiatr Nervenkr 231:283–287

Chapter 43

Spinal Abscesses

Hans-Walter Pfister

Spinal Epidural Abscess

Definition and Epidemiology

Among spinal abscesses, epidural abscesses are most frequently observed. Spinal epidural abscesses are diagnosed in approximately 0.2–2.8 cases per 10000 admissions to large tertiary-care centers. There is no seasonal trend. The male-to-female ratio is about 1:1. Spinal epidural abscesses have been reported in all age-groups; however, they are very uncommon in children. An epidural abscess requires urgent surgery and antibiotic therapy because a severe neurological deficit (e.g., paraplegia) may develop within hours.

Pathogenesis and Pathophysiology

Spinal epidural abscesses are located posteriorly in over 70% of cases. Because anteriorly the dura mater is tightly adherent to the vertebral bodies and to the ligaments, the epi-

dural space is only a potential space in the anterior region. Three to six adjacent spinal cord segments are involved in most cases, but the entire length of the spinal cord may be affected in very rare cases. Epidural abscesses and subdural empyemas are most often located in the thoracic (31–63%) and lumbar (21–44%) regions of the spine. In the cervical region of the spine the large diameter of the spinal cord virtually obliterates the epidural space. Therefore, this region is less frequently involved (14–26%).

Spinal epidural abscesses arise as a result of (a) direct extension from a contiguous infection site, including vertebral osteomyelitis (found in 35–38% of patients), spondylodiscitis, retropharyngeal, perinephritic, or psoas abscess, or decubitus ulcer infections; (b) hematogenous spread from a remote infectious focus (e.g., skin and soft tissue infection, endocarditis, respiratory tract infection, urinary tract infection, deep abdominal infection, dental infection, infected spinal hematoma); and (c) invasive spinal procedures or penetrating injuries, such as lumbar puncture or spinal epi-

Section Editor: Thomas P. Bleck

dural anesthesia, or paravertebral or peridural injections. A localized source of infection can be identified in about 75% of cases.

A spinal epidural abscess may result in direct compression of the spinal cord or nerve roots and spinal vascular involvement. Vascular involvement includes vasculitis with subsequent thrombosis, edema formation, and infarction, and mechanical compression of spinal vessels with the risk of focal ischemia.

Risk factors and underlying diseases include diabetes mellitus, malignancy, intravenous drug abuse, cirrhosis, renal failure, and alcoholism. It has been suggested that an antecedent blunt trauma (history in 17–30% of patients) may facilitate the formation of a spinal abscess. It is conceivable that a small spinal hematoma or other injured tissue may be a nidus for metastatic spread during transient bacteremia.

Staphylococcus aureus is the most common etiologic agent (50%–90%, in some reports isolation rates nearly reached 100%), followed in frequency by streptococci (10–20%) and gram-negative enteric bacilli (10–30%; Table 1). Less commonly, fungi, *Mycobacterium tuberculosis, Actinomyces*, and *S. epidermidis* may be detected. In contrast to the spectrum of etiologic agents in brain abscess, anaerobic bacteria play a minor role in the genesis of spinal abscesses.

Clinical Features
and Differential Diagnosis

Rankin and Flothow (1946) and Heusner (1948) proposed a clinical staging system for epidural spinal

Table 1. Etiologic agents in spinal epidural abscesses adapted from Danner and Hartman 1987 and Wheeler et al. 1992

Etiologic agent	Frequency (%)
Staphylococcus aureus	52–95
Gram-negative rods[a]	9–37
Aerobic streptococci	8–15
Anaerobes[b]	7
Staphylococcus epidermidis	2
Multiple organisms	10
Others[c]	5

[a] Especially *Escherichia coli, Pseudomonas* species; rarely *Enterococcus* species, *Serratia marcescens, Enterobacter cloacae, Enterobacter aerogenes*.
[b] *Fusobacterium* species, *Bacteroides* species.
[c] *Mycobacterium tuberculosis, Proteus* species, *Salmonella, Streptococcus pneumoniae, Streptococcus sanguis, Streptococcus milleri, Morganella morganii, Listeria monocytogenes, Brucella* species, *Haemophilus influenzae, Actinobacillus actinomycetemcomitans, Bacillus* species, *Actinomyces israelii, Nocardia*, fungi (*Cryptococcus neoformans, Aspergillus* species, mucormycosis, blastomycosis, coccidioidomycosis, *Pseudoallescheria boydii*), parasites (*Taenia solium, Echinococcus*, guinea worm, *Cysticercus*).

abscess: phase I – spinal ache (back pain, localized tenderness, fever); phase II – nerve root pain (radicular pain, fever, leukocytosis, headache or nuchal rigidity, abnormal deep tendon reflexes); phase III – weakness (motor impairment, sensory abnormalities, bowel and bladder dysfunction); phase IV – paralysis (complete plegia and sensory level). An emergent diagnostic evaluation is necessary when radicular pain or an incomplete neurological deficit (sensory loss, weakness, bowel or bladder dysfunction) is present which may progress to paraplegia.

The neurological symptoms and signs usually develop during a period of several days up to 14–16 days (*acute* form of the disease) or for a period longer than 14–16 days up to several weeks (*chronic* form of the disease). Surgical decompressive intervention most often reveals purulent material in the acute forms of the disease and organized granulation and fibrous tissue in the chronic forms. Acute forms of the disease are often associated with a hematogenous spread from a remote infectious focus, while in chronic forms a direct extension from a contiguous infectious focus is the predominant finding. Patients with chronic disease may be afebrile and have a normal white blood cell count.

Complications in the course of the disease are spinal vascular involvement with medullary infarctions, purulent meningitis, and septic shock.

Differential diagnoses include mainly intradural or extradural neoplasms (primary tumors or metastatic disease involving the spine) and transverse myelitis.

Ancillary Tests

Neuroimaging. Plain films of the spine may reveal a narrowed intervertebral disk space and/or lytic changes involving the adjacent vertebrae. If available, *MRI* should be the next diagnostic step. This imaging modality, if used in conjunction with paramagnetic enhancement, allows direct visualization of the inflammatory tissue (Figs 1, 2); distinction between an abscess and granulation tissue is possible. *Myelography* via a cervical approach followed by *CT* is capable only of showing the accompanying extradural mass lesion with its attending effects on CSF flow; the inflammatory tissue is shown only indirectly.

Laboratory Tests and CSF. The peripheral leukocyte count and erythrocyte sedimentation rate are usually elevated. Cerebrospinal fluid (CSF)

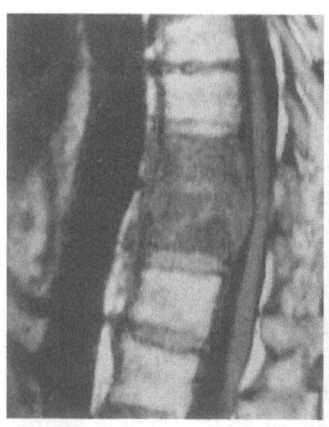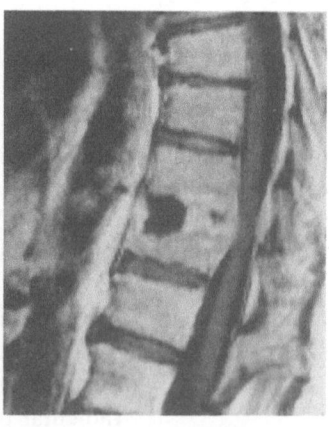

a   b

Fig. 1a,b. Spondylodiscitis in a 59-year-old man with diminished knee as well as ankle jerk on the left but no paresis. T1-weighted midsagittal MR images before (**a**) and after (**b**) IV administration of paramagnetic contrast agent are remarkable for signal abnormality of the 11th and 12th thoracic vertebrae (including the disk space) that becomes largely masked by the enhancement of the diseased bone. Granulation tissue not only occupies the disk space but also extends into the spinal canal, focally compressing the dural sac and cord. (Courtesy of Klaus Sartor and Marius Hartmann, Heidelberg)

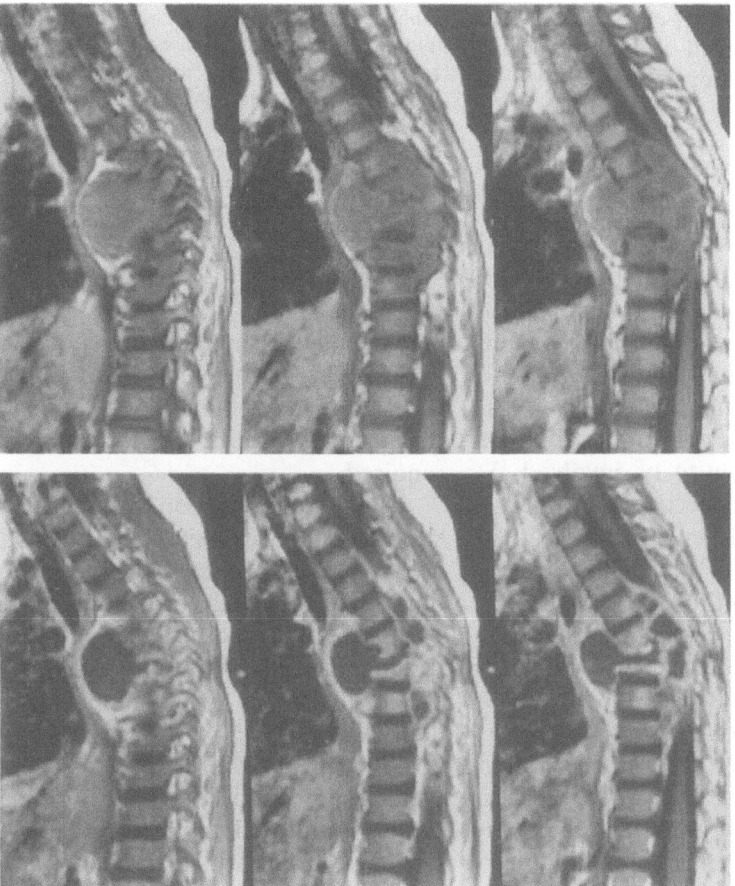

Fig. 2. Tuberculous spondylodiscitis in a 3-year-old boy with rapidly progressive paraparesis of the legs. T1-weighted sagittal MR images before (*upper row*) and after (*bottom row*) IV administration of paramagnetic contrast agent show a large soft tissue mass that surrounds several partially destroyed vertebrae of the midthoracic region, projecting both away from the spinal column and extending into the spinal canal. Abnormal enhancement is confined to the periphery of the lesion as well as sept-like formations, suggesting the lesion to consist of multiple abscesses. Note the severe compression of the cord at the level of the gibbus. (Courtesy of Klaus Sartor and Marius Hartmann, Heidelberg)

usually reveals a mixed pleocytosis of up to several hundred white blood cells per cubic millimeter, consisting of polymorphonuclear leukocytes and lymphocytes, and an elevated total protein content which may exceed several hundred mg/dl in case of a complete spinal block. However, if epidural abscess is suspected, a lumbar puncture should not be performed, because the needle may inadvertently carry infectious material into the subarachnoid space.

Positive abscess cultures have been reported in 50–90% of patients, positive blood cultures in 60–70%, and positive CSF cultures in 20%. Etiologic agents isolated from the blood are nearly always identical to those isolated from the abscess pus during surgical intervention.

Management

Urgent surgical intervention is crucial to prevent neurological dysfunction. Treatment of choice is the combination of laminectomy for decompression and drainage of the purulent material and intravenous administration of antibiotics directed against the etiologic agents most likely to be involved: *S. aureus*, streptococci, and gram-negative rods. A combination of an antistaphylococcal penicillin (e.g., oxacillin, nafcillin, or flucloxacillin), a third-generation cephalosporin (e.g., cefotaxime or ceftriaxone), and perhaps an aminoglycoside (e.g., gentamicin or tobramycin) is recommended to cover the most common pathogens (Tables 2 and 3). If a methicillin-resistant *S. aureus* is involved, vancomycin should be used instead of the antistaphylococcal penicillin. When the etiologic agent is known from cultures, the antibiotic regimen should be modified according to the susceptibility tests. Treatment duration of 3–4 weeks is usually re-

Table 2. Empiric antimicrobial therapy in epidural spinal abscess (4–6 weeks)

3rd-generation + oxacillin[b] + aminoglycoside[c] cephalosporin[a]

[a] Cefotaxime or ceftriaxone.
[b] Alternative: flucloxacillin; in methicillin-resistant staphylococci: vancomycin.
[c] Tobramycin or gentamicin.

commended; it should be extended to 6–8 weeks in osteomyelitis. Rapid surgical intervention to eliminate the primary source of infection is required.

The administration of corticosteroids is controversial. Their benefit is not proved; controlled studies do not exist. They may be administered during the first week of therapy (e.g., dexamethasone 24 mg i.v. per day in adults) in combination with antibiotics.

Successful nonsurgical management using antibiotic therapy alone has been reported in selected patients, including those with extended, multisegmental spinal abscess, slight neurological dysfunction, or complete paralysis for more than 3 days. However, the role of nonsurgical management has yet to be determined in controlled studies.

Table 3. Recommended doses of antibiotics in epidural spinal abscess

Antibiotic	Total daily dose (dosing interval)	
	Adults	Children
Cefotaxime	6 g/day i.v.	200 mg/kg/day i.v. (every 8 h)
Ceftriaxone	2(–4) g/day i.v.	100 mg/kg/day i.v. (every 24 h)
Oxacillin	12 g/day i.v.	150 mg/kg/day i.v. (every 4 h)
Vancomycin	2 g/day i.v.	40–60 mg/kg/day i.v. (every 12 h)
Tobramycin, or gentamicin	240 mg/day i.v.	5 mg/kg/day i.v. (every 8 h)

Prognosis

Spinal epidural abscess, either acute or chronic, may cause direct injury due to compression of the spinal cord or nerve roots and indirect injury secondary to vascular involvement and infarction. The widespread use of MRI offers the hope for prompt diagnosis and more rapid treatment with surgical intervention and initiation of antibiotic therapy.

In an analysis of 188 cases of spinal epidural abscesses done by Danner and Hartman (1987) the outcome was as follows: complete recovery (39%), weakness (26%), paralysis (22%), death (13%). The chance for complete recovery depends on early diagnosis and treatment and is most likely in those patients without a neurological deficit or with a deficit which has developed within 24 h before diagnosis and treatment. In patients in whom weakness or paralysis exists for a period longer than 36–48 h complete recovery is unlikely.

Spinal Subdural Empyema

Very rarely, spinal subdural empyema may occur. Signs and symptoms resemble those of spinal epidural abscess. Diagnosis is made by post-myelography CT or MRI. A spinal subdural abscess is most often caused by hematogenous spread from a remote infectious focus, with *S. aureus*, streptococci, and gram-negative rods being the most frequent etiologic agents. Therapy includes antibiotic agents directed against these bacteria (see management of spinal epidural abscess) and rapid surgical intervention consisting in laminectomy and drainage.

Suggested Reading

Baker AS, Ojemann RG, Swartz MN, Richardson EP jr (1975) Spinal epidural abscess. N Engl J Med 293:463–468

Brock DG, Bleck TP (1992) Extra-axial suppurations of the central nervous system. Semin Neurol 12:263–272

Danner RL, Hartman BJ (1987) Update of spinal epidural abscess: 35 cases and review of the literature. Rev Infect Dis 9:265–274

Del Curling O, Gower DJ, McWhorter JM (1990) Changing concepts in spinal epidural abscess: a report of 29 cases. Neurosurgery 27:185–192

Ericsson M, Algers G, Schliamser SE (1990) Spinal epidural abscesses in adults: review and report of iatrogenic cases. Scand J Infect Dis 22:249–257

Gellin BG, Weingarten K, Gamache FW Jr, Hartman BJ (1991) Epidural abscess. In: Scheld WM, Whitley RJ, Durack DT (eds) Infections of the central nervous system. Raven, New York, pp 499–514

Heusner AP (1948) Nontuberculous spinal epidural infections. N Engl J Med 239: 845–854

Hlavin ML, Kaminski HJ, Ross JS, Ganz E (1990) Spinal epidural abscess: a ten-year perspective. Neurosurgery 27:177–184

Leys D, Lesoin F, Viaud C et al. (1985) Decreased morbidity from acute bacterial spinal epidural abscesses using computed tomography and nonsurgical treatment in selected patients. Ann Neurol 17:350–355

Rankin RM, Flothow PG (1946) Pyogenic infection of the spinal epidural space. West J Surg Obstet Gynecol 54:320–323

Shulman JA, Blumberg HM (1991) Paraspinal and spinal infections. In: Lambert HP (ed) Infections of the central nervous system. Decker, Philadelphia, pp 374–391

Wheeler D, Keiser P, Rigamonti D, Keay S (1992) Medical management of spinal epidural abscesses: case report and review. Clin Infect Dis 15:22–27

Inflammatory Diseases: Viral Infections

Chapter 44

Herpesvirus Encephalitis

Uta Meyding-Lamadé, Daniel F. Hanley,
and Birgit Sköldenberg

Clinically Relevant Features of Herpesviruses

Eight herpesviruses cause human disease: herpes simplex virus 1 (HSV-1), herpes simplex virus 2 (HSV-2), cytomegalovirus (CMV), varicella-zoster virus (VZV), Epstein-Barr virus (EBV), human herpesvirus 6 and 7, and simian herpesvirus B. All of these except HSV-7 can cause devastating central nervous system (CNS) disease. All herpesviruses contain double-stranded DNA, located at a central core with a size of 120–300 nm, average molecular weight of 80–150 million, consisting of 120 000–130 000 base pairs. HSV-1 and HSV-2 have approximately 50% homology. The most common herpesviruses causing herpes encephalitis in human beings belong to the alpha subclass of herpesviruses, namely HSV-1, HSV-2, and VZV. They are characterized by a very short reproductive cycle, prompt destruction of the host cell, and the ability to establish latency, usually in sensory ganglia. During replication different gene classes are expressed, the immediate early gene such as thymidine kinase being particularly important for virus replication and current antiviral chemotherapy. Latency is characteristic for all herpesviruses. Persisting in an apparently inactive state for a variable duration of time, their reactivation occurs by provocative stimuli such as physical (e.g., surgery in trigeminal neuralgia) or emotional stress, fever, and exposure to ultraviolet light. Reactivation appears to be dependent upon an intact anterior pathway and peripheral pathway. Latent virus has been isolated from trigeminal, sacral, and vaginal ganglia in human beings. In animals HSV can become latent directly within the brain; so far this has not been found in human beings. Neurovirulence is the consequence of peripheral multiplication, invasion of the CNS, and growth in the CNS, but HSV isolated from encephalitic brains often differs genetically from HSV isolated from peripheral blood.

Section Editor: Daniel F. Hanley

Herpes Simplex Encephalitis

Epidemiology, Pathogenesis, Pathology

Epidemiology. Herpes simplex virus encephalitis (HSVE) has an incidence of 1/250 000–1/300 000. It occurs throughout the year, one third occurring in patients younger than 20 years; half of the patients are older than 50 years. Mortality without treatment is 70%. Medical costs of HSVE are considerable, being $25 million in the US in 1983. In adults and older children HSVE is usually caused by HSV-1, whereas HSV-2 causes a benign lymphocytic meningitis. However, six of 93 consecutive Swedish cases of HSVE have been found to be caused by HSV-2. In the newborn HSV-2 causes a diffuse encephalitis, with or without systemic infection by HSV-2.

Pathogenesis. One third of all cases of HSVE occur in primary infections. These patients do not have a prior exposure to HSV. The majority of HSVE occurs in patients with preexisting antibodies, though only 10% of these have clinically evident recurrent HSV infections, like herpes labialis. Patients with primary infections are usually less than 18 years of age. HSVE is not more common in the immunosuppressed patient. Access of virus along the olfactory nerve and limbic system through transneural transport seems to be a tenable hypothesis, supported by animal models. In newborns suffering from HSVE and disseminated HSV infection, HSV probably seeds the CNS by a blood-borne route.

Pathology. The encephalitic brain reveals widespread, bilateral, and usually asymmetrical necrosis associated with severe meningoencephalitis. Involvement of the temporal lobe, insular gyri, and cingulate gyri, as well as the frontobasal lobe leads in general to severe brain swelling. Midbrain compression due to uncal herniation is commonly the ultimate cause of death. Histopathologic changes of the brain include acute inflammation, hemorrhage, and, after approximately 2 weeks, frank necrosis and liquefaction. Microscopic changes are vascular congestion in the cortex and subcortical white matter, perivascular cuffing, gliosis, and neuronophagia. Intranuclear inclusions, present in 50% of cases, appear in the first week. In rare cases of chronic encephalitis, sclerosis and cyst formation, as well as subsequent wallerian degeneration are found.

Clinical Features and Differential Diagnosis

Clinical Features. Typically, a patient has a 1- to 4-day history of gradually increasing headache and fever. After this variable prodrome an extremely variable stage occurs, including alteration of consciousness, memory loss, personality changes, and confusion or olfactory hallucination; this may be present very early in the disease. Focal neurological signs such as hemiparesis, aphasia, and later focal or generalized seizures often are present at this stage of disease. Most patients have clinical signs of meningeal irritation. Subsequently raised intracranial pressure can cause transtentorial uncal herniation (Fig. 1). Past medical history of prior labial or genital herpes is not helpful. Intensive studies over the past

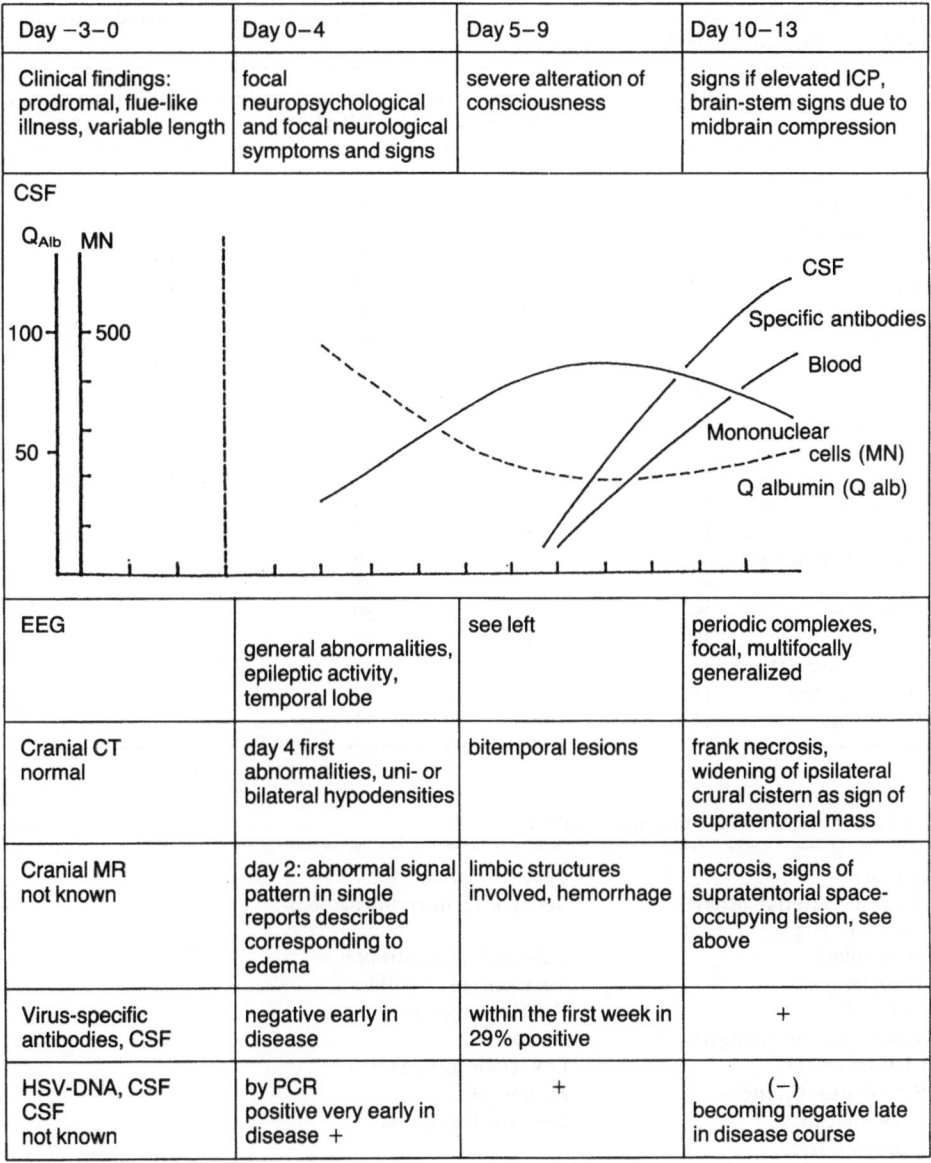

Day −3−0	Day 0−4	Day 5−9	Day 10−13
Clinical findings: prodromal, flue-like illness, variable length	focal neuropsychological and focal neurological symptoms and signs	severe alteration of consciousness	signs if elevated ICP, brain-stem signs due to midbrain compression
EEG	general abnormalities, epileptic activity, temporal lobe	see left	periodic complexes, focal, multifocally generalized
Cranial CT normal	day 4 first abnormalities, uni- or bilateral hypodensities	bitemporal lesions	frank necrosis, widening of ipsilateral crural cistern as sign of supratentorial mass
Cranial MR not known	day 2: abnormal signal pattern in single reports described corresponding to edema	limbic structures involved, hemorrhage	necrosis, signs of supratentorial space-occupying lesion, see above
Virus-specific antibodies, CSF	negative early in disease	within the first week in 29% positive	+
HSV-DNA, CSF CSF not known	by PCR positive very early in disease +	+	(−) becoming negative late in disease course

Fig. 1. Clinical course and findings with ancillary testing in HSVE (modified from Hacke and Zeumer 1986)

16 years (National Institute of Allergy and Infectious Diseases, NIAID collaborative study; Swedish study group) have documented a large overlap of clinical presentations of patients with brain-biopsy-proven herpes simplex encephalitis and those of patients with encephalitis of other origin (Table 1).

Differential Diagnosis. Any disease with rapidly increasing brain edema and focal, preferably temporobasal

Table 1. Presenting symptoms and signs in patients with herpes simplex encephalitis (data from the NIAD and the Swedish collaborative study)

	Biopsy proven (NIAID) %	Biopsy proven (Sweden) %	Not biopsy proven (NIAID) %	Not biopsy proven (Sweden) %
Historical findings				
Alteration of consciousness	97	100	98	95
Fever	90	95	78	95
Headache	81	74	77	66
Personality changes	71	87	68	41
Seizures	67	62	59	54
Vomiting	46	38	46	32
Hemiparesis	33	40	26	18
Memory loss	24		19	
Clinical presentation				
Fever	92	95	81	95
Personality changes	85	87	74	41
Dysphasia	76	36	67	15
Auton. dysfunction	60		56	
Ataxia	40		40	
Hemiparesis	38		30	
Seizures	38	62	47	54
Cranial nerve defic.	22		33	
Visual field loss	14		12	
Papilledema	14		11	

Table 2. Diseases which may mimic HSVE

Infection	*Systemic disease*
Abscess (bacterial, listerial, fungal), empyema	Systemic lupus erythematodes
Tuberculosis	Adrenal leukodystrophy
Toxoplasmosis	Toxic encephalopathies
Rickettsia	Reye's syndrome
Meningococcal meningitis	*Tumour*
EBV-infections	Low-grade astrocytoma
Enterovirus-meningitis	*Hemorrhage*
CMV infections	Subdural hematoma
Vascular disease	
End-stage ischemia	
Septic sinus venous thrombosis	

localization might mimic HSVE. Other infectious diseases such as abscesses, bacterial meningoence-phalitis, septic sinus venous throm-boses, or even toxic encephalopathies like Reye's syndrome may appear as HSVE. Of 432 patients undergoing brain biopsy because of clinically sus-picious HSVE, 55% had other, HSVE-mimicking diseases (Table 2).

Table 3. Patient clinically suspicious of HSVE – what to perform next?

Cranial CT	Normal or temporal, uni- or bilateral hypodense areas
EEG	Focal or general abnormality
CSF	Unspecific pleocytosis, lymphocytes, early in disease course granulocytes
? Cerebral angiography (MRI)	To exclude septic sinus venous thrombosis if suspected

If these criteria are fulfilled, treatment for HSVE is recommended – even if there is no proven diagnosis yet.

Testing that may prove helpful for a patient with suspicion of HSVE is shown in Table 3.

Ancillary Tests

Neuroimaging

Characteristically, the CT scan looks normal until day 4 after the onset of symptoms; thereafter, hypodense areas begin to appear unilaterally, most commonly in the left medial temporal lobe and insular region, subsequently involving the opposite temporal lobe and both frontobasal regions (Fig. 2). Space-occupying effects may be present. Hemorrhage is rarely seen on CT. Contrast enhancement is variable and of little diagnostic help.

Studies in a still small number of patients suggest that MRI reveals more extensive brain involvement. MRI may also be positive earlier than CT, with abnormalities being apparent already on day 2 after onset of symptoms rather than day 4. On MRI bilateral involvement not only of the temporal lobes, but also of limbic structures such as the cingulate gyri, is characteristic (Figs. 3, 4). Signal changes reflecting early hemorrhage (deoxyhemoglobin) may be seen. Markedly hypointense parenchymal areas on T1-weighted images and markedly hyperintensive areas on PD-and T2-weighted images cor-

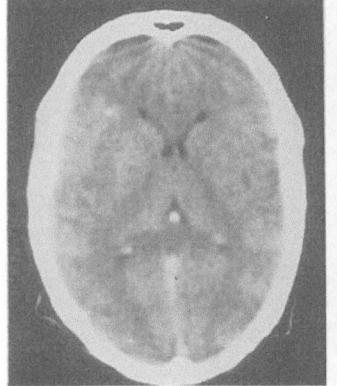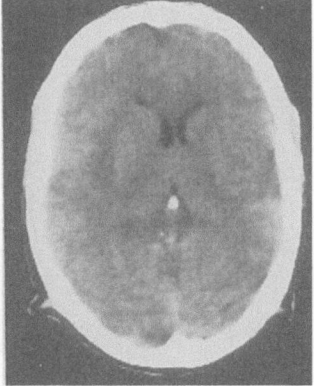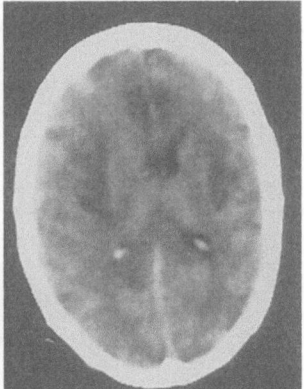

Fig. 2. Development of CT findings in proven HSVE. Scans were performed on days 4, 7, and 10 after acute onset of symptoms. First scan is normal; scan of day 7 (*middle*) shows right insular hypodensities; scan of day 10 shows bilateral insular and bifrontal hypodensities and signs of diffuse brain edema

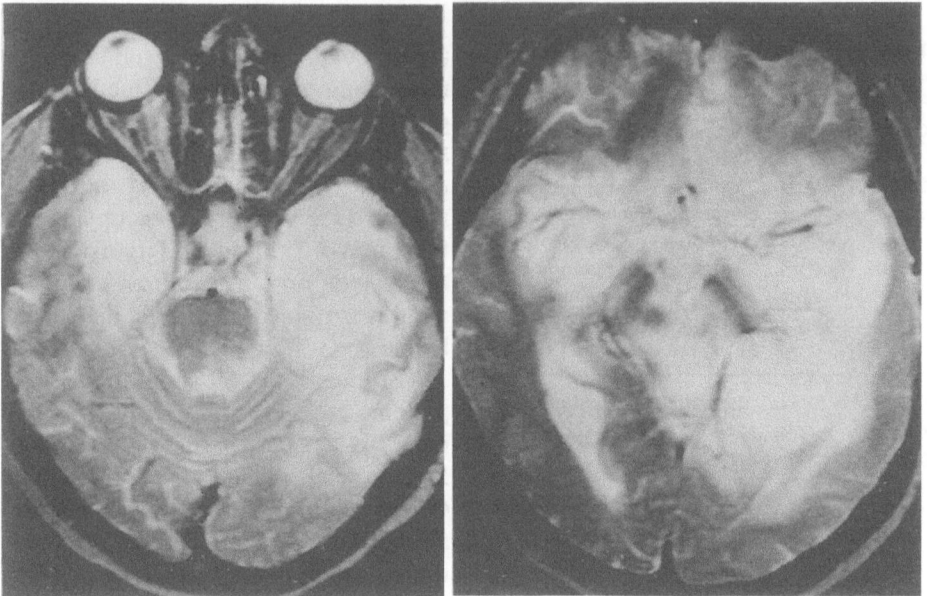

a   b

Fig. 3. MRI of a herpes simplex encephalitis in a 41-year-old woman with advanced disease. T2-weighted axial MR images demonstrate vast areas of abnormally increased signal intensity involving medial basal portions of both frontal and temporal lobes bilaterally. Small hypointensities at the lateral border of the hyperintensity in the right temporal lobe (**a**) likely represent areas of hemorrhage (deoxyhemoglobin stage). Extension of the disease onto the brain stem as seen in (**b**) is unusual. (Courtesy of Klaus Sartor and Marius Hartmann, Heidelberg)

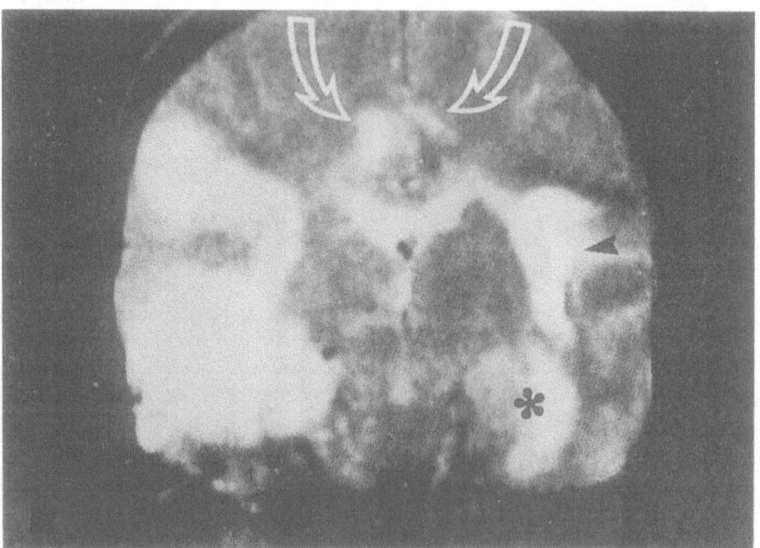

Fig. 4. MRI of a 15-year-old girl with seizures and a left temporal lobe focus (0.5 T; SE 2000/120 coronal images, 10-mm slice thickness): extensive high signal abnormality involves, in addition to right temporal/parietal lobes, medial temporal lobe (*asterisk*) and insula (*arrowhead*) on left. Both cingulate gyri (*open arrows*) are similarly affected. (From Sartor 1991, with permission)

relate with edema secondary to inflammation. Later findings of frank necrosis are present. Little experience exists regarding the use of paramagnetic enhancement. Differential diagnosis includes nonherpetic encephalitides, early cerebritis, low-grade astrocytoma, and bacterial meningoencephalitides.

Electroencephalography

Abnormal, variable findings early in the disease course have a sensitivity of approximately 84% versus a specificity of only 33%. Characteristic findings are spike- and slow-wave activity and periodic lateralized epileptiform discharges, which arise from one temporal lobe at the beginning of disease, becoming bilateral after 6–10 days. In early stages rhythmic, triphasic waves or delta waves (1.5–2/s) are typical. In later stages of disease independent pacemaker regions with characteristic periodic complexes can occur; these have been associated with a rather poor outcome.

Cerebrospinal Fluid

Cytology, Blood-brain Barrier. Even if there is a risk of increased intracranial pressure, lumbar puncture is extremely important. An early abnormal, but nonspecific finding is elevation of white blood cell count, with a predominance of lymphocytes. Mononuclear pleocytosis exists, as in other nonbacterial encephalitides, 50–500/mm^3 being encountered most commonly. Some patients have up to 2000/mm^3. This pleocytosis may be preceded by granulocytes. On day 3–6 plasma cells can be found. Erythrocytes, a slight xanthochromia, and some siderophages may be present. CSF protein is raised in over 80% of cases up to 0.5–2.5 g/l. Disturbance of the blood-brain barrier leads to an increased ratio of albumin in CSF/serum. On day 10, local production of IgG occurs. Subsequently, positive oligoclonal bands are almost always present.

Virus-specific Antibodies in CSF and Blood. As the majority of patients are seropositive prior to their presentation, only a fourfold rise in CSF antibodies is diagnostically helpful occurring in 85% of patients after the end of the first week and within 1 month. A fourfold or greater rise in CSF antibodies occurred significantly more often within a month after onset in biopsy-proven HSVE: 85% versus 29% at 1 week. Intrathecally produced virus-specific antibodies can be determined by ELISA, isoelectric focusing (IEF), and Western blotting. Whereas ELISA and isoelectric focusing are equally highly sensitive, a weak intrathecal antibody synthesis cannot be detected by Western blotting.

HSV-DNA Detection by PCR (Fig. 5). As virus-specific humoral response develops rather late in the course of disease, a reliable and sensitive HSV-DNA detection method remains important for the early diagnosis of HSVE. High sensitivity and specificity, particularly for CSF specimens with low virus content, is characteristic for the PCR, though these are still preliminary results. The occurrence of false-positive and false-negative results must be carefully considered. It proved to be positive during the early, acute stage of the disease, several days

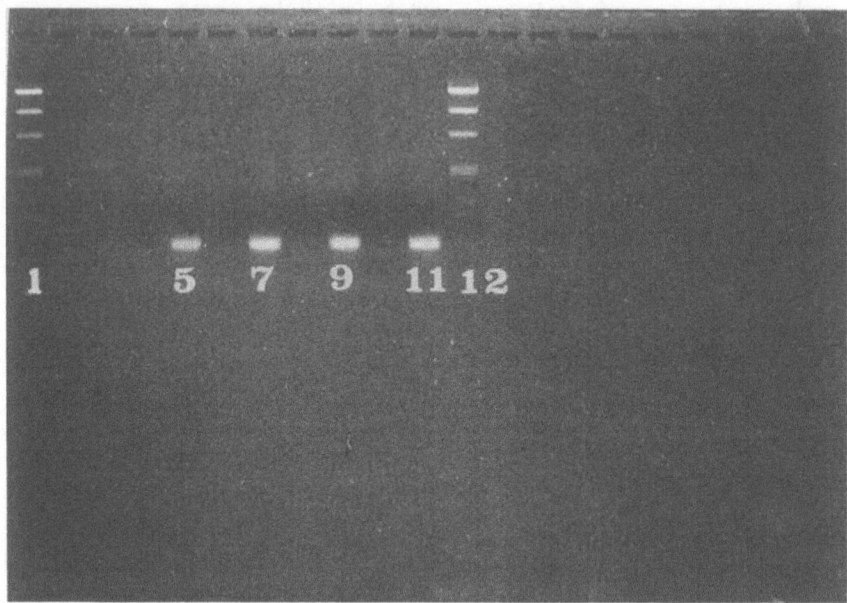

Fig. 5. PCR for herpes simplex virus type 1: *Lanes 1* and *12* represent weight markers (phage Lambda DNA). *Lanes 5, 7, 9, 11* demonstrate positive signal for HSV-1 DNA with different salt concentrations. *Lanes 4, 6, 8, 10* are negative controls without signal

before the appearance of virus-specific antibodies. Interestingly, negative PCR results may be obtained when intrathecally synthesized antibodies are detectable, suggesting that neutralization of virus by specific antibodies has occurred during the course of infection. Similar effects can be seen following the administration of acyclovir, resulting in the disappearance of HSV in the CSF samples. In the postacute phase PCR seems to be unsuitable for diagnosing HSVE, indicating the importance of the detection of antibodies during that stage of disease (Fig. 1).

Brain Biopsy

Whereas brain biopsy has been the gold standard for diagnosing HSVE, it is becoming controversial as new non-invasive, easy, and fast methods are made available. The detection of HSV in brain biopsies by either electron microscopy, immunhistochemical staining, or virus isolation in cell cultures produced positive results in about 60–70% of cases. If brain biopsy is not used initially and HSVE cannot be proven by laboratory testing, careful consideration of differential diagnosis must continue throughout that phase of illness, as well as in cases of nonresponders to acyclovir treatment.

Therapy

Specific Therapy

Large recent studies in the US and Sweden proved that *acyclovir* is the antiviral drug of choice in HSVE with respect to reduction of mortality and incidence of side effects. It is applied intravenously with a dosage of 10 mg/kg every 8 h with each infusion lasting over 1 h for a period of 10–14 days. While the elimination half-life is 2.5 h in patients with normal renal function, it increases to 20 h in anuric patients. In patients with a reduced creatinine clearance the daily number of doses has to be reduced (Fig. 6). Acyclovir may reduce the renal clearance of other drugs that are eliminated by tubular secretion (e.g., methotrexate). Acyclovir should be used during pregnancy if the potential benefit justifies the teratogenic risk to the fetus, which has been shown in animal models and cytogenetic studies. Untoward effects are rare; local phlebitis, nausea, hematuria and hypotension have been described. Obstructive nephropathy has occurred with very high dosages, as well as encephalopathy. Acyclovir has antiviral activity by inhibition of DNA synthesis essentially confined to herpesviruses, being particularly active against HSV-1 and HSV-2; VZV is less sensitive. Thymidine kinase-deficient strains of HSV which are resistent to acyclovir have so far only rarely occurred, but the frequency is increasing in patients with AIDS. Arabinoside and foscarnet have been effective as alternative treatments. The mechanism of action is demonstrated in Fig. 6.

Arabinoside (vidarabine, arabinosine monophosphate, ara-A) is administered in a dosage of 15 mg/kg as a constant intravenous infusion over a 12–24 h period. A large amount of fluid is necessary to dissolve the drug, and this causes some concern when brain edema is severe. The half-life is 3.5 h. Side effects include thrombophlebitis, hypokalemia, and inappropriate secretion of antidiuretic hormone. There is evidence that it is mutagenic and teratogenic. In HSVE acyclovir is superior to arabinoside. In neonatal HSVE arabinoside is equally effective. In acyclovir-resistent HSVE it has been used effectively.

Foscarnet is used only as an alternative treatment in acyclovir-resistent HSVE. It is administered as a bolus of 20 mg/kg over 30 min; thereafter, a continuous infusion of 230 mg/kg per day is given for 2–3 weeks. The most common side effects are reduced renal function, anemia, and hypocalcemia, as well as seizures.

General Therapeutic Strategies

Persistently raised intracranial pressure (ICP) is significantly associated with poor outcome in HSVE; therefore early and aggressive treatment of raised ICP should be considered (see Chap. 9). Steroids are controversial, as they are not effective against cytotoxic edema and may even have a permissive effect on the spread of viral infection.

Anticonvulsive therapy is indicated if seizures occur. Phenytoin is administered at an initial dosage of 250 mg intravenously over 5–10 min, thereafter, as an infusion of 750 mg over a period of 45 min. Daily administration of 3 × 250 mg or ×125 mg depends on serum levels.

Anticoagulation therapy: there is no contraindication to low-dose administration of heparin, 3 × 5000 IU subcutaneously, even though HSVE is a hemorrhagic encephalitis. Prophylactic treatment of deep venous throm-

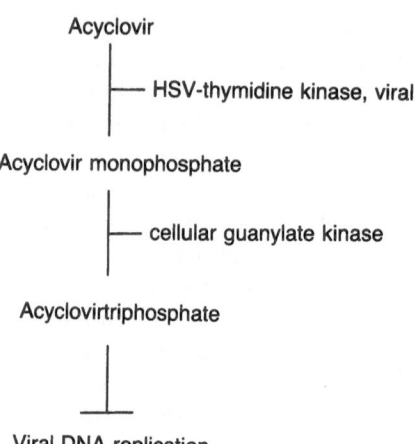

Acyclovir

├── HSV-thymidine kinase, viral

Acyclovir monophosphate

├── cellular guanylate kinase

Acyclovirtriphosphate

Viral DNA replication

Drug	Dosage	Effects	Side effects	Precaution	Alternatives
Acyclovir	10 mg/kg every 8 h intravenously, each infusion lasting over 1 h; over 10–14 days	Inhibition of viral DNA, active against HSV1, HSV2, less against VZV	Rare: local phlebitis, nausea, obstructive nephropathy in high dosages, encephalopathy	Reduced creatinine clearance; longer intervals necessary; teratogenic risk in pregnancy	arabinoside foscarnet
Arabinoside (vidarabine)	15 mg/kg/day constant intravenous infusion	HSVE if acyclovir resistance	Phlebitis, hypokalemia, rise of liver enzymes, SIADH	Mutagenic and teratogenic	Foscarnet
Foscarnet	Bolus of 20 mg/kg over 30 min; thereafter 230 mg/kg/day for 2–3 weeks, intravenous application	HSVE if acyclovir resistance	Reduced renal function, anemia, seizures, hypocalcemia	Mutagenic and teratogenic	Arabinoside

Fig. 6. Specific therapy of HSVE

bosis is discussed in detail in Chap. 14.

Close *monitoring of disease course* to check respiratory and cardiac function as well as to perform several daily neurologic examinations is part of the routine on the ICU. For a small group of critically ill patients continuous ICP measurements may be helpful to optimize therapy. More importantly, fluid limitation, diuresis, and hyperosmolar therapy are probably helpful in limiting the risk of edema and herniation. Daily EEG as well as electrophysiologic examinations, such as brain-stem-evoked potentials or somatosensory-evoked potentials, monitor disease course as well as responsive to treatment. Serial cranial CT examinations may be hazardous in patients with acutely raised ICP and therefore cannot be recommended once the diagnosis has been established during this acute phase.

New Developments and Prospects

Further development of noninvasive diagnostic procedures as well as their significance in evaluating the efficacy of treatment is under intense research at present; e.g., the appearance or persistence of viral DNA determined by PCR might have prognostic significance. But knowledge about natural course is still limited, and standardization of procedures remains to be done. Antiviral combination chemotherapy is under investigation, with the aim of reducing therapeutic failures and drug resistance. Acyclovir and arabinoside have been shown to have a beneficial additive effect when given together in vitro and in animal models. There are currently no human data available.

Prognosis and Outcome

For patients with proven HSVE but without treatment, mortality is over 70%, and only 2.5% of patients return to normal function. Patients treated with acyclovir had a mortality of 19%, 6 months after therapy; 38% of patients returned to normal function. Arabinoside reduced mortality to 44%, 6 months after initiation of therapy. Several factors are known to correlate with poor outcome: patients being older than 30 years of age, patients presenting comatose (or with a severely altered level of consciousness), or establishment of antiviral therapy after widespread bilateral HSVE proven by CT or MR. These patients do have mortality of up to 70%, even though treatment is established.

Herpes Zoster Encephalitis

Epidemiology

The actual incidence of encephalitis following varicella-zoster virus infections is not known. Clinically, two distinct entities exist: *chickenpox* is a primary infection, with over 90% of cases occurring in children less than 10 years of age. A meningoencephalitis, cerebellitis (incidence of 1/4000 children) and Reye's syndrome can occur after chickenpox. Cerebellar involvement is far more common than meningoencephalitis. *Herpes zoster (shingles)* is the consequence of reactivated latent VZV and is always a secondary infection. Patients at risk for developing shingles are immunocompromised, for example, those suffering from Hodgkin's disease as well as patients with AIDS. Encephalitis, with a mortality of 30%, as well as multifocal leukoencephalopathy, can occur. Morbidity and mortality of CNS complications are significantly higher in recurrent herpes zoster than those found in primary varicella-zoster infection (chickenpox).

Pathogenesis and Pathology

Histopathology in both herpes zoster and varicella zoster infections reveals identical intranuclear inclusion bodies (type Cowdry A). Primary VZV infection is the consequence of respiratory droplet spread. In cerebellar ataxia and meningoencephalitis associated with chickenpox two mechanisms are discussed: direct viral involvement of the CNS or a parainfectious, immunologically mediated process. In herpes zoster-associated encephalitis (HZAE) a granulomatous angiitis may be found; thus the pathogenesis may be different from that of varicella encephalitis.

Clinical Features and Differential Diagnosis

In cerebellar ataxia children may develop symptoms from several days before, to 2 weeks after the onset of rash. Nausea, vomiting and nuchal rigidity are common. Fever and seizures occur rarely. Differential diagnosis include other infectious diseases of the CNS, cerebellar tumors or obstructive hydrocephalus. Meningoencephalitis is rare but frequently more severe. Headache, fever, seizures may occur from 11 days before up to several weeks after the onset of rash. Differential diagnosis is above all Reye's syndrome, which has been associated in 30% of cases with chickenpox, occurring after concomittant salicylate therapy for fever. HZAE presents clinically like other encephalitides, altered mental state with focal neurological signs, seizures and signs of meningeal irritation are characteristic. In most cases CNS involvement begins within 1–2 weeks after cutaneous rash, but encephalitis may antedate the appearance of the rash by up to 21 days.

Ancillary Tests

Neuroimaging. There exist only few reports about cranial CT or MRI in CNS complications of VZV. In HZAE, the CT usually is normal, whereas MRI may detect more subtle changes.

Electroencephalography. In cerebellar ataxia the EEG is abnormal in 20% of cases, showing diffuse slow-wave activity. In meningoencephalitis following chickenpox, the EEG is often diffusely abnormal; epileptiform activity may persist for up to 1 year. Diffuse slowing can be found in HZAE. None of these EEG findings are specific.

Cerebrospinal Fluid. In cerebellar ataxia a mild pleocytosis as well as slightly increased protein can be found; in meningoencephalitis protein elevation is below 200 μg/l. In herpes zoster encephalitis the same findings are encountered, notably, in as many as 40% of uncomplicated herpes zoster patients. VZV has been cultured and isolated in the CSF, in contrast to the varicella-associated encephalitides in HZAE. Antibody assays to VZV membrane as well as ELISA and RIA have been utilized.

Management and Prognosis

Therapeutic management is as in HSVE, with the exception that in VZVE there have been no clinical trials so far to compare different antiviral drug regimens. HZAE has a mortality of 30%; this is in part accounted for by the underlying immunodeficiency state. The incidence of long-term sequelae is about 30%. In cerebellar ataxia mortality is low at 0–5%; most patients recover completely. In meningoencephalitis following chickenpox mortality varies between 0 and 35%, probably due to the variable incidence of Reye's syndrome.

Suggested Reading

Aurelius E, Johansson B, Sköldenberg B, Staland A, Forsgren M (1991) Rapid diagnosis of herpes simplex encephalitis by nested polymerase chain reaction assay of cerebrospinal fluid. Lancet 337:189–192

Aurelius E, Johansson B, Sköldenberg B, Forsgren M (1993) Encephalitis in immunocompetent patients due to herpes simplex virus type 1 or 2 as determined by type-specific PCR and type-specific antibody assays of cerebrospinal fluid. J Med Virol 39:179–192

Bartfei A, Stegmann B, Sköldenberg B, Aurelius E, Forsgren M (1993) Long-term cognitive effects of herpes simplex encephalitis and of encephalitis of other aetiology. J Neurol Neurosurg Psychiatry (in press)

Gordon B, Selnes OA, Hart J Jr, Hanley DF (1990) Long-term cognitive sequelae of acyclovir-treated herpes simplex encephalitis. Arch Neurol 47(6):646–647

Hacke W, Zeumer H (1986) Herpes simplex encephalitis. Dtsch Med Wochen Schr 111: 23–25

Hacke W, Buchner H (1988) Akute Virusencephalitis. In: Hacke W (ed) Neurologische Notfallmedizin, 2nd edn. Perimed, Düsseldorf, pp 124–133

Hindmarsh T, Lindkvist M, Olding-Stenkvist E, Sköldenberg B (1986) Accuracy of computed tomography in the diagnosis of herpes simplex encephalitis. Acta Radiol 209:192–196

Nahmias AJ, Whitley RJ, Visintine AN, Takei Y, Alford CA (1982) Herpes simplex virus encephalitis: laboratory evaluations and their diagnostic significance. J Infect Dis 145:829–836

Nugier F, Colin JN, Aymard M, Langlois M (1992) Occurrence and characterization of acyclovir-resistant herpes simplex virus isolates: report on a two-year sensitivity screening survey. J Med Virol 36:1–12

Pohl-Koppe A, Dahm C, Elgas M, Kühn J, Braun R, ter Meulen V (1992) The diagnostic significance of the polymerase chain reaction and isoelectric focusing in herpes simplex virus encephalitis. J Med Virol 36: 147–154

Roizman B, Sears A (1990) Herpes simplex viruses and their replication. In: Fields B, Knipe M (eds) Textbook of virology. Raven, New York, pp 1796–1828

Sartor K (1991) Viral infections. In: Sartor K (ed) MR imaging of the skull and brain. Springer, Berlin Heidelberg New York, pp 645–648

Schooley RT (1988) Encephalitis. In: Ropper A, Kennedy S (eds) Neurological and neurosurgical intensive care, 2nd edn. Aspen, Rockville, pp 289–307

Sköldenberg B, Alestig K, Burman L, Forkman A, Lovgren K, Norrby R, Stiernstedt G, Forsgren M, Bergstrom T, Dahlqvist E, Fryden A, Norlin K (1984) Acyclovir versus vidarabine in herpes simplex encephalitis. A randomized consecutive study in Swedish patients. Lancet 2:707–711

Sköldenberg B (1991) Herpes simplex encephalitis. Scand J Infect Dis [Suppl] 78:40–46

Vandvik B, Sköldenberg B, Forsgren M, Stiernstedt G, Jeansson S, Norrby E (1985) Long-term persistence of intrathecal virus-specific antibody response after herpes simplex encephalitis. J Neurol 231:307–312

Whitley RJ, Cobbs CG, Alford CA Jr, Soong S-J, Hirsch MS, Connor J, Corey L, Hanley DF, Levin M, Powell DA, and the NIAID collaborative antiviral study group (1989) Diseases that mimic herpes simplex encephalitis: diagnosis, presentation and outcome. JAMA 262:234–239

Whitley R, Schlitt M (1991) Encephalitis caused by herpesviruses, including B virus. In: Schield WM, Whitley RJ (eds) Infections of the central nervous system. Raven, New York, pp 41–86

Chapter 45

Other Viral Infections

FRANK TIECKS, HANS-WALTER PFISTER, and C. GEORGE RAY

Coxsackie and Echo Virus Infections

Introduction

Infection of the central nervous system by enteroviruses (EV) is of major epidemiological importance. About half of the annual 40 000–60 000 cases of aseptic meningitis and up to 10% of probably 20 000 cases of encephalitis in the US are likely to be caused by an EV agent, mainly Coxsackie or entero cytopathogenic human orphan (ECHO) viruses (Table 1). Usually, only a few viral strains dominate the regional incidence at a given time (i.e., 15% of strains cause more than 80% of cases). Subclinical infection is common worldwide for all subtypes and there is immunity against a particular virus after infection in immunocompetent hosts.

As with most viruses, serious CNS involvement is a complication of hematogenous spread in the course of a systemic disease, and in the case of EV

Section Editors: Karl M. Einhäupl and Werner Hacke

infection the prognosis may be limited by cardiac (Coxsackie) or hepatic (ECHO) rather than by cerebral involvement. At risk for a severe clinical course are mainly infants under 2 months of age (50% meningitis, 3% encephalitis of patients infected with EV). Males, athletes and B-cell-deficient patients are more likely to develop clinically relevant EV infection.

Pathogenesis

Enteroviruses are spread mainly by fecal-oral pathways, although respiratory spread may occur, because the virus is excreted for about 7 days after infection from the oropharynx. This might be important for the diagnosis of EV by culture from respiratory fluids, while stools are usually positive for several weeks. After initial viral replication in the intestinal epithelial and lymphoid tissues, hematogenous dissemination to susceptible organs occurs. Why a small percentage of obviously immunocompetent hosts develop clinical signs of CNS involvement, mostly aseptic meningitis, remains largely

Table 1. The human pathogenic enteroviruses

Genus	Serotype	Comment
Poliovirus	1–3	
Coxsackie	A 1–24	(except type 23)
	B 1–6	
ECHO virus	1–36	(except types 10, 28)
Enterovirus	68–71	(72 = hepatitis A virus)

unclear. Antibodies play an important role in termination of EV infections; this is illustrated by the high frequency of serious chronic EV infection in patients with agammaglobulinemia, and by reports of successful therapy with immune globulin in some cases.

Clinical Features
and Differential Diagnosis

The clinical course of EV infection varies with the patient's age and immune status. In temperate climates, epidemics occur mainly in summer and early autumn. This helps to differentiate EV infection from lymphocytic choriomeningitis or mumps, which show a peak in winter or spring. Although some of the serotypes of Coxsackie or ECHO viruses which show CNS tropism can be differentiated by their affinity to specific other organs (Table 2), identification of a specific agent on clinical grounds is not possible.

Almost all cases present – after a variable incubation period of 5–10 days – with high fever up to 40°C; this is accompanied by nonspecific symptoms and signs such as rhinitis, pharyngitis, nausea, vomiting, exanthema, lymphadenopathy, arthralgia, or myalgia. Sometimes a biphasic fever pattern with preceding nonspecific symptoms and intermediate recovery for 2–3 days is observed. Other family members frequently show similar symptoms as well. More specific presenting signs include herpangina with multiple painful papulovesicular lesions in the throat and mouth (associated with Coxsackie A strains), or the similar "hand-foot-mouth disease", often caused by Coxsackie A16 and EV 71. Coxsackie B virus strains cause Bornholm's disease, with pleurodynia and intercostal neuralgia as the striking features. They are also frequently complicated by peri- or myocarditis, which can lead to cardiomyopathy or death.

In adults and older children neurological involvement is rare. Headache, photophobia and nuchal rigidity are the common findings in this age-group, suggesting the diagnosis of meningitis, and are often accompanied by hypersomnia and increased irritability. These symptoms are usually self-limited, lasting no longer than 1 week, and lumbar puncture has been reported to relieve the symptoms in many patients, suggesting moderately elevated intracranial pressure. The syndrome of inappropriate secretion of antidiuretic hormone (SIADH) is a well known complication, while febrile seizures may be found in younger children. Focal signs are well described but rarely found. Nonpolio

Table 2. Important diagnostic features of EV disease

Diagnostic feature	Sensitivity	Specificity
1. Season (summer/early autumn)	+ +	+
2. Anamnesis		
epidemic situation	+ +	+
family involvement	+	(+)
biphasic course	+	(+)
agammaglobinemia	+	+
3. Physical examination		
headache	+ + +	(+)
photophobia	+ + +	(+)
neck stiffness	+ +	(+)
fatigue/irritability	+ +	(+)
focal deficits	+	−
fever	+ + +	(+)
flu-like symptoms	+ + +	(+)
rash	+ +	+
myalgia	+ +	+
lymphadenopathy	+ +	+
herpangina	+	+ + +
hand-foot-mouth syndrome	+	+ + +
pleurodynia	+	+ +
myo-/pericarditis	+	+ +
hepatitis (icterus, pain, hepatomegaly)	+	+

EVs are responsible for nearly all cases of paralytic poliomyelitis not caused by polioviruses and have frequently been found to cause cerebellar ataxia. They can also mimic the clinical presentation of herpes simplex or arbovirus infection. Hemiplegia, flaccid paralysis, transverse myelitis, hemichorea, and Guillain-Barré syndrome have occasionally been associated with EV infection.

In neonates, neurological and multiorgan involvement with EV infection is associated with significant acute morbidity and mortality. Nuchal rigidity, convulsions, or bulging of the anterior fontanelle may be seen, but the prognosis is also influenced by extracerebral manifestations such as hepatic, adrenal, or intestinal necrosis or myocarditis. The clinical picture in the newborn may be indistinguishable from bacterial sepsis with multiorgan failure and disseminated intravascular coagulation (DIC).

Given the wide range of clinical courses, *differential diagnosis* must include infections by other viral agents, especially herpes or arboviruses, tuberculosis, fungi (*Cryptococcus*, *Candida*, *Coccidioides*, *Histoplasma*), or bacteria. Partially treated septic meningitis, septic-embolic encephalitis, or parameningeal bacterial infection may show a similar picture.

Autoimmune disease, sarcoidosis, or neoplasm may sometimes be difficult to differentiate. In the infant, inherited metabolic diseases such as galactosemia and urea cycle enzyme deficiencies must also be considered.

Ancillary Tests

There are no specific *neuroradiological* or *neurophysiological* findings in EV infection, but they may be helpful for differential diagnosis and early detection of complications. Diffuse brain edema on cranial CT scan or MRI is a common finding in EV infection, whereas focal lesions are rare. The EEG frequently shows diffuse slowing or dysrhythmia and is helpful to differentiate from herpes simplex encephalitis, where progressive temporal lobe involvement is usually seen. EEG may also help to identify patients with a high risk for seizures. Other neurophysiological tests are usually not beneficial in establishing the diagnosis, unless unusual features like flaccid palsy or spinal symptoms occur.

Laboratory findings usually show moderate leukopenia and lymphocytosis or only slightly elevated white blood cell counts, and thrombocytopenia may occur. Erythrocyte sedimentation rate and C-reactive protein are only mildly elevated. Moderate to marked *CSF* pleocytosis of 10–1000 cells/μl (predominantly mononuclear cells) are the most typical finding in acute EV infection of the CNS, but considerably higher numbers have been described. Granulocytes may dominate the picture in early infection, but they are usually replaced by mononuclear cells within 2 days. CSF glucose and protein are mostly not markedly altered, but a wide range of extraordinary values, mimicking tuberculous meningitis, has been reported. Low CSF glucose is more frequently found than high CSF protein.

Tumor necrosis factor has been claimed to be helpful in differentiating between viral and bacterial meningitis.

It has never been detected in the course of aseptic meningitis, but it has been found in almost three quarters of patients with bacterial meningitis in major series. Interferon-alpha detection in the CSF is regarded to be a moderately sensitive, but highly specific test for viral infection, although it has been found in a few patients with *Haemophilus influenzae* meningitis and cerebral lupus erythematosus as well. Other parameters such as CSF lactate, lactate dehydrogenase, $(2'-5')$ oligoadenylate synthetase, or interleukin 1β seem to be less specific.

Thus, specific virological diagnosis is paramount for the establishment of diagnosis. It is possible to recover virus from throat, feces, and blood even before the onset of symptoms, while CSF culture will yield positive results soon after the onset of neurological symptoms in aseptic meningitis, but less frequently in other CNS manifestations. Respiratory specimens will be positive only for 1–2 weeks after clinical onset, indicating acute infection. EV culture suffers from difficulties, including an overall detection sensitivity of only 65–75% and a frequent delay in the availability of results (3.7–8.2 days, mean, for CSF growth). Blood and CSF recovery provide the strongest causative links between clinical disease and the virus detected. Hopefully, sensitivity and more rapid diagnosis will be facilitated by the introduction of polymerase chain reaction (PCR) for the detection of EV RNA.

Serological evidence of EV infection is obtained either from serum (high IgM levels or fourfold rise in IgG titers) or from CSF-antibody detection (elevated specific antibody of IgG ratio in the CSF, elevated IgG to albumin index in CSF/serum), but it may be falsely positive during the acute phase of febrile illness and does not allow rapid diagnosis in the case of acute infection. However, its sensitivity for the confirmation of a suspected disease is high.

Management

Neurological complications, requiring an ICU stay, are rare in older children or adults during EV infection and should cast doubt on a suspected EV etiology. Alternatively, B-cell defects or agammaglobulinemia should be considered. Administration of high doses of gammaglobulin has shown positive effects in such cases and may prove useful in neonates. Since no specific therapy for EV infection is available, the main aim is to provide optimal supportive care and protect the patient from potentially harmful medication, which may be considered due to the often difficult differential diagnosis.

CNS involvement is most likely to be complicated by elevated intracranial pressure, seizures, or electrolyte disturbance due to SIADH. A CT scan should be obtained wherever possible before lumbar puncture to detect elevated intracranial pressure, which may lead to herniation of cerebellar tonsils during of after LP. Measurement via epidural or intraventricular catheters may be necessary to monitor therapy.

The EEG may show signs of increased cerebral excitability or help in differential diagnosis. Temporal lobe involvement in particular may suggest a diagnosis of herpes simplex encephalitis.

The possibility of SIADH should be considered if consciousness deteriorates, and fluid and electrolyte balance may require meticulous care.

Extracerebral complications are usually due to cardiac or hepatic failure, but rarely they are also the result of lung or gastrointestinal affection. Baseline thorax radiography and echocardiography should be available, and close monitoring with respect to signs of peri- or myocarditis (Table 3) or hepatitis should be performed. Nutrition should be carefully controlled and enteral sterilization with neomycin may become necessary in cases of serious hepatic involvement. Steroids and interferons have not been shown to be effective in acute viral infection and can cause adverse effects. A new generation of drugs such as disoxaril, which inhibit uncoating or cellular receptor binding of EV viruses, has been shown to provide protection from meningoencephalitis or to cure chronic meningitis in mice, but they have not yet reached clinical trials in human beings. Finally, care should be taken to prevent further spread of the virus via stool or, in rare cases, respiratory fluid to family members or medical staff with appropriate isolation and disinfection procedures.

Prognosis and Conclusions

While EV infection with neurological involvement is common and epidemiologically relevant, the clinical course is usually benign. Only neonates, very young children, or B cell-deficient patients more frequently have a poor or fatal outcome – mostly due to non-neurological multiorgan complications. The challenge of EV

Table 3. Clinical features and complications of relevant pathogens (important serotypes)

Neurological finding	Cox. A (7, 9, 16)	Cox. B (1–5)	ECHO (not 24, 26, 27)
Meningitis/ encephalitis	+	+	+
Polio-like	+	+	(+)
Ataxia	++	++	+
Flaccid palsy	+		
Hemiplegia	+		
Hemichorea			?

General signs	Cox. A	Cox. B	ECHO
Flu-like	++	++	++
Exanthema	+	+	+
Lymphadenopathy/ splenomegaly	+	+	+
Herpangina	+		
Pleurodynia		+	

Complications	Cox. A	Cox. B	ECHO
Orchitis		+	
Myocarditis	+	++	+
Cardiomyopathy		+	
Hemolysis/uremia	+	+	
Pneumonia	+	+	+
Hepatitis	+	+	++

infection for neurological ICUs consists in differential diagnosis, early detection, management of possible complications, and prevention of further spread.

Poliomyelitis

Epidemiology

The incidence of poliomyelitis in the industrialized world has shown a dramatic decrease with the introduction of active immunization (from 1959 to 1971 > 98% reduction). Today, only 1.4 per 10 million people develop manifest poliomyelitis in countries with successful vaccination programs. Nevertheless, the disease is still a serious problem in developing countries, whereas in Europe or the U.S. most cases are caused by vaccine strains affecting immunocompromised hosts, or exposure of unvaccinated people to wild virus, e.g., tourists to endemic countries, or by the refusal of members of certain religious groups to be vaccinated. About 10% of patients with clinically manifest poliomyelitis experience life-threatening complications, requiring ICU management. Fatal cases still occur. Other viruses, especially Coxsackie, ECHO, and enterovirus 71, may mimic poliomyelitis but usually show more benign clinical courses.

Pathogenesis

The three strains of poliovirus which produce no relevant cross-reactivity belong to the group of enteroviruses which are spread by fecal-oral pathways or person-to-person contact (often by asymptomatic carriers), while the CNS (myelon *and* brain, particularly medulla oblongata) is affected in the course of viremia. Clinically inapparent infection is common (90–95%), with the remaining patients suffering from flu-like symptoms or benign aseptic meningitis; paralysis occurs in only a few cases. Neurogenic spread has been described but seems to be of lesser importance. Why some individuals are more susceptible to CNS effect is unknown.

Clinical Features and Differential Diagnosis

Infections with poliovirus show a peak in summer and early autumn, similar to other enteroviruses, whereas in the tropics the incidence remains high througout the year. The incubation period is short (3–14 days). Unspecific gastrointestinal or upper respiratory symptoms accompanied by fever are initially present in about 40% of paralytic cases; these are followed mostly by an asymptomatic interval of about 3–10 days. Thereafter, recurrent fever, headache, meningism, and muscular pain result in the clinical picture of aseptic meningitis, which is supported by the finding of CSF pleocytosis. Fasciculations may be seen already at

this stage, indicating involvement of spinal anterior horn cells for the respective limb. In most cases the disease does not progress further, the patient recovers, and the chance of diagnosis may be missed. The paralytic phase usually begins when fever has started to fall and progresses quickly in no more than 4–5 days to flaccid asymmetrical paresis. The lower limbs are generally more severely affected and a proximal pattern has often been reported, while the paucity or absence of sensory symptoms is characteristic. Sometimes the diaphragm, intercostal, or auxiliary respiratory muscles are also involved, causing respiratory distress. Lower cranial nerve paralysis, which is usually less severe, may result in impaired swallowing and aspiration. Autonomic symptoms due to brainstem or vagal disturbance are other potential life-threatening complications. Coma, tremor, and convulsions may precede a fatal outcome. Persistence of fever is associated with a poor prognosis, and further progression is considered less likely if temperature has been normal for more than 1 day. Partial or complete recovery after acute poliomyelitis is frequent, particularly for cranial nerves, but late complications, manifesting as motor neuron disease, have been described.

Differential dignosis includes Guillain-Barré syndrome, polyradiculoneuropathy (especially neoplastic or paraneoplastic), paralytic rabies, acute myelopathy, diphtheria, botulism, and tick paralysis (Table 4).

Ancillary Tests

While *neuroradiological* findings are normal, nerve conduction or electro-

Table 4. Differential diagnosis of poliomyelitis

Disease	Important differences
Guillain-Barré syndrome	No meningitic signs, symmetrical pattern, sensory symptoms, CSF: albuminocytologic dissociation; demyelinization
(Para)-neoplastic disease meningitis carcinomatosa	Sensory symptoms, progression over more than 4–5 days, different fever pattern; CSF: poss. atypical cells, low glucose; poss. reduced nerve conduction velocity
Paralytic rabies	Animal exposure, no meningitic signs, sensory symptoms
Acute myelopathy	No meningitic signs, different course, neuroradiology, CSF: no pleocytosis
Diphtheria	Early: cranial nerve palsies; late: polyneuritis syndrome
Botulism	Descending, symmetrical paralysis (except wound botulism)
Tick paralysis	History of tick exposure, symmetrical, afebrile paralysis over 4 or more days; prompt recovery if tick found and removed

Table 5. Ancillary tests for poliomyelitis

CSF		
Cells	Protein	Glucose
100–200/μl	100–200 mg/dl	normal
Cell differentiation:		
initially polymorphonuclear, later lymphocyte cell picture		

Nerve conduction velocity (NCV)/electromyography (EMG)

	NCV	SNAP	CMAP	SA	RMU
At onset	n	n	n/(−)	n	n/(−)
After 10–14 days	n	n	−	+	−

n, normal; (−), slightly reduced, −, reduced, +, increased
SNAP, sensory nerve action potential; CMAP, compound muscle action potential; SA, spontaneous activity; RMU, recruitment of motor units (full effort)

Microbiology

Viral culture:	Specimen	Timing (from onset)	Sensitivity
	Stool	−10–+20 days	+++
	Resp. fluid	−10–+3 days	++
	Blood	−7−−3 days	+
	CSF	0−+7 days	+
Antibodies:	Blood/(CSF)	0−>30 days	+++

myographic studies demonstrating isolated motor neuron dysfunction without demyelinization may be important for differential diagnosis (e.g., against acute polyneuritis) and prognosis during the course of the disease (Table 5).

CSF consistently reveals lymphocytic pleocytosis of 100–200 cells/μl in the meningitic phase of the disease, which tends to fall after the onset of paralysis. CSF protein is normal or slightly elevated in the beginning, rising to values of 100–200 mg/dl, while glucose remains normal throughout the disease. Initially, a predominance of polymorphonuclear cells may be observed, but these are soon replaced by the lymphocytes.

Virus can be recovered from the stool or respiratory fluid before and during the paralytic phase, whereas culture from blood is sensitive only before the onset of CNS symptoms. CSF cultures are very rarely positive. Other enteroviruses (Coxsackie, ECHO, enterovirus 71) should also be considered in suspected poliomyelitis. A fourfold rise in anti-polio antibodies in the course of the disease is diagnostic.

Management

Due to excretion of the virus into the feces and respiratory fluid, every patient with suspected poliomyelitis must be isolated until no more virus can be recovered from the stool, usually about 3 weeks after paralysis (Table 6). Exercise to reduce muscular pain in the meningitic stage may lead to paralysis; thus, bed rest is recommended during the first few days of suspected polio infection.

As long as no specific therapy is available the greatest risks for life in poliomyelitis derive from respiratory failure. Three possible mechanisms must be considered:

1. Impairment of the diaphragm or other respiratory muscles may lead to severely decreased vital capacity at a time when the patient's blood

Table 6. Management of poliomyelitis

1. Isolation of suspected polio patients (barrier nursing)
2. Assurance of respiratory function
   - control of vital capacity (at least daily)
   - check of swallowing function
   - monitoring of ventilation (rate, depth)
3. Monitoring of other possible hazards
   - changes in blood pressure/pulse rate
   - electrolyte imbalance
   - elevated intracranial pressure
   - convulsions
   - vigilance changes
4. Physiotherapy
   - no exercise in the meningitic stage
   - intensive exercise after the acute phase
5. Anticoagulation
   - usually low-dose heparin
   - rarely high-dose heparin

gas analysis is still completely normal. Therefore, vital capacity should be checked daily in every poliomyelitis patient, and more often if segments C3–5 are clinically involved. If it falls below approximately 1000 ml or if there is rapid deterioration the patient should be intubated.

2. Lower cranial nerve involvement may impair swallowing and lead to aspiration, with acute airway obstruction or consecutive pneumonia. Again, early intubation is warranted.

3. Polio viruses have a predilection for the medulla oblongata, including the regulatory centers for respiration. Depth or rate of ventilation may be reduced and should therefore be monitored regularly.

Other life-threatening complications resulting from spread of the virus throughout the brain, such as changes in blood pressure, raised intracranial pressure, electrolyte changes, convulsions, and coma, are possible. Thus, close monitoring during the active phase of the disease and symptomatic treatment are essential.

In the case of widespread flaccid paralysis the increased risk for deep venous thrombosis may require anticoagulation with dose-adjusted heparin. Early institution of physiotherapy is of eminent importance to avoid contractures and restore muscle function.

Prognosis and Conclusions

Although it is rare in industrial countries, poliomyelitis remains a serious disease without specific therapy once the paralytic phase has become manifest. Optimal monitoring and symptomatic ICU management, however, result in a complete or partial recovery in a substantial number of cases. Functional recovery may continue for as long as 6 months. Paralysis persisting thereafter is permanent.

Central European Encephalitis and Other Arboviral Infections

Epidemiology

Arboviruses include a variety of viruses such as togaviruses, bunyaviruses, reoviruses, and the tick-borne complex (Table 7). They are transmitted by ticks or mosquitos. Human cases show a peak incidence between July and October. Central European encephalitis, Russian spring-summer encephalitis, St. Louis encephalitis, California encephalitis, Colorado tick fever, and Japanese B encephalitis are all caused by these viruses.

The central European encephalitis (CEE) virus is transmitted by larval, nymphal, and adult ticks of the species *Ixodes ricinus* to human beings. Epidemiological studies have shown that in endemic areas 0.1% of the ticks harbor the virus. Laboratory infections with the CEE virus as well as infections after consumption of nonpasteurized milk have occasionally been reported. Person-to-person transmission has not yet been observed, but it may be theoretically conceivable if blood from a patient who is in the stage of viremia is inoculated into another person. The antibody prevalence among the European population is between 0.5% and 1.5%. Among persons living in endemic areas this shows a considerable variation, e.g., 4–8% (Germany), 14% (Austria), and 30–40% (CSFR). Risk groups for the infection are forest workers, hikers, strollers, and collectors of mushrooms and berries, with seroprevalences of 4–16% (Switzerland), 11–50% (CSFR), 30% (Denmark), and 41% (Austria). The risk of being infected with CEE virus after a tick bite in an endemic area in Germany is estimated at 1:900. The overall risk of infected persons becoming ill is approximately 10–20%. However, definite data on the risk of infection and manifest illness after a tick bite are not available because tick bites are frequently not recognized.

Pathogenesis

After inoculation by means of a tick bite, the CEE virus multiplies within the cells of the infected site and reaches the regional lymph nodes via the lym-

Table 7. Arboviruses causing encephalitis (modified from Griffin 1991)

Virus	Vector	Geographic location
Togaviridae		
Alphavirus		
Eastern equine	Mosquitoes	Eastern and Gulf coast of United States; Caribbean; and South America
Western equine	Mosquitoes	Western United States and Canada
Venezuelan equine	Mosquitoes	South and Central America; Florida; and southwestern United States
Flavivirus		
West Nile complex		
St. Louis	Mosquitoes	Widespread in United States
Japanese	Mosquitoes	Japan, China, Southeast Asia, and India
Murray Valley	Mosquitoes	Australia and New Guinea
West Nile	Mosquitoes	Africa and Mideast
Ilheus	Mosquitoes	South and Central America
Rocio	Mosquitoes	Brazil
Tick-borne complex		
Far Eastern	Ticks	Eastern USSR
Central European	Ticks	Central Europe
Kyasanur Forest	Ticks	India
Louping-ill	Ticks	England, Scotland and Northern Ireland
Powassan	Ticks	Canada and northern United States
Negishi	Ticks	Japan
Bunyaviridae		
Bunyavirus		
California	Mosquitoes	Western United States
La Crosse	Mosquitoes	Central and eastern United States
Jamestown Canyon	Mosquitoes	United States and Alaska
Snowshoe hare	Mosquitoes	Canada, Alsaska and northern United States
Tahyna	Mosquitoes	Czechoslovakia, Yugoslavia, Italy, and southern France
Inkoo	Mosquitoes	Finland
Phlebovirus		
Rift Valley	Mosquitoes	East Africa
Reoviridae		
Orbivirus		
Colorado tick fever	Ticks	Rocky Mountains of the United States

phogenous route, where again virus replication occurs. Subsequently, the virus reaches other organ systems, in particular the reticuloendothelial system by lymphogenous and hematogenous spread. A fulminant virus replication occurs, and the virus reaches the bloodstream (stage of viremia). The high virus replication is a prerequisite for passage through the blood-brain barrier. The capillary endothelial cells of the blood-brain barrier are infected intraluminally, where the virus multiplies and then enters the brain tissue.

Clinical Features

The incubation period of CEE lasts 2–28 days, with a period of 7–14 days most often observed. The first stage of the disease lasts 1–8 days and corre-lates with the stage of viremia. Non-specific clinical symptoms and signs include fever, malaise, headache, and fatigue. After this first stage a fever-free interval of 1–20 days follows. The patients are free of symptoms during this period. In the second stage of the disease symptoms and signs may develop. Neurological abnormalities include meningitis (56%), meningo-encephalitis (34%), meningomyelitis (4.5%), or meningoencephalomyelitis (4.9%). In children and young adults the course of CEE is usually milder than in adults, with a predominance of meningitis. Up to the 40th year of age meningitic courses are usually ob-served. With increasing age, especially in patients over 60 years, severe clinical courses with paralytic symptoms may develop. Approximately two thirds of persons infected with CEE virus have an inapparent infection with viremia, or have only the first stage of the dis-ease with nonspecific symptoms. Pro-gression to the second stage of the disease is observed in approximately one third of infected persons; about 50–77% of these patients have the typical biphasic course of the disease. In the remaining 23–50% the first stage of the disease is inapparent and the clinical disease begins directly with the second stage. The mortality is ap-proximately 1% of patients who have neurological manifestations. Neurolo-gical sequelae are found in 7% of the patients.

Ancillary Tests

Diagnosis is based upon the detection of CEE-IgM antibodies in the serum by enzyme-linked immunoassay. In nearly all patients with CEE serum IgM and IgG antibodies can be de-tected at the time of hospital admis-sion. The cerebrospinal fluid reveals a lymphocytic pleocytosis up to 1600 cells/μl. The total protein content is elevated and reaches 50–200 mg/dl. Patients who have suffered from a CEE infection are immune for the rest of their lives and their sera show a detectable IgG antibody titer against CEE.

Differential diagnosis of CEE in-cludes Lyme borreliosis, other viral diseases (poliomyelitis, Coxsackie virus infections, ECHO virus infec-tion, mumps infection), tuberculous meningitis, leptospirosis, and Q fever.

Management

No specific treatment exists for arthropod-borne encephalitides. Therefore, supportive care is essential in the management of patients infected with arboviruses. A vaccine is avail-able for some of these viruses, e.g., Japanese B encephalitis or CEE for prevention of human infection. Candi-dates for vaccination are persons living in or visiting endemic areas of CEE.

Prophylaxis of CEE. If a nonim-munized person recognizes a tick bite which has occurred in an area endemic for CEE, passive immunization with IgG antibodies against CEE virus is usually recommended. Within 48 h after the tick bite 0.1 ml human IgG (approximately 10–17 mg) per kg body weight is injected intramuscularly. If the tick bite is recognized on the 3rd or 4th day, 0.2 ml IgG per kg body weight is injected. If the tick bite is 4 or more days old a prophylactic effect of IgG is not to be expected. On the contrary, it may even have a negative effect on the course of the disease. The protective efficacy of CEE-IgG is approximately 75%.

Active Immunization. Active immunization is recommended for persons visiting or living in areas known to be endemic for CEE. The vaccine used contains purified, formalin-inactivated CEE virus. The primary series consists of three doses. The recommended date for the first dose is during the winter months, followed by the second within 1–3 months and a third dose 9–12 months later. The duration of the protection after the basic immunization is at least 3 years. The protection rate after two doses is 95% and after three or more vaccinations 99%. In a small number of vaccinees (<1:100000) neurological complications such as postvaccinal neuritides may develop.

Conclusion

Arboviruses which are transmitted by ticks or mosquitos may cause neurological manifestations including meningitis, meningoencephalitis, meningomyelitis, or meningoencephalomyelitis. Specific therapy for arboviral disease does not exist. Therefore, supportive therapy is the cornerstone of treatment in patients infected with arboviruses. An effective immunoprophylaxis for several clinically relevant arboviral infections is available. Active immunization is recommended for persons living in or visiting endemic areas.

Rabies

Epidemiology

Rabies is a worldwide disease (for rabies-free countries, see Table 8) which is still very common in developing countries (e.g., about 50000 cases per annum in India) but has become rare in Central Europe and the US, where less than five cases occur per year. These figures reflect the success of public health efforts to identify and control important infectious sources; these include – apart from domestic animals (especially dogs) – skunks and racoons in the US as well as foxes and bats in both Central Europe and the US (regarding worldwide important sources see Table 9). But even today rabies is an invariably fatal illness in a nonimmunized patient. ICU management has succeeded only in prolonging the course of the disease for several months, and, despite limited (serological and clinical) evidence of survival in animals, it remains unclear whether human rabies can be cured.

Pathogenesis

In contrast to most other virus species, rabies is spread to the CNS neurogenically (axoplasmatic flow in peripheral

Table 8. Rabies-free countries

Europe	Great Britain, Ireland, Norway, Sweden, Iceland
Asia	Japan, Malaysia, Singapore, Taiwan, Borneo, New Guinea
Others	Australia, New Zealand, and Antarctica
	Other smaller islands (Mediterranean, Atlantic, Pacific)

Table 9. Important animal sources (rare sources) of rabies

North America	Skunks, foxes raccoons, bats, (rodents)[a]
Europe	Foxes, bats, (wolves, raccoons)
Central/South America	Bats
Africa/Asia	Wolves, jackals, small carnivores
worldwide	Domestic dogs (cats), accounting for 90% of all cases

[a] Rodents, squirrels, guinea pigs, gerbils, rabbits and hares can all be lethally infected by rabies virus; however, they are not considered significant reservoirs for transmission to human beings – in fact, virus transmission to man by bites from these species is considered extremely unlikely. Similarly, bites by herbivores other than bats (horses, cows, deer, etc.) represent no significant risk.

neurons) from a local site. After replication in the dorsal root ganglia the virus rapidly spreads through the CNS and may be recovered from the CSF. In the last stage the virus is conveyed by efferent nerves to most other organs. Systemic hematogenous spread plays no known significant role in the pathogenesis of rabies.

Clinical Features

Infection is usually caused by direct contact with saliva or other infectious material (Table 9), most frequently as a result of a bite. Intact skin provides protection from infection, while injured skin and intact mucosa may admit viral acquisition. Other sources such as inhalation (bat excretions in caves, laboratory accidents) or cornea transplants are possible but extremely rare.

The incubation period varies between 20 and 90 days (range 4 days to several years in single cases) and tends to be shorter in the case of severe bites, particularly those of the face and scalp. Local pain, paresthesia, and itching, followed by fasciculations at the site of infection, often precede generalized symptoms, which might be explained by viral involvement of dorsal root ganglia after spread via the peripheral nerve. Flu-like symptoms including fever, increased irritability, or apathy are the first signs in most patients, before more specific symptoms occur.

Two different clinical courses of rabies may be seen. Most cases show the furious form of rabies with the characteristic symptoms of intermittent hydrophobia and aerophobia. These consist of life-threatening spasms of the diaphragm, sternocleidomastoid muscles, and accessory muscles of inspiration, which may lead to a general increase in extensor tone and spasms. Typically, these symptoms are initiated by attempts to drink water and are accompanied by panic and terror. Episodes of generalized arousal and excitation with sometimes bizarre neuropsychiatric symptoms, hyperesthesia, and vegetative disturbance may alternate with symptom-free intervals with entirely normal neurostatus. Due to the general brain involvement in furious rabies a wide range of abnormalities are seen. Meningism, cranial nerve involvement, and upper and lower motoneuron symptoms, as well as involuntary movements, seizures, or – characteristically – limbic disinhibition can be found. Autonomic symptoms such as hypersalivation, changes in heart rate and blood pressure, fever, or sweating can contribute to dangerous electrolyte disturbances, sometimes complicated by the syndrome of inappropriate secretion of antidiuretic hormone (SIADH) and respiratory and cardiac failure. Death invariably occurs within a week in the natural course of furious rabies and is prolonged for up to several months by ICU treatment.

Paralytic rabies occurs less frequently but is typical for infections acquired from bat bites in Latin America. After the nonspecific prodromata the bitten limb becomes paralytic and painful and may develop paresthesia or fasciculations, reflecting the fact that the spine is the predominant site of infection (Table 10). Progression to para- or tetraparesis is followed by the involvement of respiratory muscles and cranial nerve palsy, which leads to death within several days or weeks (longer under ICU conditions).

Furious rabies can be easily suspected, especially if the animal bite is known. Tetanus may initially be considered if pharyngeal spasms are prominent but there are no asymptomatic intervals as are seen in rabies (Table 10). Trismus, the absence of CSF pleocytosis in tetanus, and the shorter incubation period (4–14 days) may help to distinguish tetanus from furious rabies. Rarely, psychiatric disorders can mimic rabies including phobic reactions after an animal bite. Other extremely rare differential diagnostic possibilities include encephalopathy secondary to serum sickness or anaphylactic reactions to bee or wasp venoms. Paralytic rabies must be differentiated from Guillain-Barré syndrome, transverse myelitis, and poliomyelitis.

Table 10. Clinical features and differential diagnosis of rabies

Feature	Furious rabies	Tetanus
Incubation period	20–90 days	4–14 days
Animal bite	frequent	frequent
Flu-like prodrome	frequent	no
Pharyngeal spasms	frequent	frequent
Asymptomatic interval	yes	no
Trismus	no	yes
CSF pleocytosis	yes	no

Feature	Paralytic rabies	Poliomyelitis	Guillain-Barré syndrome
Incubation period	20–90 days	3–14 days	(2 weeks[a])
Flu-like prodrome	yes	yes	(yes[a])
Flaccid palsy	yes	yes	yes
Ascending course	yes	no	yes
Asymmetric distribution	sometimes	yes	no
Sensory deficit	yes	no	variable
CSF pleocytosis	yes	yes	no

[a] "Incubation" period in Guillain-Barré syndrome: time between prodromal viral infection, if reported and onset of clinical symptoms.

Ancillary Tests

If the animal from which infection was acquired is available for examination, the diagnosis can be established by histologic examination of a CNS specimen with immunofluorescence (Table 11). These methods have replaced the older stain for Negri bodies, or quarantine and observation of the animal for 10 days or longer.

In man, confirmation of the diagnosis is obtained from skin (preferably from the nape of the neck) or brain biopsies by immunofluorescence; the use of corneal smears is not adequately sensitive. Viral culture in neuroblastoma cells, requiring only 2–4 days, yields positive results from saliva and throat swabs at the onset of clinical symptoms, a few days later from CSF or brain biopsy but not from blood. Neutralizing antibodies against rabies in serum appear about 7 days after the onset of symptoms, and several days later also in the CSF, where intrathecal IgG synthesis can be found. Vaccination or passive immunization against rabies makes interpretation difficult, but high CSF/serum IgG levels suggest the presence of rabies infection.

CSF pleocytosis is usually mild, ranging from normal in a substantial number of patients, particularly at the beginning of the disease, to a few hundred lymphocytes per microliter with normal glucose and slightly elevated protein of 50–200 mg/dl. There are no specific laboratory findings in rabies, while in peripheral blood moderate neutrophil leukocytosis is evident. Neuroradiographic or electrophysiologic studies do not add specific information for the establishment of the diagnosis but may be helpful in differential diagnosis.

Management

While animal control and pre-exposure prophylaxis for risk groups have helped to make rabies a rare disease in Central Europe and the US, postexposure measures before the onset of clinical symptoms are essential in rabies and are therefore discussed here briefly. Immediate, thorough wound cleaning and disinfection should be followed as soon as possible by active and passive immunization. Active immunization consists in the injection of one standard dose of several established vaccines (Table 12) into the deltoid muscle on days 0, 3, 7, 14, and 30 after exposure. The dose is doubled in the case of delay after exposure for more than

Table 11. Confirmation of diagnosis for rabies

Method	Sensitivity	Specificity	Timing
Viral culture	Moderate	High	Early[a]
Skin biopsy	Low-moderate	High	Early
Cornea smear	Low	Moderate	Early
Antibodies (serum, CSF)	High	High[b]	1–2 weeks

[a] Saliva; throat swabs (0–10 days); brain, CSF, urine (5–14 days).
[b] Difficult after vaccination (high titers, intrathecal IgG synthesis very suggestive).

Table 12. Postexposure treatment of rabies

Wound cleaning	Immediate washing, rinsing with povidoneiodine, 70% ethanol etc., no suturing	
Active immunization	HDCSV (Institut Merieux) human diploid cell strain vacc.	1.0 ml
	or	
	PVRV (Institut Merieux) purified vero cell rabies vacc.	0.5 ml
	or	
	PCEC (Behringwerke) purified chicken embryo cell vacc.	1.0 ml

Intramuscular (*not* gluteal) injection on days 0, 3, 7, 14, 30
Standard adult dose: double dose in chronic illness, after 48 h delay, in immunocompromised or elderly hosts, if passive immunisation is not available.
After pre-exposure vaccination only on days 0, 3, 7

Passive immunization	Human (equine) hyperimmune serum	20 (40) IU/kg body weight

Administration on day 0 (not later than day 7):
50% of dose: infiltrated around the wound (not digits)
50% of dose: intramuscular (*not* gluteal) injection
Injection not at the same site as first dose of vaccine, not after pre-exposure vaccination

48 h, in chronic or immunocompromising disease, or if passive immunization is not available. For passive immunization hyperimmune human or equine antirabies serum is administered at a dose of 20 IU (human) or 40 IU (equine); half is infiltrated around the wound area and the other half is injected intramuscularly at a site separate from the vaccine dose. Patients who have previously received a full course of pre-exposure prophylaxis require only booster doses of vaccine on days 0, 3, and 7; however, it is recommended that pre- and post-vaccine sera be tested to assure that these individuals have responded adequately.

If these measures have not been performed properly or are delayed for more than 7 days, about 15–60% of people exposed to a rabid animal will develop the clinical picture of rabies. ICU management may be the only hope of achieving survival in single cases. Convulsions, cerebral edema, respiratory and cardiac problems, gastrointestinal bleeding, ileus, and electrolyte disturbance are the most common life-threatening problems encountered in the course of rabies. To counter overexcitability and vegetative crises, to prevent aspiration due to cranial nerve involvement or pharyngeal spasms, and to relieve the patient's psyche, heavy analgesia, sedation, and early intubation and tracheotomy are essential (Table 13). Due to the frequency of cardiac arrythmia, hypertension, or pulmonary edema, close monitoring of cardiac function is as important as careful fluid balance and electrolyte checks. Diabetes insipidus and SIADH are known complications of rabies and require therapy.

No specific therapy against clinically manifest rabies is known. Immunosuppressive agents including steroids, rabies hyperimmune serum, interferons, or ribavirin have failed to show positive effects. Some hope may be raised by the observation of dogs who survived after intrathecal application of highly attenuated rabies virus

Table 13. Management of manifest rabies

Problem	Measure
CNS:	
Overexcitability convulsions terror	e.g., fentanyl/midazolam; initially 0, 1 mg/ 10 mg per hour; dose rise according to response alternatively barbiturates or combinations with potent neuroleptics; avoid neuroleptics alone (seizures!)
Raised ICP	monitoring, positioning, controlled hyperventilation, osmotherapy
Cranial nerve palsy	intubation, tracheotomy
SIADH/diabetes insipidus	fluid and electrolyte balancing and therapy
Resp. failure	controlled ventilation
Cardiac failure	electrolyte and fluid balancing, invasive monitoring, antiarrhythmics, pacemaker
GI bleeding	sedation, peptic ulcer prophylaxis
Specific therapy attempt: highly attenuated virus intrathecally (no human data available)	

at the onset of clinical symptoms. Highly attenuated virus, which has shown no major side effects after intrathecal injection into monkeys, is available for use, but no experience has been accumulated with human beings. Infection of hospital staff or relative must be prevented by avoiding broken skin or mucosal contact with the patient's saliva, CSF, urine, or tissues in suspected rabies, although the risk of infection is considered to be low.

Prognosis and Conclusion

While rabies has become a rare disease due to effective pre- and postexposure measures, survival of patients with clinically manifest illness who have no pre- or postexposure vaccination has not been observed, despite ICU treat-ment. Whether elaborate nonspecific therapy or the intrathecal late administration of vaccine may offer hope for some patients remains unknown.

Rare Other Viral Infections

Introduction

Apart from the viruses previously discussed, which may be distinguished by more outstanding clinical features in many cases, the CNS may be affected by a number of other viral agents. Differentiation usually relies on the clinical picture of the initial disease, as in measles, mumps, or rubella, or on viral identification by culture or demonstration of antigen or antibodies. Helpful features for specific diagnosis are shown in Table 14.

Table 14. Relevant viral diseases with CNS involvement (not covered in the chapters before)

Virus (group)	Measles (paramyxo)	Mumps (paramyxo)	Rubella (rubi)	Lymphocytic choriomeningitis (arena)	Influenza (orthomyxo)	Epstein-Barr virus (herpes)
Clinical presentation	CNS involvement following "measles" (exanthema not obligatory) encephalomyelitis (brain more affected than myelon: coma, seizures) polyneuritis	CNS involvement may also *precede* parotitis usually meningitis rarely encephalitis (seizures, focal signs, cranial nerves)	CNS involvement following rubella acute encephalitis (drowsiness, seizures, rarely focal defects), meningitis, polyneuritis	flu-like prodromata, biphasic course encephalomyelitis, rarely encephalitis	following nonspecific "flu"-symptoms encephalitis (sometimes associated with ataxia), polyneuritis	CNS involvement may also precede mononucleosis meningitis, rarely encephalitis (cranial nerves, coma hemiparesis, seizures) myelitis; polyneuritis
Outstanding features and complications	otitis, pneumonia, cardio-resp. failure, postinfect. immuno-suppression	sensorineural deafness, orchitis, pancreatitis	congenital infection (deafness, cataract, heart)	long or chronic courses, pneumonitis	association with Reye's syndrome pneumonia	spleen rupture
Ancillary findings	CSF pleocytosis in 30% of clinically inapparent cases, mild pleocytosis	CSF pleocytosis in 50% of clinically inapparent cases, glc sometimes low		thrombopenia, lymphopenia, CSF pleocytosis; low CSF glc. often >1500 cells/ml		mononucleosis in blood – not always present
Epidemiology	*natural* measles complications 1:500–1000	winter/spring; accounting for 15–30% of cases of viral meningitis	rubella cases 1:20000	winter/spring, not rare	epidemic pattern, rare complication	spring/autumn usually inapparent

Route of infection; penetrance; incubation period	respiratory >90% 10–14 days	respiratory; about 40%; 12–25 days	respiratory; about 10%; 12–21 days	rodents; ?; 6–13 days	respiratory; high; 1–4 days	respiratory; oral; low; 8–21 days
Remarkable histological findings	usually "postinfectious" histological picture	usually "postinfectious" histol. picture	nonspec. toxic postinfectious			
Prognosis	10–20% mortality, 20–35% residual deficits	meningitis benign, encephalitis about 20–25% residual deficits	20% mortality, often complete recovery	good	good, rarely fatal	2–5% mortality. usually complete recovery
Virus (group)	RSV (paramyxo)	Adeno	CMV (herpes)	JC virus (polyoma)	SSPE and PRPE (slow viruses)	"Jakob-Creutzfeldt" (slow viruses)
Clinical presentation	CNS involvement may precede respiratory symptoms, encephalitis (drowsiness seizures), myelitis	encephalitis	may mimic mononucleosis encephalitis (cranial nerves often involved), polyneuritis	PML (progressive multifocal leukencephalopathy) encephalitis (dementia, mnestic or linguistic disorders, paresis), invariably fatal	encephalitis (dementia, personality changes, chorea, tremor, seizures), invariably fatal	encephalitis (dementia, aphasia, tremor paresis, myocloni, chorea, nystagmus), invariably fatal
Outstanding features and complications	rhinitis	cystitis, conjunctivitis immunocompromised hosts	also fetal infections; immunocompr. hosts	severely immunocompr. hosts (AIDS, sarcoidosis, leukaemia)	vegetative crises	

Table 14. *Continued*

Virus (group)	RSV (paramyxo)	Adeno	CMV (herpes)	JC virus (polyoma)	SSPE and PRPE (slow viruses)	"Jakob-Creutzfeldt" (slow viruses)
Ancillary findings			inclusion-bearing cells	CT scan: confluent hypodense areas, no space-occupying lesions	EEG: Rademecker complex CSF: IgG protein increase no pleocytosis	EEG: periodic polyphasic waves CSF: normal
Epidemiology	rare, mostly infants, children	winter/spring, commonly inapparent infection, immunocompromised hosts	commonly inapparent infection, immunocompromised hosts	immunocompromised hosts	after natural measles (5/1 million cases) childhood, adolescence, predominantly males	sporadic; main age-group 35–65 years
Route of infection; penetrance; incubation time	respiratory	orofecal; respiratory	oral, venereal, low; 2–10 weeks	respiratory ?	latency; low; 2–20 years	brain/CSF contact; low; 4 months–3 years
Remarkable histological findings			cell necrosis	demyelinating	biopsy: measle antigen panencephalitis inclusion bodies	demyelinization, inclusion bodies
Prognosis	good	usually good	variable; therapy with gancyclovir 5 mg/ kg i.v. bid; 21 gG	fatal; 3–20 months	fatal; 6–30 months	fatal; few months

Pathogenesis

With few exceptions (rabies, type-1 herpes simplex, perhaps some arboviruses), viral CNS involvement is secondary to generalized infection and follows viremia. Little is known about determinants of susceptibility, spread within the CNS, and clinical course. Some viruses show neurological symptoms only in immunocompromised hosts; others also affect obviously immunocompetent persons. While direct noxious effects of the virus appear to be mainly responsible for CNS pathology in some viruses (e.g., herpes), in others immunologically mediated damage seems more important (e.g., measles). Combinations of both are common, making a differentiation sometimes impossible. The borderline to postinfectious or postvaccinal disease often cannot be exactly drawn from the pathogenetic or histological point of view. The so-called slow viral diseases (subacute sclerosing panencephalitis, Jakob-Creutzfeldt disease) differ in their pathology and their invariably fatal, slowly progressive clinical courses after years of incubation (Table 14). They are covered elsewhere in detail.

Clinical Features and Differential Diagnosis

Nonspecific respiratory or flu-like symptoms and fever often precede viral CNS involvement, but neurological symptoms may precede other signs of infection or can be the only finding in some patients. An exanthema is very suggestive of a viral etiology. Other clues to possible causes may be found when one considers epidemiological factors such as patient age, season of onset, concomitant illness in the family and community, travel, and activity of the patient, including recreational pursuits and animal exposures.

Neurological symptoms are explained either by general effects of viral disease (signs of raised intracranial pressure due to cerebral edema, disorientation, personality changes) or by focal affected areas (hemiparesis, cranial nerve palsies, seizures, myoclonus, chorea-athetosis, neuropsychological deficits) and are only loosely correlated to a specific agent. Signs of meningitis are frequent but not obligatory. Myelitis and polyneuritis are associated with some viruses but may also be seen in other cases. Ataxia or brain-stem involvement with autonomic signs have been reported in some instances. A summary of the typical clinical presentation of relevant organisms is given in Table 14.

Differential diagnosis includes bacterial (*Streptococci, Neisseria, Listeria, Legionella, Mycoplasma, Spirochaeta,* septic-embolic abscesses, partially treated meningitis, parameningeal foci), parasitic or fungal infection, tuberculosis, sarcoidosis, malignancy, vascular disruption, or autoimmune disease. Metabolic or toxic disorders may also have to be excluded.

Ancillary Tests and Management

While there is only mild blood leukocytosis (sometimes leukopenia, usually with relative lymphoctosis) in most cases, moderate lymphocytic CSF pleocytosis will be found in about two thirds of cases. No neuroradiological or electrophysiological test is able to identify a specific agent, but their importance for early detection of complications (raised intracranial pressure, focus identification for biopsy, rarely for neurosurgical intervention), differential diagnosis, and prognosis is obvious. A cranial CT should always be obtained before lumbar puncture to detect cerebral edema and judge the risk of herniation.

ICU management is symptomatic, special attention being paid to the risks of raised intracranial pressure, seizures, and respiratory problems due to brain-stem involvement or impaired consciousness. Immunodeficiency may be the cause (cytomegalovirus, adenovirus, enterovirus, varicella, polyomaviruses) or effect (especially in measles) of viral disease, leading to a search for the reason (HIV, malignancy, malabsorption, genetic defect).

Vasculitis following viral CNS infection has been reported but seems to be a rare finding which should be considered in cases with sudden deterioration. The administration of steroids in these patients seems reasonable, but no proof of its usefulness is available, nor are there strict dose recommendations. Apart from a few exceptions shown in Table 14, no specific antiviral therapy has proved to be effective.

Prognosis

Given the heterogeneity of the diseases covered above, the prognosis varies from complete recovery after mild neurological signs to fatal outcome. The same agent may produce a wide range of clinical courses. Overall, the clinical picture is more relevant for prognosis than the identification of a specific agent, but a complete recovery may result even after extremely severe courses (Table 14).

Suggested Reading

Anderson LJ, Nicholson KG, Tauxe RV, Winkler WG (1984) Human rabies in the United States 1960 to 1979: Epidemiology, Diagnosis and Prevention. Ann Intern Med 100:728–735

Auld PAM, Kevy SV, Eley RC (1960) Poliomyelitis in children. N Engl J Med 263:1093–1100

Boe J, Solberg CO, Saeter T (1965) Corticosteroid treatment for acute meningoencephalitis: a retrospective study of 346 cases. Br Med J 5442:1094–1095

Chemtob S, Reece ER, Mills EL (1985) Syndrome of inappropriate antidiuretic hormone in enteroviral meningitis. Am J Dis Child 139:292–294

Dalakas MC, Elder G, Hallett M, Ravits J, Baker M, Papadopoulos N, Albrecht P, Sever J (1986) A long term follow up study of patients with post-poliomyelitis neuromuscular symptoms. N Engl J Med 314:959–963

Davis LE et al. (1977) Chronic progressive poliomyelitis secondary to vaccination of an immunodeficient child. N Engl J Med 297:241

Dussaix E, Lebon P, Ponsot G et al. (1985) Intrathecal synthesis of different alpha-interferons in patients with various neurological diseases. Acta Neurol Scand 71:504–509

Ecchevarria JM, Martinez-Martin P, Tellez A et al. (1987) Aseptic meningitis due to varicella zoster virus: serum antibody levels and local synthesis of specific IgG, IgM, and IgA. J Infect Dis 155:959–967

Feldman W, Larke RPB (1972) Acute cerebellar ataxia associated with isolation of Coxsackie type A9. Can Med Assoc J 106:1104–1107

Flowers D, Scott GM (1985) How useful are serum and CSF interferon levels as rapid diagnostic aid in virus infections? J Med Virol 15:35–47

Gold R, Wiethölter H, Rihs I, Löwer J, Kappos L (1992) Frühsommer-Meningoenzephalitis-Impfung. Dtsch Med Wochenschr 117:112–116

Grandien M, Olding-Stenkvist E (1984) Rapid diagnosis of viral infections in the central nervous system. Scand J Infect Dis 16:1–8

Griffin DE (1991) Viral infections of the central nervous system. In: Galasso GJ, Whitley RJ, Merigan TC (eds) Antiviral agents and viral diseases of man, 3rd edn. Raven, New York

Grist NR, Bell EJ (1984) Paralytic poliomyelitis and nonpolio enteroviruses: studies in Scotland. Rev Infect Dis 6:385–386

Grose C, Henle W, Henle G et al. (1975) Primary Epstein-Barr virus infections in acute neurologic diseases. N Engl J Med 292: 392–395

Jaffe M, Srugo I, Tirosh E, Collin AA, Tal Y (1989) The ameliorating effect of lumbar puncture in viral meningitis. Am J Dis Child 143:682–685

Johnson RT (1982) Viral infections of the nervous system. Raven, New York

Johnson RT, Griffin DE, Hirsch BL et al. (1984) Measles encephalomyelitis-clinical and immunological studies. N Engl J Med 310: 137–141

Johnstone JA, Ross CAC, Dunn M (1972) Meningitis and encephalitis associated with mumps infection: a 10-year survey. Arch Dis Child 47:647–651

Jubelt B, Wilson AK, Ropka SL, Guidinger PL, Mc Kinlay MA (1989) Clearance of persistent human enterovirus infection of the mouse central nervous system by the antiviral agent disoxaril. J Infect Dis 159:866–871

Kaplan MH, Klein SW, McPhee J, Harper RG (1983) Group B coxsackievirus infections in infants younger than three months of age: a serious childhood illness. Rev Infect Dis 5:1019–1032

Kennard CK, Swash M (1981) Acute viral encephalöitis; its diagnosis and outcome. Brain 104:129–148

Kennedy CR (1991) Acute viral infections excluding Herpes simplex, rabies, and HIV. In: Lambert HP (ed) Kass handbook of infectious diseases. Infections of the central nervous system. Decker, Philadelphia Arnold, London, pp 300–316

Koskiniemi M, Manninen V, Vaheri A et al. (1981) Acute encephalitis. Acta Med Scand 209:115–120

Kunz C, Hofmann H, Dippe H (1991) Early summer meningoencephalitis vaccination, a preventive medicine measure with high acceptance in Austria. Wien Med Wochenschr 41:273–276

Lebon P, Lyon G (1974) Non congenital rubella encephalitis. Lancet 2:468

Lin-Fangtao, Chen S, Wang Y et al. (1988) Use of serum and vaccine in combination for prophylaxis following exposure to rabies. Rev Infect Dis 10:766–770

Lumio J, Hillbom M, Roine R et al. (1986) Human rabies of bat origin in Europe. Lancet 1:378

Matthews WB (1991) Slow viruses and the central nervous system. In: Lambert HP (ed) Kass handbook of infectious diseases. Infections of the nervous system. Decker, Philadelphia, pp 329–342

Mc Cormick JB (1990) Arenaviruses. In: Fields BN, Knipe DM (eds) Virology. Raven, New York, pp 1245–1267

Mc Kinlay MA, Frank JA, Benziger DP, Steinberg BA (1986) Use of WIN 51711 to prevent echovirus type 9-induced paralysis in suckling mice. J Infect Dis 154:676–681

McKinney RE Jr, Katz SL, Wilfert CM (1987) Chronic enteroviral meningoencephalitis in agammaglobulinaemic patients. Rev Infect Dis 9:334–356

Merigan TC, Baer GM, Winkler WG et al. (1984) Human leucocyte interferon administration to patients with symptomatic and suspected rabies. Ann Neurol 16:82–87

Meyers BR, Gurtman AC (1990) The aseptic meningitis syndrome. In: Schlossberg D (ed) Infections of the nervous system. Springer, Berlin Heidelberg New York

Modlin JF (1986) Perinatal echovirus infection: insights from a literature review of 61 cases of serious infection and 16 outbreaks in nurseries. Rev Infect Dis 8:918–926

Moore M (1982) Enteroviral disease in the United States, 1970–1979. J Infect Dis 146:103–108

Moore M, Baron RC, Fiolstein MR et al. (1983) Aseptic meningitis and high school football players, 1978–1980. JAMA 249:2039–2042

Paul JR (1971) History of poliomyelitis. Yale University Press, New Haven

Peters ACB, Vielvoye GJ, Verstee GJ et al. (1979) ECHO 25 focal encephalitis and subacute hemichorea. Neurology 29:676–681

Peterslund NA, Pederson B (1982) Liquor: serum quotients of IgG and albumin in patients with meningism, meningitis and multiple sclerosis. Acta Neurol Scand 66: 25–33

Price RW, Plum F (1978) Poliomyelitis. In: Vinken PJ, Bruyn GW (eds) Handbook of clinical neurology. Elsevier/North Holland, Amsterdam, pp 93–132

Roggendorf M, Neumann-Haefelin D, Ackermann R (1989) Prophylaxe der Frühsommer-Meningoenzephalitis.   Dtsch Arztebl 86:1418–1421

Rotbart HA (1990) Diagnosis of enteroviral meningitis with the polymerase chain reaction. J Pediatr 117:85–89

Rotbart HA (1991) Viral meningitis and the aseptic meningitis syndrome. In: Scheld WM, Whitley RJ, Durack DT (eds) Infections of the central nervous system. Raven, New York

Russel WR (1947) Poliomyelitis; preparalytic stage and effect of physical activity on severity of paralysis. Br Med J 2:1023

Shohat M, Lerman-Sagie T, Levy Y, Nitzan M (1988) Cerebrospinal fluid findings in children with nonpolio enteroviral meningitis. J Med Sci 24:233–236

So YT, Olney PK (1991) AAEM case report no 23: acute paralytic poliomyelitis. Muscle Nerve 14:1159–1164

Steele JH (1988) Rabies in the Americas and remarks on global aspects. Rev Infect Dis 10:585–597

Strikas RA, Anderson LJ, Parker RA (1986) Temporal and geographic patterns of isolates of nonpolio enterovirus in the United States, 1970–1983. J Infect Dis 153:346–351

Townsend JJ, Baringer JR, Wolinski JS et al. (1975) Progressive Rubella panencephalitis. Late onset after congenital rubella. N Engl J Med 283:1505–1507

Warrell DA (1976) The clinical picture of rabies in man. Trans R Soc Trop Med Hyg 70: 188–195

Warrell DA, Warrell MJ (1991) Rabies. In: Lambert HP (ed) Kass handbook of infectious diseases. Infections of the nervous system. Decker, Philadelphia, pp 317–328

Warrell MJ, Ward GS, Elwell MR, Tingpalapong M (1987) An attempt to treat rabies encephalitis in monkeys with intrathecal live rabies virus RV 675. Arch Virol 96: 271–273

Wheeler SD, Ochoa J (1980) Poliomyelitis-like syndrome associated with asthma. Arch Neurol 37:52–53

Whitley RJ (1991) Arthropod-borne encephalitides. In: Scheld WM, Whitley RJ, Durack DT (eds) Infections of the central nervous system. Raven, New York, pp 87–111

Whitley RJ, Middlebrooks M (1991) Rabies. In: Scheld WM, Whitley RJ, Durack DT (eds) Infections of the central nervous system. Raven, New York

Wiethölter H (1988) Virale Entzündungen des zentralen Nervensystems. In: Brandt T, Dichgans J, Diener HC (eds) Therapie und Verlauf neurologischer Erkrankungen. Kohlhammer, Stuttgart, pp 373–383

Acute Disseminated Encephalomyelitis (Parainfectious and Postvaccinal Encephalitis)

BRIGITTE STORCH-HAGENLOCHER and DIANE E. GRIFFIN

Definition

Acute disseminated encephalomyelitis (ADEM) is an autoimmune inflammatory demyelinating disease of the central nervous system. It may follow a viral infection, *Mycoplasma* and bacterial infection, or immunization. The most common viruses associated with ADEM are measles, rubella, and varicella zoster. ADEM is usually a monophasic illness, but some patients may have a fulminating, progressive, or relapsing course. Histopathology shows multifocal, perivascular (mostly perivenous) lymphocytic infiltration, demyelination, and focal necrosis infrequently associated with hemorrhage. The demyelinated plaques are usually smaller than those found in multiple sclerosis (MS).

ADEM is an uncommon disease, and initially it may be difficult to distinguish it from acute viral encephalitis. Patients may have altered levels of consciousness, increased intracranial pressure, seizures, and re-

Section Editors: Karl M. Einhäupl and Werner Hacke

spiratory failure and may require neurocritical care. Special types of ADEM include acute cerebellar ataxia (children's encephalitis cerebelli et pontis), acute hemorrhagic leukencephalitis (AHL), acute transverse myelitis, monophasic variants of neuromyelitis optica (Devic's syndrome), and probably some forms of Schilder's disease.

Pathogensis

ADEM is the clinical counterpart of experimental autoimmune encephalomyelitis (EAE), a disease induced in animals by inoculation with myelin basic protein (MBP). ADEM after immunization with Semple rabies vaccine is most closely related to EAE, because the Semple vaccine is prepared from CNS tissue of sheep or goats infected with rabies and an immune response to MBP occurs. Patients with parainfectious or other postvaccinal ADEM also have an immune response to MBP, even though there is no apparent exposure to neural antigens. Viral or bacterial antigens are not detected in the CNS. Currently, it is thought that infection or immunization results in a disturbance of immune regulation that leads to an autoimmune response against MBP.

Clinical Features and Differential Diagnosis

The pattern of onset and course of disease in patients with ADEM is variable. Patients can present with diffuse encephalitis, brain-stem or cerebellar dysfunction, myelitis, or periperal nerve and cranial nerve involvement. Findings may change over time and different findings can occur at the same time. Patients with diffuse encephalitis may have headache, fever, stiff neck, and vomiting, as well as cranial nerve dysfunction, hemiparesis, seizures, depressed consciousness, and coma. In the acute phase, it may be difficult to distinguish between direct infection of the CNS and autoimmune disease. A detailed history is crucial. The antecedent illness usually occurs 1–3 weeks before the onset of neurological symptoms. It may be characterized by malaise, fever, myalgia, or symptoms of gastrointestinal or upper respiratory tract infection, or it may be nondescript. Patients should be asked about recent immunizations, medications, health of other family members, and work or social contacts. The diagnosis is easier to make when there is an interval of good health after a period of illness and before the onset of neurological symptoms. In many patients, however, the antecedent illness merges with the CNS illness.

The clinical findings of ADEM may be variable and the laboratory findings may be nonspecific; patients may have a moderate increase in leukocyte count or erythrocyte sedimention rate (ESR). The diagnosis is often made retrospectively after exclusion of other causes. For example, severe progressive encephalopathy, fatty change of the liver, and hypoglycemia after aspirin ingestion in a child should suggest Reye's syndrome. Metabolic and electrolyte abnormalities should be excluded. A CT scan is needed to rule out mass lesions, hemorrhages, or brain edema.

Bacterial and fungal infections can usually be excluded by examination of the CSF. Exclusion of viral infection is often more difficult because both patients with ADEM and those with viral encephalitis can have mononuclear pleocytosis and mildly increased protein concentration. Serological evidence for a specific infection may occasionally be discovered, although in general, viral serologies are not helpful.

It may also be difficult to distinguish patients with ADEM from those with MS, especially when there are multifocal symptoms that have developed over a long period. There are some distinguishing features, however. Patients with ADEM often have more widespread multifocal CNS disturbances than those with MS. Optic neuritis is usually bilateral in ADEM and unilateral in MS. Transverse myelitis is often complete in a few days and associated with areflexia in patients with ADEM, whereas it is usually incomplete, develops over a longer period, and is associated with hyperreflexia in patients with MS. Five to ten percent of patients die during the acute encephalitis phase of ADEM and 20–30% of patients fully recover;

the remainder have residual deficits but often can lead normal lives.

Parainfectious acute cerebellar ataxia (encephalitis cerebelli et pontis) is a special type of ADEM that occurs mainly in children days to weeks after varicella-zoster infection. The symptoms are often dramatic and most severe in the lower extremities (impaired gait). Patients may have tremor, nystagmus, speech disturbances, and brain-stem dysfunction. Ancillary studies are usually not helpful; leukocyte count, erythrocyte sedimentation rate, CSF analysis, and EEG are normal in about two thirds of patients. Patients with acute cerebellar ataxia should be hospitalized for supportive therapy, particularly to maintain hydration. Few patients die, but one fourth to one third of patients have deficits that may persist for more than 3 months.

ADEM can also present as transverse myelitis. A compressive mass should always be excluded by neuroimaging, however, in patients whose symptoms began acutely, especially in the absence of signs of widely disseminated CNS lesions. In fulminant acute transverse myelitis, the complete syndrome of transection of spinal cord function can occur in less than an hour. The preceding event is often an upper respiratory viral illness 1–3 weeks before the onset of neurological symptoms. Bacterial infections and other factors such as minor trauma and childbirth may also precede the symptoms. Most patients have sensory loss below the lesion, weakness, and sphincter dysfunction. Fever and stiff neck occur in a minority of patients. ADEM should be suspected in patients with transverse myelitis and encephalitis. Death occurs in 5–10%

of patients, usually as a result of urosepsis, deep venous thrombosis, or respiratory failure.

Acute hemorrhagic leukencephalopathy of Hurst (AHL) is a rare, acute form of ADEM. Most patients have some preceding event such as a respiratory viral infection, bacterial infection, immunization, drug reaction, or other disease. The average time between the preceding event and onset of neurological symptoms (symptom-free interval) is 4 days. The first symptoms are usually headache, malaise, and general weakness, followed by fever, depression of consciousness, vomiting, and stiff neck. Hemiparesis can be found in up to 50% of patients. AHL should be suspected in patients with infection followed by rapidly evolving hemispheric dysfunction, fever, and leukocytosis. The differential diagnosis includes cerebral abscess, meningitis, vasculitis, dural sinus thrombosis, cerebral tumors, and other space-occupying lesions. Most patients develop coma within a few days, and death from herniation occurs in 70%.

Ancillary Tests

Neuroimaging

Both CT and MRI findings can support the diagnosis of ADEM. Low-attenuation white-matter lesions, similar to those seen in MS, appear on CT 5–14 days after onset of symptoms. In rare cases the lesions are visible after 2 days; in other patients, despite a convincing clinical diagnosis, both CT and MRI may remain normal, because of the delay in the appearance of lesions. Contrast enhancement of the lesions occurs in about 25% of patients. Midbrain edema with effacement of the quadrigeminal cistern and circumscript enhancement of gyri has also been described. Clinical improvement is accompanied by complete or partial resolution of the low-attenuation lesions and disappearance of contrast enhancement. There is no correlation, however, between the abnormalities on CT and clinical outcome.

Multifocal lesions in the cerebral and cerebellar white matter, corpus callosum, or pons can be seen on T2-weighted MR images (Fig. 1); hemorrhages are extremely rare. As on CT scan, these lesions appear similar to the lesions in MS, although in MS there is usually a combination of contrast-enhancing and nonenhancing lesions, and enhancement rapidly disappears with corticosteroid treatment. Studies of enhancement in ADEM have not been done, but enhancement probably also disappears with high-dose corticosteroid therapy. It has been reported that after 3 days of treatment with corticosteroids, 51% of lesions no longer showed enhancement and 96% of patients showed a decrease in blood-brain barrier abnormalities. In general, acute MRI abnormalites in ADEM are more extensive and symmetrical than those in MS (for example, lesions in the basal ganglia are rarely observed in patients with MS). Some abnormalities may persist on MRI for 1–2 years despite full clinical recovery. In transverse myelitis, demyelinating lesions are often seen within 4–7 days. There are no exact data regarding contrast enhancement on MRI in patients with ADEM and transverse myelitis.

Cerebrospinal Fluid and Other Laboratory Tests

Results of cerebrospinal fluid analysis may be variable. Cell count and protein concentration may be normal, but often there is a mononuclear pleocytosis with up to several hundred cells and increased protein concentration (reflecting damage to the blood-brain barrier). Glucose concentration and lactate concentration are normal. Serological tests for arbovirus, varicella-zoster virus, herpes simplex virus, Epstein-Barr virus, cytomegalovirus, and measles, rubella, influenza, and mumps viruses, as well as Mycoplasma pneumoniae should be done. Virus cultures are rarely positive. Some viruses can be detected by polymerase chain reaction (PCR), but the test is not widely available. Antibodies against infectious agents are not increased in the CSF of patients with ADEM. If detected, intrathecal production and viral infection of the CNS

Fig. 1a–f. Acute disseminated encephalomyelitis in a 30-year-old man. Initial axial MR scans (**a, b**, T2-weighted; **c, d**, T1-weighted after IV administration of paramagnetic contrast material) show patchy areas of abnormally increased signal involving the perisupraventricular cerebral white matter, mostly in the parietal lobes (**a, b**). Lesions are inapparent on T1-weighted images, have no definite mass effect, and do not enhance. Corresponding T2-weighted images obtained about 9 weeks later (**e, f**), after treatment of the patient with steroids, reveal near full regression of the abnormality. (Courtesy of Klaus Sartor and Marius Hartmann, Heidelberg)

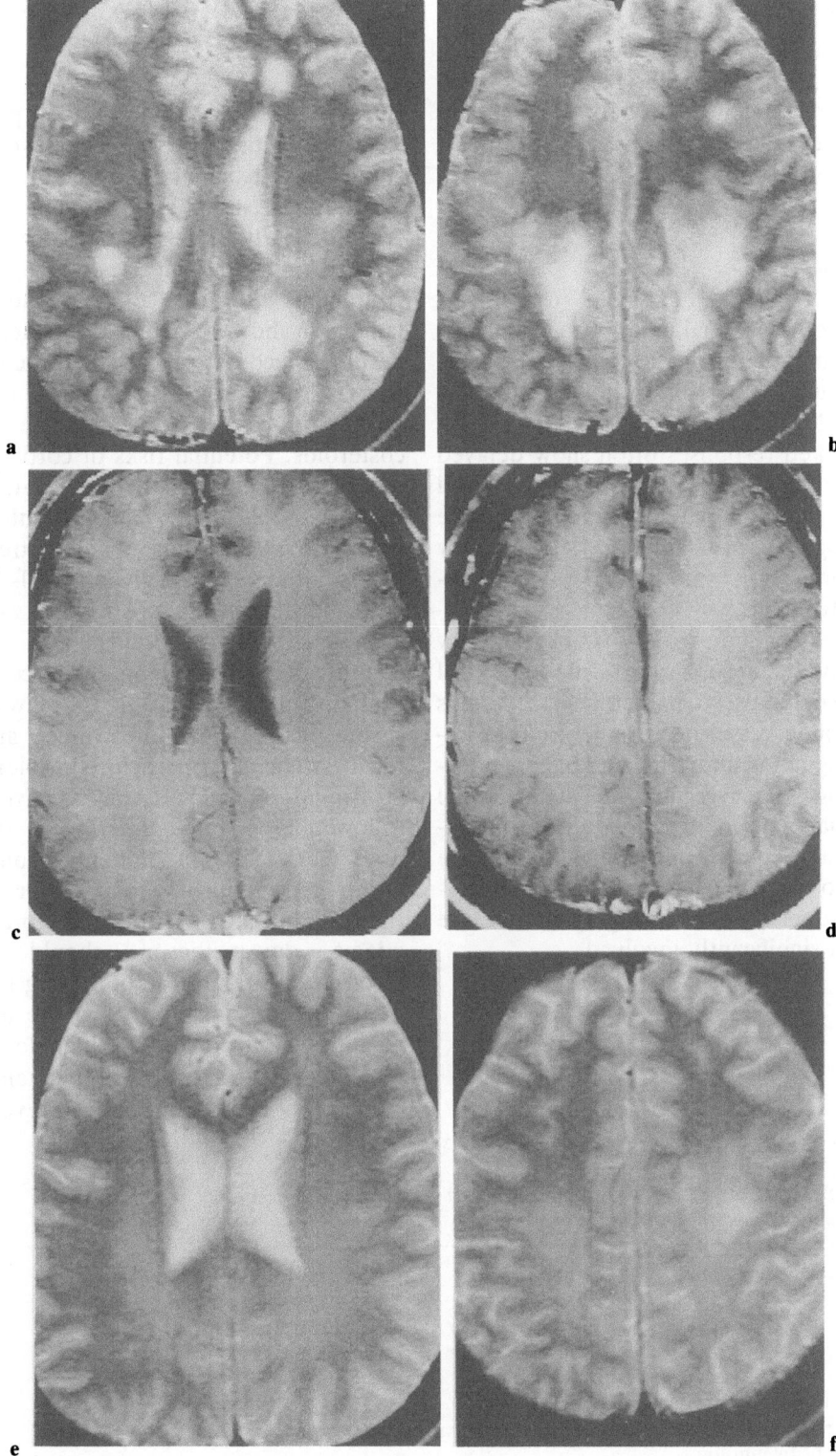

a b c d e f

is suggested. Chronic demyelinating disease such as MS is associated with oligoclonal activation of B cells and increased production of intrathecal immunoglobulins.

Other Tests

Electroencephalography may be useful in monitoring the course of disease. Visual and brain-stem auditory-evoked potentials and somatosensory-evoked responses often show delayed latencies. These tests may be used to monitor patients and may give prognostic information. EMG may demonstrate peripheral nerve involvement.

In patients with AHL, brain biopsy may be necessary to rule out viral encephalitis. Characteristic findings include vessel necrosis with fibrin impregnation and "ring and ball" hemorrhages. Perivascular and parenchymal inflammation (often polymorphonuclear), edema, and demyelination are also seen. Characteristically, white-matter U fibers and gray matter are not significantly involved.

Treatment

Because EAE can be prevented by pretreatment with corticosteroids, several studies have examined the role of corticosteroids in the treatment of ADEM. Early studies in patients with ADEM following measles were encouraging; however, later studies failed to show a significant benefit, despite anecdotal reports to the contrary. Slowly progressive disease can be interrupted by treatment with corticosteroids. Potential risks of corticosteroid treatment include amplification of virus replication, bacterial infections, hyperglycemia, and stress ulcers, although when given for 10–14 days, corticosteroids are usually well tolerated. Corticosteroids are recommended for patients with cerebral or spinal edema. In those with severe neurological impairment and focal deficits, methylprednisolone 1000 mg/d for 3 days can be given, followed by a rapid tapering of the dose (see Table 1). Patients should also receive antacid and H2-blocker therapy. In patients with severe brain edema, dexamethasone should be given at an initial dose of 100 mg i.v. There are no data regarding the use of intravenous cyclophosphamide in patients with ADEM. Rarely, hemicraniotomy may be needed to prevent

Table 1. Treatment of ADEM patients with severe neurological impairment and focal deficits

Methylprednisolone	1000 mg/d p. inf.	days 1–3
	500 mg/d p. inf.	day 4 + 5
	80 mg/d p. inf. or p.o.	for 5 days
	40 mg/d p. inf. or p.o.	for 5 days
	6 mg/d p.o.	for 5 days
then alternating therapy every 2 days		

p. inf., by infusion

lateral herniation in patients with unilateral brain edema. Children with acute cerebellar ataxia following varicella-zoster infection usually require no treatment other than maintenance of adequate hydration.

Suggested Reading

Alvord EC (1985) Disseminated encephalomyelitis: its variations in form and their relationships to other diseases of the nervous system. In: Vinken I, Koetsier JC (eds) Demyelinating diseases. Elsevier Science, Amsterdam, p 476 (Handbook of clinical neurology, vol 3)

Boos J, Esiri MM (1986) Viral encephalitis – pathology, diagnosis and management. Blackwell Scientific, Oxford

Bray PF et al. (1992) Demyelinating disease after neurologically complicated primary Epstein-Barr virus infection. Neurology 42:278–282

Chancellor AM, Glasgow GL (1986) Recovery from parainfectious encephalomyelitis. N Z Med J 99:839–840

Dun V et al. (1986) MRI in children with postinfectious disseminated encephalomyelitis. Magn Reson Imaging 4:25–32

Gendelman HE et al. (1984) Measles encephalomyelitis: lack of evidence of viral invasion of the central nervous system and quantitative study of the nature of demyelination. Ann Neurol 15:353–360

Groen De PC et al. (1987) Central nervous system toxicity after liver transplantation. N Engl J Med 317:861–866

Kesselring J et al. (1990) Acute disseminated encephalomyelitis. Brain 113:291–302

Lukes SA, Norman D (1983) Computed tomography in acute disseminated encephalomyelitis. Ann Neurol 13:567–572

Miller DH et al. (1992) High-dose steroids in acute relapses of multiple sclerosis: MRI evidence for a possible mechanism of therapeutic effect. J Neurol Neurosurg Psychiatry 55:450–453

Sartor K (1992) MR imaging of the skull and brain. Springer, Berlin Heidelberg New York

Selbst RG et al. (1983) Parainfectious optic neuritis. Report and review following varicella. Arch Neurol 40:347–350

Toyka KV (1987) Klinische Neuroimmunologie. Ed Medizin, VCH, Weinheim

Chapter 47

HIV Infection and Associated Opportunistic Infections

WOLFGANG ENZENSBERGER and WALTER ROYAL III

Introduction

Neurological involvement is a major problem in HIV patients. More than half of the patients may develop one or more neurological complications. Ten percent of patients will have a problem affecting the nervous system at initial presentation. It is often possible to effectively treat these patients as out-patients; however, it is occasionally necessary to administer care in an intensive care unit (ICU). Often those patients suffer from additional internal complications, e.g. *Pneumocystis carinii* pneumonia or generalized cytomegalovirus infection and therefore need interdisciplinary intensive care.

The duration of stay on the ICU varies between a few days and several weeks. While acute problems like seizures may quickly be controlled, chronic inflammatory complications may warrant prolonged inpatient care. At the Frankfurt University Hospital, about 10% of 700 HIV-1 seropositive

Section Editors: Karl M. Einhäupl and Werner Hacke

patients at different stages of HIV-1 disease were admitted to the ICU. At the Johns Hopkins Hospital (Baltimore), it was found in a study of patients seen in the emergency department in 1986 that 3.0% of all critically ill patients were infected with the human immunodeficiency virus. By the next year, this had increased to 7.8% of patients seen in the department; most of these cases involved penetrating trauma and were, therefore, not associated with direct complications of HIV-1 infection.

Spectrum of HIV Neurological Manifestations

Neurological complications of the acquired immune deficiency syndrome (AIDS) usually occur in full-blown AIDS, although they can also develop at earlier stages. From a systematic point of view it is possible to differentiate between primary, i.e. directly HIV-induced, and secondary neurological manifestations. At the time of HIV seroconversion, in about 1% of all cases acute HIV meningoencephalitis develops, leading to progressive loss of consciousness and seizures, which may necessitate intensive care. Chronic AIDS encephalopathy, also called AIDS dementia complex, is usually not an ICU problem unless it occurs in combination with other neurological or internal problems.

Among the secondary neuromanifestations central nervous system (CNS) toxoplasmosis is the most common cause of neurological illness. However, other opportunistic pathogens, e.g., *Cryptococcus neoformans*, *Mycobacteria*, or *Listeria monocytogenes* may also be causative agents of serious neurological disease. Furthermore, CNS lymphoma may lead to emergency situations, such as seizures, progressive stroke hemiparesis, or elevated intracranial pressure. Among those patients with known HIV-1 infection admitted to critical care units in the United States, more than two-thirds have respiratory failure due to infections (*Pneumocystis carinii*, cytomegalovirus, *Toxoplasma*, *Mycobacterium avium-intracellulare*, *Cryptococcus*, *Aspergillus*, gram-negative organisms), tumors (Kaposi's sarcoma, lymphoma), lymphoid interstitial pneumonitis, sedative overdose, and asthma. Seizures are the major neurological complication responsible for ICU admission, occurring in about 13% of seropositive ICU patients.

Finally, an important group of patients has to be considered, who have unidentified HIV-1 infection and present with HIV-independent diseases or after accidents. This last group will normally not need AIDS-specific differential diagnosis, but leads to problems of increased risk of HIV infection in hospital staff.

Risk of HIV Infection in the ICU

Intensive care procedures are often invasive and definitely raise the risk of infection for nurses and doctors. As ICU patients are normally seriously ill and not able to give a history on admission, it is recommended that unit staff practice universal precautions in handling blood and body fluids from all patients. In addition to these precautions, the indication for any invasive procedure should be checked thoroughly. Even the simple sensory examination using needles may carry a risk of infection. Therefore wooden tooth picks should be preferred in the neurological examination of any patient. On admittance to the neurological ICU, routine HIV testing should be performed for the information and security of the staff. A number of diagnostic and therapeutic decisions will also depend on knowledge of HIV seropositivity.

If despite of all precautions, a member of the staff suffers a needle-stick injury with contaminated material, the measures shown in Table 1 should be taken immediately. The needle-stick injury carries a risk of seroconversion of about 0.5%; nevertheless, case reports have been published, showing that HIV seroconversion after needle-stick injury may

Table 1. Recommended action after needle-stick injuries with HIV-contaminated material

---

Provocation of bleeding

Cleaning and disinfection of the wound (alcohol >70%)

Prophylactic zidovudine therapy (orally or ?intravenously), 5 × 250 mg daily for 2 weeks

Repeated serological HIV testing at days 0, 45, 90, 180, 365

---

occur in spite of all the measures described.

Acute HIV Meningoencephalitis

Definition and Epidemiology

Acute HIV meningoencephalitis is encephalitis due to HIV itself, which occurs in about 1% of all HIV patients before or during HIV seroconversion. In some other patients acute HIV polyradiculopathy (Guillain-Barré syndrome) has been described. Patients have been well until then and do not always belong to an obvious HIV risk group.

Clinical Features and Differential Diagnosis

Patients with acute HIV meningoencephalitis show nonspecific acute to subacute encephalitic signs and symptoms, such as headache, fever, progressive organic brain syndrome, and seizures. The differential diagnosis includes all other forms of viral encephalitis.

Ancillary Tests

Diagnosis of acute HIV meningoencephalitis is difficult and can in some cases be linked to HIV only retrospectively. HIV antigen in blood and CSF is normally detectable, whereas HIV antibodies may develop days to weeks later. Therefore repeated HIV serology tests should be performed in suspected cases. Polymerase chain reaction (PCR) studies may show the presence of HIV genome in the CSF. Inflammatory signs in CSF and general changes in the EEG are nonspecific. Computed tomography (CT) and magnetic resonance imaging (MRI) show no abnormalities.

Management

As the HIV etiology will not be clear in most cases, usually intravenous acyclovir therapy will be given, in order not to miss herpes simplex encephalitis. It is unclear whether zidovudine is helpful in patients with acute HIV meningoencephalitis.

Prognosis

Acute HIV meningoencephalitis has a good prognosis, with complete remission within several days to weeks, and will need only general intensive care during the acute phase of the disease. The significance of early neurological manifestations of HIV for the later course of the disease is still unclear.

CNS Toxoplasmosis

Definition and Epidemiology

CNS toxoplasmosis is the most frequent HIV-related cause of admittance to the neurological ICU. CNS toxoplasmosis occurs in 10%–20% of all AIDS patients and results from reactivation of dormant bradyzoites in individuals who have had toxoplasmosis previously (20%–70% of immunocompetent individuals in the United States and Germany and more than 90% of adults in France, El Salvador, and Tahiti) in the setting of advanced HIV immunodeficiency.

Clinical Features
and Differential Diagnosis

CNS toxoplasmosis develops sub-acutely within a few days or several weeks. The clinical picture depends strongly on the site of the granulomas and is therefore variable. It can consist of a progressive organic brain syndrome (>70%), focal neurological deficits [hemiparesis (>60%), aphasia, extrapyramidal signs, hemianopia, or cerebellar hemiataxia] and/or generalized or focal seizures (>30%). Patients may complain of headache if the granulomas are space-occupying. Less than half of the patients have fever.

Differential diagnosis includes CNS lymphoma and progressive multifocal leukoencephalopathy.

Ancillary Tests

Neuroimaging

Diagnosis will usually be established by cranial CT or MRI. Characteristic CT or MRI findings in patients with CNS toxoplasmosis are multiple hypodense brain lesions with ring enhancement and perifocal edema (Fig. 1). Ninety percent of toxoplasmosis lesions may be seen on CT with contrast administration, but enhanced MRI can demonstrate lesions not reliably seen on CT (Fig. 2), particularly those in the posterior fossa. It is not always possible to distinguish toxoplasmosis from lymphoma. In some cases, both can be present simulta-

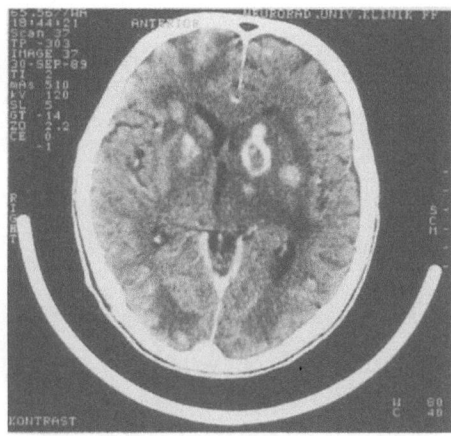

Fig. 1. Computed tomographic of the brain of a patient with acquired immune deficiency syndrome (AIDS) with central nervous system toxoplasmosis, showing multiple hypodense lesions and ring contrast enhancement with surrounding space-occupying edema. (Scan by Prof. Dr. H. Hacker, Department of Neuroradiology, University Hospital, Frankfurt am Main)

neously. Areas infected with toxoplasmosis show early normalization during treatment. Lymphoma should be suspected if no change or even growth of the lesion is present on repeated CT or MRI 1 week after the start of treatment.

Laboratory Tests, CSF Analysis, and Microbiology

Lumbar puncture and specific toxoplasmosis serology is usually not very helpful. CSF analysis shows non-specific inflammation. Serological tests will reveal low or moderately elevated specific IgG titers, due to earlier *Toxoplasma gondii* primary infection, but usually not IgM. However, in some cases active infection is indicated by a positive test for IgM, a four-fold rise in IgG titer, or a stable IgG

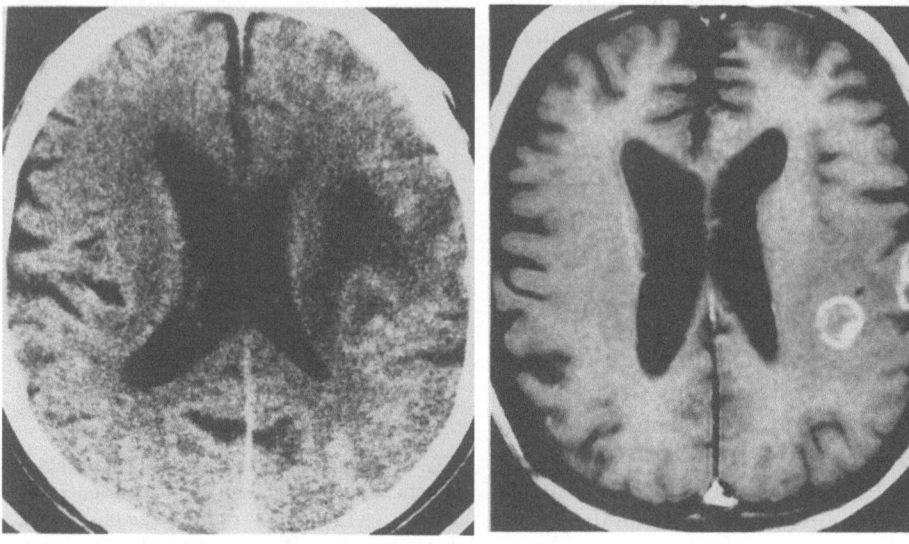

Fig. 2a,b. Cerebral toxoplasmosis with abscess formation in a 69-year-old hemophiliac man with AIDS. Axial CT scan (**a**) and MR image (**b**), both obtained after IV administration of contrast material, demonstrate two cortical and subcortical brain lesions with ring enhancement and marked perifocal edema. The edema is more obvious on CT, while lesion conspicuity is much better on MR (T2-weighted MR would have shown the edema as well as CT or better). (Courtesy of Klaus Sartor and Marius Hartmann, Heidelberg)

titer greater than 1024. Perhaps *Toxoplasma* PCR will bring diagnostic progress in the future. Definite in vivo diagnosis of toxoplasmic infection can be tried by identification of the organism in tissue sections obtained at biopsy. Organisms may be seen with Wright-Giemsa or hematoxylin-eosin stains or by immunoperoxidase staining techniques using specific antibodies to *Toxoplasma* antigens. Despite these approaches, *Toxoplasma gondii* may be difficult to detect in vivo. Therefore, the organism can be first amplified by intraperitoneal injection of infected material into nude mice.

Electrophysiology

Electroencephalography (EEG) will often show general slowing of the basal activity and in many cases additional focal and/or paroxysmal signs.

Management

If CNS toxoplasmosis is suspected, empiric anti-*Toxoplasma* therapy should be started immediately. Clinical remission will begin within a few days and normalization of CT and MRI scans can be expected within about 4 weeks. Table 2 sets out an effective drug regimen which will lead to clinical improvement in 90% of all cases. Daily administration of folinic acid is necessary to avoid thrombocytopenia. Alternatively, clindamycin may be given intravenously (4 × 600 mg), which may be preferable in acute treatment, if the patient is not able to swallow, or if the patient shows

Table 2. Treatment rocommendations in HIV-associated opportunistic infections

Infection	Recommended treatment (doses per day)
CNS toxoplasmosis	1. 50–100 (–150) mg pyrimethamine 2. (2–)4–6(–8) g sulfadiazine 3. 15 mg folinic acid
CNS cryptococcosis	1. 0.3–0.6 mg/kg amphotericin B (in glucose 5%, over 6–8 h) 2. 75–150 mg/kg flucytosine (4 divided doses) 3. 400 mg fluconazole
Progressive multifocal leukoencephalopathy	No therapy available
CNS tuberculosis	1. 5 mg/kg isoniazid 2. 10 mg/kg rifampicin 3. 15–25 mg/kg ethambutol 4. 15–30 mg/kg pyrazinamide
CNS listeriosis	6–12 g ampicillin (3–4 divided doses)

allergic or toxic adverse reactions to sulfonamides. Patients with significant cerebral edema respond well to corticosteroid treatment (prednisone 50 mg tapered over 10 days). Seizures respond to routine anticonvulsant therapy (e.g., 3 × 200 mg carbamazepine). Anticonvulsants can interfere with the pyrimethamine metabolism which can make it necessary to raise the dosages.

About 80% of patients treated for CNS toxoplasmosis will relapse if the drug therapy is stopped. Therefore, treatment of this opportunistic infection is lifelong (e.g., 50 mg pyrimethamine daily and 15 mg folinic acid 2–3 times a week).

If there is no clinical improvement following therapy within 2 weeks, and if the CT/MRI lesions do not show a reduction in size, stereotactic brain biopsy should be performed, especially if the lesions are easily accessible and the general state of the patient is still acceptable. Biopsy may yield an alternative histologic diagnosis of the lesions examined, e.g., lymphoma or other infections.

Prognosis

The degree of disturbance of consciousness on admittance and initiation of therapy is directly related to prognosis. Patients with initial seizures may have a slightly better prognosis, as treatment will be started earlier. About 80% of patients with successfully treated CNS toxoplasmosis will have neurological defects. The average survival time after CNS toxoplasmosis is about 6–12 months.

Cryptococcal Meningitis

Definition and Epidemiology

Cryptococcal Meningitis is the most common fungal infection in patients with AIDS and is normally acquired by inhalation of the microorganisms. About 2% of the AIDS patients in most European countries and up to about 10% of the AIDS patients in France, Belgium, and the USA suffer from cryptococcosis. Bird feces are the most important natural reservoir for *Cryptococcus neoformans*.

Clinical Features and Differential Diagnosis

Patients with cryptococcal meningitis usually have fever and complain of malaise and headache of insidious onset and progressive character (80%–90%): Only about 30% of the patients show meningism. If treatment is not started early, progressive disturbance of consciousness and cranial nerve deficits may develop. Differential diagnosis includes tuberculous meningitis, and meningitis from *Listeria monocytogenes* or *Treponema pallidum*.

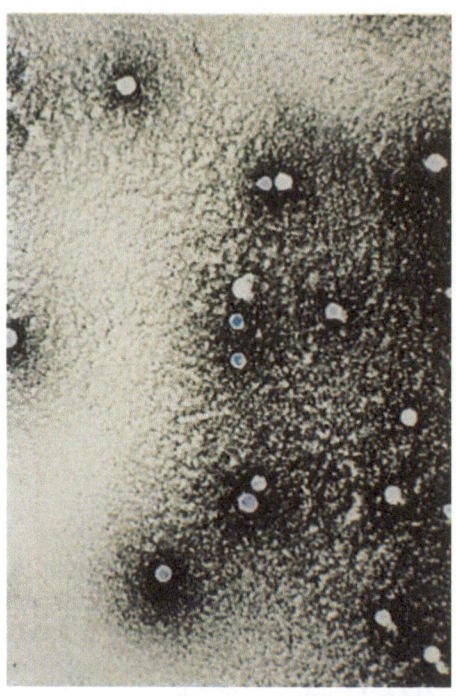

Fig. 3. India ink staining of a cerebrospinal fluid smear from an AIDS patient with CNS cryptococcosis. The cryptococcus can be identified by its typical light halo, which is due to the polysaccharide capsule surrounding the microorganism. The cryptococcus itself is blue from additional methylene blue staining

Ancillary Tests

Neuroimaging

Cranial CT or MRI are usually not helpful, except in rare cases in which CSF circulation disturbances or cryptococcoma occur.

Laboratory Tests, CSF Analysis, and Microbiology

The diagnosis is made by evaluation of CSF. Whereas usual CSF analysis techniques show only minimal inflammatory response due to the low antigenicity of the cryptococci, India ink staining of the CSF will in most cases (80%) reveal the cryptococci with their typical light halo (Fig. 3). Additionally, isolation of the organisms should be tried on special culture media (Guizotia abyssinica agar). Cryptococcal antigen titers in CSF and blood, which are positive in more than 90% of cases, should be determined.

Electrophysiology

EEG shows only nonspecific general slowing.

Management

The mainstay of acute treatment of cryptococcal meningitis is amphotericin B with flucytosine (Table 2). It is important to monitor renal function because of the nephrotoxic side effects of amphotericin B. If the serum creatinine rises above 2 mg%, amphotericin B treatment must be discontinued until creatinine levels return to the normal range. Liposomal amphotericin seems to be less toxic, but is not yet freely available. Flucytosine may induce lymphopenia and thrombopenia as side effects. Fluconazole is very well tolerated and can be given in combination (400 mg daily), especially in patients with significant adverse reactions to amphotericin B or flucytosine. Therapy should be monitored by repeated lumbar punctures and cryptococcal antigen titers in CSF and blood and isolation of the microorganisms in culture. After successful acute treatment of 4–8 weeks, permanent maintenance therapy with fluconazole at a reduced dosage (200 mg daily) has to be given orally to avoid relapse.

Prognosis

Prognosis is closely related to the progression of the underlying disease and the level of consciousness at the beginning of the antifungal treatment. If the patient is still awake at the start of the therapy, remissions up to more than 2 years are possible.

Progressive Multifocal Leukoencephalopathy

Definition and Epidemiology

Progressive multifocal leukoencephalopathy (PML) is a subacute, demyelinating CNS disease in patients with significant   immunosuppression,

caused by a reactivation of the JC virus in 2% of patients with AIDS. About 70% of all individuals have been exposed to this virus.

Clinical Features and Differential Diagnosis

The onset of PML is insidious, progressive organic brain syndrome and focal neurological deficits are the typical clinical signs. Differential diagnosis includes the entire list of focal secondary HIV neuromanifestations, i.e., CNS toxoplasmosis, CNS lymphoma, and mycobacterial CNS infection.

Ancillary Tests (Fig. 4)

Without biopsy, definite diagnosis of PML is difficult. The disease can be suspected if CT or MRI show single or multiple white matter lesions without contrast enhancement and without major mass effect.

EEG may show nonspecific focal or general changes. CSF analysis shows nonspecific inflammatory signs. Identification of the virus from the urine is sometimes possible by electron microscopy. Positive JC virus PCR in CSF may become an important diagnostic help in the future.

Management

So far no successful therapy is available for PML. Some reports have been published proposing repeated administration of cytosine arabinoside, but the effects of this rather toxic substance are not yet convincing in PML.

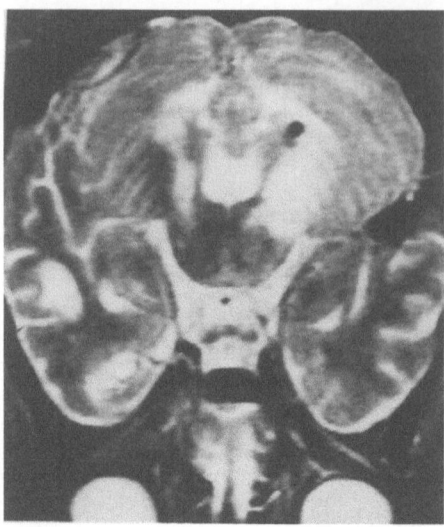

Fig. 4. Progressive multifocal leukoencephalo-pathy (biopsyproved) in a 57-year-old HIV-positive man with dysarthria and ataxic right hand movements. T2-weighted axial MR image demonstrates multiple regions of abnormal hy-perintensity without mass effect involving sub-cortical white matter of left temporal lobe as well as deep cerebral hemispheric white matter bilaterally. On IV administration of paramag-netic contrast material lesions did not enhance. *Black dot* posterolateral to fourth ventricle on right represents marker from biopsy. (Courtesy of Klaus Sartor and Marius Hartmann, Hei-delberg)

Prognosis

The disease normally leads to death within months. However, spontaneous remission has also been seen in pa-tients with less severe immunosup-pression.

Mycobacterial Infection of the CNS

Definition and Epidemiology

Infection of the CNS by *Mycobacter-ium tuberculosis* has become more

frequent in the AIDS era, but still remains a rare complication. Among patients with HIV-1 infection, inject-ing drug users are more likely to have tuberculosis infection. CNS involve-ment in tuberculosis has been reported in as many as 1%–2% of patients with AIDS.

Clinical Features and Differential Diagnosis

Mycobacterial infection can lead to the clinical picture of meningitis with sub-acute headache, fever, and stiff neck. In case of mycobacterial brain abscess focal neurological deficits, seizures, and an organic brain syndrome can result. Differential diagnosis includes other focal neuromanifestations, such as CNS toxoplasmosis, CNS lym-phoma, and PML.

Ancillary Tests

Neuroimaging

Diagnosis is difficult. CT scans may show single or multiple hypodense lesions with diffuse or ring-shaped contrast enhancement and mass effect in brain abscess. MRI can be more sensitive in demonstrating lesions and may reveal meningeal enhancement related to tuberculous meningitis.

Laboratory Tests, CSF Analysis, and Microbiology

CSF analysis reveals inflammatory signs with pleocytosis (granulocytes and lymphocytes), elevated protein concentrations, and markedly low glucose. Staining of a CSF smear is positive for acid-fast bacilli in only about 10% of cases; cultures are positive after some weeks in about 25% of cases. The diagnosis can be made by brain biopsy with tissue specimens positive for acid-fast bacilli on stains and cultures.

Electrophysiology

EEG shows nonspecific focal and/or general changes.

Management

Antituberculotic treatment should be started with a combination of three or four drugs for several months including isoniazid and rifampicin (see Chap. 37) (Table 2). Initially, corticosteroids can be co-administered to lower the risk of hydrocephalus in patients with meningitis. If the patient improves, treatment can be reduced to a two-drug regimen using isoniazid and rifampicin after 3–4 months.

Prognosis

Prognosis remains doubtful, although initial response and control of CNS tuberculosis have been published in AIDS patients.

CNS Listeriosis

Definition and Epidemiology

This is a rare CNS complication in AIDS patients, which is surprising, as *Listeriae* frequently cause meningitis in other immunocompromised hosts. The most important natural reservoirs for *Listeria* are milk and milk products, especially cheese.

Clinical Features and Differential Diagnosis

Patients usually suffer from signs of meningitis, rarely with an organic brain syndrome and focal neurological deficits in case of CNS abscess. Differential diagnosis includes other causes of meningitis in AIDS patients, such as meningitis due to *Cryptococcus neoformans*, *Mycobacterium tuberculosis*, or *Treponema pallidum*.

Ancillary Tests

Diagnosis is established by positive CSF and blood cultures and positive specific serology. Inflammatory signs in CSF are nonspecific. EEG, CT and MRI scans are not diagnostically helpful, except in patients with CNS abscess.

Management

Treatment should be done with ampicillin intravenously for 4–6 weeks (Table 2).

Prognosis

Remissions have been described, but there is little experience on which to base a general prognosis of this CNS complication.

Ethical Issues of Critical Care for HIV-1 Seropositive Patients

A final important problem is the question of limiting intensive care of HIV patients. Physicians treating HIV patients in ICUs are often faced with decisions whether to withhold or terminate treatment of the severely ill. The goal of ethical care of patients is to administer therapy which will promote good health while maintaining the patient's autonomy, or ability to choose his or her own fate, without increasing the patient's discomfort or disability. Apart from the patient's will, which should always guide the doctor's decisions, if the patient desires or refuses intensive diagnostic and therapeutic measures, a number of medical aspects will have to be considered in each individual case. Asymptomatic HIV patients with HIV-independent diseases will usually be treated like HIV-negative patients. In case of full-blown AIDS other factors such as the duration of the disease, the patient's general state, the presence of a wasting syndrome, or other lifethreatening non-CNS manifestations of AIDS will influence the decisions. Whether resuscitation, mechanical ventilation, or surgery are still indicated or not depends on several individual factors. The general prognosis of AIDS patients dependent on mechanical ventilation, according to treatment results published by several intensive care centers, is bad.

Suggested Reading

Abos J, Graus F, Miro JM, Mallolas J, Trilla A, Mercader JM (1991) Intracranial tuberculomas in patients with AIDS. AIDS 5:461–462

Baker JL, Kelen GD, Sivertson KT, Quinn TC (1987) Unsuspected human immunodeficiency virus in critically ill emergency patients. JAMA 257:2609–2611

Bartlett JG (1992) Recommendations for the medical care of persons with HIV infection. Crit Care Am 1:44–49

Berger JR, Kaszovitz B, Post JD, Dickinson G (1987) Progressive multifocal leukoencephalitis associated with human immunodeficiency virus infection. Ann Intern Med 107:78–87

Carne CA, Tedder RS, Smith A, Sutherland S, Elkington SG, Daly HM, Preston FE, Craske J (1985) Acute encephalopathy coincident with seroconversion for anti-human T lymphotropic virus type III. Lancet II:1206–1208

Centers for Disease Control (1988) CDC update: universal precautions for prevention of transmission of human immunodeficiency virus, hepatitis B virus and other bloodborne pathogens in health-care settings. MMWR 37:377–388

Chuck SL, Sande ME (1989) Infections with Cryptococcus neoformans in the acquired immunodeficiency syndrome. N Engl J Med 321:794–799

Culver CM, Gert B (1984) Basic ethical concepts in neurologic practice. Semin Neurol 4:1–8

Enzensberger W (1989) Neuromanifestationen bei AIDS. Schwer, Stuttgart

Enzensberger W, Enzensberger R, Doerr HW, Fischer P-A (1990) HIV-Infektionsrisiko in der Neurologie. Nervenarzt 61:250–251

Enzensberger W (1991) Neuro-AIDS – aktuelle Entwicklungen. Aktuel Neurol 18:42–48

Fischer P-A, Enzensberger W (1987) Neurological complications in AIDS. J Neurol 234:269–279

Grant IH, Gold JWM, Rosenblum M, Niedzwiecki D, Armstrong D (1990) Toxoplasma gondii serology in HIV-infected patients: the development of central nervous system toxoplasmosis in AIDS. AIDS 4:519–521

Haverkos HW (1987) Assessment of therapy for toxoplasma encephalitis. The TE study group. Am J Med 82:907–914

Levy RM, Bredesen DE, Rosenblum ML (1985) Neurological manifestations of the acquired immunodeficiency syndrome (AIDS): experience at UCSF and review of the literature. J Neurosurg 62:475–495

Luft BJ, Remington JS (1987) Toxoplasmic encephalitis. J Infect Dis 157:1–6

McArthur JC (1987) Neurologic manifestations of AIDS. Medicine (Baltimore) 66:407–437

Nelson WA, Bernat JL (1989) Decisions to withhold or terminate treatment. Neurol Clin 7:759–774

Parsons M (1989) The treatment of tuberculous meningitis. Tubercle 70:89–92

Rosenblum ML, Levy RM, Bredesen DE (1988) Neurosurgical implications of the acquired immunodeficiency syndrome. Clin Neurosurg 34:419–445

Rosenblum ML, Levy RM, Bredesen DE (eds) (1988) AIDS and the nervous system. Raven, New York

Snider WD, Simpson DM, Neilson S, Gold JWM, Metroka CE, Posner JB (1983) Neurological complications of acquired immune deficiency syndrome: analysis of 50 patients. Ann Neurol 14:403–418

Sugar AM, Stern JJ, Dupont B (1990) Overview: treatment of cryptococcal meningitis. Rev Infect Dis 12:S338–S348

Wachter RM, Luce JM, Hopewell PC (1992) Critical care of patients with AIDS. JAMA 267:541–547

Zuger A, Louie E, Holzman RS, Simberkoff MS, Rahal JJ (1986) Cryptococcal disease in patients with the acquired immunodeficiency syndrome. Ann Intern Med 104:234–240

Inflammatory Diseases: Others

Chapter 48

Fungal Infections

Erich Schmutzhard

Introduction

This chapter focuses on fungal infections of the central nervous system (CNS mycosis). In general, fungi cause disease by tissue invasion, by releasing toxins (for example, after ingestion), or by eliciting an immune response. Immune competence is probably the most important factor that determines susceptibility to fungal infections, although other factors such as geography, climate, urbanization, occupation, and possibly hormonal factors (95% of fungal infections occur in men) may also be important. Fungi are ubiquitous. Those that cause disease in the nervous system are Zygomycetes, Ascomycetes, Basidiomycetes, and Deuteromycetes (Table 1). Almost any fungus can invade almost any tissue in patients who are immuno-compromised. All of the following fungi, for example, have been reported to cause CNS mycosis: Alternaria, Cephalosporium species, Curvularia, Drechsleria species,

Fonsecaea species, Fusarium, Madurella, Paecilomyces species, Penicillium, Rhodotorula, Sependonium species, Torulopsis glabrata, Trichophyton, Trichosporon, and Ustilago.

Most patients with fungal infections of the CNS have symptoms of chronic meningitis and granulomas or abscesses. The diagnosis is usually made at autopsy. The differential diagnosis of patients suspected of having CNS mycosis is listed in Table 2. The list is by no means complete, since almost any inflammatory brain disease can present as CNS mycosis. Fungi relevant to critical care treatment are listed in Table 3.

Ancillary Tests

Neuroimaging

Plain films of the skull and nasal sinuses in patients with CNS mycosis may show bone destruction of the skull base, mucosal thickening, or soft tissue masses extending from the paranasal sinuses into the intracranial space. A variety of CT findings have

---

Section Editors: Karl M. Einhäupl and Werner Hacke

Table 1. Pathogenic fungi in neurocritical care

Zygomycetes	– Mucor
	– Rhizopus
	– Absidia
Ascomycetes	– Histoplasma
	– Candida
	– Blastomyces
	– Pseudallescheria
Basidiomycetes	– Cryptococcus neoformans
Deuteromycetes	– Coccidioides
	– Aspergillus
	– Cladosporium
	– Sporothrix

Table 2. Differential diagnosis

Infectious meningoencephalitis
 – Bacterial (especially partially treated)
 – Mycobacterial (tuberculous)
 – Brucellosis
 – Spirochetal
   – neuroborreliosis
   – neurosyphillis
 – Actinomycosis
 – Nocardiosis
 – Parasitic
   – toxoplasmosis
   – trypanosomiasis (sleeping sickness)
   – toxocarosis
   – cysticercosis
   – granulomatous amebic encephalitis
   – secondary cerebral amebiasis
Noninfectious meningoencephalitis
 – Parainfectious encephalitis
 – Sarcoidosis
 – Behçet's disease
 – Vogt-Koyanagi syndrome
 – Carcinomatous and leukemic meningitis

been described, including meningeal enhancement in basal meningitis, hydrocephalus, granulomas, and abscesses. Patients may have cerebral infarction with or without hemorrhagic transformation from associated vasculitis and, rarely, subarachnoid hemorrhage from a ruptured mycotic aneurysm. Most patients have ring enhancement of focal lesions. Immuno-compromised patients, however, may not have ring enhancement, reflecting failure to contain or "wall-off" the infection; this is usually associated with a poor prognosis. The CT findings are nonspecific, and other chronic granulomatous diseases such as tuberculosis, sarcoidosis, and neoplasm must be excluded. Clinical correlation (history of exposure, clinical course, extracranial fungal disease) is needed to interpret the CT findings.

The appearance of fungal infections on MRI is similar to that on CT. MRI provides better images of the soft tissues of the head and neck region, though, and it is more sensitive in detecting hemorrhagic transformation of ischemic infarcts. Both MR angiography and conventional cerebral angiography can be used to confirm vasculitis, arterial occlusion, mycotic aneurysm, and sinovenous thrombosis.

Other ancillary tests, such as EEG and evoked potentials, although also nonspecific, can often confirm clinically suspected focal lesions and may be especially helpful in patients with seizures and focal or diffuse organic brain syndrome. Transcranial doppler sonography, a simple method that can be done at the bedside, can be useful for monitoring intracranial pressure and vasculitis.

Cerebrospinal Fluid and Other Laboratory Tests

Analysis of the cerebrospinal fluid (CSF) in patients with chronic meningitis may reveal pleocytosis from a few to several thousand cells per milliliter. Although usually mononuclear, polymorphonuclear pleocytosis may be seen early and in patients with

Table 3. Fungi relevant to neurocritical care

Class	Of neurological interest	Neurological manifestation	Extracerebral manifestation	Clinical course	Diagnostic steps
Zygomycetes	*Mucor* *Rhizopus* *Absidia*	– meningitis (frontobasal) – meningo-encephalitis – cranial nerve involvement – infarction – abscess – cavernous sinus thrombosis	– paranasal sinus – lungs – skin – gastro-intestinal tract – disseminated	– rapidly progressive (coma and death within 2 weeks)	Plain X-ray – skull – paranasal sinuses – orbital structures CT scan – paranasal structures – intracerebral/-cranial involvement? – cerebral infarction MRI (see CT) – hemorrhagic transformation – cerebral hemorrhage Angiography – arterial occlusion – arterial encroachment – cavernous sinus thrombosis CSF: unspecific – polymorphonuclear pleocytosis – low glucose – raised protein Isolation of organisms is usually not possible Culture: – takes several days to become positive unrewarding Serology (antibodies and antigen): not reliable Biopsy – demonstration of fungus – histopathology: fungal elements involving arteries and veins – microbiology

Table 3. Continued

Class	Of neurological interest	Neurological manifestation	Extracerebral manifestation	Clinical course	Diagnostic steps	
Ascomycetes	*Histoplasma capsulatum*	– meningitis (mainly basal) – hydrocephalus – meningo-encephalitis – granuloma – small and multiple (perivenous/parenchymal) – large (histoplasmoma)	– acute pulmonary – disseminated pulmonary	– usually chronic, phases of dormant disease status and reactivation	Chest X-ray CT scan MRI (see CT) CSF: unspecific (rarely): Serology: Biopsy	– basal enhancement – hydrocephalus – granuloma – superior in demonstration of basal structures – mononuclear pleocytosis – low glucose – raised protein – visualization of fungi, – Cultures: (incl.blood, urine, sputum) – animal inoculation (2–4 weeks) – antibodies: unreliable – antigen (serum, urine in disseminated disease) – demonstration of fungus – histopathology – microbiology
	Candida spp.	– meningitis – basal meningitis – ventriculitis – embolism – mycotic aneurysms – cerebritis	– mucous membranes – skin – upper and lower respiratory that – myocarditis	– meningitis/abscess: subacute/chronic – vascular manifestation: abrupt onset	Culture and biopsy from any obvious source of infection (skin, mucous membranes etc., incl.i.v. catheters, shunts, blood, etc.) CSF: unspecific	– polymorphonuclear pleocytosis

- abscess
- granuloma

- pericarditis
- endocarditis
- endophthalmitis
- metastatic systemic infection
- joints, bones, muscles
- liver
- spleen,
- gallbladder
- peritoneum
- candidemia

- low glucose
- raised protein

CT-scan:
- meningeal enhancement
- granuloma
- hydrocephalus
- infarction
- subarachnoid hemorrhage

MRI (see CT): superior in demonstrating hemorrhagic transformation of infarction and subarachnoid hemorrhage due to mycotic aneurysm

Four-vessel angiography:
- mycotic aneurysm

Stereotactic biopsy of intracranial lesion

Serology:
- antibodies: difficult to interpret
- demonstration of antigen and/or cell wall constituents indicates systemic infection

Blastomyces dermatitidis
- meningitis (chronic)
- granuloma
- abscess

- lung
- skin
- subcutaneous tissue
- bones, joints
- genito-urinary tract
- reticuloendothelial tissue
- disseminated

- acute
- chronic
- recurrent

Culture and biopsy from any obvious site of infection (skin, subcutaneous tissue, lymph node etc.)

Chest X-ray, bronchoscopy

CSF: unspecific
- lymphocytic pleocytosis
- low glucose
- raised protein
- demonstration and culture of pathogens from CSF is difficult

Table 3. *Continued*

Class	Of neurological interest	Neurological manifestation	Extracerebral manifestation	Clinical course	Diagnostic steps
					CT scan: unspecific – meningeal enhancement – granuloma – abscess MRI (see CT) Stereotactic biopsy of intracranial lesion – histopathology – demonstration and – culture of fungal elements Serology: – antibodies (of little use) – antigen (Elisa relatively high sensitivity but low specificity)
Pseudalle scheria boydii		– meningitis (chronic) – abscess	– ear – paranasal sinuses – lung – disseminated	– chronic	Culture and biopsy from any obvious site of infection Chest X-ray – cavities! CSF: unspecific – mixed pleocytosis, mainly mononuclear cells – low glucose – raised protein CT scan (MRI): – meningeal enhancement – abscess Stereotactic biopsy of intracranial lesion

		Clinical forms	Course	Diagnosis
Basidiomycetes	*Cryptococcus neoformans*	– meningitis (mainly chronic) – meningo-encephalitis – hydrocephalus – cranial nerve involvement – granuloma (cryptococcoma)	– insidious – subacute – chronic	CSF: – increased pressure – mononuclear pleocytosis – low glucose – raised protein – demonstration of fungi (India ink or nigrosin) – culture – demonstration of capsular polysaccharide antigen – culture of blood, urine, sputum, bone marrow
		– lung – skin – subcutaneous tissue – disseminated		Biopsy of cutaneous and subcutaneous lesions CT scan (MRI) – meningeal enhancement – hydrocephalus – granuloma Chest X-ray Stereotactic biopsy of intracerebral lesion
Deuteromycetes	*Coccidioides immitis*	– meningitis (basal) – granuloma (rare)	– acute	History of exposure in endemic area (Americas) CSF: – mononuclear pleocytosis (in acute disease polymorphonuclear, frequently eosinophilia) – low or normal glucose – raised protein – demonstration of fungi – culture (attention: biologic hazard! for laboratory personnel)
		– lower respiratory tract (acute) – chronic pulmonary disease – skin – disseminated (mainly musculoskeletal)		

Table 3. Continued

Class	Of neurological interest	Neurological manifestation	Extracerebral manifestation	Clinical course	Diagnostic steps
					Serology: – antibodies in CSF Biopsy from any obvious site of infection
					CT scan (MRI): – basal enhancement – hydrocephalus – granuloma
					Chest X-ray Stereotactic biopsy of intracranial lesion
	Aspergillus spp.	– meningitis – granuloma – abscess – septic sinus vein thrombosis – embolic infarction – vasculitis – mycotic aneurysm	– ear – paranasal sinuses – eye – disseminated	– acute – chronic	Skull X-ray CSF: – mixed pleocytosis – low/normal glucose – raised protein – culture: rarely positive CT scan: – abscess – enhancement of meninges – infarction – subarachnoid hemorrhage MRI (MRA) see CT, superior in – hemorrhagic transformation of infarction – sinus thrombosis and SAH due to mycotic aneurysm

Cladosporium spp.	– abscess – meningitis	– usually no extracranial manifestation	– insidious – acute	Four-vessel-angiography: – mycotic aneurysm – vasculitis – sinus vein thrombosis Biopsy from any obvious site of infection: – demonstration of hyphae – culture CT scan (MRI): – abscess CSF: – no or mainly polymorphonuclear pleocytosis – normal or low glucose – raised protein – culture from aspirate/bioptic material (stereotactic biopsy)
Sporothrix schenckelii	– meningitis – abscess	– skin – subcutaneous tissue – joints – bones – lungs	– chronic	CSF: – mononuclear pleocytosis – low glucose – raised protein Culture(?) CT scan (MRI): – small, multiple abscesses Biopsy from any obvious site of infection (histopathology, culture (?))

Table 4. Mycology of fungi relevant to neurology and neurocritical care

Class	Genus/species	Polysaccharide capsule	Presentation in tissue	Ideal culture medium	Direct visualization of fungus in CSF, other body fluids, or tissue	Technique to facilitate recovery	Diagnostic value of				
							Serology	Direct visualization	Culture of CSF, other body fluid, or tissue	Histopathology	Serology
Zygomycetes	*Mucor Rhizopus Absidia*	–	hyphae		biopsy specimen: potassium hydroxide, touch slide: hyphae H+E methenamine silver PAS	potassium hydroxide 10%	investigational	+	(+) tissue	++	–
Ascomycetes	*Histoplasma capsulatum*	–	yeast		combination of H+E and methenamine silver	lysis centrifugation	antigen (+) antibodies + cave: cross-reactivity with, e.g., *Blastomyces*	+	+	+	(+)
	Candida spp.	–	yeast budding	- vented routine blood culture bottle - agar plates	Gram stain	- potassium hydroxide 10% - biphasic blood culture bottles - lysis centrifugation	antigen (+) antibody (?)	(+)	++ (blood, CSF, tissue)	+	+
	Blastomyces dermatitidis	–	yeast	Sabouraud agar - enriched agar (e.g.,	H+E methenamine silver, PAS, Mayer's mucicarmine	potassium hydroxide 10%	antigen + antibodies + cave: cross-reactivity	++	++	++	(+)

	Form	Culture (Sabhi Gormans' medium)	Stains		Serology				
Basidiomycetes									
Pseudalle-scheria boydii	hyphae	Sabouraud agar	H+E methenamine silver	–	antigen – antibodies?	(+)	+	+	–
Cryptococcus neoformans	yeast	Sabouraud agar	wet mount: India ink, nigrosine (sensitivity 50%), methenamine silver, PAS, Mayer's mucicarmine, Masson-Fontana silver		antigen + antibodies –	+	++	++	++
Deutero-mycetes									
*Coccidioides immitis**	yeast spherules containing endospores	Sabouraud agar	wet mount: lactophenol – cotton blue H+E, PAS, methenamine silver	potassium hydroxide 10%	antigen + antibodies +	+	+	++	+
Aspergillus spp.	hyphae	Sabouraud agar	H+E, PAS		antigen + antibodies –	+	+ (danger! contamination)	++	+
Cladosporium spp.	hyphae	Sabourand agar	methenamine silver	–		(+)	(+)	++	–
Sporothrix schenckii	yeast	Sabouraud agar	PAS	–		(+)	+ (skin)	+	–

PAS, Periodic acid-Schiff; H + E, hematoxylin and eosin.

abscesses close to the subarachnoid space. Rupture of a mycotic aneurysm results in hemorrhagic or xanthochromic CSF. Eosinophilia may also be present. The glucose concentration is usually decreased (CSF/serum ratio < 0.5) but never as low as in patients with bacterial meningitis. Protein concentration is usually mildy increased but may be extremely high (>1000 mg/dl) in patients with impaired CSF circulation from arachnoiditis or obstructive hydrocephalus. Other measurements, such as C-reactive protein, lactic acid, and certain aminoacids, are not helpful in the diagnosis of CNS mycosis. Increased adenosine deaminase can be seen in patients with tuberculous meningitis, but whether it is specific enough to distinguish tuberculous meningitis from CNS mycosis is not known. Cytology is helpful in excluding carcinomatous or leukemic meningitis.

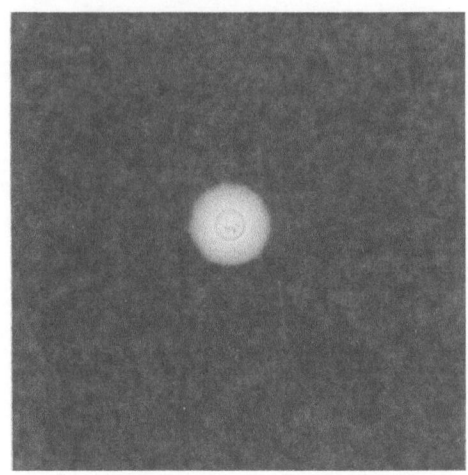

Fig. 1. *Cryptococcus neoformaus* surrounded by a polysaccharide capsule visualized with India ink

Microbiology

Aspergillus species and Zygomycetes typically appear as molds on culture, that is, with hyphae, and most of the Ascomycetes, Basidiomycetes (*Crytococcus* neoformans), and Deuteromycetes appear as yeast. In vitro, some of the Deuteromycetes can also grow as molds. Histology of a biopsy specimen, although less accurate than culture, may be more helpful clinically, given the slow growth of most fungi. Both Gomori methenamine silver reagent and periodic acid-schiff (PAS) reagent stain fungal cell walls. Typically, C. neoformans appears surrounded by a polysaccharide capsule which can be easily seen on India ink or nigrosin staining (Fig. 1). Candida

species are the only fungi seen on Gram's stain. Signs of invasion and inflammation suggest infection rather than contamination. Endotoxin is not produced by any of the fungi that cause CNS mycosis. Culture methods are described in Table 3 (those fungi that may be hazardous to laboratory personnel are marked with an asterisk). The diagnostic workup of patients suspected of having a fungal infection of the CNS is outlined in Tables 3 and 4.

Treatment

Patients with CNS mycosis are frequently immunocompromised and often have disseminated involvement or mulitiorgan failure. Thus, treatment of the CNS disease should always be in addition to treatment of the underlying disease. Supportive measures, including maintainence of adequate oxygen saturation in patients with severe pulmonary disease, should be provided.

Specific Chemotherapy and Adjuvant Therapy

Specific chemotherapy regimens for various CNS fungal infections are listed in Table 5. Treatment of CNS fungal infections may be different than treatment of disseminated fungal infections. Many of the drugs used may be associated with toxicity of the kidneys and bone marrow. Renal function and erythrocyte, leukocyte, and platelet counts need to be monitored closely. Some treatments such as in-

Table 5. Chemotherapy of CNS mycoses

Fungus species	Drug	Alternative drug	Form of administration	Dose	Duration
Mucor *Rhizopus* *Absidia*	Am B	–	i.v.	1.0–1.5 mg/kg/day	Depends on clinical course
Histoplasma capsulatum	Am B	–	i.v.	0.6 mg/kg/day	Up to 2 months
Candida spp.	Am B+ 5 Fc		i.v. p.o.	0.4–0.6 mg/kg/day } 150 mg/kg/day	} 2–4 weeks
		Fluconazole (?)	i.v./p.o.	800 mg (?)	?
Blastomyces dermatitidis	Am B	–	i.v.	0.3–0.6 mg/kg/day	30–50 days
Pseudallescheria boydii	Am B	–	i.v.	0.6 mg/kg/day	?
Cryptococcus neoformans	Am B+ 5 Fc	–	i.v. p.o.	0.3 mg/kg/day (−1.0 mg/kg/day) } 150 mg/kg/day	} 6 weeks
Coccidioides immitis	Am B+ Am B	–	i.v. i.th (lumbal, cisternal ventricular, cervical)	1.0–1.5 mg/kg/day start with 0.01–0.2 mg (increase to 0.3–0.5 mg) (three times per week slow tapering off)	30 days months ?
		Fluconazole	i.v./p.o.	up to 800 mg/day	
Aspergillus spp.	Am B		i.v.	0.6 mg/kg/day	?
		Am B+ 5 Fc	i.v. p.o.	0.6 mg/kg/day } 150 mg/kg/day	} ?
Cladosporium spp.	Am B+ 5 Fc	–	i.v. p.o.	?	Response is questionable
Sporothrix schenckelii	Am B		i.v.	0.5 mg/kg/day	40–60 days
		Am B+ 5 Fc	i.v. p.o.	0.5 mg/kg/day } 150 mg/kg/day	} 40–60 days

Am B, Amphotericin B; 5 Fc, 5-Flucytosine; ?, unknown.

trathecal amphotericin B may be complicated by local irritation, and intrathecal corticocsteroids may be useful to reduce the inflammation. Sytemic corticosteroids, however, should never be used. Anticonvulsive therapy may be necessary in some patients (see Chap. 66).

Neurosurgical Intervention

Ventriculoatrial and venticuloperitoneal shunts are essential for patients with hydrocephalus, and early shunting has been shown to improve overall outcome. Intracranial granulomas or abscesses may warrant surgical débridement, excision, or drainage. An Ommaya reservoir may also be helpful, especially in patients with coccidioidosis.

Prognosis

The prognosis of patients with fungal infections of the CNS varies, but it is generally poor, despite the availability of antifungal chemotherapy. For example, the mortality is near zero in patients with cryptococcal infections, while it approaches 80% in those with aspergillus infections. Patients often require prolonged treatment and, because fungal infections frequently relapse, they may need recurrent therapy or prophylaxis. Because the underlying disease greatly affects prognosis, an interdisciplinary approach ensures the best outcome.

Suggested Reading

Bennett JE (1987) Rapid diagnosis of candidiasis and aspergillosis. Rev Infect Dis 9:398-402

Bennett JE (1990) Mycoses: Introduction. In: Mandell GL, Douglas RG, Bennett JE (eds) Principles and practice of infectious diseases, 3rd edn. Churchill Livingstone, New York, pp 1942-1943

Bouza E, Drever JS, Hewitt WL, Meyer RD (1981) Coccidioidal meningitis. Medicine 60:139-172

Bowen BC, Post MJD (1990) Diagnostic imaging of CNS infection and inflammation. In: Schlossberg D (ed) Infections of the nervous system. (Clinical topics in infectious disease.) Springer, Berlin Heidelberg New York, pp 315-380

Buchsbaum HW, Norton TF, Valdivia FR (1985) Cisternal Ommaya reservoirs in the treatment of coccidioidal meningitis. In: Einstein HE, Catanzaro A (eds) Proceedings of the 4th international conference on coccidioidomycosis, San Diego, 1984. University of Arizona Press, Tucson, pp 444-447

Centeno RS, Bentson JR, Mancuso AA (1981) CT scanning in rhinocerebral mucormycosis and aspergillosis. Radiology 140:383-389

Daie DC (1981) Defects in host defense mechanisms in compromised patients. In: Rubin RH, Young LS (eds) Clinical approach to infection in the compromised host. Plenum Medical Book, New York, pp 35-74

Diamond R, Bennett JE (1973) A subcutaneous reservoir for intrathecal therapy of fungal meningitis. N Engl J Med 288:186

Diamond RD, Bennett JE (1974) Prognostic factors in cryptococcal meningitis. A study of 111 cases. Ann Intern Med 80:176-181

Dismukes WE, Cloud G, Gallis HA, Kerkering TM, Medoff G, Graven PC, Kaplowitz LG, Fisher JF, Gregg CR, Bowies CA (1987) Treatment of cryptococcal meningitis with combination amphotericin B and flucytosine for four as compared with six weeks. N Engl J Med 317:334-341

Emmons CW, Binford CH, Utz JP, Kwon-Chung KJ (1977) Medical mycology. Lea and Febiger, Philadeiphia

Eng RHK, Person A, Mangura C, Chmel H, Corrando M (1981) Susceptibility of

Zygomycetes to amphotericin B, miconazole and ketoconazole. Antimicrob Agents Chemother 20:688–690

Eng RHK, Bishburg E, Smith SS (1986) Cryptococcal infection in patients with acquired immune deficiency syndrome. Am J Med 81:19–23

Fetter BF, Klintworth GK (1988) Uncommon fungal diseases. In: Harris AA (ed) Microbial disease. Elsevier Science, Amsterdam, pp 479–503 (Handbook of clinical neurology, vol 8/52)

Hartsein AI, Winn RE (1988) Aspergillosis. In: Harris AA (ed) Microbial disease. Elsevier Science, Amsterdam, pp 377–384 (Handbook of clinical neurology, vol 8/52)

Horten BC, Abbott GF, Porro RS (1976) Fungal aneurysms of intracranial vessels. Arch Neurol 33:577–579

Kaps M, Burkhardt E, Krauss H, Hornig CR, Weiss R (1985) Zur Liquordiagnostik der meningealen Kryptokokkose. Fortschr Neurol Psychiatr 53:442–446

Klein BS, Kuritsky WAC, Kaufman L, Green J, Chappell WA, Davies SF, Williams JE, Sarosi GA (1986) Comparison of enzyme immunoassay, immunodiffusion and complement fixation tests in detecting antibody in human serum to the A antigen in B. dermatitidis. Am Rev Respir Dis 133:144–148

Labadie EL, Hamilton RH (1986) Survival improvement in coccidioidal meningitis by high-dose intrathecal amphotericin B. Arch Intern Med 146:2013–2018

Lazo A, Wilner HJ, Metes JJ (1981) Craniofacial mucormycosis: computed tomographic and angiographic findings in two cases. Radiology 139:623–626

Lowe JT, Hudson WR (1975) Rhinocerebral phycomycosis and internal carotid artery thrombosis. Arch Otolaryngol 101:100–103

Mandell GL, Douglas RG, Bennett JE (1990) Principles and practice of infectious diseases, 3rd edn. Churchill Livingstone, New York

Mikhael MA, Rushovich AM, Ciric J (1985) Magnetic resonance imaging of cerebral aspergillosis. Comput Radiol 9:85–89

Morgan MA, Wilson WR, Neel H, Roberts GD (1984) Fungal sinusitis in healthy and immunocompromised individuals. Am J Clin Pathol 82:598–601

Nov AA, Cromwell LD (1984) Computed tomography of neuraxis aspergillosis. J Comput Assist Tomogr 8:413–415

Rinaldi MG (1983) Invasive aspergillosis. Rev Infect Dis 5:1061–1077

Rippon JW (1988) Medical mycology. The pathogenic fungi and the pathogenic actinomycetes, 3rd edn. Saunders, Philadelphia

Sagg MS, Dismukes WE (1988) Treatment of histoplasmosis and blastomycosis. Chest 93:848–851

Salaki JS, Louria DM, Cheml H (1984) Fungal and yeast infection of the central nervous system. A clinical review. Medicine 63:108–132

Schiossberg D (1990) Infections of the nervous system. (Clinical topics in infectious disease.) Springer, Berlin Heidelberg New York

Schmutzhard E, Vejjajiva A (1988) Treatment of cryptococcal meningitis with combination amphotericine B and flucytosine, high dose and long duration. Am J Med 85:737–738

Schmutzhard E, Jitpimolmard S, Boongird P, Vejjajiva A (1987) Peripheral eosinophilia in the course of treatment of cryptococcal meningitis. Mykosen 30:601–604

Schmutzhard E, Boongird P, Gerstenbrand F, Jitpimolmard S, Ponglikitmongkol S, Vejjajiva A (1990) Is cryptococcal meningoencephalitis in the tropics a distinct entity? A retrospective study from Thailand. Trop Geogr Med 42:133–139

Sekhar LN, Dujovny M, Rao GR (1980) Carotid-cavernous sinus thrombosis caused by *Aspergillus fumigatus*. J Neurosurg 52:120–125

Weiner MH (1983) Antigenemia detected in human coccidioidomycosis. J Clin Microbiol 18:136–142

Whelan MA, Stern J, Denapoli RA (1981) The computed tomographic spectrum of intracranial mycosis: correlation with histopathology. Radiology 141:703–707

Winn RE, Ramsey PD, Mc Donald JC, Dunlop KJ (1983) Maxillary sinusitis from *Pseudallescheria boydii*. Efficacy of surgical therapy. Arch Otolaryngol 109:123–125

Wood M, Anderson M (1988) Neurological Infections. Saunders, London (Major problems in neurology, vol 16)

| **Parasitic Infections**

Erich Schmutzhard

Introduction

This chapter focuses on parasitic infections of the central nervous system (CNS parasitosis). A detailed knowledge of the epidemiology, mode of transmission, and predisposing factors of parasitic infections is necessary for timely diagnosis and treatment. Table 1 lists, by geographical distribution, the most common parasites that cause neurological disease. Some parasites are found in all parts of the world; others are found only in tropical areas, in specific tropical areas, or in areas with temperate climates. Parasites can cause disease directly – by invading tissues and causing space-occupying lesions, tissue hypoxia, and hemorrhage, or indirectly – by immune-mediated mechanisms. Diagnosis and treatment are specific for the parasite and the mechanism of disease.

Clinical Features

Symptoms and signs of CNS parasitosis vary and depend on the specific parasite, location of the infection, stage of the disease, and immune status of the patient. Nematodes that can cause CNS disease include Bailisascaris procyonis, Brugia malayi, Lagochilascaris minor, Loa loa, Onchocerca volvulus, and Wuchereria bancrofti. Fatal encephalopathy from B. procyonis and L. minor has been reported in only a few immunocompromised patients. The filarial worms (B. malayi, L. loa, O. volvulus, and W. bancrofti) can cause severe CNS disease. They are usually found only in certain geographical areas such as West Africa, southeast Asia, and Central and South America. Some patients treated with diethylcarbamazine, a microfilaricidal substance, develop local allergic reactions that can cause worsening of the neurological deficits, seizures, and even increased intracranial pressure. Trematodes (liver and intestinal flukes), on the other hand, usually do not cause serious CNS disease. Bovine and giant fish cestodes similarly do not usually cause

Section Editors: Karl M. Einhäupl and Werner Hacke

Table 1. Parasites relevant to neurocritical care

Geographical distribution	Protozoa	Helminths	Arthropods
Entire world	Acanthamoeba species Naegleria species Toxoplasma gondii	Strongyloides stercoralis Trichinella spiralis Cysticercus cellulosae Sparganum proliferum Toxocara canis	
Tropical areas	Entamoeba histolytica Plasmodium falciparum	Schistosoma species Paragonimus species	
Specific tropical areas	Trypanosoma species	Angiostrongylus Filariae Gnathostoma spinigerum Echinococcus granulosus Coenurus cerebralis	Pentastomatidae
Temperate climates	Babesia species	Anisakis species Bailisascaris procyonis Echinococcus granulosus	

serious disease, with the exception of neurological symptoms from vitamin B_{12} or folic acid deficiency. The clinical features of various parasitic infections are summarized in Table 2.

Ancillary Tests

Neuroimaging

Most CT and MRI findings are nonspecific. Occasionally, focal brain edema may be seen. In patients with cerebral malaria, trypanosomiasis, or babesiosis neuroimaging may even be normal. CNS infection with *Naegleria* species may result in meningeal contrast enhancement. Single or multiple parenchymal hypodensities without enhancement may be seen on CT with trichinosis, early toxoplasmosis, early cysticercosis, acanthamoebosis, sparganosis, and coenurosis. Ring-like contrast enhancing lesions may be seen

in infection with *Toxoplasma gondii*, *Entamoeba histolytica*, *Acanthamoeba* species, *Toxocara canis*, *Cysticercus cellulosae*, *Schistosoma* species, and *Paragonimus* species.

Plain film radiography of the skull, chest, and muscles may show calcifications or cyst formations in patients with infection by cestodes, *Paragonimus* species, or *Trichinella spiralis*. Obstructive hydrocephalus may be found in cestode and trematode diseases and in gnathostomiasis (which can also cause subarachnoid hemorrhage and eosinophilic meningitis).

Ultrasound and Electrophysiology

Ultrasound may be helpful by detecting extracranial manifestations of parasitic disease such as liver abscesses in patients suspected of having an amebic brain abscess, hydronephrosis, or hydroureter in patients with schis-

Table 2. Summary of CNS parasitoses

Pathogenic organism	Mode of transmission	Neurological clinical features	Course of disease	Typical findings	Differential diagnosis
Protozoa					
Acanthamoeba spp.	contact lens	granulomatous encephalitis, focal neurological deficit, fever, seizures (mainly in immunocompromised)	insidious	CSF and CT scan: unspecific; Biopsy of accompanying skin, sinus or lung lesion, brain biopsy	chronic meningitis, in particular granulomatous disease of CNS (tuberculosis, sarcoidosis, fungal disease)
Babesia spp. (mainly obvine)	tick, blood transfusion	hemolysis leading to hypoxemia, hypoxic encephalopathy, fever (mainly in splenectomized)	fulminant	blood smear (Giemsa stain): ring forms in erythrocytes	malaria
Entamoeba histolytica	water, food, feco-oral	brain abscess (preceded or accompanied by liver abscess), focal neurological deficits, seizures, increased intracranial pressure	subacute/acute	abscess formation in CT scan, serology	abscess of any other origin
Naegleria spp.	transnasal (water-pools)	meningoencephalitis (purulent)	fulminant	purulent CSF – neutrophilic pleocytosis, wet-mount CSF examination: amebic trophozoites	purulent meningitis
Plasmodium falciparum	Anopheles mosquitoes, Blood transfusion	fever, coma, seizures (diffuse or focal encephalopathy), multiorgan failure	acute/fulminant	*Plasmodium falciparum* – intraerythrocytic ring forms in Giemsa stain (blood smear), hemolysis, multiorgan failure, normal CSF	encephalitis, meningoencephalitis, sepsis syndrome
Toxoplasma gondii	food-borne, congenital	encephalitis, focal lesion, seizures (in immunocompromised), encephalopathy	subacute chronic	CSF: unspecific; CT scan: enhancing ring lesions, hypodensities; Serology	encephalitis, abscess, tumor (lymphoma)

Trypanosoma gambiense, rhodesiense	tsetse fly (*Glossina* spp.)	meningoencephalitis	chronic	CSF: plasmacellular pleocytosis ("morula cells") wet-mount CSF examination: motile trypanosomes Blood smear: trypanosomes	chronic meningitis (e.g., tuberculosis, fungal disease)
Trypanosoma cruzi	reduviid bugs, laboratory infection	meningitis/meningo-encephalitis, embolic cerebrovascular disease	acute/subacute	CSF: unspecific – serology blood concentration techniques Giemsa	acute/subacute meningitis bacterial endocarditis with secondary embolism
Helminths **Nematodes**					
Angiostrongylus cantonensis	ingestion of snails	meningitis	acute/subacute	CSF: eosinophilic pleocytosis larvae	meningitis of other origin
Anisakis spp.	ingestion of raw herring	diffuse and focal encephalopathy	acute/subacute	CT scan: nonspecific, eosinophilia	encephalitis
Gnathostoma spinigerum	ingestion of undercooked fish, snails, chicken, duck meat	encephalomyelitis, radiculitis, subarachnoid hemorrhage	acute, fulminant	CT scan: focal lesion, SAH CSF: high eosinophilia xanthochromia larvae	meningitis radiculitis encephalitis SAH } of other origin
Strongyloides stercoralis	skin penetration	purulent meningitis, abscess (so-called hyperinfection syndrome) accompanied by gram-negative sepsis/meningitis (only in immuno-compromised)	peracute	CSF: purulent larvae	purulent meningitis, gram-negative sepsis
Toxocara canis	incidental ingestion of toxocara eggs while playing with dogs	focal lesion cerebral, spinal cord	subacute	CSF: eosinophilia CT scan: granulomatous lesion	neoplasma, chronic/subacute granulomatous inflammatory disease

Table 2. *Continued*

Pathogenic organism	Mode of transmission	Neurological clinical features	Course of disease	Typical findings	Differential diagnosis
Trichinella spiralis	ingestion of under-cooked raw pork	encephalopathy, diffuse and focal	acute	eosinophilia, preceding diarrhea, periorbital edema, larvae in muscle-biopsies, raised muscle enzymes CT (+MRI) scan: unspecific focal lesions	encephalitis
Cestodes *Cysticercus cellulosae* (adults: *Taenia solium*)	feco-oral ingestion of eggs	space-occupying lesion (cyst) obstructive hydrocephalus diffuse encephalopathy meningitis meningovascular syndrome	chronic, occasionally acute	serology, eggs in feces, soft-tissue X-ray: calcifications/cysticerci in muscles CSF: unspecific/normal frequently no eosinophilia CT/MRI scan: cystic lesions (often multiple) calcifications obstructive hydrocephalus (intraventricular cyst) poorly defined hypodensities	cysts and chronic meningitis of any other origin encephalitis meningovascular syndrome
Echinococcus granulosus	ingestion of eggs (excreted by canines)	space-occupying lesions giant cysts obstructive hydrocephalus	chronic	CSF: normal, rarely eosinophilia CT/MRI scan: cystic lesions (scolices might be visualized)	cysts of any origin

Sparganum proliferum (adults: *Diphyllobothrium* spp.)	ingestion of infected raw snails, frogs	space-occupying lesions cysts obstructive hydrocephalus	chronic	CSF: not recommended CT/MRI scan: multiple cysts (unspecific) larva migrans visceralis/cutanea (larvae in muscles)	see *Cysticercus* above
Coenurus cerebralis (adults: *Taenia multiceps*)	ingestion of eggs (excreted by dogs)	see *Sparganum proliferum* (above)	chronic	CSF: not recommended CT: multiple cysts rarely: larvae in muscles	see *Cysticercus* above
Trematodes *Paragonimus* spp.	ingestion of raw freshwater crab/crayfish	space-occupying lesion cysts/partially calcified basal meningitis	insidious	CT: "soap-bubble" cysts (partially calcified cysts)	chronic meningitis of any other origin any space-occupying lesion cysts
Schistosoma spp.	active penetration into skin of forktailed cercariae	granuloma space-occupying lesion	chronic	CSF: unspecific, possibly eosinophilia CT: unspecific	space-occupying lesion granuloma of any other origin
Pentastomatidae *Linguatula* spp.	raw snake meat	calcifying space-occupying lesions	protracted	?	cestodes and trematodes infection

tosomiasis. None of the electro-physiologic tests provides specific results. They are generally useless in patients with parasitic disease.

Cerebrospinal Fluid and Other Laboratory Tests

The results of cerebrospinal fluid analysis in patients with CNS parasitosis are highly variable and non-specific. Patients infected with Naegleria species and Strongyloides stercoralis often have purulent meningitis and polymorphonuclear pleocytosis. Acantamoeba species and E. histolytica can also cause purulent meningitis when an abscess forms close to the subarachnoid space. CSF protein concentration is increased and glucose concentration is decreased. Patients with trypanosomiasis, and occasionally those with toxoplasmosis, have lymphocytic and plasmacellular pleocytosis. In these patients, particularly in those with African trypanosomiasis, CSF protein concentration may be markedly increased (because of high IgM levels). Eosinophilic pleocytosis is the hallmark of Angistrongylus cantonensis and Gnathostoma spinigerum infections. Other helmiths do not usually cause CSF eosinophilia. The CSF may be normal in patients with babesiosis and cerebral malaria or in patients with helminthic infections that result in chronic space-occupying lesions, calcifications, or intracranial cysts. Living parasites may be seen on a wet mount of the CSF from patients with naegleriasis, trypanosomiasis, strongyloidiasis, gnathostomiasis, angiostrongyliasis, and toxocarosis.

Patients with Plasmodium falciparum and babesiosis can develop potentially life-threatening hemolysis and multiorgan failure. Leukocytosis is present in patients with amebiasis (E. histolytica), in Naegleria infection, and possibly in Strongyloides infection. Peripheral eosinophilia can be seen in any helminthic infection, although it is not a regular feature. Filarial infestation and those helminthic infections caused by migrating larvae are more likely to show peripheral eosinophilia. Trichinella and cestode infections may cause increased creatine-kinase concentrations.

Microbiology

Plasmodium falciparum, Babesia species, Trypanosoma species, and filarial worms can be seen on a Giemsa-stained peripheral blood smear. Wet-mount examination of the CSF can be diagnostic of trypanosomiasis, naegleriasis, strongyloidiasis, gnathostomiasis, angiostrongyliasis, and toxocarosis. Muscle biopsy may be diagnostic in anisakiasis, trichinosis, cysticercosis, sparganosis, and coenurosis. Serological tests may increase the diagnostic yield; however, they are usually less important in patients with life-threatening CNS disease.

Because almost any organ can be involved, patients need a complete medical evaluation. Patients with American trypanosomiasis may have nonspecific ECG changes such as dysrhythmias or conduction abnormalities. CNS strongyloidiasis is frequently associated with gram-negative sepsis or meningitis and many patients, particularly those with cysticercosis, have seizures.

Treatment

Specific Chemotherapy

Recommendations for specific chemotherapy are listed in Table 3. Many patients with parasitic infections can be treated on the regular ward, but those with cerebral malaria (P. falciparum), primary amebic meningoencephalitis (N. fowleri), babesiosis (B. bovina), gnathostomiasis, and *Strongyloides* hyperinfection syndrome should be considered medical emergencies and should be admitted to a critical care unit. Other reasons for admission to a critical care unit include (a) increased intracranial pressure from encephalitis, hydrocephalus (aresorptive or occlusive), intraventricular cysts, granuloma, abscesses, or perifocal edema; (b) acute purulent meningitis; (c) meningovascular syndrome; (d) hypoxic encephalopathy (for example, in patients with cerebral malaria); (e) brain-stem disease; (f) granulomas or cysts of the third or fourth ventricle or posterior fossa; (g) cardiac involvement (for example, in patients with Chagas disease); and (h) multiorgan failure.

Adjuvant Therapy

Many patients, such as those with P. falciparum malaria and babesiosis, may become critically ill from hemolysis and multiorgan failure. Patients should be given an exchange transfusion if more than 10% of erythrocytes are parasitized. General supportive care should include hemofiltration or dialysis for renal failure, assisted ventilation for respiratory failure, and anticonvulsive therapy for treatment of seizures. The benefit of anticoagulation with heparin and corticosteroids has never been established. Corticosteroids may be detrimental in patients with cerebral malaria, but they may be helpful in those with helminthic diseases such as trichinosis, cysticercosis, and schistosomiasis. Corticosteroids should always be given either before or at the same time as specific antihelminthic therapy. Preliminary data suggest that treatment with pentoxifylline, a TNF antagonist, may be beneficial for patients with cerebral malaria.

Neurosurgical Intervention

Neurosurgical intervention, for diagnostic and therapeutic purposes, may be warranted in patients with abscesses, granulomas, or cysts. Surgery should generally be avoided in patients with secondary cerebral amebic abscesses. Patients with hydrocephalus from space-occupying lesions and impaired CSF circulation require ventriculoatrial or ventriculoperitoneal shunting. Patients with C. cerebralis infection may develop meningovascular disease and those with Chagas disease may develop cardiac involvement. Patients with larva migrans, especially S. stercoralis, are at risk for gram-negative sepsis and meningitis.

Table 3. Specific chemotherapies in CNS parasitoses

Drug	Dose	Duration of treatment
Cerebral malaria		
– Quinine dihydrochloride (Davis et al. 1988)	loading dose 20 mg/kg body weight maintenance dose 10 mg/kg every 8 h	over 4 h for 1 week
– Quinidine gluconate (Phillips et al. 1985)	loading dose 10 mg/kg followed by constant i.v. infusion of 0.02 mg/kg/min followed by oral quinine sulphate (650 mg/8 hourly)	over 1–2 h for 75 h for 3 days
– Mefloquine (Stuiver et al. 1989)	no parenteral formulation	
– Arthemeter (Myint et al. 1989)	300 mg i.m. 150–200 mg i.m.	on day 1 on days 2 and 3
– Artesunate (sodium) (Li et al. 1982)	60 mg b.i.d. i.v. o.d. i.v.	on day 1 on days 2 and 3
– Halofantrine (Wirima et al. 1988)	no parenteral formulation	
Babesiosis		
– Clindamycin plus Quinine (Wittner et al. 1982)	300–600 mg q.i.d. i.v. 650 mg t.i.d. p.o.	7–10 days
Secondary cerebral amebiasis (*Entamoeba histolytica*)		
– Metronidazole	750 mg t.i.d. p.o. or i.v.	5–10 days
– Dehydroemetine Schmutzhard et al. 1986)	60–80 mg i.m. o.d.	5–10 days
Primary amebic meningoencephalitis (*Naegleria fowleri*)		
– Amphotericin B (Am B) combined with	1.0 mg/kg/day i.v.	not known
Amphotericin B intrathecally (Martinez 1985)	starting with 1.0 mg and continuing with 0.1 mg on alternate days, possibly via a reservoir	
– Potential synergy:	combination of Am B with rifamycin, miconazole, or tetracyline	not known
Granulomatous amebic encephalitis (*Acanthamoeba* spp.) possible drugs		
– diamidine derivatives (Pentamidine)	?	?
– Am B	?	?
– 5 fluorocytosine (Martinez 1985)	?	?
Chagas' disease (*Trypanosoma cruzi*)		
– Nitrofurane derivative (Nifurtimox)	8–10 mg/kg/day p.o.	3–4 months
– Benznidazole (Radanil) (Marr and Docampo 1986)	5 mg/kg/day p.o.	2 months
Sleeping sickness (*Trypanosoma gambiense* and *T. rhodesiense*)		
– Suramin followed by	1 g/d p.o. 200 mg test dose (before treatment)	on days 1, 3, 7, 14, 21

Table 3. *Continued*

Drug	Dose	Duration of treatment
Melarsoprol (Mel B) (Gutteridge 1985)	3.6 mg/kg/day i.v.	for 3 days, repeat this course after 1 or 2 weeks
– Difluoromethylornithine (DFMO) followed by (Taelman et al. 1987) (Onyeyili and Onwalu 1991)	400 mg/kg/day/i.v. 4 × 75 mg/kg/day	for 2 weeks for 1 month
Angiostrongyliasis, anisakiasis, gnathostomiasis – no specific drugs available (Schmutzhard et al. 1988)		
Strongyloides stercoralis hyperinfection syndrome – Thiabendazole (Cook 1987)	25 mg/kg/b.d. p.o.	for 3 days
Toxocarosis – Thiabendazole (Medical letter 1988)	25 mg/kg/day p.o.	for 1 week
Trichinosis – Thiabendazole – Mebendazole – Flubendazole (Fröscher and Saathoff 1986)	25 mg/kg/day p.o. 5 mg/kg/day p.o. 40 mg/kg/day p.o.	for 1 week for 2 weeks for 2 weeks
Neurocysticercosis – Praziquantel (Moodley and Moosa 1989; Del Brutto 1992)	50 mg/kg/day p.o.	for 2 weeks
Echinococcosis (hydatid disease) – Albendazole (uncertain action in cerebral hydatid disease) (Horton 1989)	15 mg/kg/day p.o.	for 40 days
Coenurosis and sparganosis (Michal et al. 1977)	?	?
Paragonimiasis – Bithionil (Higashi et al. 1971) – Praziquantel (Medical letter 1988)	50 mg/kg/day p.o. 50 mg/kg/day p.o.	for 1 month, on alternate days single dose
Schistosomiasis *Schistosoma mansoni* and *S. haematobium* – Praziquantel *Schistosoma japonicum* – Praziquantel (Watt et al. 1989)	40–50 mg/kg p.o. 20 mg/kg t.i.d. p.o.	single dose in 24 h
Infection with Pentastomatidae	no specific drug available	

Prognosis

The prognosis of patients with parasitic infections of the CNS varies according to the pathogen. Almost 20% of patients with cerebral malaria die and 7% are left with neurological sequelae such as paresis, seizures, and diffuse organic brain synrome. The mortality is high among patients with cerebral amebiasis (E. histolytica) and primary meningoencephalitis (N. fowleri). If untreated, African trypanosomiasis usually results in death; treatment with diflouromethylornithine (DFMO) may be beneficial. In children, the mortality of CNS infection with T. cruzi may be as high as 12%. Angiostrongyliasis, anisakiasis, toxocarosis, and trichinosis usually do not cause death. Infection with G. spinigerum causes death in 8% of patients and neurological sequelae in 38%. The mortality associated with S. stercoralis hyperinfection syndrome is as high as 75%. Finally, the course of trematode and cestode infection depends on the stage and extent of disease.

Suggested Reading

Anonymous (1990) Exchange transfusion in *Falciparum* malaria. Lancet 1:324–325

Benach JL, Habicht GS (1981) Clinical characteristics of human babesiosis. J Infect Dis 144:481

Best H, Seitz HM (1986) Die Echinokokkus-Erkrankung des Nervensystems. Akt Neurol 13:161–164

Bia FJ, Barry M (1986) Parasitic infection of the nervous system. Neurol Clin 4:171–206

Bowen BC, Post MJD (1990) Diagnostic imaging of CNS infection and inflammation. In: Schlossberg D (ed) Infections of the nervous system. (Clinical topics in infectious disease.) Springer, Berlin Heidelberg New York, pp 315–388

Brewster DR, Kwiatkowski D, White NJ (1990) Neurological sequelae of cerebral malaria in children. Lancet 2:1039–1043

Bruce-Chwatt LJ (1985) Essential malariology, 2nd edn. Heinemann, London

Butt CG (1966) Primary amebic meningoencephalitis. N Engl J Med 274:1473–1476

Cook GC (1987) *Strongyloides stercoralis* hyperinfection syndrome: how often is it missed? Q J Med 244:625–629

Davis TME, White NJ, Looareesuwan S, Silamut K, Warrell DA (1988) Quinine pharmacokinetics in cerebral malaria: predicted plasma concentrations after rapid intravenous loading using a two-compartment model. Trans R Soc Trop Med Hyg 82:542–547

Del Brutto OH (1992) Diagnosis and management of cysticercosis. J Trop Geogr Neurol 2:1–9

Ellrodt A, Halfon P, Le Bras P, Halimi P, Bouree P, Desi M, Caquet R (1987) Multifocal central nervous system lesions in three patients with trichinosis. Arch Neurol 44:432–434

Fan KJ, Pezeshkpour GH (1986) Cerebral sparganosis. Neurology 36:1249–1251

Fröscher W, Saathof M (1986) Trichinose des Nervensystems. Akt Neurol 13:151–156

Gjerde IO, Mörk S, Larsen JL, Huldt G, Skeidsvoll H, Aarli JA (1984) Cerebral schistosomiasis presenting as a brain trumor. Eur Neurol 23:229–236

Graninger W, Thalhammer F, Locker G (1991) Pentoxifylline in cerebral malaria. J Infect Dis 164:829

Gutteridge WE (1985) Trypanosomiasis. Existing chemotherapy and its limitations. Br Med Bull 41:156–161

Higashi K, Aoki H, Takebayashi K, Movoka H, Sakata Y (1971) Cerebral paragonimiasis. J Neurosurg 34:515–528

Horowitz SL, Bentson JR, Benson F, Davos J, Gottlieb B, Pressman B (1983) Intracerebral toxoplasmosis in patients with acquired immunodeficiency syndrome. Arch Neurol 40:649–652

Horton RJ (1989) Chemotherapy of *Echinococcus* infection with albendazole. Trans R Soc Trop Med Hyg 82:97–102

Jörg ME, Freire RS, Orlando AS, Bustamante AG, Figueiredo RC, Peltier YA, Oliva R

(1972) Disfunción cerebral minima coma secuela de meningoencefalitis aguda por *Trypanosoma cruzi*. Prensa Med Argent 59:1658–1669

Kremsner PG, Grundman H, Neifer S, Sliwa K, Sahlmüller G, Hegenscheid B, Bienzle U (1991) Pentoxifylline prevents murine cerebral malaria. J Infect Dis 164:605–608

Kwiatkowski D, Molineux M, Taylor T, Klein N, Curtis N, Smit M (1991) Cerebral malaria. Lancet 1:1281–1282

Li GQ, Guo ZB, Jin H, Wang ZC, Jian HX, Li ZY (1982) Clinical studies on treatment of cerebral malaria with quinghaosu and its derivatives. J Tradit Chin Med 2:125–130

Libonatti E, Maglio F (1977) Manifestaciones neurologicas agudas en la enfermedad de Chagas-Mazza. Rev Neurol Argent 3: 420–424

Lombardo L, Alonso P, Arroyo LS, Brandt H, Mateos JH (1964) Cerebral amebiasis. Report of 17 cases. J Neurosurg 21:704–707

Looareesuwan S, Warrell DA, White NJ, Sutharasamai P, Chanthavanich P, Sundaravej K, Juel-Jensen BE, Bunnag D, Hariinasuta T (1983) Do patients with cerebral malaria have cerebral edema? A computed tomographic study. Lancet 1: 434–437

Mandell GL, Douglas RG, Bennett JE (1990) Principles and practice of infectious diseases, 3rd edn. Churchill-Livingstone, New York

Manson-Bahr PEC, Apted FIC (1991) Manson's tropical diseases, 19th edn. Baillère-Tindall, London

Marr JJ, Docampo R (1986) Chemotherapy for Chagas' disease: a perspective of current therapy and considerations for future research. Rev Infect Dis 8:884–903

Martinez AJ (1980) Is *Acanthamoeba* encephalitis an opportunistic infection? Neurology 30:567–574

Martinez AJ (1985) Free-living amebas: natural history, prevention, diagnosis, pathology and treatment of disease. CRC Press, Boca Raton

Medical letter (1988) Drugs for parasitic infections. Med Lett 30:15–24

Michal A, Regli F, Campiche R, Cavallo RJ, de Crousaz G, Oberson R, Rabinowicz T (1977) Cerebral coenurosis. Report of a case with arteritis. J Neurol 216:265–272

Molyneux ME, Taylor TE, Wirima JJ, Borgstein A (1989) Clinical features and prognostic indicators in paediatric cerebral malaria: a study of 131 comatose Malawian children. Q J Med 71:441–459

Moodley M, Moosa A (1989) Treatment of neurocysticereosis: is Praziquantel the new hope? Lancet 1:262–263

Myint PT, Shwe T, Soe L, Htut Y, Myint W (1989) Clinical study of the treatment of cerebral malaria with artemether (quinghaosu derivative). Trans R Soc Trop Med Hyg 83:72

Onyeyili PA, Onwualu JE (1991) Efficacy of combination of DFMO and diminazene aceturate in the treatment of late-stage *Trypanosoma brucei* infection in rats. Trop Med Parasitol 42:143–145

Phillips RE, Solomon T (1990) Cerebral malaria in children. Lancet 2:1355–1360

Phillips RE, Warrell DA (1986) The pathophysiology of severe *Falciparum* malaria. Parasitol Today 2:271–282

Phillips RE, Warrell DA, White NJ, Looareesuwan S, Karbwang J (1985) Intravenous quinidine for the treatment of severe falciparum malaria: clinical and pharmacokinetic studies. N Engl J Med 312:1273–1278

Pitella JEH (1984) Ischemic cerebral changes in the chronic chagasic cardiopathy. Arq Neuropsiquiatr 42:105–115

Poltera AA (1985) Pathology of human African trypanosomiasis with reference to experimental African trypanosomiasis and infections of the central nervous system. Br Med Bull 41:169–174

Punyagupta S, Juttijudata P, Bunnag T (1975) Eosinophilic meningitis in Thailand. Clinical studies of 484 typical cases probably caused by *Angiostrongylus cantonensis*. Am J Trop Med Hyg 24:921–931

Russegger L, Schmutzhard E (1989) Spinal toxocaral abscess. Lancet 2:398

Saddler M, Barry M, Ternouth I, Emmanuel J (1990) Treatment of severe malaria by exchange transfusion. N Engl J Med 322:58

Schlossberg D (1990) Infections of the nervous system. (Clinical topics in infectious disease.) Springer, Berlin Heidelberg New York

Schmutzhard E, Gerstenbrand F (1984) Cerebral malaria in Tanzania. Its epidemiology, clinical symptoms and neurological long-term sequelae in the light of 66 cases. Trans R Soc Trop Med Hyg 78:351–353

Schmutzhard E, Mayr U, Rumpl E, Prugger M, Pohl P (1986) Secondary cerebral amebiasis due to infection with *Entamoeba histolytica*. Eur Neurol 25:161–165

Schmutzhard E, Boongird P, Vejjajiva A (1988) Eosinophilic meningitis and radiculomyelitis in Thailand, caused by CNS invasion of *Gnathostoma spinigerum* and *Angiostrongylus cantonensis*. J Neurol Neurosurg Psychiatry 51:80–87

Scowden EB, Schaffner W, Stone WJ (1978) Overwhelming strongyloidiasis: an unappreciated opportunistic infection. Medicine (Baltimore) 57:527–544

Sotelo-Avila C (1987) *Naegleria* and *Acanthamoeba*. Free-living amebas pathogenic for man. Perspect Pediatr Pathol 10:51–58

Strout RG (1962) A method for concentrating hemoflagellates. Parasitol 48:100 (Research note)

Stuiver PC, Ligtheim RJ, Goud TJLM (1989) Acute psychosis after mefloquine. Lancet 2:282

Taelman H, Schaechter PJ, Marcelis L (1987) Difluoromethylornithine, an effective new treatment of Gambian trypanosomiasis. Am J Med 82:607–614

Truelle JL, Hauteville JP, Ricon P, Le Bigot P (1974) Cénurose cérébrale intraventriculaire. Nouv Press Med 1151–1153

Van Meirvenne N, Le Ray D (1985) Diagnosis of African and American trypanosomiases. Br Med Bull 41:156–161

Vazquez V, Sotelo J (1992) The course of seizures after treatment for cerebral cysticercosis. N Engl J Med 327:696–701

Warrell DA, Looareesuwan S, Warrell MJ, Kasemsarn P, Intaraprasert R, Bunnag D, Harinasuta T (1982) Dexamethasone proves deleterious in cerebral malaria. A double-blind trial in 100 comatose patients. N Engl J Med 306:313–319

Watt G, Long GW, Ranoa CP, Adapon B, Fernando MT, Cross JH (1989) Praziquantel in treatment of cerebral schistosomiasis. Lancet 2:262–263

White NJ, Looareesuwan S, Phillips RE, Chanthavomich P, Warrell DA (1988) Single-dose phenobarbitone prevents convulsions in cerebral malaria. Lancet 2:64–66

Wirima J, Khoromana C, Molyneux ME, Gilles HM (1988) Clinical trials with halofantrine hydrochloride in Malawi. Lancet 2:250–252

Wittner M, Rowin KS, Tanowitz HB, Hobbs JF, Saltzman S, Wenz B, Hvisch R, Chisholm E, Healy GR (1982) Successful chemotherapy of transfusion babesiosis. Ann Intern Med 96:601–604

Wood M, Anderson M (1988) Neurological infections. Saunders, London (Major problems in neurology, vol 16)

World Health Organization Malaria Action Programme (1986) Severe and complicated malaria. Trans R Soc Trop Med Hyg 80 [Suppl]:3–50

Chapter 50

Chronic Meningitis

ULRICH BOGDAHN and BRIGITTE WILDEMANN

Definition

Chronic meningitis causes a meningoencephalitic syndrome that may develop over weeks or even years. Abnormalities in cerebrospinal fluid (CSF) persist for more than 4 weeks. Most patients present with fatigue, headache, low-grade fever (continuous or recurrent), cranial nerve palsies and other focal deficits, seizures, and various degrees of mental alteration. Neck stiffness may be the leading symptom and papilledema may be present. Neurocritical care may be required for treatment of brain edema, hydrocephalus, seizures, vasculitis (which may cause stroke-like syndromes), difficulty in swallowing or breathing (from caudal brain stem involvement), paraplegia or hemiplegia (from spinal or radicular nerve involvement), or abscesses (subdural or epidural, central, paraspinal, or medullary).

Section Editors: Karl M. Einhäupl and Werner Hacke

Etiology and Pathogenesis

Chronic meningitis may be a primary or secondary result of many infectious and noninfectious diseases and frequently is the first clinical manifestation. Infectious causes include bacterial, viral, fungal, and parasitic infections. Noninfectious causes include autoimmune diseases, sarcoidosis, neoplasm (including paraneoplastic syndromes), and toxic disorders (Table 1). Occasionally, the cause may not be known. Predisposing factors include various exposures, depressed immune status, underlying systemic disease, and history of travel. In infectious chronic meningitis, central nervous system (CNS) involvement usually occurs by hematogenous spread (bacteria, fungi), local invasion (fungi, parasites), or along cranial nerves (viruses). Sometimes the primary disease may have occurred several months before (for example, syphilis or borreliosis) or even years before (for example, tuberculosis). CNS disease may be part of a multistage process (for example, syphilis, HIV infection, tuberculosis). Fre-

Table 1. Etiology and pathogenesis of chronic meningitis syndrome

Causative agent/pathogen	Risk group/factors	Clinical indicators
Bacterial		
Mycobacterium tuberculosis	Prior systemic exposure	Hydrocephalus, diplopia
Mycobacterium leprae	Prior systemic exposure	Skin lesions, PNS
Borrelia burgdorferi	Tick bite, open air	Erythema, radicular pain
Treponema pallidum	Exposure	Dependent upon stage
Listeria monocytogenes	Age, diabetes, neoplasia	Early impairment of consciousness
Mycoplasma	Epidemics, adolescence	"Walking" pneumonia
Legionella	Epidemics, military occupation	Pneumonia
Whipple's disease	Abdominal disease	Arthritis, parenchymal CNS lesions
Brucella	Animal contact	Lumbosacral osteomyelitis, radicular pain, PNS and CNS involvement
Ornithosis, psittacosis	Bird/animal contact	Pneumonia
Nocardia	Immunosuppression, renal transplantation	Pneumonia, subcutaneous lesions, CNS microabscess
Actinomyces	Immunosuppression, poor hygiene	Cervicofacial, abdominal, thoracic, pelvic involvement
Fungal		
Aspergillus	Immunosuppression	Pulmonary, paranasal sinus involvement, local invasion (orbit, brain)
Candida	Pregnancy, steroids, immunosuppression	Oral, mucocutaneous, GI tract symptoms, CNS abscess
Cryptococcus	AIDS, pregnancy	Pneumonia, skin lesins, CNS granuloma, hydrocephalus
Histoplasma	Endemic, AIDS, dust exposure	Pulmonary involvement, septicemia, uveitis
Coccidioides species	Endemic, dust exposure, AIDS, pregnancy	Pulmonary manifestation, hydrocephalus
Blastomyces	Male sex, endemic, dust exposure	Pulmonary and skin involvement, chest pain, anorexia
Mucormyces	Diabetes mellitus	Paranasal sinus lesion, local cavernous sinus invasion, GI tract and pulmonary manifestation
Viral		
Cytomegalovirus	AIDS, hematological neoplasms, transplants	High fever, anorexia, myalgias, retinitis, rash, lymphadenopathy
Herpes simplex virus	Immunosuppression	Bell's palsy, Mollaret's meningitis, sacral autonomic dysfunction, GBS, tansverse myelitis
Varicella zoster virus	Immunosuppression	Angiitis, myelitis, radiculitis, sacral autonomic dysfunction
Epstein-Barr virus	AIDS, epidemic	Mononucleosis, encephalitis
HIV	HIV risk groups	Concomitant disease, GBS

Table 1. *Continued*

Causative agent/pathogen	Risk group/factors	Clinical indicators
Japanese B encephalitis virus	Endemic	Rarely, meningitis
Parasites		
Cysticercus	Exposure (dog)	Calcified eye, muscle, CNS lesions, cystic lesions, hydrocephalus
Echinococcus	Exposure (canine)	CNS involvement, seizures, cystic lesions, hydrocephalus
Schistosoma	Exposure	CNS, spinal cord involvement
Paragonimus species	Exposure (crabs, crayfish)	Seizures, pseudotumor, CNS calcifications, dementia, spinal symptoms
Filaria	Exposure	CNS, seizures, pseudotumor, immune/allergic reaction, spinal cord compression
Trichinella	Exposure (meat)	Cerebral sinus thrombosis, CNS hemorrhage, seizures
Acanthamoeba	Age, immunosuppression, ocular trauma, soft contact lense	Sinus or lung involvement, CNS mass lesion
Plasmodium	Exposure	Rapid coma, retinal hemorrhage, convulsions
Toxoplasma gondii	AIDS, congenital, pregnancy	CNS mass lesion, GBS, ocular involvement
Trypanosoma	Exposure (American/Chagas' disease; African sleeping sickness)	CNS embolism (stroke), parkinsonian symptoms, chorea, fasciculations, ataxia
Autoimmune		
Connective tissue disease	Concomitant	Cerebritis, embolism from endocarditis
Systemic vasculitis	Concomitant	CNS lesions, seizures, PNS involvement
Isolated CNS vasculitis	Concomitant	Systemic features absent
Behçet's disease	Concomitant	Pseudotumor, sinus vein thrombosis, multifocal and psychiatric symptoms
Vogt-Koyanagi and Harada syndromes	Unknown	Uveiitis, deafness, vitiligo
Sarcoidosis	Unknown	CNS and PNS involvement, psychiatric symptoms, optic and other cranial nerve palsies
Neoplastic, paraneoplastic		
Neoplasia	Hematological, ovarian, oat cell, testicular, thyroid, breast or renal tumors melanoma, lymphoma	Seizures, cranial nerve palsies
Paraneoplasia	Oat cell, ovarian tumors	Dementia, limbic encephalitis

Table 1. *Continued*

Causative agent/pathogen	Risk group/factors	Clinical indicators
Toxic/chemical		
Drugs	Nonsteroid anti-inflammatory drugs	Psychosis, cognitive dysfunction
Chemical	Neuroepithelial cyst, epidermoid, dermoid, craniopharyngioma, ependymoma. Intrathecal drugs, contrast material	CNS lesions, severe headaches, seizures

CNS, Central nervous system; GBS, Gruillan-Barré syndrome; GI, gastrointestinal; PNS, peripheral nerve system.

quently, the first clinical symptoms are from CNS disease.

Clinical Features

Patients with chronic meningitis usually present with dull headaches (occipital more than frontal). There usually is no circadian rhythm. Patients may be slightly confused and nauseated, and may have a low-grade fever. Muscle cramps are also occasionally reported. Cranial nerve palsies are common and result in diplopia, impaired conjugate eye movements, impaired accommodation, facial muscle weakness, and difficulty swallowing. Papilledema may be present. Some patients may develop neuropsychological symptoms or dementia. Frequently consciousness may be only mildly impaired if at all.

Diagnosis

Once the diagnosis of meningitis is made, the underlying cause should be determined. All patients should be evaluated for underlying systemic disease. Physical examination should focus on lymph nodes, liver and spleen size, skin changes, and ophthalmological findings. Diagnostic studies include CSF analysis, special laboratory tests (Table 2), neuroimaging studies, and other ancillary tests. Among these, CSF analysis and neuroimaging are the most important.

Cerebrospinal Fluid and Other Laboratory Tests

Analysis of CSF cell count, glucose and protein concentration, and cytology should be performed. In general, polymorphonuclear pleocytosis is seen in patients with bacterial meningitis and early fungal infections. A lymphocytic or plasmacellular pleocytosis is found in patients with borreliosis and viral meningitis. A mixed polymorphonuclear and mononuclear pleocytosis is typical for meningitis caused by brucellosis, actinomycosis, tuberculosis, leprosy, and syphilis. CSF eosinophilia characteristically occurs with tuberculous, fungal, parasitic (particularly helminthic) infections or with malignancies (especially lymphomas) and sarcoidosis. High protein concentrations are seen with tuberculosis, sarcoidosis, borreliosis, and some fungal infections. Extremely low glucose concentrations are seen with tuberculous and sarcoid meningitis. The CSF should be stained with periodic acid–Schiff (PAS) reagent, Gram's stain, and India ink stain. Other studies that may be important include measurement of CSF immunoglobulins (IgG, IgM, IgA), angiotensin converting enzyme, and β_2-microglobulin.

Routine laboratory tests, although often nonspecific, should include complete blood count, erythrocyte sedimentation rate, electrolytes, liver injury tests, blood urea nitrogen and creatinine measurement, coagulation tests, serum protein electrophoresis, antinuclear antibody, angiotensin converting enzyme, and specific serologies. Cultures should be taken from blood, sputum, urine, gastric washings, and stool and should be repeated several times. The recommended tests for each disorder are summarized in Table 2.

Neuroimaging and Other Ancillary Tests

Computed tomography and magnetic resonance imaging (MRI) can show parenchymal involvement, characteristic distribution of lesions (for example, cysticercosis), brain edema, hydrocephalus, space-occupying lesions, or brain abscesses. MRI with gadolinium may show enhancement of meninges.

On electroencephalography, generalized slow wave activity can sometimes be seen as well as focal or diffuse seizure activity. Transcranial Doppler ultrasonography can be useful in detecting vasculitis. Nuclear medicine leukocyte scans may also be helpful in localizing primary lesions suitable for biopsy.

All suspicious lesions should be biopsed whenever possible. Extracranial sites should be biopsied first except in patients with progressive neurological deterioration, in whom brain or meningeal biopsies should be done. Bone marrow aspiration is frequently nondiagnostic, but may be helpful when leukemic or lymphomatous meningitis is a possibility (Table 2).

Treatment

Table 2 lists general recommendations for treatment (given the multiple causes of chronic meningitis, only general recommendations are given. Specific therapies are reviewed in Chaps. 42, 48, and 49). An interdisciplinary approach is recommended *early* in the course of the disease, involving mainly specialists in infectious disease and oncology. Surgical intervention may be necessary for drainage and extirpation of brain abscesses or for external ventricular drainage in patients with hydrocephalus. Corticosteroids should be given to patients with hydrocephalus from basal granulomatous meningitis or vasculitis. Because of allergic reactions, corticosteroids may be required with treatment of parasitic or syphilitic meningitis. Treatment of brain edema is reviewed in Chap. 9. Antiseizure medications may be necessary for control of seizures.

Table 2. Diagnosis and treatment of chronic meningitis syndrome

Cause	Diagnostic test	Treatment
Bacterial		
Mycobacterium tuberculosis	Stain, culture, PCR, ELISA	INH, RIFA, pyrazinamide, ethambutol, i.t. streptomycin, ventricular shunt
Mycobacterium leprae	Stain, biopsy, serology	Dapsone, RIFA
Borrelia burgdorferi	Serology, immunoblot, PCR	Penicillin, cephalosporin
Treponema pallidum	Serology	Penicillin, erythromycin
Listeria monocytogenes	Culture, serology	Penicillin, ampicillin, erythromycin
Mycoplasma	Isolation, CBR, NBA, WBA, cold agglutinins	Erythromycin
Legionella	Culture, DFA/IFA, NBA	Erythromycin, ciprofloxacin
Whipple's disease	Intestine biopsy, PCR	Trimethoprim, sulfamethoxazole
Ornithosis, psittacosis	Serology, group antigen	Erythromycin, chloramphenicol
Brucella	Isolation, serology, IgM	Trimethoprim, sulfamethoxazole, RIFA, abscess drainage
Nocardia	Culture, stain, histology	Trimethoprim, sulfamethoxazole, surgery
Actinomyces	Culture, histology	Penicillin G, surgery
Fungal		
Aspergillus	Biopsy, culture	Surgery, amphotericin B, flucytosine
Candida	Culture, stain, biopsy	Amphotericin B, flucytosine, fluconazole
Cryptococcus	Capsular Ag-LA biopsy, India ink stain	AIDS: amphotericin B + flucytosine, fluconazole
Histoplasma	Culture, biopsy, CF	Ketoconazole, amphotericin B
Coccidioides species	Culture, (cave), serology	Amphotericin B, fluconazole, surgery
Blastomyces	Culture, histology	Amphotericin B, ketoconazole, fluconazole?
Mucormyces	Biopsy, histology culture	Extensive surgery, amphotericin B, antidiabetics, tapering of immunosuppression
Auto-immune		
Connective tissue disease	Systemic disorder	Steroids, other immuno-suppressants, symptomatic
CNS vasculitis	Biopsy, serology	Cyclophosphamide, steroids
Behçet's disease	Biopsy, clinical features	Steroids, chlorambucil, azathioprine, cyclophosphamide, (cyclosporin A)
Vogt-Koyanagi and Harada syndromes	Clinical features	Steroids?
Sarcoidosis	Angiotensin converting enzyme, biopsy	Steriods (systemic + i.t.)

WBA, Western blot analysis; IHA, indirect hemagglutination; ELISA, enzyme-linked immunosorbent assay; IFA, indirect immunofluorescent assay; NBA, Northern blot analysis; CBR, complement binding reaction; PCR, polymerase chain reaction; DFA, direct fluorescent antibody test; CF, complement fixation; SFDT, Sabin Feldman dye test; LA, latex agglutination test; i.t., intrathecal.

If the cause of chronic meningitis remains unknown despite an extensive evaluation, symptomatic treatment of the inflammatory process is indicated. We recommend intrathecal corticosteroids (for example, 80 mg triam cinolone acetonide twice or three times a week). Each new CSF sample should analyzed as fungal, tuberculous, and sarcoid meningitis can often be diagnosed this way. If intrathecal corticosteroids are not effective, local cytosine arabinoside (40–80 mg) made be used twice weekly (cytarabine, Alexan). With this approach, either the diagnosis will be made because of exacerbation of CSF findings, or the inflammatory process will be suppressed.

Suggested Reading

Bacterial Chronic Meningitis

Jacobs RF, Sunakorn P et al. (1991) Intensive short course chemotherapy for tuberculous meningitis. Ped Inf Dis HJ 11:194–198

Krishnan VV, Mathai A (1991) ELISA to detect Mycobacterium tuberculosis antigen 5 and antimycobacterial antibody in CSF of patients with tuborculous meningitis. J Clin Lab Anal 5:233–237

Gourie DM, Satishchandra P (1991) Hyaluronidase as an adjuvant in the management of tuberculous spinal arachnoiditis. J Neurol Sci 102:105–111

Jaton K, Sahli R, Bille J (1992) Development of PCR assays for detection og Listeria monocytogenes in clinical CSF samples. J Clin Microbiol 30:1931–1936

Skogberg K, Syrjanen J, Jahkola M, Ronkonen OV et al. (1992) Clinical presentation and outcome of listeriosis in patients with and without immunosuppressive therapy. Clin Inf Dis 14:815–821

Narita M, Matsuzono Y et al. (1992) DNA-Diagnosis of CNS infection by Mycoplasma pneumoniae. Pediatrics 90:250–253

Michel D, Antoine JC et al. (1992) Lumbosacral meningoradiculitis associated with Chlamydia pneumonia infection. J Neurol Neurosurg Psychiatry 55:511

Chlamydia pneumonia infection.

Fungal Chronic Meningitis

Saag MS et al. (1992) Comparison of amphotericin B with fluconazole in the treatment of acute AIDS-associated cryptococcal meningitis. N Engl J Med 326:83–89

Pruit AA (1991) Central nervous system infections in cancer patients. Neurol Clin 9:867–888

Hutchinson DO et al. (1991) Cryptococcal meningitis in Auckland 1969–1989. N Z M J 104: 57–59

Bozette SA et al. (1991) A placebo controlled trial of maintenance therapy with fluconazole after treatment of cryptococcal meningitis in AIDS. J Engl J Med 324: 580–584

Allendoorfer R, Marquis AJ, Rinaldi MG et al. (1991) Combined therapy with fluconazole and flucytosine in murine cryptococcal meningitis. Antimicrob Agents Chemotherapy 85:726

Le Conte P et al. (1992) Tissue distribution and antifungal effect of liposomal intraconazole in experimental cryptococcosis and pulmonary aspergillosis. Am Rev Respir Dis 145:424–429

Fisher EW, Toma A, Fisher PH et al. (1991) Rhinocerebral Mucormycosis: Use of liposomal amphotericin B. J Laryngol Otol 105:575–577

Pearson GJ, Chin TW, Fong IW (1992) Treatment of Blastomycosis with fluconazole. Am J Med Sci 303:313–315

Bradsher RW, Blastomycosis (1992) Clin Inf Dis 14[Suppl]: S82–90

Williams PL, Johnson R, Pappagianis D, Einstein II et al. (1992) Vasculitis and encephalitis complications associated with Coccidioides immites infection of the CNS in humans. Clin Inf Dis 14:673–682

Wrobel CJ, Rothrock J (1992) Coccidioidomycosis meningitis presenting as anterior spinal artery sysndrome. Neurology 42: 1840

Wrobel CJ et al. (1992) MR findings in acute and chronic coccidioidomycosis meningitis. AJNR 13:1241

Thaboshi I, Casas Parera I et al. (1992) Chronic Histoplasma capsulatum infection of the CNS successfully treated with fluconazole. Europ Neurol 32:70–73

Hostetler JS, Denning DW, Stevens DA (1992) US experience with itraconazole in Aspergillus, Cryptococcus and Histoplasma infections in the immunocompromised host. Chemotherapy 38[Suppl. 1]:12–22

Lyman CA, Walsh TJ (1992) Systomically administered antifungal agents. A review of their clinical pharmacology and therapeutic applications. Drugs 44:9–35

Viral Chronic Meningitis

Rotbart HA (1991) Viral Meningitis and the Aseptic Meningitis Syndrome. In: Scheld W.M. et al. (eds) Infections of the Central Nervous System, Raven Press 19–31

Parasitic Chronic Meningitis

Overbosch D (1992) Neurocysticercosis. An over-view. Schweiz Med Wschr 122:893–898

Luft BJ, Hafner R (1990) Toxoplasmosis encephalitis. AIDS 4:593–595

Ma R, Visvesvara GS, Martinez AJ et al. (1990) Naegleria and Acanthamoeba infections: review. Rev Inf Dis 12:490–513

Joubert J, Jenni WK (1990) Treatment of Neurocysticercosis. S Afr Med J 77:27–30

Autoimmune Chronic Meningitis

Wakefield D et al. (1990) Cyclosporin therapy in Vogt Koyanagi Syndrome. Aust N Z J Ophthalmol 18:137–142

Sasamoto Y, Ohno S, Matsuda H (1990) Studies on corticosteroid therapy in Vogt Koyanagi syndrome. Ophthalmoligica 201:162–167

Gille M et al. (1990) Neurological involvement as manifestation of Beheet's disease. Acta neurol Belg 90:233–247

Idiopathic/Toxic

Okazaki H et al. (1990) A case of mixed connective tissue disease exacerbated by griseofulvin complicating aseptic meningitis. Ryumachi 30:418–423

Chapelon Z et al. (1990) Neurosarcoidosis, signs, course and treatment in 35 confirmed cases. Med Baltimore 69:261–276

Neoplastic

Phillips ME, Ryals TJ et al. (1990) Neoplastic vs inflammatory meningeal enhancement with Gd-DTPA. J Comp Ass Tomogr 14:536–541

Stroke

Chapter 51

General Therapy of Acute Ischemic Stroke

Thomas Brott, Cesare Fieschi, and Werner Hacke

Introduction

Precise strategies of therapeutic management following acute cerebrovascular occlusion are still lacking. Earlier therapeutic studies have had major methodological limitations, and in most instances patients have been treated too late. In addition, since many of the studies were planned and performed in the pre-computed tomography (CT) era, different subtypes of stroke could not be accurately distinguished. Even in the last decade, studies have been performed in which no CT was required and patients were entered into the study 24 h after stroke onset or even later. Today most stroke investigators agree that the optimal time window for treatment of patients with acute brain infarction is less than 8 h, perhaps less than 2 h in some cases. Enthusiasm for immediate treatment has developed during the past few years, including enthusiasm for an intensive care unit (ICU)-type management approach for selected subtypes of acute stroke.

Given this changing environment and the completion of several encouraging pilot therapy studies, we can anticipate practical therapeutic advances in three areas over the coming decade. The first is that of restoring blood flow to the focally ischemic brain by acute arterial recanalization. The second area is that of neuronal protection, developing medical therapies that slow the metabolic clock, widening the window of opportunity for arterial recanalization. The third area of advance will be urgent stroke treatment delivery: that is, development of specific techniques for faster recognition of symptoms by patient and family, international development of a trauma-like approach to stroke patient transport to hospital, and development within hospitals of an "every minute counts" approach to treatment administration. In anticipation of these improvements in specific therapy for ischemic stroke, we describe an intensive-care approach to diagnosis and general management.

Critical care management of acute stroke requires parallel processes at different levels of patient management. For example, acute assessment

Section Editor: Werner Hacke

of neurological and vital functions is performed while treatment for acutely endangering conditions is going on. The selection of special treatment strategies may already be under way before the final decision as to the subtype of acute ischemic stroke has been made. The time factor is important, especially during the first minutes and hours of stroke, so speed and rapid decision making may be required. For the first hours and days after onset of symptoms, the manifestations of the stroke and its primary complications are the paramount considerations in management. As the end of the first week approaches, treatment of secondary complications becomes more important. Those complications usually do not develop without some warning, so measures can be taken without the pressure of time present during the first hours after stroke. Special management problems such as treatment of hypertension may occur several times during different stages of the patient's management and are addressed in the context of both the first hours and the later hospital course.

One of the major problems in early treatment of acute stroke victims is to distinguish patients who need immediate ICU treatment from those who can be managed less aggressively. The overall mortality in acute ischemic stroke as assessed in large neurological data banks is somewhere between 12% and 20%, which indicates that the degree of acuity or severity is comparable to that in myocardial infarction. Not all patients are candidates for ICU management (Table 1). In the Heidelberg stroke data base, approximately 1200 patients a year are admitted with acute ischemic stroke. Out of 800 patients who are managed by the

Table 1. Potential indications for admission to intensive care following cerebral infarction

Neurological indications
Progressing symptoms, crescendo transient ischemic attacks
Fluctuating, hemodynamically induced infarction
Embolic intracranial internal carotid/middle cerebral artery occlusion
Multiple emboli
Septic emboli and unstable endocarditis
Elevated intracranial pressure
Arterial dissection plus embolism
Proposed thrombolytic therapy
Proposed hypervolemic therapy

Systemic indications
Multimorbidity
Serious cardiac arrhythmias
Concurrent myocardial infarction
Septic endocarditis
Hypertensive crisis
Severe hypotension
Sepsis, aspiration pneumonia
Severe dehydration
Renal failure
Electrolyte disturbances
Endocrine crisis

Department of Neurology, 135 are judged to require management in the neurocritical care unit, representing approximately 10% of all hospitalized acute stroke victims. A much higher percentage of patients with selected subtypes of stroke may benefit from ICU-type management, such as those with acute basilar thrombosis, acute proximal middle cerebral artery embolism, or cerebellar infarction.

Initial Resuscitation

During the first minutes after symptom onset, the stroke patient should be regarded as a seriously ill medical patient without an established diagnosis. Once the patient has been transported to the emergency department, the examining physician should first assess the ischemic stroke patient as having a potentially life-threatening illness, with emphasis on the ABC of resuscitation (i.e., airway, breathing, circulation). The brief medical and neurologic examination has been discussed in Chap. 1.

The ischemic stroke patient usually has a stable airway. In our experience with thrombolytic therapy and other urgent interventions, we evaluated patients within the first minutes and hours following symptom onset and have encountered the problem of a threatened airway only in the rare patient with extensive vertebrobasilar distribution infarction, or in patients with very large middle cerebral distribution infarction, hemispheric or brainstem hemorrhage, or sustained seizure activity. In those instances, endotracheal *intubation* should be carried out by an appropriately skilled and experienced physician. In the event of a pathological respiratory pattern, severe hypoxemia, or hypercarbia, and in the unconscious patient with high risk for aspiration pneumonia, early endotracheal intubation is also recommended. There are several methods for insertion of an endotracheal tube. In the emergency situation, the orotracheal method is preferred after induction of general anesthesia, if the hemodynamic status allows. The orotracheal method provides rapid control of the airway, blunts the stress response to manipulating the airway, and facilitates hyperventilation. Blind nasal and fiberoptic-guided intubations are easily performed in the spontaneously ventilating patient. Chronic nasotracheal intubation may

be more tolerable for the patient and makes nursing care of the mouth easier but carries a higher risk of inflammation of the paranasal sinuses. Because of this, most prefer transoral endotracheal intubation for the first few days.

In the great majority of stroke patients, ventilatory function is stable at the time of first evaluation by prehospital care personnel and usually remains stable throughout the time of evaluation in the emergency department. Acute airway disease is occasionally present but tends to be mild, most often in the form of slightly exacerbated chronic obstructive airway disease. Patients with asthma may have a modest increase in symptoms or signs of bronchospasm. Stroke usually occurs in the elderly, and elderly patients have lowered ventilatory reserve. Aging of the lungs, including loss of elasticity and increased physiologic shunting, results in declining mean arterial PO_2 with each decade, such that the PO_2 is usually in the 70–80 mmHg range in those over the age of 65 years. Advancing age is associated with a progressive reduction in cerebral homeostatic response to change in ventilatory function. Stroke patients have lower inspiratory power than normal subjects, and they have an impaired response to increases in airway resistance. In addition, ventilation may be particularly compromised during sleep in normal subjects and may be compromised even more in stroke patients.

When arterial blood gases are measured, the stroke patient's high oxygen saturations ($\geq 90\%$) may be misleading. The patient was likely aroused during arterial blood sampling. More important, peripheral oxygen saturation of 90% may not accurately reflect conditions within the brain, particularly within the deep white matter. Experimentally, the PO_2 in the deep cerebral hemisphere of dogs has been measured at mean of 10 mmHg and the PCO_2 at a mean of 68 mmHg under conditions in which the peripheral mean PO_2 was 81 mmHg and the mean peripheral PCO_2 was 43 mmHg. Following administration of 100% oxygen, increases in the cerebral PO_2 to a mean of 41 mmHg and decreases in the cerebral PCO_2 to a mean of 61 mmHg occurred. These dramatic changes were not reflected by significant changes in peripheral oxygen saturation. Unfortunately, measurements of oxygen concentration within the brain have not been performed in stroke patients. Future studies should address the plausible hypothesis that modest abnormalities in oxygen or carbon dioxide concentration measured peripherally may reflect significant abnormalities within cerebral tissue, particularly in the deep white matter.

Therefore, because of what very well may be a lowered reserve with respect to cerebral oxygenation and overall ventilatory function, we recommend that stroke patients be treated with supplementary oxygen, favoring 2–4 l/min via nasal prongs. Using this form of supportive therapy over the last 15 years, we have not had any significant complications (e.g., CO_2 retention in patients with chronic obstructive pulmonary disease).

Heart failure is an uncommon complication of stroke within the first few hours after symptom onset. Nonetheless, the physician must carefully rule out the presence of acute myocardial infarction, atrial fibrillation associated with an inappropriately accelerated ventricular response, or significant valvular disease. Each of these disorders may predispose to stroke, each may complicate stroke, and each may diminish cardiac function. If clinical heart failure is present, immediate treatment is indicated. Accordingly, the cardiac examination of the stroke patient should include attention to the presence of tachypnea, tachycardia, jugular venous distention, peripheral edema, rales, or a third heart sound. If any symptoms or signs suggest the possibility of heart failure, an emergency chest radiograph should be performed. Subsequent treatment measures should avoid intravascular volume contraction when feasible. Drops in systemic blood pressure should be minimized. Among the inotropic agents, dobutamine has the advantage of increasing cardiac output without substantially affecting either heart rate or blood pressure. Dopamine may be particularly useful in patients with relative hypotension. Augmentation of cardiac output has already been shown experimentally to result in modest increases in regional cerebral blood flow. In human stroke, autoregulation is impaired and so systemic increases in cardiac output may well increase cerebral perfusion in tissues which have been rendered pressure passive by acute ischemia.

Antihypertensive treatment in the ICU will be discussed below and in detail in a later paragraph. In the emergency department setting, antihypertensive drugs are best used sparingly. Drops in mean arterial blood pressure may directly reduce local cerebral blood flow (CBF) within the area of infarction. In chronically hypertensive patients with stroke, such reductions in CBF may be accentuated as the autoregulatory curve has likely been shifted to the right. Antihypertensive therapy should be used only if specific indications are present such as acute myocardial ischemia or infarction, heart failure, selected instances of acute renal failure, acute hypertensive encephalopathy, or hemorrhagic stroke shown by CT.

Management During the First Hour of Stroke

After the stroke patient has been medically stabilized with regard to airway, breathing, and circulation, a more careful history-taking and neurological examination may proceed.

An eyewitness description of the stroke onset should be sought because the history provided by the patient is frequently incomplete or inaccurate. The neurological investigator should identify any risk factors present and should seek unusual causes for stroke such as arterial dissection, venous thrombosis, illicit drug use, or severe medical illness such as hyperosmolar coma. The initial physical examination should include several measurements of blood pressure and heart rate, careful cardiac examination to supplement the brief cardiac examination performed earlier, neurovascular examination, examination for signs of trauma, and neurological examination.

After the emergency assessment, which will in part be done by emergency nurses or other staff (Table 2), the neurologist will perform a brief and focused neurological examination. During this examination, those neurological tests which are not crucial for the decision-making process may be omitted. The neurological examination will be described for the awake and the unconscious patient separately.

The Awake Patient (Table 3)

If the patient is conscious, the physician will obtain the current and past medical history and will ask simple questions regarding orientation. The patient's responses will allow assessment of cognitive function and aphasia. If the questions are answered correctly, the answers will be used to obtain information about the time of onset and the mode of onset of symptoms. The conscious patient will be asked whether any pain was experienced in connection with symptom onset. He or she will be asked to demonstrate movements of the face as well as movements of the upper and lower extremities, allowing assessment of the grade of paresis in the arms, hands, and fingers. The visual fields, the oculomotor functions, and other cranial nerve functions should be tested. Sensory functions in the face, arms, and legs should be tested, and cerebellar function should be assessed. Particularly important is testing for neck stiffness, including Lasègue's and Brudzinski's signs, and assessment of the breathing patterns. The blood pressure should be examined in both arms, the heart should be auscultated, and signs of heart failure such as a third heart sound, pulmonary rales, and distal edema should be sought.

The Unconscious Patient (Table 4)

With the unconscious patient, the grade of impaired consciousness is

Table 2. Emergency assessment of an acute stroke patient: vital signs

Variable	How to test; signs and symptoms	Actions to be taken
Respiration	Arrest? Disturbed breathing Low PO_2 Signs of aspiration pneumonia	Resuscitation, intubation O_2 administration Ventilation Nasogastric tube Antibiotics
Cardiac function	Arrest Arrhythmia Murmur Low output	Resuscitation Defibrillation Treat arrhythmia and give volume

Blood pressure	Elevated pressure
	
	 Hypertensive crisis
	
	 Low pressure
		None if <220 mmHg
		   systolic or 120 mmHg
		   diastolic
		 Give intravenous
		   labetalol or oral
		   nifedipine
		 Volume expanders
		 Dopamine, dobutamine

Metabolism	Obvious dehydration
	
	 Hyperglycemia
		Draw blood for
		   electrolyte analysis
		 Give volume
		 If blood glucose
		   >200 mg/100 ml give
		   insulin

Signs of elevated
   bleeding risk
	Petechiae,
	   ecchymoses
		Check complete blood
		   count, prothrombin
		   and partial
		   thromboplastin times

Vigilance	Reaction to verbal or
	   physiological
	   stimuli:
	 Yes → Table 3
	 No → Table 4	

estimated according to the best reaction to verbal, tactile, or painful stimuli. The latter are applied to the face, especially to the septum of the nose, the skin of the proximal arms, the nail beds, and the legs, both proximally and distally. The reactions to painful stimuli are observed carefully with respect to motor response on both the stimulated and the contra-lateral side, a maneuver which occasionally allows the identification of hemiparesis or hemisensory loss. The size of the pupils and the pupillary responses can then be assessed. Then the examiner can bring a hand under the patient's occiput and test for neck stiffness. Using the same position with the patient's eyes held open, the vertical oculocephalic response can be

Table 3. Emergency assessment of an acute stroke patient: the awake patient

Variable	How to test
Orientation and higher cortical functions	Space, time, person: where? when? who?
Speech	Spontaneous speech; commands Fluent Nonfluent Global aphasia
Neglect, extinct	Give simultaneous optical and tactile stimuli

Motor function and paresis	Test motor functions of arm, hand, hip, and leg (against resistance or gravity)
	Describe paresis according to:
	  severity
	  distribution
	  able to walk?
	  able to stand?
	Describe abnormal movements and seizure activity

Oculomotor	Visual field test using finger perimetry Spontaneous gaze? Gaze deviation? Gaze deviation? Pupillary reflexes Describe nystagmus, if present
Caudal cranial nerves	Test swallowing and tongue movement Dysarthria Meningism
Neck stiffness	Lasegue's and Brudzinski's signs
Sensory function	Test sensory function of face, arm, hand, leg Check for dissociated sensory loss Repeat test for neglect or extinction
Cerebellar function	Finger-nose and finger-finger tests Heel-knee test Able to stand? Cerebellar tremor?

tested. After moving the hand to the bregma, the examiner can test the horizontal oculocephalic response after carefully watching for spontaneous eye movements. With assessment of the corneal reflexes, the examiner may also be able to judge the presence or absence of facial weakness. The breathing pattern which has already been observed will now be documented, examining carefully for specific respiratory patterns and noting any spontaneous movements.

If relatives of the patient are present, they will be questioned regarding stroke risk factors, previous stroke, medications, previous disabilities, and other factors that might be important for management.

Table 4. Emergency assessment of an acute stroke patient: the unconscious patient

Variable	Symptoms	How to test
Vigilance	Somnolence	Best reaction to painful stimuli
		Able to wake up shortly; defense movements
	Coma	Brainstem-motor patterns (flexor, extensor)
	Confusion	Pupil size and responses
Neck stiffness		Meningismus; opisthotonus (may be lost in deep coma)
Brainstem function	Gaze	Head/gaze deviation
	Reflexes	Oculocephalic response
		Gag reflex
	Respiration	Ataxic
		Cheyne-Stokes
		Machine-like
Motor function and spontaneous movements		Muscle tone, posture
		Reaction to painful stimuli
		Brainstem patterns
		Flexor patterns
		Extensor patterns
		Pyramidal signs
Symptoms and signs of elevated intracranial pressure		Dilated, anisocoric pupils
Sensory function		Can be assessed during motor function examination (reaction to painful stimuli)

Urgent Neuroradiological Studies

Following the assessment by history and examination, assessment aimed at a specific diagnosis may proceed. CT should be performed as an emergency procedure to distinguish ischemic infarction from intracerebral hemorrhage (Fig. 1). It is important to make this distinction as soon as possible, since management of blood pressure, choice of intravenous fluids, and specific treatment (e.g., surgery) will vary depending on whether the stroke is ischemic or hemorrhagic. In this setting CT is still preferable to magnetic resonance imaging (MRI), since many patients studied in the first hour are acutely ill, often confused, and occasionally agitated.

In ischemic stroke, the emergency CT scan may suggest a particular type of cerebral infarction. For example, a history of pure motor hemiparesis may be associated with the CT finding of a small area of low attenuation within the posterior limb of the contralateral internal capsule, suggesting a small vessel occlusion. The CT scan from another patient may reveal prior infarctions in the distribution of the suspect intracranial artery, suggesting proximal large vessel disease. Alternatively, the CT scan may show prior cerebral infarctions in several arterial distributions, leading suspicion to cardiac embolization or subcortical microvascular disease.

Careful inspection of CT scans performed in the first hours after

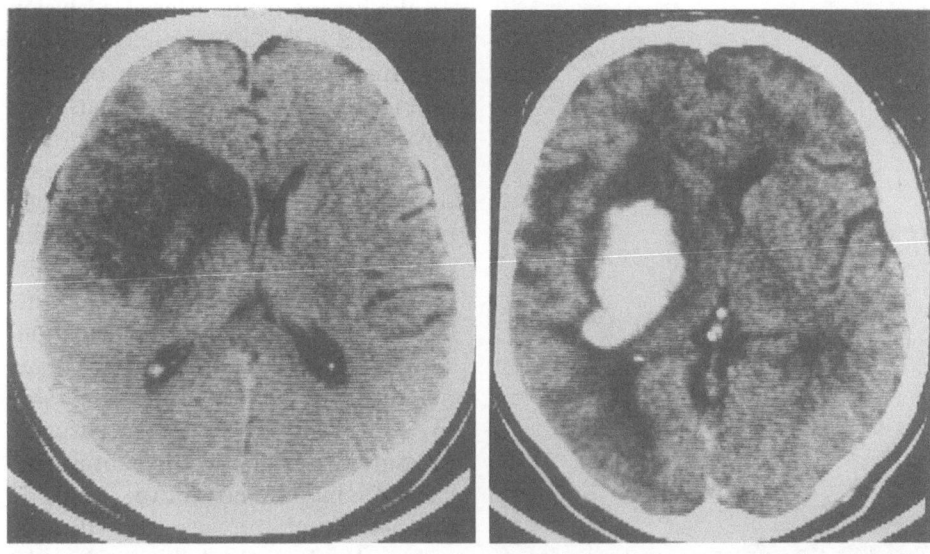

Fig. 1. a Right hemispheric medium-sized basal ganglia hemorrhage and **b** territorial middle cerebral artery infarction (partial) on the right side. Both types of stroke may present clinically with the identical syndrome, i.e. dense left hemiparesis, drowsiness, forced eye or head deviation, and gaze palsy

symptom onset may allow localization of acute thrombi. Punctate or linear foci of increased attenuation, corresponding to the locations of the larger intracranial arteries, frequently signify the presence of intraluminal thrombus (Fig. 2). This radiographic sign, the hyperdense artery sign, is detected in fewer than 5% of patients studied several days to several months after stroke onset. However, in the National Institutes of Health pilot study of tissue plasminogen activator, the hyperdense artery sign was present in the middle cerebral artery in 18 of the first 55 patients examined within 90 min by CT (33%). In a larger study of 272 unselected patients examined by CT within 12 h of cerebral infarction onset, the hyperdense sign was identified in 27% of all patients and in 41% of those with middle cerebral artery distribution infarction. In the Heidelberg stroke data base, more than 85% of patients exhibiting the hyperdense artery sign on CT showed occlusion of the suspected vessel by cerebral arteriography. Thrombi may be identified at a variety of sites, including the internal carotid terminus, the middle cerebral stem, the primary branches of the middle cerebral artery stem, the posterior cerebral artery, and the basilar artery. Bastianello et al. (1991) conclude from their studies that there is a close relation between the presence of the hyperdense artery sign and early CT hypodensity when the sign is identified within the middle cerebral artery stem. They further state that both signs, the hyperdense artery and early CT hypodensity, are early indicators of brain injury, predicting development of hemorrhagic infarction and of late brain damage. Limitations of this sign will continue to include its limited

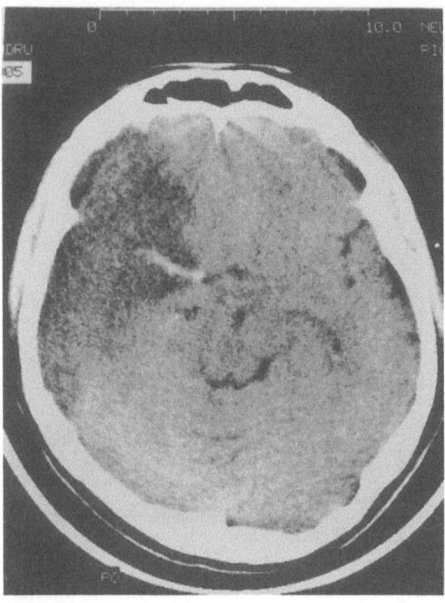

Fig. 2. The linear snake-like zone of increased attenuation can be seen in the expected location of the right middle cerebral artery, signifying the presence of intraluminal thrombus. The computed tomographic scan was performed approximately 12 hours after the onset of acute left hemiplegia and dense left hemisensory loss which were associated with forced deviation of the eyes to the right and left-sided neglect. Subsequent cerebral arteriography demonstrated occlusion of the distal right internal carotid artery and occlusion of the M1 segment of the right middle cerebral artery

sensitivity and specificity. False positives become problematic in patients with calcified vessels, particularly in relation to the internal carotid and basilar artery sites.

Management of Hypertension

Any therapy, whether surgical or medical, should be assessed critically and should be given only for specific indications.

Following acute arterial occlusion within the brain, experimental studies and human studies with positron emission tomography indicate that an early physiologic response is an increase in cerebral blood volume. This increase reflects vasodilatation within the bed of ischemic cerebral tissue. With this compensatory vasodilatation, the ischemic tissue has exhausted its capacity for further autoregulation. Accordingly, the ischemic brain tissue may be considerably more vulnerable to reductions in systemic perfusion pressure than nonischemic brain tissue. As mentioned above, drops in arterial blood pressure may directly reduce local cerebral flow within the area of infarction and to the penumbra, particularly in the elderly or in patients with chronic hypertension.

In the first hours after stroke onset, as many as 70% of patients may present with a blood pressure of 170/100 mmHg or higher, and approximately 50% of patients present with a history of pre-existing hypertension. Increases in adrenergic tone have been documented in the setting of acute stroke and such increases in adrenergic tone may explain in part the acute elevations in arterial blood pressure. They may also explain why many acute elevations in blood pressure may resolve spontaneously, without medical treatment. In the National Institutes of Health pilot study of tissue plasminogen activator for stroke, 29 of 74 patients (39%) had an initial systolic blood pressure of more than 160 mmHg. From the time of the initial blood pressure measurement to the time of treatment (<90 min), 27 of those 29 (93%) underwent a decline in systolic blood pressure. The mean decline was 28 mmHg. Of the 41 patients who had an initial diastolic blood pressure greater than 90 mmHg, 34 (83%) had a decline in diastolic pressure by the time of treatment. The mean decline was 14 mmHg. These rapid (<90 min) and spontaneous declines have two important implications. First, antihypertensive therapy is usually unnecessary if treating physicians are willing to defer therapy. Second, and more important, antihypertensive therapy administered in the first hour may be dangerous. The effects of antihypertensive medication superimposed upon a spontaneous blood decline in pressure could result in rapid induction of a relatively hypotensive state. For the stroke patient, slower and less substantial reductions are preferred.

If antihypertensive therapy is necessary, several options are available (Table 5). Labetalol may be useful. Its intravenous administration and rapid onset of effect allow the antihypertensive effects to be judged quickly. Labetalol blocks α- and β-adrenergic receptors and so matches well pathophysiologically with the increases in adrenergic tone. Labetalol also reduces

Table 5. Antihypertensive treatment in acute ischemic stroke

Cincinnati regimen (Brott and McCarthy 1989)
1. Systolic BP 180–230 mmHg[a]   Do not treat
   and/or diastolic
   <120 mmHg
2. Diastolic BP > 140 mmHg,   (a) Sodium nitroprusside 2 μg/kg per min, may be repeated with
   systolic BP slightly increased   double dose after 3–5 min
   on repeated measurements
   5 min apart
3. Systolic BP > 230 mmHg or   (a) Labetalol 10 mg i.v., may be repeated with double dose
   diastolic BP 120–140 mmHg   after 10 min as needed to max 160 mg[b]
   or both, on repeated   (b) Nifedipine 10 mg sublingually
   measurements 20 min apart

Heidelberg regimen (Hacke et al. 1990)
1. Systolic BP < 200 mmHg,   Do not treat
   diastolic BP < 120 mmHg
2. Diastolic BP > 120 mmHg,   (a) Nitroglycerin 5 mg i.v. or 10 mg orally
   systolic BP slightly increased   (b) Sodium nitroprusside (rarely)
   on repeated measurements
   15 min apart
3. Systolic BP > 220 mmHg or   (a) Nifedipine 10 mg sublingually[c]
   diastolic BP 110–   (b) Clonidine 0.075 mg s.c.
   120 mmHg, or both on   (c) Uripidil 12.5 mg i.v.[d]
   repeated measurements
   15 min apart

BP, Blood pressure.
[a] Please notice the different blood pressure thresholds in the two recommendations.
[b] Avoid labetalol in patients with asthma, cardiac failure, severe conduction abnormalities, and bradycardia.
[c] Nifedipine may cause an overly rapid decline in blood pressure.
[d] In patients with unstable conditions and rapidly fluctuating blood pressure we use alternating treatment with uripidil and Arterenol (norepinephrine).

peripheral vascular resistance and does not ordinarily reduce cardiac output. Labetalol does not cause reflex tachycardia or redistribution of coronary blood flow, both of which may occur following administration of sodium nitroprusside. We recommend 10 mg as the initial intravenous dose for stroke patients, lower than the 20 mg initial dose usually used for patients without stroke, who tend to be younger with lesser comorbidity.

In Europe, oral nifedipine (10 mg) and subcutaneous Catapresan (clonidine; 0.5 mg) are frequently used. Unfortunately, the effects of both these agents are frequently very substantial and may be more rapid and extensive than desired. With either agent, the duration of the action may be difficult to predict. Uripidil administered intravenously is an alternative agent. Finally, sodium nitroprusside will sometimes become necessary despite some major potential side effects which include reflex tachycardia, coronary ischemia, and increased intracranial pressure. For isolated elevation of diastolic blood pressure, nitroglycerine (in Europe) and sodium nitroprusside (in North America) are frequently used.

Signs of Acutely Elevated Intracranial Pressure

Early signs of elevated intracranial pressure are rare in ischemic stroke patients; they are detected more frequently in patients with acute intracerebral hemorrhage or acute subarachnoid hemorrhage. Vomiting, hiccups, increasing drowsiness, and altered pupillary reflexes are initial signs of elevated intracranial pressure.

In case of an isolated unilateral dilated pupil, whether opposite or ipsilateral to the presumed stroke, 125 ml 20% mannitol should be infused immediately. The patient should be reexamined by CT if the cause of deterioration was not previously identified. The distinction between intracerebral hemorrhage, ischemic stroke, subarachnoid hemorrhage, and even acute subdural hematoma is discussed in detail in Chap. 24 of this textbook. Management of acutely elevated intracranial pressure is addressed in Chap. 9.

Blood Glucose

Blood glucose concentration should be assessed using a dextrostrip. Elevated blood glucose over 200–300 mg/100 ml should be counteracted using intravenously administered insulin. Hypoglycemia should also be identified as it may rarely cause focal neurological deficit. Rapid normalization of blood glucose levels using 20 g oral glucose, or 10% glucose infusion (peripheral veins), or 20% glucose (central venous line) will normalize neurological function quickly if no additional reasons for the neurological deficit are present. Presently the authors see no indication for 40% glucose solutions in this phase of the patient's management.

Management During the First Day of Stroke

Additional diagnostic planning may proceed after the stroke patient has been medically stabilized, neurologically evaluated, and studied with CT. For vascular diagnosis, emergency cerebral arteriography has the advantage of providing a high diagnostic yield. In a study by Fieschi et al. (1989) arteriography was performed within 6 h in 80 patients with acute ischemic stroke. Occlusions appropriate to the focal symptoms were found in 61 patients. The arteriographic abnormalities were found within the ipsilateral carotid system in 22 cases, the ipsilateral intracranial circulation in 20 cases, and the extracranial carotid system in 19 cases. In a dose-escalation study of tPA in which arteriography was carried out before and after treatment within 8 h of symptom onset, 112 of 139 patients (80.6%) had a complete occlusion in a vessel appropriate for the presenting symptoms. Among the 93 patients who received recombinant tissue plasminogen activator (tPA), 23 (25%) had occlusion of the extracranial internal carotid artery, 12 of whom had ipsilateral middle cerebral artery occlusions (the remaining 11 did not have contralateral carotid injections). Sixty-two patients (67%) had occlusion of the middle cerebral artery stem or of one of the middle cerebral artery branches. Procedure-related cerebral infarction occurred in one of the 139 patients.

Selective angiography of the cervical and intracranial vessels may be performed today with lower risk than previously, using digital subtraction techniques. In both North America and Europe, selective digital subtraction angiography in patients with suspected cerebrovascular disease is performed with arterial injection; intravenous injections with large boluses of contrast have largely been abandoned. Cerebral angiography remains the gold standard for the demonstration of vessel stenosis or occlusion. In addition, the high frequency of acute arterial occlusion has encouraged the development of strategies to reestablish perfusion, such as local or systemic thrombolytic therapy and balloon angioplasty, which are now being investigated further in clinical trials.

Is emergency cerebral arteriography indicated for the acute management of cerebral infarction? Because the results will not usually alter acute treatment, we suggest that arteriography should be performed selectively. Potential indications for emergency cerebral arteriography are listed in Table 6. As this decade proceeds, early detection and localization of thrombi may become important if the current thrombolytic therapy trials demonstrate reasonably safe arterial recanalization and improved neurological outcome.

Doppler Ultrasound Studies

The noninvasive alternatives to cerebral angiography continue to improve. Doppler ultrasonography of the internal carotid artery can be performed within 24 h of symptom onset, in some centers within the first few hours. The degree of internal carotid artery stenosis can be measured with acceptable reliability, even in acutely ill patients with severe neurological deficits. This information is important. During the first day, therapy decisions must be made with regard to fluid management, the administration of anticoagulants or rheologic agents, and management of severe hypertension. Knowledge that one or both internal carotid arteries are occluded or severely narrowed may help guide

Table 6. Potential indications for cerebral angiography after ischemic stroke

Condition	Possible therapeutic consequences
Carotid territory	
High grade symptomatic extracranial ICA stenosis	Carotid endarterectomy
Suspected intracranial arterial stenosis	Consider anticoagulant therapy
Suspected severe vasospasm after SAH	Consider aggressive hypervolemic therapy and/or angioplasty
Acute cerebral embolism (intracranial ICA, MCA)	Thrombolysis, heparin
Arterial dissection (vertebral artery, ICA)	Consider anticoagulant therapy
Vasculitis	Consider immunosuppressive and antibiotic therapy
Vertebrobasilar territory	
Acute basilar occlusion of other etiology	Consider thrombolytic and/or anticoagulant therapy
Cerebellar infarction with mass effect, without basilar artery occlusion	Ventricular drainage, decompressive surgery

ICA, Internal carotid artery; MCA, middle cerebral artery; SAH, subarachnoid hemorrhage.

those decisions, or suggest a need for cerebral angiography. The same knowledge may later assist in judgements regarding patient positioning, the pace of patient mobilization, or the vigor of physical therapy.

Noninvasive assessment of the intracranial vascular anatomy is also improving and has become increasingly available. Transcranial Doppler sonography (TCD) may be possible during the first 24 h or even, frequently, on an emergency basis. Satisfactory recordings may be obtained in 80% or more of patients studied. When such an occlusion or stenosis is identified, the vessel may be studied serially so as to detect spontaneous recanalization. In the study by Fieschi et al., 15 patients with middle cerebral artery occlusion were followed with serial TCD; recanalization was demonstrated in 10 patients, and arterial recanalization occurred within 24 h in 4. The sensitivity of TCD in experienced hands may be 75% or higher for hemodynamically significant middle cerebral artery stenosis or occlusion. Even microemboli may be detected by TCD in selected patients.

Magnetic Resonance Imaging and Magnetic Resonance Angiography

MRI and magnetic resonance angiography (MRA) cannot be performed in all acute stroke patients because of (a) the complexity of the examination and (b) problems in monitoring the patients during MRI. Nevertheless, more and more patients are being studied early by MRI, and techniques have been developed to make MRI studies possible in unstable patients, even patients on ventilators.

In selected stroke patients, emergency MRI and MRA provide invaluable information. For patients with posterior circulation symptoms, MRI is considerably more sensitive than CT, showing signs of infarction within 2–8 h, and the flow voids and/or the MRA may show evidence of impending vertebral or basilar artery occlusion. In patients suspected of having arterial dissection, the intramural thrombus and the reduced flow void within the intracranial internal carotid or the vertebral artery may be demonstrated. In patients with suspected venous sinus occlusion, MRI, with or without MRA, is sensitive in detection of thrombotic occlusion and sensitive in detection of hemorrhage infarction. Experimentally, selected contrast agents already allow imaging of nonperfused brain areas. MRA is becoming widely available but has not yet been compared prospectively with cerebral angiography in patients during the first hours after stroke onset. MRA does not depict the vessel anatomy directly, and the information on flow provided may be subject to nonanatomical influences such as blood pressure, and to assorted artifacts such as pulsation artifact.

We foresee a development in which different MR techniques performed within minutes will give information on (a) the morphology of tissue injury, (b) the perfusion of the brain, (c) the flow state within the vessels (MRA), and even (d) cellular events (spectroscopy, diffusion weighted imaging). Theoretically, this MR information may be obtained in 30 min or less and provide a comprehensive, very early understanding of the evolving stroke

proces. This information could then be used to monitor initial treatment strategies.

Intracranial assessment is also possible with single photon emission computed tomography (SPECT). The development of improved radiopharmaceuticals allows a "snapshot" of regional cerebral blood flow, and the "snapshot" may be acquired 1 or 2 h after symptom onset. For example, a patient sustaining a right middle cerebral artery distribution with onset at 2.00 p.m. could be injected with the SPECT radiopharmaceutical at 3.30 p.m., after arrival to the hospital and prior to detailed work-up. The patient's neurological assessment could then be completed and the CT scan performed. The patient could then be taken to the nuclear medicine suite for completion of the SPECT pictures, perhaps at 5.30 p.m. The pictures, even though obtained 2 h after the radiopharmaceutical injection, would reflect regional cerebral blood flow at 3.30 p.m. A second SPECT study could be completed within the first week. For a given patient, serial SPECT studies could supplement assessment of acute intervention (e.g., intravenous streptokinase) by providing measures of regional cerebral blood flow before and after the administration of the treatment, and give early clues as to prognosis.

Ensuring Best Possible Quality of the Ancillary Tests

As a rule, the examiner must make sure that all diagnostic studies are performed without undue delay and to the best possible quality. If no skilled neurosonologist is present, one should not wait 1 h or more until he or she arrives at the hospital. Instead, one should proceed with the next diagnostic measure, e.g., angiography, if indicated, or MRI and MRA. Many patients with an acute stroke are uncooperative and restless. Quite often CT scans, MRI scans, and even angiograms are disturbed by the artifacts. Use of short-acting sedative drugs or even anesthesia and intubation may be necessary to obtain the best possible quality from a given examination in some patients.

General Management

Because the temporal course of cerebral infarction may be unpredictable and because progression of symptoms is not uncommon, admission of the patient to either a stroke unit or some other ICU should be considered (Table 1). Special care units designed for stroke patients have been in use for over 10 years and have increased in number slowly, perhaps because the value of a dedicated stroke unit has been difficult to document. The most positive study to date included 220 patients randomized either to treatment in a specialized stroke unit or to treatment in a general medical ward. At 6 weeks, 56% of the stroke unit patients were at home, compared to 33% of the general medical patients ($p = 0.0004$); and at 6 weeks, mortality was 7% among the stroke unit patients and 17% among the general medical patients ($p = 0.027$). These results are encouraging and, if replicated, would justify expanded development of dedicated stroke units.

While stroke units exist at only a few hospitals, ICUs are widely available. Admission to such a unit offers distinct advantages with regard to staffing and equipment. The nurse/patient ratio is ideal, often 1:2 or even 1:1, making for a staff density far superior to that which is possible on general hospital wards. Having more nurses allows more comprehensive nursing care. Frequent attention to the patient's airway, oxygenation, cardiovascular status, and blood pressure becomes practical. Perhaps more important, nurses working in the ICU setting are better able to assess changes in the patient's neurological function.

Minimum Requirements for Centers Dealing with Acute Stroke Patients

In order to allow early and quality care for acute stroke patients, the following must be available 24 h a day under all circumstances:

Electrocardiography
Blood chemistry tests
Hematological analysis
Urine analysis
Cranial CT
Extracranial Doppler ultrasonography
Conventional X-ray (chest, head other)

The following should be available 24 h a day:

Neurologists[1]
Cerebral angiography
Laboratory analysis of cerebrospinal fluid

---

[1] In many parts of Europe, smaller hospitals do not have neurologists who can see patients on a daily basis.

Finally, the following aids should be available at least within 24 h after admission of the patients:

MRI
Echocardiography (including transesophageal)

Transfer to the ICU

After transfer from the emergency department to the ICU, the patient should be placed in bed and supportive care should proceed. As discussed earlier, we recommend supplementary oxygen. Cerebral oxygenation may be improved, the treatment is benign, and the nasal prongs or mask used for administration will serve as a gentle restraint for confused patients and will remind family members of the gravity of stroke as an illness. For the first 12–24 h, most patients should not be fed. During that time, control of the airway will not be certain nor easily assessed, so there is a real danger of aspiration of any solid food provided. Elevations and fluctuations in serum glucose concentration following meals may be detrimental to potentially viable tissue in the penumbra of the infarction.

Intravenous fluids should be administered so as to maintain adequate hydration. Glucose-containing solutions should probably be avoided as they have not been shown to benefit stroke patients and may potentiate the development of cerebral edema. Whether or not fluid management should include volume-expanding agents during the first day remains controversial. Clinical trials have been negative, but the study designs have been less than ideal, with therapy often

beginning many hours after stroke onset. One approach would be to administer fluids so as to achieve a relatively volume-expanded state during the first several hours after symptom onset, possibly enhancing cerebral blood flow. After the first 24 h, cerebral edema becomes a potentially serious or even fatal complication for patients with large infarctions, and so fluid administration could then be cut back so as to avoid overhydration or a relatively hypoosmolar state.

General ICU Monitoring

In all ICU stroke patients, cardiac and blood pressure monitoring are required. Cardiac monitoring will be performed continuously. In most instances the electrodes for cardiac monitoring allow monitoring of the respiratory rate as well, but the accuracy of these respiratory measurements must be verified for each patient. Pulse oximetry is preferable as a technique for ventilatory function because of its safety, sensitivity, and widespread availability. Blood pressure monitoring can be done discontinuously using an automatic sphygmomanometer, or continuously with an arterial catheter and pressure transducer. If precise arterial blood pressure monitoring is required, the catheter method is preferred. The arterial line should be placed electively, not during the first half hour after the patient's admission to the ICU, but rather when adequate time is available for unhurried catheter insertion. The radial artery site is preferred after the adequacy of the ulnar collateral has been tested.

Direct evaluation of cardiac function is now available with real-time echocardiography. Transesophageal echocardiography (TEE) is an adjunct to the usual transthoracic echocardiography. The probe can be inserted in the awake (with topical anesthetic), sedated or comatose patient and two-dimensional pictures of chamber volume, valvular function, and myocardial wall motion are obtainable. The addition of the color-flow Doppler capability to TEE has facilitated the diagnosis and interpretation of right-to-left shunts in the etiology of cerebrovascular disease. Soon it will be possible to routinely measure cardiac output by this method.

Monitoring of neurological function should be frequent, but this may be difficult with the assessment tools currently in use. As mentioned earlier, standardized neurological stroke examination scales are designed for use in clinical trials. They do not allow frequent examinations during the first several hours because the briefest of such scales requires several minutes or more to administer. The nursing assessment forms currently in use are frequently insensitive and cumbersome. We recommend that for the frequent assessments one neurological sign be followed closely in addition to the level of consciousness. The sign chosen should be the one thought most likely to show change if the patient deteriorates or improves. For example, in the patient with right hemiplegia, the arm may be without movement but the leg may have preserved movement, perhaps even against gravity. Frequent testing of the arm will not be sensitive to either improvement or deterioration, whereas frequent testing of the leg will, since the borderline function of the leg is more likely to change following any changes in brain function related to the acute infarction (see Table 5). Assessment of such a neurological sign requires less than 1 min, and so truly frequent serial testing by the nurse is practicable, even as often as every 15 min in the first 3 h after stroke onset.

Despite the absence of effective specific treatments for stroke, frequent monitoring of neurological function is not an exercise in futility. For the present, early detection of any deterioration is important if the aggressive general therapeutic measures described below are to be accomplished in a timely manner. In the future – hopefully within the next few years – therapeutic trials may yield one or more effective specific treatments. Each of the treatments under current study would require close patient monitoring if it were to come into general use.

Optimizing Fluid and Electrolyte Balance

A central venous catheter and venous pressure monitoring are helpful. This relatively noninvasive technique provides indirect information on intravascular volume, cardiac function, and compliance within the venous system; the catheter provides a route for administration of fluids, nutrition, and medications requiring central administration, and access for obtaining venous blood samples. The safest route of introduction of a central venous catheter is via the basilic vein in the antecubital fossa. The risk of pneumothorax is nil; however, the catheter sometimes does not reach the superior vena cava, because of coiling within the axillary vein, passage up the jugular system, or passage beyond the heart to the inferior vena cava. If a central position of the catheter is necessary for accurate pressure measurements or the administration of concentrated fluids or vasopressors, an X-ray must be obtained to confirm its proper placement.

The femoral vein can be easily and rapidly accessed as a route for administering high volumes, concentrated fluids, and vasoactive substances for shorter periods. The elevated risk of infection makes this site less desirable. Direct application of a central venous catheter into the veins may also be accomplished through the internal jugular or subclavian veins. Pneumothorax is less frequent using the jugular vein, but jugular puncture can impede the drainage of venous blood from the brain (especially in patients with increased intracranial pressure) and carries the subsequent risk of jugular vein thrombosis. Therefore, the subclavain vein approach is often preferred. If the patient needs continuous application of fluids, vasopressors, and nutrition, or frequent administration of drugs and antibiotics, a central venous catheter with two or three lumens can be inserted. Such a catheter insures uninterrupted therapy and simultaneous monitoring of the central venous pressure.

The central venous pressure can be measured in millmeters of mercury (normal limits 1–8 mmHg) or, more often, in centimeters of water (normal limits 2–10 cmH$_2$O). There are some limitations in interpreting the central venous pressure as a measure of intravascular volume. The central venous pressure is the sum of four components: (1) volume and flow of blood in the central veins, (2) contractility of the right atrium and ventricle, (3) tone of the central veins (capacitance), and (4) intrathoracic pressure. However, serial measurements can give considerable information about the patient's fluid balance. With a stable intrathoracic pressure, comparison of the central venous pressure and the systemic blood pressure responses to fluid administration gives information on the volume and compliance of the venous system and cardiac performance, respectively. Central venous lines allow the infusion of higher volumes of fluid and higher concentrations of electrolytes.

More invasive monitoring with Swan-Ganz catheter techniques is only rarely used, usually if hypervolemic therapy is planned or if the patient is in heart failure. The Swan-Ganz catheter allows measurement of the pulmonary artery pressure, pulmonary vascular resistance, and the pulmonary capillary wedge pressure (PCWP; normal limits 5–12 mmHg) as an estimate of the filling pressure of the left ventricle. The catheter provides the added option of measuring cardiac output and deriving a value of systemic vascular resistance. The pulmonary artery catheter can be placed in the same way as a central venous catheter using the Seldinger technique. Its flow-directed introduction is easier through the right internal jugular and the left subclavian veins, but it can be placed through alternate routes to the right heart (jugular, subclavian, basilic, and femoral veins). Confirmation of the position of the tip of the catheter in the proximal pulmonary artery should be made on insertion and daily thereafter. Confirmation of the catheter location and a continuous display of the wave form will help prevent two serious potential complications: pulmonary artery infarction and rupture.

Neurological Monitoring

Intracranial pressure (ICP) monitoring may become necessary in selected patients with massive stroke. We prefer epidural probes. Many problems are associated with ICP monitoring, and the reliability of the epidural probe method is not always optimal. Multiple ICP probes – up to three or four placed over different compartments of the brain – have shown that among the different compartments, the ICP may differ significantly. Intraventricular ICP monitoring is used primarily in cases of posterior circulation stroke requiring ventricular drainage. In those instances, the ventricular shunt will be used for the ICP measurements. We prefer computing the cerebral perfusion pressure simultaneously with the ICP, calculating it as the difference between mean arterial pressure (MAP) and ICP. For further details on ICP monitoring, see Chap. 8. For discussion of specific therapies for cerebral edema and elevated ICP, see Chap. 9.

In Heidelberg, evoked potential monitoring in stroke patients has been useful. Medial nerve somatosensory evoked potentials (SEP) with both spinal and cortical leads, brainstem evoked auditory evoked potentials (BAEP), middle latency acoustic potentials, and less frequently, visual evoked potentials are all measured daily. Evoked potential measurements have been included in the decision-making process in cases of space-occupying cerebellar infarction, basilar thrombosis, and massive hemispheric stroke. For example, in patients with basilar occlusion who are already comatose, aggressive treatment will only be given if brainstem evoked potentials show at least partial function of the brainstem (see Chap. 58). Alteration of SEP and BAEP in patients still awake with space-occupying cerebellar infarction and occlusive hydrocephalus helps in the assessment for neurosurgical intervention, and absence of contralateral SEP in patients with massive space-occupying middle cerebral artery infarction will suggest that less aggressive management may be appropriate (see Chap. 57).

Most stroke patients will receive repeated CT or MRI scans. In patients in whom the infarct results in significant mass effect, daily CT scans may be useful during the first several days. Changes in the CT scan, such as progressive hydrocephalus in cases of cerebellar infarction or significant midline shift and compression of the basal cisterns in cases of hemispheric infarction, can be used together with results from clinical and electrophysiological monitoring for therapeutic decisions.

As mentioned earlier, transcranial Doppler ultrasonography may be very useful for the assessment of recanalization, particularly in patients with acute embolic occlusion of major cerebral arteries. In the Heidelberg ICU, TCD, evoked potential systems, and various ICP monitoring systems are in use, and the results of those tests are continuously evaluated in relation to the management of the patients (see Chap. 7).

Prevention and Treatment of Medical Complications

Prevention of acute pulmonary embolism should be a daily priority in the care of every patient with stroke. Pulmonary embolism may be the cause of death in up to 25% of patients dying after ischemic cerebral infarction. Pulmonary embolism can be a particularly tragic complication, as it may affect patients who otherwise would have had an excellent recovery from the stroke. Pneumatic compression boots are recommended for patients kept in bed, since they can decrease the risk of deep vein thrombosis. Subcutaneous heparin, 5000–7500 units every 12 h, should be administered. Since chest pain and dyspnea will occur in 70%–80% of those with documented pulmonary embolism, patient complaints should be paid careful attention to, particularly those of patients with abnormal language function, whose symptoms will be difficult to decipher. Nurses and physicians should be attentive to any increases in respiratory rate; tachypnea is a sensitive sign of pulmonary embolism (and of pneumonia). Examination of lower extremities should be performed daily to detect signs of deep vein thrombosis. Compressive duplex ultrasonography should be performed in patients with positive examinations and in patients at high risk for deep venous thrombosis, such as those with no movement in one or both legs. If pulmonary embolism is suspected, a ventilation-perfusion lung scan should be performed immediately. In selected patients, pulmonary angiography will be necessary. If any of those studies shows embolism, anticoagulation is indicated with full-dose intravenous heparin for 5–10 days, followed by warfarin for at least 3 months.

Bacterial pneumonia accounts for 15%–25% of stroke deaths. The majority of cases of pneumonia are caused by aspiration. Since aspiration may be detectable by video fluoroscopy in as many as 50% of patients during the initial days after stroke onset, oral feeding should be withheld until the patient has demonstrated both intact swallowing of small amounts of water and intact coughing to command. In elderly patients, the traditional symptoms and signs of pneumonia may be attenuated, particularly in those with cerebral hemispheric infarction. Subtle changes suggestive of infection should prompt sputum analysis, chest X-ray, blood cultures, and possible serologic testing for viral agents or *Mycoplasma* or *Legionella* species. Empiric antibacterial therapy should be given until a specific diagnosis is established and antibiotic sensitivities are determined.

Cardiovascular complications following stroke account for 10%–20% of the acute deaths. The patient should be questioned daily with regard to chest pain and dyspnea. Vital signs should be inspected to detect tachycardia or tachypnea. Any suspicion of cardiovascular deterioration should prompt systematic evaluation and appropriate consultation.

Urinary tract infection is the most common complication of acute cerebral infarction and is not benign, being present in as many as 40% of patients dying from stroke. The majority of hospital-acquired urinary tract infections are associated with the use of indwelling catheters. Consequently, intermittent catheterization or condom catheterization is preferable to an indwelling catheter in patients with voiding problems. Systemic antibacterial therapy should be limited to treatment of symptomatic infection.

Decubiti have been common among stroke patients, although skilled nursing and technical aids have now significantly reduced their incidence. Frequent turning of immobilized patients is useful for prevention. The skin of incontinent patients should be kept dry. For patients at particularly high risk, an air- or fluid-filled mattress system should be used. If a decubitus develops, wet-to-dry saline dressings should be applied four times daily. These dressings may provide some degree of debridement and may reduce bacterial colonization. If the decubitus does not respond to conservative therapy, antibiotic therapy may be justified for several days before proceeding to definitive surgical debridement.

Conclusion

Physicians caring for patients with ischemic stroke have been hampered in their efforts by the absence of effective specific therapies. Nonetheless, the case mortality rate for ischemic stroke appears to be falling. We suggest that more careful attention to the general medical management of the stroke patient may be responsible for part of the improvement. If an intensive-care approach were to be widely employed for the acute care of stroke patients, stroke mortality and morbidity could improve even further.

Suggested Reading

Andersen AR, Friberg HH, Schmidt JF, Hasselbalch SG (1988) Quantitative measurements of cerebral blood flow using SPECT and 99 mTc-d, 1-HM-PAO compared to Xenon-133. J Cereb Blood Flow Metab 8:S69–S81

Bastianello S, Pierallini A, Colonnese C, Brughitta G, Angeloni U, Antonelli M, Fantozzi LM, Fieschi C, Bozzao L (1991) Hyperdense middle cerebral artery sign. Comparison with angiography in the acute phase of ischemic supratentorial infarction. Neuroradiology 33:207–211

Bounds JV, Wiebers DO, Whisnant JP, Okazaki H (1981) Mechanisms and timing of deaths from cerebral infarction. Stroke 12:474–477

Britton M, Carlsson A, DeFaire U (1986) Blood pressure course with acute stroke and matched controls. Stroke 17:861–864

Broderick J, Brott T, Barsan W, Haley EC, Levy D, Marler J, Blum C (1990) Blood pressure during the first hours of acute focal cerebral ischemia. Neurology 40:145

Brott T (1991) Thrombolytic therapy for stroke. Cerebrovasc Brain Metab Rev 3:91–113

Brott T, Adams HP, Olinger CP, Marler JR, Barsan WG, Biller J, Spilker J, Holleran R, Eberle R, Hertzberg V, Rorick M, Moomaw CJ, Walker M (1989) Measurements of acute cerebral infarction: a clinical examination scale. Stroke 20:864–870

Brott T, MacCarthy EP (1989) Antihypertensive therapy in stroke. In: Fisher M (ed) Medical therapy of acute stroke. Dekker, New York, pp 117–141

Brott T, Reed R (1989) Intensive care for acute stroke in the community hospital setting: the first 24 hours. Stroke 20:694–697

Brown M, Glassenberg M (1973) Mortality factors in patients with acute stroke. JAMA 224:1493–1495

Castaldo JE, Nicholas GG, Gee W, Reed JF (1989) Duplex ultrasound and ocular pneumoplethysmography concordance in detecting severe carotid stenosis. Arch Neurol 46:518–522

Chen HJ, Lee TC, Wei CP (1992) Treatment of cerebellar infarction by decompressive suboccipital craniectomy. Stroke 23:957–961

Dantzker DR, Tobin MJ (1990) Pulmonary vascular disease. In: Andreoli TE, Carpenter CCJ, Plum F, Smith LH (eds) Cecil essentials of medicine. Saunders, Philadelphia, p 153

Delashaw JB, Broaddus WC, Kassell NF, Haley EC, Pendleton GA, Vollmer DL, Maggio WW, Grady MS (1990) Treatment of hemispheric cerebral infarction by hemicraniectomy. Stroke 21:874–881

del Zoppo GJ, Poeck K, Pessin MS, Wolpert SM, Furlan AJ, Ferbert A, Alberts MJ, Zivin JA, Wechsler L, Busse O, Greenlee Jr R, Brass L, Mohr JP, Feldmann E, Hacke W, Kase CS, Biller J, Gress D, Otis SM (1992) Recombinant tissue plasminogen activator in acute thrombotic and embolic stroke. Ann Neurol 32:78–86

Duke RJ, Bloch RF, Turpie AGG, Trebilcock R, Bayer N (1986) Intravenous heparin for the prevention of stroke progression in acute partial stable stroke: A randomized controlled trial. Ann Intern Med 105:825–828

Dyken ME, Somers VK, Adams H, Yamada T, Zimmerman B Investigating the relationship between sleep apnea and stroke. Sleep Res (in press)

Fieschi C, Argentino C, Lenzi GL, Sacchetti ML, Toni D, Bozzao L (1989) Clinical and instrumental evaluation of patients with ischemic stroke within the first six hours. J Neurol Sci 91:311–321

Frackowiak RSJ (1985) The pathophysiology of human cerebral ischaemia: a new perspective obtained with positron tomography. Q J Med 57:713–727

Gacs G, Fox AJ, Barnett HJM, Vinuela F (1983) CT visualization of intracranial arterial thromboembolism. Stroke 14:756–762

Garibaldi RA, Neuhaus EG, Nurse BA (1988) Infections in the elderly. In: Rowe JW, Besdine RW (eds) Geriatric medicine. Little Brown, Boston, p 302

Gibbs JM, Wise RJS, Leenders KL, Jones T (1984) Evaluation of cerebral perfusion reserve in patients with carotid-artery occlusion. Lancet i:310–314

Giubilei F, Luigi G, Di Piero V, Pozzilli C, Pantano P, Bastianello S, Argentino C, Fieschi C (1990) Predictive value of brain perfusion single-photon emission computed tomography in acute ischemic stroke. Stroke 21:895–900

Greenwood Jr J (1968) Acute brain infarction with high intracranial pressure: surgical indications. Johns Hopkins Med J 122:254–280

Grotta JC (1987) Current status of hemodilution in acute cerebral ischemia. Stroke 18(4):689–690

Grotta JC, Pettigrew LC, Allen S, Tonnesen A, Yatsu FM, Gray J, Spydell J (1985) Baseline hemodynamic state and response to hemodilution in patients with acute cerebral ischemia. Stroke 16:790–795

Hacke W (1985) Neuromonitoring. J Neurol 232:125–133

Hacke W, Hennerici M, Gelmers HJ, Krämer G (1990) Cerebral ischemia. Springer, Berlin Heidelberg New York

Hacke W, Krieger D, Hirschberg M (1991) General principles in the treatment of acute ischemic stroke. Cerebrovasc Dis 1:93–99

Hagan AO, DeMaria AN (1989) Left ventricular function. In: Hagan AO, DeMaria AN (eds) Clinical applications of two-dimensional echocardiography and cardiac doppler. Little Brown, Boston, pp 233–260

Harmsen P, Tsipogianni A, Wilhelmsen L (1992) Stroke incidence rates were unchanged, while fatality rates declined, during 1971–1987 in Goteborg, Sweden. Stroke 23:1410–1415

Hemodilution in Stroke Study Group (1989) Hypervolemic hemodilution treatment of acute stroke: results of a randomized multicenter trial using pentastarch. Stroke 20:317–323

Heros RC (1992) Surgical treatment of cerebellar infarction. Stroke 23:937–938

Horner J, Massey EW, Riski JE, Lathrop DL, Chase KW (1988) Aspiration following stroke: clinical correlates and outcome. Neurology 38:1359–1362

Howard G, Toole JF, Becker C, Lefkowitz DS, Truscott L, Rose L, Evans GW (1989) Changes in survival following stroke in five North Carolina counties observed during two different periods. Stroke 20:345–350

Hyers TM (1990) Venous thromboembolic disease: diagnosis and use of antithrombotic therapy. Clin Cardiol 13:23–28

Indredavik B, Bakke F, Solberg R, Rokseth R, Haaheim LL, Holme I (1991) Benefit of a stroke unit: a randomized controlled trial. Stroke 22:1026–1031

Italian Acute Stroke Study Group (1988) Haemodilution in acute stroke. Results of the
Italian Haemodilution Trial. Lancet 1:318–
321

Jaker M, Atkin S, Soto M, Schmid G, Brosch F
(1989) Oral nifedipine vs oral clonidine in
the treatment of urgent hypertension. Arch
Intern Med 149:260–265

Keller TS, McGillicuddy JE, Labond VA, Kindt
GW (1985) Modification of focal cerebral
ischemia by cardiac output augmentation. J
Surg Res 39:420–432

Kennealy JA, McLennan JE, Loudon RG,
McLaurin RL (1980) Hyperventilation-
induced cerebral hypoxia. Am Rev Respir
Dis 122:407–412

Kushner MJ, Zanette EM, Bastianello S,
Mancini G, Sacchetti ML, Carolei A,
Bozzao L (1991) Transcranial Doppler in
acute hemispheric infarction. Neurology
41:109–113

Leys D, Pruvo JP, Godefroy O, Rondepierre P,
Leclerc X (1992) Prevalence and significance of hyperdense middle cerebral
artery in acute stroke. Stroke 23:317–324

Lindenstrom E, Boysen G, Christiansen LW,
Rogvi Hansen B, Nielsen PW (1991)
Reliability of Scandinavian Neurological
Stroke Scale. Cerebrovasc Dis 1:103–107

Macdonell RAL, Kalnins RM, Donnan GA
(1987) Cerebellar infarction: natural history, prognosis, and pathology. Stroke 18:
849–855

McMahon SM, Heyman A (1974) The mechanics
of breathing and stabilization of ventilation
in patients with unilateral cerebral infarction. Stroke 5:518–527

Myers MG, Norris JW, Hachinski VC, Sole MJ
(1981) Plasma norepinephrine in stroke.
Stroke 12:200–204

Orgogozo JM, Dartigues JF (1991) Methodology
of clinical trials in acute cerebral ischemia.
Cerebrovasc Dis 1:100–111

Petty GW, Wiebers DO, Meissner I (1990)
Transcranial Doppler ultrasonography:
clinical applications in cerebrovascular disease. Mayo Clinic Proc 65:1350–1364

Phillips TJ, Gilchrest BA (1988) Skin. In: Rowe
JW, Besdine RW (eds) Geriatric medicine.
Little Brown, Boston, p 144

Phillipson EA (1977) Regulation of breathing
during sleep. Am Rev Respir Dis 115:217–
224

Plum F (1983) What causes infarction in ischemic
brain? Neurology 33:322–333

Powell-Griner E (1990) Characteristics of persons dying from cerebrovascular diseases.
Adv Data 180:1–16

Pressman BD, Tourje EJ, Thompson JR (1987)
An early CT sign of ischemic infarction:
increased density in a cerebral artery.
AJNR 8:645–648

Pulsinelli WA, Levy DE, Sigsbee B, Scherer P,
Plum F (1983) Increased damage after
ischemic stroke in patients with hyperglycemia with or without established diabetes
mellitus. Am J Med 74:540–544

Robin ED, Whaley RD, Crump CH, Travis DM
(1958) Alveolar gas tensions, pulmonary
ventilation and blood pH during physiologic
sleep in normal subjects. J Clin Invest 37:
981–989

Ropper AH, Rockoff MA (1988) Treatment of
intracranial hypertension. In: Ropper AH,
Kennedy SF (eds) Neurological and neurosurgical intensive care. Aspen, Maryland,
pp 23–41

Ropper AH, Shafran B (1984) Brain edema
after stroke. Arch Neurol 41:26–29

Scandinavian Stroke Study Group (1987) Multicenter trial of hemodilution in acute
ischemic stroke: I. Results in the total
patient population. Stroke 18:691–699

Schmidt SM, Herman LM, Koenig P, Leuze M,
Monahan MK, Stubbers RW (1986) Status
of stroke patients: a community assessment. Arch Phys Med Rehabil 67:99–
102

Sette G, Baron JC, Mazoyer B, Levasseur M,
Pappata S, Crouzel C (1989) Local brain
haemodynamics and oxygen metabolism in
cerebrovascular disease: positron emission
tomography. Brain 112:931–951

Sette G, Young AR, Miyazawa H, Hartmann
A, Dettmers C, Rommel T, Theron J,
Derlon JM, MacKenzie ET, Baron JC
(1991) Estimation of local cerebral perfusion pressure (CPP) by the CBF/CBV ratio
using positron emission tomography:
validation studies in experimental focal
ischemia in anaesthetized baboons. J Cereb
Blood Flow Metab 12:S543

Silver FL, Norris JW, Lewis AJ, Hachinski VC
(1984) Early mortality following stroke: a
prospective review. Stroke 15:492–496

Skillman JJ, Collins RE, Coe NP, Goldstein BS,
Shapiro RM, Zervas NT, Bettmann MA,
Salzman EW (1978) Prevention of deep
vein thrombosis in neurosurgical patients:
a controlled randomized trial or external

pneumatic compression boots. Surgery 83: 354–358

Sparrow D, Weiss ST (1988) Pulmonary system. In: Rowe JW, Besdine RW (eds) Geriatric medicine. Little Brown, Boston, p 266

Stumpf JL (1988) Therapy review: drug therapy of hypertensive crises. Clin Pharm 7:582–591

Tomsick T, Brott T, Barsan W, Broderick J, Haley EC, Levy D, Sheppard G, Spilker J (1992) Thrombus localization with emergency cerebral computed tomography. AJNR 13:257–263

Wallace JD, Levy LL (1981) Blood pressure after stroke. JAMA 246:2177–2180

Wilson DJ, Wallin JD, Vlachakis ND, Freis ED, Vidt DG, Michelson EL, Langford HG,
Flamenbaum W, Poland MP (1983) Intravenous labetalol in the treatment of severe hypertension and hypertensive emergencies. Am J Med 75:95–102

Wolf PA, D'Agostino RB, O'Neal A, Sytkowski P, Kase CS, Belanger AJ, Kannel WB (1992) Secular trends in stroke incidence and mortality. The Framingham study. Stroke 23:1551–1555

Yatsu FM, Zivin J (1983) Hypertension in acute ischemic stroke: not to treat. Arch Neurol 42:999–1000

Yoshikawa TT (1989) Pneumonia, UTI, and decubiti in the nursing home: optimal management. Geriatrics 44:32–43

Chapter 52

Special Aspects in the Treatment of Severe Hemispheric Brain Infarction

ANTHONY J. FURLAN, OTTO BUSSE, and
E. BERND RINGELSTEIN

Introduction

While respiratory, cardiac, nursing, nutritional, and rehabilitative management are critical in determining outcome in many patients with acute stroke, it is the emergence of several new direct treatment strategies for brain ischemia that has rekindled interest in the intensive management of acute stroke. Because there has been no proven treatment strategy available, a fatalistic or even nihilistic attitude towards acute stroke management has evolved in the medical and general communities. Patients are often admitted for "observation", "supportive care", or "physical therapy". In the past, the major immediate treatment decision often revolved around acute anticoagulation with heparin, and anticoagulation frequently was not started until worsening had actually occurred in hospital. Therapeutic trials of new agents used patient entry times exceeding 24 h from onset, and several studies indicated that only a minority of patients present to their local emergency room within the first several hours after stroke onset. Upon arrival at the hospital there are frequent logistical delays, such as obtaining brain imaging, which impede prompt initiation of therapy. Since the therapeutic window in most patients with evolving brain infarction is probably less than 8 h, perhaps as brief as 2 h in some cases, such delays are not acceptable and must be overcome through aggressive educational programs. The NINDS thrombolytic trial in acute stroke has employed novel quality-management techniques to accelerate patient flow upon arrival at hospital.

Ischemia/infarction implies a mismatch between blood flow and the metabolic needs of brain tissue. Hence, maintenance of cerebral blood flow (CBF) above the infarction threshold is critical in preventing irreversible brain damage. Normal average CBF is approximately 55 ml/100 g/min. CBF is constant between a mean arterial blood pressure (MAP) of approximately 50–150 mmHg. This phenomenon of *autoregulation* is largely due to changes in the diameter of the cerebral resistance vessels. As

---

Section Editor: Werner Hacke

MAP falls the resistance vessels dilate, and as pressure rises they constrict to maintain a constant CBF. When CBF falls to approximately 20 ml/100 g/min the ischemic threshold is crossed, which is first characterized by slowing of the EEG or change in waveform amplitude. At flows of 15 ml/100 g/min ischemia deepens and evoked potential activity is lost. It is not until CBF drops below approximately 10 ml/100 g/min that infarction, i.e., irreversibility, occurs. Sustained CBF below 10 ml/100 g/min triggers the so-called ischemic cascade, a complex series of events culminating in cell death. One goal of acute intervention, therefore, is to maintain CBF above the infarction threshold.

CBF thresholds have led to the concept of the ischemic "penumbra" – an area of brain surrounding a dead infarcted core where blood flows are between 10 and 20 ml/100 g/min. In the penumbra zone neurons are said to be "idling", i.e., functionally silent (EEG, evoked potentials) but structurally intact and potentially salvageable. Many treatment strategies are therefore aimed at preserving and expanding the penumbra zone. Positron emission tomography (PET) studies have identified certain patterns indicative of the penumbra zone. In addition to decreased CBF, jeopardized brain tissue may show increased blood volume related to compensatory vasodilatation, or an increased oxygen extraction fraction (OEF) which maintains cerebral metabolism of oxygen in the face of reduced flow. Unfortunately, PET is not widely available and is not a practical tool for urgent or repeated monitoring of CBF and cerebral metabolism in patients with rapidly evolving infarction. Single photon emission computer tomography (SPECT) has been employed in some trials of early thrombolytic therapy since the isotope can be immediately injected and the imaging delayed until therapy has been started. SPECT provides a more objective measurement of CBF and, perhaps, of tissue viability but is not quantifiable and has not yet been convincingly linked with clinical outcome. Bedside monitoring of CBF employing xenon inhalation or injection can be done, but it entails radiopharmaceuticals, is cumbersome, and is of uncertain validity. Laser probes have been used to continuously monitor microcirculatory flow, but these techniques permit analysis of only small volumes of tissue and are still experimental. Magnetic resonance (MR) diffusion imaging and functional MR imaging, combined with MR angiography, hold great promise for the early characterization of brain ischemia.

Maintaining Cerebral Perfusion

Blood Pressure Manipulation in Acute Brain Infarction

Until better bedside CBF monitoring techniques are developed, CBF is best managed by manipulating cerebral perfusion pressure (CPP) according to the formula: CPP = MAP − intracranial pressure (ICP). CPP manipulation in acute stroke patients requires an ICU setting with hemodynamic monitoring. In most patients with acute hemispheric ischemia the immediate concern is to avoid *hypotension*. CBF autoregulation is often defective in an area of evolving infarction so that flow in the critical penumbra zone is passively dependent on MAP. Furthermore, many patients with acute stroke have chronic hypertension and the CBF autoregulatory curve may be shifted to the right, so that CBF begins to fall at a relatively high MAP.

Although many patients with acute hemispheric infarction have elevated blood pressure on admission, severe elevation of blood pressure requiring emergency treatment is uncommon. Wallace and Levy (1981) found that among 334 consecutive patients admitted for acute stroke the blood pressure was elevated in 84% on the day of admission. In patients with hemispheric atherothrombotic infarction, the average admission blood pressure was 181/100, falling to 147/83 by day 10. Among 41 patients with cerebral infarction within 24 h at the University of Cincinnati, Brott and Reed (1989) found a systolic blood pressure >239 mmHg or diastolic pressure >120 mmHg in 15%; 10% of patients had sustained hypertension requiring parenteral therapy. Hence, aggressive lowering of blood pressure in patients with acute hemispheric infarction is not only dangerous but seldom necessary.

Currently, a continuous infusion of sodium nitroprusside (0.5–10 µg/kg/min) or intermittent infusions of labetalol (20 mg every 1–2 min) are most commonly employed in the United States. A continuous labetalol infusion (2 mg/min, maximal dose 150 mg) may also be employed. Sodium nitroprusside acts directly on vascular smooth muscle cells, and dilatation of cerebral vessels can raise intracranial pressure. CBF tends to increase with low doses but decreases

with high doses. If sympathetic tone is increased, CBF will fall when nitroprusside reduces blood pressure by 40%. The effects of labetalol, which has combined alpha and beta adrenergic blocking properties, on CBF in patients with acute stroke has not been well studied. Beta-adrenergic blockers produce vasoconstriction and decrease and redistribute cerebral blood flow during acute administration, although they apparently have little effect on cerebrovascular function during chronic administration. Alpha-adrenergic antagonists apparently have no major effect on basal CBF, but their effects on autoregulation are not known.

Calcium antagonists, still frequently used, may have an unpredictable effect on CBF autoregulation in the acute situation. Bertel et al. (1983) measured CBF in five patients who received 10–20 mg oral nifedipine for emergency blood pressure control. CBF increased in four cases and decreased in one case, but the mean variation was only +4 mm/100 g/min. Sublingual nifedipine is best avoided in patients with acute brain infarction as it can produce a precipitous and unpredictable fall in blood pressure. Inhibitors of angiotensin-converting enzyme (ACE) have many theoretical advantages over other medications for the treatment of hypertension in patients with evolving stroke. Treatment with ACE inhibitors quickly lowers the range of autoregulation to relatively normal levels. The shift in autoregulation occurs quickly after acute administration of ACE inhibitors and is maintained during chronic treatment. As a result, basal CBF is usually normal and blood flow can frequently be maintained satisfactorily during moderate increases and decreases in arterial pressure. ACE inhibitors may improve endothelial function by increasing the release and activation of endothelial-derived relaxation factors (EDRF). In addition to a decrease in the upper and lower limits of autoregulation, captopril may decrease the range of the autoregulatory plateau. Newer ACE inhibitors such as fosenopril shift the lower limit of autoregulation downward but have no effect on the upper limit. Drugs like fosenopril may widen the range of autoregulation and provide excellent protection to cerebral vessels during episodes of acute hypertension. Fosenopril is more lipid soluble than captopril and thus may have a greater effect on cerebral vessels. For more detailed data on the treatment of hypertension in acute stroke victims please refer to Chap. 51.

Although it is well established that hypotension can be detrimental in brain ischemia, the beneficial effects of *hypertensive therapy* in evolving cerebral infarction have been less studied. Potential risks of hypertensive therapy in acute ischemia include cerebral hemorrhage and aggravation of cerebral edema. There is no compelling experimental evidence for the assumption that raising the blood pressure improves outcome after focal ischemic insults in animal models. In one study, the response to nimodipine following experimental focal ischemia was not influenced by manipulating the level of mean arterial blood pressure. Clinical experience, however, has demonstrated a subset of patients who seemingly benefit from acute hypertensive therapy during evolving cerebral ischemia. These so-called hemodynamic strokes usually have high-grade stenosis or occlusion of a major vessel such as the internal carotid artery or basilar artery with inadequate collateral circulation. In such cases even a modest decrease in mean arterial blood pressure can result in neurologic worsening, and focal neurologic deficits may be reversed with hypertensive therapy. If cardiac output is decreased, dopamine or dobutamine infusion may be effective alone. If cardiac output is relatively normal Levophed (norepinephrine bitartrate) can be used to raise mean arterial pressure, sometimes combined with intravenous dopamine to maintain the cardiac rate.

Raised Intracranial Pressure in Patients with Hemispheric Infarction

Postischemic (infarct) brain edema starts to develop in the first hours after cessation of cerebral blood flow. The infarct edema is initially cytotoxic and later becomes vasogenic. The two phases of ischemic brain edema overlap; the cytotoxic phase takes place over the first minutes to hours and may be reversible. Infarct edema reaches its maximum between 24 and 72 h. During this period the intracranial pressure can rise but seldom is a major problem in the first 24 h after stroke onset. Infarct edema has a space-occupying effect with a shift of midline structures in 3.6% of supratentroial infarctions.

In some patients the cause of severe infarct edema may be reperfusion injury. Spontaneous lysis or fragmentation of an arterial embolus is followed by reperfusion of blood into vessels with an increased permeability caused by ischemic endothelial damage. The result can be a massive leakage of protein-rich fluid with increasing hemispheric brain swelling. Reperfusion leakage may be the cause of massive infarct edema reported after thrombolysis in some cases, but it seems not to be more frequent than in patients not treated with thrombolysis.

Young or middle-aged patients with a middle cerebral artery (MCA) distribution infarct tend to have elevated intracranial pressure more often than older patients because they have little or no underlying cerebral atrophy. Even if the infarct is not very large and involves less than half of the affected hemisphere, edema in such a setting can result in herniation and death. Therefore, treatment of raised intracranial pressure should begin early. Clinical signs are not reliable indicators of the presence of raised ICP or its level. Although controversial, continuous monitoring of ICP permits some control of treatment by attempting to keep the ICP level below 15 mmHg. In patients in whom ICP was continuously monitored, pressures below 15 mmHg were associated with survival, whereas persistently higher levels led to brain death despite pressure-lowering medical treatment. However, this may simply reflect infarct size. Nonetheless, control of increased ICP due to edema may lead to a better outcome after stroke. ICP monitoring facilitates the timing of hyperventilation and, rarely, decompressive hemicraniectomy, which has favorable results only if performed before raised ICP causes global ischemia.

The method usually employed is epidural ICP monitoring, which provides inaccurate readings in up to 50% of cases. Ventricular monitoring often is not possible because of compressed slit-like ventricles, but a timely ventriculostomy allows measurement of ICP as well as drainage of CSF in patients who are deteriorating from increased ICP (Chap. 9).

In hemispheric ischemic infarctions with raised ICP and mass effect due to edema, hyperosmolar agents are indicated but problematic. They dehydrate the normal rather than the edematous brain and may thereby produce deleterious tissue shifts. On the other hand, hyperosmolar agents are very efficient in lowering raised ICP quickly and can be lifesaving. Osmotic gradients obtained by the parenteral administration of hyperosmolar solutions tend to be short-lived. After a few hours of delay, plasma levels fall and there is the possibility of a rebound effect with a further increase of ICP. The dosage of the hyperosmolar agent depends on the ICP value. If ICP monitoring is not available, clinical and radiological signs of raised ICP are indications for antiedema medical treatment. Intravenous mannitol is the agent of choice, the initial dose being 50 g in a 20% solution over 30 min, repeated every 6–12 h depending upon ICP and an optimal serum osmolality of 300–315 mosm. Furosemide may also be given in a dosage of 20–60 mg every 6–12 h to increase diuresis. Alternatively 50 mg of 10% glycerol can be given as an oral bolus or an infusion over 30 min. The maximum dose for glycerol or mannitol is 200 mg/day. The time of action is 3–4 h for glycerol and 1.5 h for mannitol. Bolus injection with a short infusion time reduces the extent of the rebound effect. There is no evidence that corticosteroids are useful in the treatment of raised ICP due to ischemic brain edema; both large and conventional doses of dexamethasone have been ineffective or even harmful. (For more details refer to Chap. 9).

Space-occupying (malignant) hemispheric infarctions due to severe brain edema have a mortality of more than 80%. Surviving patients are often severely disabled or in a vegetative state. Clinical signs of a malignant hemispheric infarction include severe hemiparesis progressing to hemiplegia, forced eye deviation, and rapid deterioration of consciousness with the first 3 days after onset. CT usually shows a large infarction of the entire MCA territory, sometimes in combination with infarcts in the ACA or PCA territory, often due to an embolic occlusion of the intracranial ICA bifurcation, occluding in turn both the ACA and the proximal MCA. In selected cases decompressive hemicraniectomy is indicated to reduce ICP and to increase perfusion pressure. Some reports indicate that this procedure not only is lifesaving but also can provide a reasonable quality of life (Table 1). The timing of surgery is problematic because hemicraniectomy has been successful only when performed before clinical signs of uncal herniation emerge. If ICP values of more than 30 mmHg persist and can-

not be lowered by hyperosmolar agents, decompressive surgery should be considered. Resection of necrotic tissue does not seem to be necessary. Usually, patients with nondominant hemispheric infarction are selected because survivors with dominant hemispheric strokes suffer global aphasia with an extremely poor quality of life. Ethical doubts remain about whether decompressive surgery is useful with respect to the anticipated severe neurologic deficit. Before this aggressive procedure is undertaken, the patient's age, possible functional outcome, life quality, and the quality of family support should be considered.

Anticoagulation

Although heparin anticoagulation has been advocated for many years for either acute atherothrombotic progressing infarction or acute nonhemorrhagic cardioembolic infarction, the evidence supporting the use of heparin in such patients is inconclusive. Recent studies of patients with progressing infarction have failed to demonstrate a benefit from heparin. However, these studies fail to consider selection factors that are possibly im-

Table 1. Retrospective studies carried out in the past 5 years regarding hemispheric malignant infarction

Author	Year	No. of patients	Non-survivors	Survivors	Independent, or moderate disability	Severe disability
Kondziolka and Fazl	1988	5	–	5	5	–
Delashaw et al.	1988	9	1	8	4	4
Steiger	1991	8	2	6	4	2
Rieke et al.	1992	15	6	9	6	3
Total		37	9 (24%)	28 (76%)	19 (68%)	9 (32%)

portant in determining the efficacy of heparin. Conversely, earlier studies showing a benefit of heparin are hopelessly flawed, so the issue remains controversial.

Theoretically, heparin might be beneficial in the presence of a flow-altering large-vessel stenosis, or to prevent thrombus propagation and distal embolization after an acute occlusion – situations which may be unknown or absent in the patient with acute stroke. Early vascular imaging can therefore help in selecting the most appropriate candidates for heparin. Pending further study, we favor heparin anticoagulation for acute progressing stroke caused by large-vessel atherothrombosis in the absence of severe neurologic deficit and hemorrhage on CT. The duration of heparin therapy is generally 48–72 h (up to 10 days in many European centers) for carotid territory ischemia, and 7–10 days for vertebral basilar ischemia. At that point most patients have stabilized, and a long-term management plan can be formulated.

In acute cardioembolic stroke the risk of converting a bland infarct into a hemorrhage must be weighed against the risk of re-embolization. Hemorrhagic infarction is common after cardiac embolism, although clinically significant hematoma formation is infrequent. The risk of recurrent brain embolism appears to be about 1% per day for the first 2 weeks, although some studies suggest a lower risk. Heparin can be safely administered to most patients but is hazardous for patients with large infarcts, poorly controlled blood pressure, or significant hemorrhage on CT. There is suggestive, but not definitive, evidence that heparin safely reduces the risk

of recurrent embolism in carefully selected patients.

Emerging issues include the use of low-molecular-weight heparinoids in acute stroke, concomitant anticoagulant or antiplatelet therapy after thrombolysis, and the role of antiplatelet therapy in patients with acute brain ischemia. A recent pilot study by Biller et al. (1989) indicated that heparinoids may reduce the risk of hemorrhage when used in patients with acute cerebral infarction. The safety and efficacy of antithrombotic therapy following thrombolysis in very early stroke has not been established, although it will likely be required in some cases to prevent re-occlusion. There are virtually no data on antiplatelet therapy in acute stroke, which is under study in the International Stroke Trial.

When used in acute stroke, heparin is given by continuous intravenous infusion to maintain the activated partial thromboplastin time (APTT) 1.5–2 × control (usually 300–400 units/kg/ 24 h). An initial bolus injection is best avoided, as anecdotal evidence suggests that it increases the risk of brain hemorrhage. However, the optimal heparin regimen in acute progressing or cardioembolic stroke has not been established.

Thrombolysis

In the early 1980s, the evolution of imaging techniques and clot-specific agents prompted a comeback of thrombolysis for the acute treatment of basilar artery thrombosis. This approach was quickly extended to patients with acute strokes in the carotid artery territory due to middle cerebral artery occlusions. Subsequently, nearly a dozen trials of thrombolysis in acute ischemic stroke either have been published or are underway. The underlying hypothesis is that rapid restoration of blood supply within the first several hours after ictus might save that part of the ischemic brain which is nonfunctioning but still viable (penumbra) and would thus improve outcome.

Although theoretically attractive, the efficacy of thrombolysis in brain infarction remains unproven. A recent meta-analysis reviewed the six *randomized* trials of thrombolysis in acute ischemic stroke. After exclusion of the two trials conducted without the benefit of computed tomographic scanning, a 37% reduction in the odds of death and a significant 56% reduction in the odds of death or deterioration after thrombolytic treatment were calculated. On the basis of these findings, proper testing of thrombolysis in sufficiently large and well-designed randomized trials is advocated.

Identification of Appropriate Patients and Therapeutic Window. After excluding lacunar and low-flow-induced infarcts, mostly with mild deficits and good prognosis, and concentrating on large brain infarctions in major vascular distributions causing severe neurologic deficit, more than 90% are embolic in nature. Emboli originate from the heart or the ascending aorta, or from complicated atherosclerotic plaques in the large craniocervical arteries. Emboli lodge in the main stems of the large pial arteries or their major branches, predominantly the MCA. Because of the poor prognosis in terms of disability and death, it is

this group of stroke patients in whom the most aggressive type of treatment seems justified and for whom thrombolysis would be expected to work best. Since it is not possible to unequivocally identify these patients based on clinical findings alone, an initial CT scan must be done to exclude intracerebral hematoma, and (ideally) a vascular technique which identifies the site and extent of the vascular occlusion should be performed. Cerebral angiography can be done safely after acute stroke, although any diagnostic benefit may be offset by the 1 or 2 h of resulting delay. In most cases where there is occlusion of the *main stem* of the MCA, transcranial Doppler sonography (TCD) would suffice to make a reliable diagnosis.

Pretreatment tests require a considerable amount of time, during which many MCA occlusions lyse spontaneously. More importantly, reperfusion of infarcted brain tissue is clinically useless and potentially hazardous. Consequently, thrombolytic agents have to be given as early as possible, probably within 6 h for anterior circulation strokes and perhaps within up to 12 h for posterior circulation strokes. Because of such time constraints, many clinical trials have forgone pretreatment vascular imaging studies.

Thrombolytic Agents, Route of Delivery and Dosing. Despite its low costs, streptokinase is not frequently used because individual dosing is difficult and bleeding complications may be higher. Urokinase has most frequently been used because of its availability and relatively low cost, and because high local concentrations can be achieved by intra-arterial application via catheters. The intra-arterial route was initially chosen to maximize local thrombolytic effects and to avoid systemic adverse effects. More recently, recombinant tissue plasminogen activator (rtPA) has become fashionable despite its very high costs. Systemic rtPA was expected to work in a highly clot specific manner. However, none of the randomized, multi-center trials has been able to define a dosage that clearly accelerates lysis or increases the percentage of lysed arteries within a certain time limit. rtPA has been given intravenously (i.v.) for 1 h in dosages of 34–100 mg, or 15 mg intra-arterially (i.a.). Urokinase has been given i.a. in dosages ranging from 200 000 to 500 000 IU per hour over a period of 1–4 h, and i.v. in a total dosage of up to 2.5 million IU over several hours without excessive intracranial or extra-cranial bleeding complications. For comparison, the standard i.v. doses for myocardial infarction are 1.5 MU streptokinase or 100 mg rtPA. At present, a dose-dependent effect of rtPA has been demonstrated only in animal experiments with an up to 50% recanalization rate in treated animals as compared with a 5% rate in control animals. In most experimental settings, however, a clear-cut benefit of fibrinolysis was achieved only within the first 30 min after embolism and stroke.

Complications of Fibrinolytic Treatment. A low risk of intracranial bleeding – mostly clinically silent hemorrhagic transformation of the infarct, but also frank parenchymatous hemorrhage with lethal outcome – has been documented during animal ex-periments and clinical trials in patients. Spontaneous hemorrhagic transformation of brain infarction occurred in approximately 50–70% of cases studied during autopsy, and in 5–43% investigated by CT. Several prospective studies indicate that hemorrhagic transformation only rarely has an adverse effect on the clinical course, with clinical deterioration seen in only 4% of cases with hemorrhagic infarction. In contrast, parenchymal hematoma leads to abrupt clinical worsening or even death by herniation. The risk of a *spontaneous* hematoma into an ischemic infarction was found to be as low as 2%, except in a recent study by Okada et al. (1989), where it occurred in 8.6%.

Intracranial hemorrhagic complications during rtPA treatment in acute brain infarction have occurred with moderately increased frequencies. Parenchymal hematoma has occurred in 4–8.4% of cases with nearly 50% lethality. Hemorrhagic transformations occurred in 4–27% of the patients, with clinical worsening in approximately one of six. However, all of the randomized trials of fibrinolysis with serial CT scanning found massive hemorrhages slightly more often in placebo-treated patients. Frank hematomas tend to occur more often in patients with sustained hypertension if rtPA is administered later than 6 h after ictus, or if a low-density area is already visible on the initial CT. Surprisingly, an increased rate of cerebral hemorrhages in older patients was not seen in any of the studies. The risk of malignant brain edema with herniation does not appear to be increased either.

In summary, given the poor prognosis of embolic MCA occlusions, hemorrhagic complications do not appear to be a principal obstacle to fibrinolytic treatment in acute stroke patients, although the true risk remains uncertain. The *clinical benefit* of any type of fibrinolytic treatment in the anterior circulation has not yet been established. A dramatic improvement with thrombolysis alone seems highly improbable, even if applied within a very tight time window (e.g., 90 min). The efficacy of concomitant treatment (e.g., acetylsalicylic acid in combination with fibrinolytic compounds, or therapeutic heparinization shortly after fibrinolysis to prevent reocclusion) has not yet been evaluated. The features of all randomized studies of thrombolysis since the beginning of the CT era are summarized in Table 2.

Hemorrheologic Management

Hemodilution has been advocated for stroke treatment, because CBF in the normal brain increases with decreasing hematocrit (HCT). In ischemic regions CBF also increases as HCT falls. Hemodilution seems most effective in ischemia due to viscosity reduction in the microcirculation with its low shear rate. Unfortunately, most clinical trials of hemodilution have produced negative results, while experimental studies using agents such as low-molecular-weight dextran (LMWD) and LMWD in combination with nimodipine have been somewhat encouraging. The lack of success in clinical trials may in part be due to relatively delayed treatment following stroke onset, insufficient reduction of hematocrit after hemodilution treatment, and hemodynamic failure or increased brain edema with high mortality in extensive hypervolemic hemodilution. Theoretical

studies have suggested that a hematocrit of 30% is the lower limit, below which oxygen delivery is compromised, and where the trade-off between increased CBF and reduced oxygen delivery peaks. Successful laboratory studies have reduced hematocrit to 32–35% within 1–1.5 h of stroke onset, whereas most clinical trials have reached a hematocrit of 36–40% within 24 h of stroke onset. Albumin and LMWD have usually been used as hemodilutants in clinical stroke therapy trials. More recently, the complex polymer hydroxyethel starch 200/0.5 (HES) has been used in stroke therapy, since it decreases platelet and erythrocyte aggregation over administration periods of 2–3 days, in contrast to LMWD. LMWD is associated with increased viscosity with long-term administration over several days. In addition, HES does not seem to exacerbate cerebral edema.

At this time, the routine use of hemodilutant therapy cannot be recommended; however, hemodilutant therapy with or without phlebotomy can be considered in patients with a hematocrit exceeding 50%. Isovolumic hemodilution is probably preferable to hypervolemic hemodilution and can be achieved by administering 50 ml LMWD/h with sufficient 0.9% NACL (typically 50 ml/h) to keep the central venous pressure between 6 and 10, or pulmonary wedge pressure 14–16.

Emergency Vascular Surgery

Emergency carotid endarterectomy (CEA) is a controversial issue; the indications are not well defined. CEA early after cerebral infarction carries a

Table 2. Randomized trials of thrombolysis in acute ischemic stroke carried out since the beginning of the CT era

Reference/eponym	F/O	No. of patients vs. control	Compound, dose	Time window	Pretreatment angiogram	Route	Endpoints: recanal (R) at __h / clinical impr. (CI) at __h	Improved in treated vs. controls (n)
Mori et al. (1992)	F	19/12	tPA: 34–60 mg	<6 h	+	i.v.	at 1 h	47/12
Ohtomo et al. (1985)	F	189/81	UK: 60 000 IU per day	<5 days	+	i.v.	CI at 4 weeks	56/42
Abe et al. (1981)	F	54/53	UK: 60 000 IU per day	<30 days	+	i.v.	CI at 1 week and 4 weeks	63/43
Japanese Thrombolysis Study Group	F	31/47	tPA: 34 mg	<6 h	+	i.v.	CI at 4 weeks	72/55
European Cooperative Acute Stroke Trial (ECASS)	O	300/300	tPA:	<6 h	∅	i.v.	ADL at 3 months	
Donnan/et al. ASK	O	?	Streptokinase or ASA vs. placebo	<3 h	∅	?	?	?
Candelise/MAST-Italy	O	?	Streptokinase or ASA or both vs. placebo	?	∅	i.v.	?	?
NIH multi-center tPA Trial	O	?	tPA vs. placebo	<90 min <180 min	∅	i.v.	Neurologic scale	?

F, Finished; O, ongoing; S, to be started; UK, urokinase.

high risk of perioperative worsening or massive hemorrhage into the infarct due to the sudden increase of perfusion pressure after restoration of blood flow. However, in selected cases emergency CEA may be indicated, for example, in patients suffering an acute carotid occlusion during hospitalization, during angiography, or immediately after carotid surgery.

Emergency CEA should also be considered for patients with fluctuating or progressive neurologic deficits and high-grade stenosis of the internal carotid artery. This includes patients with progressive stroke, waxing and waning neurologic deficits, and crescendo TIAs despite anticoagulation. Even for a progressive stroke patient with a floating intraluminal thrombus, delay of CEA is usually advocated since immediate carotid surgery carries a high risk of perioperative embolism. If anticoagulation does not stop the attacks, CEA can be justified to prevent massive arterial embolization or acute thrombotic occlusion of the carotid artery. If fluctuating symptoms are of hemodynamic origin, CEA can restore blood flow and promptly improve or stabilize neurologic deficits. This rare clinical scenario can be confirmed by transcranial ultrasound with estimation of the vasomotor reserve using CO_2 or diamox stimulation. In the future angioplasty may be the treatment of choice in such cases, provided that the carotid stenosis is smooth and without ulceration. In rare cases with bilateral severe ICA stenoses, or occlusion on the symptomatic side with contralateral severe stenosis, immediate CEA can improve collateral flow to the hemisphere producing clinical signs of ischemia of hemodynamic origin. MCA embolectomy attempts to restore blood flow immediately, and there are some reports of favorable results if the operation is performed within 6 h after the embolic event. The operation is associated with the risk of large hematoma due to recirculation injury. Since local and systemic thrombolysis is now feasible, MCA embolectomy is only of historical interest. As in thrombolysis, the extent of collateral flow documented during pretreatment angiography is the best predictor of outcome.

Enhancement of Cellular Resistance to Metabolic Insult

General Strategies

When CBF drops below approximately 10 ml/100 g/min, a complex series of events termed the "ischemic cascade" is triggered. The hallmark of ischemic cell death is a massive increase in intracellular calcium. Disruption of calcium homeostasis is one of the central events culminating in cell death, and many new treatment strategies attempt to maintain or restore calcium balance in the cell subjected to acute ischemia.

Initially, it was hoped that the relatively central nervous system-selective dihydropyridine-type calcium entry blockers such as nifedipine, nimodipine, or nicardipine would protect neurons from calcium-induced damage. Nimodipine was shown to improve outcome after subarachnoid hemorrhage without reversal of angiographic vasospasm, suggesting a protective effect at the cellular level. Unfortunately, early positive trials of nimodipine in ischemic stroke were not supported by a recent multicenter randomized study which showed a trend favoring nimodipine, but only in patients treated less than 12 h from stroke onset.

The apparent ineffectiveness of commonly available dihydropyridine calcium entry blockers in acute cerebral infarction has been partly explained by the identification of at least six different calcium receptors in the central nervous system (Spedding 1987). Available calcium blockers interfere only with a single type of voltage-dependent channel, permitting calcium influx through several other routes. Attention has now focused on the excitatory amino acid transmitter receptors, in particular, the glutamate-dependent NMDA receptor. There is accumulating evidence that blockade of excitatory amino acid transmitter receptors, both NMDA-dependent and non-NMDA (AMPA) receptors, results in smaller infarctions and better outcome in experimental animals. Another class of agents, the so-called receptor abuse-dependent antagonists such as the GM1 gangliosides, may act by blocking the effects of calcium on cellular membrane function.

In addition to disturbed calcium homeostasis, there are a number of other important components to the ischemic cascade. The generation of free radicals may contribute to neuronal death. New free-radical scavengers which are lipid soluble and cross the blood-brain barrier, such as the 21 aminosteroids, are being developed. Increasing attention is also being focused on the blood-endothelial interface and its role in the ischemic process. The role of platelet-activating factor and white cells in the ischemic process is only now coming under scrutiny.

Reperfusion Injury

Early reperfusion of ischemic tissue leads to a secondary injurious process with cellular damage. The secondary damage results not only from edema or hemorrhagic transformation and diapedesis as a result of endothelial ischemic damage with increased permeability, but also entails calcium influx, blood cell-endothelial interactions, and the production of free radicals which oxidize and damage components of the cellular compartment and membrane. Superoxide, in the presence of iron, is converted to the hydroxyl free radical that can initiate cell membrane damage by lipid peroxidation and protein degradation. Hydroxyl radicals may also be formed by reactions between superoxide and endothelium-derived relaxing factor (EDRF). Consequently, lipid peroxidation inhibitors may play a role in the treatment of reperfusion injury. Free-radical scavengers are able to reduce the size of experimental ischemic infarction. Of special interest is superoxide dismutase, which improves cerebral blood flow and reduces ischemic cerebral edema in animal models with reperfusion after stroke. High doses of glucosteroids also inhibit lipid peroxidation. There is much interest in a new hydroxyl radical scavenger, the 21-aminosteroid tirilazad mesylate (U 74006 F), which has no corticosteroid activity but inhibits lipid peroxidation during the reperfusion period.

Following ischemia, the peptide endothelin may be produced by damaged endothelial cells. Endothelin causes severe vasoconstriction, mediated in part by PAF (endothelium-derived platelet-activating factor), which has a vasoconstrictive and neurotoxic effect. Like free radicals, PAF acts predominantly as a mediator of ischemic damage following transient ischemia. Experimental data show that PAF antagonists have vasodilatatory and cytoprotective effects which reduce infarct size following MCA occlusion in animals.

Multimodal Treatment Strategies

The so-called stroke cocktail for the treatment of brain infarction in man has not yet been mixed. However, potential ingredients have already been envisaged by many stroke researchers.

New calcium antagonists (e.g., levopamil) and NMDA-receptor antagonists (e.g., MK-801) are promising candidates to improve the ischemic tolerance of neuronal tissue, i.e., to help ischemic neurons survive longer. This could widen the therapeutic window for recanalizing or flow-improving procedures. It would seem logical to combine therapeutic strategies, e.g., rtPA or urokinase with a calcium antagonist, an NMDA-receptor antagonist, or a free-radical scavenger, or both. Recently published animal experiments in focal and global cerebral ischemia clearly demonstrate that infarct size and neurologic dysfunction were significantly reduced by combining rtPA with a glutamate antagonist, or superoxide dismutase with deferoxamine, as opposed to using a single agent.

With respect to the importance of transcortical collateral blood flow in preserving the ischemic cortex within the first hours after stroke, a combination of cellular protective compounds with a defibrinogenating drug (e.g., ancrod) would also make sense. Fibrinogen is an important plasma component related to viscosity. Promising findings during a recent multicenter randomized, double-blind acute stroke trial seem to justify such an approach.

In order to keep the number of variables as low as possible, a trial with a cocktail made of no more than two components with different mechanisms of action would seem a reasonable first approach. Two main problems remain unsolved, however, and prevent us from immediately stepping into this exciting new field: First, the choice of the number and type of drugs to be combined is uncertain, and second, legal obstacles have to be overcome. Internationally accepted rules for trials in human beings may not allow the combination of more than one drug not already registered for a particular indication. Thus, clinicians are eagerly awaiting further lessons from the animal laboratory with combined treatments of focal ischemia. Promising findings like those mentioned above may soon open the bar for the administration of such cocktails to the acute stroke patient.

Suggested Reading

Abe T, Kazama M, Naito I, Ueda M, Tanaka T, Higuchi H, Saso S, Kariyone S, Yoshimura M (1981) Clinical evaluation for efficacy of tissue-cultured urokinase (TCUK) on cerebral thrombosis by means of multi-centered double-blind study. Blood Vessels 12:321–341

Allen GS, Ahn HS, Preziosi TJ et al. (1983) Cerebral arterial spasm – a controlled trial of nimodipine in patients with subarachnoid hemorrhage. N Engl J Med 308: 619–624

Astrup J, Siesjö BK, Symon L (1981) Thresholds in cerebral ischemia – the ischemic penumbra. Stroke 12:723–725

Astrup J (1982) Energy-requiring cell functions in the ischemic brain. J Neurosurg 56: 482–497

Barnett GH, Bose B, Little JR, Jones SC, Friel HT (1986) Effects of nimodipine on acute focal cerebral ischemia. Stroke 17:5

Barry DI, Lassen NA (1984) Cerebral blood flow autoregulation in hypertension and effects of antihypertensive drugs. J Hypertens 2 [Suppl 3]:519–526

Barsan WG, Brott TG, Olinger CP, Marler JR (1989) Early treatment for acute ischemic stroke. Ann Intern Med 111:449–451

Baumbach GL, Heistad DD (1988) Cerebral circulation in chronic arterial hypertension. Hypertension 12:89–95

Bertel O, Conen D, Radu EW, Muller J, Lang C, Dubach US (1983) Nifedipine in hypertensive emergencies. Br Med J 286:19–21

Bielenberg G, Wagner G (1990) PAF antagonists reduce infarct size in focal ischemia in the rat brain. In: Krieglstein J, Oberpichler H (eds) Pharmacology of cerebral ischemia. Wissenschaftliche Verlagsgesellschaft, Stuttgart, pp 281–284

Biller J, Massey EW, Morler JR, Adams HP et al. (1989) A dose-escalation study of ORG 10172 (low-molecular-weight heparinoid) in stroke. Neurology 39:262

Biller J, Love BB (1991) Nihilism and stroke therapy. Stroke 22:1105–1107

Brott T, Reed RL (1989) Intensive care for acute stroke in the community hospital setting. The first 24 hours. Stroke 20:694–697

Brott TG, Haley EC, Levy DE, Barsan W, Broderick J, Sheppard GL, Spilkr J, Kongable GL, Massey S, Reed R, Marler JR (1992) Urgent therapy for stroke: part I. Pilot study of tissue plasminogen activator administered within 90 minutes. Stroke 23: 632–640

Brott T, Reed RL (1989) Intensive care for acute stroke in the community hospital setting. Stroke 20:694–697

Buchan A, Gates P, Pelz D, Barnett HJM (1988) Intraluminal thrombus in the cerebral circulation. Implications for surgical management. Stroke 19:681–687

Candelise L MAST-Italy personal communication

Caplan LR (1989) To heparinize or not: an unsettled issue (letter to editor). Stroke 20:968

Cerchiari EL, Hoel TM, Safar P, Sclabassi RJ (1987) Protective effects of combined superoxide dismutase and desferoxamine on recovery of cerebral blood flow and function after cardiac arrest in dogs. Stroke 18:869

Cerebral Embolism Study Group (1983) Immediate anticoagulation of embolic stroke: a randomized trial. Stroke 14:668

Cerebral Embolism Task Force (1989) Cardiogenic brain embolism (second report). Arch Neurol 46:727

Cerebral Embolism Task Force (1987) Cardiogenic brain embolism. Neurology 43:71–78

Cerebral Embolism Study Group (1984) Immediate anticoagulation of embolic stroke. Brain hemorrhage and management options. Stroke 15:779–789

Cerebral Embolism Study Group (1987) Cardioembolic stroke, immediate anticoagulation and brain hemorrhage. Arch Intern Med 147:636

deErausquin GA, Manav H, Guidotti A, Costa E, Brooker G (1990) Gangliosides normalize distorted single cell intracellular free Ca^{2+} dynamics after toxic doses of glutamate in cerebellar granule cells. Proc Natl Acad Sci USA 87:8017–8021

Del Zoppo GJ, Poeck K, Pessin MS, The Acute Stroke Study Group (1992) Recombinant tissue plasminogen activator in acute thrombotic and embolic stroke. Ann Neurol 32:78–86

Delashaw JB, Broaddus WC, Kassell NF, Haley EC, Pendleton GA, Vollmer DG, Maggio WW, Grady MS (1990) Treatment of right hemispheric cerebral infarction by hemicraniectomy. Stroke 21:874–881

Dereuck J, Vandekerckhovi T, Bosma G et al. (1988) Steroid treatment in acute ischemic stroke. Eur Neurol 28:70

Donnan GA, Davis SM, Chambers BR et al. (1993) Austrialian Steptokinase Trial (ASK). In: Del Zoppo GJ, Mori E, Hacke W (eds) Thrombolytic therapy in acute ischemic stroke II. Springer, Berlin Heidelberg New York

Duke RJ, Bloch RF, Alexander GG, Turpie MB, Trebilcock R, Bayer N (1986) Intravenous heparin for the prevention of stroke progression in acute partial stable stroke: a randomized controlled trial. Ann Intern Med 105:825–828

Estol CJ, Pessin MS (1990) Anticoagulation: is there still a role in atherothrombotic stroke? Curr Concepts Cerebrovasc Dis Stroke 25:1–6

Fayad PB, Brass LM (1991) Single photon emission computed tomography in cerebrovascular disease. Stroke 22:950–954

Frackowiak RS (1985) The pathophysiology of human cerebral ischemia, a new perspective obtained with position emission tomography. Q J Med 57:713–727

Garrido EB, Stein M (1976) Middle cerebral artery embolectomy. J Neurosurg 44:517–521

Giordano JM, Trout HH, Kozloff I, DePalma RG (1985) Timing of carotid artery endarterectomy after stroke. J Vasc Surg 2:250–254

Goldstone J, Moore WS (1976) Emergency carotid artery surgery in neurologically unstable patients. Arch Surg 111:1284–1291

Hacke W (1993) Stroke and embolus subtype. In: Del Zoppo GJ, Mori E, Hacke WY (eds) Thrombolytic therapy, in acute stroke. Springer, Berlin Heidelberg New York

Haley EC Jr, Kassell NF, Torner JC (1988) Failure of heparin to prevent progression in progressing ischemic infarction. Stroke 19:10–14

Haley EC, Levy DE, Brott TG, Sheppard GL, Wong MCW, Kongable GL, Torner JC, Marler JR (1992) Urgent therapy for stroke: part II. Pilot study of tissue plasminogen activator administered 91–180 minutes from onset. Stroke 23:641–645

Harry DJ, Kenny MA (1984) Computerized transcutaneous monitoring incorporating laser Doppler velocimetry. Med Instrument 18:121–126

Heros RC, Korosue K (1989) Hemodilution for cerebral ischemia. Stroke 20:423–427

Heros RC (1988) Carotid endarterectomy in patients with intraluminal thrombus. Stroke 19:667–668

Herpin D (1990) The effects of antihypertensive drugs on the cerebral blood flow and its regulation. Prog Neurobiol 35:75–83

Hornig CR, Dorndorf W, Agnoli AL (1986) Hemorrhagic cerebral infarction. A prospective study. Stroke 17:179–185

Italian Acute Stroke Study Group (1988) Haemodilution in acute stroke: results of the Italian haemodilution trial. Lancet 318–320

Jones TH, Morawetz RB, Cromwell RM, Marcous FW (1981) Thresholds of local cerebral ischemia in awake monkeys. J Neurosurg 54:773–782

Japanese Thrombolysis Study Group Intravenous tissue plasminogen activator in acute thromboembolic stroke: a placebo-controlled, double-blind trial. In: Del Zoppo GJ, Otis S, Mori E (eds) Proceedings of the 2nd international conference on thrombolysis in acute ischemic stroke. Springer, Berlin Heidelberg New York (in press)

Katzmann R, Clasen R, Klatzo I, Meyer JS, Pappius HM, Waltz AG (1977) Brain edema in stroke. Study group on brain edema in stroke. Stroke 8:512–540

Klatzo I (1972) Pathophysiological aspects of brian edema. In: Reulen HJ, Schürmann K (eds) Steroids and brain edema. Springer, Berlin Heidelberg New York

Kondziolka D, Fazl M (1988) Functional recovery after decompressive craniectomy for cerebral infarction. Neurosurgery 23:143–147

Korbmacher G, Ringelsteiń EB (1987) The risk of brian hemorrhage during anticoagulation of acute stroke patients. Preliminary results of a prospective study. In: Poeck K, Ringelstein EB, Hacke W (eds) New trends in diagnosis and management of stroke. Springer, Berlin Heidelberg New York, pp 103–113

Koudstaal PJ, Stibbe J, Vermeulen M (1988) Fatal ischaemic brain edema after early thrombolysis with tissue plasminogen activator in acute stroke. BMJ 297:1571–1574

Ley Pozzo J, Ringelstein EB (1990) Non-invasive detection of occlusive disease of the carotid siphon and middle cerebral artery. Ann Neurol 28:640–647

Lindsberg PJ, Hallenbeck JM, Feuerstein G (1991) Platelet-activating factor in stroke and brain injury. Ann Neurol 30:117–129

Lodder J (1984) CT-detected hemorrhagic infarction: relation with the size of the infarct, and the presence of midline shift. Acta Neurol Scand 70:329–335

594   A.J. Furlan et al.

Marder VJ, Sherry S (1988) Thrombolytic therapy: current status. N Engl J Med 318: 1512–1520

Masaryk AM, Ross JS, DiCello M et al. (1991) 3DFT MR angiography of the carotid bifurcation: potential and limitations as a screening examination. Neuroradiology 179:797–804

Meyer FD, Piepgras TG, Sundt TM, Yanagihara T (1985) Emergency embolectomy for acute occlusion of the middle cerebral artery. J Neurosurg 62:639–647

Minematsu K, Li L, Fisher M et al. (1992) Diffusion-weighted magnetic resonance imaging: rapid and quantitative detection of focal brain ischemia. Neurology 42: 235–240

Mohr JP, Caplan LR, Melski JW, Goldstein RJ, Duncan GW, Kistler JP, Pessin MS, Bleich HL (1978) The Harvard Cooperative Stroke Registry: a prospective registry. Neurology 28:754–762

Mohr JP, Dilanni M, Muschett JL et al. (1989) Nimodipine in acute ischemic stroke. Ann Neurol 26:124

Mori E, Yoneda Y, Tabuchi M, Yoshida T, Ohkawa S, Ohsumi Y, Kitano K, Tsutsumi A, Yamadori A (1992) Intravenous recombinant tissue plasminogen activator in acute carotid artery territory stroke. Neurology 42:976–982

Moseley ME, Wedland MF, Kuchorczyk J (1991) Magnetic resonance imaging of diffusion and perfusion. Top Magn Reson Imaging 3:50–67

O'Brien MD, Jordan MM, Waltz AG (1974) Ischemic cerebral edema and the blood-brain barrier. Distributions of pertechnetate, albumin, sodium and antipyrine in brains of cats after occlusion of the middle cerebral artery. Arch Neurol 6:49–55

Ohtomo E, Araki G, Itoh E, Tougi H, Matuda T, Atarashi J (1985) Clinical efficacy of urokinase in the treatment of cerebral thrombosis. Clin Eval 13:711–751

Ojemann RG, Heros RC, Cromwell RM (1987) Occlusive cerebrovascular disease. In: Ojemann R (ed) Surgical management of cerebrovascular disease. Williams and Wilkins, Baltimore

Okada Y, Yamaghucchi T, Minematsu K, Miyachita T, Sawada T, Sadochima S, Fujichima M, Omae T (1989) Hemorrhagic transformation in cerebral embolism. Stroke 20:598–603

Ott BR, Zamani A, Klefield J, Funkenstein H (1986) The clinical spectrum of hemorrhagic infarction. Stroke 17:630–637

Perez-Trepichio AD, Furlan AJ, Little JR, Jones SC (1982) Hydroxyethyl starch 200/ 0.5 reduced infarct balance after emboli stroke in rats. Stroke 23:98–103

Phillips DA, Fisher M, Smith TW, Davis MA (1988) The safety and angiographic efficacy of tissue plasminogen activator in a cerebral embolization model. Ann Neurol 23: 391–394

Raichle ME (1983) The pathophysiology of brian ischemia. Ann Neurol 13:2–10

Rieke K, Krieger D, v Kummer R, Aschoff A, Hacke W (1993) Decompressive surgery in space-occupying hemispheric infarction. Results of an open, prospective trial. (In press)

Ringelstein EB, Biniek R, Weiller C, Ammeling B, Nolte PN, Thron A (1992) Type and extent of hemispheric brain infarctions and clinical outcome in early and delayed middle cerebral artery recanalization. Neurology 42:289–298

Ringelstein EB, Korschorke S, Holling A, Brückmann H, Lambertz H, Minale C (1989) CT-patterns of proven embolic brain infarctions. A prospective study. Ann Neurology 26:759–765

Ringelstein EB, Zeumer H (1982) The role of continuous-wave Doppler sonography in the diagnosis and management of basilar and vertebral artery occlusions, with special reference to its application during local fibrinolysis. J Neurol 288:161–170

Ringelstein EB, Sievers C, Ecker S, Schneider PA, Otis SM (1988) Noninvasive assessment of CO_2-induced cerebral vasomotor response in normal individuals and patients with internal carotid artery occlusions. Stroke 19:963–969

Ropper AH (1985) In favor of intracranial pressure monitoring and aggressive therapy in neurologic practice. Arch Neurol 42:1194–1195

Ropper AH, Shafran B (1984) Brain edema after stroke. Clinical syndrome and intracranial pressure. Arch Neurol 41:26–29

Rothman SM, Olney JW (1986) Glutamate and the pathophysiology of hypoxic-ischemic brain damage. Ann Neurol 19:105–111

Sanella NA (1992) Bilateral severe carotid stenosis or occlusion and computed tomographic scan-positive hemispheric stroke with neurologic deficit: immediate contralateral carotid endarterectomy. Ann Vasc Surg 6:252–257

Scandinavian Stroke Study Group (1987) Multicenter trail of hemodilution in acute ischemic stroke. I. Results in the total patient population. Stroke 18:691–699

Scheinberg P (1989) Heparin anticoagulation. Stroke 20:173–174

Schmidley JW (1990) Free radicals in central nervous system ischemia. Stroke 21:1086–1090

Siesjo BK (1981) Cell damage in the brain: a speculative synthesis. J Cereb Blood Flow Metab 1:155–185

Siesjo BK (1984) Cerebral circulation and metabolism. J Neurosurg 60:883–908

Siesjö BK (1992) Pathophysiology and treatment of focal cerebral ischemia, part II: mechanisms of damage and treatment. J Neurosurg 77:337–354

Slivka A, Levy D (1990) Natural history of progressive ischemic stroke in a population treated with heparin. Stroke 21:1657–1662

Spedding M (1987) Three types of Ca^{2+} channel explain discrepancies. Trends Pharmacol Sci 8:115–117

Spence JD, Del Maestro RF (1985) Hypertension in acute ischemic strokes. Treat Arch Neurol 42:1000–1002

Steiger HJ (1991) Outcome of acute supratentorial cerebral infarction in patients under 60. Development of a prognostic grading system. Acta Neurochir (Wien) 111:73–79

Sterman AB, Furlan AJ, Pessin M, Kase C, Caplan L, Williams G (1987) Acute stroke therapy trials: an introduction to recurring design issues. Stroke 18:524–527

Strandgaard S, Olesen J, Skinhoj E, Lassen NA (1973) Autoregulation of brain circulation in severe arterial hypertension. Br Med H 1:507–510

von Kummer R, Hacke W (1992) Safety and efficacy of i.v. TPA and Heparin in acute MCA Stroke. Stroke 23:646–652

Wallace JD, Levy LL (1981) Blood pressure after stroke. JAMA 246:2177–2180

Walters BB, Ojemann RG, Heros RC (1987) Emergency carotid endarterectomy. J Neurosurg 66:817–823

Wardlaw JM, Warlow CP (1991) Thrombolysis in acute ischemic stroke: does it work? Stroke 23:182–1839

Williams JL, Furlan AJ (1992) Cerebral vascular physiology in hypertensive disease. Neurosurg Clin North Am 3:509–520

Wood JH, Simeone FA, Fink EA, Golden MA (1983) Hypervolemic hemodilution in experimental focal cerebral ischemia. J Neurosurg 59:500–509

Wylie FJ, Hein MF, Adams JE (1964) Intracranial hemorrhage following surgical revascularization for treatment of acute strokes. J Neurosurg 21:212–215

Xue D, Slivka A, Buchan AM (1992) Tirilazed reduces cortical infarction after transient but not permanent focal cerebral ischemia in rats. Stroke 23:894–899

Yatsu FM, Zivin J (1985) Hypertension in acute ischemic strokes. Not to treat. Arch Neurol 42:999–1000

Young W, Wojak JC, DeCrescito V (1988) 21-Aminosteriod reduces ion shifts and edema in the rat middle cerebral artery occlusion model of regional ischemia. Stroke 19:1013–1019

Yuh WTC, Crain MR, Loes DJ et al. (1991) MR imaging of cerebral ischemia: findings in the first 24 hours. AJNR 12:621–629

Zeumer H, Hacke W, Kolmann HL, Poeck K (1982) Lokale Fibrinolysetherapie bei Basilaristhrombose. Dtsch Med Wochenschr 107:728–731

Zivin JA, Mazzarella V (1991) Tissue plasminogen activator plus glutamate antagonist improves outcome after embolic stroke. Arch Neurol 48:1235–1238

Chapter 53

Vertebrobasilar Stroke, Cerebellar Stroke, and Basilar Occlusion

ANDREAS FERBERT, MICHAEL S. PESSIN, and KLAUS RIEKE

Introduction

This chapter is concerned mainly with "major" and life-threatening ischemic strokes in the posterior circulation. There is a rough correlation between the clinical severity of brain-stem strokes and the presence of large artery occlusive disease in the vertebrobasilar system. Small penetrating vessel or branch arterial disease results in restricted brain-stem and cerebellar infarcts with a relatively good functional prognosis and will not be the main focus of this discussion.

Pathogenesis

The majority of strokes in the posterior circulation are caused by arteriosclerosis. There are several locations in the posterior circulation that are particularly prone to the development of arteriosclerotic stenosis or occlusion, such as the intracranial part of the vertebral artery and the proximal

Section Editor: Werner Hacke

and middle parts of the basilar artery. It is believed that embolic events (mainly emboli from the heart) may be less common in the posterior circulation, yet this pathogenetic mechanism may be underestimated. Actually, the posterior cerebral arteries, the top of the basilar artery, and the posterior inferior cerebellar artery (PICA) are predominant recipients for arterosclerotic artery-to-artery or cardiac emboli. Coma in a patient with atrial fibrillation may be caused by an embolus to the basilar artery that resolves very quickly without leaving residual neurological signs that provide clues to the neurologist as to the origin of the coma. An embolus that enters the basilar artery usually reaches the most rostral part of the basilar artery, causing the "top of the basilar artery syndrome". It may then enter one or both posterior cerebral arteries. However, other patterns of embolic occlusion are known: The embolus may be lodged in the distal vertebral artery or even in the middle part of the basilar artery. The latter pattern is due not to the anatomy of the artery, which has a similar diameter throughout, but more likely to altered flow characteristics once occlusion of the more proximal basilar artery causes retrograde flow in the distal part of the vessel. Arteriosclerotic lesions may also produce hemodynamic insufficiency of ischemia as well as serving as substrate for artery-to-artery local embolism, thereby preventing a clear separation of the two pathogenetic mechanisms on clinical grounds alone. For example, high-grade stenosis of the intracranial vertebral artery and the proximal basilar artery are possible origins of embolization into the distal vascular bed.

Lacunar infarctions are caused by arteriohyalinosis of small perforating arteries, mostly due to long-standing hypertension. In the pons they can be found in the tegmentum and pontine base. Branch occlusions of the paramedian pontine arteries often lead to infarctions of the pontine base that are larger than lacunar infarctions, even when the vessel occlusion cannot be identified by angiography.

There are a number of other possible etiologies for strokes in the posterior circulation such as vertebral artery dissection, transient migrainous vasospasm, vasculitis (one of the first cases of basilar artery occlusion described in the literature was of syphilitic origin; see also Fig. 1 in the chapter on syphilis, Chap. 39), and tumorous vessel compression.

Clinical Features and Differential Diagnosis

(for more details refer to Chap. 30)

Lacunar infarctions of the brain stem are responsible for a variety of brainstem syndromes. Their severity, however, tends to be relatively mild and

functional outcome good, irrespective of the treatment regimen. For the purpose of this book we will therefore concentrate on patients with infarctions due to larger branch occlusions (e.g., paramedian perforating arteries) or occlusions of the large arteries like the vertebral arteries or the basilar artery.

Infarctions of the dorsolateral medulla oblongata lead to what is clinically called Wallenberg's syndrome and are caused by occlusions of the vertebral or posterior inferior cerebellar artery. Both embolic and arteriosclerotic lesions may occur; in the long term it is a relatively benign condition, leaving the patient with only mild neurological deficit. In the acute stage, however, it can occasionally lead to serious complications if the vertebral artery occlusion extends into the basilar artery. The hallmark of Wallenberg's syndrome is severe vertigo with nystagmus, sensory loss, and unilateral ataxia. In the classical case this consists of hypalgia, ipsilateral in the face and contralateral in the body, most pronounced in the leg. However, it is not uncommon to find the sensory loss purely on the contralateral side with a faciobrachial predominance. This indicates location of the infarction more mediolateral with involvement of the ventral trigemino-thalamic tract instead of the spinal trigeminal tract and nucleus. Further signs include ipsilateral Horner's syndrome. Dysphagia often endures for weeks and makes feeding through a nasogastral tube temporarily necessary. It is particularly severe in the first few days and poses the threat of aspiration pneumonia for the patient. Although hemiparesis is not part of Wallenberg's syndrome, the hemiataxia renders the

Table 1. Prodromal symptoms in 53 of 85 patients with basilar artery occlusion

Symptom	No. of patients
Vertigo, nausea	26[a]
Headache, neckache	18
Hemiparesis	9
Double vision	9
Dysarthria	9
Hemianopia	5
Hemihypoesthesia	5
Tinnitus, hearing loss	5
Drop attack	4
Confusion	3
Other	6

[a] Only four of these patients did not experience other prodromal symptoms.

patient unable to use the affected hand. Truncal ataxia including abasia is present, but its severity is dependent on an additional cerebellar infarct that often accompanies dorsolateral medullary infarction.

The term *vertebrobasilar occlusion* includes occlusion of both vertebral arteries or the basilar artery. In contrast to dorso-lateral medullary infarction, this condition is often preceded by prodromal symptoms days to weeks before the onset of the stroke (Table 1). Moreover, a majority of cases may show a progressive temporal profile different to that of strokes in the carotid territory.. A progressive stroke in the posterior circulation that may initially manifest mild signs often leads to the full clinical picture of basilar artery occlusion, and therefore early diagnosis is of paramount importance (Table 1). In such cases an extracranial and transcranial Doppler ultrasound study or angiography must be performed.

Since basilar artery lesions are often associated with unilateral or bila-

teral vertebral occlusion through thrombus extension or distal embolization, a strict separation of clinical syndromes is difficult. There are, however, some typical features of vertebrobasilar occlusion at different levels:

1. Bilateral vertebrobasilar artery occlusion is often associated with dysarthria, vertigo, nystagmus, vomiting, and paresis of caudal cranial nerves in a progressive or staggering fashion over a few days. Headache is more frequent than in carotid territory strokes and sometimes gives rise to misdiagnosis such as meningitis or subarachnoid hemorrhage. The headache is probably due to meningeal ischemia and is only rarely found in upper basilar artery occlusions. In contrast to those with Wallenberg's syndrome, patients with bilateral vertebrobasilar occlusion show hemi- or tetraparesis. Sudden respiratory arrest has frequently been observed, even in unilateral brain-stem stroke, and underlines the necessity for treatment in the ICU. Typically, patients are awake unless there is embolism to the top of the basilar artery, where coma or confusion are commonly present. If the thrombus extends from proximal occlusions into more distal vessels, slowly progressing change of consciousness is the typical clinical syndrome.

2. Occlusions of the middle part of the basilar artery often present with a sudden onset leading to posturing of the arms, sometimes mistaken as an epileptic fit. Severe tetraparesis is the rule and is a prominent feature in the locked-in

syndrome (see Chap. 30). Ocular abnormalities are dominated by disturbances of the horizontal gaze center (internuclear ophthalmoplegia, one-and-a-half syndrome, uni- or bilateral gaze palsy).

3. Occlusions of the rostral part of the basilar artery often produce coma, at least in the acute stage. The occlusion of the superior cerebellar artery is critical in this respect, whereas an embolus to the very top of the basilar artery, sparing the superior cerebellar artery, may result in drowsiness that resolves quickly. The latter case can be found as part of the "top of the basilar artery syndrome", which includes cortical blindness and disorientation. Bilateral medial thalamic infarction sparing the occipital lobe produces memory impairment and reduced drive, in its severest form as akinetic mutism. Vertical gaze palsy and/or fascicular oculomotor palsy and other oculomotor abnormalities related mainly to the vertical gaze system are common in all of the above-mentioned varieties of rostral basilar artery occlusion (see Fig. 1), whereas tetraparesis is less pronounced than in mid-basilar syndromes.

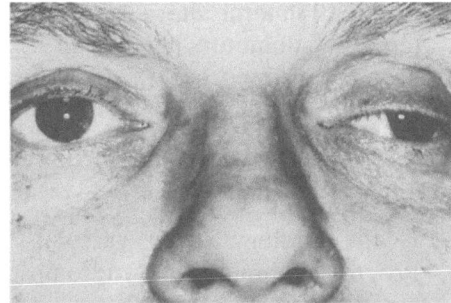

a

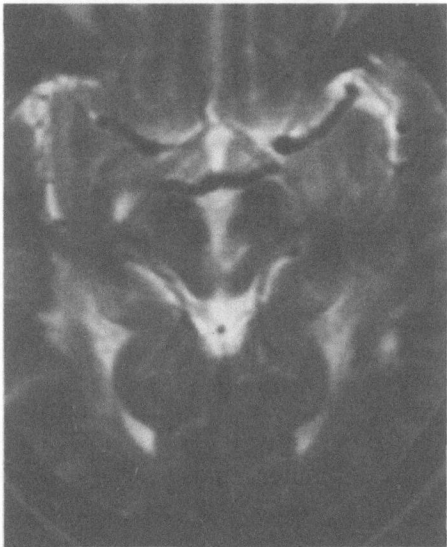

b

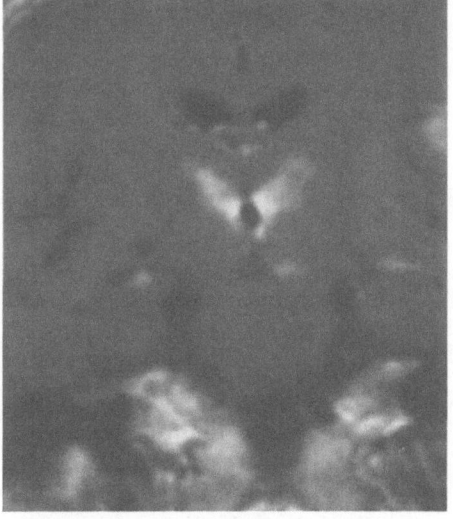

c

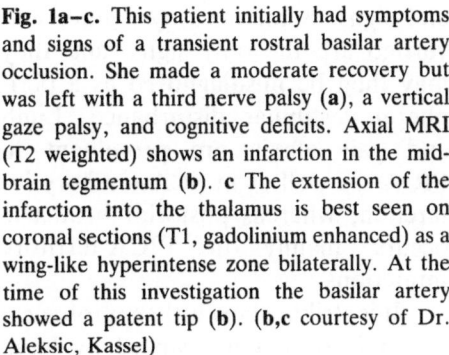

Fig. 1a–c. This patient initially had symptoms and signs of a transient rostral basilar artery occlusion. She made a moderate recovery but was left with a third nerve palsy (**a**), a vertical gaze palsy, and cognitive deficits. Axial MRI (T2 weighted) shows an infarction in the midbrain tegmentum (**b**). **c** The extension of the infarction into the thalamus is best seen on coronal sections (T1, gadolinium enhanced) as a wing-like hyperintense zone bilaterally. At the time of this investigation the basilar artery showed a patent tip (**b**). (**b,c** courtesy of Dr. Aleksic, Kassel)

Isolated bilateral internal and external oculomotor nerve palsies have been reported in patients with mesencephalic infarcts.

In the differential diagnosis three questions are of importance:

1. Is the etiology really vascular? Progressive brain-stem syndromes can also occur in brain-stem encephalitis and sometimes show few abnormallities in CSF studies. Ancillary vascular tests may be necessary to clarify the diagnosis. In patients with cardiac arrhythmia sudden onset of coma can be the result of transient cardiac arrest and global cerebral ischemia or an embolus to the top of the basilar artery.
2. Which vascular territory is involved? The predominance of oculomotor and vestibular abnormalities, as well as the presence of bilateral signs, makes this question easy to answer unless the initial presentation is only hemiplegia that occasionally heralds (mid-) basilar artery thrombosis. Bilateral carotid territory infarction can occasionally mimic upper basilar artery occlusion, including some of the oculomotor signs.
3. What is the presumed pathophysiology? Progressive syndromes are suspect for being the result of a major vessel thrombotic occlusion. Certain associated cardiac abnormalities, such as atrial fibrillation, suggest an embolic origin; occasional premonitory signs are not contradictory to this possibility. The migration of the embolus to the upper basilar artery may take from a few hours up to some days with several "arrests", caus-

ing a typical, staggering sequence of signs progressively affecting a widespread area of brain-stem function. Bilateral paresis is common in basilar artery occlusion and uncommon in branch occlusion or lacunar infarction. Preceding chiropractic maneuvers or other, even minor, traumatic events predispose to vertebral artery dissection and may require clarification by neuroimaging.

Cerebellar Stroke

Isolated cerebellar infarction may occur in the territory of one of the major cerebellum-supplying arteries: the posterior inferior (PICA), anterior inferior (AICA), or superior cerebellar artery (SCA). Most cerebellar infarctions have a benign course; however, space-occupying cerebellar infarcts are a subtype with particularly high morbidity and mortality. SCA infarcts have mostly an embolic origin, often from local diseases in the basilar artery, whereas in PICA-territory infarction the mechanism is equally divided between cardiogenic embolism and local intracranial vertebral artery disease. Infarctions in the territory of the PICA and AICA are particularly prone to inducing vestibular symptoms and signs. Sometimes nystagmus and vertigo are the only signs, and they may then be misdiagnosed as a peripheral vestibular disturbance. Limb and gait ataxia are prominent in PICA- as well as in SCA-territory infarction, whereas posterior headache occurs mainly in PICA-territory infarctions.

It is striking how little neurological deficit is sometimes caused by large

Table 2. Clinical features of cerebellar infarction

Stage	Symptoms	Clinical signs
Early	Dizziness, nausea, vomiting, lack of balance	Nystagmus, appendicular ataxia, stiff neck, dysarthria
Intermediate	Irritability, confusion, drowsiness	Pseudo sixth nerve palsy, sixth nerve palsy, gaze palsy, forced gaze deviation, Babinski's signs, seventh nerve palsy, small pupils reactive to light
Late	Stupor, coma, posturing, cardiovascular instability	Pinpoint pupils, ataxic respiration, apnea

and sometimes even space-occupying PICA-territory cerebellar infarctions before they cause secondary compressive brain-stem signs and altered level of consciousness. Slowly progressive deterioration in consciousness and a sixth nerve palsy are caused by brain-stem compression from the swollen cerebellum, a potentially life-threatening condition (Table 2). Hydrocephalus develops in the course of brain-stem compression and further complicates the increased ICP. In milder cases of hydrocephalus an external shunt operation may be sufficient to reduce ICP. However, in cases of massive brain-stem compression a posterior fossa decompressive operation with removal of the infarcted tissue is indicated to prevent herniation. Stupor and coma are important clinical indications for decompressive surgery. Studies are currently under way to test the value of neurophysiological monitoring of brain-stem auditory evoked potentials (BAEP) and somatosensory evoked potentials (SEP) as indicators for surgery and predictors of outcome. They have the advantage of not being influenced by sedative drugs, which must often be given to patients with artificial ventilation. Patients with

large PICA-territory infarcts should be transferred to the ICU, as clinical deterioration may occur rapidly. Coma of sudden onset or hemiplegia without sixth nerve palsy may be the result of basilar artery occlusion. Patients who have already sustained a major brain-stem infarction will not benefit from cerebellar decompressive surgery. Isolated SCA-territory infarcts commonly have a benign course, and massive brain-stem compression is rare.

Ancillary Tests

Neuroimaging

In patients with a permanent or progressing vascular event in the posterior circulation, neuroimaging should be carried out as soon as possible to clarify the vascular pathology; CT is still the fastest method of detecting or excluding hemorrhage. MRI is more sensitive than CT in detecting ischemic lesions in the brain stem and cerebellum. However, in the very early stage an ischemic lesion may not be detected even on MRI. If MRI is not quickly enough available in a hospital it should be postponed, and a CT scan may be sufficient for deciding on further diagnostic and therapeutic measures. MR angiography (MRA) can additionally give some information about the status of the arteries, but this technique may not be available quickly enough for the emergency case.

Doppler Ultrasound

The sensitivity of ultrasound in detecting occlusive lesions is high in the case of bilateral vertebrobasilar occlusion. Lesions of the cranial vertebral and basilar artery can be detected by transcranial Doppler. However, the exact morphology requires angiographic confirmation at the present time. The lowest sensitivity of transcranial Doppler is with emboli to the rostral tip of the basilar artery. If the Doppler studies suggest bilateral vertebral occlusion or basilar occlusion, angiography should be done immediately unless the patient has already been in coma for several hours or an infarct is visible on CT.

Neurophysiology

Neurophysiological tests include mainly BAEP and SEP, which can give objective information about brainstem function even in the noncooperative patient. In basilar artery occlusion several types of BAEP abnormalities can be found, according to the different levels of the occlusion in the craniocaudal extension. They can also be used as continuous monitoring during fibrinolytic therapy. With cerebellar infarctions, evaluation and monitoring of brain-stem compression

by the swollen cerebellum can be achieved. This condition causes increased interpeak latency of peaks I–V of BAEP. In patients with locked-in syndrome the residual sensory input can be tested by evoked potentials. Finally, in patients who do not appear well clinically, evoked potentials can give important prognostic information. Bilateral loss of cortical SEPs for more than 12 h are invariably associated with poor outcome or death.

Others

An ECG should be obtained in the acute stage to detect arrhythmia. Echocardiography should also be performed, but if angiography and fibrinolysis are planned, it should be postponed in order to avoid delay in therapy.

Lumbar puncture is usually unnecessary unless brain-stem encephalitis is suspected. In contrast to vertebrobasilar occlusive disease, this is a rare condition.

Management

Patients with symptoms and signs suggestive of vertebrobasilar occlusive disease should be investigated as soon as possible. If the clinical course is progressive, vertebrobasilar occlusion has to be assumed and the patient should be transferred to an ICU. Angiography should be performed. In cases of coma of unknown etiology an upper basilar artery occlusion should be suspected. As Doppler ultrasound diagnosis of upper basilar artery occlusion is more difficult than that of more

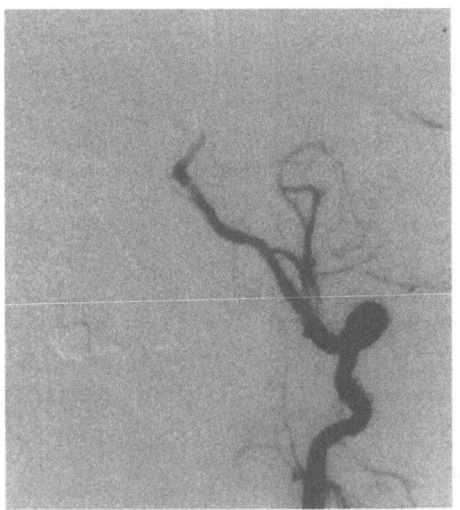

a

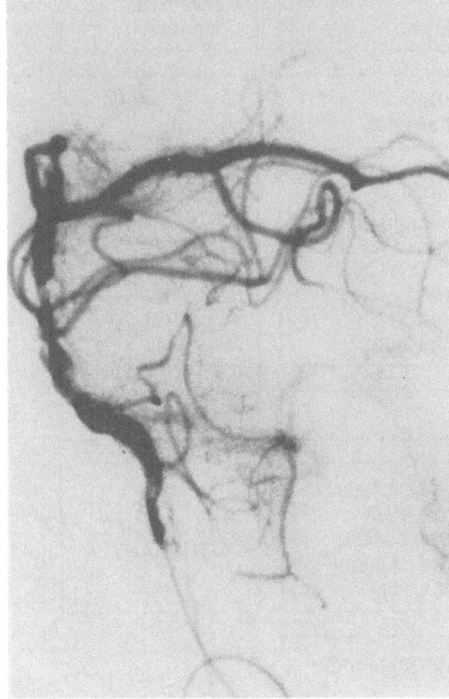

b

Fig. 2a,b. A 66-year-old man with attacks of vertigo and progressive loss of consciousness within 1 day. **a** Vertebral angiography shows complete occlusion of the basilar artery distal to the AICA. **b** After local infusion of 500 000 IU urokinase into the basilar artery via a microcatheter partial recanalization has occurred, leaving severe stenotic lesions. (Courtesy of Dr. Stephan, Kassel)

proximal bilateral vertebrobasilar occlusion, angiography may be necessary despite normal ultrasound results unless coma persists for 5 h or more. In all cases a CT scan should be obtained to exclude hemorrhage.

Since the natural course of vertebrobasilar occlusion is often unfavorable, local intra-arterial fibrinolysis is currently being investigated in several centers. It has been shown that this treatment may improve the clinical outcome. With a thin catheter in the vertebral artery, 750 000 IU urokinase is infused – 500 000 IU during the first hour, 250 000 IU during the second hour in order to achieve partial or full recanalization (Fig. 2). Prolonged fibrinolysis does not result in benefit for the patient, although recanalization can be achieved later. Heparin (1000 IU/h) should be given 30 min

Table 3. Therapeutic regimen

Local intra-arterial fibrinolysis (LIF, investigational)
– catheter position in the distal vertebral artery or proximal basilar artery
– 500 000 IU urokinase during the first hour
– 250 000 IU urokinase during the second hour
– clinical (and electrophysiological) monitoring

Intravenous fibrinolysis (investigational)
0.9–1.1 mg/kg rt-PA i.v. in case LIF is not possible for technical reasons

Anticoagulation
Acute: heparin 24 000–36 000 IU/day for high-grade stenosis of the basilar artery or embolus to the basilar artery or active embolic source
Chronic: coumarin for high-grade stenosis of the b.a.

Decompressive cerebellar craniectomy and ventricular drainage
– ICP treatment
– ventricular drainage
– large bone flap
– resection of infarcted tissue optional

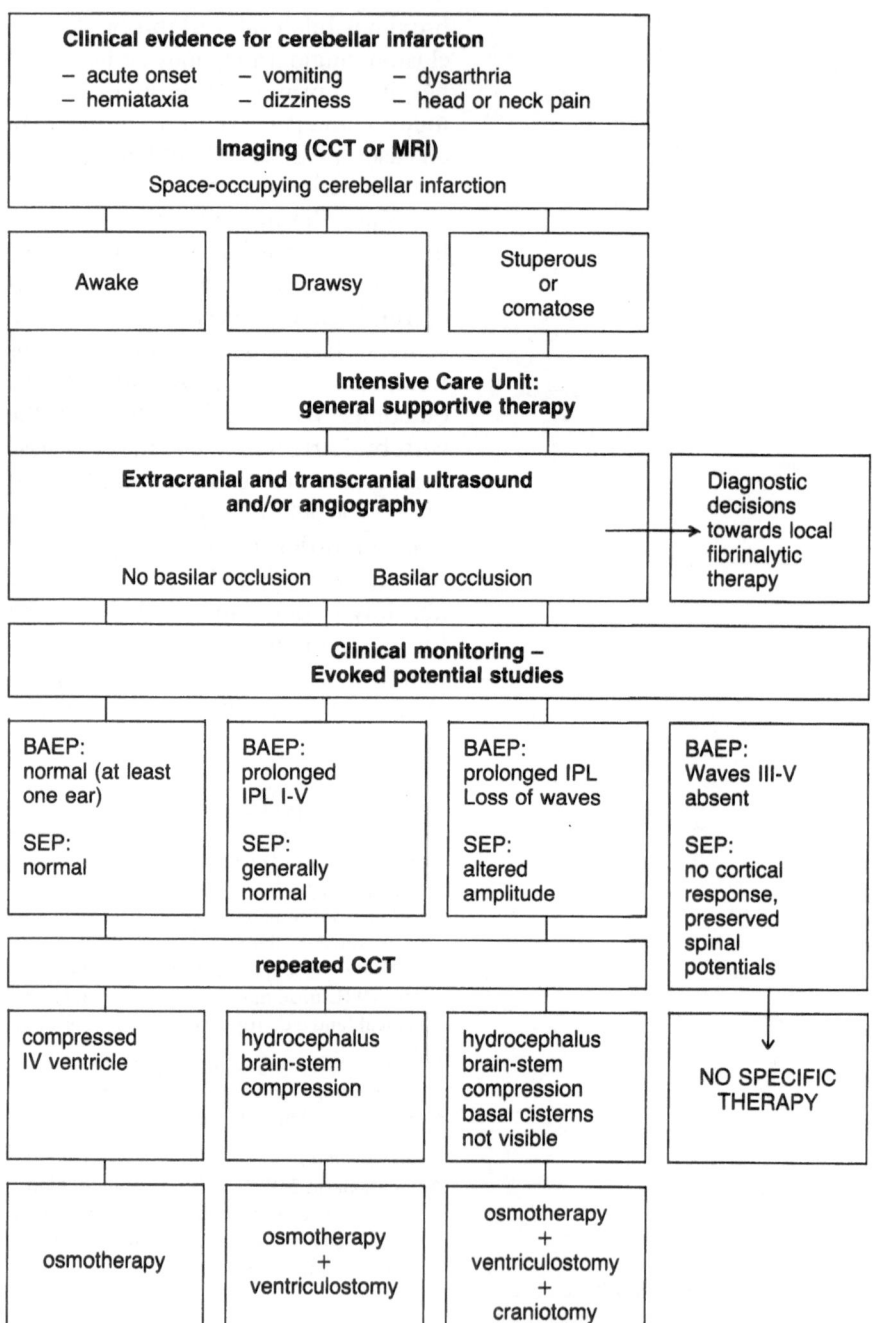

Fig. 3. Prospective protocol for therapeutic management of patients presenting with cerebellar stroke

after the catheter has been withdrawn (see also Table 3).

With pure cerebellar infarction clinical (and, if available, electrophysiological) monitoring should be performed. If the course progresses to drowsiness, CT should be repeated. If hydrocephalus is present an external ventricular CSF shunt should be inserted. Mannitol infusion and hyperventilation should be initiated. It is sometimes difficult to distinguish between deterioration due to compression of the brain stem from the cerebellar mass effect and an occlusion of the basilar artery. Continuous deterioration in the level of consciousness and a sixth nerve palsy without hemi- or tetraparesis favor brain-stem compression, whereas a sudden deterioration, one-and-a-half syndrome, and motor paresis suggest basilar artery occlusion. Angiography may be necessary to differentiate between the two conditions. If clinical deterioration occurs rapidly or the patient is already in coma, a suboccipital decompressive craniotomy with removal of the infarcted tissue should be performed. There is general agreement about the necessity of such an operation; however, the exact timing is still somewhat controversial. Furthermore, some authors deny the advantage of an external CSF shunt procedure, claiming that it might produce upward herniation of the cerebellum through the tentorial notch. They are therefore in favor of an earlier craniotomy. Figure 3 shows our proposed decision tree for stepwise management of patients with acute cerebellar infarction.

Suggested Reading

Archer CR, Horenstein S (1977) Basilar artery occlusion. Clinical and radiological correlation. Stroke 8:383–390

Brueckmann H, Ferbert A, del Zoppo GJ, Hacke W, Zeumer H (1987) The acute vertebro-basilar thrombosis. Angiological-clinical comparison and therapeutic implications. Acta Radiol [Suppl] 369:38–42

Caplan LR, Baquis GD, Pessin MS, D'Alton J, Adelman LS, DeWitt LD, Ho K, Izukawa D, Kwan ES (1988) Dissection of the intracranial vertebral artery. Neurology 38: 868–877

Caplan LR, Pessin MS, Mohr JP (1992) Vertebrobasilar occlusive disease. In: Barnett HJM, Mohr JP, Stein BM, Yatsu FM (eds) Stroke. Pathophysiology, diagnosis and management, 2nd edn. Churchill Livingstone, New York, pp 443–515

Caplan LR (1980) "Top of the basilar" syndrome. Neurology 30:72–79

Caplan LR (1983) Bilateral distal vertebral artery occlusion. Neurology 33:552–558

Castaigne P, Lhermitte F, Buge A, Escourolle R, Hauw JJ, Lyon-Caen O (1981) Paramedian thalamic and midbrain infarcts: clinical and neuropathological study. Ann Neurol 10:127–148

Castaigne P, Lhermitte F, Gautier JC, Escourolle R, Derouesne C, der Agopian P, Popa C (1973) Arterial occlusion in the vertebrobasilar system. A study of 44 patients with postmortem data. Brain 96: 133–154

Chen HJ, Lee TC, Wei CP (1992) Treatment of cerebellar infarction by decompressive suboccipital craniectomy. Stroke 23:957–961

Ferbert A, Brueckmann H, Drummen R (1990) Clinical features of proven basilar artery occlusion. Stroke 21:1135–1142

Ferbert A, Buchner H, Brueckmann H, Zeumer H, Hacke W (1988) Evoked potentials in basilar artery thrombosis: correlation with clinical and angiographic findings. Electroencephalogr Clin Neurophysiol 69: 136–147

Hacke W (1986) Clinical relevance of multimodal assessment of brainstem functions in severe vascular brainstem lesions. In: Kunze K, Zangemeister WH, Arlt A (eds) Problems of brainstem disorders. Thieme, Stuttgart, pp 101–110

Hacke W, Zeumer H, Ferbert A, Brueckman H, del Zoppo G (1988) Intra-arterial thrombolytic therapy improves outcome in patients with acute vertebrobasilar occlusive disease. Stroke 19:1216–1222

Heros R (1992) Surgical treatment of cerebellar infarction. Stroke 23:937–938

Heros R (1982) Cerebellar hemorrhage and infarction. Stroke 13:106–109

Kase CS, Norrving B, Levine SR, Babikian VL, Chodosh EH, Wolf PA, Welch KMA (1993) Cerebellar infarction: clinical and anatomic observation in 66 cases. Stroke 24:76–83

Krieger D, Busse O, Schramm J, Ferbert A (1992) German and Austrian Space Occupying Cerebellar Infarction Study (GASCIS): study design, methods, patient characteristics. J Neurol 239:183–185

Kubik CS, Adams RD (1946) Occlusion of the basilar artery. A clinical and pathological study. Brain 69:73–121

Pessin M, Lathi ES, Cohen MB, Kwan ES, Hedges TR, Caplan LR (1987) Clinical features and mechanism of occipital infarction. Ann Neurol 21:290–299

Rieke K, Krieger D, Adams HP, Aschoff A, Meyding-Lamadé U, Hacke W (1993) Therapeutic strategies in space-occupying infarctions based on clinical, neuroradiological and neurophysiological data. Cerebrovasc Dis 3:45–55

Ringelstein EB, Zeumer H, Poeck K (1985) Noninvasive diagnosis of intracranial lesions in the vertebrobasilar system. A comparison of Doppler sonographic and angiographic findings. Stroke 16:848–855

Zeumer H (1985) Vascular recanalizing technique in interventional neuroradiology. J Neurol 231:287–294

Zeumer H, Hacke W, Kolmann HL, Poeck K (1982) Lokale Fibrinolysetherapie bei Basilaris-Thrombose. Dtsch Med Wochenschr 107:728–731

Chapter 54

Septic Embolic Encephalitis

DERK KRIEGER and JOHANNES BRACHMANN

Definition and Epidemiology

Septic embolic encephalitis (SEE) results from infectious, ischemic, and hemorrhagic damage to the neuroparenchyma following infective thromboembolism from any part of the body. The heart is the most common source (infective endocarditis), followed by bacteremia and pulmonary infections. At autopsy, SEE is characterized by diffuse congestion and hyperemia of the leptomeninges, cerebral edema, and sometimes focal subarachnoid hemorrhage. Numerous microabscesses can be seen and occasionally they coalesce to form space-occupying macroabscesses. Vessel occlusion by thromboemboli and bacterial vasculopathy (including septic erosion of the vessel wall) can result in cerebral ischemia, intracerebral hemorrhage, or both. Evaluation and treatment of septic embolic encephalitis in the neurocritical care unit requires an interdisciplinary approach.

Section Editor: Werner Hacke

Pathophysiology

SEE and brain abscesses usually result from bacterial infections, or rarely fungal infections, of the neuroparenchyma. SEE occurs in 20%–56% of patients with infective endocarditis regardless of whether the infection is on native or prosthetic valves. SEE and brain abscesses occur more often after infection of the mitral and aortic valve than after infection of the tricuspid valve and are more common with *Staphylococcus aureus* infections than with *Streptococcus viridans* infections (2:1 ratio). The timing and incidence of embolization is related to the particular organism involved and the size of the vegetation.

Solitary brain abscesses are often caused by purulent pulmonary infections, such as lung abscess or empyema, bronchiectasis, arteriovenous fistula, and cyanotic congenital heart disease (especially with right-to-left shunting). Infected intravenous catheters may also occasionally cause brain abscesses. The reasons for the brain's susceptibility to abscess formation are not clear, but abscesses

Table 1. Risk factors for and principal clinical features of septic embolic encephalitis (SEE)

Cardiac disease
Rheumatic cardiovalvular disease
Mitral valve prolapse
Degenerative heart disease in the elderly
Prosthetic cardiac valves
Congenital heart disease

Others
Drug addiction
Compromised immune function (malignant
    disease)
Central venous catheters
Arteriovenous shunts (congenital and
    therapeutic)
Chronic infectious disease (mostly pulmonary)

Clinical features
Fever
Head/and or backache, stiff neck
Acute organic-type mental disturbance
Transient or permanent focal deficit
Seizures
Unconsciousness

---

usually form in areas of preexisting damage. The most common organisms in brain abscesses are *Staph. aureus, Serratia marcescens*, and group D streptococci (Table 1).

Clinical Features and Differential Diagnosis

Ischemic stroke is the most common mode of presentation of patients with SEE. About 15% of patients have symptoms of transient ischemia (presumably from emboli). Because of the anatomy of the cerebral vessels, damage most often occurs in the distribution of the middle cerebral artery, rarely in the distribution of the posterior circulation (>9:1 ratio). Other neurological manifestations include

toxic encephalopthy (20%), brain hemorrhage (5%), meningitis (4%), isolated headache (3%), and brain abscesses (<1%).

Toxic encephalopathy is characterized by mental status changes and psychosis and results from multiple scattered microinfarcts or abscesses and the resulting fever and immune response. Brain hemorrhage (intracerebral or subarachnoid) occurs as a result of vessel damage, ranging from acute pyogenic necrosis to large mycotic aneurysms. Rarely, this can occur weeks to months after cure of the infection. Ruptured mycotic aneurysms account for 1.7% of all brain hemorrhages, though the fraction of patients who could benefit from surgical repair, under ideal circumstances of detection, is small. Secondary hemorrhagic transformation can occur in patients with thromboembolic cerebral infarcts.

Patients may present with severe headache that develops rapidly, is recurrent, and is related to fever. It usually clears with antibiotic treatment. Focal or generalized seizures are uncommon, but may suggest purulent meningitis, uremia, hypoxia, or drug toxicity in the setting of infective endocarditis. Diseases that can mimic SEE include autoimmune diseases, tumors, and chronic infections, such as tuberculosis (Table 2).

Diagnosis

SEE should be suspected in all patients presenting with a focal neurological deficit or toxic encephalopathy (Table 2). Infective endocarditis can be diagnosed with echocardiography

Table 2. Differential diagnoses in relation to SEE in neurocritical care patients

Microbial disease
Septic thrombosis of the dural venous sinuses
Tuberculous meningitis
Toxic shock syndrome
Kawasaki's disease
Chagas' disease
Cerebral malaria

Viral disease
Aseptic meningitis
Acute viral encephalitis (herpes simplex encephalitis)
Reye's syndrome

Cerebrovascular ischemic disease
Drug abuse-related stroke
Nonbacterial thrombotic endocarditis-related stroke
Disseminated intravascular coagulation-related stroke
Noninfectious granulomatous angiitis of the central nervous system
Systemic lupus erythematosus-related stroke
Fat and air embolism

Cerebrovascular hemorrhagic disease
Aneurysmal subarachnoid and/or intracerebral hemorrhage
Arteriovenous malformation-related subarachnoid and/or intracerebral hemorrhage

Table 3. Principal microbes reported in infective endocarditis

Microbe	Estimated incidence
Strep. viridans	50%
Strep. faecalis	15%
Staph. aureus	20%
Staph. epidermidis	5%
Group D streptococci	4%
Haemophilus sp.	4%
Serratia marcescens	<1%
Pseudomonas aeruginosa	<1%
Candida sp.	<1%
Aspergillus sp.	<1%

predisposing factor and appears to be shifting toward rarer forms (Table 3). Fever is almost always present but may be lower in elderly patients. Blood cultures may be negative in patients with endocarditis and brain abscesses. Analysis of the cerebrospinal fluid (CSF) may reveal predominantly polymorphonuclear pleocytosis, increased protein concentration, and decreased glucose concentration. Only 16% of CSF cultures are positive.

(especially transesophageal echocardiography) and multiple blood cultures. Still, it remains unclear, even in the presence of valvular vegetations, what the exact composition of the thromboembolism is (for example, bacteria, fungi, thrombi). Use of cardiac magnetic resonance imaging (MRI) may help to distinguish infectious from thrombotic material (because of the ferromagnetic properties of thrombi). Although *Strep. viridans* has historically been the most common causative organism in infective endocarditis, today the spectrum is more dependent on the underlying

Neuroimaging

Cranial computed tomography (CCT) and MRI may identify intracranial lesions, such as infarction, abscess, or hemorrhage. Contrast studies may show areas of ring enhancement surrounding a region of lesser density (hypodensity on T1-weighted images and ring enhancement with gadolinium). Close follow-up studies are required to differentiate cerebritis from abscesses. All patients should undergo cerebral angiography to exclude mycotic aneurysms.

Table 4. Diagnostic and therapeutic procedures in SEE

Diagnostic procedure	Therapeutic option
Basic procedures in suspected SEE	
Blood cell count	Antimicrobial treatment (for at least
Erythrocyte sedimentation rate	6 weeks)
Repetitive blood cultures	
Cardiac diagnostic procedures, incl. auscultation, EKG, B – mode transthoracic and transesophagal echocardiography, cardiac MRI	
Asdominol ultrasound, chest radiography	
SEE presenting as a syndrome of meningeal irritation or mental disturbance	
All above *plus*:	
CSF puncture including cell count, cytology and protein chemistry	Admission to ICU
CSF culture	
SEE presenting as a syndrome of transient or permanent focal symptoms and/or altered state of consciousness	
All above *plus*:	
Plain and contrast CT scan or plain and contrast-enhanced MRI	Antiepileptic therapy Brain abscess drainage
Intra-arterial DSA	Aneurysm surgery (after 6 weeks) Cardiac surgery (not before day 3–4)
SEE presenting as a syndrome of massive cerebral infarction	
All above *plus*:	Consideration of thrombolytic therapy Medical and surgical decompressive therapy

Treatment

General

Treatment should focus on the causative (or most likely causative) organism and the neurological abnormality. Antibiotics should be chosen based on culture and sensitivity results. For initial empiric treatment (before culture results become available), we recommend broad-spectrum antibiotics including penicillin G (10–20 million units per day in four doses) plus a third-generation cephalosporin, such as ceftriaxone (6 g per day in three doses) plus vancomycin (30 mg/kg per day in two doses) and tobramycin (3 mg/kg once daily). See Table 4.

Cardiac Embolism

Although patients with acute stroke from a cardioembolic source are usually treated with anticoagulants to prevent further embolic events, we generally do not recommend such treatment for those with SEE. Usually, treatment of the infection is sufficient to reduce the risk of subsequent embolic events. Early anticoagulation may also increase the risk of cerebral hemorrhage. Anticoagulation is recommended, however, for those who continue to have cerebral embolization despite adequate antibiotic treatment (we recommend heparin 10–15 IU/kg per hour). Thrombolytic therapy may also be considered, depending on the time of presentation and clinical severity. In patients with angiographically proven vessel occlusion (for example, those with complete proximal middle cerebral artery stem occlusion), the cerebral infarct is the most life-threatening event and not the infective endocarditis. This is also feasible for patients who present with SEE after having recently undergone prosthetic valve replacement. The risk of cardioembolic stroke is lower in patients with bioprosthetic valves than in those with mechanical valves. Antiplatelet drugs may be used as an alternative to anticoagulation; however, their therapeutic efficacy has not been established.

Some patients may have infective endocarditis diagnosed retrospectively after presenting with a massive cerebral infarction. Those with acute space-occupying cerebral lesions may require surgical decompression just like other patients with space-occupying cerebellar or cerebral lesions.

Mycotic Aneurysms

Patients with mycotic aneurysms may be asymptomatic until rupture occurs or they may have premonitory signs such as unremitting and localized headaches, transient focal neurological deficits, and prior embolic stroke. We recommend cerebral angiography in all patients with infective endocarditis who present with focal neurological symptoms and signs. Early cerebral hemorrhage from rupture of mycotic aneurysms is associated with a high mortality rate and is not amenable to surgery. The presence of unruptured mycotic aneurysms does not necessarily indicate surgery as these sometimes resolve spontaneously with antibiotic therapy. After completion of at least 6 weeks of antibiotic therapy, patients with no symptoms from their aneurysms should undergo elective surgery for repair.

Cardiac Surgery

The timing of cardiac surgery after an embolic stroke with SEE can be particularly difficult. Complications include secondary hemorrhage and hemorrhagic transformation of infarcted tissue during anticoagulation for cardiopulmonary bypass and further worsening of edema because of hypotension (and nonpulsatile blood flow). However, if the clinical course permits, we recommend cardiac surgery within 3–5 days in patients with large infarcts, because the risk of recurrent emboli may be higher than the risk of increasing brain edema.

Brain Abscesses

Therapy for brain abscesses should be monitored by CCT and MRI. Although most abscesses resolve with medical management, occasionally large abscesses may require surgical drainage, either by a conventional burr-hole or by stereotactic aspiration.

Seizures

Generalized or focal seizures that interfere with the acute disease should be treated with clonazepam, phenytoin, or both (see Chap. 66). Once SEE has been treated, treatment with anti-seizure drugs can generally be stopped without any permanent defect, although some patients with permanent focal lesions may require long-term treatment.

Prognosis

Factors that affect survival include early diagnosis, virulence, and microbial sensitivity of the organisms as well as the type and site of damage. The overall mortality rate varies from 20% to 50%. Patients with intracerebral or subarachnoid hemorrhages and meningitis have the highest mortality rates (80%–90%).

Suggested Reading

Aronow WS (1991) Etiology and pathogenesis of thromboembolism. Herz 16:395–404 (no 6)

Dajani AS, Bisno AL, Chung KJ, Durack DT, Freed M, Gerber MA, Karchmer AW, Millard HD, Rahimtoola S, Shulman ST, Watanakunakorn C, Taubert KA (1992) Prevention of bacterial endocarditis. Heart Dis Stroke 1:53–57

Davenport J, Hart RG (1990) Prosthetic valve endocarditis 1976–1987. Antibiotics, anticoagulation and stroke. Stroke 21:993–999

David G, Sherman MD (1990) Cardiac embolism: the neurologist's perpective. Am J Cardiol 65:32C–37C

Paschalis C, Pugsley W, John R, Harrison MJ (1990) Rate of cerebral embolic events in relation to antibiotic and anticoagulant therapy in patients with bacterial endocarditis. Eur Neurol 30(2):87–90

Salgado AV, Furlan AJ, Keys TF, Nichols TR, Beck GJ (1989) Neurologic complications of endocarditis. A 12-year experience. Neurology 39:173–178

Tettenborn B, Krämer G, Erbel R (1991) Prophylaxis and acute therapy of arterial embolism with special reference to cerebral embolism. Herz 16:444–455 (no 6)

Ting W, Silverman N, Levitsky S (1991) Valve replacement in patients with endocarditis and cerebral septic emboli. Ann Thorac Surg 51(1):18–21 (discussion 22)

Chapter 55

Vasculitis of the Central Nervous System

PETER BERLIT and PATRICIA M. MOORE

Introduction and Definitions

Vasculitis restricted to the central nervous system (CNS) may be an idiopathic disorder or may be secondary to toxins, infections, or neoplasm. Alternatively, it may be part of a systemic autoimmune disease. The vasculitis may account for the majority of symptoms or represent a relatively unimportant component of another disease process. Vasculitis frequently affects both the central and the peripheral nervous (PNS) systems. There are diseases in which CNS or PNS symptoms are the only manifestations of the vasculitic process (e.g., isolated angiitis of the central nervous system and isolated angiitis of the PNS). In other diseases the neurological symptoms are part of a systemic disease. Clinically, it is important to distinguish between vasculitis in infectious and neoplastic disease and those forms in which it arises as the expression of a primary immunological process. In the latter group, in clinical practice, a distinction is usually made between primary vas-

culitis (giant cell arteritis, panarteritis nodosa, Wegener's granulomatosis, isolated angiitis of the nervous system) and secondary vasculitis (vasculitis in collagen vascular disease, hypersensitivity angiitis). Neurological involvement as part of a systemic disease is dealt with in chapter 92; we describe here the main features of forms of vasculitis that primarily or frequently affect the nervous system. For the neurologist in the emergency ward, it is important to be aware of temporal arteritis, isolated angiitis of the central nervous system and Behçet's disease.

Temporal Arteritis (Giant Cell Arteritis, Cranial Arteritis)

Temporal arteritis is a systemic form of necrotizing vasculitis histologically characterized by the formation of giant cells. This disease primarily involves the branches of the external carotid artery, in particular the superficial temporal artery and the ophthalmic and posterior ciliary arteries. There is typically inflammation in other large arteries of the body, and almost all

Section Editor: Werner Hacke

branches of the aorta and the aorta itself may be involved. The pattern of pathologic involvement is usually patchy, so that severe arteritis and normal vessel wall may be found side by side in a single biopsy specimen. Generally, different stages of the vasculitic process are found in the same patient, ranging from inflammatory infiltrates in the media, fragmentation of the internal elastic lamina, and necrosis of the total vessel wall to aneurysm formation or narrowing due to fibrosis and proliferation. The characteristic giant cells are usually to be found between the intima and the media of the vessel wall.

Epidemiology

Temporal arteritis is a disease of the elderly occurring quite frequently in the USA and in Europe, with an incidence ranging between 0.35 and 21.5 per 100 000 inhabitants per year. The seventh and eighth decades are the most common age for this disease; before the age of 50 years, temporal arteritis is very uncommon. Women are affected two to three times as often as men.

Clinical Features

The presenting symptoms of temporal arteritis are: headache, jaw claudication, polymyalgia rheumatica, and constitutional symptoms such as loss of weight and appetite, subfebrile temperatures, and fatigue. On clinical examination, patients may show a thickened and tender superficial temporal artery. Involvement of other larger vessels may be identifiable by

bruits or pulse and blood pressure differences. Claudication of the tongue and/or pharyngeal muscles and necrosis of the scalp or the tongue may also occur.

The symptom most likely to bring the patient into a neurological emergency ward is uni- or bilateral blindness due to involvement of the posterior ciliary or central retinal arteries. While this most feared complication of temporal arteritis was reported in 50% of cases in early reports, the more recent literature gives figures between 8% and 20%. At the onset of the acute blindness, the patient has often experienced symptoms of a systemic disease for several weeks or months. Only a minority of the patients with ophthalmic complications first present with temporary visual disturbances, such as diplopia, flittering scotoma, or amaurosis fugax. Ischemic lesions may be present in cranial nerves III, IV, and VI, as well as in the ocular muscles themselves. Disturbances of pupillomotor responses, ocular hypotonia, ptosis, and Horner's syndrome have all been reported.

Other neurological complications include hemispheric stroke, especially in the territory supplied by the posterior or the middle cerebral artery. Vertebrobasilar infarctions have been described, as have ischemic myelopathies, cerebral hemorrhages, and lesions of the pituitary gland and the hypothalamus. Besides these acute neurological syndromes, cognitive disturbances, depression, and/or hallucinations may be present. Peripheral neuropathies present most often as mononeuropathies, involving especially the median nerve (carpal tunnel syndrome) and the peroneal nerve. Rarely, acute polyneuritis has also been reported. Seizures are very rare.

The nonneurological complications of temporal arteritis are unusual given the systemic nature of the disease. They include claudication of the arms and legs and abdominal colic and heart pain due to involvement of the intestinal and coronary arteries. Pulmonary and renal arteries and the arteries of the uterus and the adnexa may also be involved. Temporal arteritis may imitate the aortic arch syndrome seen in young patients with Takayasu's disease.

About 50% of patients with temporal arteritis present symptoms of polymyalgia rheumatica, i.e. symmetrical muscle pain close to the large joints with morning stiffness and tenderness. The upper extremities are involved more frequently.

Ancillary Tests

An elevated erythrocyte sedimentation rate (ESR) is the most consistent laboratory finding in temporal arteritis; usually, it is above 100 mm in the 1st h. A value of less than 50 mm/h is very uncommon, although it has been described in isolated cases. Other laboratory signs are hypochromic anemia, altered iron-copper quotient, and elevation of acute phase reactants such as the C-reactive protein. An elevation of alpha-II globulin fraction and the hepatic enzymes, including alkaline phosphatase, is frequent. The level of angiotensin converting enzyme may be increased. Neuroradiological studies will show the infarcted territory and the distribution of vessel occlusions.

The diagnosis of temporal arteritis is primarily a clinical one and the cor-rect diagnosis depends largely on a high index of suspicion in patients presenting with constitutional symptoms, headache, blindness, stroke, or acute psychiatric disturbances. High ESR and hypochromic anemia support the clinical suspicion. If possible, a biopsy of one of the superficial temporal arteries should be performed rapidly, but since the serious complication of amaurosis may occur suddenly even in occult temporal arteritis, appropriate treatment must be instituted immediately upon clinical suspicion of the disease. Because of the segmental pattern of the inflammation, a biopsy specimen at least 2 cm in length should be obtained. Occasionally, biopsy of the temporal artery on the other side or one of the occipital arteries may be necessary. The overall sensitivity of the temporal artery biopsy is reported to be 70%. Since 30% of patients will thus have no specific pathologic findings in a given biopsy specimen, treatment may be given even if the biopsy shows normal results. On the other hand, a positive temporal artery biopsy is a good indicator that long-term treatment with corticosteroids will be necessary.

Treatment

Corticosteroids are the treatment of choice for temporal arteritis. The appropriate initial dose is 1 mg/kg body weight per day. This therapy must be instituted as soon as the clinical diagnosis of temporal arteritis is made. The sensitivity of biopsy decreases after institution of corticosteroid therapy from 70% to about 50% for the first 3 days.

The daily dose of corticosteroids is reduced depending on the clinical signs and the ESR. The reduction of the dose must be very cautious, with frequent checks of ESR and close clinical monitoring of the patient. Usually it is possible to reduce the corticosteroid dose to about 20–40 mg daily over a period of 8–12 weeks. Reductions by about 10 mg every 4th–8th day in general are possible. After the dose of 40 mg has been reached weekly reductions should not exceed 2 mg. As a double-blind study has shown, alternate day regimens are less effective than daily treatment. The treatment must be continued for at least 12 months. In our experience both relapses and exacerbations of the disease are much more common when treatment is terminated less than 20 months after onset.

Prognosis

Since temporal arteritis requires long-term treatment with corticosteroids, typical side effects of these drugs are often encountered. A range of immunosuppressive drugs have been tried in order to reduce the corticosteroid dosage in these patients, but in general these are ineffective and it is not possible to shorten or avoid steroid therapy. Faster reduction of the steroid dosage is possible if additional treatment with azathioprine is given. As, however, only a small reduction in steroids is achieved in this way, we suggest this combined therapy only in patients with diabetes mellitus or who suffer severe side effects from the corticosteroids.

Isolated Angiitis of the CNS

Definition and Pathophysiology

Isolated angiitis of the CNS is by definition an idiopathic recurrent inflammatory disease of the small and medium-sized vessels, confined to the brain and the spinal cord. The first reports on this disease were based on neuropathological findings and the term "granulomatous angiitis of the CNS" has often been used. Since, however, granulomas are not a constant finding, the term "isolated angiitis of the CNS" (IAC) is preferable. Pathologically, small and medium-sized vessels in the CNS are affected within the dural reflections. Choroidal and retinal vessels may also be affected. Mononuclear infiltrates with some accompanying polymorphonuclear cells are usually to be found. Different stages of the vasculitis with and without infiltrates and necrosis may be seen in the same patient at the time of examination, supporting the view that IAC is a recurrent and progressive vasculitis. In IAC there are often signs of endothelial proliferation, with inflammatory cells and some degree of scarring of vessel wall, but giant cells are not found. Immunofluorescent stains do no usually reveal evidence of immunocomplexes or antibody deposition.

IAC may be more frequent than was previously thought. While all the early reports were based on pathological findings, a clinical diagnosis is now more frequently made. Although many reports lack the diagnostic criteria necessary for the documentation of IAC (Table 1), this is not a rare disease and it should be considered in the differential diagnosis of patients with

Table 1. Diagnostic criteria in isolated angiitis of the central nervous system

1. Headaches and multifocal neurological deficits present for at least 6 months unless the onset is devastating or rapidly progressive
2. Cerebral angiography demonstrating several areas of arterial narrowing
3. No systemic infection or inflammation
4. Leptomeningeal/parenchymal biopsy to demonstrate vascular inflammation and rule out infection, neoplasia, and vasculopathies

headache, encephalopathy, recurrent stroke, or myelopathy.

Clinical Features

Persisting headaches and the signs and symptoms of encephalopathy with personality changes, cognitive disorders, and memory disturbances are the most frequent presenting symptoms of the disease. Multifocal neurological deficits result from recurrent cerebral ischemia and cranial nerve involvement. Myelopathies occur in less than 10% of the patients. Cerebral ischemic symptoms and myelopathic signs develop acutely and may bring the patient into a neurological emergency ward. The other symptoms (headache and encephalopathy) follow a more insidious course, with relapses and a slowly progressive cognitive disorder.

Ancillary Tests

Systemic symptoms and signs do not occur and serologic tests are normal. CSF studies may show some degree of pleocytosis or increase in protein, but in the majority of cases normal findings are obtained. There are no inflamma-tory signs in the peripheral blood count; the ESR is normal. There are no detectable immunocomplexes, autoantibodies, or antibodies against bacteria, fungi, or viruses.

Cranial computed tomography (CCT) and magnetic resonance imaging (MRI) may show multilocular ischemic lesions or white matter lesions. The most important neuroradiological examination in these patients is selective cerebral angiography, which may show segmental stenoses or dilatations of the smaller arteries. Occlusion of individual branches is typical, but the angiogram is frequently normal.

Since even the "typical" angiographical findings are at least nonspecific, other diseases have always to be excluded. There is a large range of differential diagnoses for CNS vasculitis, including tumors, infectious diseases, and toxic lesions. A list of important differential diagnoses is given in Table 2.

A leptomeningeal biopsy demonstrating vasculitis is the only reliable diagnostic method and is a sine qua non, because the immunosuppressive treatment is deleterious for a patient with a fungal or other infectious disease misdiagnosed as IAC. The biopsy site should be chosen in the light of CCT, MRI, and angiographic findings – we try to take the material from the nondominant hemisphere, including both leptomeningeal and parenchymal tissue.

Treatment

Since monophasic vasculitic illness – e.g., after exposure to drugs – may manifest with clinical and neuroradio-

Table 2. Differential diagnosis of central nervous system vasculitis

---

Vasculitis: idiopathic
  Systemic vasculitis (polyarteritis nodosa,
    Churg-Strauss syndrome, Wegener's
    granulomatosis)
  Behçet's disease
  Isolated angiitis of the central nervous system
Vasculitis: secondary
  Infections (fungi, viral, bacterial, treponemal,
    mycobacterial)
  Neoplasia (Hodgkin's lymphoma,
    paraneoplastic)
  Toxins (amphetamines, cocaine)
  Collagen vascular disease (systemic lupus
    erythematosus, Sjögren's syndrome,
    rheumatoid arthritis)
Vasculopathy
  Amyloidosis
  Postirradiation
  Fibromuscular dysplasia
  Neoplasia (lymphoma)
  Degenerative (systemic lupus erythematosus)
Coagulopathy
  Thombotic thrombocytopenic purpura (TTP)
  Hyperviscosity
  Antiphospholipid/cardiolipin antibody
    (systemic lupus erythematosus)
  Anti factor VII antibody
  Paraproteinemia
  Sickle cell disease

---

logical findings identical to those in IAC, the clinical development of the patient should be observed before treatment is instituted. If there is a acute course requiring urgent treatment in the intensive care unit, a leptomeningeal biopsy is necessary before the treatment of choice – cyclophosphamide and corticosteriods – is started. Treatment is instituted with a daily dose of 1–2 mg prednisone/kg body weight and 100–200 mg cyclophosphamide. The tapering of the dose depends on the clinical course of the disease; in general, at least 1 year of therapy is necessary.

Behçet's Disease

Definition and Epidemiology

Behçet's disease is named after the Turkish dermatologist Behçet, who in 1937 first described the triad of iridocyclitis, oral aphthosis, and genital ulcers. The disease is characterized by intermittent vasculitis of the capillaries and veins of the mucous membranes, the eye, and, in about 40% of cases, of the CNS vessels. The frequency of Behçet's disease follows the Silk Route, being frequent in Japan, China, and the Eastern Mediterranean countries, while the incidence in Europe and the United States is less than $1:100000$ inhabitants per year. Men are affected twice as frequently as women, with a mean age of 28 years at onset of the disease.

Clinical Features

The typical dermatological manifestations of Behçet's disease are aphthous stomatitis, genital ulcerations and ocular inflammation including iridocyclitis, hypopyon iritis, and conjunctivitis. Retinal vein thrombosis may occur. Other skin manifestations include erythema nodosum and hypersensitivity reactions. Multilocular arthralgias, involvement of the gastrointestinal tract, and abdominal or peripheral phlebitis with frequent thrombosis are symptoms of the systemic disease.

Neurological involvement has been described in 10%–49% of all patients with Behçet's disease, but neurological symptoms are the presenting symptoms of the disease in only about 5%. Thrombosis of cerebral veins may be the presenting symptom of Behçet's disease. Sinus thrombosis presents most frequently with the signs of intracranial hypertension. These patients may have none of the other clinical signs seen with isolated cerebral vein thrombosis. Meningoencephalitis may also be the clinical presentation. Headaches, disturbances of consciousness, and focal neurologic symptoms are frequent; spinal cord involvement occurs.

Ancillary Tests

If a patient presents with signs of elevated intracranial pressure, MRI and angiography are the most important studies to evaluate for cerebral venous thrombosis. In patients with other presentations, MRI may also be helpful by demonstrating hyperintense lesions in the T2-weighted images, which have a predilection for the pons and cerebral peduncles.

Treatment

The treatment of choice for Behçet's disease consists of steroids at an initial dose of 60–80 mg/day in combination with an immunosuppressive agent such as chlorambucil or azathioprine.

Primary Systemic Vasculitis

Primary systemic vasculitis, which may involve the nervous system, is discussed in Chap. 92. While polyarteritis nodosa and the Churg-Strauss syndrome most frequently involve the peripheral nervous system, CNS involvement is encountered in Wegener's granulo-matosis and in lymphomatoid granulomatosis. In the setting of the neurological emergency ward, patients with the symptoms of Guillain-Barré syndrome and laboratory findings indicative of systemic disease should particularly prompt the differential diagnosis of systemic vasculitis. In particular, if the polyneuritis is asymmetric, with painful severe paresis – the mononeuritis multiplex type – both polyarteritis nodosa and Churg-Strauss syndrome are important differential diagnoses. In lymphomatoid granulomatosis the presenting sign is usually intracranial hypertension with the formation of tumors demonstrable by CCT or MRI. Wegener's granulomatosis may also present with space-occupying granulomata, but cerebral ischemia or hemorrhage due to vasculitis may also occur. In the majority of patients with systemic vasculitis, the diagnosis is confirmed when the disease leads to sudden severe neurological symptoms. The peripheral nerve manifestations of the panarteritis nodosa group and the Churg-Strauss syndrome, on the other hand, may be the first symptom of the disease in about 20% of patients. In these cases, a biopsy specimen of the sural nerve or muscle may prove very helpful, if there is neurophysiological evidence of involvement. The treatment of choice for all these systemic diseases is the combination of corticosteroids with an immunosuppressive drug, usually cyclophosphamide.

Suggested Reading

Berlit P (1992) Clinical and laboratory findings with giant-cell arteritis. J Neurol Sci 111: 1–12

Berlit P, Storch B, Schmitt HP (1986) Diagnosis and treatment of allergic granulomatosis Churg-Strauss. Eur Arch Psychiatr Neurol Sci 235:200–205

Caselli RJ, Hunder GG, Whisnant JP (1988) Neurologic disease in biopsy-proven giant cell (temporal) arteritis. Neurology 38: 352–359

Fauci AS, Haynes BF, Costa J, Katz P, Wolff SM (1982) Lymphomatoid granulomatosis. Prospective clinical and therapeutic experience over 10 years. N Engl J Med 306:68–74

Gross WL (1993) Granulomatous vasculitides: neurological aspects. In: Berlit P, Moore PM (eds) Vasculitis, collagen vascular disease and the nervous system. Springer, Berlin Heidelberg New York

Hartmann A, Berlit P, Olbert D, Krastel H (1982) Neurologische Komplikationen bei Morbus Behçet. Aktuel Neurol 9:78–82

Hawke SHB, Davies L, Pamphlett R, Guo YP, Pollard JD, McLeod JG (1991) Vasculitic neuropathy. Brain 114:2175–2190

Hogan PJ, Greenberg MK, McCarty GE (1981) Neurologic complications of lymphomatoid granulomatosis. Neurology 31:619–620

Huston KA, Hunder GG, Lie JT, Kennedy RH, Elveback LR (1978) Temporal arteritis. A 25 year epidemiologic, clinical and pathologic study. Ann Intern Med 88:162–167

Ishikawa K, Uyama M, Asayama K (1983) Occlusive thromboaortopathy (Takayasu's disease): cervical arterial stenoses, retinal arterial pressure, retinal microaneurysms and prognosis. Stroke 14:730–735

Moore PM, Cupps TR (1983) Neurological complications of vasculitis. Ann Neurol 14: 155–167

Moore PM (1989) Diagnosis and management of isolated angiitis of the central nervous system. Neurology 39:167–173

Moore PM (1989) Immune mechanisms in the primary and secondary vasculitides. J Neurol Sci 93:129–145

Perruquet JL, Davis DE, Harrington TM (1986) Aortic arch arteritis in the elderly. Arch Intern Med 146:289–291

Rosenberg MR, Parshley M, Gibson S, Wernick R (1990) Central nervous system polyarteritis nodosa. West J Med 153:553–556

Yazici H, Pazarli H, Barnes CG et al. (1990) A controlled trial of azathioprine in Behçet's syndrome. N Engl J Med 322:281–285

Chapter 56

Spontaneous Intracerebral Hemorrhage

ALLAN H. ROPPER and HANSGEORG SCHÜTZ

Clinical and CT Findings Relevant to the Etiology of Hemorrhage

The clinical signs of cerebral hemorrhages evolve in minutes, but the incidence of clinical deterioration from rebleeding in the first few hours has probably been underestimated. A third or more of massive, nonaneurysmal hemorrhages have bled to a lesser extent in the preceding hours. Hemorrhages are best described, and therapy planned, on the basis of anatomical location and size on computed tomographic (CT) scan. One difficult clinical problem is distinguishing spontaneous hematomas from (a) single traumatic hemorrhage, (b) aneurysmal bleeding, and (c) hemorrhagic transformation of ischemic infarcts in patients receiving Coumadin (warfarin) or heparin.

Ganglionic spontaneous (hypertensive) intracerebral hemorrhages are frequently oval (Figs 1, 2). Traumatic intracerebral hemorrhages may also be spherical or oval, thus simulating

Section Editor: Allan H. Ropper

spontaneous bleeding; their favored sites, however, are the low frontal lobes and anterolateral temporal areas, but putaminal hematomas traumatic also occur. They often have an associated overlying contusion, and patients tend to be drowsier or have a more severe focal neurological deficit than expected from the CT appearance. The presence of many red blood cells in the CSF soon after the ictus also suggests trauma when the hemorrhage is deeply situated, but lumbar puncture is obviously not advisable.

Bleeding from a saccular aneurysm of the circle of Willis sometimes projects upwards into the frontotemporal parenchyma with little associated subarachnoid blood. Hemorrhages associated with apoplectic headache or stiff neck, or with the appearance on CT of any inferiorly pointing hematoma, should also suggest aneurysmal bleeding and should prompt early angiography.

Multiple hemorrhages suggest trauma, amyloid, or superior sagittal sinus thrombosis. Cerebral vascular amyloid deposition is probably a more common cause of lobar hemorrhage in the elderly patient than is usually

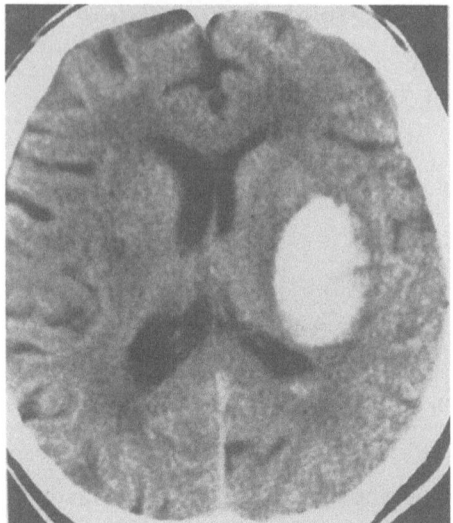

Fig. 1. Hypertensive basal ganglionic hemorrhage in a 67-year-old woman with aphasia, right hemiparesis, and history of hypertension. Axial CT scan reveals typical oval-shaped hyperintensity centered in posterolateral portion of left striatum. Mass effect has led to effacement of ipsilateral cerebral sulci/sylvian cistern, slight compression of lateral ventricle and mild displacement of midline structures toward the right side. Small amount of blood is present in left occipital horn, indicating minimal intraventricular hemorrhage. (Courtesy of Klaus Sartor and Marius Hartmann, Heidelberg)

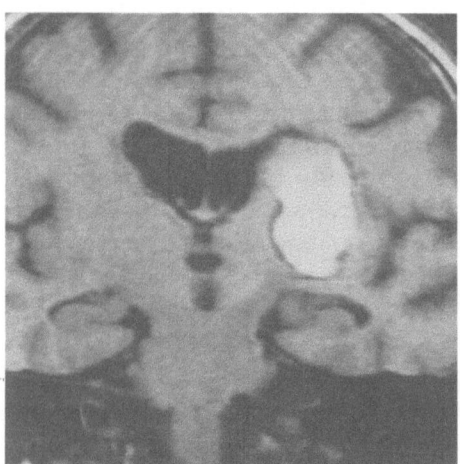
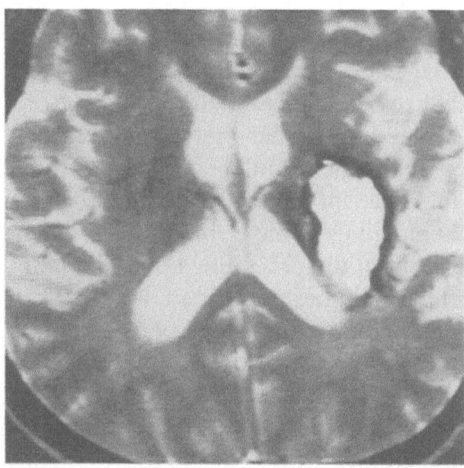

a   b

Fig. 2a,b. Hypertensive basal ganglionic hemorrhage in a 54-year-old man with severe right hemiparesis, aphasia, and history of hypertension. T1-weighted coronal MR image (**a**) shows sharply demarcated hyperintensity involving left striatum and internal capsule. T2-weighted axial image (**b**) is characterized by homogeneous hyperintensity surrounded by marked linear hypointensity. Signal pattern indicates that lesion is subacute to chronic, since central high signal in both sequences reflects presence of (extracellular) methemoglobin, while hypointense rim is evidence of hemosiderin deposition in macrophages. (Courtesy of Klaus Sartor and Marius Hartmann, Heidelberg)

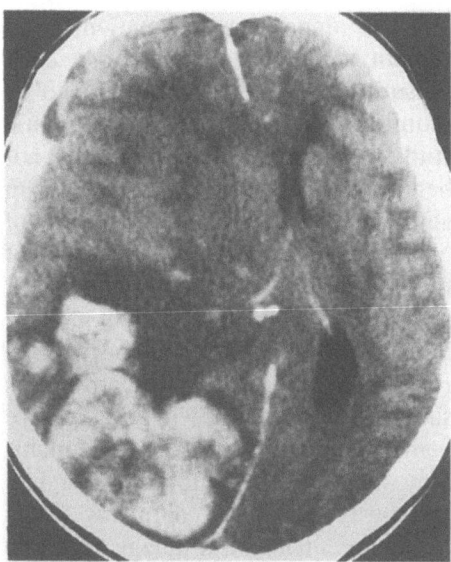

Fig. 3. Lobar occipital hemorrhage due to congophilic angiopathy in a 90-year-old woman found comatose. Axial CT scan demonstrates large lobulated mass lesion with density characteristics of acute hemorrhage accompanied by edema that extends from deep occipital white matter to cerebral surface. Note unusually severe mass effect with massive displacement of midline structures, including falx cerebri. (Courtesy of Klaus Sartor and Marius Hartmann, Heidelberg)

appreciated. Often there is preceding minor trauma. It is widely said that amyloid hemorrhages (Fig. 3) should not be operated on, because it is often difficult to stop bleeding in the hemorrhage cavity, and post-operative hemorrhages at a second site may occur, but a recent article by Green and coworkers questions this dictum.

General Comments on Acute Assessment

The major features guiding therapy are the level of consciousness, size, depth, and location of the hematoma, amount of horizontal displacement of the pineal calcification, extension of clot into the thalami, and hydrocephalus (prone to occur with hemorrhages close to the third ventricle or aqueduct). In hemorrhages uncomplicated by much ventricular blood or hydrocephalus, or by direct destruction of diencephalic reticular structures, the level of consciousness has been, in the experience of one of the authors (A.H.R.), related in a graded fashion to the horizontal pineal shift. Patients with less than 3 mm horizontal displacement are awake, those with 4–6 mm drowsy, with 6–8 mm stuporous, and above 8 or 9 mm comatose. If the level of consciousness is not commensurate with the expected pineal shift, then diencephalic extension, hydrocephalus, subarachnoid or intraventricular blood, or hypoxia at onset of the ictus are probably playing a role. A suggestion that recovery after surgery would be expected only in patients with appropriate shift has been disproved in a study by the group from San Francisco General Hospital. Compression of the lateral brainstem cisterns has consistently been associated with diminished consciousness and poor outcome. Pupillary enlargement on the side of the hemorrhage is usually associated with stupor or coma, and large pineal shift. There is a rough correspondence between loss of visualization of these cisterns on CT and pupillary changes. A common pitfall with hemorrhages extending into the nondominant parietal lobe is to assume patients are stuporous when they have only a disinclination to open their eyes.

Therapy in the First Hour

Medical therapy is the mainstay of acute treatment, with surgical evacuation considered only when worsening occurs, or when the size of the hemorrhage on CT and the clinical syndrome indicate that medical therapy is not likely to be successful in saving life. Immediate therapy for stuporous or comatose patients includes the administration of 0.5–1 g/kg mannitol intravenously, followed usually by intubation and hyperventilation to a PCO_2 of 29–34 mmHg. Vomiting and drowsiness also justify intubation but not necessarily mechanical ventilation. Corticosteroids, even if helpful, have a delayed effect and therefore play a minor role in acute management. One controlled trial failed to show benefit on outcome of dexamethasone; however, careful examination of the data shows that in the group expected to benefit from intervention steroids had a significant influence on survival. For further details of treatment of elevated intracranial pressure (ICP) see Chap. 9.

Phenytoin is generally favored as a prophylactic anticonvulsant but is not a high priority unless there have been recent seizures. If there are ecchymoses or known anticoagulant use, vitamin K 5 mg is administered. If surgery or ICP monitor placement are considered, fresh frozen plasma may be given. Hydrocephalus is significant if the adjacent cortical sulci or basal cisterns are compressed to any degree; treatment is with a ventricular drain in patients who are stuporous or worse. Bilateral ventricular drains are required if there is clot in the third ventricle.

The management of patients who remain stuporous or comatose after these interventions is greatly aided by monitoring of ICP, but a systematic study demonstrating benefit has not been done. We use a fiberoptic strain gauge device because of its ease of handling and safety, and because of the availability of a continuous ICP waveform without hydraulic coupling, but any device that has been used repeatedly by the intensive care staff is satisfactory. Patients who already have ventricular drains for hydrocephalus may have ICP monitored through a three-way stopcock allowing intermittent ventricular drainage, but the drainage system must be kept closed to prevent infection. The drain is generally opened when ICP exceeds 15–20 mmHg.

Surgical Evacuation of Hemorrhages

General Remarks

Despite several trials demonstrating no benefit from surgery in cases of typical supratentorial hemorrhages, the problem has not been studied yet in a useful way, and no definite conclusions can be drawn (see below). The indication for surgery in supratentorial cerebral hematoma is still disputed. We consider that conventional surgical treatment should still be restricted to putaminal, lobar, and cerebellar hematomas.

Many authors believe that evacuation of a hematoma is only indicated as a life-saving measure in secondary deterioration of young patients. Immediate evacuation of a putaminal or lobar hemorrhage can be occasionally life-saving in comatose patients but severe deficits must be expected. There is still no proof that evacuation of a hematoma by conventional surgery reduces residual deficits or speeds recovery. Surgery is indicated in patients with increasing ICP and secondary deterioration of consciousness, or patiens whose ICP does not normalize with appropriate medication. We believe that surgery is indicated with a Glasgow Coma Score (GCS) of at most 10 and at least 6. Possibly patients with very large hematomas (>50 ml volume) or clots with extensive perifocal edema causing increasing ICP could benefit from early surgery to prevent secondary damage to the reticular formation (Fig. 4). When the basal cisterns are open and the patient is not yet comatose, surgical outcome is better.

Signs of secondary brainstem compression by supratentorial hemorrhage, such as pupillary dilation or bilateral extensor limb posturing for more than several hours, are generally associated with poor outcome whether medical or surgical therapy is undertaken. Younger patients (especially those less than 50 years old) may still benefit from surgical evacuation in the 1st day after the ictus. Alcoholics with coagulation defects are high-risk surgical candidates and benefit from aggressive medical therapy with ICP monitoring.

By contrast, the indication for surgery in cerebellar hematomas is now undisputed (Fig. 5). Experience has shown that localization and volume of hematomas permits quite precise esti-

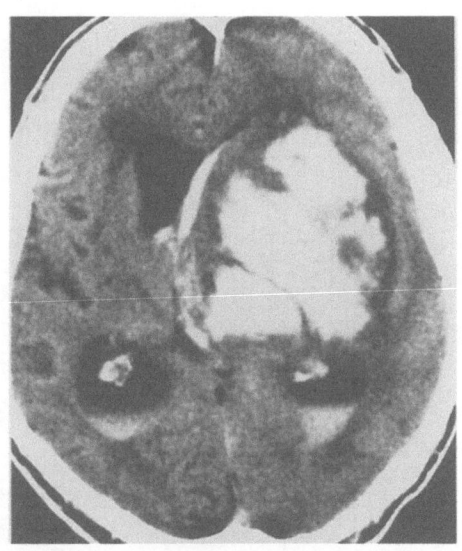

Fig. 4. Hypertensive basal ganglionic hemorrhage in a 73-year-old comatose man with bilaterally increased deep tendon reflexes, tachypnea, and long history of hypertension. Axial CT scan shows large hyperintense area typical for acute hemorrhage in region of left basal ganglia. Hematoma appears lobulated, features halo of perifocal edema, and has broken into ventricular system, with blood being present in left frontal horn, third ventricle, and both occipital horns. Severe mass effect has caused total effacement of sulc on side of lesion and marked displacement of midline structures toward right side. (Courtesy of Klaus Sartor and Marius Hartmann, Heidelberg)

mation of the patient's risk. The prognosis grows rapidly worse with a hematoma volume of 20 ml or more (i.e., mean diameter of 3 cm). Therefore almost all cerebellar hematomas with a diameter of 3 cm or more should be treated surgically without delay. Hematomas of the superior vermis are unfavorable, as early brain stem compression and aqueductal occlusion are common. Such hematomas frequently extend into the pons via the cerebellar peduncles. Displacement or com-

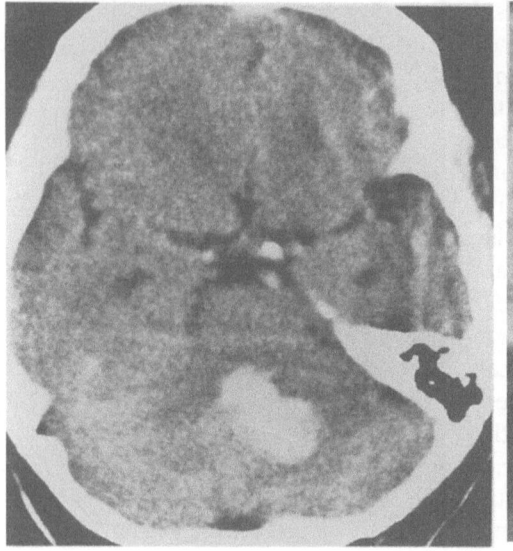
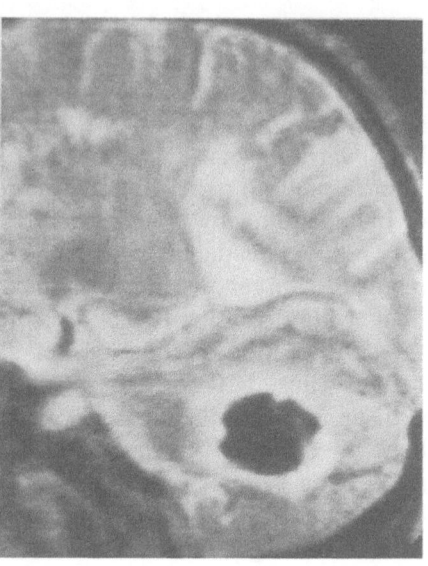

a   b

Fig. 5a,b. Hypertensive cerebellar hemorrhage in a 49-year-old hypertensive woman with rapid onset of nausea and vomiting, nystagmus, and gait ataxia. Axial CT scan (**a**) is remarkable for sharply marginated oblong hyperintensity typical for acute hemorrhage. The lesion, located in the white matter of the cerebellum, mostly left-sided, has led to compression of the fourth ventricle. T2-weighted sagittal MR image (**b**) reveals lesion to have hypointense signal reflecting predominance of deoxyhemoglobin at this stage of hematoma evolution

pression of the fourth ventricle and incipient hydrocephalus is a further indication for surgery; with small hematomas, ventricular drainage can be sufficient.

Cerebellar hematomas are classified into three stages. Patients in stage I are fully conscious and occasionally have a unilateral sixth nerve palsy and Babinski sign in addition to cerebellar symptoms. In this stage surgery is not mandatory if the hematoma volume does not exceed 20 ml. Stage II (intermediary stage) is characterized by a fluctuating level of consciousness and a combination of brain stem signs, bilateral third nerve palsy, gaze palsies, sixth and seventh nerve palsies, bilateral Babinski signs, and pupillary abnormality. Patients in stage II should be operated on immediately.

Patients in stage III are deeply stuporous or comatose and exhibit pyramidal signs and extensor spasms. Survival can be achieved only if coma is very recent; otherwise surgery is disappointing. Our surgeons have not found a role for surgical evacuation of brain stem hemorrhages but several studies of small series have been undertaken.

Randomized/Controlled Trials

The results of McKissock's trial of surgical evacuation in the pre-CT era was a harbinger of modern attempts to improve outcome. Surgery was probably viewed generously because intensive care therapy of raised ICP had not yet been refined. Despite the title of

McKissock's paper, the trial was not "controlled" in the modern sense.

The best modern trial was conducted in Helsinki in 1989, prospectively randomizing 52 patients who were mostly stuporous or comatose. At 6 months, the main criteria for comparison were similar in both groups: overall mortality (38% medical vs 46% surgical) and independent living (31% vs 27%). The mortality among stuporous and "semicomatose" patients (GCS 7–10), however, was significantly lower in the surgical group (0/4 vs 4/5). All these survivors were disabled.

A smaller, recent US study was more complicated to follow since it included three treatment groups: best medical therapy, best medical therapy with ICP monitoring, and surgery. Only patients with severe deficits and a clot diameter over 3 cm were included. The study was stopped after only 21 patients had been taken up (it took 6 years to access this number and only 8 patients had surgery). Seven of 9 patients in the best medical group died or were severely disabled, compared to 6 of 8 in the surgical group. In our opinions, this study was too small and had too poor accession rates to be conclusive, but it has been interpreted as another negative surgical trial.

In a study in Austria, evacuation of clot by endoscopy (requiring small corticectomy) vs medical therapy in 100 patients was investigated. Although among patients with putaminal or thalamic hemorrhage there was a trend to better quality of survival in the operated group, statistically outcome was no better than in the medically managed group. Among patients with subcortical (lobar) hematomas, however, mortality (30% vs 70%) and minimal deficit at 6 months (40% vs 25%) were better in the operated group.

Techniques

Operative evacuation is performed through an incision at the point where the lesion is closest to the surface. Speech areas are generally avoided and occasionally an incision through the insula is used. For temporal and putaminal clots an anterior temporal gyrus approach is used. Hemostasis must be meticulous to prevent reaccumulation of the hemorrhage.

With a recent resurgence, stereotactic procedures or endoscopic techniques as discussed above have generally been as satisfactory as, or better than, direct corticectomy, though there have been no trials comparing special techniques to conventional surgery. Hondo's group has built on previous Japanese work, particularly from Matsumoto, and has shown that almost any hypertensive clot can be evacuated safely by CT-guided aspiration. The relatively long preparation required for stereotactic procedures renders emergency evacuation impossible to date, and only between 30% and 80% of the hematoma can be aspirated. Subsequent instillation of streptokinase or urokinase and external drainage can only reduce the hematoma volume marginally.

The main advantage of the method lies in its sparing of surrounding brain tissue and in the accessibility of even thalamic hematomas to surgery. Anecdotal reports suggest that stereotactic puncture of not only large but also of small hematomas that otherwise do not need surgery achieves rapid remission of disturbance of consciousness and other neurological deficits. Mortality is approximately 10%, most studies including not only patients with vital risk, but also patients who would have survived without surgery. There are no studies comparing the results of stereotactic surgery with conventional surgery and with conservative treatment. New ultrasonic aspirators or other devices have been adapted to remove dense clot in the acute stage.

Summary

To sum up, we believe the following principles regarding conventional surgery in the treatment of spontaneous intracerebral hematomas to be reasonable:

1. Conventional surgery is not indicated for treatment of thalamic and pontine hemorrhage (Fig. 6).
2. Putaminal hemorrhages should only be evacuated if the patient's level of consciousness deteriorates rapidly (GCS between 10 and 6 points) or if the elevation of ICP cannot be controlled pharmacologically and brain stem distortion or herniation is incipient. Larger hematomas with lateral displacement of midline structures, extensive edema, and raised ICP may be evacuated in conscious patients.
3. Lobar hematomas should also only be operated on if the patient deteriorates (GCS between 10 and 6 points). Some lobar hematomas in old age are caused by cerebral amyloid angiopathy (CAA), a vascular disease with amyloid deposits in leptomeningeal and cortical arteries. CAA often leads to multiple and recurrent hemorrhage and may have a coincidence with Alzheimers' disease. If CAA is suspected, patient selection for surgery should be even more cautious, as severe postoperative hemorrhages have been observed.
4. That most patients with cerebellar hemorrhage should undergo surgery is undisputed. Small hemispheric hematomas without

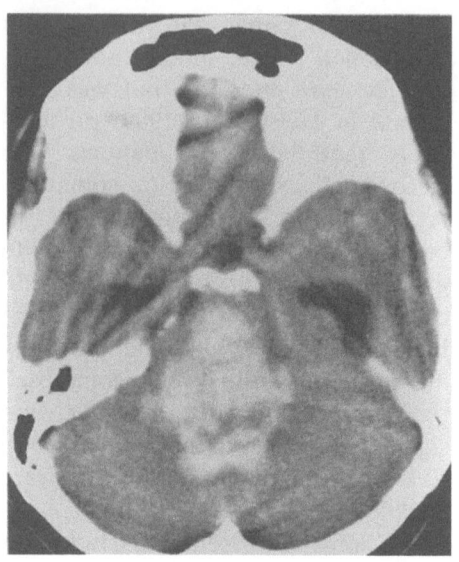

Fig. 6. Hypertensive brain stem hemorrhage in a 63-year-old hypertensive man with dilated, nonreactive pupils and absent corneal reflexes who acutely had become comatose. Axial CT scan shows large hyperdense mass lesion typical for acute hemorrhage that involves central portions of the pons, the middle cerebellar peduncle on the right, the fourth ventricle, and the cerebellar parenchyma around this ventricle. The enlarged temporal horns indicate that the mass effect of the lesion has caused obstruction of the median CSF pathways, resulting in hydrocephalus. (Courtesy of Klaus Sartor and Marius Hartmann, Heidelberg)

disturbed consciousness, clinical signs of brain stem compression, hydrocephalus, or distortion of the fourth ventricle on CT can be treated conservatively. Hematomas with 20 ml volume or more (miminum 3 cm diameter), compression of the fourth ventricle, and hydrocephalus should be surgically treated. Decompression should also be carried out if the patient reaches an "intermediate stage" of incipient brain stem herniation characterized by agitation followed by stupor, sixth or seventh nerve palsy, gaze palsy, Horner sign, progressive hemiparesis, and bilateral pyramidal signs. Our experience is that patients can survive massive cerebellar hemorrhage without major deficits with prompt ventricular drainage and evacuation of the hematoma even if they have been comatose for a short time.

5. Ventricular drainage should be performed with marked ventricular dilatation due to obstruction of the foramen of Monro or due to blood in the ventricles. Ventricular drainage can be life-saving in acute cases and in patients with primary intraventricular hemorrhage.

Management of Medical Complications of Hemorrhage

Aspiration Pneumonia

Vomiting at the onset of cerebral hemorrhage is common and often leads to adult respiratory distress syndrome, or at the least, pneumonia. To prevent passive regurgitaton the "Sellick maneuver" is useful. This consists of manual compression of the cricothyroid cartilage, occluding the esophagus while waiting for intubation. Single doses of Xylocaine 100 mg intravenously or pentobarbital 100–150 mg i.v. are useful in preventing the reflex rise in ICP associated with endotracheal manipulation. Penicillin is given for out-of-hospital or emergency room aspirations. Nosocomial pneumonia, acquired after the first 4 h in the hospital, with or without aspiration, is usually penicillin-resistant and should be treated on the basis of culture results and the Gram stain appearance of the predominant organism.

Seizures

Seizures occur in about 10% of patients with cerebral hemorrhage during the first 3 days. Because they can cause devastating rises in ICP and deleterious cardiovascular effects, prophylactic administration of phenytoin is sensible. Intractable seizures are rarely a problem but are best handled by rapid induction of general anesthesia by pentobarbital, since the loss of time involved in controlling convulsions with conventional anticonvulsants may lead to severe elevations in ICP and severe cerebral edema.

Venous Clots

We have used sequential compression air boots in almost all patients with hemorrhages who are stuporous or worse.

Feeding

It is reasonable to wait for 3–5 days before attempting nasogastric feeding. "Two-cal" or other concentrated formulas may be used to maintain serum osmolarity. Peripheral hyperalimentation generally requires large fluid volumes (>3 l/day) to establish adequate nutrition.

Management of the Stabilized and Improving Patient

Hyperventilation and mannitol are withdrawn gradually, beginning on the 4th–10th day depending on the patient's alertness. Patients with hemorrhages in unusual locations, with configurations suggesting aneurysmal rupture, or young individuals are all considered as candidates for angiography. As deep hemorrhages are absorbed, CT scans often show contrast enhancement of the rim of the clot, giving the misleading appearance of an arteriovenous malformation.

Suggested Reading

Andrews BT, Chiles BW, Olsen WL et al. (1989) The effect of intracerebral hematoma location on the risk of brain-stem compression and on clinical outcome. J Neurosurg 69: 518–522

Auer LM, Deinsberger W, Niederkorn K et al. (1989) Endoscopic surgery versus medical treatment for spontaneous intracerebral hematoma: a randomized study. J Neurosurg 70:530–535

Batjer HH, Reisch JS, Allen BC et al. (1990) Failure of surgery to improve outcome in hypertensive putaminal hemorrhage. Arch Neurol 47:1103–1106

Crowell RM, Ojemann RG, Ogilvy CS (1992) Spontaneous brain hemorrhage: surgical consideration. In: Barnett HJM, Mohr JP, Stein BM, Yatsu FM (eds) Stroke, pathophysiology, diagnosis and management, 2nd edn. Churchill Livingstone, New York, pp 1169–1188

Drake CG, Vinter HV (1985) Intracerebral hemorrhage. In: Plum F, Pulsinelli W (eds) Cerebrovascular diseases. Raven, New York

Greene GM, Godersky J, Biller J et al. (1990) Surgical experience with cerebral amyloid angiopathy. Stroke 21:1545–1549

Heros CR (1982) Cerebellar hemorrhage and infarction. Stroke 13:106

Hondo H, Uno M, Sasaki K et al. (1990) Computed tomography controlled aspiration surgery for hypertensive intracerebral hemorrhage. Experience of more than 400 cases. Stereotact Funct Neurosurg 54/55: 432–437

Juvela S, Heiskanen O, Poramen A et al. (1989) The treatment of spontaneous intracerebral hemorrhage. A prospective randomized trial of surgical and conservative treatment. J Neurosurg 70:755–758

Kase CS, Mohr JP, Caplan LR (1992) Intracerebral hemorrhage. In: Barnett HJM, Mohr JP, Stein BM, Yatsu FM (eds) Stroke, pathophysiology, diagnosis and management, 2nd edn. Churchill Livingstone, New York, pp 561–616

Little JR, Tubman DE, Ethier R (1978) Cerebellar hemorrhage in adults: diagnosis by computerized tomography. J Neurosurg 48:575

McKissock W, Richardson A, Taylor J (1961) Primary intracerebral hemorrhage: a controlled trial of surgical and conservative treatment in 180 unselected cases. Lancet 2:221–226

Mohadjer M, Braus DF, Krauss JK, Milios E, Birg W, Mundinger F (1990) CT-stereotaktische Entleerung und Fibrinolyse der spontanen, vorwiegend hypertensiven intrakraniellen Massenblutungen – Langzeitergebnisse. In: Walter W, Krenkel W, Mewe R (eds) Jahrbuch der Neurochirurgie 1990. Biermann, Zülpich, pp 189–201

Poungvarin N, Bhoopat W, Viriyavejakul A et al. (1987) Effects of dexamethasone in primary supratentorial hemorrhage. N Engl J Med 316:1299–1233

Ropper AH (1986) Lateral displacement of the brain and level of consciousness in patients with an acute hemispheral mass. N Engl J Med 314:953–958

Ropper AH, Shafran B (1984) Brain edema after stroke: clinical syndrome and intracranial pressure. Arch Neurol 41:26–29

Ross DA, Olsen WL, Ross AM et al. (1989) Brain shift, level of consciousness, and restoration of consciousness in patients with acute intracranial hematomas. J Neurosurg 71:498–502

Schütz H (1988) Spontane intrazerebrale Hämatome. Pathophysiologie, Klinik und Therapie. Springer, Berlin Heidelberg New York

Chapter 57

Subarachnoid Hemorrhage

HANS-HERBERT STEINER, MATTHEW E. FINK,
PAUL KREMER, and MICHAEL N. DIRINGER

Introduction and Epidemiology

Subarachnoid hemorrhage from intracranial arterial aneurysms occurs in 30 000 patients annually in North America, accounting for 6–10% of all strokes. The world-wide incidence of aneurysmal subarachnoid hemorrhage is 15 cases per 100 000 people. In contrast to the declining incidence of parenchymatous cerebral hematoma and brain infarction, due to improved treatment of hypertension and heart disease, the incidence of aneurysmal subarachnoid hemorrhage has remained the same over the past five decades.

The clinical importance of ruptured aneurysm is clearly shown in an article by Kassell. In the United States, yearly 10 000 of 28 000 patients suffering from an aneurysmal subarachnoid hemorrhage are not sent to a specific therapy due to their sudden death or to misjudgement of the symptoms. Further, 8000 of the remaining 18 000 patients die of complications related to the subarachnoid hemorrhage or survive with neurological deficits despite intensive therapy. Only 10 000 patients, about 35%, survive with good clinical outcome.

After 1 year survival without definitive surgery, there is a 3.5% average incidence of rebleeding for the next decade. The acute mortality from a second hemorrhage is 67%.

The overall prevalence of intracranial aneurysms in the general population is uncertain, but from a number of autopsy series, we know that unruptured aneurysms are present in 0.2–9% of brains at autopsy (the average is 2.4%). Aneurysms are rare in children.

The age range for highest probability of aneurysm rupture is 40–64 years of age, accounting for 65% of all cases of first subarachnoid hemorrhage. From the age of 20 until 70, intracranial aneurysm is the most common cause of nontraumatic subarachnoid hemorrhage. Women account for 60% of the cases. There are multiple aneurysms in 15–20% of patients with acute subarachnoid hemorrhage.

Section Editor: Michael N. Diringer

Pathophysiology

The acute subarachnoid hemorrhage shows a sudden onset of the disease in full health. The hemorrhage invades the subarachnoid space between brain surface and arachnoidea. According to the course of the cerebral arteries and the enlargements of the subarachnoid space, these bleedings prefer localizations inside the basal cisterns, sylvian fissure, and interhemispheric fissure. In severe cases, bleeding into the ventricular system can also be observed (hematocephalus); one third of the cases even present with an intracerebral hematoma.

In 80% of cases the subarachnoid hemorrhage is due to an aneurysm of the cerebral arteries; other reasons such as cerebral (10%) or spinal angiomas are less frequent. Subarachnoid hemorrhages without hemorrhagic source have a frequency of 10–15% (see Table 1). With regard to repeated bleeding, these spontaneous forms have a good prognosis.

Intracranial arterial aneurysms are classified as fusiform, saccular, or dissecting. Fusiform aneurysms, also called dolichoectasia, are usually seen in advanced atherosclerotic cerebral arteries, most commonly in the basilar artery and the intracranial segment of the internal carotid artery. Rarely, in children and young adults they may be caused by degeneration of the media and elastica of the arterial wall. Rupture of fusiform aneurysms is rare, but if sufficiently large, they may cause symptoms due to compression of the brain stem or structures in the cavernous sinus (cranial nerves II, III, IV, V, VI). Fusiform aneurysms may be a source of thromboemboli that cause transient ischemic attacks or brain infarction in the distribution of the parent vessel.

Saccular aneurysms ("berry aneurysms") are the most common type and the major cause of subar-

Table 1. Causes of subarachnoid hemorrhage other than ruptured aneurysms and arteriovenous malformations

Arteriopathy	Amyloidosis, arteritis, atherosclerosis, kongophilic angiopathy, eclampsia, embolism, hypertension, lupus, scurvey, telangiectasias
Blood disorders	Agranulocytosis, aplastic anemia, anticoagulants, aspirin, disseminated intravascular coagulation, hemophilia, Hodgkin's disease, leukemia, liver disease, lymphoma, myeloma, sickle-cell disease, polycythemia vera, thrombocytopenia
Infections	Bacterial meningitis, fungal meningitis, syphilitic meningoencephalitis, tuberculous meningitis, viral meningoencephalitis (especially herpes simplex, influenza, cytomegalovirus, hemorrhagic fevers), malaria
Intoxications	Alcohol, amphetamines, carbon monoxide, cocaine, epinephrine, lead, monoamine oxidase inhibitors, narcotic analgesics, snake venom, sympathomimetic drugs
Trauma	Altitude sickness, electrocution, epileptic seizures, heat injury, impact injuries, radiation, strangulation
Tumors	Choriocarcinoma, ependymoma, glioma, hemangioblastoma, melanoma, metastatic carcinoma
Venous thrombosis	Cardiolipin antibodies, contraceptives, infection, pregnancy, trauma

achnoid hemorrhage. Normally, an increase of the saccular aneurysm has no clinical symptoms until its sudden rupture. Local symptoms caused by the close relation to the adjacent nervous structures arise only occasionally. Disturbances of the oculomotor nerve caused by aneurysms originating at the posterior communicating artery are known.

Saccular aneurysms develop and increase slowly over years and decades. They are frequently called "congenital" aneurysms, because they rarely occur in neonates and usually develop and enlarge over years to cause symptoms in young and middle-aged adults. There is no definitive evidence that there are developmental abnormalities in the arteries of patients who develop aneurysms compared with those who do not. Other authors believe that aneurysms are acquired, and significant risk factors appear to be cigarette smoking, heavy alcohol use, oral contraceptive use, and arterial hypertension. The role of genetic factors is uncertain, but some investigators have reported familial clusters of patients with intracranial aneurysms. Biochemical abnormalities and deficiencies of type-III collagen have been described in some patients with aneurysms, and a decrease in reticulin fibers in the arterial walls of aneurysm patients has been identified at autopsy.

Congenital diseases in which the prevalence of intracranial aneurysms is greater than among the general population are coarctation of the aorta, polycystic disease of the kidneys, fibromuscular dysplasia of the renal arteries, Marfan's syndrome, and Ehlers-Danlos syndrome, all

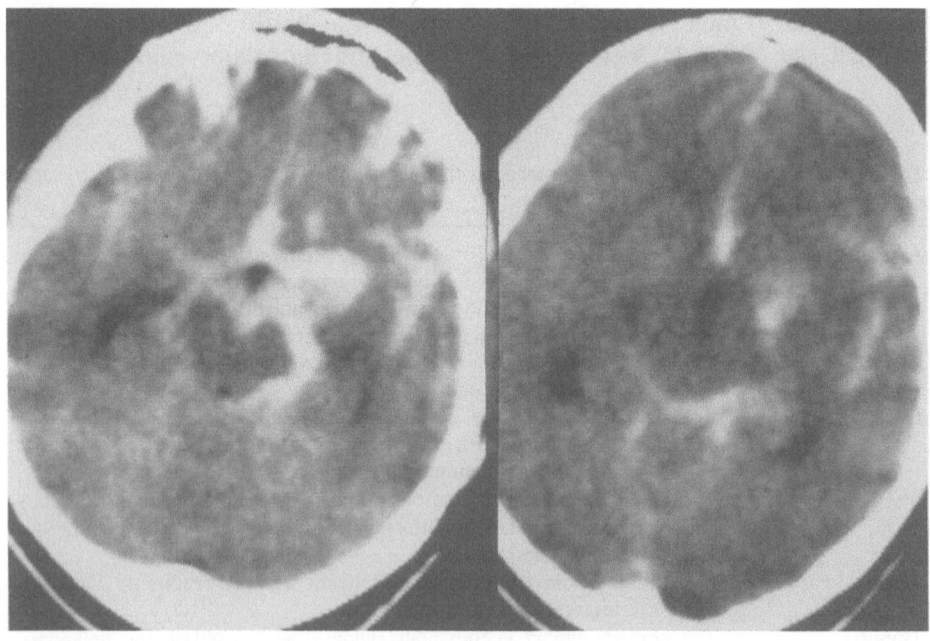

Fig. 1. CT appearance of a typical subarachnoid hemorrhage with maximum over the right hemisphere (ICA aneurysm)

Table 2. Localization of saccular intracranial aneurysms (frequency in %)

Author	Localization			
	ICA	ACA	MCA	BA/VA
Sahs et al. (1981)	40	34	20	6
Sano et al. (1987)	40	31	21	8
Yasargil et al. (1973)	34	36	21	9
Steiner and Kunze (1989)	30	36	28	6

ICA, Internal carotid artery; ACA, anterior cerebral artery; MCA, middle cerebral artery; BA/VA, basilar artery/vertebral artery.

disorders of connective-tissue biochemistry. There is an increased risk of aneurysms on the feeding arteries of congenital arteriovenous malformations.

Saccular aneurysms occur at the forks of arterial bifurcations of the major cerebral arteries of the circle of Willis. The common locations, based on the International Cooperative Study, are listed in Table 2. At the time of acute subarachnoid hemorrhage, 78% were <12 mm in diameter, 20% were 12–24 mm, and 2% were >24 mm. Saccular aneurysms form through a defect in the muscularis layer of the media at the arterial bifurcation (see Fig. 1). If there is damage to the internal elastic lamina and high arterial flow or high arterial pressure, an aneurysm may form and enlarge. Intracranial arteries are more susceptible to this process than coronary or mesenteric arteries, because intracranial arteries have no adventitial supports in the subarachnoid space. Defects in the muscularis layer of arteries are common, but these alone do not explain aneurysm formation; elastic tissue damage is required as well.

The risk of subarachnoid hemorrhage from an unruptured intracranial aneurysm found incidentally, or multiple aneurysms found during angiography for subarachnoid hemorrhage is uncertain. The best retrospective data available indicate a 1–2% average yearly incidence of rupture, with increased risk for aneurysms 10 mm or greater in internal diameter, or those associated with the feeding vessels of arteriovenous malformations. Dissecting aneurysms are not true aneurysms, rarely cause subarachnoid hemorrhage, and usually present with syndromes of focal brain ischemia due to arterial occlusion or distal embolization.

Clinical Signs and Symtpoms

Warning Symptoms of Impending Aneurysm Rupture

The classical presentation of a ruptured intracranial aneurysm is distinctive and hard to miss – sudden onset of severe headache, followed by depression in consciousness and stiff neck. However, up to 30% of patients are initially misdiagnosed, causing a delay in referral to a neurosurgeon and adding to the morbidity and mortality of a dreadful disease. In retrospective clinical series it was found that 28–59% of patients had warning symptoms and signs weeks before a major subarachnoid hemorrhage occurred. The most common symptoms and signs prior to a major aneurysm rupture, in order of frequency, are (a) symptoms due to minor bleeding, such as generalized headache, nausea, neckache, chest, back, and leg pain, lethargy and photophobia; (b) signs due to enlargement of the aneurysm, such as visual-field defects, impairment of eye movements, eye, face, or local head pains; (c) symptoms due to brain ischemia or infarction, such as loss of balance, dizziness, syncope, motor, sensory, or visual impairments, hallucinations, speech and cognitive impairments, or mood changes.

The most common *misdiagnoses* are systemic viral infection, migraine headache, hypertensive encephalopathy, cervical arthritis or disk herniation, brain tumor, aseptic meningitis, sinusitis, myocardial infarction, cerebral infarction, alcohol intoxication, toxic-metabolic encephalopathy, head trauma, otitis, vertigo, syncope, and malingering!

Symptoms and Signs of Acute Rupture

Almost pathognomonic for the acute subarachnoid hemorrhage ist the sudden onset of a violent headache at the neck with radiation to the forehead and upper part of the vertebral spine. The patients report that they have never yet experienced this symptomatology of headache. The subarachnoid hemorrhage often is accompanied by vegetative symptoms such as nausea or vomiting. Initial

unconsciousness occurs in about 50% of cases. This sudden loss of consciousness may resemble a generalized tonic seizure, with stiff extension of all limbs, opisthotonus, trismus, and apnea, leading to full cardiopulmonary arrest. Most patients spontaneously reawaken, but 10–15% remain in coma and die before reaching the hospital. Also typical of this disease is meningism, varying in its intensity and temporal appearance.

Depending on the location of the aneurysm, the distribution and amount of subarachnoid and/or intraventricular blood, the presence of intraparenchymal clot, the degree of intracranial atherosclerosis, and the magnitude of intracranial hypertension, any type and combination of neurological signs may be present. The modified Hunt and Hess Grading Scale (Table 3) is widely used to simplify and standardize the clinical classification of patients based on the initial neurological examination. Recently, the Word Federation of Neurological Surgeons proposed further modification to improve reliability.

Symptoms and Signs of Unruptured Aneurysms

About 70% of unruptured saccular aneurysms found incidentally as part of an unrelated evaluation cause no symptoms. Aneurysms greater than 8 mm in diameter, depending on their location, may cause symptoms by compressing nearby structures, such as cranial nerves and the optic nerve and chiasm. The neocortex of frontal or temporal lobes may be irritated, causing epileptic seizures. Spontaneous thrombosis of an aneurysm may cause severe, acute headache and nuchal rigidity, mimicking an acute subarachnoid hemorrhage ("thunderclap headache"). There may be inflammatory cells in the cerebrospinal fluid. An intraluminal thrombus may embolize to more distal branches of the parent vessel, causing transient ischemic attacks or embolic brain infarction. The rate of enlargement of unruptured aneurysms and the risk factors that precipitate rupture are unknown.

Diagnosis

Neuroimaging

Computerized tomography is the initial test of choice for the diagnosis of acute aneurysmal subarachnoid hemorrhage (Fig. 1). CT has high sensitivity and specificity and may be performed quickly and safely, even in patients with depressed levels of consciousness who require endotracheal intubation and mechanical ventilation. The pattern of hemorrhage in the basal cisterns may point to the location of a ruptured aneurysm or arteriovenous malformation, and intraventricular, parenchymatous, and subdural components of the blood are well visualized. Based on the pattern of blood on CT, 70% accuracy is attained in diagnosing the location of the ruptured aneurysm. Rapid-sequence, thin-section, contrast-enhanced CT (angio-CT) has been reported to show the offending aneurysm in over 90% of cases studied. A CT scan is indispensable to demonstrate possible complications of the hemorrhage, such

Table 3. Clinical grading scales for patients with acute aneurysmal subarachnoid hemorrhage

A Hunt and Hess

Grade	Examination findings
I	Normal neurological examination, mild headache, and slightly stiff neck
II	Moderate to severe headache and stiff neck; no confusion or neurological deficit except for cranial nerve palsy
III	Persistent confusion and/or focal neurological deficit
IV	Persistent stupor; moderate to severe neurological deficit
V	Coma with moribund appearance

B World Federation of Neurological Surgeons

WFNS Grade	Glasgow Coma Scale Score	Motor deficit
I	15	absent
II	13–14	absent
III	13–14	present
IV	7–12	present or absent
V	3–6	present or absent

as intracerebral hematoma (see Fig. 2) or hydrocephalus (see Fig. 3).

The sensitivity of CT depends on the time interval from acute hemorrhage to scanning, with an overall positive rate of 85%. CT on the day of hemorrhage has the highest sensitivity, with 92% of scans showing subarachnoid blood. The sensitivity falls with each subsequent day, so that by the fifth day only 58% of scans show blood. Only 5% of the initial CT scans will show the actual aneurysm after acute subarachnoid hemorrhage, usually those larger than 10 mm. Ordinary CT scanning has a low sensitivity for diagnosing unruptured, asymptomatic aneurysms, which are usually under 10 mm in diameter.

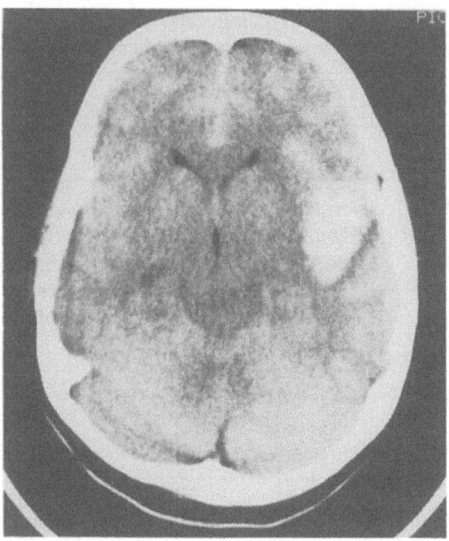

Fig. 2. CT-appearance of subarachnoid hemorrhage and additional intracerebral hematoma (left MCA aneurysm)

If CT is performed within 4 days of subarachnoid hemorrhage, there is a high correlation between the amount of blood visualized in the basal cisterns and the subsequent development of vasospasm and delayed cerebral ischemia. A thick layer of blood in the cisterns or sylvian fissures will predict vasospasm and delayed ischemia in 60–90% of patients. Early contrast enhancement of the basal cisterns, indicating vascular permeability, is highly predictive of subsequent vasospasm. Seventy percent of patients with symptomatic delayed ischemia will develop low-density lesions on CT within the first 2 weeks. The quantity of blood seen on CT also correlates with the initial clinical grade, with comatose patients (grades IV and V) having the largest amounts of blood

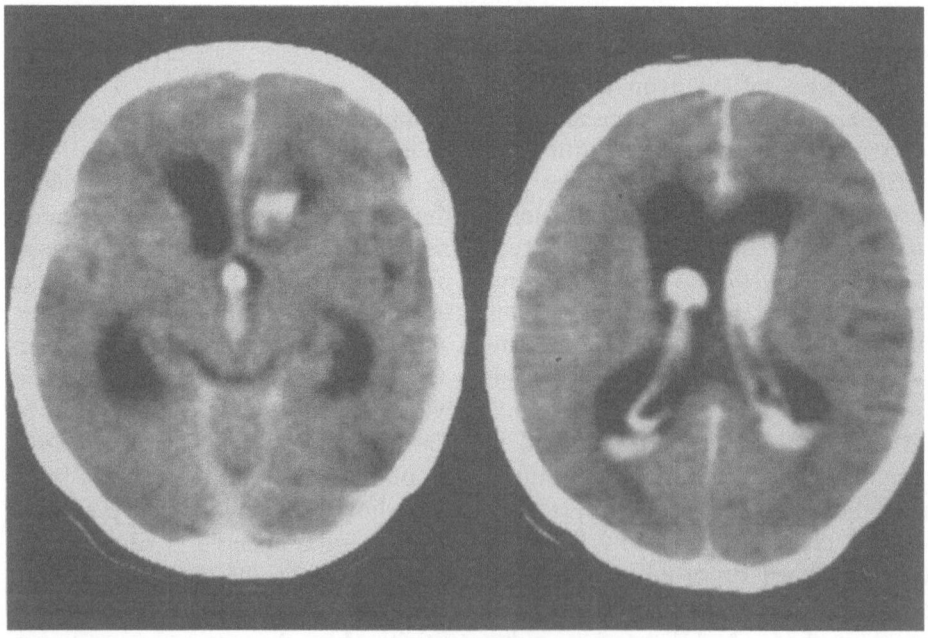

Fig. 3. Subarachnoid hemorrhage including intraventricular hemorrhage in a case of ACA aneurysm as assessed by CT-scanning

clot in the basal cisterns and subarachnoid spaces over the convexities.

Lumbar puncture is performed infrequently to diagnose subarachnoid hemorrhage, but it remains critically important in the 15% of patients who have a suspicious clinical history but a normal CT scan. Aneurysmal subarachnoid hemorrhage cannot be excluded until both normal CT and lumbar puncture are confirmed. Following aneurysm rupture, blood appears in the lumbar cerebrospinal fluid within minutes, but the primary pigment found in the supernatant, oxyhemoglobin (pink color), does not appear for 2–4 h. Red blood cell counts are maximal within the first 24 h, then fall and usually red cells disappear in 7–10 days, depending on the quantity of the initial hemorrhage. Xanthochromia does not appear for about 12 h, reaches a maximum at 48 h, and may persist for up to 4 weeks. The finding of xanthochromia in cerebrospinal fluid 2 weeks after a severe acute headache in a patient with a normal CT scan strongly suggests a recent subarachnoid hemorrhage. Because of the delay in formation of oxyhemoglobin and bilirubin, cerebrospinal fluid examined less than 4 h after subarachnoid hemorrhage may have a clear supernatant and could be confused with a traumatic lumbar puncture. If CT is positive for subarachnoid hemorrhage, a lumbar puncture should not be performed because there is a small risk of inducing rebleeding.

Angiography

Cerebral angiography has been the diagnostic standard for the diagnosis

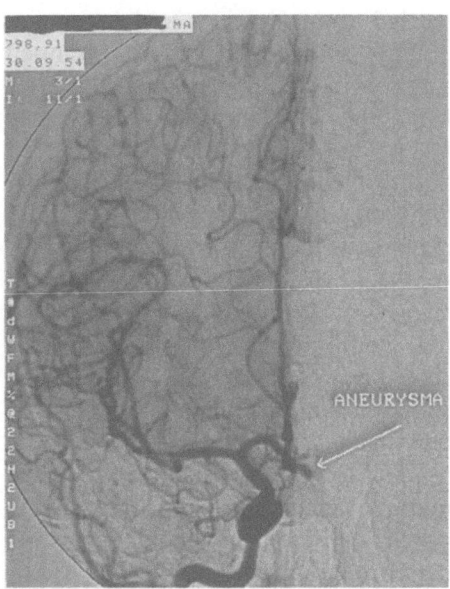

Fig. 4. Aneurysm of the ACoA in digital subtraction angiography (DSA) via selective right internal carotid artery cannulation. The a.p. view shows a typical saccular aneurysm 0.8 cm in diameter with anterior and slightly caudal projection

of intracranial aneurysms since the late 1930s. The technique of percutaneous, transfemoral catheterization with selective arterial injections has been refined to a high degree of safety, sensitivity, and specificity. If subarachnoid hemorrhage is demonstrated by CT or lumbar puncture, complete 4-vessel angiography is performed as soon as an experienced angiography team can be mobilized (Fig. 4). Angiography should demonstrate an intracranial aneurysm in at least two views, and the angiographer may need to customize the examination to confirm the presence of an aneurysm. The pressure of intra-arterial contrast injection briefly exceeds arterial blood pressure. Therefore, fear of re-rupture of the aneurysm during angiography has led some clinicians to delay angio-graphy until just before planned surgery. In the largest published series from the Cooperative Study, only seven repeat hemorrhages occurred during angiography in 5484 patients. Delayed angiography hinders accurate diagnosis because vasospasm may pre-vent clear visualization of the ruptured aneurysm. With modern technology, the neurological complication rate should be under 1% from angiography, and fatal complications should occur in less than 0.2%.

Up to 20% of patients will have multiple aneurysms, and determining which one is responsible for acute hemorrhage may be difficult. Com-bination of careful neurological history and examination, CT scan findings, and angiographic features should result in correct identification. The following features are associated with the rup-tured aneurysm: largest aneurysm (85%), irregular shape or multilobular (85%), focal vasospasm (60%), local-ized clot on CT (100%), cranial third nerve palsy (100%), hemiparesis (60%), dysphasia (80%), headache localization (30%).

To what extent conventional angiography will be replaced by MRI angiography in the future is still un-clear. Although MR visualization of small aneurysms (>3 mm $\varnothing$) is already possible, this examination has limited practicality for initial diagnosis, be-cause monitoring of patients with poor clinical grades during MRI has not yet been finally solved, and the reliability in detecting small and distal aneurysms has not been established. The diag-nostic decision tree is summarized in Fig. 5.

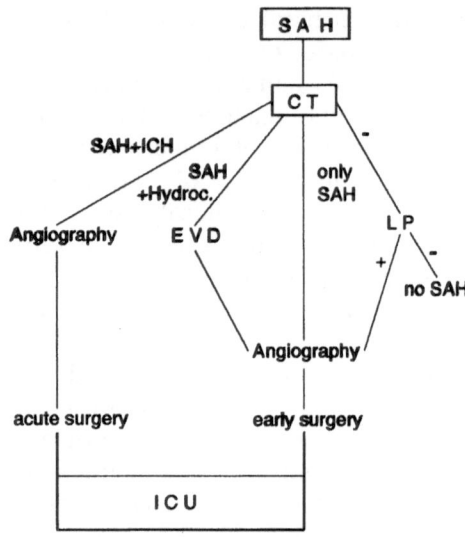

Fig. 5. Decision tree for diagnosis and treat-ment of subarachnoid hemorrhage (*SAH*). *EVD*, External ventricular drainage; *LP*, lumbar punc-ture; *CT*, computer tomography; *ICH*, intra-cerebral hemorrhage

Morbidity and Mortality after Aneurysm Rupture

Of the 85% of patients with ruptured saccular aneurysms who survive to reach the hospital, only half will leave in good neurological condition. The most common causes of morbidity and mortality after aneurysm rupture, in order of frequency, are delayed cerebral ischemia from vasospasm, acute brain injury from the initial hemorrhage, rebleeding from the aneurysm, complications of surgery, intracerebral hematoma, hydro-cephalus, and complications of medi-cal therapy.

Vasospasm and delayed cerebral ischemia following subarachnoid hemorrhage were first described in early angiographic studies in the 1950s. About 4 days after subarachnoid hemorrhage, the major arteries of the circle of Willis that are exposed to thick hematomas in the basal cisterns develop vasospasm. It may last for more than 2 weeks and is associated with cerebral ischemia. About 60% of all patients with aneurysmal subarachnoid hemorrhage develop angiographic vasospasm. One half of those (35%) develop symptomatic cerebral ischemia, which can progress to permanent neurological deficits and death. The initial Cooperative Study in the 1960s recognized that there was an association between level of consciousness and severity of vasospasm, but it was not until the 1980s that a clear relationship was observed between the quantity of blood in the basal cisterns, as measured on CT images, and the severity of vasospasm. Vasospasm follows the same time course, regardless of the timing of surgery.

In the mid 1980s, investigators in many centers recognized that vasospasm was a misleading term. Human pathology and animal models showed a proliferative arteriopathy, with structural changes in the arterial wall and fixed luminal narrowing causing a loss of cerebral autoregulation. The formation of oxyhemoglobin during red blood cell breakdown in the subarachnoid space induces arterial wall injury, probably via the production of free radicals and lipid peroxidation. Hundreds of attempts to induce arterial relaxation with vasodilator drugs failed, because the problem is not caused by smooth muscle spasm. In addition, delayed natriuresis occurs after aneurysmal subarachnoid hemorrhage, probably mediated by atrial natriuretic hormone, causing intravascular volume depletion, a fall in cardiac output, a fall in mean arterial pressure, and global brain ischemia. Current attempts at treatment focus on techniques to increase cerebral blood flow and on pharmacologic agents to prevent ischemic cell damage.

Severe intracranial hypertension follows acute aneurysm rupture, and intracranial pressure may reach diastolic arterial blood pressure. This is an important mechanism to tamponade and arrest the bleeding. It also explains the loss of consciousness that occurs in one half of patients following aneurysmal subarachnoid hemorrhage. Doppler studies showed short-term zero flow when rebleeding occurred during Doppler-monitored aneurysm surgery. A rise of intracranial pressure to levels equal to arterial pressure results in cessation of cerebral blood flow. If the volume of extravasated subarachnoid blood exceeds intracranial buffering capacity, sustained intracranial hypertension persists and brain death follows. In most cases, the acute rise in intracranial pressure resolves, but it may leave varying degrees of ischemic brain damage after recovery.

Rebleeding occurs in about 20% of patients during the 2 weeks following the initial subarachnoid hemorrhage. The clinical presentation is an acute depression in level of consciousness, or a sudden increase in headache accompanied by confusion. In a patient already in coma from the initial bleeding, there may be an alteration in breathing pattern, apnea, pupillary dilation with loss of the light reflex, or seizure-like activity. The period of highest risk for rebleeding is the first 48 h after the initial event. The mortality associated with a second hemorrhage is about 65%. CT scanning is the most accurate diagnostic tool to identify rebleeding. Prior to definitive aneurysm clipping, about two thirds of all episodes of acute clinical deterioration will have CT evidence of additional hemorrhage.

Intracranial hematomas are present in 15–20% of patients on the initial CT scan. Hematomas are usually in the sylvian or anterior interhemispheric cisterns near the ruptured aneurysm. In 5% of all patients admitted to the International Cooperative Study, emergency craniotomy was required to evacuate large hematomas which were causing life-threatening brain-stem compression. In the other patients, the hematoma was removed at the planned time of aneurysm clipping. Focal hematomas are associated with a high risk for focal vasospasm and delayed cerebral ischemia, and it is believed that clot removal may reduce the incidence of this complication.

Acute hydrocephalus occurs in 20% of patients and is associated with intraventricular as well as subarachnoid hemorrhage. Hydrocephalus causes increased intracranial pressure and depressed consciousness. Most patients require external ventricular or lumbar cerebrospinal fluid drainage, depending on the distribution of intraventricular blood, to reduce intracranial pressure prior to surgery. A clot in the fourth ventricle, causing a noncommunicating hydrocephalus, demands ventricular drainage. Lumbar puncture could be hazardous in this situation. Half of the patients with acute hydrocephalus will require permanent ventricular shunting at a later time.

Hyponatremia occurs during the first week after subarachnoid hemorrhage in up to 30% of patients. Until recently, these patients were managed with fluid restriction for treatment of a presumed "syndrome of inappropriate antidiuretic hormone" release. However, recent studies have shown that low serum sodium is usually due to renal salt-wasting and intravascular volume contraction. Neurohumoral regulation of vasopressin and atrial natriuretic hormone are deranged, so that hyponatremia will occur with either too much or too little free-water administration. Hyponatremia with volume contraction is associated with delayed cerebral ischemia. Hyponatremia with volume expansion is associated with brain edema and increased intracranial pressure. Extremely careful management of intravascular volume and serum electrolytes is critical.

Cardiac arrhythmias and electrocardiographic changes of acute myocardial ischemia (peaked T-waves, T-wave inversion, depression or elevation of the ST segment) are found in up to 50% of patients with aneurysmal subarachnoid hemorrhage. In the past, these changes were thought to represent a noncardiac electrical disturbance ("cerebral T-waves") of no clinical or pathological significance. However, high blood levels of circulating catecholamines are found in these patients, approaching the levels seen in patients with pheochromocytoma. At autopsy, examination of the heart has revealed myofibrillar degeneration and focal necrosis with subendocardial hemorrhages, accompanied by myocardial contraction-band necrosis. It appears that subarachnoid hemorrhage and other causes of increased intracranial pressure may trigger catecholamine-induced cardiac injury and cardiac arrythmias. What role this mechanism plays in the high early mortality is unknown, but it warrants further investigation.

Acute pulmonary edema was reported in 67 of 3521 patients (2%) enrolled in the Cooperative Study. In some of these patients, neurogenic pulmonary edema developed suddenly, without prior signs of cardiac failure in those without known heart disease. With the advent of hypervolemic, hypertensive, hemodilution therapy, clinically significant pulmonary edema will become a more important problem.

Epileptic-like tonic extensor spasms occur in 10–15% of patients during acute aneurysm rupture, but true epileptic seizures are unusual after the acute period. When epileptic seizures occur, re-rupture of the aneurysm must be considered. If not, there is usually an underlying structural or metabolic abnormality to account for seizures.

Management

Initial Phase (Pre-ICU)

Initial management focuses on patient stabilization, prevention of rebleeding, and observation for the development of hydrocephalus. Obtunded patients should be carefully evaluated for their ability to protect their airway. If intubation is necessary it should be performed with premedication to prevent any rise in blood pressure or intracranial pressure. Blood pressure should be aggressively managed to avoid hyper- or hypotension. Elevated blood pressure often responds to treatment of headache with analgesics and the administration of nimodipine (see below). If these measures are not rapidly effective, antihypertensives such as labetalol or nifedipine should be used. Although the risk of seizures is small, in some centers anticonvulsants are administered to avoid even the potential risk of a seizure causing rebleeding. Dilantin is preferred by some centers because it can be given parenterally and does not produce sedation. Although they are often used, the utility of steroids has not been established.

Prevention of rebleeding is attempted by avoiding hypertension and with Valsalva maneuvers. Agitated patients should be sedated. It is important to use short-acting or reversible sedatives and to avoid over sedation so as not to mask the clinical signs of hydrocephalus. Definitive prevention of rebleeding is achieved with surgical repair of the aneurysm (see below). With the advent of early surgery the use of antifibrinolytics has ceased. In addition, even the brief use of these drugs is associated with an increased incidence of vasospasm. However, antifibrinolytics have never been tested in the presence of calcium antagonists such as nimodipine. Table 4 summarizes the general critical care procedures to be followed for patients with subarachnoid hemorrhage. All procedures are detailed elsewhere in this book.

Microsurgical Intracranial Aneurysm Clipping

By the mid 1970s, the binocular operating microscope was accepted by neurosurgeons as the key to successful surgery for intracranial aneurysms,

Table 4. Critical care procedures in subarachnoid hemorrhage

Invasive procedures	Venous catheter, central venous catheter, intra-arterial catheter In comatose patients additional: intratracheal tube and ventilation, gastric tube, urethral catheter, Swan-Ganz catheter (in selected cases)
Monitoring	Cardiopulmonary monitoring (rate, MABP, CVP, PO2, PCO2, BE), X-ray chest, electrocardiogram, transcranial Doppler sonography, som.tosensory/acoustic evoked potentials In comatose patients additional: ICP monitoring (ventricular/epidural), CPP, PCWP (in selected cases)
Specific medication	Dexamethasone 24 mg/day, nimodipine 2 mg/h i.v. or 360 mg p.o. After surgery (clipping) additional: hypervolemic therapy, hypertensive therapy

MABP, Mean arterial blood pressure; CVP, central venous pressure; BE, base excess; ICP, intracranial pressure; CPP, central perfusion pressure; PCWP, pulmonary capillary wedge pressure.

and microsurgical aneurysm clipping became the treatment of choice. In conjunction with refinements in micro-surgical instrumentation, bipolar electrocautery, precise intraoperative blood pressure control, brain relaxation using spinal drainage and mannitol, and advanced intensive care facilities for postoperative care, microsurgery reduced the operative mortality of elective aneurysm surgery to as low as 2%. Nevertheless, in spite of dramatic improvements in surgical results, until recently, the overall management mortality of subarachnoid hemorrhage remained high, approaching 50% in the first month.

For decades, surgeons appreciated the advantages of operating on patients days to weeks after hemorrhage. Delay in surgery selected a population of patients with the best chance of successful operation – those who improve after the effects of the initial hemorrhage. Alert and neurologically stable patients have a much better outcome after surgery. The remainder of the patients deteriorated or died from rebleeding and delayed ischemia, or

were deemed "too unstable" for surgery.

By 1987, a number of uncontrolled neurosurgical series suggested that early surgery effectively reduces the risk of rebleeding with acceptable operative morbidity and mortality. In 1990, after considerable delay, the International Cooperative Study on the Timing of Aneurysm Surgery published its findings on the surgical and medical management of 3521 patients, enrolled from 1980 until 1983, and followed up in a prospective, non-randomized, observational survey. Patients were divided into groups according to a "planned" surgery interval. There was no difference in case mortality between early surgery (0–3 days after the bleeding) and late surgery (11–14 days). Outcome was worse if surgery was performed during the 7–10 day post-bleeding interval. Surgical results were better after day 10, and analysis of complications suggested that the reduction in rebleeding afforded by early surgery was offset by more postoperative complications. Patients who were alert at the time of surgery had the best outcome, regardless of the time interval.

The International Study findings cannot be considered definitive, however. The study was not randomized, and during the time of patient enrollment (1980–1983), medical therapies to prevent and treat delayed cerebral ischemia were not consistently used. Calcium-channel blockers were not available, and intravascular volume expansion was used in only 22% of patients. The reported 13.5% incidence of death and disability from delayed cerebral ischemia is high by today's standards and could be reduced with current treatments. Even with the use of antifibrinolytic drugs, 7.5% of patients died or became disabled from rebleeding, a complication that is eliminated with early surgery. Of the patients admitted early, 30% did not survive to undergo surgery at the later planned interval. Waiting 2 weeks for surgery was associated with a 12% risk for rebleeding and a 30% risk for focal ischemic deficits.

A more recent, prospective, randomized study from Finland enrolled 216 patients into three groups: acute surgery (0–3 days), intermediate surgery (4–7 days), or late surgery (8 or more days). After a 3-month follow-up, 92% of the early surgery group were independent, compared with 80% of the late surgery group. This difference occurred even though the investigators did not use intravascular volume expansion and 25% of the early surgery group had permanent neurological deficits from delayed cerebral ischemia.

Without a large, prospective, randomized timing-of-surgery trial, using standardized medical therapies to prevent and treat delayed cerebral ischemia, it is difficult to make definitive recommendations regarding timing of surgery. However, recent published clinical series support the position that patients in good clinical condition at the time of hospital admission (Hunt and Hess grades I and II) should undergo early surgery (0–3 days). Neurologically impaired, but alert patients (grade III) may also benefit from early surgery, but this position remains controversial and depends on the experience of the individual surgical team. Without prospective randomized data to guide us, each surgical center should evaluate its own results and apply their findings to clinical decision-making. It is our view that early surgery and intensive medical therapy to prevent and treat delayed cerebral ischemia offer the best overall outcome.

Ligation of the Parent Vessel

Extracranial carotid artery ligation (common or internal) has been used since 1885 to treat intracranial carotid aneurysms, long before intracranial clipping became technically possible. The rationale is to reduce distal arterial pressure, reduce stress on the wall of the aneurysm, reduce the risk of rupture, and promote thrombosis. However, in practice, if there is good collateral circulation the risk of aneurysm rupture remains high (0–40% depending on follow-up), and if collateral circulation is poor the risk of ischemic injury is high (25–50%). There is no difference in complication rate between rapid and slow carotid occlusion techniques using a variety of metal clamps. Preoperative angiographic features do not predict postoperative complications. Preoperative cerebral blood flow studies and temporary endovascular balloon occlusion may help to select patients who will escape ischemic complications. Microsurgical clipping remains preferable whenever possible, but carotid ligation still plays a role in the treatment of giant extradural carotid aneurysms (petrosal and cavernous).

Some neurosurgeons have combined extracranial-intracranial bypass procedures with internal carotid artery or basilar artery ligation for aneurysms deemed unclippable. The bypass is performed several days prior to artery ligation, in the hope that ischemic complications will be avoided. Unfortunately, aneurysm rupture and distal embolization with brain infarction may still occur. Bypass techniques can also be combined with intracranial ligation above and below the aneurysm ("trapping"). The advantage of trapping is that the aneurysm is completely excluded from the circulation, avoiding further risk of rupture. Ischemic complications still occur, however, depending on the adequacy of collateral circulation. These procedures are performed in small numbers in specialized centers, and it is difficult to evaluate their overall impact on the natural history of the disease.

Circulatory Arrest with Hypothermic Brain Protection

Since the 1960s, attempts have been made to surgically obliterate giant intracranial aneurysms under the protection of deep hypothermia with total circulatory arrest. Until recently, these attempts were hampered by the complexities of cardiopulmonary bypass using full systemic heparinization and intracranial vascular surgery. Postbypass coagulopathy was a serious source of morbidity. Now several investigators have organized successful programs to treat complex giant aneurysms under the protection of hypothermic circulatory arrest. With this procedure, the aneurysm is dissected as much as possible in the fully arterialized state with meticulous hemostasis. Then full heparinization, cardiopulmonary bypass, rapid cooling to 18°C, total circulatory arrest, and exsaguination are sequentially instituted. During arrest, the aneurysm can be clipped or excised and extensive arterial reconstruction performed as needed. Currently, the mortality from this technique is 10%, compared with the 50% mortality reported with standard techniques.

Endovascular Catheter Procedures to Obliterate the Aneurysm

With the development of small, flexible, directional catheters and detachable balloons, several centers have successfully obliterated unclippable intracranial aneurysms with balloon embolization. These usually include midbasilar saccular or fusiform aneurysms and cavernous-carotid artery aneurysms. An attempt is made to place the balloon directly into the aneurysm. If this is not possible, occlusion of the parent vessel is performed. The advantage of balloon occlusion is the ease of reversibility if the patient cannot tolerate vessel occlusion due to ischemia. The greatest hazard is aneurysm rupture, which may occur in up to 50% of patients where there is incomplete aneurysm occlusion by the balloon. An alternative technique is endovascular platinum coil embolization. Platinum coils have been used successfully to embolize and induce thrombosis of arteriovenous malformations. Platinum coils can pass through smaller arteries than detachable balloons and, in selected cases, can induce thrombosis of an aneurysm that is not surgically accessible. The long-term outcome of these procedures is unknown, and follow-up angiographic studies are needed to evaluate their place in the overall management of patients with intracranial aneurysms.

Prevention and Treatment of Vasospasm and Delayed Cerebral Ischemia

Calcium-Channel Antagonists

Nimodipine has been approved for use in its oral form in the USA and both orally and intravenously in Europe for patients with aneurysmal subarachnoid hemorrhage to prevent and reduce neurological deficits associated with vasospasm and cerebral ischemia. The mechanism of action in clinical situations remains uncertain. Nimodipine does not significantly change angiographic vasospasm (although single case reports documented immediate vasodilation in both vasospasm and basilar migraine), but it probably improves microvascular collateral circulation in pial arterioles and inhibits calcium entry into ischemic neurons, thereby preventing the chain reaction of calcium-activated proteases and phospholipases producing cytotoxic free-radicals and leukotrienes. Other members of the dihydropyridine class of calcium-channel antagonists, nifedi-

pine, nicardipine, and nitrendipine, have similar effects but vary in their abilities to act on brain vs. peripheral vascular circulation. Recent studies with intravenous nicardipine have shown some benefits in reducing ischemic complications and ameliorating angiographic vasospasm. Transcranial Doppler ultrasonography is frequently used for detection and monitoring of developing vasospasm.

In a series of prospective, randomized clinical trials, nimodipine reduced clinical and CT evidence of brain infarction after subarachnoid hemorrhage by 10% to 86% compared with matched control patients. Beneficial effects were seen in all clinical grades. Side effects from the drug are minimal and include headache, reversible hypotension, flushing, and peripheral edema. The recommended dose is 60 mg orally or by gastric tube every 4 h for the first 21 days after subarachnoid hemorrhage (US) or 2 mg/h i.v. for 14 days (Europe). The dose must be reduced or counteracted if hypotension occurs. Based on experimental studies in ischemic stroke, it is likely that a small dose is also effective. In Europe, many patients receiving nimodipine after SAH are also treated with vasoactive drugs such as dopamine and dobutamine to avoid critical hypotension. Intravenous nimodipine may lead to pulmonary shunting and decrease the PaO_2 in selected patients (Fig. 6). In addition, gastrointestinal side effects such as subileus and decreased gastric motility have been reported.

Hypertensive Hypervolemic Therapy

Based on clinical studies showing that patients with symptomatic vasospasm

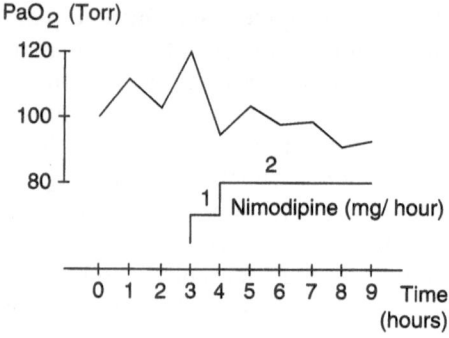

PaO$_2$ (Torr)

Nimodipine (mg/ hour)

Time (hours)

Fig. 6. Pulmonary complication of nimodipine administration: at the start of intravenous medication, the arterial oxygenation decreases. With 2 mg/h administration a further dose-related decline of PaO$_2$ is seen

have decreased blood volume due to natriuresis, many centers have adopted hypertensive hypervolemic therapy to prevent and treat delayed cerebral ischemia. In the setting of vasospasm, autoregulation is lost and blood flow is determined by physical characteristics – arterial lumen diameter, vessel length, arterial pressure gradient, blood viscosity, and oxygen-carrying capacity. Intravascular volume expansion repletes fluid deficits, increases cardiac output, increases mean arterial pressure, reduces blood viscosity, and increases blood flow to the microcirculation of ischemic brain regions.

Intravascular volume expansion therapy may be used prophylactically or for acute treatment of ischemic symptoms. Upon admission to the hospital, a pulmonary artery catheter is inserted to monitor cardiac output and left ventricular filling pressure. Prior to aneurysm clipping, euvolemia is maintained with isotonic crystalloids and 5% albumin. Following surgery, volume expansion is increased to reach a maximum cardiac output, with pulmonary artery wedge pressure moni-

toring to prevent pulmonary edema (usually 14–16 torr). Volume expansion is usually accompanied by a 10–20% rise in mean arterial pressure and a 10% fall in hematocrit. This protocol is maintained for 10–14 days, depending on symptoms and the degree of angiographic vasospasm on postoperative angiography. Other protocols use adrenergic substances to minimize the hemodilutional effect. Transcranial Doppler sonography can be used to follow the course of vasospasm and adjust therapy. If arterial blood pressure does not rise with volume expansion and the patient has symptomatic ischemia, dopamine infusion may be used to further increase cardiac output and blood pressure. Hypertensive hypervolemic therapy should be used only after definitive aneurysm clipping, because it may precipitate aneurysm re-rupture.

Although this treatment has not been evaluated with a prospective, randomized, clinical trial, broad experience in recent years at a number of centers around the world supports its use. It is notable that even with volume expansion, the frequency of ischemic events is the same, occurring in 25% of patients, but the incidence of permanent deficits is dramatically reduced. When compared with historical series, mortality in patients who develop delayed cerebral ischemia dropped from over 50% to less than 5%.

Subarachnoid Clot Removal

Since the late 1970s, Japanese neurosurgeons have stressed the importance of vigorous removal of blood clots from the subarachnoid space to reduce the severity of vasospasm and delayed ischemia. This approach is supported by strong evidence that the severity of vasospasm is proportional to the thickness of the blood clot in the basal cisterns. However, aggressive surgical removal must be balanced with the risks of brain injury from attempts to remove adherent clots. To date, there are no studies that definitely show a beneficial effect from surgical clot removal.

An alternative technique for removing a subarachnoid clot, with less trauma to the brain, is subarachnoid instillation of a fibrinolytic agent. Tissue plasminogen activator, a potent fibrinolytic agent approved for use in acute coronary thrombosis, was recently tested in primates and found to be safe and effective in lysing subarachnoid hematoma and preventing the development of vasospasm. It may also reduce the incidence of hydrocephalus. The major risk is postoperative intracranial hemorrhage. A multicenter clinical trial is now in progress and we await its findings with excitement.

Endovascular Transluminal Angioplasty

In spite of maximum therapy with calcium-channel antagonists and intravascular volume expansion, 5–10% of patients develop intractable symptoms and signs of cerebral ischemia from vasospasm. If the ischemic insult is due to focal narrowing of a large artery (internal carotid, middle cerebral, basilar) transluminal balloon angioplasty can dilate the stenosis and effectively restore perfusion. This procedure is applicable to only a small number of patients and has the potential risks of aneurysm rupture, total arterial occlusion, hemorrhagic infarction, and arterial rupture.

Other treatments for vasospasm and delayed cerebral ischemia which are still in the early stages of laboratory and clinical investigation include peptide antagonists of endothelium, platelet-aggregation inhibitors, 21-aminosteroids (U74006F), deferoxamine, ascorbic acid, cyclosporine, calcitonin gene-related peptide, and vasoactive intestinal polypeptide.

Suggested Reading

Aaslid R (ed.) (1986) Transcranial Doppler sonography. Springer, Vienna New York

Adams HP (1991) Nonaneurysmal subarachnoid hemorrhage (editorial). Ann Neurol 29: 461–462

Adams HP, Aschenbrener CA, Kassell NF et al. (1982) Intracranial hemorrhage produced by spontaneous dissecting intracranial aneurysm. Arch Neurol 39:773–776

Adams HP, Kassell NF, Torner JC, Haley EC (1987) Predicting cerebral ischemia after aneurysmal subarachnoid hemorrhage: influences of clinical condition, CT results, and antifibrinolytic therapy. A report of the Cooperative Aneurysm Study. Neurology 37:1586–1591

Adams HP, Kassell NF, Kongable GA (1988) Intracranial operation within seven days of aneurysmal subarachnoid hemorrhage. Results in 150 patients. Arch Neurol 45: 1065–1069

Allen GS, Ahn HS, Preziosi TJ et al. (1983) Cerebral arterial spasm – a controlled trial of nimodipine in patients with subarachnoid hemorrhage. N Engl J Med 308: 619–624

Andreoli A, Di Pasquale G, Pinelli G, Grazi P (1987) Subarachnoid hemorrhage: frequency and severity of cardiac arrhythmias; a survey of 70 cases studied in the acute phase. Strke 18:558–564

Andrews RJ (1979) Familial intracranial aneurysms. Arch Neurol 36:524

Andrews R, Spiegel P (1979) Intracranial aneurysms: Age, sex, blood pressure, and multiplicity in an unselected series of patients. J Neurosurg 51:27–32

Awad IA, Carter P, Spetzler RF, Medina M, Williams FW (1987) Clinical vasospasm after subarachnoid hemorrhage. Response to hypervolemic hemodilution and arterial hypertension. Stroke 18:365–372

Bailes JE, Spetzler RF, Hadley MN, Baldwin HZ (1990) Management morbidity and mortality of poor-grade aneurysm patients. J Neurosurg 72:559–566

Bailes JE, Spetzler RF, Hadley MN, Baldwin HZ (1990) Management morbidity and mortality of poor-grade aneurysm patients. J Neurosurg 72:559–566

Ballenger OM, Salcman M, Ducker TB, Perot P (1977) Prognosis of surgically treated intracranial arterial aneurysm patients. J Am Med Assoc 237:1845–1847

Baum HM, Goldstein M (1982) Cerebrovascular disease type specific mortality: 1968–1077. Stroke 13:810–817

Becker G, Winkler J, Hoffman E, Bogdahn U (1990) Imaging of arteriovenous malformation with transcranial color-coded real-time sonography (TCCS). Neuroradiology 32:280–288

Bell B, Symon L (1979) Smoking and subarachnoid hemorrhage. Br Med J 1:577–578

Black PM (1986) Hydrocephalus and vasospasm after subarachnoid hemorrhage from ruptured intracranial aneurysms. Neurosurgery 18:12–16

Brown RD, Wiebers DO, Forbes GS (1990) Unruptured intracranial aneurysms and arteriovenous malformations: frequency of intracranial hemorrhage and relationship of lesions. J Neurosurg 73:859–863

Chyatte D, Fode NC, Sundt TM (1988) Early versus late intracranial aneurysm surgery in subarachnoid hemorrhage. J Neurosurg 69:326–331

Chyatte DC, Reilly J, Tilson MD (1990) Morphometric analysis of reticular and elastin fibers in the cerebral arteries of patients with intracranial aneurysms. Neurosurgery 26:939–943

Cioffi F, Pasqualin A, Cavazzini P et al. (1989) Subarachnoid hemorrhage of unknown origin: clinical and tomographical aspects. Acta Neurochir (Wien) 97:31–39

Day JW, Raskin NH (1986) Thunderclap headache: symptom of unruptured cerebral aneurysm. Lancet 1:1247–1258

Ebeling H, Reulen HJ (1985) Cerebral vasospasm and aneurysm surgery. In: Auer LM (ed) Timing of aneurysm surgery. De Gruyter, Berlin, pp 414–419

Flamm ES (1986) The timing of aneurysm surgery 1985. Clin Neurosurgery 33:147–158

Fox AJ, Drake CG (1990) Endovascular therapy of intracranial aneurysms. AJNR 11:641–642

Fox JL (1983) The incidence of intracranial aneurysm. In: Fox JL (ed) (Hrsg) Intracranial aneurysms. Springer, Berlin Heidelberg New York, pp 15–18

Giombini S, Bruzzone MG, Pluchino F (1988) Subarachnoid hemorrhage of unexplained cause. Neurosurgery 22:313–316

Graf CJ (1971) Prognosis for patients with non-surgically-treated aneurysms: analysis of the cooperative study of intracranial aneurysms and subarachnoid hemorrhage. J Neurosurg 35:438–443

Harders AG (1986) Neurosurgical applications of transcranial Doppler sonography. Springer, Vienna New York

Harders AG, Gilsbach JM (1987) Time course of blood velocity changes related to vasospasm in the circle of Willis measured by transcranial Doppler ultrasound. J Neurosurg 66:718–728

Hart RG, Byer JA, Slaughter JR, Hewett JE, Easton JD (1981) Occurance and implications of seizures in subarachnoid hemorrhage due to ruptured intracranial aneurysms. Neurosurgery 8:417–421

Higashida RT, Halbach VV, Cahan LD et al. (1989) Transluminal angioplasty for treatment of intracranial arterial vasospasm. J Neurosurg 71:648–653

Higashida RT, Halbach VV, Barnwell SL et al. (1990) Treatment of intracranial aneurysms with preservation of the parent vessel: results of percutaneous embolization in 84 patients. AJNR 11:633–640

Hodes JE, Fox AJ, Pelz DM, Peerless SJ (1990) Rupture of aneurysms following balloon embolization. J Neurosurg 72:567–571

Hund E, Aschoff A, Tronnier V, Hampl J, Kunze St (1990) Nimodipine: evidence for clinically significant gastrointestinal side-effects. Acta Neurochir (Wien) 102:73–75

Hunt WE, Hess RM (1968) Surgical risk as related to time of intervention in the repair of intracranial aneurysms. J Neurosurg 28:14–20

Jenkins A, Hadley DM, Teasdale GM, Cordom B, Macpherson P, Patterson J (1988)

Magnetic resonance imaging of acute subarachnoid hemorrhage. J Neurosurg 68: 731–736

Kassell NF, Torner JC (1984) The International Cooperative Study on timing of aneurysm surgery – an update. Stroke 15:566–570

Kassell NF, Kongable GL, Torner JC, Adams HP, Mazuz H (1985) Delay in referral of patients with ruptured aneurysms to neurological attention. Stroke 16:587–590

Kassell NF, Torner JC, Haley EC, Jane JA, Adams HP, Kongable GL (1990) The international cooperative study on the timing of aneurysm surgery, part 1: overall management results. J Neurosurg 73:18–36

Kazner E, Sprung C, Adelt D, Ammerer HP, Karnick R, Baumann H, Böker DK, Grotenhuis JA, Jaksche H, Istaitih AR, Sachsenheimer W, Schackert G, Schramm J (1985) Clinical experience with nimodipine in the prophylaxis of neurological deficits after subarachnoid hemorrhage. Neurochirurgia (Stuttg) 28:110–113

Kurtzke JF (1985) Epidemiology of Cerebrovascular Disease. In: McDowell FH, Kaplan LR (eds) Cerebrovascular Survey Report for the National Institute of Neurological and Communicative Disorders and Stroke. National Institutes of Health, Bethesda, pp 1–34

Lennihan L, Petty GW, Mohr JP, Solomon RA, Fink ME, Beckford AR (1989) Transcranial Doppler detection of anterior cerebral artery vasospasm (abstract). Stroke 20:151

Little JR, St Louis P, Weinstein M, Dohn DF (1981) Giant fusiform aneurysm of the cerebral arteries. Stroke 12:183–188

Ljunggren B, Brandt L (1986) Timing of aneurysm surgery. Clin Neurosurg 33:159–175

Locksley HB (1966a) Report on the Cooperative Study of Intracranial Aneurysms and Subarachnoid Hemorrhage: section V, part I. Natural history of subarachnoid hemorrhage, intracranial aneurysms and arteriovenous malformations based on 6368 cases in the cooperative study. J Neurosurg 25:219–239

Locksley HB (1966b) Report on the Cooperative Study of Intracranial Aneurysms and Subarachnoid Hemorrhage: section V, part II. Natural history of subarachnoid hemorrhage, intracranial aneurysms and arteriovenous malformations based on 6368 cases in the cooperative study. J Neurosurg 25: 321–368

Mettinger KL, Ericson K (1982) Fibromuscular dysplasia and the brain: observations on angiographic, clinical and genetic characteristics. Stroke 13:46–52

Mizukami M, Takamae T, Tazawa T, Kawase T, Matsuzaki T (1980) Value of computed tomography in the prediction of cerebral vasospasm after aneurysm rupture. Neurosurgery 7:583–586

Niizuma H, Kwak R, Ohio T, Katakura R, Mizoi K, Suzuki J (1978) Complications of cerebral angiography in 939 patients with intracranial aneurysm. Neurol Surg 6: 673–679

Norris SL, Nosko M, Weir B, King EG, Grace M (1986) Acute cardiopulmonary effects of subarachnoid hemorrhage in monkeys. Crit Care Med 14:491–494

Oken BS (1983) Intracranial aneurysms in polycystic kidney disease. N Engl J Med 309: 927–928

Ostergaard J, Reske-Nielsen E, Oxlund H (1987) Histological and morphometric observations on the reticular fibers in the arterial beds of patients with ruptured intracranial saccular aneurysms. Neurosurgery 20:554–558

Peerless SJ, Kassell NF, Komatsu K et al. (1980) Cerebral vasospasm: acute proliferative vasculopathy? II. Morphology. In: Wilkins RH (ed) Cerebral arterial spasm. Williams and Wilkins, Baltimore, pp 88–96

Petruk KC, West M, Mohr G et al. (1988) Nimodipine treatment in poor-grade aneurysm patients. Results of a mulcicenter double-blind placebo-controlled trial. J Neurosurg 68:505–517

Phillips LH, Whisnant JP, O'Fallon WM, Sundt TM (1980) The unchanging pattern of subarachnoid hemorrhage in the community. Neurology 30:1034–1040

Post KD, Flamm ES, Goodgold A, Ransohoff J (1977) Ruptured intracranial aneurysms: case morbidity and mortality. J Neurosurg 46:290–295

Rinkel GJE, Wijdicks EFM, Vermeulen M et al. (1990) Outcome in perimesencephalic (nonaneurysmal) subarachnoid hemorrhage: a follow-up study in 37 patients. Neurology 40:1130–1132

Ropper AH, Zervas NT (1984) Outcome 1 year after SAH from cerebral aneurysm: management morbidity, mortality, and functional status in 112 consecutive good-risk patients. J Neurosurg 60:909–915

Ross JS, Masaryk TJ, Modic MT, Harik SI, Wiznitzer M, Selman WR (1989) Magnetic resonance angiography of the extracranial carotid arteries and intracranial vessels: a review. Neurology 39:1369–1376

Sahs AL, Perret GE, Locksley HB, Nishioka H (eds) (1969) Intracranial aneurysms and subarachnoid hemorrhage. A cooperative study. Lippincott, Philadelphia

Sahs AL, Nibbelink DW, Torner JC (eds) (1981) Aneurysmal subarachnoid hemorrhage: report of the cooperative study. Urban and Schwarzenberg, Baltimore

Sano K, Asano T, Tamura A (1987) Acute aneurysm surgery. Springer, Vienna New York

Sasaki T, Kassell NF, Colohan ART, Nazar GB (1985) Cerebral vasospasm following subarachnoid hemorrhage. In: McDowell F, Caplan L (eds) Cerebrovascular survey report for the National Institute of Neurological and Communicative Disorders and Stroke. MD: National Institutes of Health, Bethesda, pp 109–132

Säveland H, Hillman J, Brandt L, Edner G, Jakobsson KE, Algers G (1992) Overall outcome in aneurysmal subarachnoid hemorrhage. J Neurosurg 76:729–734

Seiler RW, Grolimund P, Aaslid R, Huber P, Nornes H (1986) Cerebral vasospasm evaluated by transcranial ultrasound correlated with clinical grade and CT-visualized subarachnoid hemorrhage. J Neurosurg 64:594–600

Sloan MA, Haley EC, Kassell NF et al. (1989) Sensitivity and specificity of transcranial Doppler ultrasonography in the diagnosis of vasospasm following subarachnoid hemorrhage. Neurology 39:1514–1518

Solomon RA, Fink ME (1987) Current strategies for the management of aneurysmal subarachnoid hemorrhage. Arch Neurol 44: 769–774

Solomon RA, Fink ME, Lennihan L (1988) Early aneurysm surgery and prophylactic hypervolemic hypertensive therapy for the treatment of aneurysmal subarachnoid hemorrhage. Neurosurgery 23:699–704

Solomon RA, Fink ME, Lennihan L (1988) Prophylactic volume expansion therapy for the prevention of delayed cerebral ische-

mia following early aneurysm surgery: results of a preliminary trial. Aroh Neurol 45:325–332

Solomon RA, Onesti ST, Klebanoff L (1991) Relationship between the timing of aneurysm surgery and the development of delayed cerebral ischemia. J Neurosurg 75:56–61

Solomon RA, Klebanoff LM, Lennihan L, Fink ME. Aggressive treatment for aneurysmal subarachnoid hemorrhage: comparison of a si. ndardized treatment protocol to historical controls. Arch Neurol (in press)

Spetzler RF, Hadley MN, Rigamonti D et al. (1988) Aneurysms of the basilar artery treated with circulatory arrest, hypothemia, and barbiturate cerebral protection. J Neurosurg 68:868–879

Stehbens WE (1983) The pathology of intracranial arterial aneurysms and their complications. In: Fox JL (ed) Intracranial aneurysms, vol 1. Springer, Berlin Heidelberg New York, pp 272–357

Stehbens W (1989) Etiology of intracranial berry aneurysms. J Neurosurg 70:1989

Steiner HH, Kunze S (1989) Die akute Subarachnoidalblutung: Mikrochirurgische Therapie nach Aneurysmaruptur an den Hirngefäßen. Intensivmedizin 26:438–449

Sundt TM, Whisnant JP (1978) Subarachnoid hemorrhage from intracranial aneurysms: surgical management and natural history of disease. N Engl J Med 299:116–122

Suzuki J, Yoshimoto T (1979) Distribution of cerebral aneurysms. In: Pia HW, Langmaid C, Ziersky J (eds) Cerebral aneurysms. Springer, Berlin Heidelberg New York, pp 127–133

Suzuki R, Masaoka H, Hirata Y, Marumo F (1992) The role of Endothelin-I in the origin of cerebral vasospasm in patients with aneurysmal subarachnoid hemorrhage. J Neurosurg 77:96–100

Taneda M, Otsuki H, Kumura E, Sakaguchi T (1990) Angiographic demonstration of acute phase of intracranial arterial spasm following aneurysm rupture. Case report. J Neurosurg 73:958–961

van Gijn J, van Dongen KF, Vermeulen M et al. (1985) Perimesencephalic hemorrhage. A nonaneurysmal and benighn form of subarachnoid hemorrhage. Neurology 35: 493–497

Weir B (1985) Intracranial aneurysms and subarachnoid hemorrhage: an overview. In: Wilkins RH, Rengachary SS (eds) Neurosurgery. McGraw-Hill, New York, pp 1308–1329

Whisnant JP, Phillips LH, Sundt TM (1982) Aneurysmal subarachnoid hemorrhage: timing of surgery and mortality. Mayo Clin Proc 57:471–475

Wiebers DO, Whisnant JP, O'Fallon WM (1981) The natural history of unruptured intracranial aneurysms. N Engl J Med 304:696–698

Wijdicks EP (1985) Volumne depletion and natriuresis in patients with a ruptured intracranial aneurysm. Am Neurol 18:211–216

Wijdicks EFM, Vermeulen M, Hijdra A, van Gijn J (1985) Hyponatremia and cerebral infarction in patients with ruptured intracranial aneurysms: is fluid restriction harmful? Ann Neurol 18:137–140

Wilkins RH (1976) Aneurysm rupture during angiography: does acute vasospasm occur? Surg Neurol:299–303

Winn HR, Richardson AE, Jane J (1977) The long-term prognosis in untreated cerebral aneurysms: I. The incidence of late hemorrhage in cerebral aneurysm: a 10-year evaluation in 364 patients. Ann Neurol 1:358–370

Winn HR, Richardson AE, O'Brien W, Jane J (1978) The long-term prognosis in untreated cerebral aneurysms: II. Late morbidity and mortality. Ann Neurol 4: 418–426

Zimmerman RD, Leeds NE, Goldman MJ (1985) Digital subtraction angiography in the evaluation of patients with cerebrovascular disease. In: Fein JM, Flamm ES (eds) Cerebrovascular surgery, vol 2. Springer, Berlin Heidelberg New York, pp 343–358

Chapter 58

Cerebral Sinus Venous Thrombosis

Arno Villringer, Marie-Germaine Bousser, and Karl M. Einhäupl

Definition

The traditional view of thrombosis of the cerebral veins and/or sinuses (SVT) is that of a rare disease, difficult to diagnose, difficult to treat, and with a poor prognosis. Based on a number of recent findings, this concept has been revised. SVT is more frequent than previously thought but still rare compared with arterial stroke. Diagnosis is accomplished easily and in most cases noninvasively with new neuroimaging methods, however, the crucial first step towards the diagnosis is to think of it in the differential diagnosis of many clinical signs and symptoms. Many patients with SVT present with only minor neurological symptoms; however, if undiagnosed and untreated, the disease may progress to a state requiring intensive care (approximately 20% of cases).

Epidemiology

The exact incidence and prevalence of SVT are not known. Autopsy studies have reported up to 9%. In the Paris series ($n = 110$) the mean age was 38.7 $\pm$ 14.8 SD, in the Munich series ($n = 107$) 37.0 $\pm$ 15.2 SD. It is slightly more frequent among young women due to specific causes such as oral contraceptives, pregnancy, and postpartum. The sex ratio (f/m) was 1.29 in the Paris series and 1.68 in the Munich group.

Etiology and Pathogenesis

The thrombotic process with the cerebral venous system as well as the risk factors are essentially the same as for venous thrombosis in other parts of the body. Etiological factors (Table 1) include local infections, sepsis, mechanical obstruction, hormonal alterations such as those occurring during pregnancy and puerperium, coagulation disorders, chronic inflammatory conditions such as Behçet's, disease and several others. It is impor-

Section Editor: Werner Hacke

Table 1. Etiology of sinus venous thrombosis
(Ameri and Bousser 1992)

Infective causes
Local
    Direct septic trauma, intracranial infections,
        regional infections
General
    Systemic bacterial, viral, parasitic (malaria,
        trichinosis), or fungal (aspergillosis)
        infection

Noninfective causes
Local
    Head injury
    Neurosurgical operation
    Cerebral infarction and hemorrhages
    Tumors
    Porencephaly, arachnoid cysts
    Infusions into the internal jugular vein

General causes
    Surgery with or without deep venous
        thrombosis
    Pregnancy and puerperium
    Oral contraceptives

Medical
    Cardiac disorders (congenital heart disease,
        cardiac insufficiency, pacemaker)
    Malignant tumors (any visceral carcinoma,
        lymphoma, leukemia, carcinoid)
    L-asparaginase therapy, other cytostatic
        therapy, steroid treatment
    RBC disorders (polycythemia,
        posthemorrhagic anemia, sickle cell
        disease, paroxysmal nocturnal
        hemoglobinuria)
    Thrombocythemia
    Coagulation disorders (AT III, protein C, or
        protein S deficiencies, circulating
        anticoagulants, DIC, heparin- or
        heparinoid-induced thrombocytopenia,
        epsilonaminocaproic acid treatment)
    Severe dehydration of any cause
    Digestive: cirrhosis, Crohn's disease,
        ulcerative colitis
    Connective tissue disorders: systemic lupus
        erythematosus, temporal arteritis,
        Wegener's granulomatosis
    Venous thromboembolic disease, Hughes-
        Stovin syndrome
    Others: Behçet's disease, sarcoidosis,
        nephrotic syndrome, neonatal asphyxia,
        parenteral injuctions, androgen therapy

Idiopathic

tant to note that, despite so many known reasons, the etiology remains unknown in approximately a quarter of cases. Although etiological factors and the pathophysiology of the thrombotic process itself are similar to venous thrombosis in other parts of the body, due to special properties of the brain, pathophysiological consequences differ considerably. The impaired venous outflow leads to various types of intracranial bleeding (intracerebral, subdural, subarachnoid hemorrhage), to venous infarcts which may lead to irreversible brain tissue damage, and to an increase in intracranial pressure due to (a) reduction of venous outflow, (b) impairment of CSF resorption, and (c) brain edema following tissue necrosis.

Another feature specific to brain tissue is an abnormal excitability that occurs as a consequence of various types of damage. In SVT, epileptic seizures occur frequently (37% in the Paris study, 49% in the Munich study) and may further damage brain tissue. This is indicated by the fact that epileptic seizures in SVT patients are frequently followed by a deterioration of the clinical status, such as a paresis persisting after the seizure (Todd's paresis).

Clinical Signs

The most important characteristic of the clinical picture of SVT is the great variety of clinical signs and symptoms and the variability in the mode of onset, which, in contrast to arterial stroke, is more frequently subacute (2–30 days, 50%) than acute (<48 h, 30%). Any focal neurological sign,

656   A. Villringer et al.

such as hemiparesis, hemihypesthesia, different types of aphasia, and other disorders of higher cognitive function, may occur. The main symptoms raising particular suspicion of the diagnosis SVT are (a) headache (present in approximately 90% of all patients), (b) focal epileptic seizures with a subsequent Todd's paresis, (c) a fluctuating course of the clinical signs over several days or longer, and (d) the clinical syndrome of pseudotumor cerebri.

These various signs can be grouped into two main patterns, which have distinct prognoses and require slightly different management: (a) SVT with focal signs/deficit and/or seizures, which carries a risk of neurological sequelae (comprising 66/110 = 60% in the Paris study and 71/107 = 66% in the Munich study), and (b) SVT with isolated intracranial hypertension (benign ICH, pseudotumor cerebri) (40% Paris, 34% Munich), which carries a risk of blindness if papilledema is not promptly relieved.

Ancillary Tests

Neuroimaging

Computed tomography does not permit a definitive diagnosis, although it assists in the diagnosis and allows monitoring of tissue damage. The most important direct CT signs of thrombosis are (a) the Delta sign, (b) the dense sinus sign, and (c) the cord sign. It should be emphasized that pitfalls in the interpretation of these signs do exist, rendering diagnosis based on CT alone difficult. Indirect CT signs of SVT are various types of intracranial hemorrhage (intracerebral, subdural, subarachnoid), brain swelling, and infarction.

In many cases, standard spin echo sequences show thrombosis by a lack of flow in the cerebral sinuses (Fig. 1). False-positive findings may be due to slow-flow, and false-negative findings may occur due to magnetic susceptibility effects within older thrombi.

Several groups have been able to demonstrate that MR angiography (MRA) permits the diagnosis of SVT (Fig. 2). MRA may show the venous system almost as detailed as angiography. The spatial resolution is somewhat lower than that of digital subtraction angiography. MRA has the advantage of showing the vascular tree in more projections. MRI with MRA will probably become the imaging modality of choice in the future.

Digital subtraction angiography and plain film angiography are still the gold standard in the diagnosis of SVT. They should be performed in all patients with doubtful findings in MRA and MRI, or when those methods are not available within a few hours.

Electroencephalography

EEG shows unspecific generalized or focal abnormalities in approximately 80% of the patients. Other neurophysiological methods are of no specific value in the diagnostic process.

CSF and Laboratory Findings

CSF analysis is performed in order to exclude inflammatory disease of the CNS. CSF findings in SVT are very

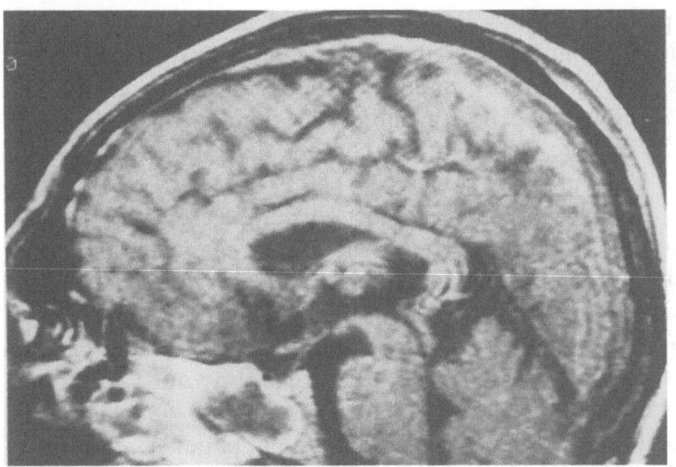

Fig. 1. MRI appearance of sagittal sinus thrombosis with loss of flow void in the sinus, hyperintense thrombosis signal, and edema fermation in the adjacent parenchyma CTZ-weighted image (courtesy of Rüdiger von Kumner, Heidelberg)

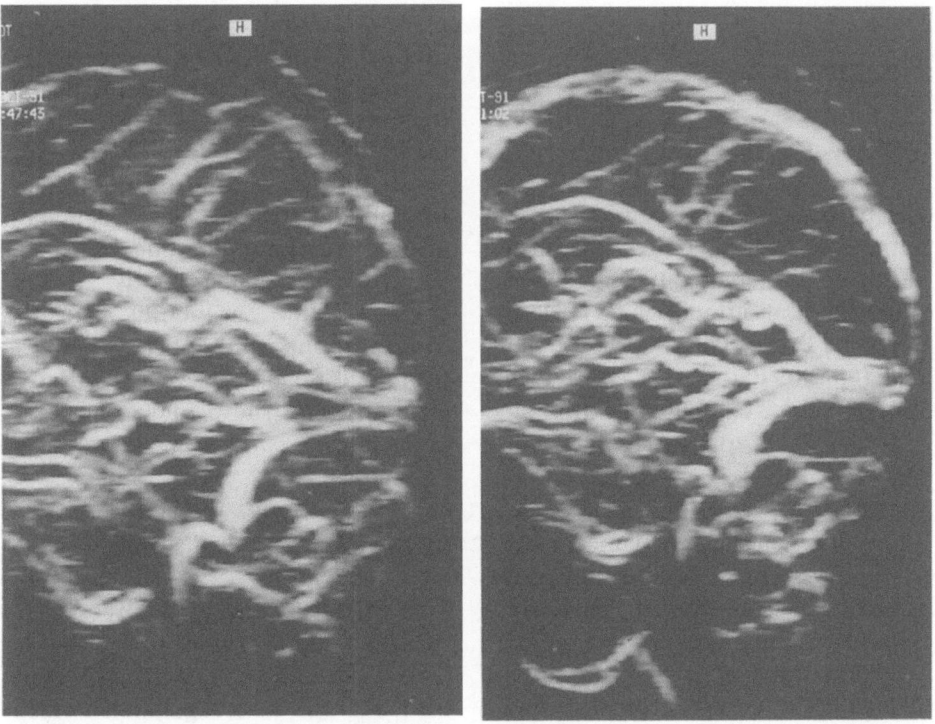

Fig. 2a,b. Magnetic resonance angiograms in the acute phase of SVT (**a**) and 1 month after heparin treatment (**b**)

heterogeneous. Many patients (34% = mean of Paris and Munich groups) showed normal findings; elevated protein was seen in 29%, elevated cell count in 26%, and in 23% there were signs of hemorrhage. CSF pressure was elevated in 62%. Lumbar puncture is of crucial importance when the patient presents with isolated signs of intracranial hypertension and normal CCT (so-called benign intracranial hypertension). It allows the measurement of CSF pressure and is the most rapidly effective treatment when vision in threatened in patients with papilledema.

A detailed analysis of coagulation factors should be performed in all patients in whom the etiology of the thrombosis is unknown.

Therapy

Anticoagulation

The basis of the therapeutic regimem in patients with SVT is dose-adjusted intravenous heparin treatment. We aim at least at a doubling of PTT; the target PTT is usually between 60 and 120 s (60–90 s Paris, 80–120 s Munich). Among the combined Paris and Munich SVT patients, 143 were treated with dose-adjusted intravenous heparin. Only four of them died. These four patients had in common an extremely rapid progression of the disease and stupor or coma when efficient heparin treatment was started. Whether this subgroup of patients might require a more aggressive treatment approach such as thrombolysis or surgical intervention is not yet clear, and the data of our groups indicate that (if at all) only a small subgroup might profit from such treatments. Anecdotal experience with thrombolytic therapy in SVT from other centers does not support this view.

Our experience with heparin treatment in SVT indicates that even in patients with intracranial bleeding or hemorrhagic infarcts, heparin is effective and indicated. Such patients have been treated by our two groups, with no worsening in 43 of 46. The three remaining patients with intracranial bleeding died. In these patients efficient heparin treatment was started only when they were already in an extremely poor clinical condition (stupor or coma). Of 13 patients with intracranial hemorrhage who did not receive heparin, nine died.

At hospital discharge, long-term oral anticoagulation with coumarins (or warfarin) is instituted for all patients (overlapping with heparin treatment). There is no general consensus yet as to the length of this treatment. In patients without any coagulation disorder requiring life-long anticoagulation, anticoagulation is usually stopped after 3 months. In the Munich group, oral anticoagulation is continued for up to 1 year if MRA at 3 months still shows signs of venous occlusion.

Elevated Intracranial Pressure

We do not recommend any specific treatment for the minor brain swelling that is observed in almost all patients with SVT. If anticoagulation is instituted early, the subsequent improvement of venous outflow is sufficient to treat these minor forms.

Antiedematous agents are given only in more severe cases when herniation is threatening. In these cases, invasive monitoring of ICP is recommended and ICP is lowered with 20% mannitol infusions. Corticosteriods are not recommended.

In patients with isolated intracranial hypertension and threatened vision one or two lumbar punctures should be performed to rapidly lower CSF pressure and improve vision before starting anticoagulation.

Antiepileptic Treatment

A significant number of patients with SVT will suffer from focal epileptic seizures during the course of the disease. Since such seizures might deteriorate the metabolic situation of certain brain regions and thus induce tissue necrosis, prophylactic antiepileptic treatment should be considered. Such treatment is systematically used in Munich, whereas in Paris anticonvulsants are used only in patients with seizures. If a seizure has occurred in an untreated patient, phenytoin therapy is started with intravenous administration in order to achieve therapeutic concentrations more rapidly. For further details of antiepileptic therapy, please refer to Chap. 66.

Other Treatment

More than 90% of all patients with SVT suffer from headache. Since the combination of antiplatelet drugs and dose-adjusted intravenous heparin carries a high risk of hemorrhage, drugs like aspirin should be avoided in patients with probable or definite SVT. We recommend paracetamol or pentazocin. We have had good experience with trifluopromazin for antiemetic treatment and haloperiodol in patients with significant agitation.

Prognosis and Conclusion

When effective heparin treatment was instituted in patients in good clinical condition (better than stupor), prognosis was always good. No fatal outcome occurred in these patients in either series. In patients presenting with stupor or coma at the beginning of effective heparin treatment, prognosis was somewhat worse; however, we have seen surprisingly good recoveries even in such patients.

In the two series together, of 171 patients receiving intravenous heparin, 129 completely recovered (75%), 32 (19%) were left with neurological sequelae, and ten (6%) died. In many of these cases death was related to the underlying cause such as malignancy, subdural empyema, etc., and not to the SVT itself. In conclusion, of all stroke syndromes, SVT is the variety which can be most effectively treated. Early diagnosis and treatment are therefore absolutely crucial.

Suggested Reading

Ameri A, Bousser MG (1992) Cerebral venous thrombosis. Neurol Clin 10;1:87–111

Bousser MG, Chiras J, Bories JB, Castaigne P (1985) Cerebral venous thrombosis – a review of 38 cases. Stroke 16:199–210

'Buonanno FS, Moody DM, Ball RM (1978) Computed cranial tomographic findings in cerebral sino-venous occlusion. J Comput Assist Tomogr 2:281–290

Einhäupl KM, Villringer A, Haberl RL et al. (1990) The clinical spectrum of sinus venous thrombosis. In: Einhäupl KM, Kempski O, Baethmann A (eds) Cerebral sinus thrombosis: experimental and clinical aspects. Plenum, New York, pp 149–156

Einhäupl KM, Villringer A, Meister W, Mehraein S, Pellkofer M, Haberl RL, Pfister HW, Schmiedek P (1991) Heparin treatment of sinus venous thrombosis. Lancet 333:597–600

Macchi PJ, Grossmann RI, Gomori JM, Goldberg HI, Zimmerman RA, Bilianuk LT (1986) High-field MR imaging of cerebral venous thrombosis. J Comput Assist Tomogr 10:10–15

Villringer A, Seiderer M, Bauer W, Laub G, Haberl RL, Einhäupl KM (1989) Diagnosis of superior sagittal sinus thrombosis by three-dimensional magnetic resonance flow imaging. Lancet 1:1086–1087

Villringer A, Mehraein S, Einhäupl KM (1993) Treatment of cerebral sinus venous thrombosis – beyond the recommendation of anticoagulation. J Neuroradiol (in press)

Chapter 59

Spinal Vascular Malformations and Ischemic Lesions of the Spinal Cord

Johannes Jörg, Thorsten Steiner, and Michael Forsting

Acute Spinal Cord Ischemia

Introduction and Epidemiology

Acute paraplegia of vascular origin is one of the most serious emergencies in neurology. It is usually the result of spinal cord ischemia rather than bleeding. The ratio of cerebral ischemia to spinal ischemia varies from center to center (depending on whether open heart surgery is done at the center) but in general is 10:0.3. For neurocritical care, the most important syndromes are the anterior spinal artery syndrome and the radicular magna artery syndrome.

Pathogenesis

Ischemia of the spinal cord is relatively rare because the arteries supplying the spinal cord arteries are less affected by atherosclerosis even when severe in other parts of the body. In addition, collateral blood flow is well established

---

Section Editor: Werner Hacke

in the spinal cord, in contrast to the cerebral circulation.

Regulation of spinal blood flow is similar to that of cerebral blood flow and is dependent on hemodynamic and metabolic factors. For example, in spinal cord compression from a neoplasm, blood supply depends only on the systemic blood pressure, cardiac output, and degree of local compression.

Spinal cord ischemia can be classified by site, time course, and cause. It occurs mainly in watershed areas in the mid cervical, upper thoracic, and thoracolumbar spinal cord (Fig. 1). Without collateral blood supply, the interruption of spinal blood flow for 15–20 min leads to irreversible ischemic damage. To minimize the risk of spinal cord ischemia during suprarenal aortic surgery, blood pressure in the aorta should be kept higher than 50–60 mmHg. Infrarenal aortic surgery rarely leads to paraplegia because the origin of the radicular magna artery is at T-9 to L-2.

Vascular syndromes can be divided into two groups: Primary vascular disease and secondary vascular disease due to aortic surgery, heart disease,

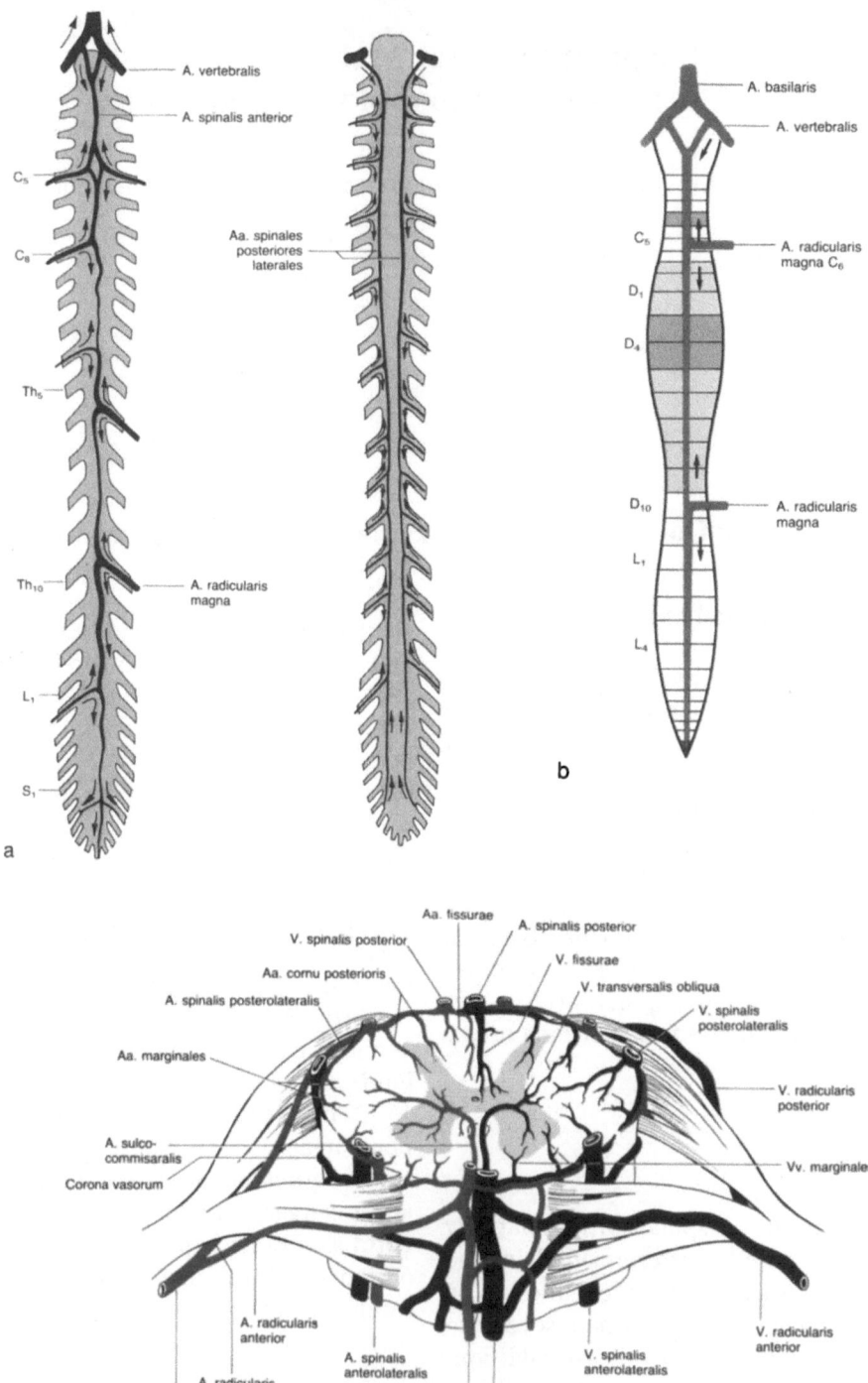

Fig. 1a–c. Spinal blood supply. **a** Anatomy of arterial territories of the spinal cord; *arrows* point in direction of blood flow. **b** Hemodynamic circulation of the spinal cord with zones of insufficient blood supply. **c** Arterial and venous blood supply – cross section

Table 1. Etiology of spinal vascular syndromes

1. Primary vascular diseases of the spinal cord
   - Fibrosis
   - Arteriosclerosis (rare)
   - Thrombosis (for example, of the anterior spinal artery, rare)
   - Emboli (for example, gas emboli in caisson disease, cardial or parts of nucleus pulposus, rare)
   - Arteriitis (for example, post-/ parainfectious, in syphilis, periarteriitis nodosa, lupus erythematosus)
2. Secondary ischemias of the spinal cord
   - Compression of vessels: tumor, cervical herniation of intervertebral disk, extramedullary inflammation, spine trauma, nippers mechanism in cases of whiplash trauma
   - Disease of the aorta: dissection, aneurysm, stenosis of the coarctation, Leriche's syndrome
   - Hemodynamic: hypotension in stenosis of segment arteries, resuscitation, congestive heart failure

neoplasm, or spinal disease (Table 1). The most frequent causes of severe vascular disease include aortic dissection (with occlusion of the respective segment artery), aortic aneurysm, Leriche's syndrome, and angiography-related complications. Metastases in the vertebral column can lead to acute compression of the outer spinal cord vessels. Progressive infarctions of the spinal cord can occur in patients with spinal angiomas or tumors (via both physical and vascular mechanisms).

Clinical Features

Patients with acute spinal cord ischemia, like those with acute cerebral ischemia, present with acute or progressive symptoms. Rarely, they may have intermittent symptoms. Myelo-

malacia usually results from occlusion of the anterior spinal artery or main radicular artery. It occurs from middle to old age and equally in both sexes. Symptoms usually occur in the morning to noon, developing over 1–2 h (rarely over 1–2 days). They occur independent of physical exercise. Progressive onset of symptoms over a longer period or acute onset within seconds, the so-called spinal stroke, are exceptions. Occasionally, a history of a spinal TIA may indicate a spinal angioma as the underlying cause.

Anterior Spinal Artery Syndrome

The anterior spinal artery supplies the anterior two thirds of the spinal cord in a variable number of segments. Patients with ischemia usually have segment paresthesias, pain, or both at the upper limit of the lesion, followed by paraparesis or tetraparesis with decreased muscle tone and areflexia (spinal shock). Pyramidal signs may initially be absent. Patients have pure dissociative disturbances of sensation below the affected segment, though symptoms may differ over segments between the right and left sides of the body. They may also have disturbances of the urinary and rectal sphincter tone and skin (because of decreased perfusion). Patients have a higher risk of decubital ulcers.

Spasticity develops after the initial spinal shock depending on the sight of the lesion. Damage of the motor neuron results in floppy paresis of the upper extremity. The extent of the paresis correlates with the number of destroyed segments. Extended infarctions of the lumbar and sacral spinal cord occur rarely and are associated with nonspastic paresis. Pain and paresthesias disappear after symptoms have reached their maximal extent. Occasionally, patients may have hyperpathia above the area of disturbed sensation. The segment of the lesion is presented by a sharp limited disturbance of sensitivity. This is because the lesion leads to damage of the anterior commissure and the posterior horn neuron that conducts temperature and pain.

The differential diagnosis of symptoms suggestive of anterior spinal artery syndrome includes:

1. Spinal angioma with steal phenomenon; in these cases pains last for longer than 2–3 h
2. Herniation of cervical intervertebral disk with compression of the anterior spinal artery
3. Psychogenic paraplegia
4. Myelitis
5. Spinal metastases (mechanical compression and circulatory effects)
6. Sulcocommissural artery syndrome
7. Acute spinal ischemia during aortography or with spinal angioma
8. Spinal intermittent claudication based on steal phenomenon rising from occlusion or stenosis of the aorta

Radicular Magna Artery Syndrome

Patients with infarction in the territory supplied by the radicular magna artery ("Adamkiewicz") usually have an abrupt onset (though not sudden or apoplectic) of motor and sensory deficits. The deficits are often ascending. Prodromal symptoms almost never occur. The affected segment is usually in the lower thoracic or upper lumbar spine, and patients often have trophic disturbances of the lower extremity with decubital pressure ulcers, and bladder and stool incontinence. If the *epicone* is affected, the lesion typically leads to a floppy palsy that does not recover. In one quarter of patients, the posterior root artery descends from the radicular magna artery. In these patients, the sensory loss is complete; that is, there is loss of protopathic and epicritic function. Anesthesia may be the reason for extended necrosis through pressure. When the lesion is above T-6, failure of sympathetic tone leads to hypotension and eventually to life-threatening reflex bradycardia.

The acute occlusion of the bifurcation of the aorta (Leriche's syndrome) with myelomalacia is characterized by pulselessness of the feet and coldness and marmoration of the skin of the legs.

The differential diagnosis of symptoms suggestive of radicular magna artery syndrome includes:

1. Acute myelitis with paraplegia: often with recurring fever, and pleocytosis
2. Leriche's syndrome through occlusion of the bifurcation of the aorta and ischemia of the extremities with consecutive motor sensory paresis ("vascular polyneuropathy")
3. Secondary vessel syndromes with tumor
4. Disease of the vertebra, fracture of the spine
5. Epidural hematoma of the spine
6. Spinal angioma
7. Epidural abscess: raised ESR, fever, severe pain

8. Hematomalazia (intraspinal hemorrhage)
9. Polyradiculitis
10. Venous infarction of the spinal cord caused by sepsis, neoplasm, or generalized thrombosis

Ancillary Tests

Electrophysiology. In patients with radicular magna artery syndrome, the amplitude of the cortical somatosensory evoked potential (SEP) is either zero or decreased. This can result in a slight reduction of latencies, a sign of severe damage to the dorsal column. In those with anterior spinal artery syndrome, the cortical SEPs are usually normal. Spinal sensory evoked potentials are not useful to locate a cervical lesion. Motor potentials cannot be evoked in patients with complete paraglegia of the lower extremities. F-waves are absent only in the affected segment.

Neuroimaging. All patients suspected of having spinal cord ischemia should have a plain X-ray of the vertebral column to exclude a mechanical or bony cause. If this reveals any abnormalities, the next step may be a myelogram or a CT scan, though in general, MRI is the method of choice for imaging the spinal cord. In ischemic lesions, the T2 signals increase within 12 h of symptom onset. An additional signal increase on contrast-enhanced T1-weighted images occurs 3–5 days later because of disruption of the blood-brain barrier (Fig. 2a,b). Spinal angiography is indicated only if myelography or MRI is suspicious for a vascular malformation.

Ultrasound. Abdominal ultrasound and transesophageal echocardiography can demonstrate diseases of the aorta, especially aneurysms.

Cerebrospinal Fluid Analysis. Analysis of the CSF shows a normal cell count and a normal to slightly increased protein concentration. Pleocytosis may occur in those with angiitis or myelitis. Those with vasculitis or Sjögren's syndrome may have increased IgG levels and oligoclonal bands. Definite signs of blood-brain barrier disturbance essentially exclude a primary vessel disease and suggest a space-occupying tumor.

Treatment

Before Admission to the Neurocritical Care Unit

– Stabile positioning of spine and extremities to avoid decubital ulcers or deterioration of pathologic vertebral fractures. To transport patients with cervical spinal injuries, a throat splinting hand grip can be used. A cervical collar should be used. If available, a vacuum mattress provides the greatest degree of safety.
– Urinary bladder catheterization should be done in those with urinary retention. This protects the bladder from hyperextension and allows accurate urine output measurements.
– Sufficient oxygenation and ventilation should be ensured with the use of oxygen and, if necessary, endotracheal intubation.
– Patients with Caisson or decompression disease with gas emboli

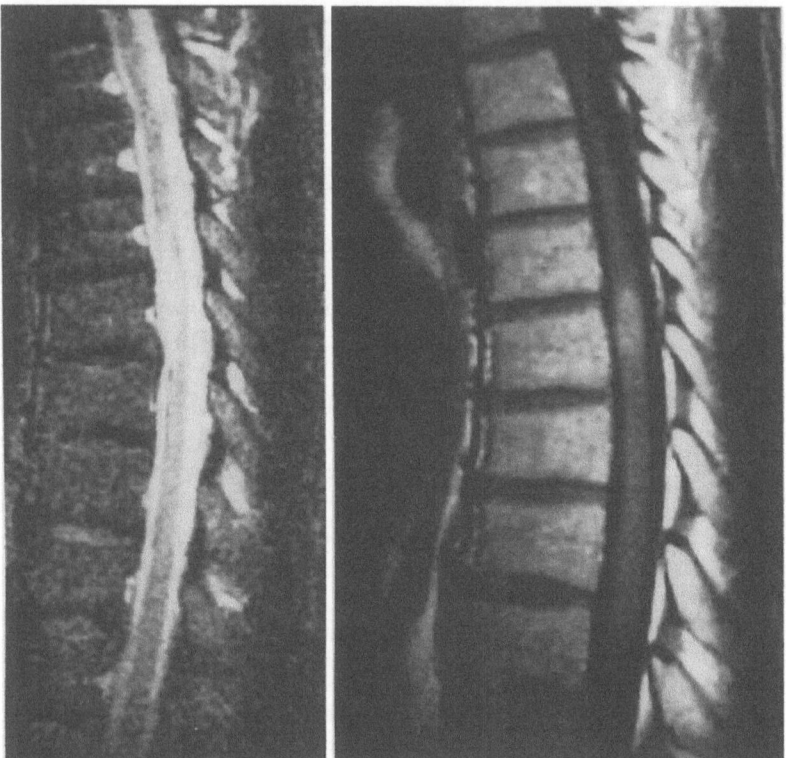

Fig. 2a,b. MRI 7 days after acute onset of paraplegia in a 67-year-old woman with a typical ischemic infarction in the territory of the anterior spinal artery. **a** Sagittal T2-weighted MRI with a zone of hyperintensity in the midthoracic region, representing the ischemic area plus perifocal edema. **b** Sagittal T1-weighted contrast-enhanced MRI clearly delineates the area of blood-brain barrier disruption

should immediately receive 100% oxygen.

In the Neurocritical Care Unit

Treatment of the underlying cause comprises:

- Surgical decompression for spinal cord ischemia from mechanical compression, for example in those with herniation of a cervical intervertebral disk or epidural neoplasm. In patients with complete paraplegia, the cause must be determined and treated in 3–6 h (Table 2). If paraplegia lasts for more than 8–12 h the patient with spinal metastasis does not benefit from surgical decompression.
- An aortic prosthesis for occlusion of the bifurcation of the aorta.
- Surgery for dissection, ascending thrombosis, or ruptured aneurysm of the aorta.
- Surgery of the intervertebral disk or foraminotomy for compression of the anterior root arteries.
- Operation at the sight of the ostium of the vessel for stenosis of the radicular magna artery.

Table 2. Diagnostic strategies in acute paraplegia

---

1. Clinical examination with definition of the lesion level
2. Radiologic workup of this part of the vertebral column

Plain X-rays to rule out bony abnormalities
If bony abnormalities: CT scan or (if available) MRI; if no bony abnormalities: myelography and CT, if available MRI
Angiography only if myelography or MRI reveals vascular abnormalities

---

– Embolization or extirpation of an angioma.
– Penicillin G for neurosyphilis with angiitis.
– Immunosuppressive therapy (occasionally with 7-S immunglobulin) for immunovasculitis.
– Immediate recompression to the starting pressure level, then slow decompression (watch for symptoms of de novo decompression) for caisson or decompression disease with gas emboli. Treatment with dexamethasone to prevent vasogenic edema is controversial.

Treatment to improve perfusion includes:

– Improvement of circulatory function: if the lesion is located above T-6, then arterial hypotension and reflex bradycardia should always be expected.
– Osmotherapy should be given to counteract ischemic edema.
– Rheological therapy and hemodilution.
– Early therapy with dexamethasone is controversial, but it appears to be effective when given between the 4th and 8th h. Because side effects of short-term therapy are minimal compared with the severity of the disease, if the cause of paraplegia remains unclear, therapy with dexamethasone in the first 24 h is always indicated.

Symptomatic treatment is directed at the following:

– High cervical spine injuries: measurement of vital capacity, oxygenation, and occasionally expiratory CO_2; if necessary, endotracheal intubation and assisted ventilation
– Intermittent bladder drainage or suprapubic catheterization (initial drainage for accurate urine output measurements)
– Early rehabilitation: positioning in bed, specialized physiotherapy; if necessary, treatment with antispastic drugs (baclofen, dantrolene, benzodiazepine, Tizanidin). Physiotherapy in upright bed position to prevent orthostatic hypotension and reflex bradycardia
– Prophylaxis of deep venous thrombosis: massage, positioning, low-dose heparin
– Prophylaxis of decubitous ulcers: change of bed position every 2–3 h, bolstering, use of special air-flotation beds ("Clinitron bed")
– Prophylaxis of pneumonia: secretolytics, bed positioning, intermittent CPAP, respiratory exercises
– Ileus prophylaxis: initial discontinuation of food, laxatives
– Prophylaxis of stress ulcer: H_2-blockers, anticholinergic drugs, psychological care

The time interval between the initial lesion and the onset of symptoms is not correlated with prognosis. The prognosis is determined by whether there is a treatable cause of ischemia, complications, and the tendency of recovery within the first 3 weeks after onset of the disease. Complications such as decubitous ulcers, pneumonia, and DVT occur more often in patients with radicular magna artery syndrome because paraplegia is more severe. Patients with primarily motor deficits have a better chance of recovery than those with primarily sensory deficits. Relapses can occasionally occur.

Spinal Angioma

Definition and Epidemiology

Spinal angiomas are vascular malformations that cause arteriovenous shunts between vessels of the spinal cord or meninges. They are classified according to their location: intradural, dural, or extradural angioma.

Most spinal angiomas are located in the thoracolumbar transition zone (T8–12). They are located in the dorsal part of the cord and cover several segments. Intradural angiomas, especially intramedullary AV angiomas and perimedullary fistulas, may sometimes be found in the cervical spine and in the ventral part of the cord. In these cases, the intramedullary angiomas are typically located at the sight of the intumescence.

About 2–10% of all intraspinal space-occupying tumors are spinal angiomas. They occur five times more often in men than in women. Intradural angiomas appear in childhood and adolescence, whereas dural fistulas occur in those older than 40 years.

Pathogenesis

An angioma is a defect of the primitive embryonic vessels. Decompensation and degeneration lead to growth of these insufficient vessels and progressive damage to the spinal cord. In some cases, these defects extend to extramedullary structures like skin, bones (vertebral angioma), and intra-abdominal organs.

In intradural angiomas, the arteriovenous shunt (nidus) is either intramedullary or extramedullary. It is supplied by spinal arteries (especially the anterior spinal artery) and drained by perimedullary veins. In spinal dural fistulas, the nidus lies within the dura and is supplied by branches of a radicular artery that otherwise does not participate in the supply of the spinal cord. The fistula is drained retrogradely by perimedullary veins to intradural veins. The small drainage capacity of these veins can contribute to congestion and edema of the spinal cord. Extradural angiomas may penetrate into the spinal cord, but they are always supplied and drained by extramedullary arteries and veins.

In dural fistulas, the main problem is increased pressure in the spinal veins, which can disturb the venous drainage even in more distant segments. In intradural angiomas, it is the high shunt volume that leads to a steal phenomenon and subsequent ischemic myelopathy.

Clinical symptoms are the result of (a) direct compression through space-occupying effects (thoracolumbar dorsal compression syndrome), (b) steal phenomenon ("arteriovenous shunt"), (c) ischemia caused by thrombosis of vessels of the spinal cord or the angioma itself, (d) rupture of vessels resulting in subarachnoid bleeding (SAB) or, in rare cases, hematomyelia, (e) arachnoiditis caused by bleeding through venous congestion, or (f) rupture of the angioma causing an epidural hematoma.

Clinical Features

Intradural angiomas usually appear between the 2nd and 3rd decades. Symptoms derive more from circulatory insufficiency than from mechanical compression. In most patients, symptoms present chronically progressive or "thrust"- or "wave"-like with or without progression. Occasionally, patients with spinal angiomas present with acute paraplegia or initially severe radicular or spinal signs. In contrast to multiple sclerosis, spinal angiomas may present with a rapid change of symptoms in the same segment over days. Quadraplegia occurs when an angioma is located in the cervical spine.

In the neurocritical care unit, it is important to be aware of the complications of spinal angiomas, i.e., rupture of the vessel and subarachnoid hemorrhage with rapid development of paraplegia, severe headache, and possibly increasing disorientation. Floppy palsies are more frequent than spastic signs. The combination of floppy and spastic signs is typical for thoracolumbar angiomas. Sensory deficits often precede motor deficits. The leading symptom is often spinal apoplexy, i.e., acute onset.

Four clinical courses may be observed: (a) prolonged progressive with medullary and radicular symptoms, (b) progressive, occasionally "thrust"-like with remission, (c) spinal apoplexy with relapsing ischemic or thrombotic episodes, and (d) spinal SAB, possibly with relapse.

About 30% of patients have spinal SAB with acute pain at the sight of the angioma (especially lumbosacral) with consecutive spreading to the lower extremities and neck (meningismus). Local pain is less often reported in cervical angiomas.

Spinal injuries, physical effort, and pregnancy have been reported to be predisposing factors. Casual trauma is usually the most common cause. The symptoms are worsened by physical effort, hot baths, hypotension, and upright position.

Spinal dural fistulas occur after the 4th decade and never lead to SAB. Patients initially present with back pain and then slowly progressing paraparesis. Eventually, patients develop both floppy and spastic symptoms that worsen with exercise. The differential diagnosis includes:

1. Spinal multiple sclerosis
2. Spinal tumor
3. Myelitis
4. Hematomyelia
5. Epidural hematoma
6. Protrusion or herniation of intervertebral disk with radicular lumbosacral symptoms
7. Cerebral versus spinal SAB: headache and meningismus are secondary signs in spinal SAB, whereas acute backache is a primary sign
8. Hemangioblastoma

Diagnosis

Neuroimaging. In some patients, a plain X-ray of the vertebral column reveals a cavernous angioma of a ver-

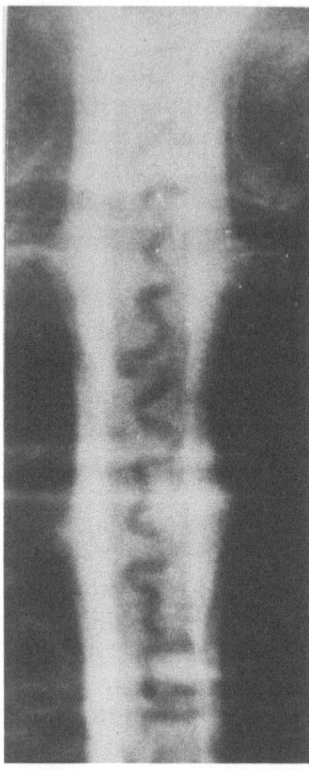

Fig. 3. Myelography in a patient with acute onset of tetraplegia. Myelography of the cervical spine clearly shows pathologic intrapinal vascular structures. The diagnosis of an intramedullary AVM was confirmed by angiography

location of the arterial feeders and draining veins (Fig. 3). MRI shows typical signal voids on spin-echo images. In dural fistulas, these are typically combined with a slight thickening and signal increase of the cord due to venous congestion.

Electrophysiology. On EMG, the floppy paretic muscles show chronic peripheral and neurogenic patterns with pathological spontaneous activity. The lower extremities or paravertebral muscles are affected in most cases. Sensory and motor neurography are normal. F-waves and H-reflex may be abnormal concerning the affected root. Spinal SEP from L-1 may be absent. In general, cortical SEP cannot be differentiated from results that are found in vascular myelopathy; if cortical tibialis SEP can be evoked, latencies are prolonged and/or the waveform is abnormal.

Cerebrospinal Fluid Analysis. The total protein concentration is typically increased up to 900 mg/l, reflecting blood-brain barrier disturbance. Pleocytosis rarely occurs. CSF contains blood or is xanthochromic in those with SAB.

tebral body. In intradural AVMs, myelography shows vascular structures in more than 90% of the patients, if done in prone *and* supine positions. In extradural AVMs myelography is sometimes nonspecific, but it usually shows a space-occupying (extradural) lesion with an incomplete stop of the contrast column. In general, CT is non-diagnostic in AVMs. If the myelogram is positive, the next step should be spinal angiography. This is the only way to differentiate between pial and dural AVMs and to show the type and

Treatment

Patients with spinal angiomas (especially those with cervical angiomas) should be treated in the neurocritical care unit. Treatment does not differ from treatment of anterior spinal artery syndrome. Insufficiency of breathing muscles and insufficient coughing increase the risk of pneumonia and frequently lead to intubation and assisted ventilation.

The specific therapy of vascular malformations depends mainly on the type, location, and arterial feeding pattern. Intramedullary AVMs with feeding arteries from the anterior spinal artery often cannot be cured with either endovascular or surgical procedures. In some patients, the combination of both procedures may be effective. Dural fistulas are easier to treat. In some patients, endovascular therapy with permanent occlusive agents is possible. New microcatheter systems allow superselective catheterization of even small feeding arteries. If the endovascular approach fails, surgery can be performed with clipping of the radicular artery. In general, treatment of spinal AVMs is a team approach that involves interventional radiologists and neurosurgeons. As in cerebral AVMs, the target of therapy is the nidus, which has to be removed completely. Treatment of angiographically proven angiomas depends on their extension, location, and arterial supply.

Prognosis

The prognosis in individual cases is difficult to determine, since it is not possible to anticipate the degree of postoperative or spontaneous regression of the spinal cord. The prognosis of early stages can be improved if embolization or operative extirpation of the fistula is possible. Progression of the disease may be stopped through repeat angiography and, if needed, repeat embolization.

Extirpation and embolization of a dural fistula does not improve the prognosis if complete paraplegia already exists.

Spinal Bleeding

Bleeding within the spinal cord or within its channels occurs in patients with coagulopathies, angiomas, or trauma. In general it is rare, and clinically it presents similar to space-occupying spinal tumors. Spinal bleeding may be located in the epidural and sometimes subdural, subarachnoid, or intramedullary (hematomyelia) spaces. Prognosis depends on three factors: (a) cause of the bleeding, (b) persistence of paresis before surgery, and (c) development of paresis before surgery.

Epidural Spinal Hematoma

Definition and Etiology

Epidural spinal hematomas occur in the epidural space between periosteum and dura mater. In contrast to cerebral epidural hematomas, spinal epidural hematomas bleed from the peridural venous plexus. For anatomical reasons, hematomas of the spinal epidural space develop quickly and are normally limited to a few vertebrae. They are usually located in the upper lumbar or lower thoracic and lower cervical spine.

About half of epidural spinal hematomas are caused by coagulopathies (especially in anticoagulated patients). Alcoholics also have a higher incidence of bleeding. Other causes include trauma, leukemia, pressure imbalances during pressing maneuvers, and vessel lesions from lumbar puncture or epidural anesthesia. Immunovasculitis has also been reported as an underlying cause. Spinal bleeding after manual therapy is extremely rare. Spontaneous epidural hematomas are rare and bleeding from the epidural venous plexus is suspected to be the source, although arterial bleeding can also occur.

Clinical Features

Epidural spinal hematomas occur in all age-groups, but most patients are between 50 and 70 years. They occur slightly more often in men. The first sign is usually severe acute pain at the height of the lesion with radicular radiation. Additionally, paresthesia in the areas of the affected roots can occur. Spinal compression with paraplegia develops in hours to 1–2 days, without signs of vascular disease. If the hematoma is located at the typical site (between T-10 and L-1), the patient presents with sensorimotor paresis, bladder and stool incontinence, and local spontaneous pain.

The differential diagnosis includes:

1. Epidural abscess: pain through percussion and local pressure is more severe; typical reflective fixation of the spine; serum analysis points towards bacterial infection
2. Neoplasm: especially metastases are found in epidural location
3. Acute or subacute myelitis
4. Spinal angioma: may lead to SAB, but not to epidural bleeding
5. Acute vascular myelomalacia: no local pain to percussion; the symptoms develop faster
6. Lumbar herniation of intervertebral disk with cauda equina syndrome
7. Myocardial infarction or lung emboli
8. Dissection of the aorta

Diagnosis

Neuroimaging. Plain X-rays of the vertebral column showing a cavernous angioma of a vertebral body are suggestive of epidural bleeding. Myelography usually reveals an epidural space-occupying mass. Only large hematomas are visible on CT scan. Smaller ones are visible on MRI, but unfortunately only after 3–5 days. At this time methemoglobin shortens the T_1-signal on spin-echo images and the hematoma is visible as a clot of bright signal.

Cerebrospinal Fluid Analysis. CSF analysis shows blood-brain barrier disturbance, even "stop liquor". A mild pleocytosis often occurs 2–3 days after the bleeding.

Treatment

The prognosis depends on early surgical removal of the bleeding and tissue decompression. Coagulopathies should be corrected first, for example, substitution of prothrombin complex and treatment with phytonadione in anticoagulated patients. A PTT of 40–50% is sufficient for operation. Platelet transfusion is indicated if platelet count is less than 20 000.

Subdural Spinal Hematoma

Subdural spinal hematomas are rare because there are no large subdural blood vessels below the foramen magnum; the main location is thoracic or thoracolumbar. They usually develop as a complication of anticoagulation therapy, hemophilia, or thrombocytopenia. Patients with vertebral fractures or mild trauma are also at risk. Lumbar puncture should be avoided, or performed only in life-threatening situations in those with platelet counts less than 20 000 (or rapidly falling platelet counts), during high-dose-heparin, or anticoagulation therapy. Clinical course and therapy are the same as in epidural spinal hematoma.

Spinal Subarachnoid Bleeding

Introduction

Spinal subarachnoid bleeding accounts for less than 1% of all SAB. Occasionally, the bleeding can extend intracranially, in which case a spinal SAB cannot be differentiated from bleeding from an aneurysm at the base of the brain.

Pathogenesis

- Intradural vascular defect, von Hippel-Lindau hemangioma
- Trauma to the spinal cord (for example, from boxing)
- Increased bleeding risk, for example hemorrhagic diathesis or anticoagulation therapy
- Aneurysm of the anterior spinal or radicular magna artery, for example, stenosis of the coarctation of the aorta or arteriitis
- Spinal tumor (ependymoma)
- Iatrogenic, lumbar or suboccipital puncture: clinically irrelevant because the bleeding stops spontaneously in almost all cases; however, in patients with hemorrhagic diathesis, lumbar puncture

may lead to severe SAB and subdural hematoma

Clinical Features

Patients present with acute back pain with hard, tense muscles at the height of the bleeding source, ischalgia, and secondary meningismus. Further meningeal irritation, medullary symptoms, and occasionally disorientation can occur. Later, signs of increasing intracranial pressure such as papilledema may be seen.

An intracranial bleeding source is almost always suspected, although bleeding from a spinal tumor may also result in increased intracranial pressure and papilledema. Clinically, patients with spinal SAB may present similar to those with cerebral SAB.

The differential diagnosis includes:

1. Intracranial SAB: no primary back pain
2. Vertebral fractures
3. Spondylitis
4. Epidural bleeding or abscess

Diagnosis

Normal CT does not exclude blood in the CSF. Although MRI is not the method of choice for diagnosis of spinal SAB, it can reveal a vascular malformation as the cause of the bleeding. In these patients spinal angiography is necessary.

Treatment

Therapy is directed towards the cause of the bleeding. Patients with bleeding from neoplastic hematomas have a better prognosis than those with bleeding from angiomas.

674   J. Jörg et al.

Hematomyelia

Definition and Epidemiology

Hematomyelia, or bleeding into the substance of the spinal cord, almost always extends to several segments and destroys the gray matter. There are no reliable data about the frequency of this disease.

Clinical Features

Only extended bleeding leads to complete paraplegia that is often initially associated with severe spinal shock syndrome and vegetative dysregulations. In most patients, hematomyelia presents like anterior spinal artery syndrome or as syringomyelia with dissociative sensory disturbances and floppy palsy. Severe back pain occurs only in the initial phase. In the acute phase, patients with hematomyelia have the same risks as those with paraplegia.

If during the clinical course symptoms of anterior horn disease appear at the height of the bleeding, the occurrence of dissociative sensory disturbances at the same site is typical. The remaining symptoms may clinically present as "syringomyelia-like" syndrome.

The differential diagnosis includes:

1. Anterior spinal artery syndrome
2. Bleeding spinal astrocytoma
3. Syringomyelia

Diagnosis

CSF rarely contains fresh blood, though it is usually xanthochromic. CSF may be normal if the hematomyelia does not communicate with the CSF space. CT or MRI can show the bleeding and may indicate the bleeding source.

Treatment

Surgical decompression and microneurosurgical extirpation are indicated if the time between onset of symptoms and diagnosis is within hours or if further extension of the bleeding is expected. Coagulopathy must be treated immediately (for example, substitution of prothrombin complex, transfusion of platelets if fewer than 20 000).

Prognosis

Since severe paresis and sensory disturbances remain in many cases, long-term complications of paraplegia must be expected.

Suggested Reading

Aminoff MJ, Logue V (1974) The prognosis of patients with spinal vascular malformations. Brain 97:211–218
Aminoff MJ, Barnard RO, Logue V (1974) The pathophysiology of spinal vascular malformations. J Neurol Sci 23:255–263
Anderson DK, Behbehani MM, Means ED (1983) Susceptibility of feline spinal cord energy metabolism to severe incomplete ischemia. Neurology (NY) 33:722–731
Bien S, Voigt K (1993) Spinale vaskuläre Malformationen und interventionelle Neuroradiologie im Spinalbereich. In: Therapie und Verlauf neurologischer Erkrankungen (Hrgb.: Th Brandt, J Dichgans, H CH Diener) Kohlhammer Stuttgart, 2. Auflage, pp 451–460
Brandt M (1980) Spontaneous intramedullary haematoma as a complication of anticoagulant therapy. Acta Neurochir (Wien) 52:73–77
Brosch T, Kölmel HW, Christe W (1990) Akute spinale Ischaemie bei Erkrankungen der Aorta. Nervenarzt 61:231–234

Brückmann H (1992) Vaskuläre Erkankungen des Spinalkanals. In: Uhlenbrock D (ed) Kernspintomographie der Wirbelsäule und des Spinalkanals. Springer, Berlin Heidelberg New York, pp 389–401

Buchan AM, Barnett HJM (1986) Infarction of the spinal cord. In: Barnett HJM, Mohr JP, Stein BM (eds) Stroke: pathophysiology, diagnosis and management. Livingstone, New York, pp 707–719

Bühlmann AA (1985) Dekompressionskrankheit des Rückenmarks. Resultate der Früh- und Spätbehandlung. Schweiz Med Wochenschr 115:796–800

Byrne ThN, Waxman SG (1990) Spinal cord compression. Davis Company, Philadelphia

Caroscio JT, Brannan T, Budabin M et al. (1980) Subarachnoid hemorrhage secondary to spinal arteriovenous malformation and aneurysm. Arch Neurol 37:101–103

Collmann H, Rimpau W (1978) Raumforderndes spinales subarachnoidales Hämatom nach Lumbalpunktion. Nervenarzt 49:605–608

Critchley E, Eisen A (1992) Diseases of the spinal cord. Springer, Berlin Heidelberg New York

Djindjian R (1972) Neuroradiological examination of spinal cord angiomas. In: Vinken PJ, Bruyn GW (eds) Handbook of clinical neurology, vol 12/2. Elsevier, Amsterdam, pp 631–643

Djindjian M (1978) Clinical symptomatology and natural history of arteriovenous malformations of the spinal cord. In: Pia HW, Djiandjian R (eds) Spinal angiomas – advances in diagnosis and therapy. Springer, Berlin Heidelberg New York, pp 75–83

Ferbert A (1986) Akute Rückenmarkskrankheiten. In: Hacke W (ed) Neurologische Intensivmedizin. Perimed, Erlangen, pp 194–201

Flaschka G, Sutter B, Ebner et al. (1990) Das spinale Epiduralhämatom. Nervenarzt 61:629–633

Foo D, Rossier AB (1983) Anterior spinal artery syndrome and its natural history. Paraplegia 21:1–10

Groen RJM, Ponssen H (1990) The spontaneous spinal epidural hematoma. A study of the etiology. J Neurol Sci 98:121–138

Harik SI, Raichle ME, Reis DJ (1971) Spontaneously remitting spinal epidural hematoma in a patient on anticoagulants. N Engl J Med 284:1355

Hassler W, Thron A, Grote EH (1989) Hemodynamics of spinal dural arteriovenous fistulas. J Neurosurg 70:360–370

Henson RA, Parsons M (1967) Ischemic lesions of the spinal cord: an illustrated review. Q J Med NS 36 142:205–222

Holdorff B, Bradac GB (1987) Thorakolumbosakrale Lähmungen bei sakraler extraduraler arteriovenöser Fistel. Aktuel Neurol 14:187–191

Hughes JT (1971) Venous infarction of the spinal cord. Neurology 21:794–800

Jellinger K (1967) Spinal cord arteriosclerosis and progressive vascular myelopathy. J Neurol Neurosurg Psychiatry 30:195–206

Jellinger K (1980) Morphologie und Pathogenese spinaler Durchblutungsstörungen. Nervenarzt 51:65–77

Jörg J (1985) Neurologische Allgemein- und Intensivtherapie. Springer, Berlin Heidelberg New York

Jörg J (1992) Rückenmarkerkrankungen. Edition medizin, Weinheim

Koenig E, Thron A, Schrader V, Dichgans J (1989) Spinal arteriovenous malformations and fistulae: clinical, neuroradiological and neurophysiological findings. J Neurol 236:260–266

Konttinen YT, Kinnunen E, von Bonsdorff M (1987) Acute transverse myelopathy successfully treated with plasmapheresis and prednisone in a patient with primary Sjögren's syndrome. Arithritis Rheumatol 330:339–344

Koyama T, Igaraski S, Hamakita J, Handa J (1982) Das spinale epidurale Hämatom – Zur Ursache der Blutung. Neurochirurgia 25:11–13

La Torre E, Fortuna A (1971) Syndrome of anterior spinal artery from cervical spondylosis relieved by surgery. Minerva Neurochir 15:22–23

Lazorthes G (1972) Pathology, classification and clinical aspects of vascular diseases of the spinale cord. In: Vinken PJ, de Bruyn GW (eds) Handbook of neurology, vol 12/2. Elsevier, Amsterdam, pp 492–506

Logue V (1979) Angiomas of the spinal cord: review of the pathogenesis, clinical features and results of surgery. J Neurol Neurosurg Psychiatry 42:1–11

Maeda S, Miyamoto T, Murata H, Yamashita K (1989) Prevention of spinal cord ischemia by monitoring spinal cord perfusion pres-

676   J. Jörg et al.: Spinal Vascular Malformations and Ischemic Lesions

sure and somatosensory evoked potentials. J Cardiovasc Surg 30:565–571

Meinecke FW (1990) Querschnittlähmungen. Springer, Berlin Heidelberg New York

Odom GL (1962) Vascular lesions of the spinal cord: malformations, spinal subarachnoid and extradural hemorrhage. Clin Neurosurg 8:196

Oliver AD, Wilson CB, Boldrey EB (1973) Transient postprandial paresis associated with arteriovenous malformations of the spinal cord. J Neurosurg 39:652–655

Pia HW (1973) Diagnosis and treatment of spinal angiomas. Acta Neurochir (Wien) 28:1–12

Pia HW (1985) Spinale Angiome. In: Schirmer M (ed) Querschnittslähmungen. Springer, Berlin Heidelberg New York, pp 395–408

Pou Serradell A, Aragones JM, Oliveras C (1990) Lumbosacral spinal cord infarction. Data provided by magnetic resonance im-

aging. Rev Neurol 146:293–296

Ropper AH (1992) Neurological and neurosurgical intensive care, 3rd edn. Raven, New York

Schirmer M (1985) Querschnittlähmungen. Springer, Berlin Heidelberg New York

Schulze HAF (1988) Neurologische Intensivbetreuung. VEB Thieme, Leipzig

Stöhr M, Brandt T, Einhäupl KM (1991) Neurologische Syndrome in der Intensivmedizin. Kohlhammer, Stuttgart

Vogelsang H (1980) Neuroradiologische Untersuchungen und Befunde bei spinalen Gefäßerkrankungen. Nervenarzt 51:81–86

Wildemann B, Storch-Hagenlocher B, Hacke W (1991) Zerebrale Vaskulitiden. Aktuel Neurol 18:8–14

Wolman L, Bradshaw P (1967) Spinal cord embolism. J Neurol Neurosurg Psychiatry 30:446

Neurotrauma

Chapter 60

Cranial Trauma

JONATHAN GREENBERG and ALEXANDER BRAWANSKI

Epidemiology of Cranial Trauma

Cranial trauma and its sequelae are a major public health problem throughout the industrialized world. The incidence of head injury depends on cultural and socioeconomic factors, including poverty, crime, locality, alcohol or drug abuse, the use of seat belts, occupational safety requirements, and recreational pastimes. In the United States, approximately 500 000 people (an incidence of approximately 200/100 000) require medical attention for evaluation of cranial trauma each year. Of those, approximately 150 000 sustain severe head injuries, and 50 000–60 000 die every year as a result.

The peak incidence of head injury occurs in the 15- to 24-year age-group. It is the leading cause of death in men under the age of 35, and, depending on the location, men outnumber women by 2:1–4:1.

Overall, approximately 50% of multisystem traumas involve injury to the central nervous system, and brain injury is present in 75% of patients who die as a result of motor vehicle accidents. Motor vehicle accidents remain the major cause of cranial trauma, with alcohol or drug abuse and the failure to wear seat belts and shoulder restraints implicated in a major proportion of resulting fatalities. Violence is a major source of blunt and penetrating cranial trauma, particularly in inner-city environments, where penetrating injury can surpass motor vehicle accidents as a cause of head injury. Each year in the United States, approximately 10 000 people die as a result of gunshot wounds, whether self-inflicted, accidental, or as a result of criminal assault. Other causes of cranial trauma include industrial accidents, falls, and such dangerous recreational activities as hang-gliding or mountain climbing.

Pathophysiology of Brain Injury

Primary Brain Injury

Section Editors: Thomas P. Bleck and Alan H. Ropper

Recognition of the different pathophysiologic processes following cranial trauma is essential for directing appropriate medical management and for a realistic appreciation of the potential for neurologic recovery. Primary brain injury results from forces impacting on the cranium within the first few milliseconds of injury; direct crush injuries to neurons and supporting glial cells, synaptic disruptions, evulsion, or thrombosis of cerebral vessels all occur long before any rescue arrives at the scene of the injury. Thus, the only effective treatment for primary brain injury is prevention.

Secondary Brain Injury

Secondary brain injury is the delayed consequence of the initial mechanical injury to brain tissue and its supporting structures, and it may be exacerbated by systemic injuries. At the cellular level, the cerebral hypermetabolic response to trauma and subsequent ischemia reduces intracellular ATP concentration and increases both Monophosphate (MP) and adenosine levels, promoting hypoxanthine-mediated free radical formation and lipoperoxidation. The latter two are thought to cause further cellular damage, allowing Ca^{2+} influx and ultimate Na^+/K^+ pump dysfunction and, finally, cytotoxic edema due to intracellular water accumulation.

Cytotoxic edema increases intracranial pressure (ICP), if it cannot be compensated by reduction of intracranial blood volume or cerebrospinal fluid shift (Monro-Kellie doctrine, see Chap. 9). Increased ICP reduces cerebral perfusion pressure (CPP). Reduced CPP results in a reduction of cerebral blood flow (CBF). Significant decrement in CBF from normal values (approximately 80 ml/ min/100 g for the cortex and 20–30 ml/ min/100 g for the white matter) results in progressive ischemia, leading to an increase in cytotoxic edema. It ultimately creates a downward spiral, which leads to brain-stem compression, focal and global ischemia, and brain death. The goal of management of secondary brain injury is to prevent further damage by interfering with this cascade at the earliest possible time. The following is a distillation of clinical and experimental work that suggests that there are some secondary phenomena amenable to therapy after head trauma has occurred.

Exacerbating Factors in Secondary Brain Injury

Systematic cardiovascular or cardiopulmonary instability jeopardizes cerebral perfusion, resulting in ischemia, hypoxemia, and metabolic acidosis, which facilitate anaerobic metabolism, intracellular lactic acidosis, increased free-radical formation, and lipoperoxidation. Airway compromise or obstruction can further promote hypercarbia, which leads to cerebral vasodilatation and increased ICP. Hyperthermia increases systemic and cerebral metabolic requirements by 8%/°C; fevers of only a few degrees above normal may rapidly outstrip the metabolic reserves of injured but viable brain tissue. Mechanical obstruction of cerebrospinal fluid (CSF) outflow, either by intraventricular/extrinsic hemorrhage, compression, or obstruction to CSF flow may cause axial distortion of the brain stem, increased ICP, or both. Traumatic subarachnoid hemorrhage may result in delayed cerebral vasospasm, enhancing ischemia and cytotoxic edema. Occult systemic injuries, such as retroperitoneal hematomas and pelvic fractures, produce hypotension from intravascular depletion. Undiagnosed cervical spine injuries associated with cranial trauma may produce cardiovascular collapse as a result of a traumatic sympathectomy. Long bone fractures (e.g., femur fractures) lead to fat emboli, which can result in generalized prostaglandin release, lipoxygenation, and free-radical formation or, in rare circumstances (where the patient has a patent foramen ovale), multifocal cerebral fat emboli. Finally, restoration of oxygenation and perfusion after a period of significant ischemia may be associated with reperfusion injury and free-radical formation.

Central Nervous System Response to Brain Injury

Humoral Surge

The body's response to multisystem and central nervous system trauma further complicates the management of the patient who sustains significant cranial trauma. The hypothalmic-pituitary axis is the primary mediator of the neurohumoral response to major trauma. Antidiuretic hormone (ADH), produced in the preoptic and paraventricular nuclei of the hypothalamus, preserves intravascular volume by mediating resorption of water from the distal renal tubules. Failure to recognize the frequent hypersecretion of ADH may predispose to iatrogenic water intoxication (SIADH – the syndrome of inappropriate ADH secretion) from excess fluid administration or the use of hypotonic fluids. Conversely, cranial base trauma with direct injury to the pituitary infundibulum or the basal hypothalamus may result in impaired synthesis or release of ADH, resulting in diabetes insipidus and hypernatremia.

The pituitary response to head injury includes the release of somatostatin and adrenal cortical-stimulating hormone (ACTH); both induce hyperglycemia, and the latter stimulates release of glucocorticosteroids, which induce protein mass catabolism to promote gluconeogenesis. Sympathetic (hypothalamic-mediated) stimulation of the adrenal cortices leads to catecholamine release, and stimulation of the pancreas causes glucagon release, both of which promote hyperglycemia and insulin resistance, which in turn can worsen ischemic brain damage.

Release of exitatory neurotransmitters such as glutamate or aspartate within the brain itself increase cerebral metabolic activity and is thought to promote ischemia and increase the risk of seizures.

Neuronal Surge (Sympathetic Nervous System Response)

As noted above, catecholamine release is part of a generic central nervous system response to injury or stress; it increases CPP and CBF, glucose uptake, and cerebral metabolism and has profound effects on many organ systems and systemic metabolism that may ultimately reduce host immune defenses. Early electrolyte changes include hypokalemia and catecholamine release, which may be associated with tachyarrhythmias and subendocardial ischemia.

Generalized, Nonspecific Biochemical Response

Significant cranial trauma and penetrating head injury in particular can result in release of biochemical substances that initiate multiple organ system dysfunction as a result of non-specific biochemical cascades. Conversely, these nonspecific cascades may result from systemic trauma but may nonetheless affect cerebral function. Tissue thromboplastin, with highest concentrations located in the subfrontal and anterior temporal cortices, and tissue plasminogen activator, located in the choroid plexus and meninges, can leak into the systemic circulation if brain tissue and cerebral veins are disrupted, resulting in acute or subclinical disseminated intravascular coagulation (DIC) or fibrinolysis. The presence of multiple intravascular microthrombi affects multiple target organs. This ultimately leads to the "multiorgan system failure" syndrome encountered in many patients who sustain severe cranial injuries: progressive respiratory distress syndrome, renal insufficiency, hepatocellular dysfunction, and pancreatitis. Consumptive coagulopathy may increase the risk of delayed traumatic intracerebral hemorrhage.

Following severe head injury, tumor necrosis factor and interleukin-1 are released and may be mediators of protein catabolism and alteration of serum zinc, copper, and albumin levels.

Secondary Mechanisms Complicating Brain Injury

Loss of Voluntary Control

An impaired sensorium places the head trauma victim at increased risk for oropharyngeal airway obstruction, resulting in hypoxemia and hypercarbia, and in aspiration pneumonia.

Immobilization

Prolonged immobilization, as a consequence of an impaired sensorium or neurologic function, represents one of the greatest risks to long-term recovery because of its effects on multiple organ systems. Disorders of calcium metabolism lead to bone mass resorption, loss of protein bone matrix, hypercalcemia and hyperphosphatemia, and increased risk of nephrolithiasis and heterotopic ossification with joint dysfunction. Inactivity facilitates muscle catabolism, atrophy, and tendon shortening with muscle contractures. Fixed joint deformities may result in decubitus formation over bony prominences, leading to further nitrogen loss from tissue necrosis and serum weeping, impaired host defenses, and sepsis. Atrophy or hypotonia of respiratory muscles, together with hypophasphatemia following early depletion of phosphorylated adenosine compounds (ATP, AMP), predisposes to progressive respiratory insufficiency. Most importantly for clinical work, immobilization of the legs promotes pelvic and lower extremity venous thrombosis with the risk of pulmonary embolism.

Clinical Features

History

The patient's level of consciousness and neurologic stability influence the emergency head trauma evaluation sequence. A conscious and cooperative patient is clearly better able to assist in the diagnostic assessment than is the agitated patient with an impaired sensorium or with progressive neurologic deficit. The critical issues which must be adressed in obtaining a useful history are the following:

1. What was the mechanism of the injury (acceleration, deceleration, blunt, penetrating, fast or slow impact time)?
2. How great was the kinetic energy of the injury?
3. What was the course of neurologic function (including, if available, pre-injury status and condition at the time of initial medical evaluation)?
4. What factors might complicate medical or surgical management of the patient (e.g., antecedent medical problems, medications, allergies, associated injuries, and the time of last oral intake)?

The amount of kinetic energy, its rate of transfer to the cranial vault and its contents, and the actual biochemical mechanism of impact are critical factors in determining the potential for significant intracranial injury and the types of lesions to evolve later. Direct blows such as falls and assaults produce focal cranial compression and may lead to skull fractures, dural lacerations, extra-axial hematomas, or cerebral contusions, Acceleration-deceleration injuries create a shearing-torsion of the mass centers in the brain, causing deep white matter axonal and vessel disruption within the cerebral hemispheres, the cerebellar peduncles, and the brain stem. Penetrating injuries cause not only local tissue disruption, but also an expanding cone of destruction from shock waves, which create a large, temporary vacuum cavity, leading to transient focal elevations in ICP.

Vital Signs

Respiratory abnormalities can result from impaired airway patency, gastric or oropharyngeal secretion aspiration, or impairment of neurogenic respiratory function. Cheyne-Stokes respiration may be present with bifrontal or diencephalic injury and may precede transtentorial herniation. Direct injury to the rostral midbrain tegmentum, hypoxia, pulmonary edema, or aspiration may produce central neurogenic hyperventilation. Lesions of the dorsolateral pontine tegmentum may produce apneustic breathing, ataxic or gasping respiration, or yawning; hiccups and projectile vomiting are caused by medullary lesions. Associated rostral cervical spine injuries may interrupt afferent respiratory reflex arcs. The sympathetic nervous system-mediated response to severe head injury typically produces hypertension and tachycardia. This should be distinguished from hypotension and tachycardia, seen with loss of intravascular volume from occult intra-abdominal or retroperitoneal hemorrhage or congestive heart failure. Centrally mediated hypotension and bradycardia is most often as-

Table 1. Glasgow Coma Scale

Item	Points
Eye-opening responses	
Spontaneous	4
To voice	3
To pain	2
None	1
Best verbal response	
Oriented	5
Confused	4
Inappropriate words	3
Incomprehensible sounds	2
None	1
Best motor response	
Obeys commands:	6
Localizes (pain)	5
Withdraws (pain)	4
Flexion (pain)	3
Extension (pain)	2
None	1
Total	3–15

Neurologic Examination

The initial neurologic evaluation of the patient who has sustained cranial trauma allows for an informed assessment of the severity of the injury, facilitates the organization of initial clinical management, and provides a guideline for prognosis regarding survival and neurologic outcome.

The ideal neurologic assessment is comprehensive yet simple, minimizes interobserver reliability, and is reproducible over time; no such ideal scale exists. The development of the Glasgow Coma Scale in 1974, however, was a significant advance because of its simplicity and degree of interobserver reliability and reproducibility (Table 1). Evaluation of eye-opening, verbal, and motor responses, using a scale ranging from 3 to 15, allows rapid assessment. Coma, indicative of severe cranial trauma, corresponds to a GCS score <8; moderate head injuries are associated with a GCS score between 9 and 13, mild head injuries with a GCS score of 14 or 15. Obvious limitations of the GCS include the inability to score differences between right- and left-sided motor function (usually the best motor response is scored), to assess verbal function in an intubated patient, òr to evaluate eye opening in the patient with significant orbito-facial injury with swelling. Another major drawback is the failure to include brain-stem reflex function and pupillary function in the Glasgow scoring system. Generally, serial exams of a head-injured patient are essential and mandatory. Here the GCS is of value, despite the above-mentioned draw backs.

sociated with cervical spine injury but may be found in terminal medullary failure. The classic Kocher-Cushing reflex, i.e., hypertension with bradycardia, results from lower brain-stem compression or severe intracranial hypertension, which presumably impairs cerebral perfusion to this region. The sympathetic response which increases systemic blood pressure to improve CPP, stimulation of the carotid body receptors, consequently induces vagal stimulation and resultant bradycardia.

Disorders of temperature regulation in association with cranial trauma are unusual. Instead, more common causes of hyperthermia (infection, aspiration, anticholinergic medications) and hypothermia (barbiturates, spinal cord injury, hypoglycemia, alcohol intoxication, or phenothiazine overdose) should be considered.

The pupillary light reflex remains the most important brain-stem reflex to be assessed in the head-injured patient. By virtue of the anatomic course of the oculomotor nerve, compression or distortion results in ipsilateral pupillary dilation and anisocoria. Anisocoria resulting from oculomotor compromise should be distinguished from direct orbital trauma, from contralateral miosis due to traumatic Horner's syndrome, or from optic nerve or retinal injury with pupillary dilation reacting to contralateral light. Absent previous eye surgery and an oval or irregular pupil indicates incomplete third nerve dysfunction. A hippus reaction suggests tectal dysfunction, and pinpoint reactive pupils suggest interruption of sympathetic influence at the pontine level.

Pupillary dilation resulting from oculomotor stretching occurs approximately 80–85% of the time on the side ipsilateral to a mass lesion.

In 10% of cases of subdural hematoma, pupillary enlargement occurs contralateral to the mass, probably from distortion of the third nerve on the side opposite the brain-stem torsion. This paradoxical sign seems less common with other types of mass lesions. An additional feature as tissue shifts progress is "Kernohan's notch" phenomenon of compression of the contralateral cerebral peduncle against the territorial edge, creating hemiplegia and posturing ipsilateral to the mass.

Other brain-stem reflexes, including the oculocephalic, oculovestibular, corneal, and gag reflexes, may be tested to provide additional information with regard to the integrity of brain-stem function once cervical spine stability has been ascertained

and spinal cord injury ruled out (Table 2).

Cranial and Spinal Examination

Once the neurologic evaluation has been performed, a rapid but orderly examination of the craniofacial structures and spine should be performed. The scalp is visually assessed for contussions, lacerations, or bleeding points. Both hands of the examiner are gloved and the cranial vault is palpated bilaterally to identify bony step-offs, depressions, or asymmetries; scalp lacerations are lifted to assess for partial degloving injuries, which may be associated with depressed fractures and CSF leakage or foreign body contamination at a distance from the site of the laceration. The orbital rims, nasion, zygomatic arches, maxillae, and hard palate are palpated for crepitus or instabillity suggestive of bony injury. The periorbita and the mastoids are inspected for evidence of subcutaneous eccymosis (the "racoon's eyes" of nasoorbitoethmoidal fractures or "Battle's sign" of mastoid fractures, respectively) suggestive of basilar skull fractures. The external auditory canals and the nares are inspected with an otoscope for evidence of bleeding (otorrhagia or rhinorrhagia) or CSF leak (otorrhea or rhinorrhea). The remainder of the oropharynx and mandible may be palpated manually to check for hemorrhage, lacerations, or bony instability. Finally, the neck is assessed for evidence of tracheal deviation, if not previously inspected during intubation, and the cervical spinous processes are palpated manually for evidence of bony step-offs, angulation, or insta-

Table 2. Adjunctive measures for systemic stabilization

1. Suspected alcohol or drug abuse:
   - Naloxone 0.4–0.8 mg i.v. bolus (must be repeated every hour for opiate overdose)
   - Serum and urine toxicology samples obtained
   - Thiamine 100 mg i.v. infusion (if alcoholism suspected)
   - MgSO₄ 50% solution 2 ml i.m. (if alcoholism suspected)
   - Patient observed for evidence of drug or alcohol withdrawal. If withdrawal suspected, treatment for opiate withdrawal (methadone, Dilaudid, clonidine transderm patch) or alcohol or CNS depressant withdrawal (lorazepam, phenobarbital, clonidine, thiamine/multivitamin therapy) is initiated.
   - Flumazenil 0.2 mg i.v. over 15 s, with 0.2 mg i.v. every 60 s up to 1 mg (if benzodiazepine overdose is suspected)
   - Patient observed for evidence of benzodiazepine withdrawal, seizures, or resedation (Flumazenil is contraindicated in patients showing evidence of cyclic antidepressant overdose or where benzodiazepines are used for ICP control or anticonvulsant treatment.)
2. Open or penetrating wounds:
   - Tetanus toxoid i.m. (unit dose) (if no tetanus immunization within 10 years)
   - Hypertet 250–500 units i.m. (if recent tetanus immunization)
3. Hypoglycemia suspected:
   - Obtain Hemostix or blood glucose level *first* (Hypoglycemia is extremely rare following head injury, except following insulin administration.)
   - Dextrose 50% solution 50 ml i.v. infusion
   - Thiamine 100 mg i.v. infusion if any question regarding nutritional status
4. Systemic acidosis:
   - Arterial blood-gas determination to differentiate metabolic from respiratory acidosis
   - Correct underlying cause with standard resuscitative efforts if possible
   - If *metabolic* acidosis persists, NaHCO₃ i.v. for pH < 7.1 (1/2 calculated total base deficit [mEq] over 1 h)
5. Crush injuries:
   - Stabilization of bony fractures with splinting/casting
   - Bladder catheterization for urine output and urine sample for hemoglobinuria or myoglobinuria
   - If (+) for myoglobinuria, mannitol 0.5 g/kg i.v. bolus, followed by continuous infusion (25–50ml/h) and NaHCO₃ (55 mEq added to each liter of maintenance i.v. fluids)

bility; with the vertebral column maintained in a neutral position, this palpation should be continued down the entire spine where circumstances warrant.

Differential Diagnosis

It is sobering to note that 10–12% of patients who eventually died of their head injuries in one study were awake and responsive at the time of their initial assessments. Preventable factors in this "talk and die" syndrome included unrecognized hypoxia, hypotension, and delayed diagnosis of intracranial pathology. Some of the significant pitfalls in delayed diagnosis include the following:

1. Failure to recognize a delayed traumatic intracerebral hemorrhage. Because improved emergency medical systems are able to deliver the head-injured patient to medical centers within a short time following injury in many localities, initial evaluations (both neurologic and radiologic) may be per-

formed too early to demonstrate a delayed or slowly evolving mass lesion, particularly one overlying the floor or the frontal fossa, where bony artifacts obscure computed tomographic images. Intracranial hemorrhage may present isodense on very early CT scans.

2. Failure to recognize posterior fossa lesions. Although the abducens nerve is most likely to be injured following head trauma, presumably because of its long intracranial course, other signs such as dysconjugate gaze, nystagmus, or ocular bobbing should lead one to suspect a posterior fossa or brain-stem lesion.

3. Failure to recognize focal intracranial lesions in noneloquent cortex – the right frontal and right temporal lobes in particular – may produce a not very impressive clinical picture with mild confusion, disorientation, or diffuse headache, until a sudden deterioration occurs from distortion of the brainstem, obstruction of CSF outflow with acute hydrocephalus, or generalized increase in intracranial pressure.

4. Inadequate appreciation of posttraumatic cerebral edema. Even without expansion of cerebral contusions or intracerebral hematomas, the development of cerebral edema can increase the effective size of mass lesions by 30–40%. Hyperemia occurs during the initial phase of head injury, and edema usually develops within the first 24 h after the injury, peaking within 48–72 h. Hyperemia associated with significant elevations of ICP can persist for up to 8 days, predisposing to further exacerbation of brain edema, reducing intracranial compliance, and potentiating the mass effects of contusions or hematomas.

5. Failure to recognize delayed posttraumatic hydrocephalus. Communicating hydrocephalus may be delayed following traumatic subarachnoid or intraventricular hemorrhage. It is frequent following penetrating head injuries and may account for late deterioration following initial improvement, or failure to improve despite favorable prognostic preconditions.

6. Failure to recognize delayed cardiovascular or pulmonary instability. The multisystem trauma patient who also suffers from severe cranial trauma may develop hemodynamic instability resulting from intra-abdominal, retroperitoneal, or intrathoracic injury. Pulmonary contusion, flail chest, or tension pneumothorax may result in delayed respiratory insufficiency and hypoxemia. Once intracranial causes of progressive dysfunction have been excluded, potential systemic causes should be sought. Myocardial failure resulting from subendocardial ischemia and neurogenic pulmonary edema should also be considered.

Ancillary Tests

Computed Tomography

Computed tomography (CT) has supplanted cerebral angiography as the neuroradiologic procedure of choice for evaluation of cranial trauma. Third- and fourth-generation CT scanners are capable of imaging cerebral parenchyma, hemorrhagic lesions and brain edema, and bony injuries to the cranium and the facial bones in great detail. CT gives far more information than plain skull films. Plain skull films are still of some use in evaluating depressed or basilar skull fractures or penetrating injuries, especially if a CT scan is not readily available. Except for patients who are cardiovascularly unstable, all neurotrauma patients should undergo emergency CT evaluation. It is the method of choice for the detection of major intracerebral contusions (Figs. 1 and 2) and acute epidural (Fig. 3) or subdural hematomas (Fig. 4). In extemely rare situations, where a CT scanner is not available, direct craniotomy of a deteriorating patient may become necessary. In infants with open fontanelles or in patients with large cranial defects, ultrasonography may be considered as an alternative to CT studies.

For patients at risk of delayed intracerebral hemorrhage or edema, serial CT studies must be performed; a reasonable rule of thumb for serial evaluation of patients is to repeat studies at 24 h, 72 h, and 7 days following the initial CT study. Later studies may be necessary to rule out delayed post-traumatic hydrocephalus in patients who fail to improve or who regress. Recent data from the National Traumatic Coma Data Bank, classifying head injury based on initial CT evaluation using the status of the mesencephalic cisterns, the degree of midline shift, and the presence of masses amenable to evacuation, demonstrate the usefulness of CT in as-

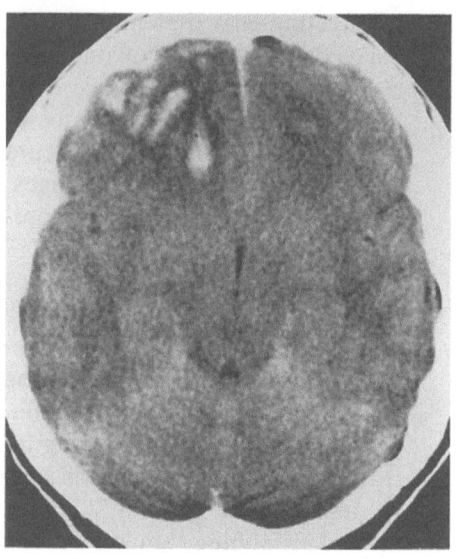

Fig. 1. Hemorrhagic cerebral contusions in a 34-year-old man with severe headaches, meningismus and a history of a bicycle accident a few hours previously. Axial CT scan demonstrates multiple round to oval hyperdensities in the frontal lobes bilaterally, right more than left. These lesions are cortical as well as subcortical and surrounded by rim of hypodensity, reflecting edema or nonhemorrhagic contusion. Hyperdensity of rostral interhemispheric fissure is due to accompanying traumatic subarachnoid hemorrhage. (Courtesy of Klaus Sartor and Marius Hartmann, Heidelberg)

sessing the risk of raised ICP and fatal outcome.

Magnetic Resonance Imaging

MRI offers unique advantages over CT in the evaluation of brain injury. Its resolution of cortex, white matter, and deep nuclear structures and its multiplanar imaging capability makes it the superior method, especially in the posterior fossa and in spinal cord trauma. However, MRI is not well established in the management of

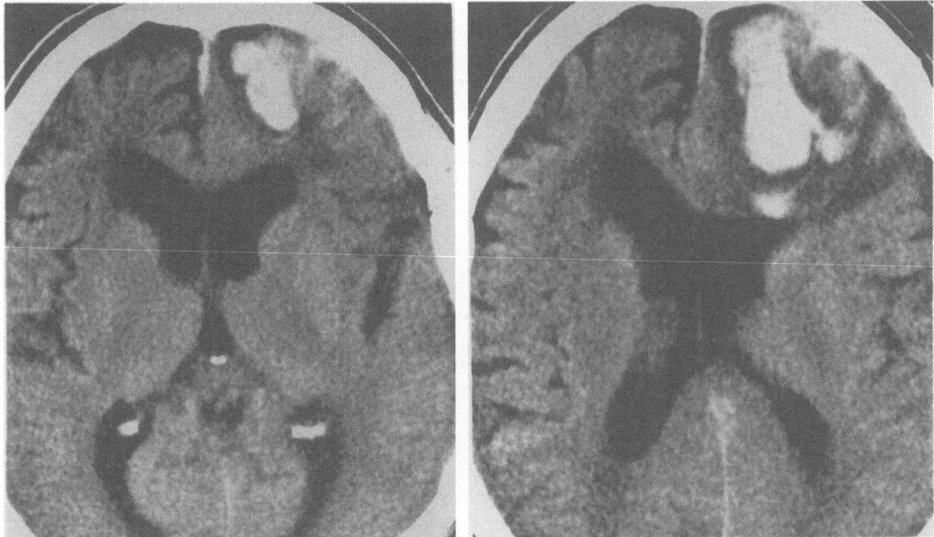

Fig. 2. Hemorrhagic cerebral contusion in a 75-year-old man with nausea and vomiting starting 4 h after bicycle accident. Axial CT scans show hyperdense intracerebral mass lesion typical for acute hematoma that involves left frontal lobe, extending from cortex to ventricle. Surrounding hypo-intensity represents edema and nonhemorrhagic contusion. Mass effect is confined to injured lobe. (Courtesy of Klaus Sartor and Marius Hartmann, Heidelberg)

acutely head injured patients. MRI studies may be limited by the presence of ventilator and monitoring equipment, although new monitoring devices are in use. The scanner design presently in use limits patient observation and access for prolonged periods of time. MRI does not image bone calcium matrix, which appears as a void, rendering it unsuitable for evaluation of cranial base injury or craniofacial trauma. Acute intracranial hemorrhage is also poorly delineated by MRI. After approximately 72 h, however, hemoglobin breakdown makes MRI a suitable choice for follow-up neuroradiologic assessment of brain-stem involvement or for detecting small parenchymal lesions (Figs. 5 and 6).

Cerebral Angiography

Cerebral angiography still plays a role in the assessment of post-traumatic neurovascular lesions such as those associated with penetrating injury, high-velocity bullet trauma, depressed fractures over major venous sinuses, traumatic dissections, or occlusions of extracranial carotid or vertebral arteries associated with hyperextension injuries, blunt or penetrating trauma, or cervical vertebral injury, and suspected carotid-cavernous fistulae. Digital subtraction angiography has the advantage of providing high-resolution assessments of the cerebral vasculature, with a minimum of time and contrast-medium injection. Interventional neuroradiologic

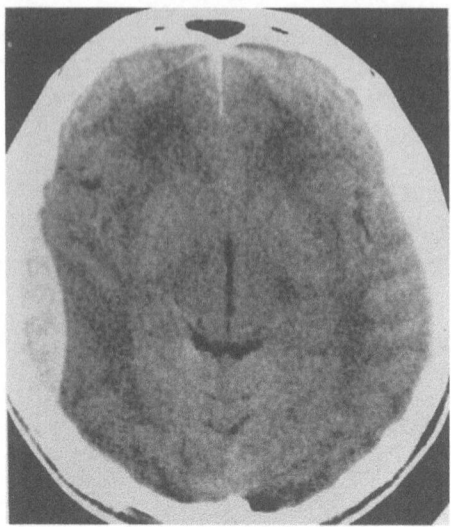

Fig. 3. Acute epidural hematoma in a 22-year-old man with a history of having fallen on the back of his head; plain radiographs were remarkable for temporal fracture. Axial CT scan shows biconvex extra-axial mass lesion with density of acute hematoma that compresses brain focally. (Courtesy of Klaus Sartor and Marius Hartmann, Heidelberg)

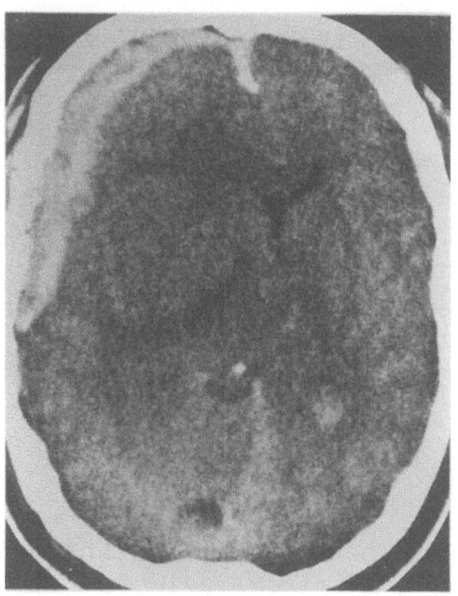

Fig. 4. Acute subdural hematoma in a 23-year-old comatose person who had been involved in a car accident. Axial CT scan shows extra-axial mass lesion with density characteristics of acute hematoma and irregular contours that covers mainly right frontal and temporal lobes but extends into rostral interhemispheric fissure. Note marked displacement of midline structures to opposite side, with compression of the ipsilateral ventricle. (Courtesy of Klaus Sartor and Marius Hartmann, Heidelberg)

occlusions of post-traumatic lesions such as carotid-cavernous fistulae, false aneuryms, and the like may provide definitive treatment at the same session.

Further developments in noninvasive magnetic resonance angiography (MRA) suggest that this modality may further reduce the value of cerebral angiography in the diagnosis of post-traumatic neurovascular lesions.

Intracranial Pressure Monitoring

The neurosurgery literature contains extensive documentation of the fact that intracranial hypertension has an adverse effect on survival and on neurologic outcome. Because ICP determines CPP, and – at least qualitatively – CBF, measurement of ICP is essential to an informed and controlled management regimen to prevent and treat intracranial hypertension. Recent studies suggest that maintaining CPP, rather than controlling ICP, is an acceptable alternative course of therapy for severely head injured patients. Nonetheless, measurement of ICP remains an important intermediate determinant affecting management and outcome.

A wide variety of ICP monitoring devices are available, each with par-

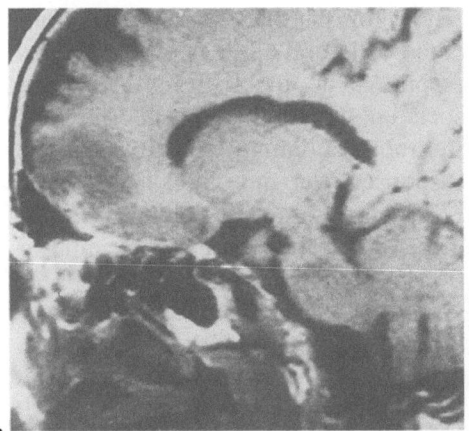

a

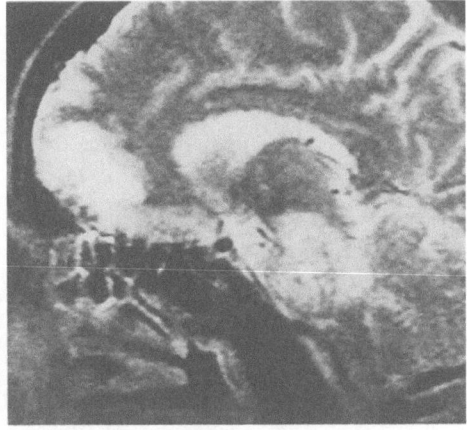

b

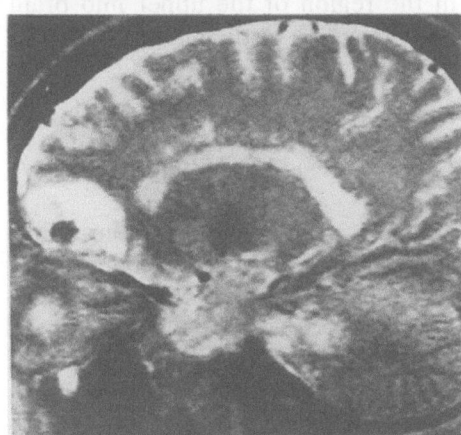

c

Fig. 5a-c. Cerebral contusion with involvement of the frontal lobe and brain stem in a 58-year-old comatose woman, victim of a severe car accident. Sagittal MR images (a, T1-weighted; b,c, T2-weighted) show areas of abnormal signal intensity consistent with edema or contusion in basal portions of the frontal lobe and in the pons. No evidence of hemorrhage is noted in the pons (a,b), whereas classic signs of hemorrhage are present in the frontal lobe, with hyperintensity representing methemoglobin at the undersurface (a) and focal hypointensity representing deoxyhemoglobin within the lesion. (Courtesy of Klaus Sartor and Marius Hartmann, Heidelberg)

ticular advantages and disadvantages. Ease of placement, accuracy of ICP readings with a minimum of drift, risk of infection or hemorrhage, and the ability to aspirate CSF for further analysis are factors that must be considered in the system.

All nonmoribund patients who sustain severe head injuries (GCS score ≤ 8) with abnormal initial CT studies should be considered candidates for ICP monitoring. In addition, patients with moderate head injuries (GSC score 9–13), CT lesions associated with focal mass effects, and shift of midline structures >5 mm should be evaluated on a case-by-case basis to determine whether they should have their ICP monitored.

Electrophysiologic Parameters in Neurocritical Care

The conventional EEG is useful in the early diagnosis of ischemic lesions, epileptic patterns, and depth and type of coma, as well as in monitoring of barbiturate coma or demonstrating the efficacy of drugs aimed at protecting the brain. EEG monitoring assists in finding the correct dose of sedatives for drug therapy of post-traumatic coma. An isoelectric EEG corre-

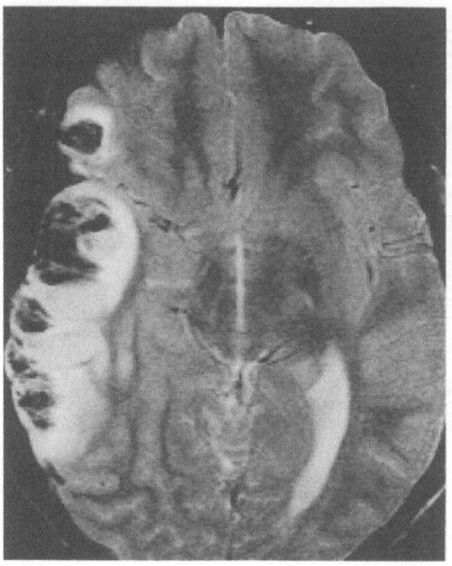

Fig. 6. Hemorrhagic cerebral contusions in a 24-year-old man with change in mental status following bicycle accident, T2-weighted axial MR scan reveals signal abnormalities involving lateral portions of the right temporal lobe, with some additional involvement of the frontal lobe. The appearance of these lesions – which display a mixture of hyper- and hypointensity – is characteristic for acute hemorrhagic contusions, with the dark components representing acute hemorrhage (deoxhemoglobin state) and the bright components edema or nonhemorrhagic contusion. (Courtesy of Klaus Sartor and Marius Hartmann, Heidelberg)

sponds to maximal reduction in cerebral oxygen metabolism. Computerized techniques to analyze the EEG (compressed spectral array, spectral edge frequency) may in future show trends in the functional status of the brain. EEG is essential to some criteria for determining brain death and is of prognostic value if sleep activity or reactions to external stimuli can be observed.

Evoked potentials (EP) have a stronger prognostic power than do EEGs. SEPs have an excellent corre-

lation for good as well as bad outcome. Bilateral absence of the cortical responses in the SEPs is always associated with a bad prognosis. Furthermore, a diminution of the cortical responses over time indicates secondary deterioration in clinical status. The value and therapeutic implications of motor evoked potentials or visual evoked potentials in head-injured patients remain to be proven. Wave V of the BAEP has been used to detect mass effect from raised ICP in the region of the upper mid brain and may be valuable if followed serially.

Cerebral Blood Flow Studies

Noninvasive blood flow studies allow serial evaluation of cerebral perfusion. Radionuclide isotope flow scans give qualitative "snapshot" assessment of CBF, albeit with poor resolution, but they may detect flow decrements in major vascular territories. Single positron emission computed tomography (SPECT) has the advantage of assessing regional blood flow and, in part, cerebral metabolism. Jugular bulb catheters have also been used to monitor cerebral O_2 extraction, but the clinical value of any of these studies remains uncertain.

Cerebral blood flow in the post-traumatic state is often associated with a considerable variability in CBF values. There is only a poor correlation of CBF to neurologic state and outcome. Autoregulation and CO_2 vasoreactivity of CBF have been shown to be affected by head injury. It is reported that a severe reduction of CO_2 reactivity is associated with a poor prognosis. Real-time quantitative bedside monitoring of blood-flow velocity of the major intracranial arteries can be accomplished by serial transcranial Doppler (tcD) studies. The continuous monitoring of blood-flow velocity by tcD allows the detection of increased vascular resistance or changes of CBF. The increase of the pulsatility of the Doppler spectrum is associated with elevated ICP. New experimental modalities, such as transcranial laser photospectroscopy, may allow bedside quantitative assessments of cortical perfusion.

Cerebrospinal Fluid Studies

Numerous biochemical CSF studies have been performed following closed head injury. CSF pH and lactate levels seem to have some prognostic value, as do levels of neuron-specific enolase. Excitatory neurotransmitter and catecholamine levels are used in clinical investigations, but not for routine ICU monitoring. In fact, nowadays lumbar puncture is only rarely indicated after neurotrauma.

Systemic Monitoring

ECG and blood pressure monitoring are required in every patient following significant cranial trauma. Other monitoring modalities include central venous or right-heart/pulmonalis catheterization, measurement of mixed venous saturation, and pulse oxymetry. Pulmonary function can be monitored with serial blood-gas analyses and ventilator peak airway pressure. Bladder catheterization allows for assessment of fluid excretion and balance. Daily weights, not easily measured in an ICU environment, are helpful in maintaining fluid balance, especially if insensible water losses vary significantly due to ventilation, fever, or profuse diaphoresis.

Management Prior to Admission to the Intensive Care Unit

Airway

Airway compromise may result from direct craniofacial trauma with edema, hemorrhage, or bony injury such as mandibular or palatal fractures, neck injuries, chest trauma, aspiration, or loss of voluntary control and depression of caudal-cranial reflexes. Rapid establishment of an adequate airway is essential for maintaining adequate oxygenation and preventing hypercarbia and respiratory acidosis. The patient with evidence of upper airway stridor, impaired respiration, severe cranial trauma (GCS score ≤ 8), or significant maxillofacial trauma should be endotracheally intubated. Failure to establish an adequate airway prior to transfer from the emergency room may lead to cardiorespiratory arrest and death in the CT suite or in transit to patient care areas.

If cervical spine injury has not been excluded radiographically at the time of initial assessment, and emergency intubation is required, manual in-line stabilization of the patient's head and neck should be performed by a second person while the patient is intubated. The oropharyngeal airway should be cleared manually, and an oral airway inserted to prevent obstruction by the tongue. Blood or vomitus should be suctioned, and an

Ambu bag with oxygen placed to pre-oxygenate the patient.

Short-acting muscle relaxants should be used only with caution, since the inability to obtain an adequate airway in a patient who is pharmacologically paralyzed can be catastrophic. Furthermore, acute elevations of blood presure, ICP, and heart rate have been observed, which have been partially attributed to succinylcholine and to the mechanical stimulation caused by intubation. A small dose of intravenous lidocaine may abort the spike in ICP associated with endotracheal intubation. Fiberoptic laryngoscopy may facilitate nasal or oropharyngeal endotracheal intubation. The endotracheal tube should be sufficiently large to accommodate endotracheal suction catheters, usually 8.0-mm internal-diameter cuffed tubes or larger. A tracheostomy tray should be readily available; if circumstances permit, a controlled tracheostomy may be performed should severe facial injury prevent nasal or oral intubation. However, if an airway must be established in a life-and-death situation, a cryothyroidotomy should be performed as the procedure of choice, since a secured endotracheal airway can be established within a matter of seconds. Following intubation, the patient should be (re)placed in a firm collar to prevent cervical subluxation or airway kinking.

Breathing

Once an adequate airway has been secured, effective ventilation becomes the next priority, both to provide oxygenation and to allow initial hyperventilation for control of suspected intracranial hypertension, pending definitive diagnosis. Hyperventilation with arterial pCO_2 levels of 25–30 mmHg is an effective level; however, care should be taken to avoid overhyperventilation, which can potentially produce cerebral ischemia. Chest injuries which can prevent effective ventilation (pneumothorax or hemothorax, or flail chest with underlying pulmonary contusion) should be treated with appropriate measures like tube thoracostomy or positive airway pressure. Ventilatory insufficiency due to impaired sensorium, intoxication, or cervical spine injury with quadriplegia mandates respiratory support with physiologic parameters necessary to maintain oxygen saturation $\geq 95\%$. At this time, pharmacologic paralysis may be necessary to reduce agitation and "fighting" the respirator.

Circulation

Cerebral perfusion depends on adequate systemic circulation. Occult sources of hemorrhage such as long bone fractures, pelvic fractures, retroperitoneal hemorrhage, intra-abdominal injury with splenic capsular or liver laceration, or hemothorax should be excluded with appropriate examinations. Pericardial tamponade as cause of circulatory failure is frequently overlooked. Scalp lacerations can be significant sources of hemorrhage. Particularly in infants, intracranial hematoma can cause hypovolemic shock. Occult spinal cord injury in association with cranial trauma may impair cardiac function, blood pressure, and right-heart venous return. Replacement of intravascular volume using Ringer's solution, saline, or hetastarch solutions, colloid or albumin should aim at euvolemia and avoid overhydration. Myocardial failure or systemic hypotension may require inotropic substances such as dopamine, dobutamine, or even arterenol derivatives.

Systemic Stabilization with Ancillary Measures

Following initial resuscitation and stabilization, the patient will be transported for additional tests and secondary survey for evidence of multisystem trauma. Occasionally, cardiovascular instability may necessitate exploratory surgery. For this reason, all patients with severe cranial trauma should have a 12-lead ECG, cervical spine and chest plain films, complete blood counts, serum electrolytes, clotting parameter tests (PT, aPTT, fibrinogen, and, if possible, fibrin split products), a urinanalysis, and a blood-bank sample taken. Blood counts and clotting parameters should be repeated within the next 1–2 h. Abdominal lavage should be performed if there is any sign of abdominal trauma. Additional serum chemistry, including liver function tests, amylase, calcium, and magnesium levels may be sent to assess baseline values for later comparison and for calculating nutritional support values. Additional adjunctive measures are listed in Table 2.

CSF leaks from depressed fractures with dural lacerations or from penetrating injuries should be cleaned and dressed with sterile gauze, pending definitive closure in the operating room. Skull-base fractures with CSF leaks should be treated with head posi-tioning that minimizes fluid pressure at the putative site of leakage and with sterile dressings. If the leak persists in the acute phase and no intracranial mass lesion is present, lumbar spinal drainage (80–100 ml/8 h), with the bag just below head level, is recommended by some centers. The patient should be monitored for evidence of early meningitis. We do not administer prophylactic antibiotics. Nursing protocols should include at least hourly monitoring of vital signs and neurologic functions of severely head injured patients.

Management of Intracranial Hypertension

Effective resuscitation, as described above, is a prerequisite for controlling ICP. Where cerebrovascular CO_2 responsiveness has been preserved, decreasing the arterial pCO_2 produces, for each 2–4 mmHg, an approximately 1-mmHg decrease in ICP. Hyperventilation is therefore the fastest means of initially reducing ICP. Endotracheal intubation is usually necessary, and pharmacologic paralysis may be required. Head elevation to 30° generally reduces jugular venous pressure resistance to cerebral venous outflow and, consequently, ICP. Osmotic and loop diuretics shift fluid from the intracellular and perivascular compartments into the intravascular space, transiently increasing cerebral perfusion but dramatically reducing ICP. Mannitol is very effective as an osmotic diuretic. Loop diuretics are effective adjunctive agents, although they can cause fluid and electrolyte disorders. Acetazolamide reduces CSF production and promotes diuresis, but, as a carbonic anhydrase inhibitor, it also promotes tissue and metabolic acidosis and is generally not used in acute situations. Analgesia and sedative therapy reduce patient discomfort and agitation; local anesthetic instillation may reduce tracheal irritation during endotracheal suctioning, and early tracheostomy should be considered for patients who still require long-term ventilatory support. Hyperthermia, which promotes cerebral vasodilatation and hypermetabolic injury, should be treated aggressively with appropiate hypothermia techniques. Similarly, medications which induce or promote cerebral vasodilatation or reduce systemic arterial pressure, and therefore CPP, should be avoided.

Cerebrospinal fluid drainage, via an intraventricular catheter, in some situations remains an effective method for controlling intracranial pressure and measuring ICP and intracranial compliance. Surgical mass lesions which contribute significantly to intracranial hypertension and reduction in intracranial compliance should, of course, be evacuated, provided the patient is cardiovascularly stable and does not have an active and correctable coagulopathy. Standard methods for controlling ICP and medications that may worsen ICP are listed in Tables 3 and 4 and Chap. 9.

Alternative methods for controlling elevated ICP are effective for a short term, but their efficacy for long-term management remains unknown. Dimethylsulfoxide (DMSO) is an osmodiuretic which may also reduce cerebral venous resistance. However, it promotes fluid overload, induces significant electrolyte abnormalities (primarily hypernatremia), and may

Table 3. Standard methods for controlling intracranial hypertension

---

Endotracheal intubation
Hyperventilation (pCO_2 between 25 and
  30 mmHg)
Head elevation to 30°
Osmotic diuretics
  Mannitol (loading: 1 g/kg i.v. over 15–30 min;
    maintenance: 0.25–0.7 g/kg i.v. every 4 h)
  Glycerol (0.5–1.0 g/kg p.o. or n.g. every
    3–4 h)
  Sorbital (0.25–0.5 g/kg p.o. or n.g. every 4 h)
Loop diuretics (optional)
  Furosemide (0.5 mg/kg i.v. following osmotic
    diuretic administration)
  Ethacrynic acid (0.5–1.0 mg/kg i.v. following
    osmotic diuretic)
Carbonic anhydrase inhibitor (optional)
  Acetazolamide (250–500 mg p.o., n.g., or
    i.v. every 6–12 h)
Muscle paralysis (with ventilatory support)
  Pancuronium (4–6 mg/h every hour or i.v.
    infusion)
  Vecuronium (6–10 mg/h i.v. infsuion)
  Atracurium (50–75 mg/h i.v. infusion)
Analgesics
  Codeine (30–60 mg i.m. every 3–4 h)
  Morphine sulfate (0.1–0.15 mg/kg i.m. every
    4 h, or 1–2 mg/h i.v. infusion)
  Fentanyl (0.5–2.0 mg/h i.v. infusion)
  Nalbuphine (5–10 mg i.m. every 3–6 h)
Sedatives
  Diazepam (5–10 mg i.v. or i.m. p.r.n.)
  Lorazepam (0.5–2.0 mg/h p.r.n. or i.v.
    infusion)
Cerebrospinal fluid drainage (intraventricular
  catheter)
Surgical decompressive procedures
  Evacuation of mass lesions
  Decompressive craniectomy with expansile
    duroplasty
  Decompressive frontal or temporal lobectomy
Hypothermia (hyperthermia prevention)
Tracheostomy
Lidocaine pretreatment for endotracheal
  suctioning (25–50 mg i.v. or through tube)

---

dissolve tubing and equipment not designed for DSMO administration. Although corticosteroids are effective in reducing peritumoral edema, their

Table 4. Substances that may cause intracranial hypertension

Calcium channel blockers
  Nifedipine
  Nimodipine
  Verapamil
Primary peripheral vasodilators
  Nitroprusside
  Nitroglycerine
  Amiodarone
  Hydralazine
Catecholamine receptor/re-uptake blockers
  Chlorpromazine
  Reserpine
Anesthetic agents
  Propofol
  Phenoperidine
  Ketamine (primary vasodilatation)
  Droperidol
  Inhalation anesthetics including isoflurane

Table 5. Alternative methods for controlling intracranial pressure

General anesthetic agents
  Althesin (alfaxalone plus alfadolone)
  Midazolam
  Barbiturates
Local anesthetic agents
  Lidocaine (1.5 mg/kg i.v. bolus)
Prostaglandin (cyclo-oxygenase) inhibitor
  Indomethacin (30 mg i.v. bolus)
Hypertonic saline (NaCl 5 mM/ml i.v.)
DMSO (20% solution at 1–8 g/kg/day)
Steroids

efficacy in the management of elevated ICP is doubtful. Clinical trials of a new generation of steroids, the 21-aminosteroids, the so-called lazaroids, are under way to determine their role in the mangement of intracranial hypertension. Other alternative methods for the treatment of raised ICP are listed in Table 5.

Like other general anesthetic agents, short-acting barbiturates decrease the cerebral metabolic rate (CMRO$_2$) and CBF in a dose-dependent fashion. At a dose sufficient to produce an isoelectric EEG, CMRO$_2$ and CBF are decreased by approximately 50%. Barbiturates induce cerebrovascular vasoconstriction, decreasing intracranial blood volume and ICP, and induce hypothermia. High-dose barbiturate therapy has drawbacks including myocardial depression, systemic hypotension, increased venous capacity, impaired gastrointestinal motility, and reduced host immune response. They render the neurologic monitoring unreliable. Induction of barbiturate therapy for control of raised ICP requires extensive ICU monitoring (Table 6).

Although intermittent boluses of barbiturates may be administered for transient elevation in ICP, induction of barbiturate coma requires a clear appreciation of indications, goals, and end points of the therapy. In many centers barbiturate coma is not used. It is believed that repeated boluses are equally effective and do not bear the extensive risks of barbiturate coma. Barbiturate coma can be discussed when the patient is considered to have a potentially survivable injury, there is no surgically treatable lesion, other standard treatment methods have failed, and the ICP is greater than 25 mmHg for more than 20 min, or greater than 40 mmHg for any shorter period of time. Other potential indications include unilateral cerebral edema with significant midline shift, a low GCS score, and absent or blunted basal cisterns. The therapy should be stopped if the ICP remains uncontrollable despite EEG burst-suppression pattern or electrical silence, or if intolerable side effects such as severe hypotension uncontrollable by cate-

Table 6. Critical care monitoring for high-dose barbiturate therapy

Cardiovascular
  Arterial line: systemic arterial blood pressure
  Swan-Ganz catheter:
    Cardiac output (CO)
    Cardiac Index (CI)
    Stroke Volume (SV)
    Systemic vascular resistance (SVR)
    Pulmonary vascular resistance (PVR)
    Right-heart filling pressures[a]
    Pulmonary capillary wedge pressure
      (PCWP)
  Bladder catheter: urinary output
Cerebrovascular and neurophysiologic
  Intracranial pressure (ICP) monitor
    (ventriculostomy/fiberoptic/subdural/
    subarachnoid/epidural)
  Cerebral perfusion pressure (CPP)
  Brain temperature monitoring (optional)
  Jugular bulb O_2 monitoring/oximeter
    catheter (optional)
  Somatosensory or brain-stem auditory
    evoked potentials (SSEP, BAEP)
    (optional)
  Electroencephalogram (EEG)
General monitoring
  Nasogastric catheter (pH and output)
  Core body temperature probe
  Arterial blood gas
  Intake and output
  Serum barbiturate levels

[a] May be measured by central venous pressure catheter.

Table 7. Dosing regimens for barbiturate coma therapy

A. Pentobarbital intravenous therapy
    High dose
      Loading: 30–40 mg/kg over 4 h
      Maintenance: 1.8–3.3 mg/kg per hour
    Mid-level dose
      Loading: 10 mg/kg over 30 min, with
        25–25 mg/kg over the first 4 h
      Maintenance: 5 mg/kg per hour × 3 h,
        then 2.0–2.5 mg/kg per hour, with
        5 mg/kg boluses as needed if
        pentobarbital serum level is ≤ 3.0 mg/dl
    Low dose
      Loading: 3–6 mg/kg over 30 min
      Maintenance: 0.3–3 mg/kg per hour
    Therapeutic serum level: 2.5–4.0 mg/dl
      (= 25–40 μg/ml); serum levels as high as
      6.0 mg/dl may be required
    Therapeutic EEG response: Burst-
      suppression pattern or cortical electrical
      silence (with preservation of SSEP and
      BAEP)
    Weaning: Dosage is halved every 24 h
      (pentobarbital half-life = 12–24 h in the
      head-injured patient)
B. Thiopental intravenous therapy
    Loading: 3 mg/kg bolus, followed by
      10–20 mg/kg over 1 h
    Maintenance: 3–5 mg/kg per hour
    Therapeutic serum level: 6.0–8.5 mg/dl
    Therapeutic EEG response: same as for
      pentobarbital
    Weaning: same as for pentobarbital, but
      detectable serum levels of pentobarbital, a
      metabolite of thiopental, may be present
      during weaning

cholamines, progressive pulmonary edema, or sepsis develop. Barbiturate dosing regimens are outlined in Table 7. Barbiturate coma may be required for 7 days or more, although some authors believe that it may lose its effect on cerebral blood volume after 2–3 days. In Europe ethomidate bolus therapy is occasionally used instead of barbiturates. Ethomidate should not be used longer than 24 h.

Newer protocols have been designed to improve CPP by affecting the pressure rather than the resistance side of the CPP/ICP equation, with the goal of increasing CPP and inducing cerebral vasoconstriction, resulting in reduced cerebral blood volume and ICP. A particular protocol has been established at the University of Alabama; it is detailed in Table 8. The essential elements of this protocol are the use of CSF drainage for reducing ICP, maintenance of normal intravascular volume and total body sodium, the use of vasopressive agents to drive CPP, and minimization of blood viscosity to improve microvascular circulation. This approach derives from work showing that plateau waves and raised ICP may be aborted or reduced by elevating blood pressure, and from the assumption that hypertension does not greatly exaggerate edema, a position that is not unanimously shared by other investigators. There are similar protocols with minor modifications. Ventricular drainage is not used everywhere. Head elevation up to 30° is used frequently, although the effect on ICP can be counteracted by the reduction of perfusion pressure due to head elevation.

Intensive Care Unit Management

Management of Secondary Systemic Effects

Cardiovascular. The massive catecholamine surge following severe cranial trauma can cause direct myocardial injury, with elevation of CPK-MB fraction serum levels and subendocardial necrosis, hemorrhage, and ischemia with electrocardiographic changes – largely repolarization abnormalities. Acute hypokalemia following catecholamine release is capable of exerting an independent, synergistic arrhythmogenic effect. Metabolic acidosis, whether the result of hypoxemia or sympathetically mediated increases in metabolic activity, further potentiates cardiac irritability and arrhythmias. Peripheral vasoconstriction increases cardiac afterload, which can impair left ventricular function. Direct sympathetic neurogenic sti-

Table 8. University of Alabama ICP protocol

1. Ventriculostomy with CSF drainage *first*
2. Fluid therapy replacement of all output and insensible losses; follow intravascular volume with CVP or PCWP.
3. Minimize prolonged periods of positive sodium balance or total body water (follow urine electrolytes).
4. Systemic pressors: dopamine and phenylephrine
5. Mannitol 0.5–1.0 g/kg when CPP is less than 50–60 mmHg; furosemide is *not* routinely used.
6. Head of bed 0°.
7. F_iO_2 to maintain arterial oxygen saturation greater than 90% and pCO_2 at 35 mmHg; muscle relaxants and pharmacologic paralysis as needed
8. Maintain CPP ≥ 70 mmHg; many patients may require a CPP of 90–100 mmHg, with a CPP of approximately 84 mmHg optimal.
9. Packed cell transfusions to maintain a hematocrit between 30 and 35%
10. Wean off pharmacologic paralysis and ventilatory support only after the patient is independent of mannitol and arterial pressors.

mulation of the pulmonary vascular bed may result in significant increases in right-heart afterload, predisposing to right-heart failure, which may be further aggravated by administration of osmotic diuretics.

All patients who have sustained significant cranial trauma should have ECG and CVP monitoring. Some require more invasive cardiovascular monitoring, such as Swan-Ganz catheterization. The use of catecholamine-blocking agents – and those with antiarrhythmic effect, in particular – should be considered part of the early management regime for severe cranial trauma.

Pulmonary. The catecholamine surge also alters pulmonary vascular bed function, exaggerating normal physiologic ventilation-perfusion mismatches, either directly or as a result of inducing left-heart dysfunction. Direct sympathetic effects of the pulmonary capillary bed may produce neurogenic pulmonary dysfunction and neurogenic pulmonary edema. The adult respiratory distress syndrome (ARDS) in head-injured patients may result from various pathophysiologic mechanisms, including (a) aspiration pneumonitis (bacterial or chemical) secondary to airway, pharyngeal, or gastroesophageal dysfunction, (b) brain-tissue thromboplastin and tissue plasminogen activator release (DIC-fibrinolysis), (c) fat embolization from long bone fractures, with induction of a lipoperoxide-prostaglandin cascade, infarction of lung tissue, and further release of tissue thromboplastin, and (d) direct catecholamine injury to pulmonary capillary endothelium.

Alterations in pulmonary vascular compliance, alveolar-capillary permeability, and atelectasis increase intrapulmonary shunting of desaturated blood, reducing arterial oxygen saturation and increasing the arteriovenous oxygen gradient (A-VO$_2$). Decreasing pulmonary compliance signalled by rising peak inspiratory pressures (PIP) may signal tracheobronchial obstruction, interstitial thickening of the pulmonary parenchyma, pneumothorax, or decreased chest-wall compliance. Close monitoring of a variety of pulmonary function indices (Table 9) is therefore essential when treating cranial trauma patients.

Various methods for ventilatory support of severely head injured patients have been used with success. Small, more frequent ventilator-driven inspirations more closely approximate

Table 9. Desired values for pulmonary function in head injury

O$_2$ saturation	>95%
PaO$_2$	>100 mmHg
A-V$_{O_2}$ gradient	2–4 ml%
SvO$_2$	60–80%
Pulmonary shunt	<15%
PIP	<20 mmHg

PIP, Positive inspiratory pressure; PaO$_2$, arterial oxygen partial pressure; SvO$_2$, systemic venous oxygen saturation; A-V$_{O_2}$ gradient, arteriovenous oxygen volume difference.

normal ventilation physiology (e.g., 10–12 ml/kg at a rate of 10–12 breaths/min) with fewer adverse effects on intrathoracic, intracranial, and right-heart filling pressures. However, even with a sigh mode, progressive atelectasis and pulmonary shunting may ensue. An alternative approach is to deliver larger tidal volumes at a lower rate (e.g., 15 ml/kg or more at a rate of 8–10 breaths/min. This method allows for recruitment of more alveoli, preventing atelectasis, but increases ICP. If pulmonary shunting develops and arterial saturation does not respond to nontoxic levels of inspired oxygen, higher values of positive end-expiratory pressure (PEEP) may become necessary. PEEP levels higher than 15–20 cm H$_2$O increase the risk of barotrauma to the lung and increase ICP, but PEEP levels as high as 30–40 cm H$_2$O may be necessary to adequately oxygenate patients with ARDS or neurogenic pulmonary edema, with an increased risk of pneumothorax. High PEEP levels adversely affect right-heart filling pressures. Swan-Ganz monitoring should be considered; significant right-heart compromise may require inotropic support (e.g., dopamine 3–

$10\,\mu g/kg/min$, dobutamine $1-3\,\mu g/kg/min$, or isoproterenol $0.25-0.5\mu g/kg/min$). If prolonged ventilation is necessary, an elective tracheostomy should be performed to reduce the risk of aspiration, facilitate pulmonary toilet, and reduce the risk of vocal cord injury.

Immobilization increases the risk of occult pelvic or lower extremity phlebitis and pulmonary embolism, which may be more difficult to diagnose in the head-injured patient. Prevention of pulmonary embolism is the best defense: sequential compression devices (SCD) on the lower extremities and early placement on kinetic therapy treatment tables offer the best protection, while Ace-wraps offer somewhat less protection. Subcutaneous heparin can probably be used safely in small doses in most head-injured patients. Fever, tachycardia, and an increase in end-tidal CO_2 may be the presenting signs of embolism in a ventilated patient, as opposed to the more classic signs of transient hypoxemia, ECG right-axis deviation or right bundle branch block, and tachypnea. A ventilation-perfusion scan or pulmonary angiography is needed to establish the diagnosis. If the patient is at increased risk for intracranial hemorrhage with full-dose anticoagulation therapy (usually within the first $10-14$ days of injury), a Greenfield filter in the infrarenal inferior vena cava is the treatment of choice. Symptomatic fat embolism, presenting with transient truncal petechia and progressive respiratory insufficiency within $24-72\,h$ following long bone fractures, should be treated with high-dose corticosteroids, presumably to reduce the free-radical/lipoperixidation response.

Renal. Renal function may be affected by sympathetic and catecholamine-induced vasoconstriction of the renal arteries, producing prerenal azotemia, but more often there is prerenal azotemia from the therapy. Overuse of mannitol may result in mannitol nephropathy, including crystallization of mannitol within the renal cortex. Urinary spot electrolytes and 24-h urine collections for creatinine clearence provide additional information with regard to renal function. Prerenal azotemia is treated with repletion of intravascular volume, but it may also require use of renal-dose dopamine ($3-6\,\mu g/kg/min$).

Gastrointestinal. Catecholamine surge causes vasoconstriction of gastric mucosal and submucosal vessels, resulting in mucosal stress ischemia and ulceration (Cushing's ulcer), which can lead to upper gastrointestinal hemorrhage, pyloric obstruction, or perforation. Sympathetic neurogenic effects include gastric dilatation (which may cause regurgitation and aspiration), ileus, biliary stasis, and sphincteric dysfunction. Lower esophageal sphincter dysfunction allows gastric acid reflux and esophagitis or gastroesophageal ulceration.

Early decompression of the stomach with a nasal or orogastric tube reduces the risk of regurgitation and aspiration and allows for monitoring and control of gastric pH. Antacids (e.g., Maalox or Amphogel $30\,ml/h$ p.r.n.) and sucralfate (Carafate $1\,g/6\,h$) should be used to keep gastric pH 3.5 until the patient can be fed enterally. H_2-blockers, including cimetadine ($900-1200\,mg$ i.v./24 h), ranitidine ($100\,mg$ i.v./24 h), or famotidine ($40\,mg$ i.v./24 h), are effective in reducing gastric acidity, but they sacrifice the bactericidal activity of gastric acid and may predispose to sepsis, should aspiration of gastric contents occur. Ultimately, early enteral feeding (within 24–48 h, if possible) is the best protection against gastric dysfunction, once ileus is resolved. Pancreatitis is frequent in patients with cranial trauma. Serum amylase levels may be inadequate alone, and urinary amylase determinations and serum lipase levels may provide additional sensitivity, with ultrasonography or abdominal CT confirming the diagnosis. Pancreatitis is treated in the standard fashion.

Hematopoietic/Coagulation System. The patient who sustains a head injury may have additional risk factors, including medications, pre-injury disease states, or iatrogenic interventions, which can affect the development of a coagulation disorder. Early post-injury changes include significant decreases in alpha 2-plasmin inhibitor, moderate decreases in antithrombin III, slight decreases in fibrinogen levels, and significant increases in fibrin degradation products; in post-surgery patients, there is decreased platelet survival, a transient increase in fibrinogen (at 48–72 h), and elevated fibrinolytic activity and fibrin degradation products. This normal hyper-coagulable response to injury is magnified by injuries that allow release of brain-tissue thromboplastin or tissue plasminogen into the systemic vasculature – as may occur following penetrating head injury, predisposing to thromboembolism and delayed traumatic intracerebral hematoma. Platelet count, PPT/APPT, and PT are the least sensitive indices for detecting coagulation disorders. Quantitative assays of fibrinogen, fibrin, and fibrin degradation (or split) products remain the most reliable tests for uncovering early or subclinical coagulation disorders. The treatment of these disorders is outlined in Table 10.

Metabolism

Metabolic rate increases by 115–215% over the pre-injury basal metabolic rate after severe head trauma, with daily nitrogen excretion rates increasing from 12 to 30–50 g/day and protein metabolism increasing from 75 to 200–300 g/day. Pharmacological paralysis reduces energy metabolism associated with decorticate posturing. Hypothermia associated with barbiturate treatment further reduces energy expenditures.

Depleted energy stores must be restored as early as possible. If the patient cannot be fed enterally, parenteral alimentation should be initiated within the first 24 h. Because of the high dextrose concentrations and the fluid volumes involved in providing hyperalimentation, hyperglycemia and overhydration are potential risks. Blood glucose levels should be monitored closely, and insulin-infusion therapy should be started if glucose serum levels exceed 150–200 md/dl. Multivitamins, Mg^{2+}, carnitine, and phosphate should be added. Amino acids have to be given immediately; lipids after 2–3 days. Enteral feeding should be started early if possible. Patients who require long-term tube enteral feeding may require placement of a percutaneous gastrostomy.

Table 10. Treatment of coagulopathy in acute head injury

I. Platelet disorders
  A. Thrombocytopenia (dilutional, hemorrhagic, secondary to DIC)
     Platelet concentrate (1 donor unit = 20 000/mm³ in vivo):
     Transfuse 3–5 donor units every 6–8 h to maintain platelet count of 75 000–100 000/mm³
  B. Thrombocytopenia (heparin or hetastarch induced):
     If no new thrombosis:
        Discontinue heparin or hetastarch (Hespan)
        Platelet concentrate if bleeding still not controlled
     If heparin-induced thrombosis or abnormal platelet aggregation:
        Discontinue *all* heparin (including i.v. flushes, etc.)
        Begin antiplatelet aggregation therapy:
        – Dextran 25 ml/h i.v. infusion
           (Acetylsalicylic acid, dipyramidole, sulfinpyrazone not recommended for head-injured
           patients)
  C. Impaired platelet function:
     If irreversible (e.g., recent aspirin ingestion):
        Platelet concentrate transfusions to replace inactive platelets
     If reversible (e.g., after hetastarch):
        DDAVP (desmoarginine vasopression) infusion (But N.B.: DDAVP releases
           plasminogen and induces SIADH)
        Cryoprecipitate (Factor VIII and ristocetin co-factor) infusion
II. Clotting factor deficiencies
  A. Fresh-frozen plasma 2–4 units for initial control or 1 unit FFP/5 units of packed cells
     transfused; repeat every 6–12 h as needed
     – replaces all clotting Factors I–XIII, vWF, antithrombin III)
  B. Cryoprecipitate infusion (1–10 Unit concentrates)
     – replaces Factors I, VIII, XI, XIII, vWF
  C. Phytonadione (vitamin K₁/Aquamephyton) 2.5–10 mg i.m./s.c. every 8–12 h × 2 (for
     vitamin K₁ deficiency, repeat up to 7 days) or 2.5–25 mg i.m./s.c. (for reversing Coumadin).
     N.B.: may cause anaphylaxis if administered i.v.
     – enables liver synthesis of Factors II, VII, IX, X (N.B.: requires functioning liver and
        12–24 h for effect)
  D. Menadiol sodium diphosphate (vitamin K₃/Synkayvite) 5–15 mg i.v./i.m./s.c. every 12 h
     (for reversing vitamin K deficiency or Coumadin); may be repeated as needed.
     – action similar to that of phytonadione
  E. Protamine sulfate (reversal of 90–115 units of heparin/mg) SLOW i.v. infusion (no more
     than 50 mg over 10 min), based on heparin dose-time
     – Acts within 5 min to reverse heparin activity on antithrombin III
     – If thrombin time remains prolonged, may be repeated
     – Overdosage may cause anticoagulation
  F. Antihemophilic factors (purified):
     Pasteurized (Monoclate-P, Humate-P) 15–50 I.U./kg, then 10–25 I.U./kg every 8 h (N.B.:
        May cause a hypersensitivity reaction)
     – replaces Factors VIII: C and (in lesser amounts) vWF: Ag
     Proplex-T (Factors VII, IX), similar dosing
     Monoclonal antihemophilic factor (Hemofil-M) 1 I.U./cc plasma (40 I.U./kg)
     – genome-produced Factor VIII
     – dosage adjusted by serial assessment of factor activity (%)
III. Disseminated intravascular coagulation (DIC)
   Eliminate underlying cause (débride brain injury, treat sepsis, etc.)
   Supportive therapy for cardiovascular system if function is compromised
   – whole blood, packed cells, crystalloid as needed
   – reverse acidosis or hypothermia

Table 10. *Continued*

    Replace depleted coagulation factors if hemostatic failure is present
    – Fresh-frozen plasma 2–4 units initially, then as needed
    – Cryoprecipitate (for fibrinogen) as needed
    – Platelet concentrate as needed
    If DIC is not controlled by definitive therapy and coagulation factor replacement,
    – Heparin 100–500 units i.v./h infusion (initial bolus = 2000–5000 units i.v.)
    – Conjugated steroids (e.g., Premarin 2.5–10 mg i.v. every 12 h)
      – anecdotal efficacy, particularly with DIC secondary to malignancy
    – If DIC associated with acute fat embolism syndrome, consider glucocorticoids (e.g.,
      methylprednisolone 1–2 g i.v. loading, followed by 250–500 mg i.v. every 6 h for 24–48 h) for
      membrane stabilization and lipoperoxidation inhibition
IV. Fibrinolysis associated with disseminated intravascular coagulation (DIC/F) Treat in same
     manner as for DIC alone
 V. Primary fibrinolysis
     Antifibrinolytic agents (N.B.: absolutely contraindicated if DIC present)
     – ε-Aminocaproic acid (Amicar) 4–5 g i.v. loading, followed by 1–2 g i.v. every hour × 3 h,
       then 1–2 g i.v. every 2 h i.v./p.o.
     – Tranexamic acid (alternative to Amicar) 10 mg/kg i.v. every 4 h or 30–50 mg p.o. every 4 h

---

Fluid and Electrolyte Balance

Fluid and electrolyte disturbances occur as a result of the neurohumoral and sympathetic responses to injury, fluid, electrolyte, and diuretic administration, and certain other medications. Catecholamine release produces transient hypokalemia. Sympathetic nervous system stimulation induces adrenal release of aldosterone, causing sodium retention, kaliuresis, and activation of the renin-angiotensin system, which affects glomerular filtration. Antidiuretic hormone (ADH) secretion causes sodium and water retention and decreased urine output, whereas diabetes insipidus causes the opposite.

Normal serum osmolality ranges between 285 and 305 mOsm/l. Serum osmolality is modulated by hypothalamic osmoreceptors. Competing goals of fluid and electrolyte management, of maintaining an euvolemic or hypervolemic state for CPP and CBF management, and of inducing osmotic diuresis to reduce ICP can complicate care. For the detailed management of fluid and electrolyte disturbances please refer to Chap. 87.

Anticonvulsant Therapy

Anticonvulsants are clearly indicated in the early management of cranial trauma patients, largely because of the risk for secondary brain injury caused by post-traumatic seizure activity. Post-traumatic seizuries are frequent following penetrating injures (30–34%), intracranial hematoma, depressed skull fractures, or dural laceration. Except for these patients, anticonvulsive prophylaxis has not been associated with benefit concerning the development of post-traumatic epilepsy. Anticonvulsants used for early treatment of seizures after cranial trauma include diazepam, phenytoin, and carbamazepine. For dosages and other details please refer to Chap. 66.

Prognosis of Cranial Injuries

Predicting outcome for severely brain injured patients remains problematic. Many neurosurgeons can recall anecdotal cases of very old patients with acute subdural hematoma and low GCS scores who had a good outcome after surgery. Nevertheless, there are general principles which affect prognosis for survival (Table 11), albeit not with 100% accuracy. Poor prognosis for survival is associated with lower GCS scores, impaired pupillary responses of both eyes, and increasing age. Intracranial hypertension that cannot be controlled is associated with increased mortality. Initial CT scans demonstrating midline shift >5 mm at septum level, compressed or absent perimesencephalic cisterns, or high-density lesions >25 mm^3 in volume are associated with increased mortality and poorer neurologic outcome. However, early surgical intervention may significantly reduce mortality associated with certain lesions. Absent or severely impaired BAEPs – with

Table 11. Estimated mortalities for various head injuries

Evaluation		Mortality (%)
1. Glasgow Coma Scale score:		
GCS > 8		12
GCS < 8 (for >24 h)		30–50
GCS = 5		27
GCS = 4		78
2. Initial CT findings:		
No visible injury (diffuse injury-I)		9.6
Midline shift 0–5 mm and/or lesion densities present (DI-II)		13.5
Cisterns compressed or absent, with midline shift 0–5 mm (DI-III)		34
Midline shift > 5 mm (DI-IV)		56
Evacuated mass lesion		38.8
Nonevacuated mass lesion		52.8
Brain-stem injury		66.7
3. Intracranial pressure:		
ICP > 25 mmHg		69
ICP < 15 mmHg		15
ICP < 20 mmHg and not reducible		92
4. Pathological entity:		
Epidural hematoma		10–12
Subdural hematoma		
Simple		21–25
Complicated		40–75
Bilateral		77–100
Cortical laceration(s)		
Single		43
Multiple		62
Diffuse axonal injury		30–60
5. Neurometric findings:		
Severe attenuation or absence of BAEP or	SSEP	50–75
6. Hypotension associated with elevated ICP		80–100

intact cochlear function – predict poor outcome, as do progressive decreases and loss of the median nerve SEPs.

In summary, neurocritical care for the patient who has sustained significant cranial trauma requires comprehensive multisystem assessment, monitoring, and treatment in order to optimize survival and neurocognitive outcome. Because of the profound effects critical care management of cranial trauma can have on mortality and neurologic rehabilitation, effective management not only saves lives, but also reduces long-term costs to the patients, their families, the community, and society at large. On the other hand, survival without a considerable quality of life, for example, in a persitent vegetative state, cannot be considered the optimal therapy result. In severe cranial trauma, as in other devastating CNS diseases, the physicians have to be aware of the danger of overusing their technical skills at the expense of the patients and their relatives.

Suggested Reading

Anderson DC, Bundlie S, Rockswold GL (1984) Multimodality evoked potentials in closed head trauma. Arch Neurol 41: 369–382

Brenner RP, Schwartzmann RJ, Richey ET (1975) Prognostic significance of episodic low-amplitude or relatively isoelectric EEG patterns.Dis Nerv Syst 10: 582–586

Bricolo A, Turella G (1973) EEG patterns of acute traumatic coma: diagnostic and prognostic value. J Neurosurg Sci 17: 278–285

Compton JS, Teddy PL (1987) Cerebral arterial vasospasm following severe head injury: a transcranial Doppler study. Br J Neurosurg 1:435–439

Dauch WA (1991) Prediction of secondary deterioration in comatose neurosurgical patients by serial recording of multimodality evoked potentials. Acta Neurochir (Wien) 111:84–91

Dearden NM, Miller JD (1989) Paired comparison of hypnotic and osmotic therapy in the reduction of intracranial hypertension after severe head injury. In: Hoff JT, Bets AL (eds) ICP VII. Springer, Berlin Heidelberg New York, pp 474–481

Frobes AM, Dally FG (1970) Acute hypertension during induction of anesthesia and endotracheal intubation in normotensive man. Br J Anaesth 42:618–624

Greenberg RP, Newlon PG, Becker DP (1982) The somatosensory evoked potentials in patients with severe head injury: outcome prediction and monitoring of brain function. Ann NY Acad Sci 388:683–688

Hansotia P, Gozzschalk P, Green P, Zais D (1981) Spindle coma: incidence, clinicopathologic correlates and prognostic value. Neurology 31:83–87

Holzschuh M, Brawanski A, Meixensberger J, Ullrich W (1992) Transcranial Doppler sonography with assessment of CO_2-reactivity in head injury. Ultraschall Med 13:208–212

King BD, Harris LC Jr, Griefenstein FE et al. (1964) Reflex circulatory responses to direct laryngoscopy and tracheal intubation performed during general anesthesia. Anesthesiology 43:201–208

Lindsay KW, Carlin J, Kennedy I, Fry J, McInnes A, Teasdale GM (1981) Evoked potentials in severe head injury – analysis and relation to outcome. J Neurol Neurosurg Psychiatry 44:796–802

Maynard DE, Jenkinson JL (1984) The cerebral function analysing monitor. Anaesthesia 39:678–690

Messeter K, Nordström CH, Sundbärg G (1986) Cerebral hemodynamics in patients with acute severe head trauma. J Neurosurg 64:231–237

Nagao S, Kuyma H, Honma Y, Momma F, Nishiura T, Murota T, Suga M, Tanimoto T, Kawauchi M, Nishimoto A (1987) Prediction and evaluation of brain-stem function by auditory brain-stem responses in patients with uncal herniation. Surg Neurol 27:81–86

Newell DW, Aaslid R (1992) Transcranial Doppler: clinical and experimental uses. Cerebrovasc Brain Metab Rev 4:122–143

Newlon PG, Greenberg RP, Hyatt MS, Enas GG, Becker DP (1982) The dynamics of neuronal dysfunction and recovery following severe head injury assessed with serial multimodality evoked potentials. J Neurosurg 57:168–177

Obrist WD, Gennareli TA, Segawa H et al. (1979) Relation of cerebral blood flow to neurological status and outcome in head injured patients. J Neurosurg 51:292–300

Pampiglione G, DaCosta AA (1975) Intravenous therapy and EEG-monitoring in prolonged seizures. J Neurol Neurosurg Psychiatry 38:371–377

Prior PF (1985) EEG monitoring and evoked potentials in brain ischemia. Br J Anaesth 57:63–81

Prior PF, Maynard DE (1986) Monitoring cerebral function. Elsevier, Amsterdam

Riffel B, Stöhr M, Rost E, Ullrich A, Graser W (1987) Frühzeitige prognostische Aussage mittels evozierter Potentiale beim schweren Schädel-Hirn-Trauma. Z EEG EMG 18:192–199

Rumpl E, Prugger M, Gertenbrandt F, Hackl JM, Pallua A (1983) Central somatosensory conduction time and short-latency evoked potentials in post-traumatic coma.

Electroencephalogr Clin Neurophysiol 56:583–596

Schalen W, Messeter K, Nordström CH (1991) Cerebral vasoreactivity and the prediction of outcome in severe traumatic brain lesions. Acta Anaesthesiol Scand 35:113–122

Starr A, Hamilton AE (1976) Correlation between confirmed sites of neurologic lesions and abnormalities of far-field auditory brain-stem responses. Electroencephalogr Clin Neurophysiol 41:595–608

Takeshima K, Noda K, Higaki M (1964) Cardiovascular response to rapid anesthesia induction and endotracheal intubation. Anesth Analg (Cleve) 43:201–208

Westmoreland BF, Klass DW, Sharbrough FW, Reagan TJ (1975) Alpha coma. Arch Neurol 32:713–718

Wise B, Perkins R, Stevenson E et al. (1964) Penetration of ^{14}C-labelled mannitol from serum into cerebrospinal fluid and brain. Exp Neurol 10:264–270

York DH, Pulliam MW, Rosenfeld JG, Watts C (1981) Relationship between visual evoked potentials and intracranial pressure. J Neurosurg 55:909–916

| # Spinal Trauma

JÜRGEN PIEK, WOLFGANG J. BOCK, and DENNIS G. VOLLMER

Epidemiology

The true incidence of spinal cord injuries (SCI) is unknown, since most patients either have only mild impairment of neurological function or short-lasting effects and most are treated as outpatients or are never referred to specialized centers. In industrialized countries, the incidence of SCI is estimated to be about 50 cases per million population per year. The incidence of acute traumatic paraplegia or quadraplegia is about 10 cases per million population per year. In the neurosurgical critical care unit in Dusseldorf, Germany, SCI represents approximately 4.5% of all trauma cases. It is frequently assossiated with cranial trauma (Fig. 1). SCI is largely a problem of industrialized countries. It occurs mainly in traffic accidents, work-related accidents, or sporting and recreational activities. Most patients are in their mid twenties and are male. During wartime, the rate of spinal cord injury increases substantially. The economic consequences

of these injuries are striking; the expenses of a quadraplegic patient may be as high as several hundred thousand dollars, including costs for life-long medical care, rehabilitation, and equipment. The cost to society from lost productivity is also significant.

With the exception of associated traumatic injuries, pulmonary complications are the main reason why patients with spinal cord injuries require neurocritical care (especially those with lesions at the high cervical and thoracic cord levels).

Pathogenesis and Classification of Spinal Cord Injuries

The mechanism of injury to the spine and spinal cord may be purely vertical compression, flexion, extension, rotation, or distraction, but usually, the injury occurs because of a combination of two or more of these forces. The severity, direction, and site of the forces detemine whether ligamentous or bony injury of the spinal column occurs, and to what degree the spinal cord itself is involved.

Section Editor: Thomas P. Bleck

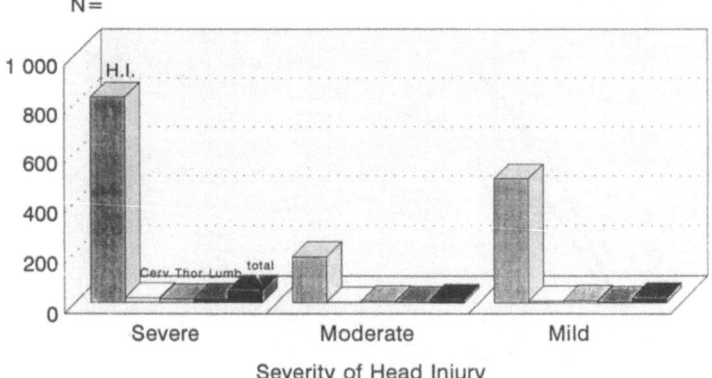

Fig. 1. Incidence of spinal cord injuries in patients with head injuries. Analysis of 1672 patients with head injuries admitted to our intensive care unit from 1981–1989

Spinal cord injuries may be classified according to whether they are open or closed, according to the tissues involved (bony or ligamentous), and according to the neurological symptoms that result usually described by the highest spinal cord level involved. There have been numerous attempts to classify fractures of the spine according to morphological and biochemical viewpoints. According to the fundamental work of Louis (1977) and of Roy-Camille and co-workers in the late 1970s, each vertebral segment can be divided into three main parts: anterior, median, and posterior.

The anterior part (A) consists of the vertebral body itself (without its posterior margin), the anterior ligament, and the intervertebral disk. The median part (B) is the so-called osteo-ligamentous complex, including both facettes. The posterior part (C) consists mainly of the lateral and dorsal processes with all the connecting ligaments and muscles. Fractures that involve only the anterior part (A) are usually stable, while those that involve both the anterior part (A) and the median part (B) are potentially unstable. Those fractures that involve all three parts are definitely unstable (Fig. 2).

Clinical Assessment of a Patient with a Spinal Cord Injury

Clinical assessment of a patient suspected of having a spinal cord injury should not focus on the spinal cord alone. Regardless of how they were characterized before referral, all patients must be presumed to have multiple trauma until proven otherwise. A complete physical examination of the head, chest, abdomen, and extremites, as well as plain chest films should be performed to exclude additional injuries. Abdominal ultrasonography or a diagnostic paracentesis should be considered for all patients with abdominal sensory dysfunction. Circulation and respiratory functions must be stabilized before additional diagnostic procedures are done.

The initial assessment of patients with acute SCI includes: (a) analysis of

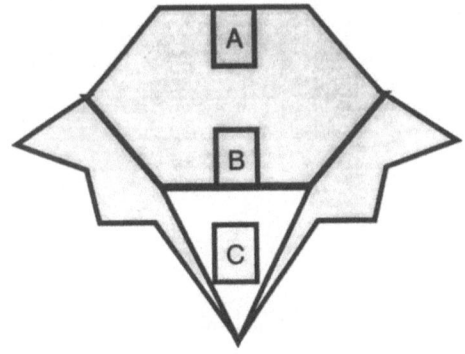

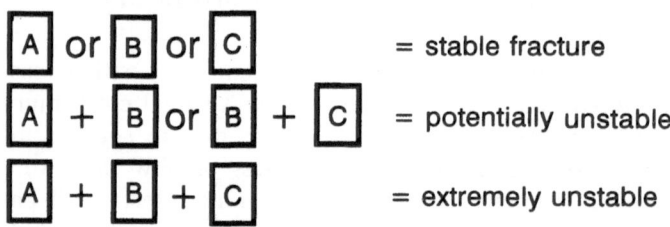

A   vertebral body (without posterior margin)
     anterior longitudinal ligament
     intervertebral disc

B   posterior longitudinal ligament
     posterior margin of vertebral body
     pedicle

C   transverse process
     spinous process
     articular capsule
     interspinous ligament
     supraspinous ligament
     ligamentum flavum

A or B or C   = stable fracture

A + B or B + C   = potentially unstable

A + B + C   = extremely unstable

Fig. 2. Simple classification of spinal injury stability

the nature of the injury (i.e., the biomechanical forces involved), (b) evaluation of the level and degree of spinal cord involvement by a careful neurological examination (to guide additional diagnostic steps, serve as a baseline for neurological follow-up, and provide early prognostic information regarding recovery of neurological function), and (c) determination of the stability of the spinal column; this factor plays an important role in establishing the diagnostic and therapeutic plan for the individual patient.

These aims must be achieved without causing further neurological injury to the patient. Therefore, unless stability of the spine has been proven, immobilization of the spinal column is mandatory before any further investigation is done.

Trauma History

Assessment of the patient with a suspected spinal cord injury starts with a short but careful history of the mechanism and forces involved in the trauma. Certain mechanisms tend to result in typical fractures at specific sites of the spine. Analysis of the forces involved may guide further diagnosis and management of the patient. Those with falls from great heights, or pedestrians hit by a car, usually have fractures of the lower thoracic and lumbar levels. Those with diving injuries or high-speed motor vehicle accidents often have cervical fractures.

Neurological Examination

Important signs elicited during the neurological examination may be grouped under six major headings:

1. Local signs of injury
2. Changes in motor functions
3. Changes in sensory perception
4. Changes in reflex activity
5. Changes in sphincter control
6. Cardiovascular and respiratory changes

These changes may not be permanent, and may vary from hour to hour. Thus, the neurological examination must be repeated frequently, especially shortly after the injury, so as not to overlook worsening from causes amenable to neurosurgical intervention (for example, dislocation of fractures, developing spinal hematomas). It is important to document and follow these signs on a flow chart (Fig. 3).

Local Signs of Injury

Because most SCIs are combined with injuries of the spinal column, pain is the leading local sign of the injury. Pain may be caused by muscular or ligamentous injuries, stiffness at the site of the injury, or nerve entrapment resulting in radicular pain. Slight pressure on the midline and the paravertebral muscles may elicit tenderness or radicular pain, thus indicating the site of the spinal column injury.

Changes in Motor Function

Localization of the spinal cord lesion is based primarily on the correct identification of the segmental level of paralysis. Cross-innervation of voluntary muscles by two or more nerve roots occurs, and this may make it difficult to define the exact level of injury. Normally, a level of total paralysis can be identified by careful motor examination, together with a sensory level one or two segments above, where incomplete paralysis occurs.

The neurological examination should focus not only on testing the full range of upper and lower limb function, but also on the breathing pattern of the patient, to detect involvement of intercostal muscles and the phrenic nerves after cervical and thoracic spinal cord injuries.

Changes in Sensory Perception

The sensory examination includes tests of painful stimuli, light touch, palesthesia, thermesthesia, and coordination. Most of these tests can be performed only with conscious and

Spinal Cord Injury Assessment
Neurosurgical Clinic, Heinrich-Heine-Universität, Düsseldorf

Time	1200 L / R	1300 L / R	1400 L / R	1500 L / R	
Shoulder Abduction (C5)					
Elbow Flexion (C5/6)					**Motor**
Wrist Dorsiflexion (C6/7)					5 = normal 4 = weak
Elbow Extension (C7)					3 = against gravity 2 = on blanket
Hand Grasp (C8)					1 = contraction only 0 = none 1 = on
Hip Flexion (L2/3/4)					
Knee Extension (L3/4)					
Foot Dorsiflexion (L5)					
Foot Plantiflexion (S1)					
Upper intact sens. level					
Lower intact sens. level					

Fig. 3. Spinal cord injury follow-up sheet

cooperative patients. Testing of the sacral sensory function should also be performed in all patients, as preservation of sacral sensory function is often overlooked in those with lesions at much higher levels.

Changes in Reflex Activity

Following acute spinal cord injury, there is usually a change in reflex activity at and below the level of injury. The alterations found may vary in pattern and degree, from complete absence of all reflexes to exaggeration of reflexes. The term "spinal shock" describes a state of complete depression of motor reflex activity combined with paralysis of the limbs; this usually occurs after severe spinal cord lesions. Some reflexes, however may be preserved, indicating a less severe spinal cord lesion. Increased reflex activity can occasionally be observed immediately after the injury, often combined with spasticity and withdrawal response to skin stimuli. These observations are usually made with patients with less severe lesions and may be associated prognostically with functional recovery.

Changes in Sphincter Control

Alterations in sphincter control, not always recognized during the initial examination, should be suspected even in patients with incomplete lesions. If loss of bladder control is supected, a sonographic study of bladder capacity should be performed. Bladder catheterization for the *diagnosis* of urinary retention can thereby be avoided, although it may be necessary to *therapeutically* catheterize some patients for the first few days after their injury. If transurethral catheterization is performed and the patient cannot feel the passing of the catheter, loss of sphincter control is likely. Retention of urine with bladder overflow is the most common bladder disturbance found in patients with acute spinal trauma.

Paralytic ileus is usually the first manifestation of changes in bowel activity and sphincter control. Abdominal distension, absent or impaired bowel sounds, and vomiting may indicate these complications of the injury. Perianal sensory loss, impaired anal sphincter tone, and loss of anal reflexes are usually found in these patients.

Cardiovascular and Respiratory Changes

Cardiovascular and respiratory changes may be observed in patients with cervical or high thoracic lesions. Pulse and blood pressure should be checked in all patients with spinal cord trauma. Bradycardia (less than 60 bpm) and hypotension (systolic blood pressure less than 90 mmHg) indicate neurogenic shock and should not be confused with hemorrhagic shock, in which tachceardia is generally present.

Respiratory insufficiency is most commonly due to paralysis of the intercostal muscles, the diaphragm, or to injuries to the ribs and lungs.

Complete loss of voluntary respiration occurs with lesions above the C-4 level and usually leads to death at the scene of the accident. Preservation of diaphragmatic breathing and loss of intercostal muscle activity occurs with lesions between the C-5 and T-1 levels. The degree of isolated loss of intercostal muscle function depends on the thoracic segments involved. Techniques for intubating patients with cervical spine injuries are discussed below.

If severe respiratory distress is present, arterial blood gases should be obtained and intubation and assisted ventilation should be started. In acutely injured patients, the O_2 saturation should be kept above 90%, the PaO_2 should be above 70 mmHg, and the pCO_2 should be kept at less than 40 mmHg.

Ancillary Tests

Anterior and Lateral Radiography of the Spine

Following the physical examination, additional information should be obtained with diagnostic neuroradiology, provided that the patient is hemodynamically stable and has an adequate airway, and that life-threatening associated injuries have been excluded. Injured patients should be transported carefully, especially if cervical injury is suspected. Movement of potentially unstable fractures may cause further neurological damage to the patient. All patients should be transported from the resuscitation area to radiology in the supine position, with the cervical spine fixed by two sandbags lateral to the head to avoid further dislocation.

Initial plain-film radiography should be performed while the patient is in this position.

Anterior-posterior and lateral films of the whole spinal column should be obtained initially as a routine to rule out multilevel trauma, even if a specific level of injury is suspected. Because most cervical fractures occur between C-5 and T-1, it is necessary to obtain full lateral visualization of the cervical spine down to T-1. If T-1 cannot be completely visualized with lateral films, it may be necessary to put traction onto both arms by two helpers, or to perform the so-called swimmers view radiograph. These routine X-rays should be completed with mouth-open views of the odontoid process.

Oblique Radiography and Conventional Tomography

Special views, such as oblique radiography or lateral and anterior-posterior tomography, may be necessary to establish the diagnosis of injuries to the facets or pedicles, whereas flexion-extension views may be required for those with ligamentous injuries only.

Computed Tomography

Computed tomography (CT) is indicated if the anatomic site of the lesion must be determined. It also provides additional information about the structures involved, including bone and surrounding soft tissues. CT may give further information about narrowing of the spinal cord by bone fragments, disk material, and extramedullary

hematomas (usually epidural). It may be complemented by intrathecal contrast enhancement to clarify lesions in the lower cervical and thoracic regions. The advantage of CT is that patients do not need to be moved from their initial position, though unstable cervical fractures should be stabilized by traction tongs before patients are taken to the CT suite (see below).

Myelography

Diagnostic myelography is rarely indicated for patients with acute SCI. It should be performed, however, if spinal cord damage is present without any bony or ligamentous injuries on radiography or CT. It should also be considered when the level of bony or ligamentous injury does not correlate with the neurological findings on examination. Traumatic disk protrusion or subdural or epidural hematomas may be present in these cases. CT myelography provides more information than conventional myelography and requires much less movement of the patient.

Magnetic Resonance Imaging

The value of magnetic resonance imaging (MRI) in acute spinal injury remains to be defined. It appears that MRI shows all the lesions that can be seen on myelography and that it provides additional information on intraparenchymal lesions, such as cord contusions, small intramedullary hemorrhages, and spinal cord swelling. MRI is not invasive and is less stressful to the patient than ascending myelography. Disadvantages are that it takes longer than myelography, it is not available on a 24-h basis in many centers, and monitoring and management of patients (especially those requiring assisted ventilation or those who are hemodynamically unstable) requires special equipment.

Other Tests

Examination of the CSF is useless in acute spinal cord injury. It does not provide any additional information.

Somatosensory evoked potentials are usually not diagnostic in the initial assessment of acute SCI. They have prognostic value, however, and may even be used in comatose patients to monitor spinal cord function when SCI is suspected. Complete loss of somatosensory evoked potentials indicates complete loss of function and a poor prognosis. Preserved somatosensory evoked potentials in clinically complete lesions may indicate a better prognosis for functional recovery. During surgical procedures, somatosenory evoked potentials can serve as an additional tool to monitor spinal cord function. Magnetic or electric transcranial or spinal motor stimulation (TCMS) is increasingly being used to assess motor function of the spinal cord.

Management of the Patient with Acute Spinal Cord Injury

Acute management and initial assessment of the patient with acute SCI are summarized in Fig. 4.

Pre-ICU Treatment

Aspiration and shock are factors contributing to death in patients with acute spinal cord injury. Circulatory support and airway control are crucial in the prehospital management of these patients.

The best way to reduce morbidity and mortality of spinal cord injuries is to anticipate such injuries in trauma patients and thereby reduce secondary insults to the spinal cord. This is especially important in unconscious patients, in whom the frequency of associated spinal cord injuries may be as high as 5%. SCI should be suspected particularly after high-speed motor vehicle accidents, falls from great heights, and diving accidents.

The neck of any trauma patient should not be moved from the neutral position. Transportation should preferably be done by stabilizing the neck with specially designed collars and on vacuum mattresses or rigid backboards. Intubation and central catheter placement must be performed with minimal movement of the head. Circulatory and respiratory problems should be treated accordingly.

If there are no additional injuries and there is no obvious blood loss, then blood volume is usually normal and infusion of fluid should be minimized. Large volumes of intravenous fluid may result in pulmonary edema, which can be worsened by insufficent cardiovascular function in those with cervical injuries. Loss of sympathetic nerve function below the level of injury usually results in dilatation of arterioles, increased peripheral pooling of blood volume, and hypotension. Elevating the legs to 45° may help to

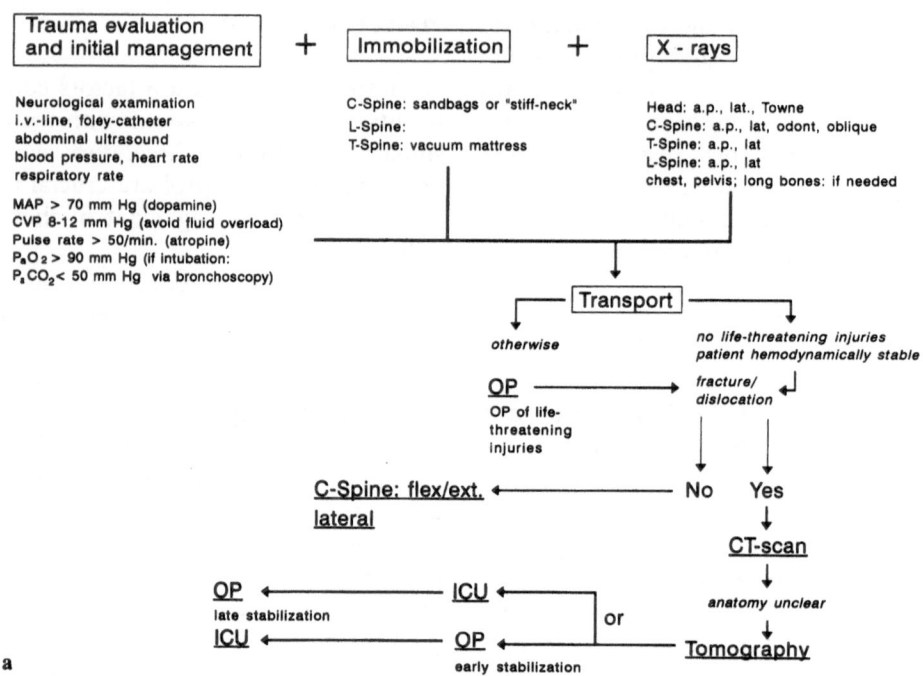

a

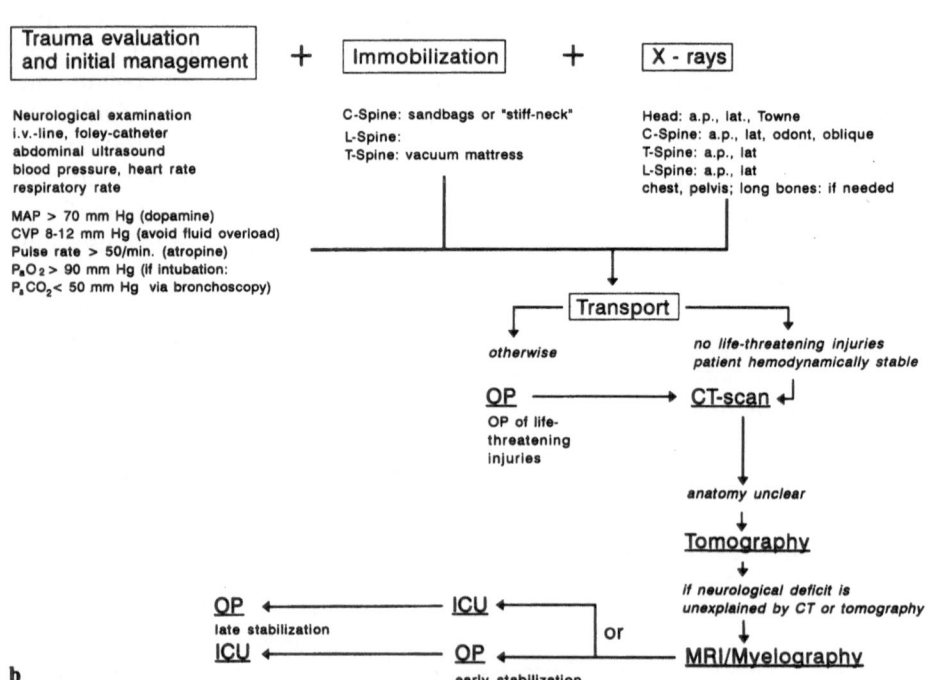

b

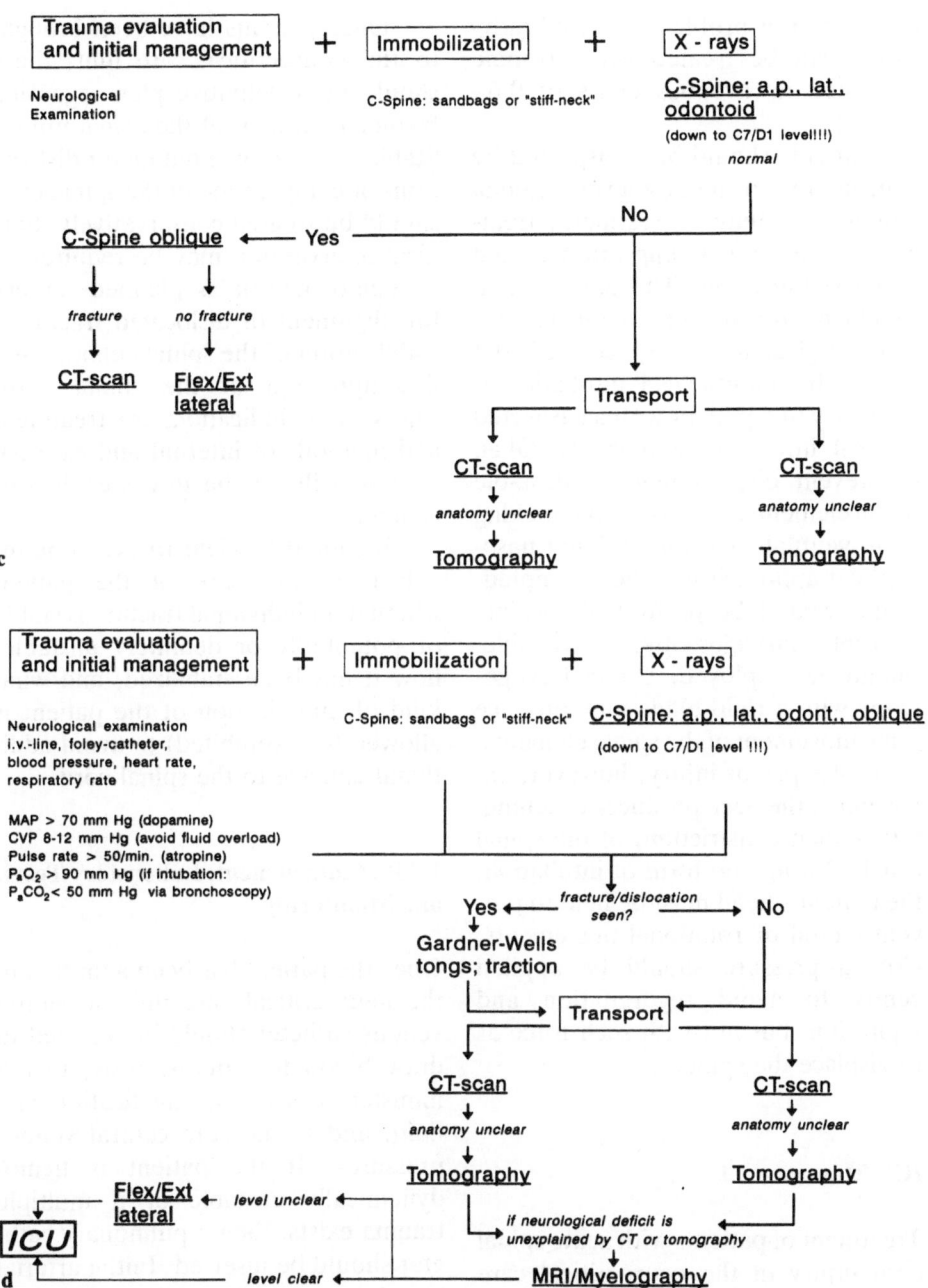

Fig. 4. a Algorithm for the patient with multiple trauma and additional spinal injury without neurological deficit. **b** Algorithm for the patient with multiple trauma and additional spinal injury with neurological deficit. **c** Algorithm for the patient with suspected cervical spine injury without neurological deficit. **d** Algorithm for the patient with suspected cervical spine injury with neurological deficit. *C-Spine*, cervical spine; *a.p.*, anteroposterior; *lat.*, lateral; *odont.*, odontoid process; *MAP*, mean arterial pressure; *CVP*, central venous pressure; *Flex/Ext*, flexion/extension; *CT*, computed tomography; *MRI*, magnetic resonance imaging; *ICU*, intensive care unit

overcome this problem. Severe brady-cardia can be treated with atropine (repeated intravenous doses of 0.6–1.0 mg).

Patients should be transported by helicopter to the nearest level-I trauma unit for the initial assessment, treatment of life-threatening injuries, and initial stabilization. The patient then should be transferred to the nearest neurosurgical unit or specialized SCI center. If endotracheal intubation is necessary in a patient with a suspected cervical injury, care must be taken to prevent displacement of unstable spinal elements. If the patient is making some ventilatory effort, a blind naso-tracheal approach may be attempted. If this cannot be performed, flexible fiberoptic laryngoscopy, if available, should be employed. Direct laryngo-scopy with a rigid blade may produce some movement of the spinal elements. In most types of injury, however, extension of the neck produces widening, rather than constriction, of the spinal canal. During and form of intubation, the patient's head must be held to prevent lateral or rotational movements. Cricoid pressure should be applied gently to avoid regurgitation and aspiration, but not with such force as to displace the spine.

ICU Management

Treatment of patients with acute spinal cord injury in the neurocritical care unit has the following goals:

1. Avoidance of additional damage to the spinal cord
2. Stabilization of the spine
3. Prevention of secondary complications

Once patients have been brought to the neurocritical care unit, there should be a definitive plan regarding further treatment of the spinal injury. Stable fractures without major dislocations or compression of the spinal cord should be treated conservatively. Surgical intervention may be required as an emergency or as planned surgery for alignment of dislocated fractures, stabilization of the spinal column, and decompression of the spinal cord. The various indications for treatment and methods of internal and external fixation will not be discussed in this chapter.

It should be clear to everyone involved in the care of the patient whether an individual fracture is stable or potentially or definitely unstable, how it has been stabilized, and what kind of mobilization of the patient is allowed (or prohibited) to avoid additional damage to the spinal cord.

Initial Management, Laboratory Tests, and Monitoring

Once the patient has been admitted to the neurocritical care unit, a central venous catheter should be inserted to draw blood for routine tests, to administer intravenous medication and fluid, and to measure central venous pressures. If the patient is hemodynamically unstable or if multiple trauma exists, then a pulmonary catheter should be inserted. Initial arterial blood gases should be drawn from an arterial cannula in patients with severe pulmonary dysfunction and in those requiring assisted ventilation. Otherwise, transcutaneous oxygen saturation can be determined and monitored by a finger-tip pulse oximeter.

Initially, Foley catheterization of the bladder should be performed under sterile conditions to facilitate measurements of urine output in patients unable to void voluntarily. Once the condition of the patient allows, sterile intermittant catheterization should be started.

Assisted ventilation is usually indicated if the respiratory rate is greater than 30 breaths per minute or if the pCO_2 is greater than 50 mmHg. Tracheostomy is generally indicated initially only in patients with severe mid-face fractures. Anterior stabilization of lower cervical and upper thoracic fractures is extremely difficult in patients with tracheostomies. Close neurological observation is essential, especially in the early stages of the disease or postoperatively, so that neurological worsening as a complication of surgery is not overlooked.

Prevention and Treatment of Secondary Complications

Cardiovascular

The most important hemodynamic complication in patients with higher thoracic or cervical lesions is complete sympathectomy combined with intact vagal efferents and afferents. Usually mild hypotension (mean arterial pressure of 70–75 mmHg, together with a pulse less than 70 bpm) is observed. Hypotension is not due to hypovolemia, since central venous pressures are normal to high. The cardiac index is usually 50–100% above normal and associated with decreased systemic vascular resistance. The injured sympathetic nervous system is not able to shift volume from the musculoskeletal compartment to the renal-splanchnic compartment. Renal perfusion is usually impaired despite nearly normal arterial, central venous, and pulmonary capillary wedge pressures. Fluid administration that results in a CVP greater than 8 mmHg or a PCWP greater than 15 mmHg should be avoided.

We try to keep patients' MAP greater than 70 mmHg. If, despite adequate volume (that is, a CVP of 8 mmHg), urine output is still low, then a low-dose dopamine infusion ("renal-dose dopamine") should be started (2 μg/kg per min) Alpha-stimulating agents such as phenylepinephrine should be used only in patients with profound hypotension.

Pulmonary

Pulmonary complications, including pulmonary edema, pneumonia, atelactsis, and pulmonary embolus, are extremely common in patients with acute spinal cord injury. Overall, the incidence of pneumonia in patients with spinal cord injuries of all levels varies from 4% to 10%. The higher the level of injury, the greater the risk of pneumonia. In patients with quadriplegia, the incidence of pneumonia approaches 100%. Contributing causes are paresis of respiratory muscles, prolonged immobilization, and impaired immunological competence because of nutritonal depletion.

Early mobilization can be achieved by definitive surgical stabilization of the spine. If prolonged immobilization is required, then a self-rotating bed allows mobilizaton of secretions and optimizes lung perfusion. Aggressive respiratory therapy should be performed at least every 4 h. Supplementary therapy includes adequate hydration of the patient, intravenous drugs and inhalation therapy for secretolysis, avoidance of aspiration, and treatment of ileus to support diaphragm movements. Sputum should be cultured at least twice weekly to monitor bacterial colonization. If pneumonia develops, it must be treated vigorously with adequate antibiotic therapy and additional physiotherapy. Our routine program for pulmonary care of patients with cervical cord injuries is listed in Table 1.

Table 1. Pulmonary care of the patient with acute cervical/thoracic spinal cord injury

---

Monitoring
  Respiratory rate and rhythm (should be <35/min)
  Fingertip pulse oximetry (should be >90% saturation)
  Arterial blood gases if needed
  Lung auscultation twice daily
  Chest X-ray if needed
  Sputum cultures twice per week

Maintaining effective breathing pattern
  If fracture stable or stabilized: mobilize patient; turn at least every 2 h (left/right/upright)
  If fracture unstable: use self-rotating, self-inflating beds
  Avoid subileus/ileus

Maintaining open airways, avoiding infection
  Administer CPAP via face mask every 2 h
  Administer inhalation therapy with alternating schemes (below) every 4 h

Ipratropium bromide	3 ml	Mesna	9 ml
+Fenoterol	1 ml	+NaCl	9 ml
+NaCl	14 ml		
(every 8 h)		(every 8 h)	

  Facilitate coughing by use of abdominal thrusts

[Additional physiotherapy should be provided by physiotherapists (twice daily)]

CPAP, continuous positive airway pressure.

Gastrointestinal

Gastrointestinal complications usually are either ileus or peptic ulcers. Atony of the small intestine is regularly observed in patients following acute spinal cord injury. Therefore, bowel sounds should be checked at least twice daily. If subileus occurs, intravenous medications such as Ceruletid (2 ng/kg per minute) and Distigminbromid (0.01 mg/kg per day i.m.) may stimulate bowel activity. If bowel sounds are present, stool softeners (magnesium sulfate, oleum ricini) can be used to ensure regular bowel movements. A silicone nasogastric tube should be inserted in all patients with acute spinal cord injury for at least 3–4 days to prevent aspiration by draining gastric output. When bowel sounds and stool production have resumed, oral or nasogastric feeding can be started with increasing volumes.

About 10% of patients develop peptic ulcers. Diagnosis can be extremely difficult because of loss of abdominal sensation, even in the setting of perforation. Massive gastrointestinal hemorrhage from a peptic ulcer can be easily diagnosed but recurrent bleeding from an ulcer may be overlooked. Thus, all patients with chronic anemia should be suspected of having recurrent bleeding and should undergo endoscopy. H-2 blocking agents, e.g., ranitidine 300 mg/day by continuous infusion or sucralfate orally or via a nasogastric tube plus pirencepin (30–60 mg/day i.v.) may be effective in reducing the incidence of peptic ulcers in these patients.

Thromboembolic

Deep venous thrombosis (DVT) occurs because of immobilization and decreased venous return from the legs due to paralysis. The incidence in all patients with spinal cord injury is approximately 10–20%. Prophylaxis with low-dose heparin (5000 IU every 12 h by subcutaneous injection) is effective in reducing the incidence of DVT and is routinely used in our unit. Systemic anticoagulation, with PTT values twice the normal range, is indicated only in patients with acute pulmonary embolism and should be avoided as a routine method of prophylaxis. Early physiotherapy, regular movement of the legs, and graduated elastic compression stockings should also be used with low-dose heparin.

Urinary Tract

Urinary tract infection is the most common complication of acute spinal cord injury. It occurs in as many as 70% of all patients. During the acute phase, an areflexic bladder with urine retention and bladder overdistension is the most commonly observed picture of neurogenic bladder dsyfunction. To avoid this complication, regular drainage of the bladder should be performed. Although often necessary for the first few days after the injury, indwelling Foley catheters damage uroepithelium, induce inflammation, and lead to tissue colonization with bacteria. Therefore, a catheter-free status should be reached as soon as possible.

Sterile, intermittent catheterization with urine volumes of about 500 ml has proved to be the best method of avoiding urinary tract infections. Prophylactic use of antibiotics may reduce the incidence of positive cultures but not that of clinical infection. The urine should be regularly cultured and aggressive antibiotic treatment should be started in patients with clinical infection.

Pressure Sores

Decubitus ulcers can develop both in the early and in the late stages of acute spinal cord injury. Impaired skin perfusion is the underlying cause, resulting from low regional perfusion and decreased systemic blood pressure. Nutritional depletion and immobilization are also contributing factors. Risk factors for developing early pressure sores are unrelieved pressure before admission to the neurocritical care unit, older age, and decreased systolic blood pressure. Nurses and medical personnel should turn patients (as long as spinal stability is present) as least every 2 h. Specially designed low-flow inflating beds may further reduce the incidence of decubitus ulcers. If pressure sores develop, they should be treated by standard procedures.

Nutritional

Nutritional requirements of patients with acute spinal cord injury do not differ from those of other trauma patients. Nutritional deficiency should therefore be treated by established methods of nutritional therapy. During the atonic phase, total parenteral nutrition is indicated, but once stool production has resumed, enteral feeding via nasogastric tube can be performed, or oral nutrition can be given.

Pharmacological Treatment of Acute Spinal Cord Injury

Only one pharmacological agent – methylprednisolone – has been proven to be effective in reducing neurological deficits. In the past, interest focused on corticosteroids and naloxone as agents to reduce the neurological damage in acute SCI. Although beneficial in preventing secondary damage in experimental spinal trauma, both agents were ineffective in smaller series of injured patients. Bracken and co-workers (1990), in a prospective, double-blinded, multicenter trial, demonstrated that high-dose methylprednisolone was effective in acute SCI. Naloxone was not effective in this study. According to this protocol, all patients with acute SCI should be given a bolus injection of 30 mg/kg methylprednisolone followed by infusion at 4 mg/kg per hour during the next 23 hours. Because this treatment notably depends on the oxygen free-radical scavenging effect of methylprednisolone, other glucocorticoids should not be substituted, as the appropriate doses are not established.

Treatment of Spasticity

Early spasticity rarely occurs in acutely injured patients. In addition to early mobilization and physiotherapy, application of cold to the spastic muscles reduces spasticity by diminishing gamma motoneuron activity. Two agents are available to reduce spasticity. Baclofen increases the presynaptic inhibition of motor reflex activity and may be given in doses up to 100 mg/day. Dantrolene has a direct effect on extrafusal fibers and may be given in a maximal dose of 200 mg/day. In patients with refractory spasticity, either intrathecal baclofen delivery via a programmable pump or a longi-

tudinal myelotomy may be the treatment of choice.

Suggested Reading

Angelo CM, van Gilder JC, Taub A (1973) Evoked potentials in experimental spinal cord trauma. J Neurosure 38:332–336

Bailes JE, Herman JM, Quigley MR et al. (1990) Diving injuries of the cervical spine. Surg Neurol 34:155–158

Bhatt K, Cid E, Maiman D (1987) Bacteremia in the spinal cord injury population. J Am Paraplegia Soc 10:11–14

Black P, Markowitz R (1971) Experimental spinal cord injury in monkeys: comparison of steroids and hypothermia. Surg Forum 22:409–411

Black P, Markowitz R, Keller S et al. (1986a) Naloxone and experimental spinal cord injury: part 1. High-dose administration in a static load compression model. Neurosurgery 19:905–908

Black P, Markowitz R, Keller S et al. (1986b) Naloxone and experimental spinal cord injury: part 2. Megadose treatment in a dynamic load model. Neurosurgery 19:909–913

Blissitt PA (1990) Nutrition in acute spinal cord injury. Crit Care Nurs Clin North Am 2:375–384

Böhler J (1974) Verletzungen der Wirbelsäule – operative Behandlung, Indikation und Technik. Z Orthop 112:894–896

Bracken MD, Freeman DH, Hellenbrand K (1981) Incidence of acute traumatic hospitalized spinal cord injury in the United States, 1970–1977. Am J Epidemiol 113:615–622

Bracken MB, Collins WF, Freeman DF et al. (1984) Efficacy of methylprednisolone in acute spinal cord injury. JAMA 251:45–52

Bracken MB, Shepard MJ, Collins WF et al. (1990) A randomized, controlled trial of methylprednisolone or naloxone in the treatment of acute spinal cord injury. Results of the Second National Acute Spinal Cord Injury Study. N Engl J Med 322:1459–1461

Chakeres DW, Flickinger F, Bresnahan JC et al. (1987) MR imaging of acute spinal cord trauma. Am J Neuroradiol 8:5–10

Curry K, Casady L (1992) The relationship between extended periods of immobility and decubitus ulcer formation in the acutely spinal cord-injured individual. J Neurosci Nurs 24:185–189

De la Torre JC, Johnson CM, Goode DJ et al. (1975) Pharmacological treatment and evaluation of permanent experimental spinal cord trauma. Neurology 25:508–514

Dimitrijevicz MR, Prevec TS, Sherwood A et al. (1980) Somatosensory perception and cortical evoked potential in established paraplegia. In: Symposium international. Application cliniques des potentiels evoques en neurologie. Resumes, Lyon, p 101

Ducker TB (1976) Experimental injury of the spinal cord. In: Vinken P, Bruin G (eds) Handbook of clinical neurology, vol 25. Elsevier, Amsterdamm, pp 9–26

Ducker TB, Hamit HF (1970) Experimental treatment of spinal cord injury. J Neurosurg 33:554–563

Ducker TB, Salcman M, Daniell HB (1978) Experimental spinal cord trauma, III. Therapeutic effect of immobilization and pharmacologic agents. Surg Neurol 10:71–76

Ertekin C, Mutlu R, Sarica Y et al. (1980) Electrophysiological evaluation of the afferent spinal roots and nerves in patients with conus medullaris and cauda lesions. J Neurol Sci 48:419–433

Faden AI, Jakobs TP, Holaday J (1981a) Endorphins in experimental spinal cord injury: therapeutic effects of naloxone. Ann Neurol 10:326–332

Faden AI, Jabobs TP, Holaday J (1981b) Opiate antagonists improve neurological recovery after spinal injury. Science 211:493–494

Faden AI (1984) Opiate antagonists and thyrotropin releasing hormone. JAMA 252:1452–1454

Hall M (1843) New memoir on the nervous system. Balliere, London

Holdsworth F (1963) Fractures, dislocations and fracture-dislocations of the spine. J Bone Joint Surg [Br] 45:6–20

Holdsworth F (1970) Fractures, dislocations and fracture-dislocations of the spine. J Bone Joint Surg [Am] 52:1535–1551

Kraus JF, Franti CE, Riggins RS et al. (1975) Incidence of traumatic spinal cord lesions. J Chronic Dis 28:471–492

Krebs M, Halvorsen RB, Fishman JJ et al. (1984) Prevention of urinary tract infection during intermittent catheterization. J Urol 131:82–85

Leyendecker K, Schirmer M (1985) Traumatische Rückenmarksschädigungen. In: Schirmer M (ed) Querschnittlähmungen. Springer, Berlin Heidelberg New York, p 236

Lob A (1954) Die Wirbelsäulenverletzung und ihre Ausheilung. Thieme, Stuttgart

Longe RL (1986) Current concepts in clinical therapeutics: pressure sores. Clin Pharm 5:669–681

Louis R (1977) Les théories de l'instabilité. Rev Chir Orthop 63:423–426

Marshall SB, Marshall LF, Vos HR, Chesnut RM (eds) (1990) Neuroscience critical care. Saunders, Philadelphia

Mawson AR, Biundo JJ Jr, Neville P et al. (1988) Risk factors for early-occurring pressure ulcers following spinal cord injury. Am J Phys Med Rehabil 67:123–127

Maynard FM, Diokno AC (1984) Urinary infection and complications during clean intermittent catheterization following spinal cord injury. J Urol 132:943–946

Mesard L, Carmody A, Mannarino E et al. (1978) Survival after spinal cord trauma: a life-table analysis. Arch Neurol 35:78–83

Mirvis SE, Geisler FH, Jelinek JJ et al. (1988) Acute cervical spinal trauma: evaluation with 1.5-T MR imaging. Radiology 166:807–816

Nicoll EA (1949) Fractures of the dorsolumbar spine. J Bone Joint Surg 31:376–395

Rosner MJ (1990) Medical management of spinal cord injury. In: Pitts LH, Wagner FC Jr (eds) Craniospinal trauma. Thieme, Stuttgart, pp 213–225

Roy-Camille R, Zerah JC (1970) Osteosynthèse des fractures du rachis dorsal et lombaire – actualités de chirurgie orthopédique de l'Hopital R Poincaré VIII. Masson, Paris, pp 196–203

Roy-Camille R, Roy-Camille M, Saillant G et al. (1972) Des indications thérapeutiques chirurgicales dans les traumatismes vertébraux avec syndrome médullaire ou syndrome medullaire ou syndrome de la queue de cheval. Nouv Press Med 1:2165

Roy-Camille R, Berteaux D, Saillant J (1977) Synthèse du rachis dorso-lombaire traumatique par plaques vissées dans les pédicules vertébraux. Rev Orthop 63:452–465

Roy-Camille R, Saillant G, Saillant MA et al. (1980) Behandlung von Wirbelfrakturen und -luxationen am thorako-lumbalen Übergang. Orthopade 9:63-68

Schirmer M (1980) Die lumbale longitudinal Myelotomie – eine Möglichkeit in der Behandlung schwerster spinaler spastischer Lähmungen – klinische und experimentelle Untersuchungen. Habilitationsschrift, University of Düsseldorf

Schramm J (1985a) Evozierte Potentiale in der Praxis. Springer, Berlin Heidelberg New York

Schramm J (1985b) Spinal cord monitoring: current status and new developments. Cent Nerv Syst Trauma 3:207-227

Sedgwick EM, El-Negamy E, Frankel H (1980) Spinal cord potentials in traumatic paraple- gia and quadriplegia. J Neurol Neurosurg Psychiatr 43:823-830

Shimoij K, Kano T, Morioka T et al. (1973) Evoked spinal electrogram in a quadriple- gic patient. Electroencephal Clin Neuro- physiol 35:659-662

Stover SL, Fine PR (1987) The epidemiology and economics of spinal cord injury. Para- plegia 25:225-228

Tator CH, Edmonds VE (1979) Acute spinal cord injury: analysis of epidemiological factors. Can J Surg 22:575-578

Young JS, Northrup EN (1979) Statistical infor- mation pertaining to some of the most commonly asked questions about SCI. Spinal Cord Inj Dig 1:11-31

Central Nervous System Neoplasms, Metastases, and Earcinomatous Meningitis

Chapter 62

General Treatment of Brain Tumors

GABRIELE SCHMITZ-SCHACKERT and THOMAS P. BLECK

Definition

The annual incidence of primary intracranial tumors is estimated at 12.3 per 100 000 population. The average annual age-adjusted mortality for nervous system neoplasms ranges between 3.8 and 5.4 per 100 000 standard population. Fifty-eight percent of cerebral tumors recorded are primary. The most common intracranial tumors in adults are gliomas (50%), followed by meningiomas (20%), pituitary adenomas (10%), neurinomas (6%), and craniopharyngiomas (4%). The incidence of brain metastases ranges between 3.7 and 11.1 per 100 000 inhabitants. The mortality of patients with brain tumors amounts to five deaths in every 100 000 inhabitants per year among males and four among females. The relation of brain tumors to all other tumors is 2–3%.

The incidence of cerebral tumors is related to age. In children, CNS malignancies occur with a relatively high frequency. In this age-group they are the second most common form of cancer. Nineteen percent of all cancers in persons below the age of 15 are derived from the central nervous system, and 15–20% of all intracranial tumors occur in childhood. Thereafter, the incidence of intracranial tumors increases with age.

The incidence of primary cerebral tumors seems to be the same for most races, with the exception of the black population, in whom it is lower than in whites.

The treatment of choice for intracranial tumors is surgery. All brain tumor patients should be admitted postoperatively to an intensive care unit. They stay for about 12–24 h before they can be transferred back to the neurosurgical ward. Should complications arise, e.g., tumor bleeding, postoperative hemorrhage, or excessive brain swelling, intensive care is needed for a much longer period of time. In addition, a few patients will be admitted to the ICU because of coma of unknown origin with signs of evolving herniation. In these patients neuroimaging reveals the brain tumor as the underlying disorder.

Section Editor: Thomas P. Bleck

Pathogenesis

Oncogenes and growth factors play an important role in brain tumor development and progression. The mutation of normal genes into oncogenes results in many human tumors. Proto-oncogenes, identified by retroviral transduction, encode for aberrant proteins, of which normal homologues are involved in growth control. A high expression of the epidermal growth factor (EGF) receptor in glioma cells and an amplification of the EGF receptor gene have been described. Glioblastoma cell lines produce a platelet-derived growth factor (PDGF)-like growth factor. The presence of these proteins has been correlated with the expression of c-sis-mRNA oncogene.

The Rous sarcoma virus (RSV), discovered in 1912, was the first recognized oncogenic virus. The avian sarcoma virus (ASV, 1936) produces sarcomas in brains of chickens in 75% of cases. Many experimental models of DNA and RNA virus-induced CNS tumors have since been developed. The role of viruses as etiologic agents for human tumors is under investigation. The most studied neuro-oncogenic viruses are the papovaviruses. Epidemiologic studies have found a correlation between in utero exposure to SV40-contaminated polio vaccines and an increased incidence of CNS tumors. SV40 and BK DNA sequences have been detected in a number of CNS tumors. This suggests a possible role for papovaviruses in the development of human CNS tumors. Viral induction of brain tumors may also follow infection with herpesviruses.

Immunosuppression increases the incidence of malignant lymphomas, which occur in 30% of cases as primary CNS lymphoma. This is true for patients with AIDS and organ transplants, who frequently develop malignant lymphomas.

To date, there is no evidence that terrestrial radiation induces brain tumors. However, radiation of the brain can induce secondary tumor growth, e.g., meningiomas, astrocytomas, gliomas, and fibrosarcomas.

Chemicals are other exogeneous stimuli for tumor induction in the brain. A high incidence of glioblastoma has been observed among workers in contact with vinyl chloride. In laboratory animals, the chemical substances methylcholantren and ethylnitrosourea cause gliomas.

The presence of receptors for steroid hormones (receptors for glucocorticoids, estrogens, progesterone, and androgens) has been demonstrated in malignant gliomas. Glucocorticoid receptors are found in about 40% of cases, androgen receptors in 25%. In meningiomas combinant receptors for progesterone and glucocorticoids are present in 70% and 60%, respectively.

Endogeneous factors are genetically determined. In von Recklinghausen's disease, a high incidence of brain tumors is known; these are predominantly neurinomas, meningiomas, or gliomas. Concerning the familial incidence, among relatives of patients with gliomas brain tumors occur almost nine times more frequently than among the general population.

Clinical Features and Differential Diagnosis

Neurological Symptoms

The development of tumor growth in the brain is associated with elevated intracranial pressure and focal neurological deficits. The most common signs are headaches (65%), seizures (30%), and motor and sensory deficits (25%). Tumors of the brain parenchyma lead to neurological deficits at an early stage, when the developing tumor is located in functionally important neurological areas. The symptoms correspond to the area of presentation. Even lesions with a diameter of less than 1 cm may produce hemiparesis, when located directly in the central gyrus of the cerebrum. Conversely, tumors may reach a size of more than 4 cm in diameter when located in an area of the brain which is functionally less important – e.g., the right frontal lobe in right-handed patients. Here, the tumor can reach a huge size before symptoms of elevated intracranial pressure – e.g., headache, nausea, vomiting – occur and lead to the diagnosis of tumor growth. In most cases, patients present with both symptoms of elevated intracranial pressure and neurological deficits.

The acute onset of general symptoms or focal neurological deficits may be a sign of tumor bleeding. In some brain lesions, tumor bleeding is a common complication (e.g., metastases of the malignant melanoma, or oligodendroglioma).

Tumors of the cerebellum often lead to an obstructive hydrocephalus by occluding the cerebrospinal fluid pathways, (e.g., by compressing the fourth ventricle). In these cases, symptoms of elevated intracranial pressure are present. In childhood, most crebral tumors are located in the posterior fossa. Vomiting and headache present in the morning should always be investigated. Tumors of the brain stem are less frequent. However, even very small lesions can cause major neurolo-gical deficits. In childhood, gliomas are often located in the brain stem.

Adenomas of the pituitary gland lead either to hormonal deficits or to overproduction of certain hormones, e.g., gigantism in childhood or acromegaly in adulthood. Craniopharyngiomas also affect the hormonal regulation. Compression of the optic chiasm by adenomas or craniopharyngiomas causes the characteristic symptom of bitemporal hemianopsia and loss of vision. Metastases to the pituitary gland usually become apparent by symptoms of diabetes insipidus before other hormonal dysfunctions occur.

Tumors which develop from the dura, e.g., metastases of meningiomas, and are located at the skull base become symptomatic by causing pain or compressing cranial nerves, venous sinuses, and occasionally the brain parenchyma. Leptomeningeal metastases lead to neoplastic meningitis. Such patients develop hydrocephalus or suffer from paresis of cranial nerves.

The patient's history and clinical examination allow the diagnosis in most cases. Whenever patients present with neurological deficits or the first onset of epileptic seizures, computed tomography (CT scan) or magnetic resonance imaging (MRI) is mandatory.

Differential Diagnosis

The differential diagnosis of parenchymal lesions includes infarct, brain abscess, venous sinus thrombosis, and intracerebral hemorrhage due to cavernomas, arteriovenous malformations, and coagulopathy. In leptomeningeal tumors infectious meningitis must be considered. Tumors of the dura have to be differentiated from chronic epidural hematomas.

Ancillary Tests

Electroencephalography

Electroencephalography reveals focal abnormalities or spikes and waves as signs of seizures. Since the sensitivity and specificity of this test is very low, EEG is almost obsolete in the diagnosis of brain tumors. It remains useful in the diagnosis of transient neurological dysfunction in patients with brain tumors.

Neuroradiology

Obviously, conventional radiography of the skull is not the investigation of choice in patients who are expected to be suffering from a brain tumor. Several findings suggesting neoplasm or elevated ICP should raise the suspicion of tumor, however. In early childhood, an X-ray of the skull can reveal splitting of the sutures or increased dipital markings as signs of long-lasting elevated intracranial pressure. Metastases of the skull may manifest as destruction of the diploë or the inner or outer tables of the skull. Meningiomas can cause focal hyperostosis. Macroadenomas of the pituitary gland are associated with enlargement or asymmetry of the sella turcica. Intracanalicular growth of neurinomas of the eighth cranial nerve causes enlargement of the internal auditory canal and meatus, which can be diagnosed on Stenvers views. Optic gliomas cause an enlargement of the optic canal, visible on Rhese views. In calcifying tumors, such as oligodendrogliomas and meningiomas, the calcification may be apparent as a direct tumor sign.

Computed Tomography

CT enhanced with i.v. contrast dye is able to show lesions of a minimal size of 2–3 mm in diameter. In the case of larger tumors, the actual lesion and its peritumoral edema can be grossly distinguished. Malignant tumors, such as glioblastomas or metastases, frequently show a ring enhancement due to central necrosis. Meningiomas are well-circumscribed lesions attached to the meninges. After contrast injection they usually enhance homogeneously and have sharp margins. In small lesions mild edema may be the only sign of beginning neoplasm.

Magnetic Resonance Imaging

The ability of MRI to distinguish between normal tissue and tumor is much greater than that of CT; lesions less than 2 mm in diameter may be detected, depending on their relative signal. MRI enhanced with Gd-DTPA is mandatory in the search for cerebral metastases, as only by enhanced MRI can the number of lesions be determined accurately.

Especially for tumors of the pituitary gland, the brain stem, and tumors in the posterior fossa MRI is the most reliable method. Multiplanar sectioning allows exact localization of the tumor.

Angiography

Angiography has lost importance in the diagnosis of brain tumors since the advent of CT, and later MRI. It is still necessary for surgical planning in meningiomas and to clarify the possibility of embolization before surgery.

Cerebrospinal Fluid Examination

Examination of the cerebrospinal fluid by lumbar puncture is dangerous in patients with brain tumors. In patients suspected to have an intracranial mass, lumbar puncture should never be performed before CT or MR scanning. If the scan shows no evidence of shift or obstruction, an LP may be performed if neoplastic meningitis is a consideration. Only in patients with neoplastic meningitis or tumors close to the ventricular pathways can tumor cells be obtained.

Management

Pre-ICU Treatment

The most urgent aim of treatment is to relieve elevated ICP (Table 1). Tumors of the brain are usually accompanied by vasogenic edema. The disruption of the blood-brain barrier with its tight junctions initiates edema. Plasma proteins and fluid then pass the barrier into the extracellular space. In malignant gliomas, endothelial cells are substituted by tumor cells. Also, the neovascularization of tumors is without a blood-brain barrier. In addition, meningiomas and metastases, which do not derive from ectodermal brain tissue, do not have a blood-brain barrier. The tumor itself, as well as the peritumoral edema, causes a major mass effect. Since the brain is enclosed in the skull, there are only two compartments for compensating increasing intracranial pressure: The ventricular system and the subarachnoid space containing the cerebrospinal fluid, and the blood volume. According to the Monro-Kellie doctrine, the enlargement of one compartment of the brain is possible only with diminishing of the others. In case of tumor growth the augmentation of the tissue results in a reduction of the space of the cerebrospinal fluid (compression of the ventricular and subarachnoid space) and the blood volume (vasoconstriction). Normal intracranial pressure is about 10 mmHg. After exhaustion of the compensating mechanisms the

Table 1. Management prior to admission to the ICU

Tumor diagnosis	CT or MRI
Treatment	
Tumor with moderate edema and mild neurological symptoms	Dexamethasone: 3×1.5 mg/day
Tumor with excessive edema, neurological deficits, somnolence	Dexamethasone: bolus – 40–80 mg; 6×4 mg/day
	Osmodiuretics: glycerin – 2×250 ml/day or mannitol – 0.25 g/kg q 4 h
Tumor bleeding plus loss of consciousness	Corticosteroids:[a] bolus – as above
	Hyperventilation: to pCO_2 of 30 torr
	Osmodiuretics:[a] glycerin or mannitol as above
	Surgery: with additional mannitol and with barbiturates as needed to control ICP

[a] In critical cases the administration of corticosteroids can be increased up to tenfold and the osmodiuretics up to threefold.

intracranial pressure increases significantly, which becomes apparent with neurological symptoms of elevated intracranial pressure, e.g., headache, nausea, vomiting. Thereafter, a midline shift occurs, followed by transtentorial herniation, causing the midbrain syndrome, and finally herniation into the foramen magnum, responsible for brain death.

Corticosteroids

Corticosteroids are the most important method of reducing intracranial pressure; they work by diminishing the peritumoral edema. The antiedematous effect of corticosteroids is produced by sealing the blood-brain barrier. They alone are of remarkable benefit in patients with advanced tumor disease. Initially, 10–80 mg dexamethasone, followed by 4 mg every 4 h, usually results in evident clinical improvement within 12 h in most patients. Short-term side effects of high-dose treatment with steroids are relatively few. In patients with diabetes mellitus, additional insulin may be necessary. In patients with stomach ulcers an increased frequency of bleeding is possible. Ulcer prophylaxis using an H_2-blocker is usually instituted. Common long-term side effects include myopathy, diabetes, osteoporosis, and infections by opportunistic organisms. Besides the increasing susceptibility to infections, the immunodeficiency resulting from the prolonged use of corticosteroids may adversely influence the course of the tumor itself.

Osmotherapy

In some instances of dramatically increased intracranial pressure corticosteroids are not sufficient. Osmotherapy by intravenous infusion of hyperosmolar solutions causes an osmotic gradient between blood and tissue and leads to a reduction of fluid in the extracellular space of the whole body, including the brain. The drugs most commonly used are glycerol and 20% mannitol. In some cases the additional administration of furosemide is useful. For a detailed description of ICP treatment, please refer to Chap. 9.

Antiedematous treatment with corticosteroids or osmodiuretics is not only effective in reducing intracranial pressure; it is also of diagnostic benefit. Many patients present with neurological deficits, e.g., hemiparesis or aphasia caused by the developing tumor with its peritumoral edema. On MR, these lesions are located very close to the central gyrus or in the left frontal or temporal lobe. After treatment with .corticosteroids the symptoms disappear. This gives an important hint to the neurosurgeon that the tumor is not situated in functionally important gyri of the brain and that the operation can be done without causing or aggravating neurological deficits. In cases with evidence for primary lymphoma the corticosteroids are also of diagnostic value, as they reduce the tumor mass itself to a great extent, suggesting the diagnosis of a lymphoma.

Surgery

The aims of surgery in brain tumors are: (a) to obtain tumor tissue for histological classification, (b) to relieve symptoms resulting from compression of brain structures adjacent to the tumor, and (c) to enable the patient to tolerate and gain greater benefit from radiotherapy, chemotherapy, or immunotherapy. Surgery is indicated in all cases of tumor growth which can be removed without causing major neurological deficits. Especially in malignant tumors, e.g., glioblastomas, in which the life expectancy averages about 1 year, surgery should be performed only if the patient will not have to suffer from iatrogenically induced neurological deficits in the time that remains to him.

With brain metastases, the essential questions are the spread of metastases and the number of intracranial lesions. The incidence of solitary lesions ranges between 40 and 60%. The more precise diagnosis with MRI is shifting the number of cerebral metastases toward multiple lesions, getting closer to autopsy data of only 30% solitary lesions. Patients with multiple metastases are only rarely operated on, for example if there are two lesions in easily accessible areas, no further systemic metastases are present, or one of the metastases is situated in the cerebellum, causing an obstruction of the fourth ventricle.

Access to the tumors is gained via craniotomy or craniectomy. Progress in surgical approaches using the microscope and microsurgical techniques allow the preservation of functionally important brain structures. The employment of intraoperative ultrasound makes it possible to locate deeply situated tumors and to choose an approach by incision of the cortex in a manner avoiding neurological deficits. Meningiomas usually grow by displacing brain tissue, whereas malignant glioblastomas infiltrate normal tissue. Usually, the removal of benign tumors such as meningiomas can be done curatively, without destroying normal tissue. In cases of infiltrating tumor growth, e.g., glioblastomas or low-grade astrocytomas, the extirpation of the lesions has to be considered subtotal, as demonstrated by recurrent tumor growth in situ. Metastases are well circumscribed against the surrounding brain tissue and may allow total removal. Intrasellar tumors of the pituitary gland are approached by the transnasal transsphenoidal pathway.

Posterior fossa tumors are approached by craniectomy. Tumors which develop close to the ventricular system or in the posterior fossa are likely to cause an obstruction of the cerebrospinal fluid pathways, which results in an obstructive hydrocephalus. In cases of dramatic widening of the ventricular system with a life-threatening increase of intracranial pressure, external drainage of the cerebrospinal fluid is necessary. An internal shunt has to be considered in tumor growth of the midbrain or brain stem, in which removal of the tumor mass is not possible and obstructive hydrocephalus has developed. In tumors which can not be operated on, the histological diagnosis has to be gained by means of a stereotaxic biopsy.

ICU Management

The common postoperative course involves admission of the patient to the intensive care unit overnight and transfer to the neurosurgical ward on the day after. All patients should be in an elevated position; a 30° raised position of the bed is effective prophylaxis against raised intracranial pressure in that it optimizes venous outflow. In the early postoperative phase monitoring of the ECG, blood pressure, and the state of consciousness of the patient are essential. One of the most important parts of postoperative surveillance is the clinical examination. Examination of the pupils is mandatory as soon as the patient awakens after the operation. The aim of postoperative surveillance of patients is early detection of excessive brain swelling or occurrence of a hemorrhage.

Airway Control

Patients who require intubation should receive lidocaine 1 mg/kg and thiopental 3 mg/kg to diminish the ICP elevation associated with laryngoscopy. This should be followed by frequent blood pressure monitoring, as the thiopental may produce transient hypotension.

Blood Pressure

An excessive rise of the blood pressure has to be strictly avoided. High blood pressure, even lasting for only some hours, can significantly enhance edema formation in brain tumor patients. With a disrupted blood-brain barrier, fluid passes from the capillaries into the extracellular space according to the gradient between the blood pressure and the resistance of the surrounding tissue. Hypertension can not only initiate brain edema, but also increase the incidence of postoperative hemorrhage.

Cerebral Perfusion and Elevated ICP

Cerebral perfusion depends on the intracranial pressure. The elevation of intracranial pressure leads to a decrease of cerebral perfusion, and causes a compression of the thin-walled venules. Despite the diminished cerebral perfusion pressure, capillary blood flow initially remains unaltered on account of the compensatory dilatation of the cerebral arterioles (autoregulation). If the cerebral perfusion pressure is reduced to below 50 mmHg, the autoregulation is exhausted by maximal dilatation of the arterioles and cerebral ischemia develops. If the intracranial pressure is as high as the blood pressure, the circulation stops and brain death occurs.

The treatment of elevated ICP is detailed in Chap. 9. Some of the special aspects of ICP treatment after surgery include hyperventilation, barbiturates, cooling, and surgical procedures.

Hyperventilation affects the brain by alkalosis, causing vasoconstriction of the arterioles with reduction of the intracranial blood volume and decrease of intracranial pressure. The arterial CO_2 partial volume should be about 30 mmHg. Lower values should be avoided, as they may cause acidosis of the tissue, with resulting hyperemia.

Cerebral O_2 utilization, brain perfusion, and intracranial pressure are diminished after treatment with barbiturates. They may have a protective effect against dramatic pressure elevation. A sufficient O_2 supply of the edematous brain tissue and maintenance of a normal arterial pO_2 are extremely important. Often hypercapnia results in addition to hypoxia in patients who cannot control their airways or ventilation. Hypercapnia and hypoxia each cause dilatation of the cerebrovascular system. The increased blood volume further elevates intracranial pressure. Hyperventilation reduces systemic venous return, which may prompt hypotension requiring volume administration (with isotonic saline).

Table 2. Management in the ICU

Postoperative management:	Elevation of the head to 30°, blood pressure: systolic: 120–160 mmHg pupil check every 30 min corticosteroids: 6 × 4 mg/day dexamethasone
Postoperative brain edema with unconsciousness	Elevation of the bed to 30°, sedation, relaxation for optimal hyperventilation hypocapnia – arterial CO_2 30 mmHg blood pressure: systolic 120–160 mmHg corticosteroids: 6 × 4 mg/day dexamethasone osmodiuretics: 2 × 250 ml glycerol, or mannitol 20% (0.15–0.3 mg/kg body weight) q 4 h furosemide: 1 mg/kg/body weight
	Intracranial pressure >30 mmHg: thiopental or pentobarbital: bolus: 5–10 mg/kg body weight, then: 1–3 mg/kg body weight/h
Brain edema resistant to medication (ICP > 30 mmHg)	Craniectomy, duraplasty, ICP monitor

The O_2 utilization of brain tissue is highly dependent on the body temperature. When fever occurs the tissue needs more O_2. Existing brain edema will increase, and the intracranial pressure will be elevated. Cooling of the body surface by a fan, ice, and alcohol, antipyretic drugs, and infusions in order to restore the intravascular volume may be helpful.

Craniectomy is indicated as soon as conservative treatment fails to sufficiently reduce existing intracranial pressure. Extended craniectomy with implantation of a duraplasty provides enough space for excessive brain edema, when it is resistant to drug treatment. An ICP monitor should be installed for optimal postoperative surveillance; in cases where an internal hydrocephalus has developed, an external ventricular drain will be necessary. Table 2 summarizes ICP treatment strategies following brain surgery.

Table 3. Management of special problems and complications

Postoperative hemorrhage	Surgery: evacuation of the hematoma
Brain edema not responding to medication	Craniectomy, duraplasty, ICP monitor
Occlusive hydrocephalus	External drainage

Management of Special Complications

Causes of postoperative ICP elevations which may necessitate reoperation include: (a) postoperative hemorrhage, (b) postoperative brain swelling, (c) postoperative occlusive hydrocephalus, (d) tumor bleeding, and (e) occlusive hydrocephalus by tumor growth, e.g., in the posterior fossa (Table 3).

Sudden, excessively elevated blood pressure and bradycardia, as well as a dilated pupil, indicate a post-operative complication, such as a hemorrhage into the tumor cavity or excessive brain swelling. Surgery must follow immediately. In case of bleeding, the hemorrhage has to be evacuated. In case of excessive brain edema, in which medication has failed, the ultimate measure should be a large decompressive craniectomy with duraplasty and implantation of an ICP monitor.

Prognosis and Rehabilitation

In most cases brain tumors can be extirpated without causing additional neurological deficits. The prognosis depends on the biological behavior of the tumor. The life expectancy of patients with glioblastomas averages about 1 year. The tumor will recur locally. Patients with benign tumors can be cured by operation. Patients suffering from neurological deficits should be admitted to a rehabilitation center.

Suggested Reading

Kornblith PL, Walker MD (eds) (1988) Advances in neuro-oncology. Futura, Mount Kisco

Paoletti P (1991a) New aspects of brain tumor biology. Crit Rev Neurosurg 1:35–45

Paoletti P (1991b) New aspects of brain tumor therapy. Crit Rev Neurosurg 1:248–262

Suzuki J (ed) (1988) Treatment of glioma. Springer, Berlin Heidelberg New York

Chapter 63

Lymphomas of the Central Nervous System

MARTIN HUTSCHENREUTER and RICHARD HERRMANN

Introduction

Lymphomas of the central nervous system (CNS) make up a heterogeneous group of malignant tumors that involve mainly the brain parenchyma but can also involve the spinal cord, meninges, and cranial nerves or spinal roots. From a neurological perspective, primary non-Hodgkin's lymphomas of the CNS represent the most important subgroup.

They do not occur frequently but the incidence is increasing. Without underlying immunological disease, they account for approximately 1.5% of all intracranial tumors and fewer than 2% of all malignant lymphomas. Immunocompromised patients, such as transplant recipients, those with congenital immunodeficiency syndromes, and those with human immunodeficiency virus infection (HIV), have a 100- to 1000-fold increased risk of developing a primary lymphoma of the CNS. The development of a primary CNS lymphoma is an AIDS-defining illness. The age at onset varies widely and they are slightly more common in men.

Pathogenesis and Classification

The tumors are found where lymphoreticular tissue is normally absent. Several theories provide interesting but unproven explanations. Exogenous factors, especially Epstein-Barr virus, may play a role. Most of the lymphomas are of the B-cell type and are classified histologically according to the "Working Formulation" classification or the "Kiel classification." They are multicentric and diffusely infiltrating in more than 60% of cases. Regardless of whether they are generalized or associated with HIV, they are usually high-grade malignancies. "Lymphomatoid granulomatosis," or "malignant angioendotheliomatosis," is a rare form of lymphoma that can occlude small vessels of the brain.

Section Editor: Thomas P. Bleck

Clinical Features and Differential Diagnosis

Patients with an intracerebral lymphoma usually develop symptoms and signs of a rapidly growing intracranial mass. Depending on the location of the mass, patients may have headache, neuropsychological changes, focal deficits, or seizures. Rapidly progressive dementia and stroke-like symptoms are also possible. Patients with uveal or vitreous deposits of the eye may or may not be symptomatic. Involvement of cranial nerves and spinal roots may occur because of meningeal infiltration, but involvement of the spinal cord is extremely rare.

For diagnostic, therapeutic, and prognostic purposes, CNS lymphomas can be divided into four groups: (a) primary lymphomas in immunocompetent patients, (b) primary lymphomas in immunocompromised patients, (c) CNS involvement of systemic lymphomas, and (d) a small subgroup of other different etiologies. In an otherwise healthy patient with a CNS lymphoma, the probability of detecting a systemic lymphoma is less than 5%. All patients should be questioned about the use of immunosuppressive drugs for autoimmune diseases or after organ transplant, risk factors for HIV infection, and symptoms of an underlying systemic disease such as fever, night sweats, weight loss, gastrointestinal symptoms, or bone pain. Physical examination should be directed to the lymph nodes (including Waldeyer's ring), liver and spleen size, and signs of opportunistic infections or neoplasms of the skin, lung, or mucous membranes. Some patients, for example those with AIDS, can have lympadenopathy and hepatosplenomegaly for reasons other than lymphoma.

The differential diagnosis of patients with symptoms and signs of a CNS lymphoma is listed in Table 1. Because of their frequent multiple sites and some morphological features, solid tumor metastases and abscesses are especially important. In patients with AIDS, toxoplasmosis is the most important disease that can present in the same way as a primary CNS lymphoma, and the two diseases may co-exist.

Ancillary Tests

Neuroimaging

Lymphomas appear as isodense or slightly hyperdense lesions on CT scan

Table 1. Differential diagnosis of intracerebral lymphomas

Neoplastic	Inflammatory	Others
Primary tumors of the brain and meninges (high-grade gliomas, meningiomas, sarcomas)	Abscesses, granulomas, focal encephalitis Bacterial, viral, fungal, parasital	Low-flow vascular malformations
Metastases of carcinomas and sarcomas	Sarcoidosis Multiple sclerosis	

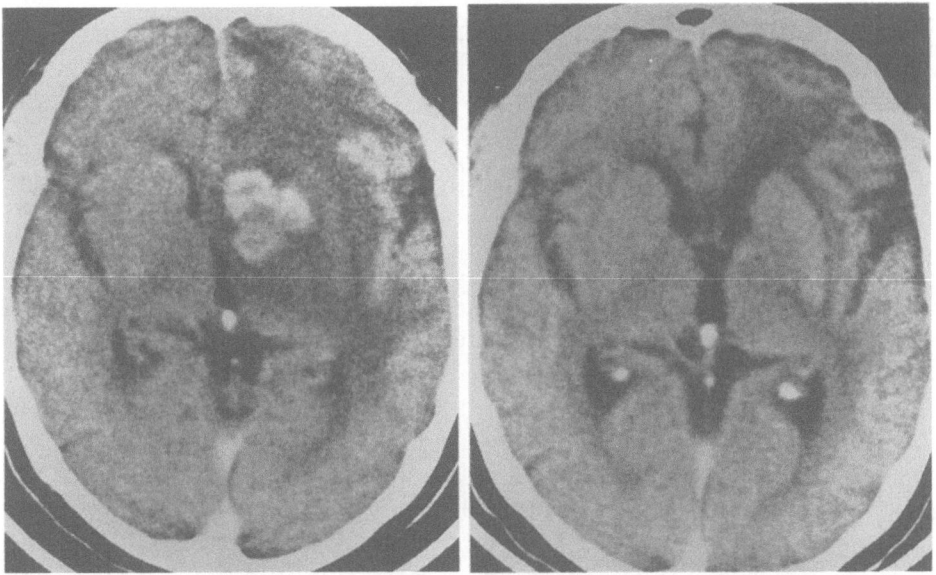

Fig. 1a,b. CT appearance of a primary lymphoma of the brain in a 44-year-old man with poor concentration and recurrent mild right hemiparesis. Inital axial CT scan obtained after IV administration of iodinated contrast material (**a**) shows trilobed enhancing mass lesion surrounded by extensive edema that involves anterior left striatum near frontal horn. Corresponding scan obtained 2 weeks later, after treatment of the patient with high doses of steroids (**b**), reveals disappearance of the abnormal enhancement plus marked reduction of the perifocal edema. (Courtesy of Klaus Sartor and Marius Hartmann, Heidelberg)

without contrast and show strong homogeneous enhancement when contrast is used. The surrounding edema is moderate compared with that of other masses. Multiple masses are found in more than 30% of patients. They are more frequently supratentorial and usually develop next to ventricular or subarachnoid spaces (Fig. 1); ocular infiltration can occasionally be detected. Despite their relatively characteristic appearance, these features are nonspecific.

MRI is more sensitive than CT (Fig. 2). It may detect small intracerebral nodules and meningeal or ependymal involvement and may be helpful in finding superficial lesions for biopsy. As with patients in the neurocritical care unit, these diagnostic advantages are outweighed by problems in managing these patients during the study. MRI is not more specific, and signal intensities vary widely. This applies to AIDS-associated lymphomas, too, which are often associated with ring-enhancing lesions or irregular patterns. For the correct interpretation of all imaging studies, it is important to remember that lymphomas grow along cerebral blood vessels, and their histological borders lie far beyond the visible limits.

Angiography occasionally may provide additional information in cases of very difficult differential diagnosis including vascular malformations. In patients with "lymphomatoid granulo-

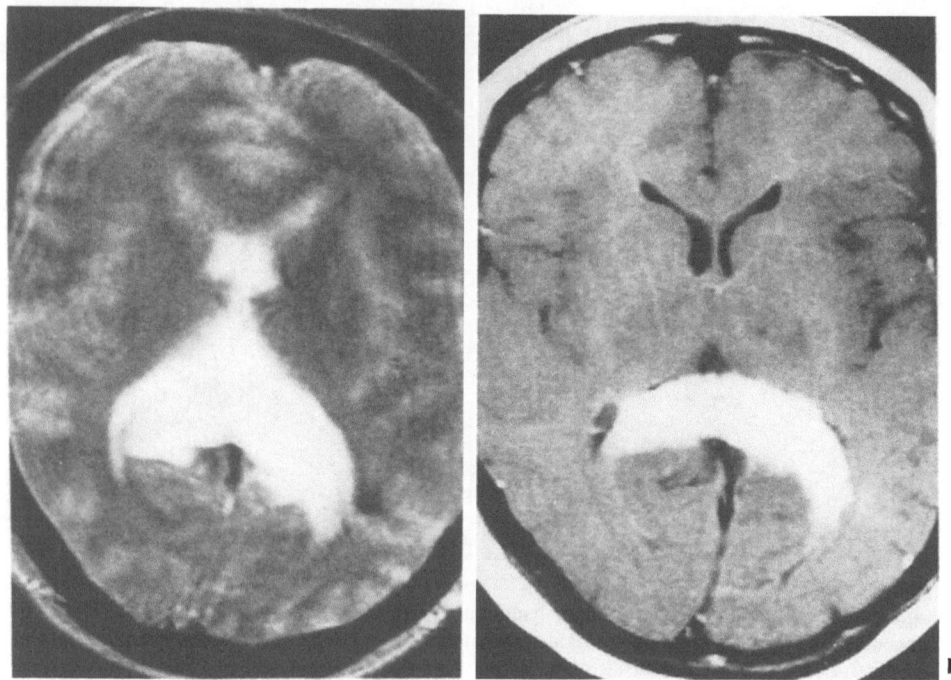

a   b

Fig. 2a,b. Primary lymphoma of the brain in a 52-year-old woman with headaches, poor volition, and change in mental status. T2-weighted axial MR image (**a**) shows abnormally increased signal intensity in swollen-appearing splenium of the corpus callosum. Corresponding T1-weighted image after IV administration of paramagnetic contrast material reveals dense homogeneous enhancement of splenium, with some extension of enhancement into left parietal white matter. (Courtesy of Klaus Sartor and Marius Hartmann, Heidelberg)

matosis," the results of angiography may be falsely negative because occlusion of capillaries cannot be detected.

Cerebrospinal Fluid and Other Laboratory Tests

A lumbar puncture should be done on all patients, excepting those with clinical signs of increased intracranial pressure. Atypical lymphocytes bearing B-cell immunocytological markers are detected in 10% of patients. Most patients have nonspecific changes such as an increased protein concen-tration and pleocytosis. An increase in beta-2 microglobulin concentration may be a helpful marker in patients without HIV infection.

Other laboratory tests should include a complete blood count, liver enzymes, lactate dehydrogenase, serum alkaline phosphatase, serum protein, and immunoelectophoresis, serolgic evaluation for HIV antibodies and, as needed, for other viruses and parasites. The significance of the latter should not be overestimated, especially if there are no former baseline results available. A paralleled CSF evaluation may lead to better interpretation.

Biopsy

If CSF studies are negative, then a CT-guided stereotactic biopsy should be done whenever prognostic and therapeutic implications are suffcient; there is no other way to prove the diagnosis. With the aid of immunohistochemistry, diagnostic results are comparable to those of larger surgical specimens. Biopsies should be done, whenever possible, with the patient not taking corticosteroids (ideally, after a steroid-free interval of 2 weeks).

Staging

Neurological staging, including a lumbar puncture, ophthalmological examination, and careful neuroradiological CNS imaging, is essential. If systemic lymphoma is suspected, at least a chest X-ray, an abdominal CT scan, and a bone marrow biopsy are recommended.

Management

General ICU therapy should focus on symptoms of increased intracranial pressure and seizures. Following the basic therapeutic and diagnostic management, it should be decided whether immediate surgical intervention (tumor resection and/or ventricular shunt) is needed. If the neuroradiological evaluation suggests an intracerebral lymphoma, conservative treatment should exclude the use of corticosteroids whenever possible; their cytotoxic effects can obscure the biopsy results. Nevertheless, if there are major space-occupying effects and signs of transtentorial herniation, dexamethasone should be given immediately. After removal of a histological specimen, treatment with corticosteroids can be started at once – for example, dexamethasone 100 mg i.v., followed by 24 mg/day. Complete tumor resection is not part of the treatment strategy. Because radiotherapy, formerly the standard treatment, is not always effective as desired, several groups have combined it with chemotherapy. Increasing evidence suggests that with this approach, results can be improved. This applies to both patients who undergo surgery and those who do not. Current recommendations are listed in Table 2. Drugs, doses, and ways of administration are still controversial.

For patients with a poor prognosis (older age, widely disseminated tumor, and other multiple medical problems) the cytotoxic effects of steroids may be sufficient, possibly supplemented by radiation therapy for palliation. In these patients, rapid regression or disappearance of a mass lesion on CT is felt to be sufficient for a diagnosis of brain lymphoma, although some radiation therapists still require biopsies. In patients with AIDS in whom the diagnosis is not clear, additional treatment for toxoplasmosis can be justified. If the mass does not resolve with this regimen, then lymphoma-specific management can be started. In organ-transplant recipients, it sometimes may be sufficient to decrease the dose or discontinue the immunosupressive drugs.

Table 2. Therapy of intracerebral lymphomas

Primary non-Hodgkin's lymphomas in immunocompetent patients	Hochberg et al. (1991): Dexamethasone 24 mg/d. Pre-irradiation i.v. MTX ($1-3$ g/m^2 every $7-21$ days). Intrathecal MTX as needed (12 mg twice a week). Whole-brain irradiation (25×180 cGy). Orbit and spine included as needed. Recurrent tumors: intravenous MTX (3.5 g/m^2 or ARA-C 3 g/m^2). De Angelis et al. (1992): Dexamethasone 16 mg/d. Pre-irradiation i.v. MTX (1 g/m^2 weekly for two doses) plus six doses of intraventricular (Ommaya) MTX (12 mg/dose). Whole-brain irradiation (20×200 cGy with 8×180 cGy boost). Two doses of i.v. cytosine arabinoside (3 g/m^2 every 3 weeks post-irradiation). Neuwelt et al. (1991): Intra-arterial MTX after blood-brain barrier disruption, combined with i.v. and oral chemotherapy
Primary non-Hodgkin's lymphomas in AIDS patients	Hochberg et al. (1991) – whole-brain irradiation in a range of 4000 cGy with single doses of $180-200$ cGy, or 150 cGy plus a boost of 2000 cGy
Cerebral manifestations in systemic lymphomas	According to the detailed treatment recommendations in generalized Hodgkin's and non-Hodgkin's lymphomas dependent on histology and staging
Lymphomatoid granulomatosis	Established therapeutic rules do not exist. Radio- and chemotherapies are under discussion.

Prognosis

In general, the prognosis is poor. Without therapy most patients live weeks to months, and with appropriate, quick, and aggressive therapy, the median survival is about 40 months.

Suggested Reading

DeAngelis LM, Yahalom J, Thaler HT, Kher U (1992) Combined-modality therapy for primary CNS lymphoma. J Clin Oncol 10:635–643

Hochberg FH, Miller DC (1988) Primary central nervous system lymphoma. J Neurosurg 68:835–853

Hochberg FH, Loeffler JS, Prados M (1991) The therapy of primary brain lymphoma. J Neurooncol 10:191–201

Levine AM, Sullivan-Halley J, Pike MC, Rarick MU, Loureiro C, Bernstein-Singer M, Willson E, Brynes R, Parker J, Rasheed S, Gill PS (1991) Human immunodeficiency virus-related lymphoma. Cancer 68: 2466–2472

Moormeier JA, Williams SF, Golomb HM (1990) The staging of non-Hodgkin lymphomas. Semin Oncol 17:43–50

Neuwelt EA, Goldman DL, Dahlborg SA, Crossen J, Ramsey F, Roman-Goldstein S, Braziel R, Dana B (1991) Primary CNS lymphoma treated with osmotic blood-brain barrier disruption: prolonged survival and preservation of cognitive function. J Clin Oncol 9:1580–1590

Chapter 64

Carcinomatous and Leukemic Meningitis

Brigitte Storch-Hagenlocher, Richard Herrmann, and Martin Schabet

Introduction

Because patients with malignancies are now surviving for longer periods, carcinomatous and leukemic meningitis is becoming more common. The most frequent solid malignancies to involve the meninges are those of the breast, lung, gastrointestinal tract, and genitourinary tract, and malignant melanomas (Table 1). In most patients, neoplastic meningitis occurs late in the course of the disease when the cancer is far advanced. Patients with acute lymphocytic and acute myelogenous leukemia and patients with high-grade non-Hodgkin's lymphoma are also at high risk of meningeal infiltration, which can be reduced by prophylactic intrathecal chemotherapy and radiation of the CNS. Primary brain tumors such as germinoma, ependymoma, and medulloblastoma may also invade the meninges.

Clinical Features

A history of cancer and signs of multiple lesions in the nervous system should suggest the diagnosis. The most common symptoms of neoplastic meningitis are confusion, headache, nausea, vomiting, gait dysfunction, back pain (with or without radicular radiation), double vision, and photophobia. Neurological examination may reveal cranial nerve abnormalities including disorders of ocular motility, nystagmus, facial weakness, impaired hearing, and dysphagia. Central or radicular palsies, especially of the lower limbs, are also frequently present and deep tendon reflexes may be decreased or absent. Patients may have ataxia, stiff neck, and altered states of consciousness.

Diagnosis

Cerebrospinal Fluid and Other Laboratory Findings

Cytological examination of cerebrospinal fluid reveals tumor cells in 60%

Section Editor: Thomas P. Bleck

Table 1. Incidence of neoplastic meningitis

	%
Leukemia, non-Hodgkin's lymphoma	5–15
Breast cancer	5
Malignant melanoma	5–15
Lung cancer	10–20
Small cell carcinoma of the lung	≥25

of patients and is the single most important test for the diagnosis of neoplastic menigitis. The presence of tumor cells in the CSF (which often requires several examinations of large volumes of fluid) confirms neoplastic meningitis; however, the absence of tumor cells does not exclude the diagnosis. The best technique for detecting the tumor cells begins with centrifuging the CSF mildly. The sediment is then centrifuged again in a protein-containing culture medium and stained with May-Grünwald-Giemsa stain. This stain is often sufficient to allow differentiation of carcinoma cells and malignant melanoma cells from normal cells. In about 20% of patients, particularly those with malignant lymphomas and leukemia, it may be difficult to distinguish malignant cells from inflammatory cells and additional immunochemical staining is needed.

Cell count and lactate concentration may be mildly elevated and protein concentration may be markedly increased. Glucose concentration and pH may be decreased. An increased IgG index and oligoclonal bands are detected in 40% of patients with leukemic meningitis (less frequently in patients with carcinomatous meningitis). Specific tumor markers, such as intrathecally produced carcinoembryonic antigen (CEA), may be helpful especially in patients with carcinomatous meningitis. Because CEA crosses the blood-brain barrier like IgG, the ratio of CEA in the CSF to CEA in the serum must be calculated like the IgG index (CEA index). Other markers include β_2-microglobulin in patients with leukemic meningitis or lymphoma, and β-human chorionic gonadotroin (β-HCG) and α-fetoprotein (AFP) in patients with germ cell tumors. Tumor markers, CSF lactate levels, and pH are useful in monitoring the patient's response to treatment. It can be difficult, especially in immunocompromised patients, to distinguish neoplastic meningitis from subacute or chronic meningitis caused by viruses, fungi, mycobacteria, spirochetes, or parasites. In these cases, special stains (Gram's stain, India ink, and methenamine silver) need to be done.

Neuroimaging and Other Ancillary Tests

CT and MR findings are nonspecific. CT is usually ordered first to exclude a space-occupying primary tumor, intracerebral metastasis, or hydrocephalus. It should be done before lumbar puncture. Mild ventricular enlargement is often seen on both CT and MRI as a result of impaired resorption of CSF. Contrast enhancement of the meninges (mainly in the cisternal area, sulci, and tentorium) can be seen on MRI (Fig. 1) and less often on CT.

Electrophysiologic studies are less important for the diagnosis of neoplastic meningitis. Diffuse slowing may be seen on EEG and spontaneous activity in the paravertebral muscles can sometimes be seen on EMG.

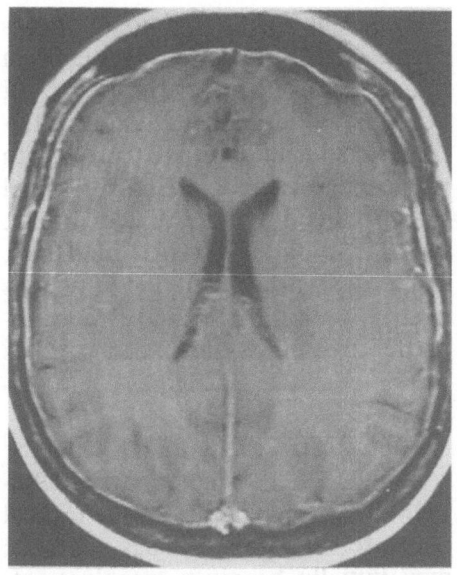

Fig. 1. Meningeal carcinomatosis in a 42-year-old woman with metastatic carcinoma of the breast, headaches, nausea and vomiting, and abnormal CSF findings (neoplastic cells). T1-weighted axial MR image obtained after IV administration of paramagnetic contrast material is remarkable for abnormal linear enhancement of the dural–arachnoidal complex over both cerebral hemispheres. More nodular enhancement would be more specific for neoplastic meningeal involvement, since linear enhancement itself is nonspecific, potentially occurring even after lumbar puncture. (Courtesy of Klaus Sartor and Marius Hartmann, Heidelberg)

Treatment

Treatment of patients with neoplastic meningitis includes radiation and chemotherapy. Both methotrexate (MTX) and cytosine arabinoside (ara-C), can be given intrathecally. MTX is usually preferred except in patients with leukemic or lymphomatous meningitis, for which a combination of MTX and ara-C is given (using the recommended single dose of each drug). For patients with neoplastic

meningitis from solid tumors, especially breast cancer, thiotepa can be used. Little information is available, however, about the efficacy or toxicity of other chemotherapeutic agents when given by intrathecal injection (for example, dacarbazine (DTIC), interferon, or IL-2). Promising results have been reported of treatment with ^{131}I-labeled monoclonal antibodies against tumor cell surface antigens.

Children with neoplastic meningitis require a special management, which is not discussed in this context. Therapy in adults too must consider individual clinical situations, the primary tumor, and prognostic factors. Once the diagnosis of neoplastic meningitis has been made and obstruction of CSF circulation has been excluded, intrathecal treatment with MTX should be started immediately. An Ommaya device should be implanted in patients whose overall condition is good and whose systemic metastases are controlled. This device allows easier delivery of drugs with more even distribution in the CSF. Patients may also benefit from systemic treatment with corticosteroids such as dexamethasone 4 mg/day intravenously.

MTX should be given in single doses of 10 mg by intraventricular injection or 15 mg by lumbar puncture (Table 2). Treatment with ara-C should be given in single doses of 40 mg by intraventricular injection or 40–80 mg by lumbar puncture. Cytotoxic drugs need to be dissolved in water, diluted in artificial CSF, or both, to a total volume of 15–20 ml. Solutions that are hyperosmolar to CSF, such as 0.9% normal saline, should not be used. The drug must be instilled slowly, over at least 10 min, with re-

Table 2. Recommended single dose (mg) of antineoplastic drugs for intrathecal instillation

Drug	Ventricular	Lumbar
Methotrexate	10	15
Ara-C	40	40–80
Thiotepa	5–10	10

peated aspiration. Folinic acid should be given 24 h after each MTX dose (four doses of 15 mg given over 48 h). Monitoring of leukocyte and platelet counts is needed and treatment must be stopped if the leukocyte count is less than $3000/mm^3$ or the platelet count is less than $100\,000/mm^3$.

After patients have received about four doses of intrathecal MTX (or ara-C), radiation therapy, directed towards the sites of major involvement (based on clinical and radiological findings), is started (Fig. 2). Patients with intracranial lesions require whole-brain radiation. Those treated intrathecally with cytotoxic drugs should also receive whole-brain radiation, even in the absence of documented intracranial lesions. Multilocular spinal lesions are treated with whole-spine radiation. Smaller spinal seedings need to be radiated focally. Usually 30 Gy are given to the skull, spine, or both in 2-Gy daily fractions over 3 weeks. Patients are concomitantly treated with corticosteroids (dexamethasone 4 mg/day intravenously).

Intrathecal chemotherapy may be continued after completion of radiation therapy depending on the clinical response and CSF findings. Patients may initially be given weekly treatments, followed by monthly treatments. Treatment may be stopped once CSF is free of tumor cells and protein and lactate concentrations have become normal again. A cumulative dose of 150 mg MTX or 700 mg ara-C should not be exceeded.

C	C	C	C	5R	5R	5R	C	C	C	C
Day 1	4	8	12	14	21	28	35	42	49	56

Intrathecal chemotherapy (C)	Radiation (R)
Ommaya (MTX, ara-C, thiotepa) folinic acid substitution after each MTX instillation	Focal lesion(s) (30 Gy) 4–8 mg dexamethasone
or	
LP (MTX, ara-C, thiotepa) folinic acid substitution after each MTX instillation	Focal lesion(s) (30 Gy) whole brain (30 Gy) 4–8 mg dexamethasone

LP, lumbar puncture

Fig. 2. Therapeutic plan for treatment of neoplastic meningitis

Side Effects of Treatment

When drugs are given repeatedly by intrathecal injection, there is a risk of extradural instillation, although small amounts of the drug are probably not harmful. The infection rate is less than 1% when drugs are given by lumbar puncture, but it is 5%–10% when given by intraventricular injection. Both MTX and ara-C are potentially neurotoxic drugs. Within 2–4 h of treatment, patients can develop acute arachnoiditis with headache, backache, vomiting, fever, stiff neck, and mild pleocytosis. Nosocomial meningitis needs to be excluded. Symptoms of acute arachnoiditis usually resolve in 2–3 days and treatment can be restarted. Patients may also have seizures. In fewer than 1% of patients, acute encephalopathy may develop in minutes to hours, with fever, mental status changes, and paresis. An acute radiculopathy can also occur with radicular pain, paraparesis, and disturbed micturition. These patients require neurocritical care and the chemotherapy regimen must be changed.

The most serious complication of intrathecal or intraventricular chemotherapy is toxic leukoencephalopathy. This usually develops months to years after treatment and is characterized by rapidly progressive dementia, seizures, disturbances of consciousness, and coma. The risk is increased in patients treated with more than 150 mg MTX and in those treated simultaneously with radiation therapy.

Prognosis

Neoplastic meningitis is a frequent, life-threatening complication of systemic malignancies. It must be recognized early. Treatment is invasive and is associated with serious side effects but should, nevertheless, be given because without treatment patients have a dismal prognosis (median survival is about 1–2 months). With combined chemotherapy and radiation therapy, the median survival is about 7 months. In most patients, the prognosis is determined by the underlying systemic disease. Approximately 60% of those with neoplastic meningitis will die from systemic manifestations of their disease. Patients with lung cancer and malignant melanoma have the worst prognosis, whereas those with leukemia and non-Hodgkin's lymphoma have a median survival of about 2 years.

Suggested Reading

Bamborschke S, Huber M (1992) CSF cytology in leukemia and malignant lymphoma involving the CNS. Definite diagnosis by immunocytochemistry. Nervenarzt 63: 218–222

Bleyer WA, Byrne TN (1988) Leptomeningeal cancer in leukemia and solid tumors. Curr Probl Cancer 12:181–238

Boogerd W et al. (1988) CSF cytology versus immunocytochemistry in meningeal carcinomatosis. J Neurol Neurosurg Psychiatry 51:142–145

Brown MJ et al. (1987) Infectious complications of intraventricular reservoirs in cancer patients. Pediatr Infect Dis J 6:182–189

Croghan MK, Booth A, Meyskens FL (1988) A phase I trial of recombinant interferon-alpha and alpha-difluoromethylornithine in metastatic melanoma. J Biol Response Mod 7:409–415

Gasecki AP, Bashir RM, Foley J (1992) Leptomeningeal carcinomatosis: a report of 3 cases and review of the literature. Eur Neurol 32:74–78

Herrmann R (1991) Behandlung der Meningeosis neoplastica beim Mammacarcinom. In: ZNS-Metastasierung des Mammacarcinoms. Springer, Berlin Heidelberg New York, p 115

Kaplan RS, Wiernik PH (1982) Neurotoxicity of antineoplastic drugs. Semin Oncol 9:103–130

Krol G, Sze G, Malkin M, Walker R (1988) MR of cranial and spinal meningeal carcinomatosis: comparison with CT and myelography. AJR 151:583–588

Mackintosh FR, Colby TV, Podolsky WJ, Burke JS, Hoppe RT, Rosenfelt FP, Rosenberg SA, Kaplan HS (1982) Central nervous system involvement in non-Hodgkin's lymphoma: an analysis of 105 cases. Cancer 49:586–595

Moseley RP et al. (1991) Carcinomatous meningitis: antibody-guided therapy with I-131 HMFG1. J Neurol Neurosurg Psychiatry 54:260–265

Obbens EAMT, Leavens ME, Beal JW, Lee Y (1985) Ommaya reservoir in 387 cancer patients: a 15 year experience. Neurology 35:1274–1278

Schabet M et al. (1986) Diagnosis and treatment of meningeal carcinomatosis in ten patients with breast cancer. Eur Neurol 25:403–411

Schabet M, Bamberg M, Dichgans J (1992) Diagnosis and therapy of leptomeningeal metastasis. Nervenarzt 63:317–327

Sze G, Soletsky S, Bronen R, Krol G (1989) MR imaging of the cranial meninges with emphasis on contrast enhancement and meningeal carcinomatosis. AJNR 10:965–975

Theodore HT, Gendelman S (1981) Meningeal carcinomatosis. Arch Neurol 38:696–699

Visser de BWO et al. (1983) Intraventricular methotrexate therapy of leptomeningeal metastasis from breast cancer. Neurology 33:1565–1572

Wasserstrom WR, Glass JP, Posner JB (1982) Diagnosis and treatment of leptomeningeal metastasis from solid tumors. Cancer 49:759–772

Weller M, Stevens A, Sommer N, Schabet M, Wiethölter H (1992) Tumor cell dissemination triggers an intrathecal immune response in neoplastic meningitis. Cancer 69:1475–1480

Yuill GM (1980) Leukaemia: neurological involvement. In: Vinken PJ, Bruyn GW (eds) Handbook of clinical neurology, vol 39: Neurological manifestations of systemic diseases, part II. Elsevier/North Holland Biochemical, New York, p 1

Chapter 65

Metastatic Spinal Cord Compression

ELLEN S. LATHI

Introduction and Epidemiology

Metastatic epidural spinal cord compression is a medical emergency which occurs in 5–10% of all cancer patients, or approximately 15 000 each year in the United States. Over half of adult patients presenting with an acute myelopathy will be found to have metastatic spinal cord compression. In addition, spinal cord compression or cauda equina syndrome will be the initial manifestation of cancer in 50% of cases, and half of these will have lung primaries.

Especially in this common disorder, timely diagnosis and treatment have the greatest impact on both quality and length of survival. Over the past decade, there have been important advances in the management of these patients. The more widespread availability of MRI scanning has led to a revision of guidelines for acute management.

Pathogenesis

The vertebral column is the most common bony structure to be involved by metastatic disease, and autopsy studies report that 70% of patients dying with disseminated cancer have vertebral metastases. Hematogenous metastasis to the vertebral body accounts for 90% of cases of epidural compression in patients with solid tumors.

Cord or root compression then results either from direct infiltration by tumor (generally anterior to the spinal cord) or from destruction of the vertebral body with vertebral collapse and secondary cord compression. In a minority of cases, there is infiltration of tumor through the intervertebral foramina from a paravertebral mass. This occurs in 75% of lymphoma patients, but in only 15% of patients with solid tumors. In such cases, bony destruction is often absent, making the diagnosis problematic. A third and even less common mechanism is retrograde venous spread of tumor from Batson's paravertebral plexus, which drains the vertebrae and intervertebral spaces.

Section Editor: Thomas P. Bleck

More than 95% of spinal metastases are epidural. Intradural and intramedullary metastases are exceptionally rare, accounting for less than 1% of the total group. MRI scanning represents a great advance in the diagnosis of intramedullary lesions. Prior to MRI, diagnosis of this syndrome was difficult and often one of exclusion. The actual incidence may be somewhat higher.

In 1983 Constans et al. reported 600 cancer patients with acute cord or root syndromes. Ninety-four percent had bony metastasis – 45% of the vertebral body, 41% of the posterior arch, and 14% involving the entire vertebra. Only 5% had spinal cord compression without bony metastasis, and only 1% had intradural lesions.

Epidural compression often occurs at the site of vertebral involvement, especially if there is vertebral collapse. Involvement of multiple vertebral levels is common. On plain X-rays alone, one third of patients have bony metastases at more than one level. If one combines plain films, CT scanning, and surgical findings, 90% of pateints have bony metastases at more than one level. This is particularly true in breast and prostate cancer. Multiple levels of epidural compression are less common, occurring in about one third of patients.

Epidural compression most commonly occurs in the thoracic region (70%). Compression affects the cervical region in 10% and the lumbosacral region in 20% of cases. Several series demonstrate that neurological outcome produced by an epidural metastasis does not vary with the spinal level of the lesion, i.e., that prognosis does not vary for lesions above and below the conus medullaris.

The most common primary tumors are in the breast and the lung. Patients with breast cancer are more likely to have known bony metastases, a long interval between onset of pain and neurological complaints, evidence of tumor at multiple vertebral levels, and gradual progression. Patients with lung carcinoma are less likely to have widespread bony disease and often have a more rapid course. Other primary tumors include lymphoma, prostate, myeloma, sarcoma, and renal cell carcinoma. These account for 75% of all cases.

Findings

Local or radicular pain is the initial symptom in over 95% of patients. Pain may precede neurological symptoms by days to more than 1 year. The median duration of pain prior to neurological signs is reported to vary from 1 to 6 months, but is usually 4–8 weeks. Pain is typically constant, progressive, aggravated by the Valsalva maneuver and by exercise, and maximal in the recumbent position. Spinal tenderness is almost always present and is often severe. Radicular pain is common and is present in 90% of lumbosacral lesions, 80% of cervical lesions, and 50% of thoracic lesions. Root pain is often bilateral in the thoracic region.

Motor weakness is present in 80% of patients at diagnosis. In this group, 50% will be ambulatory, 35% paraparetic, and only 15% paraplegic. One third of patients with objective weakness at diagnosis will become paraplegic within the first week. Bowel and bladder symptoms or signs are found in 50% of patients at diagnosis and are usually associated with moderate to severe weakness. The presence of these symptoms probably does not represent an independent variable for prognosis, as has been suggested in the past. Lesions at T-12 or L-1 which effect the conus may present with early isolated autonomic symptoms.

Sensory abnormalities are reported by 80% of patients and also tend to be proportional to the degree of motor weakness. However, an ascending sensory level can be an early sign and should not be discounted.

Patients with cervical or thoracic lesions typically present with signs of myelopathy. Examination reveals upper motor neuron paralysis, sensory level, and sphincter involvement. Long duration of pain and associated radiculopathy are characteristic of cervical lesions. Thoracic lesions tend to present with earlier myelopathy and a more rapid course. In these cases, radicular pain is often bilateral. Lower thoracic vertebral lesions may present with a conus medullaris syndrome characterized by early sphincter dysfunction and symmetrical saddle-type anesthesia. Radicular pain is relatively infrequent with conus lesions. Sacral sparing may be seen in patients with either conus or intramedullary lesions. Lesions below the L-2 vertebral body present with radiculopathy or cauda equina syndrome. This common syndrome is characterized by early lumbar and radicular pain and sensory and motor signs in a nerve root distribution. Motor examination reveals lower motor neuron signs, i.e., a flaccid, hyporeflexic, hypotonic paralysis. In contrast to the conus lesions, sphincter problems are a late manifestation.

Patients with lesions between T-11 and L-2 may present with components of both the conus medullaris and cauda equina syndromes, making diagnosis difficult. There may be upper motor neuron dysfunction relative to the affected cord segments and lower motor neuron signs referable to the affected spinal roots. One may see, for example, ankle clonus and an extensor plantar response in association with a depressed knee jerk and asymmetric weakness and sensory loss in a root distribution. Although even the most seasoned clinicians experience difficulty in differentiating myelopathy, conus and cauda equina syndromes, and lumbar plexopathy from one another, these clinical differentiations are extremely important in planning the timing and choice of diagnostic investigations.

Differential Diagnosis

Other important causes of acute compressive myelopathy in cancer patients include spinal subdural hematoma and spinal epidural abscess. The presence of coagulopathy and/or treatment with chemotherapy put patients at greater risk for these syndromes. A short interval between the onset of pain and the neurological syndrome should raise the question of hematoma. Involvement of the disk space occurs with infection but is rare with compression due to tumor. Spinal compression can also result from excessive epidural fat in patients taking corticosteroids, or in obese individuals receiving no medications.

Important causes of noncompressive radiculopathy or myelopathy include carcinomatous meningitis and intramedullary metastasis. The most common manifestations of carcinomatous meningitis include alteration in cognitive function and headache, often related to increased intracranial pressure. These features help to differentiate this disorder from epidural compression. Other symptoms and signs relate to isolated cranial nerve or root dysfunction, particularly in the lumbosacral region. Seizures indicate the likelihood of co-existent cerebral metastases.

Other considerations include viral, spirochetal, or fungal meningitis, herpes zoster radiculopathy, postradiation myelopathy, myelopathy following treatment with intrathecal methotrexate, and spinal infarction related to a hypercoagulable state. Rarely, patients with parasagittal brain metastasis or sagittal sinus thrombosis can present with an upper motor neuron-type paraparesis, although the weakness is usually asymmetric and other cortical deficits or seizures are often present. Paraneoplastic necrotic myelopathy is a diagnosis of exclusion, since the cause of this syndrome is unknown and no diagnostic test is available at present. This is the rarest of the paraneoplastic syndromes and tends to occur in patients with small-cell lung carcinoma or Hodgkin's disease. Intramedullary metastasis should be excluded (by MRI scanning) before this diagnosis is made. The syndrome presents with a subacute, painless, progressive myelopathy. There is no effective treatment.

Ancillary Tests

Conventional radiography of the spine is positive in 70–85% of all patients with metastatic epidural compression at the time of diagnosis. Lymphoma is the only exception, only one third presenting with abnormal plain films. In patients with solid tumors the test has 91% sensitivity and 86% specificity. Of the large group of patients with symptoms and signs, or abnormalities on routine plain films or bone scan, however, only a small proportion will have epidural disease.

The selection of patients for definitive imaging should be based on determination of risk for epidural disease. In more than 60% of patients with solid tumors, the onset of back pain which correlates with a lesion on plain film is associated with epidural tumor. Radiculopathy is associated with epidural tumor in over 60% of cases, regardless of the plain film results. If the plain films are abnormal and the patient has radiculopathy, there is a greater than 90% likelihood of epidural compression. In the patient with local pain, abnormal plain films, and no symptoms or signs of radiculopathy, the probability of epidural tumor is only 36%.

These figures suggest an opportunity for treatment before the onset of myelopathy and irreversible cord damage. Patients who present with only local pain and/or radiculopathy are nearly always ambulatory, and epidural tumor is generally less extensive. More than 90% of these patients remain ambulatory after treatment.

The risk of epidural disease also varies with the type of abnormality seen on plain films. Vertebral collapse has been found to be highly specific as a marker for epidural disease. Cord compression was found in 87% of patients with >50% collapse, in 30% of those with pedicle erosion without collapse, but in only 7% of those with vertebral body tumor but no collapse.

Radionuclide bone scans will be abnormal in the vast majority of patients with bony spinal metastases, but this test has a specificity of only 50%. The addition of a negative bone scan to a normal plain X-ray further reduces the probability of epidural disease.

Spine CT is particularly useful in the cancer patient with local spine pain but with a normal neurological exam and normal plain films or bone scan. CT reveals bony metastases in up to two thirds of this group. Only 15% of patients, however, will have epidural extension of tumor. Cortical disruption on CT predicts the presence of epidural tumor in 90% of cases.

The gold standard for diagnosis is myelography (Fig. 1) (with or without subsequent CT) or MRI. To date, there have been no adequate prospective trials comparing these two modalities. Myelography is likely to be available in all hospitals and is relatively inexpensive and quick. It has the added advantage of yielding spinal fluid and can be combined with postmyelographic CT.

Myelography, however, has definite disadvantages: (a) With a complete block, there remains a need for cervical puncture or postmyelograhic CT to visualize the upper limit of the block and to exclude asymptomatic secondary lesions, present in 10–30% of patients; (b) myelography is generally not useful for diagnosis of intradural and intramedullary disease; (c) cancer patients may have coagulopathy

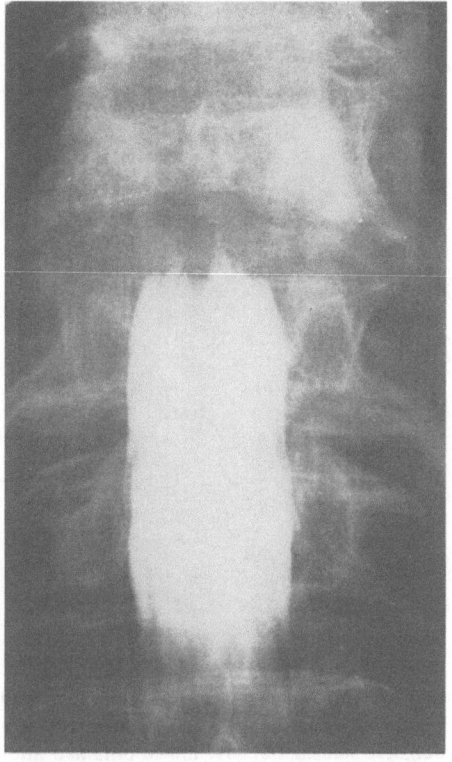

Fig. 1. Compression of dural sac due to metastasis of thoracic vertebra with neoplastic involvement of epidural space (surgically proved) in a 71-year-old man with acute paraparesis. Frontal view of ascending myelogram reveals complete block (extradural type) just below partially collapsed vertebral body. (Courtesy of Klaus Sartor and Marius Hartmann, Heidelberg)

or brain metastasis, both of which increase the risk of spinal puncture; (d) neurological deterioration following lumbar puncture below a complete block has been reported.

MRI is noninvasive and without risk for patients with coagulopathy or concurrent intracranial lesions. MRI is useful for defining both extradural and intradural lesions, and is clearly the best test available for imaging neural structures. Sagittal scanning can be

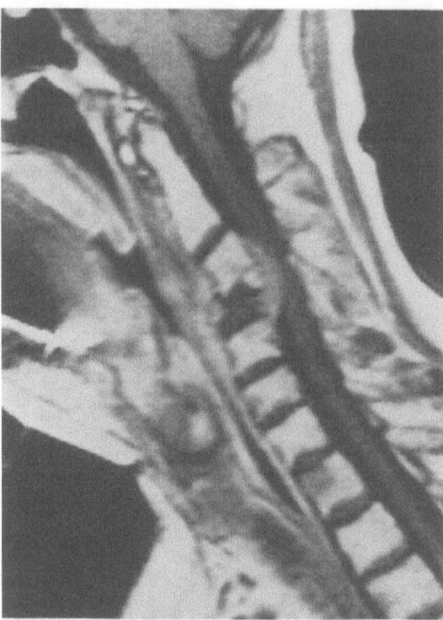

Fig. 2. Metastatic cord compression in a 52-year-old woman with acute quadriparesis and history of carcinoma of the hypopharynx. T1-weighted midsagittal MR image obtained after IV administration of paramagnetic contrast agent shows nearly complete destruction of body of fourth cervical vertebra. Enhancing abnormal soft tissue protrudes into epidural space, causing compression of dural sac and spinal cord made worse by posterior displacement of third vertebra. Note additional metastatic involvement of body of first thoracic vertebra. (Courtesy of Klaus Sartor and Marius Hartmann, Heidelberg)

used to identify asymptomatic secondary lesions (Fig. 2). Although most clinicians agree that MRI is currently the preferred test for both urgent and elective evaluation, individual decisions should be made based upon availability, imaging time, and quality of the procedure at a given institution, as well as on the ability of a patient to remain still. Paramagnetic enhancement with gadolinium compounds is useful for delineating the extent of tumor involvement.

Treatment

Steroids

Corticosteroids are warranted in the vast majority of patients. There is no question that steroids have a potent analgesic effect. Prompt institution of steroids may, in addition, prevent cord ischemia and resultant irreversible neurological dysfunction. Furthermore, there is some evidence that corticosteroids may have a direct oncolytic effect. In 1977, Posner's group first began to use a "high-dose" steroid regimen (100 mg dexamethasone bolus followed by 24 mg every 6 h), based on the observation that some patients with brain tumors improve when treated with higher doses of corticosteroids, as well as on animal evidence showing improvement in the signs of spinal cord compression with higher doses.

In 1980, Greenberg et al. further studied this regimen and showed that high-dose steroids result in pain relief in greater than 65% of patients within the first 24 h but are less likely to improve neurological status or to prevent acute deterioration. Based on the available data, it is reasonable to use dexamethasone as a 100 mg bolus followed by 24 mg every 6 h for patients with neurological dysfunction. Steroids can usually be tapered by 4 mg per dose every third day until lower dosage levels are achieved. Dexamethasone is generally continued through the end of radiation and then tapered.

In patients with local spine pain, a normal examination, and abnormal plain films, bone scan, or CT, a lower dose schedule (Decadron, 4 mg every 6 h) is recommended. This dosage schedule affords pain relief while the workup is underway.

Chemotherapy

Chemotherapy has no role as a primary treatment for metastatic spinal cord compression. There may be a future role for patients who have had maximal radiation, are not surgical candidates, or have widespread systemic disease. There have been isolated reports of resolution of paraparesis following chemotherapy in breast cancer patients who have failed radiation.

Radiation and Surgery

Before the mid 1970s, treatment with radiotherapy alone was largely unheard of, and most patients were treated with decompressive laminectomy alone. Numerous studies compared the results of decompressive laminectomy alone with the same procedure followed by radiation. All investigators reported better results with the latter group. In 1978, a retrospective nonrandomized study of 235 patients with metastatic epidural spinal cord compression was published by Gilbert and co-workers. This was the first study to show that radiation alone is as effective or more effective than surgery followed by radiation.

Today, radiation remains the treatment of choice for the vast majority of patients. The most radiosensitive tumors include lymphoma, myeloma, seminoma, and neuroblastoma. Breast and prostate cancer are also radiosensitive tumors. Lung, renal cell, colon cancer, and melanomas are commonly radioresistant. Retrospective analyses of large groups continue to show that even radioresistant tumors do equally well with radiation alone compared with standard laminectomy and radiation. Most centers use 30 Gy in 10 fractions of 300 cGy each, treating two vertebral levels above and two below the radiographic lesion. Secondary (asymptomatic) lesions are often treated because of the risk of future symptomatic epidural compression, but convincing data supporting this practice are lacking.

Several factors explain the failure of standard decompressive laminectomy. The majority of epidural tumors arise in the vertebral body, invade the epidural space anteriorly, and remain largely anterior to the spinal cord. Posterior laminectomy fails to adequately debulk an anteriorly situated tumor. In addition, laminectomy often aggravates or leads to future spinal instability. New techniques in spinal surgery over the past decade have allowed for new approaches to spinal tumors. A number of studies have reported successful results using an anterior approach to the spine in small series of highly selected patients. Anterior decompression is now being performed somewhat more routinely and clearly warrants more study in larger groups.

Anterior decompression allows for direct vision and accessibility to the anterior spinal cord, affording a safe method for direct decompression of neural structures and wider debulking. Simultaneous stabilization is possible for single- or multiple-level procedures using new techniques and instrumentation. Patients presenting with cord compression due to retropulsed bone or angulation can also be treated with this approach.

A growing number of authors believe that the anterior approach should be offered as initial treatment for patients with radio-insensitive tumors. These techniques warrant further study in larger groups with comparisons with both laminectomy and radiotherapy.

Today, potential indications for surgery include (a) absence of a tissue diagnosis, (b) spinal instability, (c) neurological deterioration during or following maximal radiation, (d) highly radioresistant tumors, (e) the possibility of an epidural abscess, (f) intractable pain despite maximal radiation, steroids, and analgesics, and (g) purely posterior lesions. Intravascular embolization of vertebral lesions which have not yet produced significant neurological symptoms is under investigation.

Prognosis

The histology of the primary cancer is probably as important in predicting outcome as the treatment employed. Lymphoma, myeloma, and breast cancer have the best prognosis and a combined 80% initial response rate; 75% of breast cancer patients alive at 1 year remain ambulatory. Patients with lung or renal cell cancer, or melanoma have the worst prognosis. Fewer than 25% of these patients respond to any treatment modality. Rate of progression of the clinical syndrome also relates to outcome; rapid onset and quick progression are associated with a poor prognosis.

Most importantly, outcome relates directly to the degree of weakness and the neurological status before treatment, regardless of the treatment modality chosen. Seventy-five to eighty percent of patients ambulatory at initial presentation remain so after treatment. Of those patients ambulatory but paraparetic prior to treatment, only 20–45% will be ambulatory upon completion of therapy. Finally, less than 5% of paraplegic patients will become ambulatory following treatment.

Summary

Metastatic epidural spinal cord compression is an urgent and common problem for which the best treatment is still unknown. The deficiencies of retrospective studies are obvious, and recent advances in imaging as well as in radiotherapy and surgical techniques have made earlier studies outdated. A prospective, large study which separates patients by age, primary tumor, and pretreatment neurological status is warranted and should offer better guidelines for the acute management of these patients.

Suggested Reading

Barcena A, Lobato RD, Rivas JJ et al. (1984) Spinal metastatic disease: analysis of factors determining functional prognosis and choice of treatment. Neurosurgery 15:820–828

Constans JP, DeDivitis E, Donzelli R, Spaziante R, Meder JF, Haye C (1983) Spinal metastases with neurological manifestations: review of 600 cases. J Neurosurg 59:111–117

Delattre JY, Arbit E, Thaler HT et al. (1989) A dose-response study of dexamethasone in a model of spinal cord compression caused by epidural tumor. J Neurosurg 70:920–924

Findlay GFG (1984) Adverse effects on the management of malignant spinal cord compression. J Neurol Neurosurg Psychiatry 47:761–766

Gilbert RW, Kim JH, Posner JB (1978) Epidural spinal cord compression from metastatic tumor: diagnosis and treatment. Ann Neurol 3:40–46

Greenberg HS, Kim JH, Posner JB (1980) Epidural spinal cord compression from metastatic tumors: results with a new treatment protocol. Ann Neurol 8:361–368

Hagen N, Stulman J, Krol G, Foley KM, Portenoy RK (1989) The role of myelography and magnetic resonance imaging in cancer patients with symptomatic and asymptomatic epidural disease. Neurology 39:309–314

Harrington KD (1984) Anterior cord decompression and spinal stabilization for patients with metastatic lesions of the spine. J Neurosurg 61:107–114

Portenoy RK, Lipton RB, Foley KM (1987) Back pain in the cancer patient: an algorithm for evaluation and management. Neurology 37:134–139

Portenoy RK, Galer BS, Salomon O et al. (1989) Identification of epidural neoplasm: radiography and bone scintigraphy in the symptomatic and asymptomatic spine. Cancer 64:2207–2211

Posner JB (1987) Back pain and epidural spinal cord compression. Med Clin North Am 71:185–196

Posner JB, Howieson J, Cvitkovic E (1977) "Disappearing" spinal cord compression: oncolytic effect of glucocorticoids (and other chemotherapeutic agents) on epidural metastases. Ann Neurol 2:409–416

Rodichok LD, Harper GR, Ruckdeschel JC et al. (1981) Early diagnosis of spinal epidural metastases. Am J Med 70:1181–1187

Rodichok LD, Ruckdeschel JC, Harper GR et al. (1986) Early detection and treatment of spinal epidural metastases: the role of myelography. Ann Neurol 20:696–703

Ruff RL, Lanska DJ (1989) Epidural metastases in prospectively evaluated veterans with cancer and back pain. Cancer 63:2234–2239

Siegal T, Siegal T, Robin G, Lubetski-Korn I, Fuks Z (1982) Anterior decompression of the spine for metastatic epidural cord compression: a promising avenue of therapy? Ann Neurol 11:28–36

Sorensen PS, Borgesen SE, Rohide K et al. (1990) Metastatic epidural spinal cord compression: results of treatment and survival. Cancer 65:1502–1508

Stark RJ, Henson RA, Evans SJW (1982) Spinal metastasis: a retrospective survey from a general hospital. Brain 105:189–196

Sundaresan N, DiGiacinto, Hughes JEO (1986) Surgical treatment of spinal metastases. Clin Neurosurg 33:503–510

Vecht CRJ, Haaxma-Reiche, van Putten WLJ, deVisser M, Vries EP, Twijnstra A (1989) Initial bolus of conventional versus high-dose dexamethasone in metastatic spinal cord compression. Neurology 39:1255–1262

Epilepsy

Chapter 66

Status Epilepticus

Thomas P. Bleck and Hermann Stefan

Definitions

Seizures are the clinical or electrographic manifestations of abnormal, excessive cortical neuronal synchrony. They are classified according to the inferred anatomy (partial vs generalized) and their effects on awareness (simple vs complex). *Epilepsy* is the tendency to experience repeated seizures as a consequence of an intrinsic abnormality of cerebral excitability. Based on these definitions, it is clear that many seizures which occur in intensive care unit (ICU) patients are not manifestations of true epilepsy, but rather reflect trauma, infection, or metabolic disturbances.

The term *status epilepticus* (SE) refers to either continuous seizure activity or serial seizures without recovery between them. For convenience, 30 min is typically used as the duration which defines SE, but pathophysiologic studies suggest that 20 min of seizure activity may represent a temporal threshold after which the ictal electrochemical activity itself

begins to damage the brain. Therefore, we will use 20 min as the defining duration in this chapter.

SE can be classified according to its clinical or its electrographic manifestations. The system of Gastaut, based on the International Classification of Epileptic Seizures, is the standard clinical classification and is presented in Table 1.

Epidemiology

Status epilepticus is one of the most common emergencies encountered in neurologic critical care, and one of the least well understood by nonneurologic intensive care physicians. In the United States, and probably other industrial nations, at least 24 patients per 10 000 head of population are affected each year; a more recent, community-based study yielded an estimate of about 1 in every 1000 head of population. Conservatively estimating that the incidence in less industrialized countries is at least as high as in the United States, about 5 million cases of status epilepticus probably

---

Section Editor: Thomas P. Bleck

Table 1. Clinical classification of status epilepticus (SE)

I. Generalized SE
  A. Generalized convulsive SE (GCSE)
    1. Primarily generalized SE
      (a) Tonic-clonic SE
      (b) Myoclonic SE
      (c) Clonic-tonic-clonic SE
    2. Secondarily generalized SE
      (a) Partial seizure with secondary generalization
      (b) Tonic SE
    3. Nonconvulsive SE (NCSE)
      (a) Absence SE ("petit mal status")
      (b) Atypical absence SE (e.g., in the Lennox-Gastaut syndrome)
      (c) Atonic SE
      (d) NCSE as a sequel of partially treated GCSE
II. Partial SE
  A. Simple partial SE
    1. Typical simple partial SE
    2. Epilepsia partialis continua (EPC)
  B. Complex partial SE (CPSE)
III. Neonatal SE

---

occur in the world each year. The mortality rate from status epilepticus among US adults is about 25%, but it is lower in children (3.6% in the study of Maytal et al.). This contrast probably reflects differences in both etiology and cardiorespiratory reserve.

Pathogenesis

The most common causes of SE are drug withdrawal (including alcohol, anticonvulsants, and other hypnosedative agents), drug ingestion (primarily central nervous system stimulants such as cocaine), and central nervous system infection. In already hospitalized patients, anoxic brain damage following cardiac or respiratory arrest is an important cause of SE.

The therapeutically relevant physiologic aspects of the pathogenesis of SE can be summarized in terms of their effects at three levels: neuronal, brain, and systemic.

Neuronal Aspects

The major physiologic distinction between a single seizure and SE is most probably failure of the inhibitory mechanisms which usually terminate a seizure. Generalized convulsive SE (GCSE) and complex partial SE (CPSE) represent circumstances in which the usual systems responsible for inhibiting repetitive synchronous neuronal firing (which are predominantly GABAergic) fail to control the excitatory amino acid (EAA) systems [involving both N-methyl-D-aspartate (NMDA) and nonNMDA receptors]. Absence SE appears to represent the converse: excessive synchronous inhibition halts many cortical functions, with an excitatory "escape" occurring throughout the cortex approximately every 300 ms.

The neuropathologic consequences of SE are currently thought to be a manifestation of *excitotoxicity*, resulting from excessive activation of EAA systems. This suggests a number of potentially useful therapies, including blockade of the channels opened by these transmitters and interference with the metabolic consequences of their actions. The high levels of free intracellular calcium produced by excessive neuronal activity activate many enzyme systems which normally mediate learning. However, in the setting of SE these systems sustain seizure activity and produce neuronal damage, which may culminate in necrosis. Drugs which control these systems may be truly *antiepileptogenic*, preventing the development of epilepsy in patients who have experienced SE.

Absence SE is devoid of these pathologic consequences, presumably because its inhibitory nature does not produce excitotoxicity.

Brain Aspects

At the onset of SE, the metabolic demands of the brain increase 200%–300%. These requirements are initially met by an increase in cerebral blood flow, which is produced by both cerebral vasodilation and systemic hypertension. After 20–60 min, however, substrate delivery becomes inadequate for the metabolic needs of the brain, and autolysis begins. This process is temperature-dependent and is likely to be accelerated in hyperthermic patients. Hypoxemic patients probably begin to experience this complication sooner.

Intracranial pressure (ICP) increases during SE, even if the patient has been paralyzed and mechanically ventilated. This is in part due to an increase in the intracranial blood volume, but another portion reflects cerebral edema. This edema is vasogenic, probably reflecting a leak in the blood-brain barrier.

Systemic Aspects

GCSE engages all systems of the body simultaneously. Blood pressure rises immediately, then declines over the 1st h, with hypotension a late manifestation. The marked increase in muscular activity produces large volumes of CO_2 to be excreted, while ventilation is impaired, producing both respiratory acidosis and hypoxemia. Aspiration of oral and gastric contents may occur and produce an initial chemical pneumonitis often followed by bacterial pneumonia. The excessive muscular work results in metabolic acidosis. The arterial blood pH early in the course of SE often reaches 6.9 or lower; this represents CO_2 accumulation and lactate excess, both of which will rapidly return to normal when SE is terminated and should not be treated with buffers. Hyperthermia is also a consequence of the motor phenomena.

Patients may develop either neurogenic or cardiogenic pulmonary edema during SE.

Musculoskeletal complications of GCSE are ubiquitous. Most patients experience muscle injury, with elevation of the serum creatine kinase concentration. If GCSE continues for several hours, especially if hyperthermia and volume depletion supervene, frank rhabdomyolysis may occur, raising the possibility of acute renal failure. Fractures, dislocations, and tendon avulsions occur rarely.

Clinical Features and Differential Diagnosis

Features of GCSE

GCSE begins with a generalized convulsion, which may arise de novo, or may reflect the secondary generalization of a partial seizure (producing the so-called clonic-tonic-clonic form of SE). The patient experiences

Table 2. Stages in the evolution of generalized convulsive status epilepticus (from Treiman et al. 1990)

Stage	Typical clinical manifestations[a]	Electrographic features
1	Tonic-clonic convulsions; hypertension and hyperglycemia commonly present	Discrete ictal rhythm with interictal slowing
2	Low or medium amplitude clonic activity, with rare generalized convulsions	Waxing and waning of ictal discharges
3	Slight, but frequent or continuous, tonic or clonic activity, often confined to the eyes, face, or hands	Continuous ictal discharges
4	Rare episodes of minor clonic activity; hypotension and hypoglycemia common	Continuous ictal discharges, puncruated by flat periods
5	Coma, without other manifestations of ictal activity	Periodic epileptiform discharges on a flat background

[a] The clinical manifestations may vary considerably, depending on the underlying neuropathophysiologic process (and its anatomy), systemic diseases, and medications.

waxing and waning seizure intensity during the first 30–60 min of GCSE. Early in the episode, there may be tonic resurgences, but these diminish after a few cycles. The patient neither regains consciousness nor reacts to noxious stimuli during the episode, although motor activity intermittently ceases. Electroencephalography reveals that early GCSE is characterized by well-defined seizure activity followed by postictal slowing. As GCSE continues, the seizures become increasingly disorganized and more difficult to distinguish from the intervening activity. Treiman and associates have characterized five stages in the electrographic evolution of GCSE (Table 2). The clinical manifestations listed in this table are quite variable, however, and should only be considered a rough guide; they are taken from personal observations, and from work reviewed by Lothman.

The electroclinical correlation shown in Table 2 has important diagnostic and therapeutic implications:

cessation of visible seizure activity, either spontaneously or after anticonvulsant administration, does not mean that SE has been controlled. The patient may have developed subclinical (nonconvulsive) SE. If the patient does not begin to awaken within 15–20 min, one should begin EEG monitoring to determine whether SE is still present and, if so, to direct its treatment.

Features of Other Types of SE

The nonconvulsive types of SE include CPSE, absence SE, and subtle SE. CPSE, formerly called "psychomotor status" or "temporal lobe status," induces a state of impaired responsiveness, usually with aphasia but without other evidence of focal brain dysfunction. The EEG typically shows runs of rhythmic slow activity, often alternating between the hemispheres. Spikes or sharp activity may be seen early in the episode, but are usually absent by the time the diagnosis is considered. The response to treatment, both electroencephalographically and clinically, is usually dramatic. CPSE occasionally produces permanent memory deficits, making emergent treatment mandatory. The patient typically does not have a history of epilepsy, and often does not suffer from seizures subsequently.

Absence SE resembles CPSE clinically, although in the former condition there are often small myoclonic movements of the eyes, face, and hands. EEG reveals a spike-and-wave pattern which waxes and wanes in both amplitude and frequency. These patients often have a history of seizures, but are commonly older than is typical for the absence epilepsies. The response to treatment is rapid. In contrast to the other forms of SE, absence SE is not associated with neuronal destruction, regardless of its duration, which lessens the pressing immediacy of its treatment.

"Subtle" SE describes the condition of patients who manifest EEG patterns resembling SE after a cardiac or respiratory arrest. Some authors use the term to describe patients who are in nonconvulsive SE following a period of more obvious convulsive movements.

Patients may also manifest simple partial SE, in which their consciousness is preserved. This is most commonly motor in type, with clonus of an extremity or one side of the face. However, it may involve the somatosensory or special sensory systems. A special case of simple partial SE is *epilepsia partialis continua*, which consists of repetitive movements confined to a small portion of the body.

Differential Diagnosis

GCSE has a very brief differential diagnosis. Disorders producing decerebrate or decorticate posturing pose the most difficulty to clinicians attempting to elicit descriptions, but are generally easily distinguished when observed. Generalized tetanus can produce movements resembling the tonic phase of a seizure, but the tetanus patient remains conscious. Sometimes psychogenic seizures mimic status epilepticus (e.g., as GCSE), often with "tonic" motor phenomena.

CPSE and absence SE are sometimes difficult to distinguish from psychiatric disturbances or drug intoxication. The EEG, with a confirmatory benzodiazepine challenge if necessary, is the only reliable diagnostic technique.

Ancillary Tests

Electroencephalography

The EEG is the only important procedure for the diagnosis of SE. Continuous EEG (or video-EEG) is valuable for monitoring the patient's response to treatment. The EEG characteristics of different phases of GCSE are outlined in Table 2. Unfortunately, the EEG during SE is often not helpful in determining the etiology of the patient's condition.

Other Ancillary Studies

Electrocardiographic monitoring and blood pressure measurement are necessary during the treatment of SE. Patients who require the therapy outlined below for refractory SE will often require invasive monitoring of systemic and pulmonary arterial pressures, cardiac output, and urine flow.

Diagnostic studies are aimed at determining the etiology of SE, and should usually be postponed until SE has been terminated and the patient stabilized. Magnetic resonance imaging (or computed tomography if magnetic resonance imaging cannot be obtained) and cerebrospinal fluid analysis are frequently required.

Management

The initial treatment of SE patients can begin in the field if rescue personnel are adequately trained to recognize the condition and administer the first line of treatment.

Basic Life Support

Airway maintenance is a crucial aspect of the care of all convulsing patients. Adequate oxygen delivery and ventilation must be provided, by placement of an endotracheal tube if necessary. Patients should have continuous ECG monitoring, and the blood pressure should be measured at least every 2 min during drug administration. Glucose (1 mg/kg as D50/W or D20/W) and thiamine (1 mg/kg) should be given after blood is obtained for glucose determination.

Terminating the SE

Treatment should begin with a benzodiazepine, e.g., lorazepam 0.05–0.2 mg/kg at 2 mg/min (Table 3). The maximum suggested adult dose is 8 mg. Lorazepam is effective against SE for several hours, allowing more time for etiologic investigation and the choice of subsequent therapy than diazepam. In Europe diazepam or clonazepam are chosen as alternatives. The maximum dose of clonazepam is 16–20 mg/day. Clonazepam treatment should begin with a 2-mg bolus followed by continuous infusion of 10 mg over 24 h. Loading with a longer-acting agent (e.g., phenytoin) should start as soon as the SE is controlled.

If the benzodiazepine fails, loading with phenytoin should be begun at a dosage of 20 mg/kg given at a rate no faster than 50 mg/min. In Europe, an initial loading dose of 10 mg/kg is usually employed, with a second 10 mg/kg dose if necessary. Many patients cannot tolerate this infusion rate, usually because of hypotension. Phenytoin should thereafter be continued with 5 mg/kg per day in three short infusions. Phenytoin should not be dissolved in large volumnes of saline, as this will lower the pH and make the drug come out of solution.

If phenytoin fails, many recommend phenobarbital (5–10 mg/kg); others suggest lidocaine (2–3 mg/kg) or paraldehyde (0.1–0.2 ml/kg, rectally). Alternatively, midazolam can be used at this stage; it provides more rapid and definitive control of SE than does phenobarbital or paraldehyde, and is becoming more and more popular in Europe, where it is already used as drug of first choice in some centers. Midazolam should be given at a load-

Table 3. Steps in the termination of SE

Steps	European approach[a]	United States approach[b]
1. Begin treatment of 1st choice	Clonazepam 1–2 mg/i.v. (5–10 min), then infusion of 10 mg/24 h (in 30 ml glucose 5%) 1 h 20 ml/h then 5 ml/h (if i.v. injection not possible, midazolam i.m. or diazepam by rectal tube)	Lorazepam (0.05–0.2 mg/kg) at 2 mg/min (max. 8 mg)
2. If benzo-diazepine fails:	Phenytoin load 10 mg/kg in 30 min and a second 10 mg/kg dose if necessary after 1 h	Phenytoin load 20 mg/kg (max. 50 mg/min)
3. If phenytoin fails:	Phenobarbital (5–10 mg/kg) or thiopentone or sodium pentobarbital narcosis	Midazolam 0.2 mg/kg loading, then infusion 0.1–0.4 mg/kg/h or phenobarbital (5–10 mg/kg) or lidocaine (2–3 mg/kg) or paraldehyde (0.1–0.2 ml/kg rectally)
4. If steps 1–3 fail:	Paraldehyde or lidocaine or isoflurane inhalation or clomethiazole (alcohol)	Pentobarbital narcosis 12 mg/kg loading dose, initial infusion rate 5 mg/kg per hour

[a] This example is the Erlangen approach.
[b] This example is the Charlottesville approach.

ing dose of 0.2 mg/kg, followed by an infusion of 0.1–2.0 mg/kg per hour as determined by EEG monitoring. Patients who have not yet been intubated should undergo intubation at this stage.

Should midazolam fail, the next step is to proceed to pentobarbital 12 mg/kg loading dose, with an initial maintenance infusion rate of 5 mg/kg per hour; the infusion rate should be titrated to obtain complete seizure control *and* to obtain a burst-suppression EEG. This EEG goal has become traditional, but whether one needs to achieve this depth of drug effect has not been tested. Maintain this EEG pattern with continuous monitoring for 12 h, and then begin to decrease the dose. If electrographic (or clinical)

seizures recur, restart the pentobarbital for another 12-h period. To maximize success in weaning patients from pentobarbital insure that they have phenytoin concentrations of 20 µg/ml, and phenobarbital concentrations over 40 µg/ml (sometimes as high as 120 µg/ml). Most patients adjust to these high phenobarbital concentrations and begin to breath spontaneously and awaken within 1–3 days.

Preventing Recurrences

The key to prevention of recurrences is to understand the etiology of SE in the particular patient. If, for example, SE was due to alcohol withdrawal, anticonvulsants may not be indicated. If SE followed inadvised discontinuation of an effective anticonvulsant regimen, that same regimen might be reinstituted if the patient will agree to follow it. For patients requiring pharmacotherapy, phenytoin is the major drug for prevention of recurrence in the immediate post-SE period. The phenytoin concentration should be kept near $20 \mu g/ml$. Phenobarbital is often necessary as well. In Europe oral carbamazepine is frequently given even at this stage.

Treating Complications

Patients with rhabdomyolysis should be rehydrated, and consideration given to alkalinzing their urine with sodium bicarbonate.

Hyperthermia should be treated with external cooling. If the fever is due to SE, the patient will usually cool rapidly once the seizures have stopped. Patients receiving high-dose pentobarbital usually become poikilothermic, and often require external warming.

Cerebral edema, if sufficient to raise intracranial pressure, may be treated with mannitol. Whether corticosteroids are useful in this setting is unknown, but they are commonly used in other forms of vasogenic cerebral edema.

Prognosis

The prognosis of patients with GCSE who are rapidly and appropriately treated depends predominantly on the etiology of their condition. Patients in whom treatment is delayed or inadequate may suffer prolonged or permanent deficits of cognitive or motor function. In CPSE, isolated cases of severe memory deficits underscore the possibility of hippocampal damage and thus the need for rapid diagnosis and treatment.

Suggested Reading

Bleck TP (1991) Status epilepticus. Clin Neuropharmacol 14:191–198

Bleck TP (1991) Tetanus. In: Scheld WM, Whitley RJ, Durack DT (eds) Infections of the central nervous system. Raven, New York, pp 603–624

DeLorenzo RL, Towne AR, Pellock JM et al. (1993) Mortality in a community-based study of status epilepticus. Epilepsia 29 [Suppl]:35–47

Gastaut H (1983) Classification of status epilepticus. In: Delgada-Escueta AV, Wasterlain CG, Treiman DM, Porter RJ (eds) Advances in neurology, vol 34, Status epilepticus. Raven, New York, pp 15–35

Hauser WA (1990) Status epilepticus: epidemiologic considerations. Neurology 40 [Suppl 2]:9–13

Kumar A, Bleck TP (1992) Intravenous midazolam for the treatment of refractory status epilepticus. Crit Care Med 20:483–488

Leppik IE, Derivan AT, Homan RW, Walker J, Ramsay RE, Patrick B (1983) Double-blind study of lorazepam and diazepam in status epilepticus. JAMA 249:1452–1454

Lothman E (1990) The biochemical basis and pathophysiology of status epilepticus. Neurology 40 [Suppl 2]:13–23

Lowenstein DH, Alldredge BK (1993) Status epilepticus at an urban public hospital in the 1980s. Neurology 42:483–488

Maytal J, Shinnar S, Moshe SL, Alvarez LA (1989) Low morbidity and mortality of status epilepticus in children. Pediatrics 83:323–331

Stefan H (1990) Status epilepticus. In: Biemond A (ed) Handbook of electroencephalography and clinical neurophysiology, vol 4. Amsterdam: Elsevier, pp 331–360

Towne AR, McGee FE, Mercer EL et al. (1990) Mortality in a community-based status epilepticus study. Neurology 40 [Suppl 1]: 299

Treiman DM, Walton NY, Kendrick C (1990) A progressive sequence of electroencephalographic changes during generalized convulsive status epilepticus. Epilepsy Res 5: 49–60

Neuromuscular Diseases

Chapter 67

Acute Inflammatory Polyneuropathy (Guillain-Barré Syndrome)

ERNST F. HUND, VOLKER SCHUCHARDT, and
ALLAN H. ROPPER

Definition, Epidemiology, and Relevance to ICU Treatment

Acute inflammatory polyneuropathy, or Guillain-Barré syndrome (GBS), is an acutely or subacutely paralyzing disorder which typically has a monophasic course and remits spontaneously. Weakness is thought to result from an immune-mediated inflammation of the peripheral nerves, leading to disruption of the surrounding myelin and secondary axonal loss. The incidence of GBS is roughly the same throughout the world, with approximately 1.0–1.5 cases per 100 000 persons per year and a possible slight preponderance for males. Most cases follow an infection. The clinical core features include a relatively symmetric muscle weakness, areflexia, and distal paresthesias. The diagnosis is usually confirmed by a characteristic spinal fluid formula of raised protein with no or few cells, and by electrodiagnostic findings indicative of demyelination. Respiratory failure due to weakness

of the diaphragm and cardiovascular instability due to autonomic dysfunction are the main reasons for intensive care. After admission to the ICU, most serious complications result from mechanical ventilation, hemodynamic or cardiac disturbances, venous thrombosis, or sepsis. This chapter focuses on the management and treatment of severe GBS, emphasizing the skilled nursing and medical care required to reduce morbidity and mortality in this fundamentally self-limited disease.

Pathogenesis

A considerable body of data now supports the view that the basic disease process in GBS is immunologic in nature. The mechanisms thought to be involved include both antibody-mediated and cell-mediated reactions to peripheral nerve myelin. However, despite numerous efforts, neither the mechanism that triggers the abnormal immune response nor the antigen against which the autoimmune response is directed have been precisely described as yet. A variety of events

Section Editors: Daniel F. Hanley and Allan H. Ropper

can initiate the abnormal immune process, suggesting a nonspecific action. Similarly, several myelin antigens are likely to be involved, varying between patients and triggering mechanisms. In experimental allergic neuritis (EAN), injection of myelin components such as protein P_0 or protein P_2 induces inflammatory lesions indistinguishable from those seen in GBS. In the clinical disease, demyelinating factors, antibodies to myelin, and activated T cells have all been found. The pathogenesis of GBS may be heterogeneous, with some patients having antibody production to myelin glycolipids or gangliosides and others having T-cell-mediated reactions to myelin P_2 protein.

Table 1. Diagnostic criteria for typical GBS (adapted from Asbury and Cornblath 1990)

Features required for diagnosis:
- Relatively symmetric progressive muscle weakness
- Loss of tendon jerks (areflexia)
- Absence of other causes of acute neuropathy, e.g.,
    porphyria
    toxin exposure
    recent diphtheria

Features strongly supportive of GBS:
- Progression of symptoms over days to 4 weeks
- Only mild sensory symptoms or signs
- Cranial nerve involvement, usually in the form of bilateral facial palsy
- Absence of fever at the onset of neuritic symptoms
- Involvement of the autonomic nervous system
- Elevated CSF protein in the presence of few or no cells (after the first week)
- Electrodiagnostic findings supportive of demyelination
- Recovery beginning 2–4 weeks after progression ceases

Clinical Features and Differential Diagnosis

Typical GBS presents as a combination of generalized weakness, mild sensory symptoms, and sometimes pain. Muscle weakness is usually the leading feature, often proximally pronounced and rather symmetric, but it may be asymmetric (however, not unilateral) in early stages of the disease. In the majority of cases, weakness begins and is more severe in the lower limbs, but atypical cases with predominant affection of the upper limbs occur. Symptoms are accompanied by areflexia in nearly all cases, although distal areflexia with definite hyporeflexia of the biceps and knee jerks will suffice for diagnosis if other features are consistent. Table 1 summarizes the diagnostic criteria currently in use.

Sensory symptoms include distal paresthesias and mild sensory loss in nearly 80% of patients. Pain described as diffuse aching in the back or the proximal limbs may be the presenting symptom and is more common than previously recognized. The cranial nerves are involved in many cases, with bilateral facial palsy being the most characteristic sign. The oropharyngeal, trigeminal, and oculomotor nerves are less frequently compromised, and cranial nerves I, II, and VIII are generally spared. Widespread peripheral nerve demyelination may also affect autonomic fibers, such as vagal, glossopharyngeal, and preganglionic sympathetic nerves. Involvement of these nerves results in dysautonomia, which is discussed below in more detail. Papilledema is a

Table 2. Preceding events thought to play a causative role in the pathogenesis of GBS

Viruses:
  Epstein-Barr virus
  Cytomegalovirus
  Varicella-zoster virus
  Human immunodeficiency virus

Vaccines:
  Swine influenza (artifact of reporting?)
  Rabies (Semple rabbit brain or suckling
    mouse brain)
  Vaccinia

Other agents:
  Campylobacter jejuni
  Mycoplasma pneumoniae

Diverse:
  Surgery?
  Drugs?

---

rare complication of GBS and may be due to impaired CSF absorption, probably related to the increased protein concentration of the CSF.

In nearly two thirds of patients with GBS, some form of infection precedes the onset of the disease, most often pulmonary and gastrointestinal illnesses. Agents that have been commonly associated with GBS include cytomegalovirus, Epstein-Barr virus, varicella-zoster virus, and – more recently – human immunodeficiency virus (Table 2). In addition, antibodies to *Mycoplasma pneumoniae* and *Campylobacter jejuni* have been found in the sera of GBS patients. In rare instances, GBS was reported to be preceded by surgical procedures, but this association may be simply coincidental. An association between Semple (containing dried formalized rabbit brain) or suckling mouse brain rabies vaccination seems to be established, whereas the association with the US swine influenza vaccine program of the

1970s, though likely, may have been overestimated. To support the diagnosis of GBS, manifestations of a preceding infection should have clearly subsided by the time neuropathy appears. Otherwise, a systemic disorder or intoxication accompanied by polyneuropathy is more likely to be the primary diagnosis.

The time course and severity of muscle weakness are quite variable. Some patients exhibit a dramatic course, requiring mechanical ventilation within a few days or even hours of onset, whereas in others symptoms may evolve gradually. Patients with a progression of symptoms longer than 4 weeks are, by an arbitrary definition, classified as having chronic idiopathic demyelinating polyneuropathy (see Chap. 68). A phase of worsening is followed by a plateau of variable duration, after which the disease slowly resolves spontaneously. The maximum motor deficit ranges from minimal weakness of the legs to paralysis of all voluntary muscles, including the extraocular muscles. Recovery may be complete or incomplete, depending on the degree of axonal damage. Fifteen to 20% of survivors may have some disability preventing them from returning to work, and 5–10% remain severely disabled. Reported mortalities have varied from 3 to 10% in the modern ICU era, but mortality should be in the lower end of this range. The median time for returning to work is between 3 and 6 months after the onset of the disease. Beyond 2 years, there is generally no further improvement. An "axonal" variant of GBS occurs in the extremely rapid onset, inexcitable motor nerves, and evidence of primary demyelination in some patients. These cases often re-

Table 3. Clinical variants of GBS (for details see text)

- Fisher's syndrome (ataxia, ophthalmoplegia, areflexia)
- Pure motor GBS
- Pure sensory GBS
- Pure pandysautonomia
- Regional variants:
  polyneuritis cranialis
  pharyngeal-cervical-brachial variant
  paraparetic variant

---

quire mechanical ventilation, and many have dysautonomia. Most eventually have widespread denervation and a poor outcome.

Several clinical variants are regarded as part of the spectrum of GBS, including Fisher's syndrome, pure sensory loss with areflexia, polyneuritis cranialis, and pure pandysautonomia (Table 3). In Fisher's syndrome, the combination of ophthalmoplegia, ataxia, and areflexia suggests brain-stem involvement, but CNS lesions have not been demonstrated in most well-documented cases. In pure sensory loss with areflexia, symptoms evolve rapidly, are widespread and symmetrical, with complete resolution. Polyneuritis cranialis, usually including bilateral facial palsy, may also be a variant of GBS. The cranial nerves I and II are uninvolved. Although autonomic dysfunction is frequently encounterd in GBS, it rarely presents in an isolated fashion. For such cases of pure pandysautonomia to be acceptable, onset must be relatively rapid and recovery complete. Before attributing any of these cases to GBS, the typical patterns of time course, electrodiagnosis, and spinal tap described above are required. For details, the interested

reader is referred to the monographs of Hughes (1990) and Ropper and collegues (1991).

Depending on the clinical history and examination, the differential diagnosis covers a broad spectrum of diseases. These include brain-stem lesions, spinal cord compression, transverse myelitis, myasthenia gravis, myopathies, neoplastic meningitis, neuropathies of various causes, and many more. Conversely, there are well-documented cases of fulminant GBS which have been misdiagnosed as coma of unknown origin or locked-in syndrome. In hysterical persons, a pretense of weakness may be so convincing that artificial ventilation is instituted. The acute axonal polyneuropathy occurring during severe illnesses should no longer be called GBS, but should be referred to as critical illness polyneuropathy (Chap. 70). Recently, several lower motor neuron syndromes have been identified that are associated with high titers of antiglycolipid antibodies and respond to immunosuppressive therapy (see Chap. 15). The asymmetrical pattern of muscle weakness and the clinical and electrophysiological absence of sensory abnormalities set these syndromes apart from GBS.

Laboratory Findings

CSF Examination. An increased CSF protein concentration in the presence of few or no cells is characteristic of GBS. However, this "albuminocytological dissociation" is often found only after the first week of symptoms. Occasionally, the CSF protein may remain within the normal range thoughout the illness, whereas other patients may have up to 50 lymphocytes/ml. The presence of CSF pleocytosis should always cast suspicion on whether the diagnosis of GBS is correct, with the one exception that GBS may be associated with human immunodeficiency virus infection, where CSF pleocytosis is frequent.

Electrodiagnostic Findings. Electrodiagnostic studies typically reveal an evolving pattern of multifocal demyelination. In general, they are more sensitive and yield abnormalities earlier than CSF examination. Characteristic features include slowing of motor nerve conduction, conduction block, temporal dispersion, increased latencies of distally evoked compound muscle action potentials, and delayed or absent F-responses. With progression of the disease, many patients show fibrillation potentials and positive sharp waves, indicative of multifocal axonal damage. Cases with primary axonal degeneration have been reported, but, as noted above, their categorization as GBS is ambiguous. A reduction of mean compound muscle action potential amplitude to less than 20% of the lower limit of normal is the most powerful predictor of a poor outcome. Electrodiagnostic studies usually confirm the clinical diagnosis of GBS and are indispensable in puzzling or variant cases.

Biopsy Findings. Pathologic examination of sural nerve biopsies usually reveals an inflammatory demyelinating peripheral neuropathy, characterized by sheets of lymphocytes and macrophages that split myelin away from axons. However, pathologic changes are often relatively mild, and if clinical and laboratory features are typical of GBS, biopsy is infrequently performed.

Clinical Management Prior to the ICU

To avoid emergency situations and unwarranted deaths, we observe any patient ill enough to be bed-bound closely for respiratory and autonomic cardiovascular dysfunction. In the following paragraphs, our guidelines are given.

Monitoring Respiratory Functions

Ventilatory performance depends on effective inspiratory effort, expiratory effort (cough), and maintenance of the airway patency (Chap. 12). Impairment of inspiratory forces due to weakness of the diaphragm is usually the main problem. It manifests as an increased respiratory rate and recruitment of accessory respiratory muscles. If alveoli become hypoventilated, there is a substantial risk of atelectasis, pneumonia, and hypoxia. Weakness of forced exhalation impairs cough and renders clearance of tracheal secretions difficult, thereby causing an additional risk for atelectasis and pulmonary infections. A third and often neglected cause of ventilatory dysfunction in the patient with GBS is weakness of the laryngeal and glottic muscles with subsequent difficulty in swallowing and coughing, and the risk of aspiration. Finally, weakness of the tongue and retropharyngeal muscles can cause positional airway obstruction leading to hypoxemia, acidosis, and even sudden death. Although these mechanisms may work independently, they usually exert their detrimental effects together in acute respiratory failure.

Respiratory muscle function should be assessed by specific evaluation of respiratory parameters. A first impression of the respiratory state is given by simple observation of the breathing pattern. In the absence of acidosis, anxiety, pneumonia, or a mechanical hindrance to breathing, activation of accessory muscles suggests weakness of the major respiratory muscles, especially the diaphragm. Weakness of the diaphragm is also suggested if paradoxical inward movement of the upper abdominal wall is present during inspiration in the supine position. The strength of cough can be assessed by simply observing the patient. Measurement of the forced expiratory volume with a bedside spirometer and of inspiratory force allows a more precise assessment. If the vital capacity falls below 20 ml/kg, we consider the patient to have a substantial risk for respiratory failure and transfer him to the ICU. The same approach applies to patients unable to generate more than $-25 \, cm \, H_2O$ of inspiratory force. The respiratory rate is another index of ventilatory function, since, as outlined above, tachypnea is an early response to increased inspiratory work. Monitoring arterial blood gases is a simple method for assessing the ventilatory state. However, hypoxia, hypercarbia, and acidosis occur only late in respiratory failure, when respiration has already been substantially compromised or is decompensated. Thus, we regard arterial blood gases as not useful for identifying patients at risk for ventilatory failure. Finally, we examine the

patient carefully with regard to the ability to protect his airway. Once speech becomes nasal, or difficulty with swallowing and protruding the tongue occur, oropharyngeal muscle involvement is obvious and referral to the ICU is indicated.

Monitoring Autonomic Functions

Signs of autonomic dysfunction are found in approximately two thirds of patients with GBS. Well-documentated manifestations include a wide range of cardiac arrhythmias, blood pressure fluctuations (hypertension, hypotension, or labile blood pressure), abnormal hemodynamic responses to drugs, electrocardiographic abnormalities, pupillary dysfunction, sweating abnormalities, urinary retention, and gastrointestinal dysfunction. Although autonomic dysfunction is often of minor clinical relevance, patients ill enough to require intensive care can develop life-threatening cardiovascular complications, mostly at the end of the progressing phase or during the plateau. In modern ICU series, death due to acute cardiovascular collapse occurs in 3–10% of patients, but these figures include deaths from sepsis and pulmonary embolism.

For clinical assessment of autonomic performance, a variety of tests are available, most using analysis of heart rate or blood pressure in response to deep breathing, changes in position, or forced expiration. However, standardization has not been achieved so far. In 1982, Ewing and Clarke proposed five tests for evaluation of diabetic autonomic neuropathy (Table 4). Recently, an alternative battery has been suggested as superior (Ryder

Table 4. Battery of tests proposed by Ewing and co-workers (1982) for assessment of cardiovascular autonomic dysfunction

Test	Description	Normal range	Pathologic range
Valsalva ratio	Ratio of the longest to the shortest R-R interval during and after forceful breathing with an expiratory pressure of 40 mmHg for 10–15 s	greater than 1.21	less than 1.1
E:I ratio (maximum-minimum ratio)	Ratio of the maximum to the minimum HR during deep breathing	more than 1.5	less than 1.1
30:15 ratio	Ratio of the HR at beat 30 to the HR at beat 15 after standing or vertical tilt	greater than 1.04	less than 1.0
BP response to standing	Measuring BP while lying down for at least 15 min and again on standing	Fall in diastolic BP of less than 10 mmHg	Fall in diastolic BP of more than 15 mmHg
Isometric exercise	Maintaining handgrip at 30% of maximum for up to 5 min	Increase in diastolic BP of more than 16 mmHg	Increase in diastolic BP of less than 10 mmHg

BP, Blood pressure; E:I, expiration:inspiration; HR, heart rate.

and Hardisty 1990). However, although each of these batteries seems useful for detecting cardiovascular reflex abnormalities in patients with mild GBS, severely affected GBS patients are unable to perform them in an appropriate fashion. For this reason, we use the response of heart rate to carotid sinus massage or to pressure on the eyeballs, and regard the occurrence of profound bradycardia or atrioventricular block as abnormal. The study of heart rate variation during deep breathing at six breaths a minute is another simple bedside test. Physiologically, heart rate variation is more than 15 bpm during this maneuver. A variation between 11 and 14 bpm is considered borderline, and a variation of less than 11 bpm is clearly abnormal. Passive tilting and calculation of the standard deviation of R-R intervals during normal breathing are more sophisticated procedures that require special equipment not available for routine purposes.

Signs of autonomic dysfunction ofter than cardiovascular should also be carefully sought and treated, if necessary. For example, hyperhidrosis may occasionally be severe enough to require additional fluids. Gastrointestinal function is assessed by noting gastric contents, bowel movements, abdominal wall tension, and defecation pattern. If ileus occurs, enteral feeding should be stopped, gastric and colonic tubes should be placed, and prostigmine should be given. Transient bladder dysfunction may occur during the evolution of symptoms, but severe and persistent bladder paresis should always render the diagnosis of GBS doubtful. Pupillary dysfunction is uncommon in typical GBS, but it may occur with complete external ophthalmoplegia, quadriplegia, and respiratory failure, or in patients with Fisher's syndrome.

Due to the life-threatening risks of cardiovascular dysfunction, the patient with GBS should be tested on a regular basis. If any one of the cited tests is abnormal, transfer to the ICU seems mandatory for closer monitoring and treatment.

ICU Management

General Management

The importance of sophisticated intensive care in GBS patients is underscored by the fact that deaths due to medical complications continue to occur. Passive limb movement is applied to prevent contractures and leg vein thrombosis. Deep vein thrombosis and pulmonary embolism are further prevented by administration of heparin or the use of intermittent pneumatic calf compression. We currently favor continuous infusion of heparin in a dose high enough to prolong partial thromboplastin time to values of 2–2.5 times of normal. Chest physiotherapy is applied to avoid mucous plugging of large airways and segmental pulmonary collapse. Urine and tracheal secretions should be cultured twice a week for early detection of infections. High-topped sneakers can be used to overcome shortening of the Achilles tendons. Effective pro-

phylaxis against decubiti in tetraplegic patients requires frequent position changes and meticulous care of already compromised skin areas. Positioning should furthermore be adequate to avoid secondary nerve damage. In patients with facial diplegia, thorough attention to eye care is mandatory to prevent corneal ulceration.

Management of Cardiovascular Autonomic Dysfunction

If major arrhythmias occur, such as symptomatic bradycardia, atrioventricular block, or cardiac arrest, insertion of a demand pacemaker is indicated. Atropine may be administered in some cases but seems inappropriate when bradycardia is intermixed with periods of tachycardia. In addition, administration of this agent increases the viscosity of tracheal secretions. A transcutaneous demand pacemaker has recently become available which avoids the complications of intravenous pacing. Due to its noninvasive nature, this system can be used in a broad range of borderline indications often met in patients with temporary autonomic failure. In our experience, safe and effective cardiac stimulation is achieved with such a system in both emergency and standby situations. However, painful muscle contractions may occasionally occur, with the need for sedation or analgesics, especially in obese patients. In such cases, we prefer intravenous systems. An intravenous pacemaker may also be inserted when the transcutaneous device has been activated several times for severe atrioventricular blocking or sinus arrest.

Volume therapy should be carefully guided because of the inability of patients with GBS to increase cardiac output in an appropriate fashion. Likewise, vasodepressor drugs, including anesthetics, should be used with caution. The pattern of cardiovascular autonomic dysfunction may change within seconds in patients with demyelinating neuropathies. When severe hemodynamic instability occurs or fluid and volume therapy becomes difficult, Swan-Ganz catheterization is indicated to facilitate hemodynamic management. Administration of beta-adrenergic blocking drugs may precipitate acute cardiovascular collapse. When such agents are needed for control of hypertension or tachycardia, they must be employed with extreme caution. It should be stressed in this context that pulmonary embolism, pneumothorax, myocarditis, and sepsis all continue to occur in intensively treated patients with GBS and thus must be anticipated with a high index of suspicion before cardiovascular complications are attributed to autonomic dysfunction.

Respiratory Management

Acute respiratory failure due to respiratory muscle denervation is a life-threatening but manageable complication of GBS. After transfer to the ICU, the patient should be carefully monitored with respect to ventilatory status to determine the need for intubation and institution of mechanical ventilation. In general, we advocate early intubation, a strategy that has been reinforced by recent reports. This approach is likely to prevent pulmonary complications as well as emergency intubation with its inherent risks. We intubate patients with or without mechanical ventilation if anyone of the following criteria is met: (a) arterial blood-gas analysis reveals ventilatory failure, i.e., arterial pO_2 less than 60 mmHg, or pCO_2 greater than 50 mmHg; (b) forced vital capacity is below 15 ml/kg; (c) paresis of bulbar muscles, with positional airway obstruction or aspiration after swallowing; (d) radiological evidence of major aspiration or atelectasis; or (e) inability to generate a forced inspiration pressure of 20 cm H_2O or more. Table 5 summarizes intubation criteria followed in our units.

Application of criteria b–e assures that intubation is performed before respiratory failure is established. Of these, a steady fall in serially measured vital capacity is the most powerful predictor for the need of mechanical ventilation. Respiratory failure may develop more quickly than limb weakness from underlying neuropathy when pulmonary infection, atelectasis, or sepsis are superimposed on the neuropathic process. If mechanical ventilation is needed, both synchronized intermittent mandatory ventilation (SIMV) and pressure-supported ventilation (PSV) are appropriate to overcome respiratory muscle weakness. However, with these modes, patients must be closely observed to assure delivery of sufficient tidal volume. If fatigue, hypoxemia, or CO_2 retention are encountered, ventilatory support must be increased or controlled mechanical ventilation must be started.

In general, early tracheotomy seems desirable. However, we do not advocate ultra-early tracheotomy because some patients require intubation only for a few days and thus can be

Table 5. Criteria for intubation of the patient with Guillain-Barré syndrome

- $PaCO_2 > 50$ mmHg
- $PaO_2 < 60$ mmHg despite supplemental O_2
- O_2 saturation < 95% on supplemental O_2
- Forced vital capacity <15 ml/kg body weight
- Forced inspiration pressure <20 cm H_2O
- Radiological evidence of pneumonia, aspiration, or atelectasis
- Loss of airway protection (aspiration, positional obstruction)

spared the operation and its associated risks. At present, our practice is to wait until the end of the second week of mechanical ventilation. By this time, approximately one third of patients no longer need intubation. Once clinical assessment shows improvement of the respiratory state, weaning from mechanical ventilation begins. Usually, it can proceed quickly, as soon as vital capacity exceeds 7 ml/kg. Both PSV and SIMV are effective modalities for weaning the patient off the ventilator; neither one has proven to be superior to the other. The details of weaning techniques are given in Chap. 12.

Nutrition

The goals of nuritional support include (a) maintenance of fluid and electrolyte balances, (b) prevention of starvation-induced muscle wasting and potential compromise of the immune system, (c) maintenance of skin integrity, and (d) minimizing the effects of metabolic stress (Chap. 11). The optimal regimen in different stages of GBS has not been satisfactorily defined. Unless more accurate data are available, we use serum retinol-binding protein and transferrin to detect malnutrition and to monitor nutritional repletion. Total calorie requirement is best determined by indirect calorimetry, but it may be estimated using the Harris-Benedict formula. Weekly measurements of nitrogen and creatinine excretion (in 24-h urine samples) are done to calculate protein catabolism. Despite therapy guided by these parameters, GBS patients do become hypermetabolic and hypercatabolic. The reasons for this are not clear.

Psychological Support and Pain Management

Like any patient in the ICU, the patient with severe GBS may exhibit demoralization, sadness, fear, and anxiety. In the most severely affected patients, the experience of sensory deprivation and total physical dependence may result in episodes of dream-like or oneiric states. Factors that cause psychological stress include loss of the normal day and night cycle due to around-the-clock nursing care, acoustic alarms often mistakenly interpreted by patients as indicative of a problem, and loss of orientation due to new surroundings. In addition, paralyzed ventilated patients frequently fear becoming accidentally disconnected from the ventilator or, when being weaned, being unable to obtain another breath.

Adequate and frequent communication is therefore mandatory for patients who are physically helpless but mentally alert. In most instances, simple codes can be arranged to assure communication via alphabetical boards or lists of frequent requests and concerns. Electrical devices operated by chin, lip, tongue, finger, or toe movements may also be used. Another cornerstone of psychosocial support is early education of both the patient and family regarding the nature of the disease and its usually favorable outcome. A world-wide GBS Foundation International is available to provide information to patients and families, and to arrange visits by former patients (P.O. Box 262, Wynnewood, PA 19096; telephone (001) 215-667-0131). In Germany, a similar service is provided by the GBS *Selbsthilfegruppe Sinsheim e.V.* (Hans-Thoma-Straße 13, 74889 Sinsheim, telephone 07261-4205). A third major concern is pain relief. Pain in GBS may be related to pressure areas or to feelings of cold in the extremities. Lambskins, changes in position, socks, and warming devices may be used for relief, in addition to nonsteroidal anti-inflammatory drugs. Unfortunately, these measures are frequently ineffective, so that narcotics are necessary for adequate pain control. Although usually given intravenously, oral or subcutaneous administration is perferable due to a lower risk of ventilatory suppression. In selected cases, epidural morphine analgesia has been employed to control pain that is unresponsive to analgesics or other therapeutic maneuvers. Finally, nursing care and laboratory examinations should be arranged and coordinated in a way that allows sleep, rest, and privacy. A room with TV, radio, and calendar, displaying photos and other personal objects, is useful to create a familiar atmosphere and reduce psychological distress.

Fear and anxiety are best treated by medication and by quiet reassurance. Unless panic is overt, benzo-diazepines are the drugs of first choice. If the patient appears to be in a state of panic or psychosis, neuroleptics such as haloperidol may be administered in oral or parenteral form. Predisposing factors such as sleep deprivation, metabolic abnormalities, medications, hypoxia, and sepsis should be eliminated. For selected patients, brief psychotherapy may be indicated.

Therapies

Plasmapheresis

Plasmapheresis (plasma exchange) permits the removal of plasma and its constituents from the circulation (see also Chap. 11). To provide hemodynamic stability, replacement fluids are needed in adequate amounts. Usually, diluted solutions of albumin or fractionated albumin are used with normal saline. Alternatively, fresh-frozen plasma (FFP) has been used, but it has not proved superior to albumin. More importantly, the use of FFP carries risks for transmission of infections including hepatitis and HIV.

The rationale for the use of plasmapheresis in the treatment of GBS is the removal or dilution of circulating factors implicated in the pathogenesis of the disease. Favorable results with plasmapheresis in GBS have been shown in several uncontrolled trials, as well in EAN. Two small controlled trials also yielded positive results of plasmapheresis in patients with severe GBS. To further evaluate the role that plasmapheresis plays in GBS, several large collaborative studies were initiated, particularly in North America, Sweden, and

France, all demonstrating beneficial effects.

Taken together, the available data provide evidence that early plasmapheresis is most beneficial. However, procedural variations of exchange, such as volume exchanged per procedure, frequency, total number, and other factors influencing outcome have not yet been defined. In the North American study, a total of 250 ml/kg within 7–14 days was exchanged with a typical schedule of 40 ml/kg every other day or 20 ml/kg daily. In the French study, four plasmaphereses, each with two plasma volumes, were done on alternate days. Currently, we use a schedule adopted from the North American study.

Unfortunately, it is not clear when to start plasmapheresis. On the one hand, plasmapheresis should be done early in the disease course to be effective. On the other hand, costs, risks, and patient discomfort would not justify this procedure to be done in mildly affected patients, with the consequence that plasmapheresis should be delayed until the patient develops a more severe deficit. We observe patients with early disease closely. If weakness develops more rapidly than usual or the patient becomes unable to walk unassisted, we consider therapeutic plasmapheresis. Plasmapheresis is not instituted in patients with stable disease for more than 1 week or in those with a mild course.

Plasmapheresis is a safe, but not completely innocuous procedure. Major side effects are either device related or procedural, and include cardic arrhythmias, episodes of hypotension, bacteremias, allergic reactions, complications with vascular access, citrate toxicity, and bleeding due to the need for anticoagulation. Plasma exchange should therefore not be performed in patients with severe uncontrolled infection, sepsis, or unstable hemodynamics. By 1985, more than 50 deaths associated with plasmapheresis had been reported. It is estimated that there were three deaths per 10 000 procedures. For these reasons, plasmapheresis should be performed only in ICUs experienced with the procedure.

Immunoglobulins

Recently, the results of a Dutch multicenter trial comparing plasmapheresis and intravenous immunoglobulins (IVIG) were published. The authors concluded that daily infusions of immunoglobulins (0.4 g/kg body weight for 5 days) are at least as effective as plasma exchange. The outcome of the plasma exchange control group was poor, however, compared with the results of similar studies. The mode of action of high-dose IVIG in immune-mediated demyelinating polyneuropathy remains unclear. Both nonspecific and specific mechanisms have been suggested, including competitive macrophage Fc receptor blockade, interference with regulation of B and T cells, and anti-idiotypic binding to autoantibodies presumed to be involved in pathogenesis of the disease. In contrast to plasmapheresis, immunoglobulins are readily available and easy to administer without the need and risks of extracorporeal circulation. Their use also seems to be safe, because modern processing techniques exclude transmission of infectious agents. Although immunoglobulin treatment is expensive, the costs are not higher than that for plasmapheresis. We currently use immunoglobulins for patients in whom plasmapheresis is contraindicated, and within prospective study protocols. Currently, a European multicenter trial is under way to further determine the effectiveness of IVIG.

Steroids

In contrast to chronic inflammatory demyelinating polyneuropathy, where corticosteroids are of substantial therapeutic value, their use in GBS is no longer justified since randomized controlled trials have failed to show any beneficial effect with conventional or high doses.

vention and management of such complications. In addition, psychological support is mandatory for patients who are often physically helpless for weeks or months. Of the available immunomodulatory therapies, both plasmapheresis and intravenous administration of immunoglobulins have been shown to be beneficial in younger patients, when administered early in the disease course. In contrast, corticosteroids are of no therapeutic value. With modern ICU techniques, the mortality has declined to 3–5% in the subgroup of severely afflicted patients, i.e., those who lose their ablility to walk unassisted during the course of the illness. Of the survivors, 10–20% may have some disability and 5–10% remain unable to return to work.

Summary

Guillain-Barré syndrome is an acutely or subacutely evolving immune-mediated inflammatory disorder of the peripheral nerves, leading to myelin damage and scattered demyelination. Areflexia and a rather symmetrical, self-limited flaccid muscle weakness, evolving over a period of 2–4 weeks, are the clinical hallmarks of the disease. Respiratory failure due to weakness of the respiratory muscles and cardiovascular instability due to involvement of the autonomic nervous system are the main reasons for the intensive care. During the stay in the ICU, most serious complications result from mechanical ventilation, cardiocirculatory disturbances, and general medical conditions like pulmonary embolism and sepsis. Skilled nursing and medical care are essential for pre-

Suggested Reading

Albers JW, Kelly JJ (1989) Acquired inflammatory demyelinating polyneuropathies: clinical and electrodiagnostic features. Muscle Nerve 12:435–451

Arnason BGW (1984) Acute inflammatory demyelinating polyradiculoneuropathies. In: Dyck PJ, Thomas PK, Lambert EH, Bunge R (eds) Periperal neuropathy, 2nd edn, vol 2. Saunders, Philadelphia, pp 2050–2100

Asbury AK, Cornblath DR (1990) Assessment of current diagnostic criteria for Guillain-Barré syndrome. Ann Neurol 27 [Suppl]: S21–S24

Borel CO, Tilford C, Nichols DG, Hanley DF, Traystman RJ (1991) Diaphragmatic performance during recovery from acute ventilatory failure in Guillain-Barré syndrome and myasthenia gravis. Chest 99:444–451

Chevrolet JC, Deléamont P (1991) Repeated vital capacity measurements as predictive parameters for mechanical ventilation need and weaning success in the Guillain-Barré Syndrome. Am Rev Respir Dis 144:814–818

Cornblath DR, Mellits ED, Griffin JW, McKhann GM, Albers JW, Miller RG, Feasby TE, Quasky SA, and the Guillain-Barré Syndrome Study Group (1988) Motor conduction studies in Guillain-Barré syndrome: description and prognostic value. Ann Neurol 23:354–359

Dalos NP, Borel C, Hanley DF (1988) Cardiovascular autonomic dysfunction in Guillain-Barré syndrome. Therapeutic implications of Swan-Ganz monitoring. Arch Neurol 45:115–117

De Jager AEJ, Minderhoud JM (1991) Residual signs in severe Guillain-Barré syndrome: analysis of 57 patients. J Neurol Sci 104: 151–156

Drury I, Westmoreland BF, Sharbrough FW (1987) Fulminant demyelinating polyradiculopathy resembling brain death. Electroencephalogr Clin Neurophysiol 67:42–43

Editorial (1982) Hazards of apheresis. Lancet 2:1025–1026

Eisendraht SJ, Matthay MA, Dunkel JA, Zimmerman JK, Layzer RB (1983) Guillain-Barré syndrome: psychosocial aspects of management. Psychosomatics 24:465–475

Ewing DJ, Clarke BF (1982) Diagnosis and management of diabetic autonomic neuropathy. Br Med J 285:916–918

Fuller GN, Jacobs JM, Lewis PD, Lane RJM (1992) Pseudoaxonal Guillain-Barré syndrome: severe demyelination mimicking axonopathy. A case with pupillary involvement. J Neurol Neurosurg Psychiatry 55: 1079–1083

Greenland P, Griggs RC (1980) Arrhythmic complications in the Guillain-Barré syndrome. J Neurol Neurosurg Psychiatry 44:983–990

Griswold K, McKenna-Guanci M, Ropper AH (1984) An approach to the care of patients with Guillain-Barré syndrome. Heart Lung 13:66–72

Hacke W, Hassel M, Schuchardt V, Englert D (1985) Autonome Regulationsstörungen und Schrittmacherversorgung bei der akuten Polyneuritis Guillain-Barré. Aktuel Neurol (Stuttgart) 12:199–203

Henschel EO (1977) The Guillain-Barré syndrome: a personal experience. Anesthesiology 47:228–231

Hughes RAC (1990) Guillain-Barré syndrome. Springer, London Berlin Heidelberg

Hughes RAC (1991) Ineffectiveness of high-dose intravenous methylprednisolone in Guillain-Barré syndrome. Lancet 338:1142 (letter)

Kleyweg RP, van der Meché FGA, Loonen MCB, De Jong J, Knip B (1989) The natural history of the Guillain-Barré syndrome in 18 children and 50 adults. J Neurol Neurosurg Psychiatry 52:853–856

Loh L (1986) Neurological and neuromuscular disease. Br J Anaesth 58:190–200

Madson JK, Meibom J, Videbak R, Pedersen F, Grande P (1988) Transcutaneous pacing: experience with the Zoll noninvasive temporary pacemaker. Am Heart J 116:7–10

McLeod JG, Tuck RR (1987) Disorders of the autonomic nervous sytem: part 2. Investigation and treatment. Ann Neurol 21:519–529

Newton-John H (1985) Prevention of pulmonary complications in severe Guillain-Barré syndrome by early assisted ventilation. Med J Aust 142:444–445

Pollard JD (1987) A critical review of therapies in acute and chronic inflammatory demyelinating polyneurolpathies. Muscle Nerve 10:214–221

Ropper AH (1992) Current concepts: the Guillain-Barré syndrome. N Engl J Med 326:1130–1136

Ropper AH, Wijdicks EFM, Truax BT (1991) Guillain-Barré syndrome. Davis, Philadelphia

Roubenoff R, Borel CO, Hanley DH (1992) Hypermetabolism and hypercatabolism in Guillain-Barré syndrome. J Parenter Enteral Nutr 16:464–472

Ryder REJ, Hardisty CA (1990) Which battery of cardiovascular autonomic function tests? Diabetologia 33:177–179

Schmidt-Degenhard M (1986) Oneiroides Erleben bei intensivbehandelten panplegischen Polyradikulitis-Patienten. Nervenarzt 57:712–718

Singh NK, Jaiswal AK, Misra S, Srivastava PK (1987) Assessment of autonomic dysfunction in Guillain-Barré syndrome and its prognostic implications. Acta Neurol Scand 75:101–105

The French Cooperative Group on plasma exchange in Guillain-Barré syndrome (1987) Efficiency of plasma exchange in Guillain-Barré syndrome: role of replacement fluids. Ann Neurol 22:753–761

The Guillain-Barré Study Group (1985) Plasmapheresis and acute Guillain-Barré syndrome. Neurology 35:146–148

Triggs WJ, Cros D, Gominak SC, Zuniga G, Beric A, Shahani BT, Ropper AH, Roongta SM (1992) Motor nerve inexcitability in Guillain-Barré syndrome. Brain 115:1291–1302

Truax BT (1984) Autonomic disturbances in the Guillain-Barré syndrome. Semin Neurol 4:462–468

Van der Meché FGA, Schmitz PIM, and the Dutch Guillain-Barré Study Group (1992) A randomized trial comparing intravenous immune globulin and plasma exchange in Guillain-Barré syndrome. N Engl J Med 326:1123–1129

Vincken W, Elleker MG, Cosio MG (1987) Determinants of respiratory muscle weakness in stable chronic neuromuscular disorders. Am J Med 82:53–58

Weiß H (1991) Psychische Veränderungen bei intensivbehandelten Patienten mit akutem Guillain-Barré-Syndrom – tiefenpsychologische Aspekte des Kommunikationsverlustes und seiner Bewältigung. Fortschr Neurol Psychiatr 59:134–140

Winer JB, Hughes RAC, Osmond C (1988) A prospective study of acute idiopathic neuropathy. I. Clinical features and their prognostic value. J Neurol Neurosurg Psychiatry 51:605–612

Chapter 68

Chronic Inflammatory Demyelinating Polyneuropathy

ERNST F. HUND, HANS-PETER HARTUNG, and ALLAN H. ROPPER

Definition, Pathogenesis, and Epidemiology

Approximately 3% of inflammatory demyelinating polyneuropathy cases progress for longer than 4 weeks, the arbitrary cut-off point for the diagnosis of GBS, or they relapse and fluctuate. Such cases are referred to as chronic inflammatory demyelinating polyneuropathy (CIDP). In CIDP, the nadir of illness is usually reached after several months, either after a chronic monophasic, a stepwise progressing, or a relapsing course. In contrast, the even rarer recurrent GBS, in which acute relapses appear after complete recovery, is usually considered to be more closely tied to GBS than to CIDP by most authorities, since time course and treatment response of single recurrences are identical to typical monophasic GBS.

It is not entirely clear whether CIDP simply represents a variant of GBS or constitutes a different disease. Differences in temporal evolution, his-

Section Editors: Daniel F. Hanley and Allan H. Ropper

tory of preceding infections, and response to therapy separate CIDP from GBS, but this separation may be arbitrary and ultimately prove not to have a pathogenetic basis. The pathologic findings in CIDP and GBS are similar, but generally more heterogeneous in CIDP. They comprise endoneural or subperineural edema, demyelinated and thinly myelinated nerve fibers, macrophage-mediated phagocytosis of myelin, and secondary axonal degeneration. Segmental demyelination and remyelination with mononuclear cell infiltration of nerve roots and peripheral nerves, although considered the hallmarks of pathologic abnormalities in CIDP, are present in only half the sural nerve biopsies. Inflammatory cell infiltration is more sparse and axonal degeneration more prominent than expected from the electrodiagnostic studies. Repeated episodes of demyelination and remyelination lead to onion-bulb formation in up to one third of cases, thereby causing confusion with hypertrophic forms of hereditary neuropathy. For unclear reasons, CIDP is associated with CNS demyelination in 5% of cases.

Because CIDP is an uncommon condition, its incidence and prevalence are difficult to assess. According to rough estimates, CIDP occurs in only 3–5 cases per million population per year, i.e., four times less frequently than GBS. The disease may occur at any age, but the average is 35 years. Men are more commonly affected than women. As is known from multiple sclerosis, which is regarded by some as the CNS counterpart of CIDP, the chronic relapsing form of CIDP is more likely to start at younger age (mean 27 years), whereas the chronic progressive form begins at an average age of 51. Although respiratory failure and life-threatening autonomic dysfunction are less frequent than in GBS, they do occur and contribute to mortality in CIDP. In the series of Dyck et al. (1975), six (11%) of 53 patients died of complications of the disease within 2–19 years after its onset. More recent series report a mortality of 3–6%.

Clinical Features and Differential Diagnosis

The clinical features, other than the tempo of evolution are similar to those described for GBS, and include relatively symmetrical proximal and distal weakness of both the upper and lower limbs, loss or diminution of tendon reflexes, and sensory symptoms such as numbness, paresthesias, and aching muscle pain. Involvement of the cranial nerves and preceding infections or immunizations occur less frequently than in GBS, but there is an associated underlying illness in up to 20% of patients. The severity of CIDP varies widely. Although progression to a bed-bound state is not uncommon, weakness is rarely severe enough to cause respiratory failure. Similarly, in our experience autonomic dysfunction, a major cause of complications in GBS, is seldom a serious problem in CIDP, and significant autonomic involvement has not been recorded in several larger surveys. Since autonomic dysfunction and respiratory muscle weakness may nevertheless be life threatening, we look carefully for signs of respiratory or autonomic failure in any patient with CIDP. When the criteria outlined for GBS (see Chap. 67) are met, the patient is transferred to the ICU.

It is essential for the diagnosis of CIDP that other causes of demyelinating neuropathy or associated systemic diseases be excluded. Such disorders include hereditary, paraproteinemic, metabolic, toxic, and infectious neuropathies (Table 1). Of these, demyelinating hereditary neuropathy (HMSN-type I) is a fairly common disorder, with a wide range of clinical manifestations. Suspicion of this disease is raised when family history is positive for neuropathy, or when deformities of the feet or spine are present. The presence of paraproteins must be carefully excluded in every case of presumed CIDP, by immune electrophoresis or immune fixation of both serum and urine. Refsum's disease and metachromatic leukodystrophy are metabolic disorders in which cerebral involvement is usually prominent. The acute hepatic porphyrias usually produce a proximally pronouced neuropathy of the axonal type and are discussed in more detail in Chap. 69. Diabetes, alcohol, chemicals, and drugs may also cause axonal damage. Amiodarone and perhexiline are important

Table 1. Differential diagnosis of chronic demyelinating polyneuropathy

---

Hereditary motor and sensory neuropathy (type I and type III)
Chronic demyelinating polyneuropathy associated with monoclonal gammopathies:
  Multiple myeloma
  Osteosclerotic myeloma
  Waldenström's macroglobulinemia
  Monoclonal gammopathy of undetermined significance
Multifocal motor neuropathy with conduction block and elevated anti-GM1 titers
Refsum's disease
Leukodystrophies:
  Metachromatic leukodystrophy
  Globoid cell leukodystrophy
  Cockayne syndrome
Neuropathy due to amiodarone and perhexilene
Neuropathy due to HIV infection or borreliosis

---

exceptions, insofar as neuropathy produced by these agents is typically demyelinating. In rare cases, vasculitis may present as isolated neuropathy without involvement of visceral organs, requiring nerve biopsy for diagnosis. Multifocal motor neuropathy with conduction block and elevated anti-GM1 antibody titers has recently been added to the list of differential diagnoses. CIDP may also occur in the context of HIV infection and borreliosis.

Ancillary Tests

Cerebrospinal fluid examination typically reveals an albuminocytological dissociation, with slight to moderate elevation of protein concentration and few or absent cells. In HIV-associated CIDP, pleocytosis may be present, however. Electrodiagnostic examination is of paramount importance in demonstrating underlying demyelination. At least three of the following electrophysiologic changes should be found: slowing of motor conduction velocities to values of 70% of normal, presence of conduction block not related to common sites of nerve entrapment and marked dispersion of the compound muscle action potential, prolonged distal latencies exceeding 130% of normal, delayed or absent compound sensory action potentials, and prolonged F-wave latencies or F-wave failure. The presence of conduction block and multifocal slowing of motor nerve conduction velocity helps to distinguish CIDP from hereditary demyelinating neuropathy, where conduction slowing is uniform and conduction block is not seen.

Treatment

Steroids

One of the most conspicuous features of CIDP is the response to steroids. This clearly distinguishes CIDP from GBS, and also differentiates it from hereditary motor and sensory neuropathy, which responds to steroids only in exceptional cases. Initial improvement is often minor and followed by relapses in about half of the cases. Of the various dosage schedules employed, none is generally accepted as best. We start with prednisone/methylprednisolone 100 mg/day for 1 month, after which the dosage is tapered by 20 mg every 4 weeks (Table 2). It is also possible to initiate treatment with a 3- to 5-day intravenous pulse of 0.5–1.0 g prednisone/methylprednisolone and then switch to

Table 2. Treatment for chronic inflammatory demyelinating polyneuropathy

Disease severity	Treatment
Mildly affected patients	No treatment
Moderately affected	Prednisone/prednisolone 100 mg daily for 4 weeks, tapered by 20 mg each following month
Severely affected	Prednisone/prednisolone as above (or i.v. pulses of 0.5–1.0 g for 3–5 days) plus Plasma exchange, 2 liters 3 times weekly, for 2 weeks or Intravenous immunoglobulins (IVIG) 0.4 g/kg daily for 3–5 days
Frequent relapses	Prednisone/prednisolone 8 mg on alternate days plus Azathioprine 2 mg/kg daily, titrated to a WBC of 3000–3500/mm^3 and a lymphocyte count of 600–800/mm^3
Otherwise uncontrolled patients	Prednisone/prednisolone 60–80 mg on alternate days plus Cyclophosphamide 2 mg/kg per day orally (or i.v. pulse therapy, see text for details) or Cyclosporin A 8–10 mg/kg, tapered to 5 mg/kg by 3 months

oral medication. Troublesome side effects must be taken seriously when high doses are used for a prolonged time; they include hyperosmolar diabetic coma, peptic ulcer, hemorrhage and perforation of stomach or duodenum, intercurrent infections, osteoporosis, cataracts, aseptic necrosis of the femoral head, arterial hypertension, and cushingoid gain in body weight. Close clinical monitoring is therefore mandatory, including blood glucose levels, white blood cell counts, blood pressure, bone mineral content, split-lamp examinations of the lenses, and careful surveillance of possible infections or gastric discomfort. We perform weekly blood tests for the first 4 weeks, then monthly. Ophthalmologic examinations are done every 6 months, and bone densitometry and X-rays of the femoral heads are performed on a yearly basis.

Immunosuppressants

In addition to corticosteroids, various immunosuppressant drugs, including azathioprine, cyclophosphamide, and cyclosporin A, have proven to be beneficial in CIDP.

Azathioprine. Azathioprine is established as having relatively little toxicity and is still used by many clinicians as a steroid-sparing agent, although a clinical trial has not found it effective in CIDP. Apart from gastrointestinal dysfunction (anorexia, diarrhea, vomiting), leukopenia, liver dysfunction, and allergic reactions are the most commonly encountered adverse effects of this drug. An additional risk to be weighed is the occurrence of late neoplasms, mostly non-Hodgkin's lymphoma or skin cancer. We administer azathioprine when treatment with steroids fails, frequent relapses occur, or unwanted side effects preclude further use of steroids. We then taper prednisone/methylprednisolone to a maintenance dose as low as 8 mg on alternate days and add azathioprine 2–2.5 mg/kg, the dose being adjusted to a white blood cell count of 3000–3500/mm^3 and a lymphocyte count of 600–800/mm^3 (Table 2). Liver and bone marrow functions are monitored on a weekly basis for the first 8 weeks and then at monthly intervals.

Cyclophosphamide. Cyclophosphamide, even in the moderate dose of 2 mg/kg orally, is relatively toxic and requires careful monitoring of the WBC, along with frequent analyses of the urine because of the drug's potential for hemorrhagic cystitis and bladder cancer. The patients are obliged to increase fluid intake, and 100 mg mesna t.i.d. orally is added for bladder protection. Repeated i.v. pulse therapy as is used in the treatment of chronic progressive multiple sclerosis may be better tolerated. Such a regimen entails daily i.v. pulses of 350 mg/m^2 for 3 consecutive days, followed by repeated cycles every 6, later every 8 weeks. WBC should be kept at 3000–3500/mm^3 and lymphocytes at 600–800/mm^3.

Cyclosporin A. More recently, anecdotal reports and two small series have emphasized the beneficial effect of cyclosporin A, which is widely used in transplantation medicine. Cyclosporin A may be started at 8–10 mg/kg per day, and reduced to 5 mg/kg by 3 months. Whole blood levels of the drug, creatinine clearance, serum creatinine levels, and blood pressure should be carefully monitored. Dose-dependent nephrotoxicity with malignant arterial hypertension is the major side effect and limits the use of this agent. We consider cyclosporin A an add-on medication for patients who are unresponsive to steroids and azathioprine.

Plasma Exchange

Since humoral factors such as antibodies, cytokines, and mediators of inflammation are involved in the pathogenesis of CIDP, plasma exchange would be expected to be of therapeutic value. In fact, plasmapheresis was shown to be effective in some small series and several anecdotal reports. A controlled trial has confirmed these positive results. However, patients may show only temporary improvement, and others become dependent on plasma exchange, in that cessation is followed by a relapse. Since improvement, if it occurs, is often rapid, plasmapheresis is a useful means of treating some rapidly worsening patients. We currently combine plasma exchange with steroids in such patients, using 2–3 l exchanged on alternate days. In severe cases or those of recent onset, we perform plasmapheresis daily. For procedural details and risks of plasma exchange, see Chap. 15.

High-dose Intravenous Immunoglobulins

Recently, the administration of high doses of intravenous immunoglobulins (IVIG) has become popular in immune-mediated diseases, and it has been successfully used in patients with CIDP. These observations were supported by a placebo-controlled crossover trial in patients who were judged to be IVIG responsive and who needed repeated IVIG infusions to maintain their improved condition. In a consecutive randomized multicenter trial, however, the improvement in the treatment group did not differ from that in the placebo group. Usually, 0.4 g/kg body wt. per day is given over 3–5 days, but many patients depend on repeated cycles to maintain improvement. In contrast to treatment with immunosuppressive drugs, including steroids, no long-term complications are known even with prolonged use of IVIG. In comparison with plasma exchange, administration of IVIG is easier to perform and more convenient for the patient. Side effects have included fever, hypertension, and anaphylaxis (if the patient is IgA deficient) during infusion, and proteinuria or aseptic meningitis delayed days or weeks after the infusion. There is evidence that plasma exchange and IVIG are also effective in chronic demyelinating neuropathies associated with monoclonal gammopathy. The major drawback of both plasmapheresis and IVIG is their high cost, which becomes especially important when prolonged use of either is necessary.

Prognosis and Conclusions

CIDP differs in time course, therapeutic approach, and prognosis from GBS. Weakness develops over months, and after initial remission, relapses occur in up to half the patients. Preceding infections or immunizations are less frequently encountered than in GBS. Although respiratory failure and autonomic dysfunction rarely bring the patient to the ICU, the disease is sometimes severe enough to result in significant neurological deficits, respiratory failure, or even death, the latter usually attributable to intercurrent infections. Corticosteroids and plasmapheresis have been established as useful to induce remissions and to delay relapses. More recently, benefit has also been shown from IVIG administration in selected patients. The criteria for the selection of patients who may benefit from IVIG treatment remain to be clarified, however.

Immunosuppressive drugs such as azathioprine, cyclophosphamide, and cyclosporin A are used, despite the absence of demonstrated benefit in controlled trials, if the disease activity is not sufficiently controlled with the combination of prednisone and either plasmapheresis or IVIG, or when side effects of steroid treatment have become no longer tolerable. The prognosis is unpredictable at the onset of the disease. Patients with a relapsing course tend to have a more favorable outcome than those with a chronic progressive course. With steroid treatment, 30% of Barohn and co-workers' patients recovered completely, and 43% were only mildly disabled 10 years after the onset of symptoms. Data on long-term follow-up with other treatments are too scarce to allow for definite conclusions.

Suggested Reading

Ad hoc Subcommittee of the American Academy of Neurology AIDS Task Force (1991) Research criteria for diagnosis of chronic inflammatory demyelinating polyneuropathy (CIDP). Neurology 41:617–618

Albers JW, Kelly JJ (1989) Acquired inflammatory demyelinating polyneuropathies: clinical and electrodiagnostic features. Muscle Nerve 12:435–451

Barohn RJ, Kissel JT, Warmolts JR, Mendell JR (1989) Chronic inflammatory demyelinating polyradiculoneuropathy. Arch Neurol 46:878–884

Bromberg MB, Feldman EL, Albers JW (1992) Chronic inflammatory demyelinating polyradiculoneuropathy: comparison of patients with and without an associated monoclonal gammopathy. Neurology 42:1157–1163

Cook D, Dalakas M, Galdi A, Biondi D, Porter H (1990) High-dose intravenous immunoglobulin in the treatment of demyelinating neuropathy associated with monoclonal gammopathy. Neurology 40:212–214

Cornblath DR, Chaudhry V, Griffin JW (1991) Treatment of chronic inflammatory demyelinating polyneuropathy with intravenous immunoglobulin. Ann Neurol 30:104–106

Dyck PJ, Lais AC, Ohta M, Bastron JA, Okazaki H, Groover RV (1975) Chronic inflammatory polyradiculoneuropathy. Mayo Clin Proc 50:621–637

Dyck PJ, O'Brien P, Swanson C, Low P, Daube J (1985) Combined azathioprine and prednisone in chronic inflammatory demyelinating polyneuropathy. Neurology 35:1173–1176

Dyck PJ, Daube J, O'Brien P, Pineda A, Low PA, Windebank AJ, Swanson C (1986) Plasma exchange in chronic inflammatory demyelinating polyradiculoneuropathy. N Engl J Med 314:461–465

Dyck PJ, Low PA, Windebank AJ, Jaradeh SS, Gosselin S, Bourque P, Smith BE, Kratz KM, Karnes JL, Evans BA, Pineda AA, O'Brien PC, Kyle RA (1991) Plasma exchange in polyneuropathy associated with monoclonal gammopathy of undetermined significance. N Engl J Med 325:1482–1486

Dyck PJ, Prineas J, Pollard JD (1993) Chronic inflammatory demyelinating polyradiculoneuropathy. In: Dyck PJ, Thomas PK, Griffin JW, Low PA, Poduslo JF (eds) Peripheral neuropathy, 3rd edn. Saunders, Philadelphia, pp 1498–1517

Grand'Maison F, Feasby TE, Hahn AF, Koopman WJ (1992) Recurrent Guillain-Barré syndrome: clinical and laboratory features. Brain 115:1093–1106

Hartung HP, Heiniger K, Schäfer B, Fierz W, Toyka KV (1988) Immune mechanisms in inflammatory polyneuropathy. Ann NY Acad Sci 540:122–161

Hartung HP, Reiners K, Schmidt B, Stoll G, Toyka KV (1991) Serum interleukin-2 concentrations in Guillain-Barré syndrome and chronic idiopathic demyelinating polyradiculoneuropathy: comparison with other neurological diseases of presumed immunopathogenesis. Ann Neurol 30:48–53

Hartung HP, Stoll G, Toyka KV (1993) Immune reactions in the peripheral nervous system. In: Dyck PJ, Thomas PK, Griffin JW, Low PA, Poduslo JF (eds) Peripheral neuropathy, 3rd edn. Saunders, Philadelphia, pp 418–444

Hodgkinson SJ, Pollard JD, McLeod JG (1990) Cyclosporin A in the treatment of chronic demyelinating polyradiculoneuropathy. J Neurol Neurosurg Psychiatry 53:327–330

Hughes RAC (1987) Chronic polyneuropathy of undetermined cause. In: Matthews WB (ed) Neuropathies. Elsevier Science, Amsterdam, pp 529–541 (Handbook of clinical neurology, vol 7/51)

Krendel DA, Parks HP, Antony DC, St Clair MB, Graham DG (1989) Sural nerve biopsy in chronic inflammatory demyelinating polyradiculopathy. Muscle Nerve 12:257–264

Lewis RA, Sumner AJ (1982) The electrodiagnostic distinctions between chronic familial and acquired demyelinative neuropathies. Neurology 32:592–596

McCombe PA, Pollard JD, McLeod (1987) Chronic inflammatory demyelinating polyradiculo-neuropathy. Brain 110:1617–1630

Pollard JD (1987) A critical review of therapies in acute and chronic inflammatory demyelinating polyneuropathies. Muscle Nerve 10:214–221

Ropper AH, Wijdicks EFM, Truax BT (1991) Guillain-Barré syndrome. Davis, Philadelphia, pp 128–145

Thomas PK, Walker RWH, Rudge P, Morgan-Hughes JA, King RHM, Jacobs JM, Mills KR, Ormerod IEC, Murray NMF, McDonald WI (1987) Chronic demyelinating peripheral neuropathy associated with multifocal central nervous system demyelination. Brain 110:53–76

van Doorn PA, Vermeulen M, Brand A, Mulder PGH, Busch HFM (1991) Intravenous immunoglobulin treatment in patients with chronic inflammatory demyelinating poly-neuropathy. Arch Neurol 48:217–220

Vermeulen M, van Doorn PA, Brand A, Strengers PFW, Jennekens FGI, Busch HFM (1993) Intravenous immunoglobulin treatment in patients with chronic inflammatory demyelinating polyneuropathy: a double-blind, placebo-controlled study. J Neurol Neurosurg Psychiatry 56:36–39

Chapter 69

The Porphyrias

ERNST F. HUND and VOLKER SCHUCHARDT

Definition, Epidemiology, and Relevance for ICU Treatment

The porphyrias are a group of inherited disorders of heme biosynthesis with clinical effects primarily on the nervous system, skin, and liver. Each of the porphyrias has specific biochemical features and a well-defined enzyme defect. The nervous system is involved only in the acute hepatic forms, i.e., acute intermittent porphyria (AIP), variegate porphyria (VP), and hereditary coproporphyria (HCP). The acute hepatic forms are all inherited by an autosomal dominant trait, with AIP being the most common variety in northern countries. The frequency of the abnormal gene is between 1 : 10 000 and 1 : 50 000, with females more often affected than males. The disease rarely manifests before puberty. Neurologic crises consisting mainly of generalized paralysis from a polyneuropathy are the most challenging problem in management of acute hepatic porphyrias and a major cause of death. In a survey

comprising 206 adult Finnish patients with AIP and VP, 47 (23%) had a total of 117 acute attacks during a 22-year observation period (Kauppinen and Mustajoki 1992). Of these, six died, and 21 had attacks accompanied by pareses (13% and 45% of the symptomatic patients, respectively). Most pareses and deaths occurred because of a delay in diagnosis and inappropriate treatment.

Pathogenesis

The pathogenetic mechanisms by which the accumulated metabolites cause nervous dysfunction are poorly understood. It is believed that neuropathy is caused by a "dying-back" degeneration, but short fibers are usually more involved than long ones, which is in contrast to classic dying-back neuropathy. The few pathological studies done in this field have revealed axonal loss, with some degree of secondary demyelination. Two mechanisms have been proposed to explain the disturbance of neurologic function: diminished heme synthesis within the

Section Editor: Daniel F. Hanley

neuron, and a toxic effect of accumulated metabolites. In persons carrying
the defect gene, an acute attack is most
often precipitated by the use of certain
drugs. Among these, barbiturates are
the most dangerous. Several other
agents known to provoke attacks and
those considered to be safe or probably
safe are listed in Table 1. In Germany,
a yearly updated list of dangerous
drugs, as well as recommendations for
anesthesia in patients with known
porphyria, is provided by the Rote
Liste, a manufacturer-edited manual
of commercially distributed drugs. A
second precipitating factor is the level
of hormones. Pregnancy, puerperium,
menstruation, and oral contraceptives
are known to increase the risk of exacerbation. In the Finnish survey,
nearly one third of women had symptoms associated with the menstrual
cycle, and 4% of pregnancies were associated with acute attacks. Additional
states that have been associated with
exacerbation include infection, starvation, and dieting. In AIP, the risk of
attacks correlates with the excretion of
porphobilinogen in the urine during
remission; a low rate of excretion
usually implies a lower risk of acute
attacks. Relatives of identified patients
should be screened for abnormalities
in heme production so that they may
avoid potentially fatal drugs.

Clinical Presentation

Porphyric neuropathy usually begins
with abdominal or lower back pain,
followed by limb weakness. The
proximal muscles are frequently more
involved than the distal ones, creating
the misleading impression of a myo-

Table 1. Drugs known to be fatal and those considered to be safe (or probably safe) in patients with acute hepatic porphyria (adapted from Moore 1980)

Drugs known to be fatal:	Drugs considered to be safe (or probably safe):
Analgesics:	
pentazocin	opiates
pyrazolone	salicylates
lidocaine	procaine
	ibuprofen
	paracetamol
Antibiotics:	
griseofulvin	streptomycin
sulfonamides	tetracycline
	penicillin
	cephalosporins
	aminoglycosides
Antiepileptics:	
phenytoin	bromides
suximides	clonazepam (in low doses)
carbamazepine	valproate (in low doses)
barbiturates	
Antihypertensives:	
methyldopa	propranolol
clonidine	thiazides
	reserpine
Narcotics and muscle relaxants:	
barbiturates	ether
enflurane	nitrous oxide
etomidate	cyclopropane
pancuronium	tubocurarine
meprobamate	succinylcholine
Psychoactive drugs:	
barbiturates	chloralhydrate
glutethimide	phenothiazines
imipramine	
chlordiazepoxide	
Micellaneous:	
theophylline	atropine
metoclopramide	prostigmine
alcohol	digoxin
estrogens	antihistamines
	corticosteroids
	heparin
	insulin
	cimetidine

pathy. Weakness is usually symmetrical, but asymmetry has been reported. Many cases progress to flaccid paraplegia or quadriplegia, and a few patients have respiratory failure. Tendon reflexes are depressed or absent, but the ankle jerks are characteristically preserved, reflecting predominant damage to short nerve fibers. Sensory disturbances are usually minor and, like muscle weakness, more prominent proximally than distally, thereby producing a characteristic "bathing-trunk" or suspended distribution of sensory loss. An autonomic neuropathy is common and may account for fever, tachycardia, labile hypertension, urinary retention, vomiting, constipation, and abdominal pain. There are often signs of CNS involvement, including a wide variety of mental disturbances such as confusion, irritability, psychosis, depression, and coma. In addition, about 10% of patients have seizures during the acute attack. The skin is never involved in AIP, rarely in HCP, but frequently in VP. Typical electrolyte disturbances include hyponatremia and hypomagnesemia. Table 2 summarizes the clinical features of the acute porphyric attack.

Diagnosis, Laboratory Findings, and Differential Diagnosis

The diagnosis of paralysis from porphyric polyneuropathy depends on the quantitative analysis of porphyrins and their precursors in urine and stool. Simple qualitative testing of urine is provided by the Watson-Schwartz test, which includes the condensation of Ehrlich's reagent with porphobilin-

Table 2. Clinical manifestions of the acute porphyric attack

Neuropathy:
Peripheral:
  muscle weakness
  respiratory failure
  sensory disturbances
  neuritic pain
  diminution of deep tendon reflexes
Autonomic:
  gastrointestinal: abdominal pain, vomiting,
    constipation
  cardiovascular: sinus tachycardia, labile
    hypertension, postural hypotension
  others: excessive sweating, urinary retention

Central nervous system:
Seizures, delirium, coma, psychosis, depression,
  hyperthermia

Skin:
Never involved in acute intermittent porphyria
Rarely involved in hereditary coproporphyria
Frequently involved in variegate porphyria

Electrolytes:
Hyponatremia (due to SIADH, excessive fluid
  therapy, salt-depleting nephropathy, or
  gastrointestinal sodium loss)
Hypomagnesemia

ogen. The stool should be examined as well, since even during the acute attack, urinary excretion of porphobilinogen may be low in VP. Direct enzyme activity measurement allows identification of gene bearers during symptom-free intervals. For more details, interested readers are referred to the corresponding chapters of standard medical textbooks.

Neuroradiologic findings are not helpful in establishing the diagnosis. The EEG may show diffuse or rhythmical slowing and sometimes spike- or sharp-wave activity, reflecting CNS involvement. Electrodiagnostic studies are usually consistent with a mixed axonal neuropathy, but they cannot differentiate porphyric from other axonal neuropathies.

The two main differential diagnoses of neuropathic porphyrias are Guillain-Barré syndrome (GBS) and lead poisoning. Mental disturbances and paradoxical preservation of ankle jerks are very unusual in GBS, while tachycardia and spinal fluid protein elevation are more marked in GBS. Electrodiagnostic studies should make it possible to distinguish GBS from porphyria, since GBS is primarily a demyelinating disease. The acute "axonal" GBS variant, which typically has an explosive onset, may, however, closely simulate porphyria. Plumbism may be regarded as an acquired disorder of heme synthesis, thus clinically and biochemically similar to the inherited porphyrias. A blue line on the gum-tooth border and anemia with basophilic stippling suggest lead poisoning; examination of urine and blood for lead will give the correct diagnosis. Fever, vomiting, and abdominal pain can mimic any abdominal disease, and exploratory laparotomy has not been rare in patients with porphyria. However, the abdominal wall is usually soft in porphyria, and tenderness is not marked.

Treatment

Treatment of the acute attack includes discontinuation of precipitating agents, provision of a high carbohydrate load (thought to suppress synthesis of delta-aminolevulinic acid, a major metabolite), and management of the complications of immobilization and respiratory failure, as in GBS. The infusion of hematin is an additional

Table 3. Management of the acute porphyric attack

Discontinuation of potentially hazardous drugs

Suppression of porphyrin synthesis
High carbohydrate intake: 500–600 mg/day of glucose p.o. or i.v.
Hematin or heme arginate: 4 mg/kg body weight every 12 h, for 3–6 days

Management of complications
Abdominal pain: chlorpromazine 50 mg i.m., repeated as needed, opiates if necessary (be careful not to depress respiration)
Psychosis: chlorpromazine and other phenothiazines
Seizures: Look for treatable causes and correct them first.
  Diazepam 5 mg i.v., with repeated doses when required
  Clonazepam in low doses (0.5 to 1.0 mg t.i.d.), to assure blood levels in a mid-therapeutic range
  Bromides 3–5 g/day, to assure serum levels in the range of 60–90 ng/dl
Hyponatremia: treated as outlined in Chap. 87
Hypomagnesemia: repletion with magnesium
Tachycardia: propranolol
Hypertension: propranolol and other antihypertensive drugs, with the exception of methyldopa and clonidine. Be careful not to overtreat the patient, because hypertension is often labile.
Postural hypotension: i.v. fluids as needed

---

approach in life-threatening crises, but side effects such as peripheral thrombophlebitis and disturbances of hemostasis limit the use of this agent. A new compound, heme arginate, may have some advantages over hematin, particularly as it causes fewer disturbances of blood coagulation. Recently, administration of tin (Sn)-substituted porphyrins has been shown to decrease the excretion of natural porphyrins and porphyrin precursors. A number of drugs widely used in critical care medicine cannot be used in patients with porphyria (Table 1).

Treatment of seizures may be particularly difficult. If hyponatremia is associated, it should be corrected immediately. Clonazepam and valproate are probably safe in low doses. If these agents fail, the use of bromides is the main alternative. Pain may be satisfactorily managed with phenothiazines or, if more severe, with opiates. With these, the risk of addiction must be considered, however. Table 3 gives an overview of management of the acute porphyric attack.

Conclusions

Acute hepatic porphyrias are a group of autosomal dominantly inherited disorders that may present with life-threatening peripheral and central nervous dysfunction. Peripheral neuropathy is predominantly motor; autonomic involvement may account for fever, abdominal pain, and cardiovascular instability. CNS involvement may manifest as any type of delirium, psychosis, depression, or seizures. The main ICU issues concern the management of generalized paralysis and, in some patients, respiratory failure. Acute attacks are most often precipitated by the use of drugs and have a substantial mortality if the diagnosis is missed. Other provoking factors include states with increased estrogen levels, infection, starvation, and dieting. Management of the acute attack includes prompt discontinuation of precipitating agents, provision of a high carbohydrate intake, and control

of complications. Intravenous administration of hematin, heme arginate, or Sn-substitued porphyrins are additional therapeutic choices.

Suggested Reading

Bonkowsky HL, Sinclair PR, Emery S, Sinclair JF (1980) Seizure management in acute hepatic porphyria: risks of valproate and clonazepam. Neurology 30:588–592
Case records of the Massachusetts General Hospital (1984) Case 39. N Engl J Med 311:839–847
Eales L (1979) Porphyria and the dangerous life-threatening drugs. S Afr Med J 56:914–917
Galbraith RA, Kappas A (1989) Pharmacokinetics of tin-mesoporphyrin in man and the effects of tin-chelated porphyrins on hyperexcretion of heme pathway precursors in patients with acute inducible porphyria. Hepatology 9:882–888
Kauppinen R, Mustajoki P (1992) Prognosis of acute porphyria: occurrence of acute attacks, precipitating factors, and associated diseases. Medicine 71:1–13
Moore MR (1980) International review of drugs in acute porphyria. Int J Biochem 12:1089–1097
Mustajoki P, Heinonen J (1980) General anesthesia in "inducible" porphyrias. Anesthesiology 53:15–20
Ridley A (1984) Porphyric neuropathy. In: Dyck PJ, Thomas PK, Lambert EH, Bunge R (eds) Peripheral neuropathy, 2nd edn, vol 2. Saunders, Philadelphia, pp 1704–1763
Simionatto CA, Cabal R, Jones RJ, Galbraith RA (1988) Thrombophlebitis and disturbed hemostasis following administration of intravenous hematin in normal volunteers. Am J Med 85:538–540
Straka JG, Rank JM, Bloomer JR (1990) Porphyria and porphyrin metabolism. Annu Rev Med 41:457–469
Volin L, Rasi V, Vahtera E, Tenhunen R (1988) Heme arginate: effects on hemostasis. Blood 71:625–628

| # Critical Illness Neuropathy

CHARLES F. BOLTON

Definition and Epidemiology

Critical illness polyneuropathy is a complication of the sepsis and multiple organ failure syndrome (critical illness). The syndrome may occur in at least 50% of patients in major medical or surgical intensive care units. It is important to diagnose this polyneuropathy, which occurs in 70% of patients with the syndrome, since it is a common cause of difficulty in weaning from the ventilator and often explains prolonged, generalized weakness in patients who recover from the syndrome.

Pathogenesis

The pathogenesis is unknown but it is probably related to the same fundamental defect that affects all organ systems in the septic syndrome. Antibiotics, steroids, and neuromuscular blocking agents may be contributing factors. The somewhat complex mech-

anisms in the pathogenesis are shown in Fig. 1. It is important to define the mechanism(s) of the polyneuropathy more clearly, since this will affect treatment strategies. For example, if the polyneuropathy is related entirely to the septic syndrome, newer methods of treating sepsis such as the use of anticachectin tumor necrosis factor monoclonal antibodies, which has been shown to be effective in preliminary studies, may also treat the polyneuropathy. If it is due mainly to medications such as antibiotics or neuromuscular blocking agents, the use of these drugs would have to be appropriately monitored.

Clinical Features and Differential Diagnosis

The polyneuropathy almost always occurs in critical or intensive care units, although we have seen two patients who were severely septic and developed the polyneuropathy on a general hospital ward. It is frequently preceded by septic encephalopathy. Just as the encephalopathy and the septic syn-

Section Editor: Daniel F. Hanley

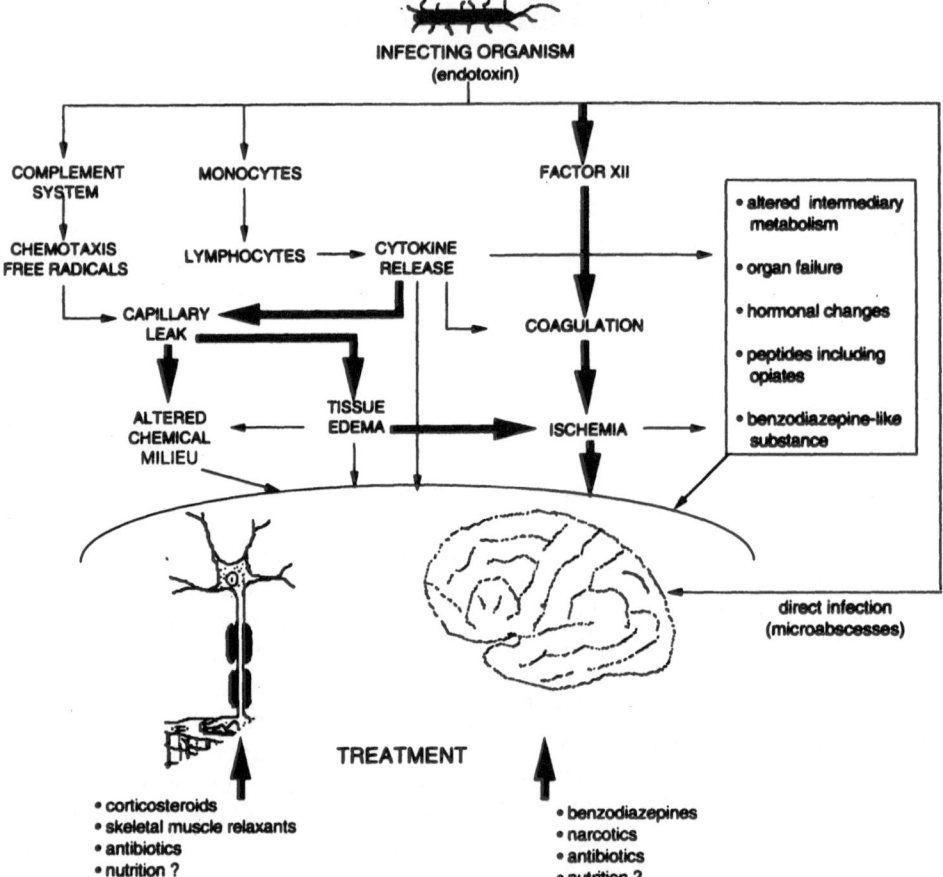

Fig. 1. Possible mechanisms for septic encephalopathy and critical illness polyneuropathy. *Arrows* pointing to the *curved line* indicate mechanisms that may apply to both the central and peripheral nervous systems. The *lower arrows* designate treatments which may affect these systems independently. The *heavy arrows* highlight the most likely mechanism. These hypotheses are complex, but involve the infecting organism inducing chemical, microvascular, metabolic, or treatment effects which may act independently or in concert. The release of cytokines from macrophages and thence from T-lymphocytes may directly affect the brain or act indirectly on the blood-brain barrier and microcirculation. Such vascular effects are abetted by activation of the complement system and factor XII. The encephalopathy may also be due to the failure of other organs or to direct infection of the brain with formation of microabscesses. Critical illness polyneuropathy may be due to disturbances of the microcirculation of peripheral nerve through vascular effects similar to those affecting brain. Various treatments used in the critical care unit may play an additive role for both the encephalopathy and the polyneuropathy. [Reproduced with permission from Bolton CF, Young GB, Zochodne DW (1993) The neurological complications of sepsis. Ann Neurol 33:94–100]

drome seem to be coming under control, and the patient should be recovering, it is noted that there is difficulty in weaning from the ventilator. The time course may be weeks or months. Careful neurological examination at this time may disclose diffuse muscle weakness, sometimes severe, which is usually confined to the limbs, particularly distally. Thus, painful distal stimulation of the limb will evoke only weak or absent movement of the limbs but will induce fairly strong facial grimacing, indicating that the painful impulses are arriving at the brain and are able to activate cranial musculature. The deep tendon reflexes may be reduced or absent, and in severe cases the plantar responses will be absent. Sensory testing is unreliable.

In at least half of all cases, these clinical signs will be absent and it will be necessary to do electrophysiological studies to establish the diagnosis (see below).

Ancillary Tests

Electrophysiological studies in the context of the clinical situation should establish the diagnosis and no further tests are usually needed. These studies will show normal or near normal conduction velocities and distal and proximal latencies but reduced muscle and sensory nerve compound action potential amplitudes. Needle electromyography will reveal fibrillation potentials and positive sharp waves in muscle as a sign of denervation. Motor unit potentials will fire in decreased numbers, either due to the neuropathy or to poor recruitment due to septic encephalopathy. In some cases, the motor unit potentials appear somewhat small and polyphasic, suggesting an associated polymyopathy as a complication of the sepsis. At times, involvement of the motor axons is more severe than that of sensory axons. Repetitive stimulation studies should be utilized in electrophysiological testing, to make certain that there is no defect in neuromuscular transmission. If there is still doubt about the nature of the neuromuscular problem, muscle, and occasionally nerve, biopsy may be necessary.

The cerebrospinal fluid examination, if carried out, is normal or shows a mild elevation in protein.

These tests will help to sort out the various conditions that may be considered in the differential diagnosis.

Differential Diagnosis

There are a wide variety of disorders of peripheral nerve, neuromuscular junction, and muscle which should be considered in the differential diagnosis of critical illness polyneuropathy (Table 1). Many of these conditions will antedate admission to the critical care unit, such as Guillain-Barré syndrome or diabetic polyneuropathy. Others will be obvious complications that occur after admission to the unit, such as paralysis due to neuromuscular blocking agents. This broad differential diagnosis must always be kept in mind and appropriate tests instituted, such as those to detect porphyria or toxicity from antibiotics. However, in our experience, the commonest cause of neuromuscular weakness in patients in the critical care unit is critical illness polyneuropathy.

Table 1. Differential diagnosis of neuromuscular signs in critically ill patients

---

Encephalopathy
  Septic
  Anoxic-ischemic, etc.
Myelopathy
  Anoxic-ischemic
  Trauma, etc.
Neuropathy
  Critical illness polyneuropathy
  Thiamine deficiency
  Vitamin E deficiency
  Nonspecific nutritional deficiency
  Pyridoxine abuse
  Hypophosphatemia
  Aminoglycoside toxicity
  Penicillin toxicity
  Guillain-Barré syndrome
  Motor neurone disease
  Porphyria
  Carcinomatous polyneuropathy
  Compressive neuropathy
  Diphtheria
Neuromuscular transmission defects
  Anesthetic drugs
  Aminoglycoside toxicity
  Myasthenia gravis
  Eaton-Lambert syndrome
  Hypomagnesemia
  Organophosphate poisoning
  Wound botulism
  Tick bite paralysis
Myopathy
  Sepsis
  Water and electrolyte disturbances –
    potassium, phosphate, calcium, magnesium
  Steroid myopathy
  Muscular dystrophy
  Polymyositis
  Acid maltase deficiency

Reproduced with permission from Bolton CF (1987) Electrophysiological studies of critically ill patients. Muscle Nerve 10:129–135.

It may be difficult, however, to distinguish particular conditions from critical illness polyneuropathy and these conditions will be briefly discussed.

Septic Myopathy

Since the septic syndrome affects all organ systems throughout the body, it seems logical that muscle would also be primarily affected. However, its presence has been difficult to detect because polyneuropathy is often associated. Thus, the presence of fibrillation potentials and positive sharp waves and reduced muscle compound action potential amplitudes could be due to either an axonal neuropathy or a primary myopathy. Creatinine phosphokinase levels have been normal or only mildly elevated in our prospective study of septic patients. Muscle biopsy or examination of muscle at autopsy has almost always shown denervation atrophy but in some of our cases there has been scattered necrosis of muscle fibers. In a heterogenous group of patients in a critical care unit who had muscle biopsy, necrosis was a prominent feature. We remain suspicious that septic myopathy is a definite entity and is probably a common complication of the septic syndrome. Only further systematic studies, combining electrophysiological and morphological studies of nerve and muscle, will help to sort out this question.

Cachexia

Osler originally described muscle weakness in association with sepsis and it is probably a significant contributing factor to muscle wasting in the septic syndrome. However, cachexia alone should produce no abnormalities on electrophysiological studies and the creatinine phosphokinase would be normal. Moreover, muscle biopsy should show only the nonspecific finding of type II muscle fiber atrophy.

Panfascicular Muscle Necrosis

This is a rare complication of infection or trauma and is probably the same process that underlies the various mechanisms causing myoglobinuria. Due to the high incidence of infection in intensive care units, it would be expected to occur somewhat more frequently in that setting. However, it apparently remains a rare complication of sepsis, since it did not occur in any of the cases studied in our prospective series of septic patients. When it does occur, it manifests as sudden onset of very severe, generalized muscle weakness accompanied by marked elevations of the creatinine phosphokinase and occasionally by myoglobinuria. Emergency dialysis may be necessary to treat acute renal failure. The condition often resolves completely and sometimes remarkably quickly, such that muscle biopsy may appear normal, even when a few hours earlier the creatinine phosphokinase levels were markedly elevated. In more prolonged and severe cases, muscle biopsy will show panfascicular muscle fiber necrosis. Thus, this syndrome may be readily diagnosed by the clinical features and laboratory tests.

Neuromuscular Blocking Agents

Competitive neuromuscular blocking agents are sometimes used for prolonged periods to facilitate mechanical ventilation. A few reports have suggested that these agents are responsible for a pure axonal motor polyneuropathy which causes difficulty in weaning from the ventilator and a severe, generalized muscle weakness. However, most, if not all, of these patients were in a state of sepsis and it is still not possible to be certain whether the neuromuscular blocking agents or the sepsis were responsible for the polyneuropathy.

A second distinct syndrome involves the patient with acute, severe asthma being treated with high-dose steroids, prolonged neuromuscular blocking agents, and assisted ventilation. After several days of this treatment, when weaning is attempted, it is found that there is a severe, generalized muscle weakness and electrophysiological studies show either an axonal polyneuropathy or a primary myopathy. Some, but perhaps not all, of these patients have been septic and there is a strong indication that the neuromuscular blocking agents, possibly in combination with steroids, will induce this syndrome. The exact relationship to septic polyneuropathy or polymyopathy is still uncertain.

Treatment and Prognosis

Since sepsis is likely the cause of critical illness polyneuropathy, measures to treat sepsis are most important. Recent reports indicate that anticachectin or tumor necrosis factor monoclonal antibodies may specifically reverse severe systemic effects. More established methods are antibiotics, drainage of abscesses, volume replacement, inotropic drugs, and mechanical ventilation, as indicated. Specific organ failure must be vigorously treated, such as dialysis for renal failure. With this aggressive treatment, at least 50% of patients will recover. If the sepsis and multiple organ failure can be successfully treated, the polyneuropathy will gradually improve, over a period of weeks in milder cases and over months in more severe cases. In extremely severe polyneuropathy, recovery from the neuropathy may not occur.

Conclusions

Critical illness polyneuropathy is a common complication of sepsis and multiple organ failure, which in turn is a common occurrence in major critical care units. Clinical and electrophysiological observations are necessary for accurate diagnosis. Once this diagnosis is made, difficulty in weaning from the ventilator and rehabilitation during the recovery process can be better managed. Investigating more thoroughly the pathophysiology of critical illness polyneuropathy may provide further insights into the basic nature of the septic syndrome and how it may be treated. The differential diagnosis is broad but, in particular, should include the potential toxic effects of neuromuscular blocking agents, steroids, and antiobiotics. If patients survive the critical illness, recovery from the polyneuropathy may be expected in all but the most severe cases.

Suggested Reading

Bolton CF (1987) Electrophysiological studies of critically ill patients. Muscle Nerve 10:129–135

Bolton CF (1988) Polyneuropathy as a cause of respiratory failure in critical illness. Intensive Crit Care Digest 7;1:7–9

Bolton CF, Laverty DA, Brown JD et al. (1986) Critically ill polyneuropathy: electrophysiological studies and differentiation from Guillain-Barré syndrome. J Neurol Neurosurg Psychiatry 49:563–573

Bolton CF, Young GB, Zochodne DW (1993) The neurological complications of sepsis. Ann Neurol 33:94–100

Coronel B, Mercatello A, Couturier J-C et al. (1990) Polyneuropathy: potential cause of difficult weaning. Crit Care Med 18:486–489

Danon JD, Carpenter S (1991) Myopathy with thick filament (myosin) loss following prolonged paralysis with vecuronium during steroid treatment. Muscle Nerve 14:1131–1139

Gooch JL, Suchyta MR, Balbierz MJ, Petajan JH, Clemmer TP (1991) Prolonged paralysis after treatment with neuromuscular junction blocking agents. Crit Care Med 19:1125–1131

Helliwell TR, Coakley JH, Wagenmakers AJM, Griffiths RD, Campbell IT, Green CJ et al. (1991) Necrotizing myopathy in critically ill patients. J Pathol 164:307–314

Osler W (1982) The principles and practice of medicine. Appleton, New York, pp 114–118

Penn AS (1986) Myoglobinuria. In: Engel AG, Banker BQ (eds) Myology. McGraw-Hill, New York, pp 1792–1793

Tran DD, Groeneveld AAJB, van der Meulen J et al. (1990) Age, chronic disease, sepsis, organ system failure, and mortality in a medical intensive care unit. Crit Care Med 18:474–479

Witt NJ, Zochodne DW, Bolton CF et al. (1991) Peripheral nerve function in sepsis and multiple organ failure. Chest 99:176–184

Young GB, Bolton CF, Austin TW et al. (1990) The encephalopathy associated with septic illness. Clin Invest Med 13:6:297–304

Ziegler EJ, Fisher CJ, Sprung CL, Straube RC, Sadoff JC, Foulke GE et al. (1991) Treatment of Gram-negative bacteremia and septic shock with HA-1A human monoclonal antibody against endotoxin. N Engl J Med 324:429–436

Zochodne DW, Bolton CF, Wells GA et al. (1987) Critical illness polyneuropathy: a complication of sepsis and multiple organ failure. Brain 110:819–842

Chapter 71

Myasthenia gravis and Lambert-Eaton Myasthenic Syndrome

KLAUS V. TOYKA and WOLFGANG MÜLLGES

Myasthenia gravis

Definition and Epidemiology

Myasthenia gravis (MG) is an auto-immune disease of the neuromuscular junction caused by antibodies against nicotinic acetylcholine (ACh) receptors. It is characterized by fluctuating skeletal muscle weakness and fatigue. The incidence of MG is 2–4 per 100 000 per year. The prevalence is higher and is increasing as patients live longer. It is slightly more common in women and usually occurs between the ages of 10 and 30. It is rare in children younger than 10 years of age.

Patients with MG require neuro-critical care for the management of myasthenic crisis, in which they are unable to swallow or breathe because of bulbar and respiratory muscle weakness. Previously, myasthenic crisis occurred in about 20% of all patients and in 50% of patients with malignant thymomas. Today, because of earlier recognition and treatment,

myasthenic crisis occurs in fewer than 2% of patients.

Pathogenesis and Pathophysiology

Myasthenia gravis is caused by an antibody and complement-mediated reduction in the number of postsynaptic acetylcholine receptors. The role of autoantibodies in the pathogenesis of myasthenia gravis was first shown by passive transfer experiments and later, indirectly, by plasmapheresis and antibody depletion. They can now be measured by double immunoprecipitation assays using alpha-bungarotoxin as a radiolabeled ligand.

The exact mechanism that results in the formation of autoantibodies is not completely understood, but a break in immunological tolerance, controlled by T lymphocytes in the thymus, has been postulated. Abnormalities of the thymus are common; about 10–15% of patients have thymomas and one fourth of these patients have thymus carcinomas (paraneoplastic type of MG).

Patients have muscle weakness and fatigue because of decreased

Section Editor: Daniel F. Hanley

neuromuscular transmission. Normally, the end-plate potential, generated by the release of discrete packets (quanta) of acetycholine, is several times greater than the threshold potential needed for generation of a muscle action potential ("safety margin"). Even though the amount of acetycholine released normally decreases somewhat with sustained muscle activity, the threshold potential can still be reached because of the "safety margin." In patients with myasthenia gravis, however, because the number of available post-synaptic ACh receptors is reduced, the "safety margin" is lost and the threshold potential cannot be reached. This is accentuated with sustained activity.

Most emergency treatments of myasthenia gravis restore the "safety margin." Plasmapheresis and immunoadsorption, for example, result in an increase in the number of available Ach receptors, and cholinesterase inhibitors increase the amount of acetylcholine in the neuromuscular junction. Other drugs lower the "safety margin" by directly or indirectly interfering with Ach receptors (for example, the early effect of corticosteroids and some antibiotics).

Diagnosis

The diagnosis of myasthenia gravis, especially in emergencies, can sometimes be difficult to make. Most importantly, one needs to consider myasthenia gravis in the differential diagnosis.

Repetitive nerve stimulation is the best way to confirm the diagnosis of myasthenia gravis. It can be done at the bedside and has a high sensitivity, even in patients treated with cholinesterase inhibitors. The best nerve to stimulate is the accessory nerve of the trapezius muscle (stimulated over the sternocleidomastoid muscle in the posterior triangle of the neck). Alternatively, the axillary nerve (deltoid muscle) or the ulnar nerve (abductor digiti quinti muscle) can be used, but it may be associated with a lower sensitivity. In most patients, a repetitive stimulation frequency of 3–5 Hz results in a normal muscle action potential at first, followed by muscle action potentials of progressively decreasing amplitudes. Most patients (except those with cholinergic toxicity) have a temporary improvement of their muscle weakness when given a cholinesterase inhibitor, such as edrophonium chloride (Tensilon; Table 3). This "Tensilon test" should be performed cautiously, however, and with ventilatory assistance available for patients with difficulty in breathing.

Treatment

Myasthenic Crisis in Patients Known to Have MG

Myasthenic crisis almost always occurs in patients with generalized muscle weakness, although occasionally it may occur in those with only bulbar and facial muscle weakness. Patients or their relatives should be questioned specifically about previous treatments, the presence of infections, toxin exposures, or medication changes before the onset of the crisis (Table 1). Other factors that can contribute to muscular weakness include emotional stress and anxiety. Hyperthyroidism or hypothyroidism, both not uncommon in

Table 1. Warning signs and preceding events in myasthenic crisis

Rapid fluctuations in myasthenic signs
Continuous reduction of daily activities
Continuous loss of body weight (often 5–10 kg over a few months)
Steady increase in the anticholinesterase dose
Head dropping (severe neck extensor weakness)
Progressive dysarthria, swallowing problems, and shortness of breath
Febrile infections, in particular upper respiratory tract infections with feeble coughing
Medication with drugs that may impair neuromuscular transmission (cf. Table 2; Oosterhuis 1993)[a]

[a] Occasionally, patients and relatives do not report overdoses of anticholinesterases or dangerous treatments by nonmedical health providers.

Table 2. Therapeutic agents that may worsen myasthenic weakness

Antibiotics:	Gentamicin
	Tobramycin
	Streptomycin
	Polymyxin B
	Clindamycin
	Lincomycin
	Tetracycline
	Sulfonamides
Antiepileptic drugs:	Phenytoin
	Carbamazepine
	Trimethadione
	Quinine
	Quiridine
	Others
Antiarrhythmics:	Local anesthetics (lidocaine, procainamide, etc.)
	Verapamil
	Propranolol
	Others
Antirheumatic drugs:	Muscle relaxants
	D-Penicillamine[a]
	Chloroquine
	Resochine (Malaria Rx)
	Quinine
	Others
Antipsychotic drugs:	Lithium salts
	Chlorpromazine
Tranquilizers:	Diazepam
	Opioids
Hormones:	Corticosteroids[b]
	Triiodothyronine
	Thyroxine
Laxatives:	Magnesium salts
Hypnotics:	Barbiturates
	Others

[a] In rare cases, D-penicillamine may cause or worsen myasthenia, possible by an immune-mediated mechanism.
[b] The myasthenic end-plate is more sensitive to corticosteroids than the normal neuromuscular junction. The effect is clinically relevant only in moderate or severe myasthenia and with high doses.

patients with MG, can also worsen muscle weakness. Several medications affect neuromuscular transmission. Although the effects are usually minor, they can become more important in patients with compromised neuromuscular transmission (Table 2). Nevertheless, patients who are doing well clinically or are in remission do not necessarily need to discontinue these medications if they require them. Occasionally, an overdose of cholinesterase inhibitors can precipitate myasthenic crisis. These patients have both generalized muscle fasciculations and cramps (nicotinic signs) and copious secretions, sweating, and tachycardia (muscarinic signs).

Respiratory failure can occur within minutes in patients with impending myasthenic crisis. In these patients, vital capacity (VC) should be evaluated immediately. This can be done with a hand-held spirometer that has a wide mouthpiece or a mask to occlude the patient's nose. Repeated measurements of negative inspiratory force (NIF) can also be used to detect respiratory muscle weakness. Normal

Table 3. Emergency management in the pre-ICU setting

Severe progressive weakness with respiration and swallowing still compensated:
– Pharmacological testing with i.v. Tensilon (edrophonium chloride), 5–10 mg through an intravenous catheter access, preferably after 0.5 mg of atropine sulphate. If patient improves, add 0.5 mg of prostigmine sulphate over 60 s.
– Provide i.v. drip with prostigmine sulphate, 0.5–1.0 mg/h or 0.1–0.5 mg Mestinon (pyridostigmine bromide)/h. This drip may be increased slowly to titrate strength. *Tensilon should not be given when there are overt signs of cholinergic toxicity.*
– The patient should be comfortably positioned to allow voiding of secretions.
– Admit patient to specialized neurology unit within a few hours.
– Monitor vital capacity at regular intervals. Be prepared for emergency intubation if VC falls below 1.5–1.2 l.[a]

[a] Depending on respiratory status the patient should be accompanied by a physician with experience in artificial ventilation.

Table 4. Warning signs of imminent respiratory failure

One or several of the following may be present:
– Inability to swallow secretions
– Dyspnea, often associated with swallowing problems
– Orthopnea, anarthria
– Inability to erect head and trunk
– Abnormal arterial blood gases (oxygen saturation without oxygen breathing below 90–85%)

values from age-matched controls should be referred to when interpreting these measurements. Intubation and assisted ventilation are needed in male patients with vital capacities of less than 1.5 l and in female patients with VC of less than 1.2 l. Further guidelines for the care of patients with impending myasthenic crises are given in Table 3, and signs of respiratory failure are listed in Table 4, the general treatment stratagies in MG are covered in Tables 5 and 6.

Plasmapheresis, in which plasma is separated from blood cells by centrifugation or plasma filtration, should be started as soon as possible in patients with myasthenic crisis. A plasma volume of 1.5–2 l should be exchanged three to five times over 6–8 days.

Patients of all ages can be treated with plasmapheresis. Some patients may not tolerate the accompanying volume changes (for example, some elderly patients or those with heart failure, multiorgan failure, and sepsis). High-dose immunoglubulin (IgG) infusions can be substituted at a dosage of 20–30 g/day over 5 days. Selective immunoadsorption by tryptophan-linked polyvinyl alcohol gels is a new alternative to plasmapheresis available in some European countries and does not require plasma replacement with protein solutions.

Most patients with myasthenic crises need assisted ventilation for 3–6 days after treatment with plasmapheresis has been started. Some patients may require assisted ventilation for a longer time, but tracheostomy is rarely needed. Weaning from the ventilator should be attempted when patients have increased muscle strength that is stable for at least 48 h. Although not widely available, maximal expiratory static pressures and maximal transdiaphragmatic pressures closely correlate with the recovery of diaphragmatic strength. To facilitate weaning, patients should have no pulmonary infections, an arterial oxygen saturation greater than 96% while

Table 5. Management of myasthenic crises in the ICU (cf. Hohlfeld and Toyka 1993)

A. Severe weakness, with respiration and
swallowing still compensated:
   1. Have patient in bed with an at least 45°
   upright position.
   2. Have nasal oxygen tubing in place with
   1–2 l/min.
   3. Give i.v. prostigmine sulphate at
   8–12 mg/24 h as a starting dose; add a
   bolus of 0.5 mg if needed. [Higher doses
   (12–20 mg/24 h) may occasionally be
   required if the patient has been on oral
   Mestinon above a dose of 900 mg for a
   prolonged period of time.]
   4. Give atropine sulphate s.c., 0.5 mg 3–5
   times daily, or ipratropium bromide 2–3
   times daily.
   5. Emergency laboratory tests should
   include serum electrolytes (check for
   low potassium, high magnesium,
   hematocrit, abnormal thyroid
   hormones, neuromuscular toxins); treat
   appropriately.
   6. Treat infections vigorously with
   antibiotics (preferably cephalosporins)
   after taking appropriate samples for
   microbiology; avoid aminoglycosides if
   not absolutely required.
   7. Monitor vital capacity every 4 h or when
   needed.

8. Monitor arterial oxygen saturation
continuously by pulse oximeter.
9. Prepare for therapeutic plasmapheresis.
10. Start corticosteroids at 100 mg or higher
– this may occasionally worsen
myasthenic weakness with a delay of
2–48 h! (Miller et al. 1986; Arsura et al.
1985).
11. If sepsis is likely, IgM/IgG preparations
(5–10 g/d) may be added to the regular
management of sepsis. Sepsis with DIC/
toxic shock is the only contraindication
for plasmapheresis.
B. In patients with overt respiratory failure (see
Table 3, Warning signs):[a]
   1. Clear airways.
   2. Prepare for transnasal intubation
   (transoral only if transnasal is not
   possible).
   3. Initiate artificial respiration.
   4. Use assisted ventilation with CPAP mode
   and PEEP setting of about 3–5 cm H_2O.
   5. Do not discontinue Prostigmine but
   reduce dose to 6–8 mg/24 h (patients may
   be terrified by complete discontinuation
   due to severe limb weakness).
   6. Use only mild sedation; try to
   communicate verbally; ask about
   dyspnea, pain, and anxieties.

[a] No controlled study has been done on the emergency treatment of myasthenic crisis. All recommendations are empirical.

Table 6. Further treatment in the ICU[a]

1. Use "assisted ventilation" mode.
2. Avoid sedation except for 20–40 mg of
haloperidol per day.
3. Continue corticosteroids at 100 mg/d (or
higher dose).
4. Start azathioprine after 3–4 days at 4 mg/kg
body weight; taper to 3 mg/kg after 1 week.
5. Monitor blood cell counts; white blood cells
are usually elevated above 10 000/µl with
corticosteroids; with concomitant
azathioprine they may decrease to 6000–
8000/µl.
6. Treat infections vigorously; use bronchial
lavage as needed (see chapter on long-term
artificial ventilation, Chap. 12).

[a] All recommendations are empirical.

breathing, and they should not require more than 5 cm H_2O of positive end-expiratory pressure (PEEP). Further guidelines for weaning are given in Table 7.

Myasthenic Crisis in Patients not Known to Have MG

Myasthenic crisis can occasionally occur in patients not known to have myasthenia gravis. These patients may have had subtle symptoms and signs that were unrecognized or thought to be from conversion disorder, malin-

Table 7. Weaning from the respirator[a]

A. Artificial ventilation less than 4 days, CPAP mode:
1. Avoid analeptic drugs.
2. Use haloperidol 20–40 mg/d if a tranquilizer is needed.
3. Give special attention to the patient's anxieties by interacting verbally.
4. Reduce airway pressure stepwise by 2 cm H_2O with continuous monitoring of arterial oxygen saturation until 8–10 cm H_2O is reached.
5. Discontinue the respirator on a trial basis for short times (e.g., when washing the patient). If longer discontinuation seems feasible, leave the machine near the patient for psychological reassurance.
6. After 24 h, check for swallowing ability and try extubation.

B. Artificial ventilation longer than 4 days or in patients with bronchopulmonary infection or prolonged weakness:
1. SIMV frequency below 6/min, respiratory volume according to body weight, PEEP around 16–18 cm H_2O.
2. Stepwise reduction of PEEP to 12–14 cm H_2O.
3. Stepwise reduction of SIMV frequency to 2/min.
4. Change to CPAP and continue steps 1–6, above.

---

[a] All recommendations are empirical.
CPAP, Continuous positive airway pressure;
PEEP, positive end-expiratory pressure.

---

gering, chronic fatigue syndrome, "old age," or multifactorial conditions. Diagnosis of myasthenic crisis may be particularly difficult in patients seen in the emergency department, already sedated or intubated by the resuscitation team. In industrialized Western countries, the most common causes of acute paralysis are acute demyelinating inflammatory neuropathy (acute polyneuritis), acute polymyositis/dermatomyositis, and drug overdoses (accidental or suicidal). A more com-plete differential diagnosis is listed in Table 8.

Transferring Patients from the Neurocritical Care Unit to the Regular Ward

Patients may be transferred to a regular ward when they have had no fluctuation in muscle weakness for 48 h, have remained stable without assisted ventilation for at least 24 h, and can take oral pyridostigmine bromide (Mestinon). The usual starting dose is 60 mg every 4 h during the daytime, for a total of five doses. Long-acting pyridostigmine bromide can also be given at bedtime at a dose of 180 mg (Mestinon time-span in the US and Mestinon retard in Europe). Patients recovering from myasthenic crisis still need to be closely monitored, and VC should be measured two to three times daily for the first few days.

In general, medical treatment of myasthenia gravis includes corticosteroids (in tapering doses) and azathioprine (3 mg/kg per day). Symptoms of myasthenia gravis should be either stable or remitting for at least 8 weeks before thymectomy is considered. The same recommendations apply for patients suspected of having thymomas, unless the tumor is especially large or invasive and needs to be resected urgently.

Elective Operations and Other Emergencies in Patients with MG

Because some patients with moderate (or mild) generalized weakness have worsening of their symptoms and even myasthenic crisis after elective surgery, patients should delay any surgery until their disease is stable or in remission.

Table 8. Differential diagnosis of acute paralytic disease[a]

Lower motor neuron
1. Acute demyelinating inflammatory polyneuropathy: prodromal illness, hyporeflexia, sensory involvement, rarely extraocular muscles
2. Acute (myelo-)meningoradiculitis: meningism, often pain and fever, hyporeflexia
3. Poliomyelitis and poliomyelitis-like disorders: prodromal enteritis, often asymmetric, no sensory signs
4. Heavy metal intoxication (e.g., lead, mercury, thallium, *cis*-platin): exposure?, skin signs, psychosis etc.
5. Diphtheria: prodromal tonsillitis or severe wound infection, weakness often asymmetric, cranial nerves involved
6. Insect bite or sting (tick, spider, scorpion, snake): only in endemic areas, may be difficult to distinguish from myasthenia
7. Acute porphyria: previous hyporeflexia, colics, history

Neuromuscular junction
1. Myasthenia gravis
2. Lambert-Eaton myasthenic syndrome (see Table 9)
3. Botulinum toxin (botulism): ingestion of home-canned and home-smoked food, gangrenous wound, muscarinic signs – accommodation paralysis, dry mouth
4. Organophosphate intoxication: suicidal or homicidal attempt, profound muscarinic signs, erythema, CNS signs

Skeletal muscle
1. Polymyositis/dermatomyositis: eye muscles not affected, skin changes, elevated creatine kinase
2. Hypokalemic periodic paralysis: history, areflexia, no muscle twitch on electrical stimulation
3. Acute toxic myopathy: drug history, elevated creatine kinase, myoglobinuria
4. Neuroleptic malignant syndrome: high body temperature, rigidity and akinesia, elevated creatine kinase

[a] Note: Electrical stimulation of motor nerves with nerve conduction measurements and repetitive nerve stimulation are extremely helpful when performed in the emergency situation. Several disorders listed in Table 8 can be distinguished.

Patients should be switched before surgery from oral pyridostigmine bromide to intravenous neostigmine bromide (Prostigmine; Table 3). Patients with MG require only small doses of muscle relaxants. The regular dose of some nondepolarizing muscle relaxants (for example, *d*-tubocarine, pancuronium bromide, gallamine) can cause prolonged apnea, and as little as 20% of the regular dose can cause complete paralysis.

Lambert-Eaton Myasthenic Syndrome

Definition and Epidemiology

The Lambert-Eaton myasthenic syndrome (LEMS) is an autoimmune disease of the neuromuscular junction caused by antibodies against calcium channels in the presynaptic membrane. The incidence is less than 1 in 1 million (20 times rarer than myasthenia gravis). Most patients are older than 40 years; however, isolated cases of patients younger than 20 years have been reported (one of Lambert's original patients was 2 years old). Most patients have cancer (50–65%), mainly small cell cancer of the lung. Occasionally, LEMS may precede the development of cancer by many years and the diagnosis of "idiopathic LEMS" may be made erroneously.

In general, muscle weakness and fatigue are similar to myasthenia gravis, with the exception that patients with LEMS almost always have lower extremity weakness, and extraocular muscle weakness is usually mild or absent. In patients with LEMS, muscle strength improves for a few seconds after maximal effort before fatigue occurs. LEMS is also frequently associated with signs of cholinergic dysautonomia. Myasthenic crisis is less common in patients with LEMS and usually occurs only in those with a long history of weakness and fatigue. Patients may, however, have respiratory failure after surgery or general anesthesia.

Table 9. Laboratory testing for Lambert-Eaton myasthenic syndrome

1. Single and repetitive nerve stimulation (see text)
2. X-ray, CT, MRI of the thorax
3. Autonomic testing (ECG with R-R-interval analysis, sweating tests, Schirmer test, etc.)
4. Autoantibodies to calcium channels (see text); rule out antibodies to AChR
5. Tests for other autoimmune disorders

Pathogensis and Pathophysiology

The Lambert-Eaton myasthenic syndrome is caused by circulating IgG antibodies against the beta subunit of presynaptic calcium channels. The antibodies can cross-react with calcium channels in other tissues and in some tumor cells. They can be detected by their binding to omega-conotoxin. Decreased influx of calcium into the presynaptic motor terminals results in decreased quantal ACh release and reduced end-plate potentials. With more frequent impulses, ACh release can be increased until eventually the supply is exhausted. Thus, muscle strength improves with sustained contraction and tendon reflexes become more brisk with repetitive tapping. Acetylcholine release can also be improved by medications such as guanidine, 3,4-diaminopyridine, which increases ACh release, and cholinesterase inhibitors.

Diagnosis

Lambert-Eaton myasthenic syndrome is initally misdiagnosed as myasthenia gravis in about one third of patients. All patients presenting with muscle weakness and fatigue should undergo a thorough evaluation for malignancy. Ancillary tests for the workup of patients suspected of having LEMS are listed in Table 9. Repetitive nerve stimulation should be done immediately. The best sites for stimulation are the ulnar, median, and peroneal nerves. Stimulation at a frequency of 3 Hz often results in decreasing amplitudes, while higher frequencies (for example, 10 Hz) or sustained muscle contraction results in increasing amplitudes in most patients. Weakness improves, as in patients with myasthenia gravis, in more than half of patients given edrophonium chloride. Rarely, the diseases may co-exist. Antibodies to calcium channels can be measured in some laboratories, but these measurements are not as sensitive or specific as those for antibodies to ACh receptors.

Treatment

Treatment of patients with LEMS is similar to that of patients with myasthenia gravis. Pyridostigmine bromide should be given to all patients. Drugs such as 3,4-diaminopyridine or 4-aminopyridine can be used in countries where they are available. As in patients with myasthenia gravis, measurements of vital capacity and negative inspiratory force are helpful in assessing the need for assisted ventilation. Corticosteroids and plasmapheresis (but not selective immunoadsorption) should also be used. Medications that affect the neuromuscular junction should be avoided whenever possible. Recovery in patients with LEMS (regardless of whether associated with cancer) is less dramatic and generally takes longer than in patients with myasthenia gravis.

Suggested Reading

Arsura E, Brunner NG, Namba T, Grob D (1985) High-dose intravenous methylprednisolone in myasthenia gravis. Arch Neurol 42:1149–1153

Borel CO, Tilford C, Nichols DG, Hanley DF, Traystman RJ (1991) Diaphragmatic performance during recovery from acute ventilatory failure in Guillain-Barré syndrome and myasthenia gravis. Chest 99:444–451

Chalk CH, Murray NMF, O'Neill JH, Spiro SG (1990) Response of the Lambert-Eaton myasthenic syndrome to treatment of associated small-cell lung carcinoma. Neurology 40:1552–1556

Fateh-Moghadem A, Wick M, Besinger U, Geursen RG (1984) High-dose intravenous gammaglobulin for myasthenia gravis. Lancet 1:848

Heininger K, Hartung HP, Toyka KV, Gaczkowski A, Borberg H (1987) Therapeutic plasma exchange in myasthenia gravis: semiselective adsorption of anti-AChR autoantibodies with tryptophan-linked polyvinyl alcohol gels. In: Drachman DB (ed) Myasthenia gravis: biology and treatment. Ann NY Acad Sci 505:898–900

Hohlfeld R (1989) Neurological autoimmune disease and the trimolecular complex of T-lymphocytes. Ann Neurol 25:531–538

Hohlfeld R, Toyka KV (1993) Therapies in myasthenia gravis. In: de Baets NH, Osterhuis HJGH (eds) Myasthenia gravis. CRC Press, Boca Raton, pp 235–261

Laroche CM, Mier AK, Spiro SG, Newsom-

Davis J, Moxham J, Green M (1984) Respiratory muscle weakness in the Lambert-Eaton myasthenic syndrome. Thorax 44:913–918

London SF, Ringel SP (1992) Neuromuscular emergencies. In: Weiner WJ (ed) Emergent and urgent neurology. Lippincott, Philadelphia, pp 59–78

Lundh H, Nilsson O, Rosén I (1984) Treatment of Lambert-Eaton syndrome: 3,4-diaminopyridine and pyridostigmine. Neurology 34:1324–1330

McEvoy KM, Windebank AJ, Daube JR, Low P (1989) 3,4-Diaminopyridine in the treatment of Lambert-Eaton myasthenic syndrome. N Engl J Med 321:1567–1571

Miller RG, Milner-Brown HS, Mirka A (1986) Prednisone-induced worsening of neuromuscular function in myasthenia gravis. Neurology 36:729–732

Newsom-Davis J, Leys K, Vincent A, Ferguson I, Modi G, Mills K (1991) Immunological evidence for the co-existence of the Lambert-Eaton myasthenic syndrome and myasthenia gravis in two patients. J Neurol Neurosurg Psychiatry 54:452–453

O'Neill JH, Murray NMF, Newsom-Davis J (1988) The Lambert-Eaton myasthenic syndrome. Brain 111:577–596

Oosterhuis HJGH (1993) Myasthenia gravis: Clinical aspects. In: de Baets NH, Oosterhuis HJGH (eds) Myasthenia gravis. CRC Press, Boca Raton, pp 14–42

Sher E, Gotti C, Canal N, Scoppetta C, Piccolo G, Evoli A (1989) Specificity of calcium-channel autoantibodies in Lambert-Eaton myasthenic syndrome. Lancet II: 640–643

Swift T (1981) Disorders of neuromuscular transmission other than myasthenia gravis. Muscle Nerve 4:334–353

Toyka KV (1990) Myasthenia gravis. In: Johnson RT (ed) Current therapy in neurological diseases, vol 3. Decker, Philadelphia, pp 385–395

Toyka KV, Hartung HP (1992) Circulating immune factors. In: Asbury AK, McKhann GM, McDonald WI (eds) Diseases of the nervous system – clinical neurobiology. Saunders, Philadelphia, pp 1396–1408

Younger DS, Braun NMT, Jaretzki III A, Penn AS, Lovelace RE (1984) Myasthenia gravis: determinants for independent ventilation after trans-sternal thymectomy. Neurology 34:336–340

| # Polymyositis and Dermatomyositis

REINHARD HOHLFELD and WILLIAM W. HOFMANN

Introduction

Polymyositis and dermatomyositis belong to the group of inflammatory muscle diseases. This chapter deals only with the "idiopathic" polymyositis and dermatomyositis syndromes; parasitic, bacterial, spirochetal, and viral infectious myopathies will not be discussed. For recent reviews of the general subject, the reader may wish to refer to Banker and Engel (1986), Dalakas (1991, 1992), Engel (1992), and Hohlfeld and Engel (1992).

There is increasing evidence that the term polymyositis refers to a heterogeneous group of myopathic conditions, the various clinical presentations differing to some extent in their pathogenesis. The term dermatomyositis, on the other hand, indicates a more homogeneous group of combined cutaneous and muscular disorders, including a specific form in children.

The incidence of polymyositis and dermatomyositis is estimated at approximately 1 case in 100 000 population per year. In both conditions there may be a fulminant, life-threatening course, or the patient may worsen gradually and progressively in spite of treatment. Furthermore, these types of inflammatory myopathy may be accompanied by cardiac and pulmonary complications (see below).

Pathogenesis

Polymyositis appears to be a cell-mediated autoimmune disorder (reviewed by Hohlfeld and Engel 1992). Immunohistochemical analysis of muscle biopsy specimens shows typical lesions in which CD8+ cytotoxic T cells surround, indent, invade, and eventually destroy segments of the muscle fiber. At the electron-microscopic level, these autoaggressive cytotoxic T cells are seen to extend spike-like processes into the muscle fibers. By contrast, dermatomyositis appears to be an antibody-mediated disease (Griggs and Karpati 1991). It is presently thought that autoantibodies against an endothelial component of the intra-muscular capillaries initiate the chain

Section Editor: Daniel F. Hanley

of pathogenetic events leading eventually to muscle weakness in this disorder. Consistent with this hypothesis, the inflammatory exudate in dermatomyositis typically contains B cells and CD4+ helper T cells, while CD8+ T cells invading non-necrotic muscle fibers are rarely found (Banker and Engel 1986).

Clinical Features and Differential Diagnosis

Both polymyositis and dermatomyositis are characterized by proximal, often symmetric muscle weakness which typically develops over weeks to months and may be associated with transient muscle pain. Extraocular and facial muscles are typically spared. In severe cases pharyngeal and respiratory involvement leads to difficulty of swallowing and breathing, each requiring special care and management by skilled personnel.

The clinical feature that differentiates dermatomyositis from polymyositis is a typical skin rash consisting of a blue-purple discoloration of the upper eyelids and erythematous lesions on the face, upper trunk, knuckles, and other joints. Later in the course of the disease, these lesions may result in scaling, depigmentation, and/or hyperpigmentation of the involved skin, leaving telltale scars. In dermatomyositis, extramuscular manifestations are more frequent in children than in adults, and may include subcutaneous calcifications and joint contractures.

Polymyositis may be associated with retrovirus (HIV, HTLV-1) infections. In these cases there is good evidence that the virus does not directly infect the muscle, but triggers a T-cell-mediated cytotoxic process similar to that seen in other forms of the disease (Illa et al. 1991). It is important to note that zidovudine, an agent used to treat HIV-infected patients, can itself cause a toxic myopathy which may be difficult to distinguish from the primary, virus-associated polymyositis (Dalakas et al. 1990; Dalakas 1991, 1992).

As many as 40% of patients with polymyositis or dermatomyositis have cardiac involvement, which may lead to conduction defects and dilated cardiomyopathy. Pulmonary involvement occurs in up to 50% of patients as the result of respiratory muscle weakness, pneumonitis as a result of methotrexate treatment, or interstitial lung disease. The latter condition is associated with anti-Jo-1 antibodies and develops in up to 10% of patients with polymyositis (Tazelaar et al. 1990). Sometimes the features of dermatomyositis overlap those of certain connective tissue diseases, such as systemic lupus erythematosus, Sjögren's syndrome, rheumatoid arthritis, systemic sclerosis, or mixed connective tissue disease ("overlap syndrome").

The possible association of myositis with malignant tumors has been the subject of a long-standing debate. A recent epidemiological study (Sigurgeirsson et al. 1992) concluded that the incidence of cancer was increased both in patients with dermatomyositis and in those with polymyositis. The mortality from the malignancy was increased only in the patients with dermatomyositis, however. A thorough search for an occult neoplasm is advisable in any inflammatory myopathy, especially in patients with dermatomyositis.

The diagnosis of polymyositis rests on the history and clinical findings, and on the results of laboratory tests, electromyography, and muscle histology as ancillary tests (see below). The differential diagnosis includes:

1. Inclusion body myositis, which shows a typical pattern of histologic changes, namely rimmed vacuoles, eosinophilic intranuclear and cytoplasmic inclusions, small groups of atrophic fibers without fiber-type grouping, and an inflammatory exudate involving endomysial and, to a lesser extent, perivascular tissue sites
2. Acid maltase deficiency, in which the muscle biopsy demonstrates a vacuolar myopathy with high glycogen content and acid-phosphatase reactivity in the vacuoles
3. Limb-girdle dystrophies, which develop more slowly and lack inflammatory changes in the muscle biopsy
4. Glucocorticosteroid-induced myopathy, in which the serum creatine kinase level is normal and the muscle biopsy shows selective type-II muscle fiber atrophy
5. Zidovudine-induced mitochondrial myopathy with "ragged-red fibers"
6. Myopathy induced by cholesterol-lowering agents, e.g., inhibitors of 3-hydroxy-3-methylglutaryl coenzyme A (HMG-CoA)
7. A wide variety of other inflammatory, degenerative, metabolic, and toxic myopathies (see reviews by Dalakas 1991, 1992; Engel 1992)

Ancillary Tests

The single most useful laboratory test is the serum level of the muscle enzyme creatine kinase (CK). The enzyme is released from necrotic muscle fibers, and the serum level usually parallels disease activity. Immunological tests may be done for rheumatoid factor and for antinuclear and anticytoplasmic autoantibodies.

Needle electromyography shows a myopathic pattern with low-voltage muscle action potentials, abnormal spontaneous activity, usually in the form of increased insertional activity, fibrillation potentials, and positive sharp waves (Robinson 1991). This pattern can be seen in a variety of myopathies and is not diagnostic for those associated with autoimmune or any other inflammatory process.

The most important ancillary investigation is the muscle biopsy. On light microscopy, the most obvious changes include the presence of inflammatory cells, necrosis and regeneration of muscle fibers, and an increase in connective tissue. A finding that is highly characteristic of dermatomyositis, but not of polymyositis, is "perifascicular atrophy" (atrophy of the muscle fibers at the periphery of fascicles). Small zones of muscle infarction may be observed in dermatomyositis of childhood, but not in the usual adult forms of either polymyositis or dermatomyositis. In dermatomyositis, in contrast to polymyositis, the intramuscular blood vessels show endothelial hyperplasia and sometimes obliteration of capillaries. Further characteristic changes that have provided important clues to the pathogenesis of both polymyositis and dermatomyositis have been reviewed by Hohlfeld and Engel (1992; see above).

Management

Prednisone is the first-line drug for the treatment of polymyositis and dermatomyositis (Banker and Engel 1986; Dalakas 1991; Engel 1992). Therapy is started with 1 mg/kg prednisone in a single daily dose. This dose is maintained for 4 weeks or longer, until the CK *and* the clinical status improve. After this, the dose is tapered slowly over approximately 10 weeks to 1 mg/kg every other day. If improvement continues, the dosage is further reduced by 5–10 mg every 4 weeks until the maintenance dose (the lowest possible dose that controls the disease) is reached. In a favorable case, the dose will eventually be 10–20 mg every other day.

A problem in treatment is that the long-term use of corticosteroids may, itself, induce a myopathy ("steroid myopathy") that is difficult to distinguish from an exacerbation of the inflammatory component. If the increase of weakness follows tapering of steroids and is accompanied by an increase of the CK, the clinical deterioration is probably due to exacerbation of myositis. Lacking clear evidence suggesting exacerbation of myositis, it may nevertheless be advisable first to increase the dose of steroids temporarily. If the patient then fails to improve, steroid myopathy is more likely than exacerbation of the inflammatory process (Dalakas 1991).

An objective increase in muscle strength usually occurs by the third month of therapy (Dalakas 1991). If prednisone fails to produce a clear benefit after this period, or if the patient requires >25 mg/day or develops steroid side effects, then a second-line drug is required. It is reasonable first to try the least toxic immunosuppressive drug, azathioprine (2.5–3 mg/kg daily for 4–6 months) and then, if treatment is still ineffective, to use methotrexate (15–25 mg/week orally). Cyclosporine may be a useful alternative or adjunctive third-line drug (reviewed in Dalakas 1992). High-dose intravenous immunoglobulins may be useful as an adjunctive immunomodulatory agent for acute exacerbations or for selected cases of severe chronic disease refractory to conventional therapy (reviewed in Dalakas 1991, 1992).

Polymyositis in HIV-positive patients presents a special therapeutic challenge. Although this form of polymyositis is probably triggered by the virus, there is no evidence that muscle cells are directly infected (Illa et al. 1991). In fact, it appears that the virus initiates a T-cell-mediated cytotoxic response against muscle fibers. In such cases, the therapeutic dilemma derives mainly from two considerations (Dalakas et al. 1990). First, treatment with prednisone is itself potentially dangerous in immunocompromised patients. Second, the anti-virus agent zidovudine can cause a mitochondrial myopathy (Dalakas et al. 1990), which may add to the muscular dysfunction.

Dalakas et al. (1990) have recommended the following strategy for the management of HIV-associated polymyositis. Before using prednisone, a nonsteroidal anti-inflammatory agent should be tried in these patients. If this fails, zidovudine should be discontinued for 3–4 weeks and the clinical response (muscle strength, CK) observed. If the strength increases, another retroviral agent should be substituted for zidovudine. If the strength decreases or does not change, prednisone should be started at a dose of 40–60 mg per day.

Patients with polymyositis or dermatomyositis may require intensive care under certain circumstances, particularly when the disease takes a fulminant course with marked initial respiratory and/or pharyngeal involvement, or if frank respiratory failure develops at any time. The latter may be precipitated suddenly, even in patients with long-standing, slowly progressive disease, by pulmonary infections or aspiration. In the presence of any severe systemic complications, especially cardiac disease and interstitial lung disease, it is safe practice to provide at least temporary treatment in the ICU.

In patients with an acute course in whom oral corticosteroids have failed, high-dose corticosteroids (e.g., 500 mg methylprednisolone per day) should be given intravenously for 5–10 days in combination with methotrexate, 25 mg/week orally. In addition, high-dose intravenous immunoglobulin (0.4 g/kg/per day) should be administered for 4–5 days (Jann et al. 1992). There is no convincing evidence that plasmapheresis or leukapheresis are effective in either polymyositis or dermatomyositis (Miller et al. 1992), although this view has been debated (Dau 1992). The response to therapy with cyclophosphamide and cyclosporine also is generally disappointing (Dalakas 1991).

Patients with chronic disease in whom respiratory failure has been precipitated by an infection should be treated with appropriate antibiotics plus high-dose intravenous immunoglobulin (see above). Further, the original treatment plan should be revised, depending on the presumed cause of the deterioration. If the pulmonary infection appears to be a complication of immunosuppression, cytotoxic drugs may have to be stopped entirely or sharply reduced. In some cases it will be necessary to change to another immunosuppressive agent. If the infection occurred as a consequence of aspiration in a severely weak "undertreated" patient, more aggressive immunosuppressive treatment is required, and it may be necessary to provide mechanical respiratory assistance for a time.

In patients with cardiac and pulmonary complications, except for interstititial lung disease, the myositis is treated according to the same principles as in patients without these complications. In patients with interstitial lung disease, cyclophosphamide may be beneficial (Al-Janadi et al. 1989; Tazelaar et al. 1990).

In patients failing to respond to these treatments, a second muscle biopsy may be needed to make sure that the diagnosis is correct and that the patient does not have, for example, inclusion body myositis, which is generally resistant to therapies.

Prognosis and Conclusions

Polymyositis and dermatomyositis are considered to be autoimmune diseases of muscle. Accordingly, the therapeutic aim is to suppress the autoimmune process. Life-long immunosuppressive treatment may be required in some patients. Intermittent respiratory failure due to neuromuscular weakness can often be managed successfully, provided it is detected early. Cardiac complications and interstitial lung disease are serious complications associated with a high mortality.

Suggested Reading

Al-Janadi M, Smith CD, Karsh J (1989) Cyclophosphamide treatment of interstitial pulmonary fibrosis in polymyositis/dermatomyositis. J Rheumatol 16:1592–1596

Banker BQ, Engel AG (1986) The polymyositis and dermatomyositis syndromes. In: Engel AG, Banker BQ (eds) Myology. McGraw-Hill, New York, pp 1385–1422

Dalakas MC (1991) Polymyositis, dermatomyositis, and inclusion body myositis. N Engl J Med 325:1487–1498

Dalakas MC (1992) Inflammatory and toxic myopathies. Curr Opin Neurol Neurosurg 5:645–654

Dalakas MC, Illa I, Pezeshkpour GH, Laukaitis JP, Cohen B, Griffin JL (1990) Mitochondrial myopathy caused by long-term zidovudine therapy. N Engl J Med 322:1098–1105

Dau PC (1992) Plasma exchange in polymyositis and dermatomyositis. N Engl J Med 327:1030

Engel AG (1992) Inflammatory myopathies. In: Wyngaarden JB, Smith LH, Bennett JC (eds) Cecil textbook of medicine. Saunders, Philadelphia, pp 2256–2258

Griggs RC, Karpati G (1991) The pathogenesis of dermatomyositis. Arch Neurol 48:21–22

Hohlfeld R, Engel AG (1992) Immune responses in muscle. Semin Neurosci 4:249–255

Illa I, Nath A, Dalakas MC (1991) Immunocytochemical and virological characteristics of HIV-associated inflammatory myopathies: similarities with seronegative polymyositis. Ann Neurol 29:474–481

Jann S, Beretta S, Moggio M, Adobbati L, Pellegrini G (1992) High-dose intravenous human immunoglobulin in polymyositis resistant to treatment. J Neurol Neurosurg Psychiatry 55:60–62

Miller FW, Leitman SF, Cronin ME, Hicks JE, Leff RL, Wesley R, Fraser DD, Dalakas MC, Plotz PH (1992) Controlled trial of plasma exchange and leukapheresis in polymyositis and dermatomyositis. N Engl J Med 326:1380–1384

Robinson LR (1991) AAEM case report no. 22: polymyositis. Muscle Nerve 14:310–315

Sigurgeirsson B, Lindelöf B, Edhag O, Allander E (1992) Risk of cancer in patients with dermatomyositis or polymyositis – a population-based study. N Engl J Med 326:363–367

Tazelaar HD, Viggiano RW, Pickersgill J, Colby TV (1990) Interstitial lung disease in polymyositis and dermatomyositis: clinical features and prognosis as correlated with histologic findings. Am Rev Respir Dis 141:727–733

Chapter 73

Rhabdomyolysis and Acute Presentations of Myopathies

Klaus Rieke and Ralph W. Kuncl

Rhabdomyolysis

Definition, Epidemiology, and Relevance To Neurocritical Care

Rhabdomyolysis is defined as acute widespread necrosis of muscle tissue and results in the delivery of myoglobin, creatine kinase (CK), aldolase, creatine, potassium, phosphate, amino acids, and uric acid into the blood. The syndrome was first described in 1910 by Meyer-Betz. Incidence and prevalence are not well defined. However, known risk groups include patients with muscle diseases (e.g., myositis, McArdle syndrome, muscular dystrophy), crush syndromes due to severe trauma (e.g., after earthquakes or mining accidents) or to prolonged coma with ischemic muscle necrosis (e.g., cocaine and barbiturate overdose, "coma/muscle crush syndrome"), and toxic or drug-induced rhabdomyolysis (e.g., due to lovastatin). Because one- to two-thirds of patients with rhabdomyolysis will develop life-threatening hyperkalemia or will de-

velop acute prolonged renal failure caused by severe myoglobinuria, these patients have to be referred to neurocritical care units (NCCU).

To the pathologist, the interchangeable use of the words *rhabdomyolysis, necrosis, hyperkalemia*, and *myoglobinuria* is erroneous. The muscle pigment myoglobin and the enzyme CK may leak into serum and urine in high quantity and still be unassociated with cell necrosis, as in phencyclidine toxicity. Necrosis may be focal, without widespread rhabdomyolysis (as in calcium-mediated, agonist-induced myopathy at neuromuscular junctions), yet cause myoglobinuria if a sensitive enough assay is used. Rhabdomyolysis, or widespread necrosis, may or may not be associated with the clinical syndrome of myoglobinuria.

Pathogenesis

Myoglobin is a small protein with a molecular weight of approximately 18 kDa and is filtered through the renal glomeruli. In case of severe damage to muscle tissue, myoglobinuria occurs, and the urine is of a brown color if

Section Editor: Daniel F. Hanley

more than 1 g/l myoglobin is present. The major complication of rhabdomyolysis is acute renal failure from tubular necrosis. The precise mechanism by which this occurs is unknown. In very severe cases, respiratory failure can occur, and fatal cardiac arrhythmias secondary to disturbances of electrolyte balance are possible.

Clinical Features and Differential Diagnosis

Symptoms of rhabdomyolysis include severe muscle pain, swelling of extremities, and pigmenturia. Urgent diagnosis is required. The swelling can proceed to compartment syndromes with peripheral nerve compression or ischemic contracture, and rapid fasciotomy is necessary in such patients. Weakness and pain regularly involve the extremity and truncal muscles, whereas involvement of cranial muscles appears rarely. Metabolic coma can occur in spectacular cases. In the beginning, urine will become dark (red to brown in color). However, myoglobinuria is only present in the early phase of the syndrome, and in 50% of patients with rhabdomyolysis myoglobinuria will be missed, especially when the onset is protracted. One must always suspect a toxin in such cases.

The differential diagnosis of myoglobinuria includes other causes of pigmenturia, such as hemoglobinuria. Some of the innumerable known causes of rhabdomyolysis and myoglobinuria are organized according to mechanism and in approximate order of frequency in Table 1. The first four categories represent by far the majority of cases when myoglobinuria is an isolated event. Primary myopathies are by comparison less common causes, unless myoglobinuria is recurrent or familial. Unfortunately, a large minority of cases remain idiopathic.

Ancillary Tests

Laboratory Tests

Laboratory tests reveal a severe increase in serum CK activity (usually more than 200-fold increased). The urine should first be screened for myoglobin by looking for a positive orthotolidine reaction (e.g., Hemastix) in an erythrocyte-free urine. For confirmation and serial follow-up, urine myoglobin can be sensitively quantitated by radioimmunoassay, ELISA, or a latex test (Behring Werke, Marburg, Germany). Disturbances of electrolyte balance may occur, with an increase in serum potassium and phosphate related to cellular necrosis. A secondary decrease of calcium linked to hyperphosphatemia may occur, with the risk of cardiac dysfunction. Electromyography or muscle biopsy play only minor roles in confirming acute destruction of muscle tissue.

Electrophysiology

Electromyography shows showers of fibrillations and positive sharp waves, and muscle biopsy reveals necrosis. If the intent of biopsy is to search for a preexisting, underlying neuromuscular disease (especially an enzyme deficiency), the biopsy must be delayed for 6–12 weeks to allow the overriding picture of acute degeneration and regeneration to pass. Imaging of the affected extremities can only show nonspecific findings, such as areas of

Table 1. Causes of myoglobinuria in humans

Trauma	*Drug and toxin-induced*	*Myositis*
Crush syndrome (earthquakes,	*rhabdomyolysis*	Polymyositis
other major disasters)	Lipid-lowering agents	Dermatomyositis
High voltage injuries	Clofibrate (and its	Viral myositis (influenza,
Burning injuries	analogues; for example,	Coxsackie, echovirus,
Freezing injuries	bezafibrate)	adenovirus, herpesvirus,
	Lovastatin (potentiated by	Epstein-Barr)
Ischemic alterations	cyclosporine or	Bacterial myositis (typhus,
Muscle infarcts due to arterial	gemfibrozil)	*Staphylococcus aureus*)
occlusions	Gemfibrozil	
Compartment syndromes, e.g.,	Biological toxins	*Metabolic myopathies*
anterior tibial syndrome	Tetanus toxin	Myophosphorylase deficiency
Prolonged tourniquet use	Coral, tiger, sea snake	Phosphofructokinase deficiency
Sickle cell disease	venoms	Myoadenylate deaminase
Disseminated intravascular	Haff disease	deficiency
coagulation	Hypokalemia	Carnitine deficiency
Coma with ischemic muscle	Laxatives	Carnitine-palmityl transferase
necrosis ("coma/muscle	Thiazide diuretics	deficiency
crush syndrome"):	Glycyrrhizate (licorice)	Phosphoglycerate mutase/
Barbiturate sedatives;	Amphotericin B	kinase deficiency
cocaine; heroin;	Lithium	
amphetamine; tricyclic	Necrosis	*Muscular dystrophies*
antidepressants; carbon	Ethanol	e.g., Duchenne muscular
monoxide; ethanol;	Toluene	dystrophy
many others (some	Epsilon aminocaproic acid	When tourniquets used during
occasionally cause	Ischemic or compartment	tenotomy
myoglobinuria unrelated	syndrome	
to coma or muscle crush)	Vasopressin	*Metabolic alterations*
	Other	Hypokalemia
Exercise induced rhabdomylysis	Succinylcholine	Hyponatremia
Exercise in untrained persons		Hypophosphatemia
("march myoglobinuria")	*Hyperthermia*	Conn syndrome
Convulsions, status epilepticus	Heat stroke	Thyrotoxic crisis
Status asthmaticus (especially	Malignant hyperthermia	Diabetic acidosis
with use of β-agonists)	(central core disease)	
Tetanus	Neuroleptic malignant	*Idiopathic myoglobinuria*
Delirium with excess motor	syndrome	
activity (e.g., phencyclidine,	Severe infections with sepsis,	
LSD, amphetamine,	fever, or lactic acidemia	
strychnine)		

reduced echogenicity using myosonography, swelling, and hypodense areas on computerized tomography, or an intense signal of the muscle tissue on magnetic resonance imaging.

Management

Since renal failure and cardiac arrhythmias are the major complications of rhabdomyolysis, all patients presenting with this disorder should be considered for critical care. Emergency management is outlined in Table 2. Simultaneous with the initial evaluation of the patient for NCCU management, life-threatening electrolyte imbalances of hyperkalemia, hypocalcemia, and hyperphosphatemia should be corrected with sodium bicarbonate, glucose-insulin infusions,

Table 2. Emergency management of myoglobinuria

Treat life-threatening hyperkalemia
Evaluate for management in a neurocritical care unit
Hydrate adequately
Alkalinize urine (sodium bicarbonate)
Monitor: cardiac rhythm, K^+, Ca^{++}, PO_4^{--}, creatinine, blood urea nitrogen, fluid intake and output
Hemodialyze, as indicated

Table 3. Neuromuscular disorders which can *present* with severe respiratory muscle weakness

Polymyositis, dermatomyositis (see Chap. 71)
Adult-onset acid maltase deficiency
Amyloid myopathy
Myasthenia gravis (see Chap. 71)
Guillain-Barré syndrome (see Chap. 67)
Amyotrophic lateral sclerosis

or dialysis. Sufficient hydration and alkalinization of the urine is one of the first tasks on admission to NCCU. Serum CK, creatinine, and electrolytes including calcium and potassium must be monitored serially. Potentially toxic agents and drugs should be removed immediately. Hemofiltration or hemodialysis is required if renal failure progresses. Patients with malignant hyperthermia or the neuroleptic malignant syndrome are treated with dantrolene, other muscle relaxants, or bromocriptine (see Chap. 83).

Acute Presentations of Other Myopathies

Certain neuromuscular disorders are of special interest to neurointensivists because they may present abruptly with severe respiratory weakness even though they may inherently cause more widespread weakness and may have a chronic or subacute course. In contrast to rhabdomyolysis, these muscular disorders do not necessarily present with myoglobinuria. This short list of disorders bears special consideration (Table 3). Three of them are myopathies.

Polymyositis and Dermatomyositis (see Chap. 72)

Inflammatory myopathies such as polymyositis and dermatomyositis can also cause acute, but more often subacute muscle weakness. In these cases, the weakness is the leading symptom, is pronounced in the proximal muscles of the extremities, and evolves over a longer period (like months). Dysphagia occurs in about 15%–20% of patients. Respiratory musculature can be affected, and respiratory insufficiency may even be a presenting feature. It is important to note that significant muscle pain or tenderness occurs *infrequently* (25% of patients) with polymyositis or dermatomyositis. Serum CK activity is elevated in most of the patients but does not extend to such high values as seen in rhabdomyolysis. Electromyography reveals spontaneous activity with small amplitude, brief duration, polyphasic motor unit potentials. Muscle biopsy shows autoreactive T lymphocytes and macrophages surrounding and invading muscle fibers, with resultant necrosis and regeneration. Initial treatment of myositis depends on corticosteroids (prednisone 1 mg/kg per day). When steroids fail, or for steroid-sparing when toxicity is excessive, immunosuppressive therapy is carried out using azathioprine, methotrexate, cyclosporine, human immunoglobulin, or other immunomodulating therapies. The degree of weakness and serum CK elevation guides the duration of steroid and immunosuppressive therapy.

Other Myopathies

Adult onset acid maltase deficiency may present in the fifth or sixth decade with diaphragmatic weakness. The diagnosis is made by biochemical assay of muscle biopsy tissue for glycogen and acid and neutral maltase. Amyloid myopathy is rare and recently recognized as also able to present with prominent respiratory muscle involvement. It is recognized clinically by the finding of muscle hypertrophy, paraproteinemia, and weakness. Diagnosis is by muscle biopsy. In rare cases, inclusion body myopathy (IBM) limited to the proximal muscles can lead to ventilation problems and may require ventilation and later out-of-hospital ventilation.

Suggested Reading

Barloon T, Zachar C, Harkens K, Honda H (1988) Computed tomography findings. J Comput Tomogr 12:193–195

Corse AM, Kuncl RW (1993) Polymyositis. In: Johnson RT, Griffin JW (eds) Current therapy in neurologic disease 4. Decker, Philadelphia (in press)

Fornage B, Nerot C (1986) Sonographic diagnosis of rhabdomyolysis. J Clin Ultrasound 14:389–392

Gabow P, Kaehny W, Kelleher S (1982) The spectrum of rhabdomyolysis. Medicine (Baltimore) 61:141–152

Grau A, Pomes J, Davalos A, Gomez E, Sola P, Genis D (1988) Computed tomography in acute alcoholic myopathy. J Comput Tomogr 12:161–164

Jerusalem F, Zierz S (1991) Muskelkrankheiten, 2nd edn. Thieme, Stuttgart, pp 341–342

Kaplan G (1980) Ultrasonic appearance of rhabdomyolysis. Am J Roentgenol 134: 375–377

Kuncl RW, Wiggins WW (1988) Toxic myopathies. Neurol Clin 6:593–619

Lamminen A, Hekali P, Tiula E, Sumaro I, Korhola O (1989) Acute rhabdomyolysis: evaluation and magnetic resonance imaging compared with computed tomography and ultrasonography. Br J Radiol 62:326–330

Lamminen A, Jaaskelainen J, Rapola J, Sumaro I (1988) High frequency ultrasonography of skeletal muscle in children with neuromuscular disease. J Ultrasound Med 7: 505–509

Lane RJM, Mastaglia FL (1978) Drug induced myopathies in man. Lancet 2:562–565

Layzer RD (1985) Neuromuscular manifestations of systemic disease. Davis, Philadelphia

Mastaglia FL (1982) Adverse effects of drugs on muscle. Drugs 24:304–321

Meyer-Betz F (1910) Beobachtungen an einem eigenartigen mit Muskellähmung verbundenen Fall von Hämoglobinurie. Dtsch Arch Klin Med 101:85–127

Penn AS (1986) Myoglobinuria. In: Engel AG, Banker BQ (eds) Myology. McGraw-Hill, New York, pp 1785–1805

Pongratz D, Reimers C, Hahn D, Nägele M, Müller-Felber W (1990) Atlas der Muskelkrankheiten. Urban & Schwarzenberg, Munich, pp 124–125

Sauvain J, Blanc P, Delacour J, Wagschal G, Daoudal P (1985) Apport de l'echographie dans le diagnostic et la surveillance des rhabdomyolyses aiguës. Presse Med 36: 1885–1886

Chapter 74

Acute Dyskalemic Periodic Paralysis

Uta Meyding-Lamadé, Robert Stingele, and
Michael N. Diringer

Definition and Epidemiology

The periodic paralyses are rare disorders of skeletal muscle characterized
by transient, often acute attacks of
muscle weakness. The associated
alterations of serum potassium concentration have led to a classification
into hypo-, hyper-, and normokalemic
forms (Table 1). These occur as primary
disorders, mostly transmitted as an
autosomal dominant trait with variable
expressivity, which have to be distinguished from secondary or acquired
periodic paralysis, e.g., associated with
thyrotoxicosis. Electrolyte changes are
less marked in primary periodic
paralysis than in secondary periodic
paralysis.

Since the attacks, although devastating, are infrequent, diagnosis
often depends on the induction of attacks with provocative testing. This
potentially hazardous procedure should
be done in an ICU setting in order to
monitor continuously ECG, repiratory
function, muscle strength, and electrolyte changes.

Section Editor: Daniel F. Hanley

Pathogenesis

In the periodic paralysis the normal
excitation process fails to develop and
thus prevents the spread of action
potentials along the muscle surface
membrane, due to an abnormally increased membrane sodium conduc-
tance. The shifts in serum potassium
ion concentration probably reflect
coupling to sodium movements through
the Na-K-ATPase pump system. The
molecular base of Gamstorp's disease
has recently been documented as a
dysfunction of a sodium channel.

Clinical Features and Differential Diagnosis

The clinical features for differential
diagnosis are summarized in Table 2.

Hypokalemic Periodic Paralysis

Attacks almost invariably begin by the
first or second decade and typically
occur at night. Normally, attacks last

Table 1. Periodic paralysis – classification

Primary periodic paralysis	Secondary periodic paralysis
Hypokalemic	Diuretics
Hyperkalemic:	
Adynamia episodica	Alcohol
hereditaria	Endocrinopathy
Gamstorp	(e.g., thyrotoxicosis)
Paramyotonia	
congenita	
Eulenberg	
Normokalemic	Alcohol, endocrinopathy

4–24 h. Limb musculature is most commonly involved. Rarely respiration, mastication, phonation, and eye movements may be impaired. Then involvement of accessory respiratory and intercostal muscles may cause acute respiratory insufficiency. Rarely, a myotonic lid lag is present. ECG findings concomitant with potassium level changes often exist. Symptomatic cardiac involvement is rare but has been reported to occur in some families; acute dilatation of the heart is the most frequently reported finding. The frequency and severity of attacks vary greatly among patients, above the age of 30 years the attacks usually diminish. Provoking factors are carbohydrate-rich meals, and rest after exertion, whereas mild exercise (walking-off) appears to be preventive. Less important provoking factors are cold, emotions, intake of alcohol, trauma, or infection. In some patients, above all

Table 2. Clinical features of periodic paralysis

	Hypokalemic periodic paralysis	Hyperkalemic periodic paralysis, normokalemic periodic paralysis	Paramyotonia congenita
Inheritance	autosomal dominant female: minor penetrance	autosomal dominant	autosomal dominant
Age at onset	second decade, usually puberty, variable	first decade, occasionally infancy	infancy
Pre-disposing factors	rest after excercise, high carbohydrate intake, cold, emotion	rest after excercise, low carbohydrate intake, cold	rest after excercise, cold
Time of day	early morning	daytime or early night	early morning
Ictal serum K+	2–3 mEq/l, occasionally only slightly lowered	usually slightly elevated, during attack, occasionally up to 8 mEq/l	normal or slightly elevated
Attack severity	+++, usually plegia or severe paresis	+, often only mild weakness	++
Duration	often prolonged (1–8 days), average 12 h	10 min to 1 h	variable

in males, permanent muscle weakness develops, involving predominantly the proximal muscles.

Attacks of hypokalemic periodic paralysis associated with thyrotoxicoxis occur predominantly among young Asian males, often coinciding with the onset of thyrotoxicosis.

Hyperkalemic Periodic Paralysis or Adynamia Episodica Hereditaria Gamstorp

Attacks begin in the first decade of life in most cases. Compared with hypokalemic periodic paralysis, attacks are more frequent (daily or at least weekly) and of shorter duration (minutes to hours). No palsy-associated deaths have been reported, although weakness of cranial and respiratory musculature is frequent. Provoking factors are rest after exercise, cold, steroid or potassium ingestion (cola beverages). Some patients develop interictal myopathies, as in hypokalemic periodic paralysis. As potassium levels do not necessarily rise above the normal range and occasionally rise only very early in the attack, provocative testing frequently is necessary to establish the diagnosis.

Hyperkalemic periodic paralysis can occur as a distinct entity, called paramyotonia congenita Eulenberg. In this disease patients suffer from myotonia precipitated by cold and excercise in addition to periodic paralysis.

Normokalemic Periodic Paralysis

Most likely, normokalemic periodic paralysis is a variant of hyperkalemic periodic paralysis. Potassium chloride can initiate an attack, and sodium chloride can be used to treat the attacks. The clinical symptoms as well as diagnostic and therapeutic procedures are as in hyperkalemic periodic paralysis.

Secondary Hypo- and Hyperkalemic Periodic Paralysis

Numerous factors, including diuretics, alcohol, corticosteroids, and certain endocrinopathies, can present with the clinical picture of periodic paralysis. In these secondary forms alterations of potassium levels are more obviously abnormal, often present in the interictal phase.

Ancillary Tests

Patient history is often indicative of the diagnosis, but particularly in sporadic cases without family history it is imperative to definitely establish the diagnosis. During the attacks continuous monitoring of respiratory function, ECG, and serum electrolytes is important. Provocative testing in the attack-free interval can be performed only if renal function is normal. During each of the loading tests ECG, muscle strength, respiratory function, and serum electrolytes should be monitored in an ICU setting. Occasionally, creatine phosphokinase can be elevated after an attack of periodic paralysis. Muscle biopsies reveal vacuolar muscle fiber changes. Ancillary tests are summarized in Table 3.

Table 3. Summary of ancillary tests

	Provocative tests	Electromyography	Muscle biopsy
Hypokalemic periodic paralysis	Oral/i.v. glucose/insulin load (see text) attention: hypoglycemia	no action potentials evocable (directly and indirectly)	vacuolar changes in muscle fibers; proliferation of T-tubules, dilation of sarcoplasmic reticulum components
Hyperkalemic periodic paralysis	oral/i.v. KCl load (see text) attention: symptoms may be aggravated	see hypokalemic periodic paralysis; no specific findings	no specific findings; after prolonged paralysis, as in hypokalemic periodic paralysis
Paramyotonia congenita	limb cooling	see hypokalemic periodic paralysis; during attack additional myotonic findings	see hyperkalemic periodic paralysis

Hypokalemic Periodic Paralysis

Provocative Testing. The administration of oral glucose (1.5 g/kg body weight) in children and adults may precipitate an attack. If no weakness is produced the glucose load can be raised up to 2 g/kg. In addition, insulin is administered either subcutaneously or intravenously (dosage: 0.1 U/kg) at 30 and 60 min. In adults the provocative testing can be potentiated by 4 × 2 g NaCl orally in an aqueous solution. Minimum levels of potassium are seen 90–150 min after initiation of the test, depending on the route of administration. Hypoglycemia often occurs 15–60 min following glucose and insulin administration and must be anticipated. Serum osmololality and volume balance can be altered markedly by this test.

Electromyography. In the acute attack action potentials can be evoked neither by direct nor by indirect stimulation. In the interictal phase a normal or slightly decreased action potential and occasionally spontaneous activity is seen.

Muscle Biopsy. Degenerative changes can be found after a series of attacks and in cases of chronic myopathy. Vacuolated changes are located near or in the center of the muscle fibers. Ultrastructural analysis of specimen reveals proliferation of T-tubules as well as dilation of sarcoplasmic reticulum components.

Hyperkalemic Periodic Paralysis

Provocative Testing. Oral potassium loading should begin with a minimum dose of 40 mEq KCl for children and 60 mEq KCl for adults. If no effect has been seen after 24 h, an increase in dosage up to a maximum of 120 mEq KCl can be administered. As an alternative to oral loading i.v. loading can be used, administrating the above dosages in glucose infusions. Possibly

Table 4. Current concepts of treatment in periodic paralysis

	Acute attack	Prophylaxis
Hypokalemic periodic paralysis	ICU: ECG, monitoring of respiratory function, serum electrolytes	Mild, infrequent attacks: avoidance of predisposing factors
	Potassium salts (orally or i.v.)	Severe, frequent attacks: acetazolamide, spironolactone
Hyperkalemic periodic paralysis	"Walking off", carbohydrate intake. If ineffective hydrochlorothiazide, salbutamol inhaler, or i.v. glucose/insulin administration	Mild, infrequent attacks: avoidance of predisposing factors
		Frequent, severe attacks: acetazolamide, chlorothiazide

associated myotonic or paramyotonic symptoms of periodic paralysis may also be worsened.

Electromyography. During the attacks the action potentials have a decreased duration and reduced amplitudes. Sometimes spontaneous activity and increased prick activity (*Einstichaktivität*) can be found even interictally.

Muscle Biopsy. In most cases structure of the muscle is normal. With prolonged paralysis changes similar to those described in hypokalemic periodic paralysis have been found.

Management

Table 4 summarizes current concepts of treatment for patients with periodic paralysis.

Hypokalemic Periodic Paralysis

Acute Attacks. Patients with a severe acute attack should be admitted to an ICU. ECG, respiratory function, and serum electrolytes should be monitored continuously. Ventilatory support should be readily available, as respiratory arrest is the most common cause of death in hypokalemic periodic paralysis. Potassium salts abort attacks and should be given orally (60–120 mEq). If oral administration is impossible due to vomiting, intravenous potassium can be delivered by a cental venous catheter at a maximum rate of 20 mEq KCl/h in 5% mannitol. Saline or glucose infusions are contraindicated as they may cause worsening of hypokalemia.

Prophylactic Treatment. Avoidance of predisposing factors like carbohydrate-rich meals is recommended. Patients with only mild, infrequent attacks do not need further medical treatment, but for those with severe, recurring attacks medical treatment is indicated. If the attacks regularly occur in the early morning an oral intake of potassium late in the evening is an effective treatment, though, in general, the prophylactic intake of KCl in hypokalemic periodic paralysis does not reduce frequency and duration of attacks. Acetazolamide at a dose of

125 mg–1.5 g daily is effective within 24 h as a prophylactic therapy. The mechanism of action is not known; it may be related to the production of acidosis or lowered insulin and glucose levels. Side effects include nausea, paresthesias, dysgeusia, and renal calculi. Spironolactone at a dose of 2 × 100 mg daily has been shown to be effective, but gynecomastia and hirsutism are common side effects.

The acute attacks of periodic paralysis in thyrotoxicosis are treated as indicated above. In general, if patients return to normal thyroid function the attacks do not recur.

Hyperkalemic Periodic Paralysis

Acute Attacks. Medical treatment is rarely necessary, as patients often are able to terminate attacks by themselves by "walking off", or prompt intake of carbohydrate-rich meals or sweet drinks. If patients take 25 mg hydrochlorothiazide or inhale a puff of salbutamol the attack often can be shortened. In general, ICU treatment is not necessary.

Prophylactic Treatment. As in hypokalemic periodic paralysis, avoidance of provoking factors is the best and often sufficient prophylaxis. If patients experience a high frequency of attacks acetazolamide at a dose of 250–750 mg daily may be effective. Thiazides (e.g., chlorothiazide 25–75 mg daily) are effective; in both the mechanism of action is still unclear.

The prophylactic treatment of hyperkalemic periodic paralysis as-

sociated with paramyotonia remains controversial; some authors recommend acetazolamide prophylactically. Treatment of the acute attack is as indicated above.

Suggested Reading

Barchi RL, Furman RE (1992) Pathophysiology of myotonia and periodic paralysis. In: Ashbury AK, McKhann GM, McDonald WI (eds) Diseases of the nervous system, clinical neurobiology, vol 1. Butterworths-Heinemann, Sevenoaks, pp 146–163

Buruma OJS, Schipperheyn JJ (1979) Periodic paralysis. In: Vinken PJ, Bruyn GW (eds) Handbook of clinical neurology, vol 41. Elsevier, New York, pp 147–174

Dalakas MC, Engel WK (1983) Treatment of permanent muscle weakness in familial hypokalemic periodic paralysis. Muscle Nerve 6:182–186

Griggs RC, Resnick J, Engel WK (1983) Intravenous treatment of hypokalemic periodic paralysis. Arch Neurol 40:539–540

Jerusalem F, Zierz S (1992) Episodische Lähmungen. In: Jerusalem F, Zierz S (eds) Muskelerkrankungen – Klinik – Therapie – Pathologie. Thieme, Stuttgart, pp 311–316

Riggs JE, Griggs RC (1979) Diagnosis and treatment of the periodic paralyses. Clin Neuropharmacol 4:123–138

Riggs JE, Griggs R, Moxley RT (1984) Dissociation of glucose and potassium arterial-venous differences across the forearm by acetazolamide. Arch Neurol 41:35–38

Ricker K, Rohkamm R, Böhlen R (1986) Adynamia episodica and paralysis periodica paramyotonica. Neruology 36:682–686

Rüdel R, Lehmann-Horn F, Ricker K, Küther G (1984) Hypokalemic periodic paralysis: in vitro investigation of muscle fibre parameters. Muscle Nerve 7:110–120

Torres CF, Griggs R, Moxley RT, Bender AN (1981) Hypokalemic periodic paramyotonica. Neurology 31:1423–1428

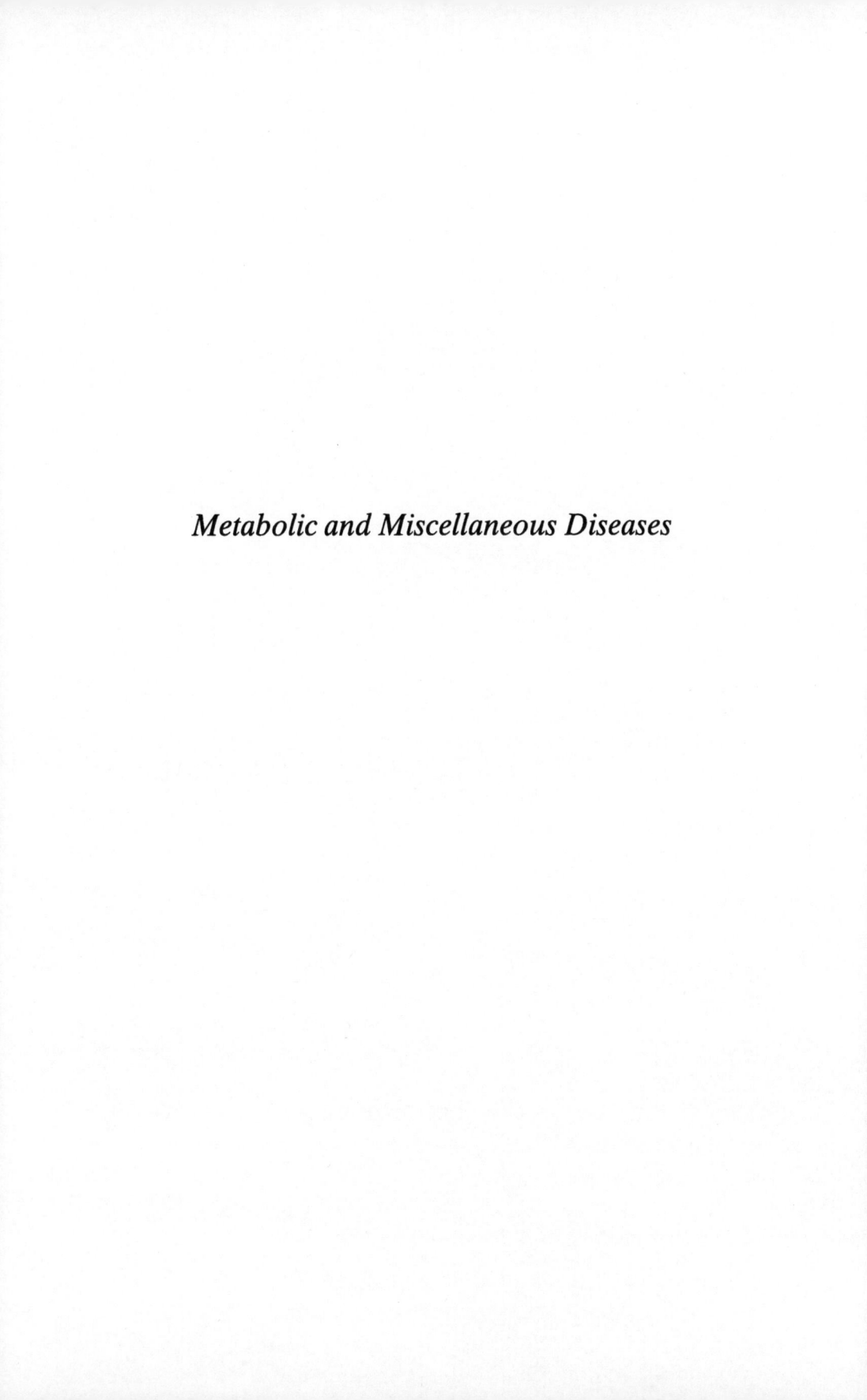

Metabolic and Miscellaneous Diseases

Chapter 75

Metabolic Encephalopathies

Klaus Kunze and Michael N. Diringer

Introduction

Metabolic encephalopathies are diffuse mutifocal cerebral states characterized by confusion, stupor, or coma with variable clinical courses. There are no specific focal neurological signs which permit a clear-cut diagnosis; however, different patterns of neurological signs and neuropsychological findings suggest the diagnosis. Because a number of different pathophysiological states can produce encephalopathy, careful serial clinical neurological examinations and extensive laboratory testing are often necessary for diagnosis and successful treatment.

Etiology

Among the many causes of metabolic encephalopathy are hypoxic or ischemic diseases, organ dysfunction including the liver, kidney, and lung, systemic diseases, and a large group of

---

Section Editor: Michael N. Diringer

toxic agents (Table 1). Although many single and distinct factors or diseases may cause encephalopathy, a combination of factors must be considered in patients in the neurocritical care unit. There are no special figures regarding the frequency of metabolic encephalopathies but cardiovascular, liver, and renal dysfunction are commonly found. Alcohol is the single most frequent exogenous factor. Multiple trauma, intoxication, and endocrine diseases are other important factors.

Pathophysiology

Brain metabolism depends almost completely on the metabolism of systemically derived substrates. About 75% of hepatic glucose production is used in the brain and about 90% of cerebral glucose metabolism takes place by the Krebs cycle and the gamma-aminobutyric acid shunt. In addition, amino acids and ammonia are taken from the blood during high metabolic rates, which vary in different regions of the brain.

Table 1. Important causes of metabolic encephalopathies

Hypoxia
- Anemia
- Pulmonary disease
- Alveolar hypoventilation
Ischemia
- Cardiovascular disease (including cardiac arrest)
- Stokes-Adams syndrome, cardiac arrythmias
- Hypersensitive carotid sinus
- Microvascular diseases
- Hyperviscosity syndrome
- Hypotension
Systemic diseases
- Hepatic disease
- Renal disease
- Pancreatic disease (gastrointestinal)
- Malnutrition (vitamin deficiency)
- Endocrine dysfunction (hypoglycemia or hyperglycemia and hyperosmolar state)
- Acid-base, electrolyte, and fluid balance
- Vasculitis
- Infection and sepsis
- Malignancy (paraneoplastic syndromes)
Toxic agents
- Alcohol, sedatives (barbiturates, narcotics, tranquilizers)
- Psychiatric medications (tricyclic antidepressants, anticholinergic drugs, phenothiazine, MAO inhibitors)
- Heavy metals
- Organic phosphates, solvents
- Other drugs (corticosteroids, penicillin, anticonvulsants)

Morphological changes in brain tissue do not always occur in patients with encephalopathies. However, those with vascular encephalopathies may have signs of tissue hypoxia and tissue edema. Tissue necrosis may be found in those with severe hepatic encephalopathy. On the cellular level, morphological changes of astrocytes (resembling Alzheimer type-II cells) may be found in patients with hepatic encephalopathy.

It is clear that metabolic encephalopathies are frequently related to systemic diseases (Table 1). The main factors are *hypoxia*, such as from vascular and immunoinfectious diseases; *endotoxins*, such as in hepatic, renal, pancreatic, and septic encephalopathies; and *exotoxins*, such as in various drug and toxic encephalopathies.

Patients requiring neurocritical care frequently have comorbidity. In many cases one of the factors, such as hypoxia-ischemia, dysregulation of fluid and electrolytes, renal or liver dysfunction, would be enough to cause encephalopathy. Brain injury especially can cause decompensation of those metabolic factors finally leading to encephalopathy. There is no single underlying pathophysiology; rather, a number of different pathogenic factors are responsible for the development of encephalopathy. There are no primary structural changes leading to signs of encephalopathy, so clinical findings are reversible if they are detected early.

Clinical Features

Two groups of clinical signs are found in those with metabolic encephalopathies: *global cerebral signs* and *focal cerebral signs* (Tables 2 and 3). Both types of signs may be found together, but generally signs of diffuse organic brain dysfunction precede focal signs. It is important to recognize global signs as early as possible, as they are warnings of impending clinical deterioration and therefore are important for treatment and development of new treatment strategies.

Global cerebral signs (Table 2) are not uniform. Their expression is

Table 2. Global cerebral signs

Disturbances of consciousness
- Somnolence
- Stupor
- Coma
Seizures
Vegetative signs
- Respiration (Cheyne-Stokes)
- Cardiac arrythmias, cardiac arrest
- Vertigo, nausea, vomiting
Vasomotor and sudomotor disturbances
Neuropsychological changes
- Agitation
- Hallucination
- Delusions
- Delirium
Brain-stem signs
- Oral and facial automatisms
- Palmomental and grasp reflexes, snouting reflexes
- Paratonia
- Decorticate and decerebrate posturing
- Tremor
- Asterixis
- Myoclonus (multifocal)

Table 3. Focal cerebral signs

Hemispheric signs
- Visual disturbances
- Aphasia-apraxia
- Hemispastic, hemiatactic, hemisensory syndromes
- Reflex and muscle-tone changes
- Focal or generalized seizures
Brain-stem signs
- Cranial nerve disturbances (oculovestibular pupillomotor)
- Nystagmus, gaze deviations
- Brain-stem reflex disturbances
- Dysarthria, dysphagia, respiratory disturbances Atactic, paretic, sensory syndromes (hemi-, quadri-, alternating)
- Quadrispastic syndromes, reflex changes
- Myoclonus

Table 4. Neuropsychological signs

Disturbance of	
Consciousness	Diminished arousal, different degrees of coma
Orientation	Time, place, situation, and self
Attention and memory	Short- and long-term memory
Form and contents	Perseveration, incoherence, flight of ideas, thinking abstraction
Perception	Illusions and hallucinations
Affect	Emotion and anxiety
Psychomotor activity	Increased or decreased motor drive, restlessness, apathy

variable in terms of quality and quantity. They can include autonomic dysfunction, altered consciousness, confusional states, and psychomotor hyperactivity. Delirium and agitation are commonly seen with or without altered levels of consciousness (Table 4).

Focal cerebral signs (Table 3) may be combined with global cerebral signs. Although there may be quite clear-cut signs from the hemispheres or the brain stem, sometimes the clinical signs do not permit a clear topographic assignment. Brain-stem signs are especially important in patients with severe encephalopathies. In this context, brain-stem signs in brain injury are much more severe and more often irreversible compared with those in metabolic encephalopathies. In metabolic encephalopathies, pupillary light reflexes are often preserved, even in severe cases. This can be an important clue for the differential diagnosis.

Ancillary Tests and Differential Diagnosis

Diagnosis of metabolic encephalopathy depends on careful and repeated neurological examinations, based on a detailed history. Underlying diseases must be considered. This requires the availability of extended data from clinical chemistries including electrolytes, glucose, liver and renal status, and acid-base status. Different types of metabolic coma, especially those resulting from endocrine and electrolyte disturbances, need to be considered. CNS and systemic infections should always be considered in the evaluation as well.

Neuroradiology

CT and MRI should be used to rule out other underlying causes. Cerebral angiography is rarely performed.

Table 5. Brain-stem reflexes

Reflex	Localization[a]
Pupillary light	II/Midbrain/III
Cornea	V/Pons/VII
Orbicularis oculi	V/Pons-medulla/VII
Oculocardiac	V/Medulla/X
Vestibulo-ocular	VIII/Pons-mesencephalon/V
Tongue-jaw	IX, X/Medulla/V
Spinocilial	Spinal cord/T1–2/cervical sympathetic ganglia
Oculocephalic	VIII, afferents from the neck/lower brain stem/ oculomotor system

[a] Roman numerals indicate cranial nerves as afferent and efferent parts of the reflex arc, in the middle the brain stem or spinal level of the reflex arc.

Other Tests

CSF analysis usually shows only minor and nonspecific changes, if any. Positron emission tomography studies are only of academic interest. EEG is frequently very useful and may show general changes and sometimes characteristic patterns that may be helpful for the diagnosis. Evoked potentials (VEP, SEP, and SEP) are of minor value. Examination and monitoring of brain-stem reflexes (Table 5) are helpful for following the clinical course.

The differential diagnosis includes brain tumors, CNS infections, vascular diseases of the brain, intracranial hemorrhages, sinus venous thromboses, and other causes of increased intracranial pressure. As neuropsychological changes may be early signs of these diseases, a correct diagnosis can be difficult to make.

Treatment

There is no specific neurocritical care treatment for patients with metabolic coma. Management should include treatment of underlying diseases, monitoring, and general supportive measures. Respiration, heart rate, and fluid balance should be carefully monitored. In come cases, brain edema may develop and ICP monitoring may become necessary. If the ICP is increased, the patient should be treated appropriately. In Europe, anticonvulsants are frequently used prophylactically.

Suggested Reading

Fischer CM (1969) The neurological examination of the comatose patient. Acta Neurol Scand 45 [Suppl 36]:1–56

Heiss WD, Beil C, Herholz K, Pawlik G, Wagner R, Wienhard K (1985) Atlas of positron emission tomography of the brain. Springer, Berlin Heidelberg New York

Kunze K (ed) (1992) Lehrbuch der Neurologie. Thieme, Stuttgart, pp 540–564

Plum F, Posner JB (1982) The diagnosis of stupor and coma, 3rd edn. Davis, Philadelphia

Chapter 76

Wernicke's Encephalopathy (Wernicke-Korsakoff Syndrome)

KLAUS KUNZE and MICHAEL A. DEGEORGIA

Introduction

Wernicke's encephalopathy is a common disease characterized, in its classic form, by oculomotor abnormalities, ataxia, and global confusion. It is caused by a deficiency of thiamine (vitamin B_1), an essential coenzyme for carbohydrate metabolism, and occurs mainly in patients with chronic alcoholism. Patients with malnutrition from other causes also develop the disease (Table 1). Thiamine deficiency in alcoholics results from a combination of inadequate dietary intake, impaired gastrointestinal absorption, and decreased hepatic storage. Decreased activation of thiamine to thiamine pyrophosphate (TPP) also occurs in alcoholics.

Pathophysiology

The exact mechanism by which thiamine deficiency causes Wernicke's encephalopathy is not known. Thiamine is a coenzyme for enzymes in the Krebs cycle (pyruvate decarboxylase and alpha-ketogluterate dehydrogenase) and the pentose phosphate pathway (transketolase; Fig. 1). Deficiency produces a marked decrease in cerebral glucose utilization, slowed axonal conduction and synaptic transmission, and impaired DNA synthesis. Excitotoxicity from release of glutamic acid may also be important. Damage to ascending norepinephrine-containing neurons in the brain stem and diencephalon and an increase in beta-endorphins may account for the amnesia in patients who later develop Korsakoff's syndrome. It remains unclear why only a small number of thiamine-deficient individuals (alcoholics and nonalcoholics) develop the disease. Although low activity of transketolase has been suggested as a possible genetic predispostion, this has not been generally accepted.

Epidemiology

Wernicke's encephalopathy is diagnosed in 0.4–0.13% of all hospital

Section Editor: Michael N. Diringer

Table 1. Causes of Wernicke's encephalopathy

- Chronic alcoholism
- Hyperemesis
- Anorexia nervosa
- Starvation or fasting (including refeeding)
- Prolonged total parenteral nutrition
- Hemodialysis or peritoneal dialysis
- Cancer
- Gastrointestinal surgery (gastric plication)
- Malnutrition from any cause

admissions. The disease is under-recognized, however, and autopsy studies have shown an incidence of 0.8–2.8% in the general population and 12.5% in alcoholics. Reasons for this under-recognition may include the emphasis that clinicians place on chronic alcoholism as an underlying cause and the absence of the classic triad of symptoms in most patients. In the Australian autopsy series of 37 cases, only 20% had been correctly diagnosed during life. Thirty-seven percent had only one symptom of the classic triad. Mental symptoms were present in 86% of patients (Fig. 2).

Clinical Features

In 1881, Wernicke first described three patients with acute onset of ophthalmoplegia, gait ataxia, and confusion. Two of the patients were alcoholics hospitalized for delirium and the third was a patient with protracted vomiting after severe intoxication. In 1887, Korsakoff described 20 patients with chronic alcoholism and global amnesia ("psychosis polyneuritica"). It is now known that Wernicke's encephalopathy and Korsakoff's psychosis are different stages of the same disease (with Wernicke's encephalopathy representing the early, acute stage and Korsakoff's psychosis representing the later, chronic stage). Thus, the term

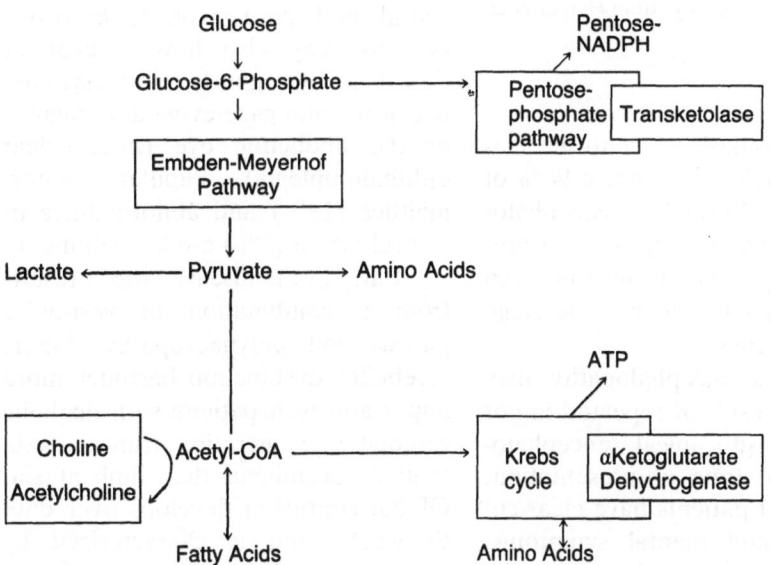

Fig. 1. Impaired enzyme activity in thiamine deficiency (from Schenker et al. 1980)

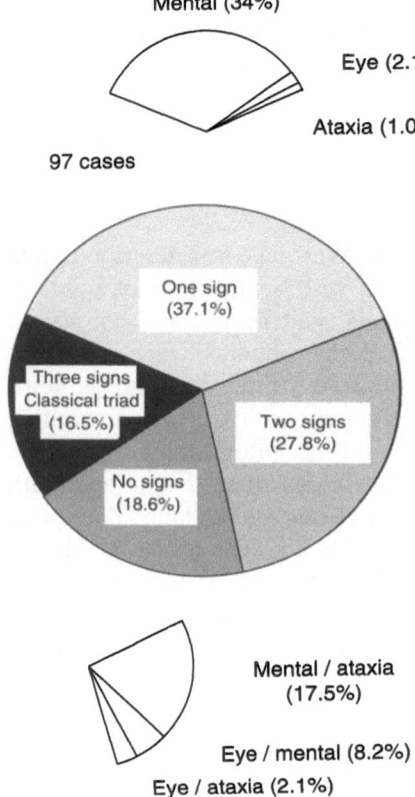

Fig. 2. Incidence of clinical signs in 97 cases of Wernicke's encephalopathy (from Harper et al. 1986)

Table 2. Initial symptoms of 163 patients with Wernicke's encephalopathy (adapted from Victor et al. 1989)

Symptom	n	(%)
Confusion	108	(66)
Staggering gait	84	(51)
Ocular ("cross-eyed")	65	(40)
Polyneuropathy	59	(36)
"Collapse", "exhaustion"	33	(20)
Other	25	(15)
Alcohol withdrawal	21	(13)

nosis can be masked by the presence of stupor or coma. Other conditions that can mimic the disease include intoxication, ischemia or hemorrhage (especially in the brain stem), encephalitis, meningitis, brain tumor, seizure disorders, and other kinds of encephalopathies.

The most frequent oculomotor abnormalities are nystagmus (85%), bilateral sixth cranial nerve palsy (54%), and conjugate gaze palsy (45%). The nystagmus is usually horizontal and gaze evoked; however, patients may also have upbeat or downbeat nystagmus, or an asymmetric horizontal gaze-evoked nystagmus of the abducting eye (internuclear ophthalmoplegia). Pupillary abnormalities (19%) and abnormalities of central vision (3%) are less common.

Early in the disease, ataxia results from a combination of vestibular paresis and polyneuropathy. Later, cerebellar dysfunction becomes more important. As in patients with alcoholic cerebellar degeneration, truncal ataxia is more prominent than limb ataxia. Global confusion develops over days to weeks and is characterized by apathy, mental sluggishness, and restlessness. Patients may be inattentive

Wernicke-Korsakoff syndrome is used. Nevertheless, as almost 90% of patients with Wernicke's encephalopathy have mental symptoms on presentation, a gradual transition from the acute stage to the chronic stage most likely occurs.

Wernicke's encephalopathy may develop as a result of repeated minor episodes of subclinical encephalopathy. At the time of presentation, however, most patients have clear-cut neurological and mental symptoms. Onset of symptoms may be acute, subacute, or chronic (Table 2). The diag-

Table 3. Clinical findings of polyneuropathy in 230 patients with Wernicke's encephalopathy (adapted from Victor et al. 1989)

Legs (189 patients)			Arms (57 patients)		
Sensory, motor, and reflex loss	66	(35)[a]	Sensory, motor and reflex loss	17	(30)
Reflex loss alone	45	(24)	Sensory loss	10	(18)
Reflex + sensory loss	40	(21)	Sensory + motor loss	10	(18)
Sensory loss alone	10	(5)	Reflex loss alone	6	(11)
Sensory + motor loss	2	(1)	Motor loss alone	5	(9)
Motor loss alone	0		Reflex + sensory loss	2	(4)
Data in complete	26	(14)	Data incomplete	7	(12)

[a] Numbers in parentheses indicate percent.

and disoriented with regard to place and time. Stupor and coma may occur and occasionally can dominate the clinical picture. Other frequent findings include hypothermia and hypotension as a result of damage to the hypothalamus and brain-stem autonomic pathways. Patients may also have tremor and tachycardia from acute alcohol withdrawal, or other signs of thiamine deficiency such as high-output cardiac failure ("wet beriberi") and polyneuropathy (Table 3).

Pathological Findings

The neuropathological changes in patients with Wernicke's encephalopthy are specific for the disease and include lesions in the thalamus (dorsal medial nucleus), hypothalamus (mamillary bodies), midbrain (oculomotor nucleus and periaqueductal areas), and pons and medulla (abducens and medial vestibular nuclei). Histopathological changes include necrosis of both nerve cells and myelinated structures, hypertrophy and hyperplasia of small blood vessels, and fresh hemorrhages in the subependymal gray matter of the wall

of the third ventricle. Some of the changes resemble those seen in anoxic necrosis, although the more gradual drop-out of neurons (particularly in the thalamus) is more characteristic of Wernicke's encephalopathy. Severe loss of Purkinje cells occurs in the anterior superior vermis of the cerebellum.

Diagnosis

The diagnosis of Wernicke's encephalopathy is made clinically. Ancillary findings are inconsistent and nonspecific. Analysis of the cerebrospinal fluid is normal or shows only a modest increase in the protein concentration. Patients may have an increased blood pyruvate concentration and a decreased erythrocyte transketolase concentration. About half of the patients have diffuse slowing on EEG. Computed tomography occasionally reveals low-density abnormalities in the diencephalon, and MR imaging often can identify atrophy of the mamillary bodies early in the course of the disease. Abnormalities have also been demonstrated on both brain-stem auditory evoked responses (BAERs, prolonged I–III intervals) and visual evoked responses (VERs, prolonged latency and reduced amplitude of the P100 component). Treatment should never be withheld while waiting for the results of these studies.

Treatment

Wernicke's encephalopathy is potentially reversible if the diagnosis is made early. Treatment should be started in all patients with symptoms and signs suggestive of the disease. Although 2–3 mg thiamine may improve the oculomotor signs, much larger doses are needed to replenish depleted stores. Fifty to 100 mg should be given immediately by intravenous or intramuscular injection. Glucose infusions should always be given after or at the same time as thiamine, since glucose can precipitate Wernicke's encephalopathy in thiamine-deficient patients. Daily infusions should include 500 mg thiamine until patients can resume a normal diet. If oral treatment is considered, 100 mg thiamine three times daily (lipid soluble) is sufficient. Other deficiencies of vitamins, minerals, and electrolytes (especially magnesium, a transketolase co-factor) should also be corrected.

With treatment, oculomotor abnormalities improve within hours and generally resolve within a week. A fine horizontal gaze-evoked nystagmus may persist indefinately in one third of patients. Ataxia improves slower than other symptoms and almost half of the patients are left with a wide-base shuffling gait.

Prognosis

Wernicke's encephalopathy is fatal without treatment, and death occurs in 10–20% of patients even with treatment. The most common causes of death in hospitalized patients are infection (pneumonia, pulmonary tuberculosis, and sepsis) and end-stage liver disease. Of those who survive, almost 80% develop Korsakoff's syndrome, characterized by retrograde amnesia (the inability to recall information) and anterograde amnesia (the inability to learn new information). In most patients, the amnesia emerges as the other symptoms begin to resolve. Patients may be disoriented with regard to place and time and have decreased spontaneity and initiative. Confabulation, the fabrication of stories, may or may not be present. The prognosis of patients with Korsakoff's syndrome is variable. Amnesia may not improve at all or may improve only slowly. Complete or nearly complete recovery occurs in fewer than 20%.

Suggested Reading

Blass IP, Gibson GE (1977) Abnormality of a thiamine requiring enzyme in patients with Wernicke-Korsakoff syndrome. N Engl J Med 297:1367–1370

Chan YW, McLeod JG, Tuck RR, Feary PA (1985) Brain-stem auditory evoked responses in chronic alcoholics. J Neurol Neurosurg Psychiatry 48:1107–1112

Chan YW, McLeod JG, Tuck RR, Walsh JC, Feary PA (1986) Visual evoked responses in chronic alcoholics. J Neurol Neurosurg Psychiatry 49:945–950

Charness ME, Delapaz RL (1987) Mammillary body atrophy in Wernicke's encephalopathy: antemortem identification using magnetic resonance imaging. Ann Neurol 22:596–600

Choi DW (1988) Glutamate neurotoxicity and diseases of the nervous system. Neuron 1:623–634

Donnan GA, Seemann A (1980) Coma and hypothermia in Wernicke's encephalopathy. Aust NZ J Med 10:438–439

Ghez C (1969) Vestibular paresis: a clinical feature of Wernicke's disease. J Neurol Neurosurg Psychiatry 32:134–139

Goto I, Nagara H, Tateishi I, Kuroiwa Y (1986) Thiamine-deficiencies encephalopathy in rats: effects of deficiencies of thiamine and magnesium. Brain Res 372:31–36

Hakim AM, Pappius HM (1983) Sequence of metabolic, clinical, and histological events in experimental thiamine deficiency. Ann Neurol 13:365–375

Harper CG (1983) The incidence of Wernicke's encephalopathy in Australia – a neuropathological study of 131 cases. J Neurol Neurosurg Psychiatry 46:593–598

Harper CG, Giles M, Finlay-Jones R (1986) Clinical signs in the Wernicke-Korsakoff complex: a retrospective analysis of 131 cases diagnosed at necropsy. J Neurol Neurosurg Psychiatry 49:341–345

Iwata H (1982) Possible role of thiamine in the nervous system. Trends Pharmacol Sci 3:171–173

Kitaguchi T, Kobayashi T, Tobimatsu ST, Goto I, Kuroiwa Y (1987) Computed tomography and magnetic resonance imaging in a young patient with Wernicke's encephalopathy. J Neurol 234:449–450

Korsakoff SS (1887) Disturbance of psychic function in alcoholic paralysis and its relation to the disturbance of the psychic sphere in multiple neuritis of nonalcoholic origins. Vestn Psichiatr IV, fasc 2

Mcdowell JR, Leblanc HJ (1984) Computed tomography findings in Wernicke-Korsakoff syndrome. Arch Neurol 41:453–454

McEntee WJ, Mair RG (1980) Memory enhancement in Korsakoff's psychosis by clonidine: further evidence for a noradrenergic deficit. Ann Neurol 7:466–470

Nixon PF, Kaczmarek MI, Tate I, Kerr RA, Price I (1984) An erythrocyte transketolase isoenzyme patern associated with the Wernicke-Korsakoff syndrome. Eur J Clin Invest 14:278–281

Reuler IB, Girard DE, Cooney TG (1985) Wernicke's encephalopathy. N Engl J Med 312:1035–1039

Summers IA, Pullman PT, Kril II, Harper CG (1991) Increased central immunoreactive beta-endorphin content in patients with Wernicke-Korsakoff syndrome and in alcoholics. J Clin Pathol 44:126–129

Thompson AD, Ryle PR, Shaw GK (1983) Ethanol, thiamine, and brain damage. Alcohol Alcohol 18:27–43

Torvik A, Lindboe CF, Rogde S (1982) Brain lesions in alcoholics: a neuropathological study with clinical correlations. J Neurol Sci 56:233–248

Torvik A (1985) Two types of brain lesions in Wernicke's encephalopathy. Neuropathol Appl Neurobiol 11:179–190

Victor M, Adams RD, Collins GH (1989) The Wernicke-Korsakoff syndrome and related neurologic disorders due to alcoholism and malnutrition. Contemporary neurology series, vol 3. Davis, Philadelphia

Wallis WE, Willoughby E, Baker P (1978) Coma in the Wernicke-Korsakoff syndrome. Lancet 2:400–401

Wernicke C (1881) Lehrbuch der Gehirnkrankheiten für Ärzte und Studierende. Fischer, Kassel

Chapter 77

Alcoholic Delirium and Other Withdrawal Syndromes

VOLKER SCHUCHARDT and DENNIS L. BOURKE

Delirium Tremens

Definition and Epidemiology

Alcoholism is a major public health problem causing various neurological diseases (Table 1), the most frequent and most important of them being delirium tremens (DT). In our experience, more than 20% of 1720 patients admitted to the neurological intensive care unit (ICU) during a 7-year period were alcohol dependent. Of these, 78 admissions (4.5%) were because of delirium tremens. Three distinct scenarios associated with alcoholism are frequently encountered in the neurological ICU:

1. A known alcoholic is admitted because of an illness not directly caused by alcohol; prophylactic treatment to avoid DT is required.
2. An alcoholic is admitted with clear signs of alcohol withdrawal (impending delirium tremens); development of full-blown delirium tremens must be prevented.
3. A patient is admitted specifically because of active delirium tremens or has developed DT while being treated for another disease.

Pathogenesis

As early as 1813, Sutton suggested that chronic alcohol abuse was the cause of delirium tremens. However, the existence of an alcohol withdrawal syndrome was not generally accepted until 1953, when Victor and Adams demonstrated clearly that DT develops after alcohol withdrawal. Although interruption of daily alcohol intake is the usual etiology of DT, the syndrome can occur following a relative decline in blood alcohol concentration or occasionally during an alcoholic binge. About 5% (3–15%) of heavy drinkers suffer from DT one or more times in their lives. After an initial episode, repeated episodes of DT occur in 12–23% of cases. The natural course of untreated DT is self-limited and runs usually 5–7 days, if the patient does not die. Withdrawal of ethanol is a model to explain DT and to formulate its therapy on a molecular basis.

Section Editor: Michael N. Diringer

Ethanol is a general depressant of all CNS function. In established alcoholism, several compensatory mechanisms develop. However, they are maladaptive in acute alcohol withdrawal and lead to the clinical signs of the withdrawal syndrome and DT. The most important mechanisms are:

1. Increased number of glutamate receptors during chronic alcholism; in alcohol withdrawal seizures occur because of disinhibition of increased glutamate receptor activity.
2. Down-regulation of the gamma-aminobutyric acid (GABA) system because of chronic alcohol intake when alcohol is withdrawn, resulting mainly in agitation and seizures.
3. Reduction of alpha-2 inhibitory receptors in chronic alcoholics, with sympathetic hyperactivity ("noradrenaline storm") in withdrawal.
4. Reduction of dopamine receptors during alcoholism; in alcohol abstinence compensatory augmentation above normal as a rebound phenomenon causes psychosis.
5. Additionally, cholinergic insufficiency.

Clinical Features

Categories of Clinical Signs

The signs of delirium tremens are psychotic, neurological, and autonomic. From a clinical point of view they may be divided into three categories:

1. Signs of organic brain dysfunction are memory deficits and disorienta-

Table 1. Alcohol-related neurological diseases

Alcohol intoxication
Alcohol-induced seizures
Isolated hallucinosis, depression
Delirium tremens (DT)
Wernicke-Korsakoff syndrome
Central pontine myelinolysis
Cerebellar degeneration

tion, hyperexcitability, agitation, and sleep disturbances, affective instability with euphoria or fear, disturbances of consciousness, including coma, and epileptic seizures ("rum fits"). These signs are caused primarily by decreased GABAergic control and cholinergic insufficiency.
2. Schizophreniform psychotic manifestations: delusions, visual and tactile hallucinations, and suggestibility. These manifestations reflect mainly dopamine hyperactivity.
3. Signs of autonomic imbalance with sympathetic hyperactivity and parasympathetic insufficiency, including hyperpyrexia up to 38.5°C, hypertension up to 180/110 mmHg, tachycardia, sweating, tremor, and increased deep tendon reflexes. A temperature higher than 38.5°C is suggestive of a bacterial infection, a blood pressure above 180/110 mmHg is usually not explained by DT alone.

Most patients display some obvious signs of alcoholism: alcohol on the breath and elevated blood alcohol level at admission, enlarged liver, muscle wasting, and multiple subcutaneous hemorrhages. Laboratory findings usually include elevated blood alcohol level, raised mean red cell volume, increased GGT, SGOT, SGPT, and alkaline phosphatase activity; additionally, increased BUN, chloride, total bilirubin, creatinine; and a low carbon dioxide. In many cases, the history from friends or relatives and, occasionally, self-admitted alcohol use helps to establish the diagnosis of alcoholism.

Stages of Delirium Tremens

For clinical purposes, it is useful to define three stages of DT. The first stage is impending DT, which is synonymous with withdrawal syndrome. It is alternatively characterized by vegetative hyperactivity including tremor, tachycardia, and profuse sweating, or by psychotic signs with ephemeral hallucinations. Epileptic seizures occur in 3–10% of cases, usually within the first 2 days after alcohol withdrawal. Reinstituting alcohol intake during this stage may prevent progression to the next stage, completed DT. Although these symptoms may subside spontaneously within several days, if they continue or progress, single-drug treatment with oral carbamazepine, a benzodiazepine, or clomethiazole is usually sufficient. A more severe course can be anticipated when there is a concurrent somatic illness, or an especially long history of alcohol abuse, a previous history of DT, abstinence convulsions, or hallucinations.

The second stage is completed DT, with elements of all three groups of signs described above: signs of organic brain dysfunction, psychotic manifestations, and evidence of autonomic dysfunction. Completed DT represents a "point of no return," from which DT runs its own course; resumption of alcohol intake will no longer influence its course. Treatment in an ICU is advisable. Drug therapy is best provided with combined drugs (see below); oral administration is effective for most patients.

The third stage is life-threatening DT, which occurs in about 7% of all patients who develop DT. Together with the symptomatology of completed DT, there is a more severe autonomic deterioration, with primarily cardiac and pulmonary complications and, in some instances, a decreased level of consciousness or even coma. In stage III, ICU admission is essential.

Differential Diagnosis

Differential diagnosis of DT includes any condition producing a delirious state (Table 2). Since the incidence of alcoholism is so high in the general population, the diagnosis of another somatic illness does not rule out simultaneous DT; for example, DT following alcohol withdrawal due to hospitalization for head trauma. Conversely, in any atypical or protracted DT courses, especially with withdrawal seizures or focal neurological signs, other CNS diseases must be considered.

Table 2. Differential diagnosis of delirium tremens

Wernicke-Korsakoff syndrome
Isolated hallucinosis
Schizophrenia
Drug or opioid withdrawal
Drug-induced delirium (dopa)
Intoxication with cholinesterase inhibitors
Bacterial or viral meningoencephalitis
Epilepsy
Confusion in cerebral atherosclerosis
Endocrine diseases (hyperthyroidism)
Hepatic encephalopathy

Therapy

General Treatment

DT is a medical emergency. A thorough physical examination, complete history from relatives and, if possible, from the patient is necessary. Additional laboratory tests including a CSF tap and CT scan are strictly recommended to rule out other diseases presenting with a delirious state. Patients with completed DT should be treated in an ICU, where appropriate monitoring and treatment are available. The comorbidity of alcoholics has to be considered, particularly pneumonia, pancreatitis, hepatitis, and trauma.

Most DT patients suffer from dehydration because of hyperhidrosis, hyperpyrexia, vomiting, and insufficient fluid intake during the days of abstinence before admission. Fluid supplementation is needed and should be continued for several days. Typical requirements are 3000–4000 ml/day. However, careful evaluation is important since some patients will be overhydrated and hyponatremic because of excessive ADH secretion; in these cases free water should be restricted to avoid development of cerebral edema. Regardless of serum magnesium concentration, the majority of alcoholics are magnesium deficient as the result of deficient intake, malabsorption, and excessive renal losses. The symptoms of DT resemble those of experimental magnesium deficiency. Enteral and parenteral feeding should contain supplemental magnesium, for example, 500–1000 mg intravenous magnesia aspartate or 2–4 g intravenous magnesium sulfate per day. Hypokalemia may occur in severe DT, and Korsakoff's syndrome may ensue. Intravenous replacement of potassium must not exceed 20 mEq/h. Profound hyperhidrosis can result in hyponatremia. Rapid correction or overcorrection can lead to the development of central pontine myelinolysis. Therefore, correction of hyponatremia should be done with a maximal increase of serum natrium of 0.6 mEq/h. Vitamin B_1 deficiency is found in about 50% of alcoholics. Because of the risk of Wernicke's encephalopathy, administration of 100 mg per day i.m. is indicated; vitamin B_1 must be given before administration of glucose. With clear signs of Wernicke's syndrome, larger doses of B_1, up to 1000 mg for the first day, are needed. More than 10% of alcoholics are vitamin B_6 deficient; therefore, B_6 and other vitamins should be supplemented. Alkalosis can occur because of hyperventilation or vomiting. Alternatively, acidosis may result from prolonged or repeated epileptic seizures, shock, or lactic acidosis. Acidosis or alkalosis should be diagnosed and treated carefully. Because they are often agitated, disoriented, and anxious, DT patients should be treated in quite, well-illuminated rooms.

Drug Therapy

More than 135 medications and drug combinations have been described for specific treatment of DT. The required properties of appropriate drugs include sedation without depression of protective reflexes, elevation of convulsive threshold, suppression of autonomic hyperactivity, and antipsychotic action. Currently, no single drug meets all these criteria.

Clomethiazole has cross-tolerance with ethanol and is the drug of choice in Europe and Australia. Clomethiazole causes sedation and autonomic stabilization, and it has an anxiolytic effect. It is an anticonvulsant, but it has only limited effect on psychotic symptoms. Oral therapy is accomplished with two 192-mg capsules 4–8 (to a maximum of 16) times a day and tapered as soon as the patient's condition permits (tablets with 500 mg are equivalent, but sometimes cause gastric bleeding). Intravenous therapy with a 0.8% solution is possible in severe cases and should be restricted to the ICU. After an initial bolus to establish sedation, continuous infusion is performed with a maximal daily dose of 2000 ml (16 g). As there is a risk of secondary dependence, clomethiazole should be administered only to inpatients and therapy should be terminated before the patient is discharged. Side effects of clomethiazole are hyperbronchorrhea, respiratory depression, tachycardia, and hypotonia, mainly occurring with insufficiently monitored i.v. use. When correctly administered and monitored, clomethiazole is an effective and safe drug. With oral therapy the risk of hyperbronchorrhea is minor; however, an alternative drug should be used for patients with severe pulmonary diseases. Sedation with clomethiazole, alcohol, and benzodiazepines is cumulative, and doses should be adjusted accordingly, especially in patients whose blood alcohol levels are still elevated.

Benzodiazepines are the most important drugs for controlling DT in the USA, as clomethiazole is not available there. Benzodiazepines are cross-tolerant to alcohol; they also carry the risk of secondary dependence. As with clomethiazole, cumulative sedation, the possibility of respiratory depression, and an increased risk of aspiration exist. There is no evidence to support the superiority of any one particular benzodiazepine. Since their sedative effect is limited by the saturation of GABA-benzodiazepine receptors, benzodiazepines may be somewhat safer than clomethiazole; however, they may be less effective for single-drug therapy. Generally, the long-acting benzodiazepines, chlordiazepoxide and diazepam, are preferable. Because of their long half-life, a single loading dose of 300 mg of chlordiazepoxide or 60 mg of diazepam may be given. As an alternative, chlordiazepoxide (25–50 mg 4–6 times a day) or diazepam (10 mg 4–6 times a day) can be administered for several days, with reduction of the dose by 20% daily according to the patient's condition. For intravenous use, doses of diazepam range up to 240 mg a day and of midazolam up to 20 mg an hour. Higher doses may be needed for heavy smokers.

Clonidine is an alpha-2 receptor agonist, effective in controlling sympathetic hyperactivity. In mild withdrawal syndrome, DT stage I, oral clonidine (0.2 mg 1–3 times a day) has a more favorable effect on hypertension and tachycardia than chlordiazepoxide. Yet clonidine PO seems to be less effective than oral clomethiazole. As it is neither anticonvulsive nor antipsychotic, nor sufficiently sedative, in completed DT clonidine should be combined with other substances. Up to 2.3 mg a day of i.v. clonidine (not yet available in USA) have been reported, but in most patients much lower doses will adequately control sympathetic hyperactivity. An initial dosage of 0.025 mg/h is recommended; that is equivalent to three 0.15-mg vials per day, to be titrated according to the patient's need.

Carbamazepine p.o. is as effective as oral benzodiazepines or oral clomethiazole in controlling agitation and seizures, but only in uncompleted DT, stage I (withdrawal syndrome). There is some advantage in using carbamazepine for alcohol withdrawal syndrome, since it is more effective than benzodiazepines in controlling psychotic symptoms. The recommended dose is 200 mg 4 times a day for the first two days, 3 times a day for 2 days, and 2 times a day for the last 2 days.

Single-drug therapy with barbiturates, beta blockers, or calcium-channel blockers is seldom effective. Paraldehyde or neuroleptics used alone can be dangerous.

Ethanol itself is effective in preventing DT or improving mild withdrawal symptoms. However, it is without effect once completed delirium has begun. Ethanol therapy, however, defeats the purpose of abstinence and permits the continuance of all the processes that finally culminate in severe delirium tremens.

Treatment Schedules

In impending DT (withdrawal syndrome), single-drug therapy with oral carbamazepine, clomethiazole, or a benzodiazepine is adequate (Table 3). In very mild withdrawal syndromes, medication is not even required if the patient is under competent staff care.

With completed DT (stage II) oral combined-drug therapy is usually necessary. The GABAergic substances clomethiazole, chlordiazepoxide, and diazepam are effective against agitation and seizures (category of signs of organic brain dysfunction) and against autonomic imbalance (the third category of signs), whereas their action on psychotic symptoms (the second category of signs) is limited. Neuroleptics, hazardous for single-drug therapy because of extrapyramidal effects and lowered epileptic threshold, are effective as part of a combined drug therapy in controlling psychotic manifestations. When used in combination with GABAergic substances, the side effects are of minor clinical importance. The recommended daily dose is haloperidol up to 60 mg.

In severe cases of DT (stage III), intravenous combined-drug therapy is indicated. A 0.8% solution of clomethiazole can be infused; alternatively, diazepam or midazolam, in combination with haloperidol or droperidol, can be used. This mode of therapy should be provided only in the ICU. Intravenous clomethiazole is not indicated for patients with pulmonary diseases or for patients who develop hyperbronchorrhea.

Autonomic hyperactivity can be treated with a beta blocker or with the alpha-2 agonist, clonidine. Up to 2.3 mg/day of clonidine have been reported, but a much lower dosage is sufficient for most patients. We recommend starting with 0.025 mg/h (equivalent to three 0.15-mg vials per day).

The prophylactic use of phenytoin in alcohol withdrawal is controversial. Despite the anticonvulsive properties of benzodiazepines and clomethiazole, a few patients will need additional anticonvulsive treatment with intravenous hydantoin or barbiturates because of seizures or status epilepticus

Table 3. Treatment schedules for delirium tremens (starting dosages)

Withdrawal syndrome, DT stage I

Carbamazepine	one 200-mg tablet, 4 times a day
or	
Clomethiazole	two 192-mg capsules 3–6 times a day
or	
Diazepam	single loading dose 60 mg (3 times 20 mg every 2 h) or 10-mg tablet, 4–6 times a day, reduction by 20% daily
or	
Chlordiazepoxide	single loading dose 300 mg (3 times 100 mg every 2 h) or 25 to 50-mg tablets 4–6 times a day, reduction by 20% daily

Completed DT, stage II; ICU treatment recommended

Clomethiazole and	two 192-mg capsules 6–8 (maximal 12) times a day
Haloperidol	i.v., possibly PO, 5–10 mg, 3–6 times a day
or	
Diazepam and	one 10-mg tablet, 6 times a day
Haloperidol	i.v., possibly PO, 5–10 mg, 3–6 times a day

Life-threatening DT, stage III; ICU treatment essential

Clomethiazole and	0.8% solution i.v., 20–80 ml/h, maximal dosage 2000 ml a day
Haloperidol	i.v., 10 mg, 6 times a day
or	
Diazepam and	i.v., 120–240 mg a day, continuously or as multiple boluses
Haloperidol	i.v., 10 mg, 6 times a day
or	
Diazepam and	i.v., 120–240 mg a day, continuously or as muliple boluses
Droperidol	i.v., up to 200 mg a day
or	
Midazolam and	up to 20 mg/h, to be titrated
Droperidol additionally	i.v., up to 200 mg a day
Clonidine	recommended initial dose 0.025 mg/h, to be titrated accodding to the sympathetic hyperactivity (oral administration not recommended in severe DT)

occurring after the very early phase of withdrawal syndrome or in completed DT.

Since information about medical treatment and doses for completed or life-threatening DT is sparse, the recommendations in Table 3 partly reflect our clinical practice and personal experience. Drug dosages needed for different individuals may differ widely. Therefore, strict recommendations cannot be given, and in every individual case the medication must be chosen and monitored thoroughly.

Table 4. Complications of delirium tremens

Pneumonia
Cardiac arrhythmia
Dehydration, circulatory shock
Hypertension
Hepatic coma
Renal insufficiency
Pancreatitis
Rhabdomyolysis
Multiple organ failure

Because co-morbidity is high in alcohol-dependent persons, complications are frequent in DT patients (Table 4). Cardiac or pulmonary complications are seen most often. Therapy is specific and symptomatic.

Prophylaxis of Delirium Tremens

Prophylactic treatment of a known alcoholic admitted to the hospital for a condition other than DT is in general not indicated. If the patient should show signs of alcohol withdrawal, carbamazepine is given in the dosage mentioned above. With early carbamazepine, the risk of developing an active delirium tremens is low.

Alcoholic patients suffering from head trauma, intracranial hematoma, and other CNS diseases like meningitis and encephalitis are difficult to monitor. Signs of the acute condition, of a developing delirium tremens, and the effects of a sedative treatment can not be discriminated exactly. Therefore, sedative drugs (benzodiazepines, clomethiazole) should be used cautiously; frequent clinical examinations are needed, as well as repeated additional investigations, including CT scans, EEG, and, in inflammatory diseases, spinal taps. Nevertheless, the treatment of delirium tremens compli-

cating acute CNS diseases essentially follows the same rules as the therapy of primary delirium.

Prognosis

Until the early 1960s, the mortality associated with DT ranged from 10% to 20%. With the introduction of clomethiazole in Germany, the mortality fell to 1.7%. In our own series of 103 patients treated in an ICU because of life-threatening stage-III DT, only two died. One of these patients had been admitted in unresponsive shock and the other developed pancreatitis and died of multiple organ failure.

Thus, the medical prognosis for patients with DT has greatly improved during the past two decades. However, in terms of recovery from alcoholism, the prognosis remains poor. Less than 20% of DT patients maintain abstinence. Amnesia regarding the DT period and lack of social support systems probably contribute to poorly motivated long-term rehabilitation.

Other Withdrawal Syndromes

CNS-Depressant Withdrawal

Barbiturates and benzodiazepines are the most commonly abused CNS depressants. Withdrawal closely resembles that of alcohol withdrawal and can be life threatening. Nutritional and electrolyte disturbances are less frequent complications of CNS-depressant withdrawal, and seizures are also less likely. Before the development of delirium, substitutive treatment with a long-acting cross-tolerant drug and supportive therapy followed by drug-tapering detoxification are indicated. Once delirium develops, the withdrawal syndrome can become life threatening, and combined-drug therapy in an ICU is necessary.

Opioid Withdrawal

Depending of the half-life of the particular opioid, withdrawal symptoms begin to occur as early as 8 h after stopping chronic use. Symptoms begin as anxiety, drug craving, sweating, and rhinorrhea. The symptoms progress through insomnia, abdominal cramps, and tremors to, at around 36 h, nausea, vomiting, hyperpyrexia, hypertension, tachycardia, and tachypnea. Opioid withdrawal does not include seizures or delirium and is seldom, if ever, life threatening. Treatment at any time during withdrawal with the substitution of a long-acting oral opioid is effective. Methadone is the treatment of choice. Due to its slow uptake and long half-life, drug highs and lows are minimized. If the abused drug dose is known, equivalency tables can be consulted. Methadone given as one third of the equivalent daily dose of the abused opioid is usually sufficient. Otherwise, 10 mg of methadone is given orally and the patient is evaluated 4 h later. The treatment is repeated at 4-h intervals until symptoms are controlled. Seldom is more than 40 mg of methadone per day required. When stabilization is established methadone can be tapered by 5 mg per day. Clonidine, an alpha-2 agonist, can be effective in suppressing the autonomic symptoms of withdrawal. However, clonidine may be less effective since it does not prevent the other symptoms of withdrawal.

Hallucinogens, Phencyclidine, and Marijuana Withdrawal

Both the minor and major hallucinogens, primarily because of their abuse pattern (i.e., intermittent rather than continual use), do not produce physical dependency. Withdrawal symptoms are psychological and do not require medical treatment. Although very heavy users of marijuana occasionally develop a mild physical withdrawal syndrome characterized by insomnia and gastrointestinal disturbances, medical treatment is not needed. Reassurance and supportive care are sufficient.

CNS-Stimulant Withdrawal

Cocaine and amphetamines constitute virtually all of the stimulant abuse. Both drugs enhance the central effects of dopamine and norepinephrine and are themselves peripheral sympathomimetics. Withdrawal does not entail medical or life-threatening consequences. Symptoms progress from craving, irritability, lassitude, nausea, and tremulousness to psychomotor retardation, depression, and, occasionally, suicidal ideation. Medical therapy is seldom required. If severe depression develops during withdrawal, drugs such as desiprimine and lithium have been advocated.

Summary

Of the various abused drugs, only alcohol and CNS depressants present potentially life-threatening problems in withdrawal that must be treated expertly and aggressively. With any withdrawal syndrome, the practitioner must be alert for symptoms of withdrawal of a second abused drug and/or of a concurrent medical illnesses. These can be very difficult and obscure diagnoses that can test any physician's expertise. Finally, treating the acute phase of withdrawal is only a small fraction of the job; far more important is setting the patient on the road to a lasting recovery.

Suggested Reading

Athen D (1986) Comparative investigation of clomethiazole and neuroleptic agents in the treatment of alcoholic delirium. Acta Psychiatr Scand 329 [Suppl]:167–170

Ballenger JC, Post RM (1978) Kindling as a model of alcohol withdrawal syndromes. Br J Psychiatry 133:1–14

Baumgärtner GR (1988) Clonidine vs. chlordiazepoxide in the management of acute alcohol withdrawal: a preliminary report. Southern Med J 81:56–60

Braun U (1991) Therapie des perioperativen Alkoholdelirs. Dtsch Med Wochenschr 116:501–503

Busch H, Frings A (1988) Pharmacotherapy of alcohol-withdrawal syndrome in hospitalized patients. Pharmacopsychiatry 21:232–237

Castaneda R, Cushman P (1989) Alcohol withdrawal: a review of clinical management. J Clin Psychiatry 50:278–284

Chick J (1989) Delirium tremens. Br Med J 298:3–4

Feuerlein W, Reiser E (1986) Parameters affecting the course and results of delirium tremens treatment. Acta Psychiatr Scand 329 [Suppl]:120–123

Hansbrough JF (1989) Massive doses of midazolam infusion in delirium tremens. Crit Care Med 17:597

Hemmingsen R, Kramp P (1988) Delirium tremens and related clinical states: psychopathology, cerebral pathophysiology, and psychochemistry: a two-component hypothesis concerning etiology and pathogenesis. Acta Psychiatr Scand 345:94–107

Jaffe JH, Martin WR (1985) Drug addiction and drug abuse. In: Godman C, Gilman A (eds) The pharmacological basis of therapeutics. McMillan, New York, pp 548–550

Pfitzer F, Schuchardt V, Heitmann R (1988) The treatment of severe alcoholic delirium. Nervenarzt 59:229–236

Ritola E, Malinen L (1981) A double-blind comparision of carbamazepine and clomethiazole in the treatment of alcohol withdrawal syndrome. Acta Psychiatr Scand 64:254–259

Robinson BJ, Robinson GM, Maling TJ, Johnson RH (1989) Is clonidine useful in the treatment of alcohol withdrawal? Alcoholism 13:95–98

Rommelspacher H, Schmidt LG, Helmchen H (1991) Pathobiochemistry and pharmacotherapy of alcohol withdrawal. Nervenarzt 62:649–657

Schied HW, Kimmerle K, Braunschweiger M (1986) A retrospective comparision of delirium tremens cases before and after the availability of clomethiazole. Acta Psychiatr Sand 73 [Suppl]:157–161

Schuchardt V (1988) Der Alkoholiker als Intensivpatient – Erfahrungen einer neurologischen Intensivstation. Intensivmedizin 25:55–62

Schuckit MA (1991) Alcohol and alcoholism. In: Braunwald E (ed) Harrison's principles of internal medicine. McGraw-Hill, New York, pp 2146–2151

Schuckit MA, Segal DS (1991) Opioid drug use. In: Braunwald E (ed) Harrison's principles of internal medicine. McGraw-Hill, New York, pp 2151–2154

Sellers EM, Naranjo CA (1986) New strategies for the treatment of alcohol withdrawal. Psychopharmacol Bull 22:88–92

Sullivan JT, Sykora CHB, Schneiderman J, Naranjo CA, Sellers EM (1989) Assessment of alcohol withdrawal: the revised Clinical Institute Withdrawal Assessment for Alcohol scale (CIWA-Ar). Br J Addict 84:1353–1357

Sutton T (1813) Tracts on delirium tremens, on peritonitis, and some other internal inflammatory affections and on the gout. Underwood, London

Victor M, Adams RD (1959) The effect of alcohol on the nervous system. Res Publ Assoc New Ment Dis 32:526–573

Chapter 78

Leigh's Disease (Subacute Necrotizing Encephalomyelopathy)

MATTHIAS SPRANGER

Introduction

Leigh's disease is a rare neurodegenerative disease caused by disorders of pyruvate metabolism. Most cases occur sporadically but autosomal recessive inheritance has been reported. Respiratory failure is the most important manifestation in patients requiring neurocritical care.

Etiology and Pathology

The exact cause of Leigh's disease is unknown, but some patients have decreased activity of pyruvate carboxylase and pyruvate dehydrogenase complex. Other patients have been shown to have cytochrome C oxidase deficiency and an inhibitor of thiamine pyrophosphate adenosine triphosphate (ATP) transferase. The lesions of Leigh's disease are similar to those of Wernicke's encephalopathy: symmetrical necrotic foci in the gray and

white matter of the brain stem, spinal cord, basal ganglia, and cerebellum. The mamillary bodies, however, are not involved. Microscopically, myelin and dendrites are more damaged than axons or neuronal cell bodies.

Clinical Features and Differential Diagnosis

The disease usually begins in infancy or childhood but can begin in adulthood. The clinical features vary depending on where the lesions are located and do not indicate the underlying biochemical abnormality. Infants may have failure to thrive and developmental retardation. Later, other signs may appear including nuclear and supranuclear oculomotor paralysis and other cranial nerve palsies, hypotonia, ataxia, hemiparesis or quadriparesis, myoclonic jerks, nystagmus, focal or generalized seizures, optic atrophy, and demyelinating peripheral neuropathy. Patients with lesions in the respiratory center of the medulla may present with clusters of irregular breathing alternating with apnea.

Section Editor: Michael N. Diringer

Rarely, patients may develop cirrhosis of the liver or cardiomyopathy.

Patients with Wernicke's encephalopathy have similar clinical features but usually have a history of malnutrition or chronic alcoholism. Mamillary body atrophy is frequently seen on magnetic resonance imaging (MRI) and microhemorrhages are seen microscopically. In infants and children, leukodystrophies and congenital lactic acidosis must also be excluded.

The course can be slow, rapidly progressive, or chronic relapsing, and cannot be predicted from the patient's symptoms, biochemical, or radiological findings. Infections and metabolic changes can trigger sudden deterioration.

Diagnosis

Laboratory Findings

Lactate and pyruvate concentrations are increased in the blood and cerebrospinal fluid (increased lactate: pyruvate ratio), especially after exercise or glucose administration.

Neuroimaging

On computed tomography (CT), patients have symmetrical, non-enhancing, low-density lesions in the basal ganglia and thalamus. MRI is more sensitive than CT and shows signs of edema and demyelination with low signal intensity on T1-weighted images and high intensity on T2-weighted images. Lesions in multiple sclerosis, Wilson's disease, amino aciduria, anoxia, and carbon monoxide poisoning may have a similar appearance. The increased lactate concentration can be visualized with MRI spectroscopy (Fig. 1a–c).

Other Studies

Patients may have generalized background slowing and spike waves on electroencephalography. Slowing of the nerve conduction velocity can occasionally be seen on electromyography. Activities of cytochrome oxidase C, pyruvate carboxylase, and pyruvate dehydrogenase complex can be measured in muscle, liver, and skin biopsies and in leukocytes. Occasionally, patients with Leigh's disease may have "ragged red fibers" on muscle biopsy, a finding that is more typical for other mitochondrial disorders such as Kearns-Sayre syndrome and myoclonus epilepsy and ragged red fibers (MERRF) syndrome. Demyelination may be seen on nerve biopsy.

Treatment and Prognosis

No treatment is curative. Patients may benefit, however, from a low-carbohydrate diet to reduce the production of pyruvate. High doses of thiamine (2 g/day orally), aspartate (0.5 g/day orally), and the coenzyme lipoic acid have been given in an attempt to activate the pyruvate dehydrogenous complex and decrease the accumulation of pyruvate. Symptomatic treatment includes anticonvulsants for patients with seizures and assisted ventilation for those with respiratory failure.

Almost 80% of patients die within 2 years of symptom onset, although

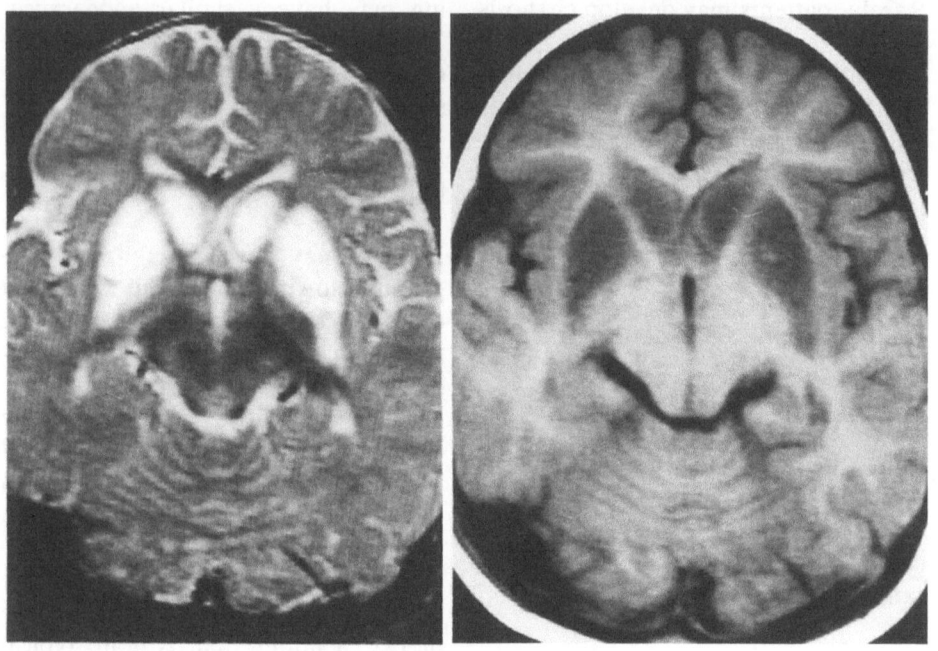

a

b

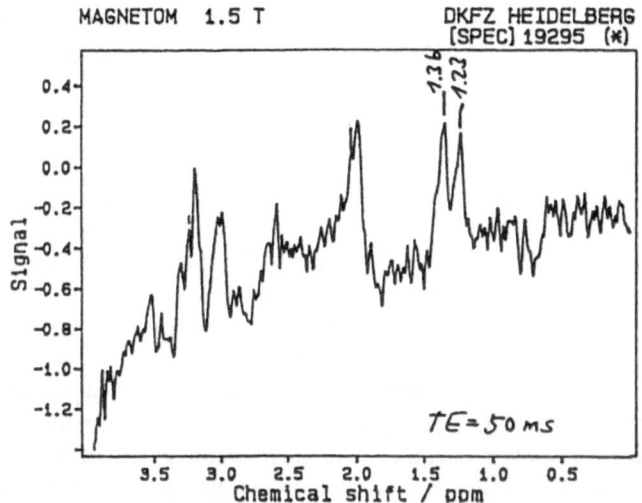

c

Fig. 1. Leigh disease (presumed) in a 15-month-old boy with psychomotor retardation. T2-weighted (a) and T1-weighted (b) MR images show bilateral, homogeneous, and almost perfectly symmetric signal abnormality in the caudate head and putamen. Both portions of the striatum appear slightly swollen, particularly evident in the caudate heads. Lesions are confined to gray matter. (Courtesy of Klaus Sartor and Marius Hartmann, Heidelberg). (c) Water suppressed ^{1}H magnetic resonance spectra (MRS) obtained from a patient with Leigh syndrome as diagnosed clinically and by MRI. Lactate levels (1.36 and 1.23 doublet peak), which are hardly detectable in normal brain, are markedly elevated in the patients MRS. The increase in lactate is consistent with a deficiency in oxidative substrate utilisation. (Courtesy German Cancer Research Institute)

some can live for more than 10 years. Respiratory failure is the most frequent overall cause of death. Genetic counseling should be provided to parents of children with Leigh's disease. Prenatal diagnosis may be possible for future pregnancies if the exact enzymatic defect is known.

Suggested Reading

Davis PC et al. (1990) MR of Leigh's disease (subacute necrotizing encephalomyelopathy). AJNR 8:71–75

Leigh D (1951) Subacute necrotizing encephalopathy in an infant. J Neurol Neurosurg Psychiatry 14:216–221

Taccone A et al. (1989) Leigh disease: value of CT in presymptomatic patients and variability of lesions with time. J Comput Assist Tomogr 13(2):207–210

Chapter 79

Reye's Syndrome*

ROBERT W. KATZ and LARRY E. DAVIS

Definition

Reye's syndrome is primarily a childhood disease and is defined by characteristic signs, symptoms, and laboratory tests. There is no specific diagnostic test. Most physicians in the United States use the criteria of the Centers for Disease Control in Atlanta, Georgia, criteria to diagnose Reye's syndrome: an acute, noninflammatory encephalopathy documented by the clinical picture of alterations in the level of consciousness and liver dysfunction. The cerebrospinal fluid (CSF) should contain no more than 8 leukocytes/mm^3. Histologic sections of the brain, when available, should demonstrate cerebral edema without perivascular or meningeal inflammation. The encephalopathy must be associated with either (1) fatty metamorphosis of the liver diagnosed by biopsy or autopsy or (2) a three-fold or greater increase in the levels of serum alanine aminotransferase (ALT), serum aspartate aminotransferase (AST), or arterial ammonia. There must be no other possible or reasonable explanation for the cerebral or hepatic abnormalities. As many of the children with this disease become comatose and require respirators, the quality of physician and nursing care in the intensive care unit plays a major role in the mortality and morbidity of this disease.

Epidemiology

Reye's syndrome occurs worldwide and has been strongly associated with the consumption of aspirin in individuals infected with influenza B, influenza A, and varicella-zoster viruses. In the United States, the illness reached its peak incidence from 1970 to 1980, occurring at a rate as high as 0.88 cases per 100 000 individuals under 18 years of age. Since 1980 the world incidence has decreased dramatically, possibly due to education programs resulting in a decrease in childhood aspirin consumption. Although Reye's syndrome occurs primarily in children between 5

* Supported by the Research Service, Department of Veterans Affairs.
Section Editor: Michael N. Diringer

and 14 years of age, cases have been recognized in adults and neonates.

Pathogenesis

The pathogenesis of Reye's syndrome remains unclear. Most children have a prodromal viral infection that is usually influenza or chicken pox. However, neither virus is usually isolated from the liver, brain, or CSF. Furthermore, the pathology does not suggest hepatitis or encephalitis. Some scientists feel that liver damage from a virus, aspirin, or unknown toxin produces the early vomiting and the encephalopathy. Elevated blood ammonia and free fatty acids have been considered as metabolic toxins capable of causing cerebral edema and coma. Other scientists have implicated mitochondrial abnormalities in liver and brain due to viruses or toxins as the cause. In liver biopsies, electron microscopy has demonstrated morphologic changes in mitochondria and biochemical studies have found the majority of enzymatic abnormalities to be mitochondrial enzymes. The role of salicylates in the pathogenesis is also unclear, but salicylates may further compromise mitochondrial function as they have been shown to uncouple mitochondrial respiration, impair ATP formation, and induce mitochondrial swelling.

Clinical Features

The clinical manifestations can be divided into a prodromal illness, the vomiting stage, and full Reye's syndrome. Up to 87% of patients experience an upper respiratory illness, commonly due to influenza B or A virus. Other children have a prodrome of chicken pox. In general the prodromal illness has no unusual characteristics or severity. Often the children have taken aspirin for the fever and aches. As the child is beginning to recover from the prodromal illness, the vomiting stage of Reye's syndrome begins (Fig. 1). Most individuals develop severe repetitive vomiting that lasts hours to several days and is difficult to control with antiemetic drugs. Fever may or may not be present. Jaundice is not seen and hepatomegaly is uncommon. However, liver function studies are abnormal. Occasional patients stop at this stage (stage 0) and never develop alterations of their mental status or have neurologic signs. Most, however, progress and experience neurologic signs and symptoms. In stage 1, the patient is lethargic, abnormally quiet, and irritable. The patient responds appropriately to verbal commands and may have a normal motor, sensory, and reflex examination.

In stage 2, the patients become agitated, restless, and disoriented. Children may not recognize family members and often are combative. Their speech may be dysarthric and not make sense. Yet, they can follow simple commands. The sympathetic nervous system may be overactive with sweating, tachycardia, tachypnea, and dilated pupils. Deep tendon reflexes are brisk and Babinski signs may be present. Generalized seizures may develop but are usually brief. This stage usually lasts several hours.

In stage 3, the child becomes comatose, which tends to follow a rostral-caudal pattern. To painful

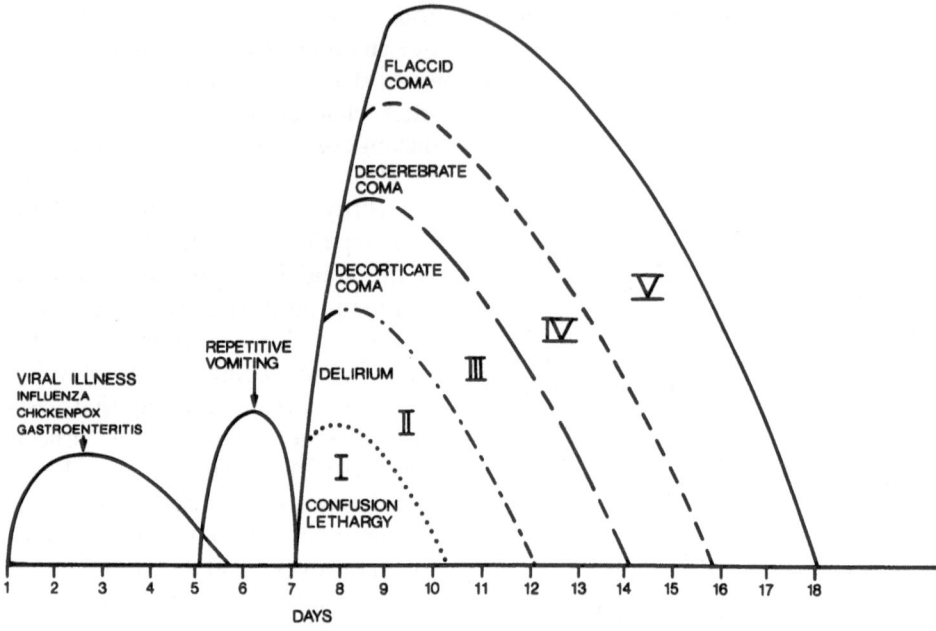

Fig. 1. Typical time course for patient with Reye's syndrome. Stages I–V of Reye's syndrome represent possible worsening of the disease. However, a given patient may stop at any stage

stimuli, the child may move limbs in a semi-purposeful manner or experience decorticate posturing. Deep tendon reflexes are hyperactive and Babinski signs are usually present. Lateralizing neurologic signs are uncommon. Seizures develop in 1/3 to 1/2 of patients. In stage 4, there is decerebrate posturing. Respirations become disorganized with the development of periodic breathing, ataxic breathing, or respiratory failure. Brainstem reflexes are abnormal. The pupils may be large, fixed, or demonstrate hippus. The oculo-vestibular reflex becomes sluggish or intermittently absent. The coma deepens in stage 5. The patient becomes flaccid with absent responses to painful stimuli and respirations cease. Deep tendon reflexes are depressed or absent. Brainstem reflexes

are very abnormal. Patients may stop progression at any stage or relentlessly progress to stage 5 over one to several days. Few patients who reach stage 5 survive.

Differential Diagnosis

Reye's syndrome should be suspected when a child experiences an upper respiratory illness or chicken pox followed by vomiting and marked alterations in mental status. The presence of elevated serum ALT or AST levels and arterial ammonia levels heightens the suspicion. Other diseases to consider fall into 3 types: general illnesses, genetic diseases, and intoxications. General illnesses include shock, hypoxic encephalopathy, ketotic hypo-glycemia, septicemia, encephalitis, acute hepatic failure, and acute pancreatitis. Genetic diseases include urea cycle enzyme defects such as orthine carbamoyltransferase deficiency, carbamoylphoephate synthetase deficiency, citrullinemia, argininosuccinic aciduria and arginase deficiency as well as several organic acidemias and abnormalities of carnitine metabolism. Intoxications include aflatoxin, endotoxin, salicylate, valproic acid, methyl bromide, camphor, pyrrolizidine, margoss oil, hypoglycin A, lead, chlordane, disulfiram, acetaminophen, and isopropyl alcohol.

No single laboratory test is diagnostic for Reye's syndrome but a liver biopsy is often very helpful. The biopsy should be considered in infants, children with recurrent encephalopathic spisodes, familial cases, sporadic patients without antecedent infection or vomiting and children with jaundice or elevated bilirubin levels. Part of the liver specimen should be frozen, cryostat sectioned and stained for the presence of fat by oil red O or Sudan black reagents. Other parts of the biopsy should be studied by light and electron microscopy and, in some patients, analyzed for enzyme abnormalities.

Ancillary Tests

Laboratory Tests and CSF Analysis

The majority of abnormal laboratory studies involve the liver and brain. Serum ALT and AST become elevated to 3–40 times above normal values. Serum bilirubin levels remain normal or only slightly elevated. Arterial ammonia levels become elevated to three or more times normal and may exceed $1000 \mu g/dl$. Arterial ammonia levels are usually highest early in the clinical course and later normalize. Arterial blood gases usually show a reduction in PCO_2, with normal oxygen saturation and pH unless respiratory failure is present. Blood lactic acid and organic acids are elevated. Hypoglycemia is present in 40% of children under 3 years of age. Insulin levels may be normal or slightly low. A generalized aminoacidemia is commonly present. Early in the clinical course, the CSF pressure may be normal or slightly elevated. As the coma deepens, the pressure elevates, often to extremely high levels. The CSF usually contains less than 8 white blood cells/mm^3 and has normal protein and glucose levels. Elevated CSF glutamine levels may be present.

Electrophysiological Tests

The electroencephalogram (EEG) is always abnormal but the changes are nonspecific. The EEG may show slowing of background activity, seizures, and a burst-suppression pattern. In stage 5, electrocerebral silence may develop. Triphasic EEG waves that have been associated with hepatic coma are rare.

Neuroimaging

The computed tomographic (CT) head scan may be normal early in the clinical course. Later, evidence of cerebral edema may be seen with low-density areas in the deep white matter, decreased gray-white matter contrast and ventricular compression. Magnetic resonance imaging (MRI) scans are similar and have shown diffuse cerebral edema.

Virology

Viral cultures taken from the respiratory tract, gastrointestinal tract, or skin vesicles have often grown viruses, especially influenza B, influenza A, and varicella-zoster viruses. However, specimens from blood, CSF, liver, or brain have almost never grown viruses, bacteria, or fungi.

Management

The management of children with Reye's syndrome ranges from basic interventions such as supplying glucose to those with stage I findings to complex management in an intensive care unit.

Children who are in stage I require close neurologic monitoring, frequent determinations of glucose concentrations, and daily measurements of ammonia, liver enzymes, and electrolytes. Glucose given as 10%–15% in maintenance amounts should prevent hypoglycemia.

Presentation in or progression to stage II or worse mandates admission to an intensive care unit. Controversy exists in regards to the role of aggressive neurointensive therapy for patients entering stage II. At the minimum they should be in an intensive care unit, have arterial lines and good venous access in place, and be very closely monitored. Any deterioration

beyond stage II requires aggressive therapy to reduce intracranial pressure and levels of ammonia. The essentials of neurointensive care are outlined below.

Intracranial Pressure Management
(see Chaps. 8, 9)

There are numerous methods for monitoring intracranial pressure. Although intraventricular catheters are probably the most reliable, decisions on monitoring type are largely determined by institutional experience. The main goals of controlling intracranial pressure are (a) maintenance of adequate cerebral perfusion and (b) prevention of cerebral herniation. Clinically, the goal is to maintain the cerebral perfusion pressure above the lower limit of autoregulation or approximately 50 mmHg. Prevention of cerebral herniation involves therapy to reduce the amount of cerebral edema; a variety of approaches are used in the intensive care setting (Chap. 9).

Reduction of Ammonia Concentrations

The elevation of ammonia concentrations is an almost universal finding in Reye's syndrome. The preponderance of evidence is that the elevated levels of ammonia are related to the pathophysiology of the encephalopathy of Reye's syndrome. A variety of therapeutic approaches have been used to reduce the ammonia, including peritoneal dialysis, exchange transfusion, total body washout, and charcoal hemoperfusion. None of these measures have been shown to be consistently effective, nor is there any evidence that the outcome of the disease has been altered by these interventions.

General Intensive Care Measures

The aggressive neurointensive care that is required in children in Reye's syndrome involves the whole spectrum of pediatric critical care medicine that is beyond the scope of this chapter. The reader is referred to several available texts on pediatric intensive care (see Suggested Reading).

Prognosis

With the advent of patient treatment in intensive care units, mortality in Reye's syndrome has fallen but is still about 30%. Factors that suggest a poor outcome include young age, rapid progression of stages, development of stage 5, and arterial ammonia levels above 300 μg/dl on admission. Patients who survive may occasionally be left with marked neurologic sequelae including hemiparesis, quadriparesis, dysarthria, cortical blindness, and epilepsy. Some children who survive are left with subtle deficits that include psychomotor retardation and visual-motor integration difficulties.

Suggested Reading

Brown RE, Forman DT (1982) The biochemistry of Reye's syndrome. Crit Rev Clin Lab Sci 17:247–297

Davis LE (1989) Reye's syndrome. In: Viral Disease, McKendall RR (ed) Handbook of clinical neurology, vol.12(56). Elsevier Science, New York, pp. 149–177.

DeVivo DC (1985) Reye syndrome. Neurol Clin 3:95–115

Jeubi JE, Partin JC, Partin JS, Schubert WK (1987) Reye's syndrome: current concepts. Hepatology 7:155–164

Hurwitz ES, Barret MJ, Bregman D, Gunn WJ, Pinsky P, Schonberger LB, Drage JS, Kaslow RA, Burlington D, Quinnan GV, LaMontagne JR, Fairweather WR, Dayton D, Dowdle WR (1987) Public Health Service study of Reye's syndrome and medications. Report of the main study. J Am Med Assoc 257:1905–1911

Mickell JJ, Cook DR, Reigel DH, Painter MJ, Safar P (1976) Intracranial pressure monitoring in Reye-Johnson syndrome. Crit Care Med 22:175–229

Pranzatelli MR, DeVivo DC (1987) Pharmacology of Reye syndrome. Clin Neuropharmacol 10:96–125

Rogers MC (ed) (1992) Textbook of pediatric intensive care. Williams and Wilkins, Baltimore.

Shaywitz BA, Rothstein P, Venes JL (1980) Monitoring and management of increased intracranial pressure in Reye syndrome: results of 29 children. Pediatrics 66:198–204

Shaywitz BA, Lister G, Duncan CC (1986) What is the best treatment for Reye's syndrome? Arch Neurol 43:730–731

| # Central Pontine Myelinolysis

HANS-WALTER PFISTER

Definition

Central pontine myelinolysis (CPM) is a rare disorder characterized by symmetrical demylinating lesions in the central pons with relative sparing of neuronal cell bodies and axons. Additional lesions occur in about 10% of patients, usually in the basal ganglia, thalamus, internal capsule, cerebellum, and spinal cord. CPM can occur at any age and primarily occurs in patients with chronic alcoholism and malnutrition. Patients with severe CPM may develop "locked in syndrome" and may require neurocritical care.

Pathogenesis

The exact cause of CPM is unknown. The results of experimental and clinical studies suggest that rapid correction of hyponatremia plays a major role (that is, greater than 25 mmol/l during the first 24–48 h). In animal studies, intravenous infusion of hypertonic saline to correct chronic hyponatremia results

---

Section Editor: Michael N. Diringer

in demyelinating lesions of the CNS. Hyponatremia without correction or hyponatremia that is slowly corrected does not cause demyelination. It has been speculated, that hypertonic saline causes osmotic endothelial damage, vasogenic edema, and the release of myelinotoxic factors (thus the term "osmotic demyelination syndrome").

Clinical Features

CPM is usually diagnosed in patients with chronic alcoholism and delirium tremens (60%–80% of patients). The reason for this association is unknown. CPM can also occur in patients such as those with syndrome of inadequate secretion of antidiuretic hormone (SIADH), adrenal insufficiency, liver disease, malnutrion, or Wilson's disease. In 30% of patients, CPM is associated with Wernicke's encephalopathy and it is occasionally seen in patients with Marchiafava-Bignami disease. Patients with CPM may have a variety of signs including oculomotor dysfunction, abducens and facial nerve palsies, latent signs of pyramidal tract lesions, quadriparesis, and being in

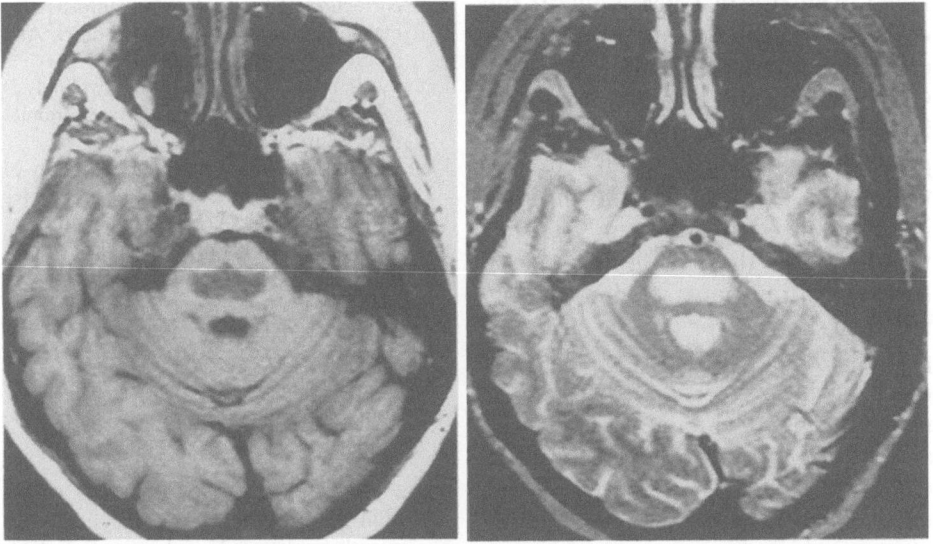

a

b

Fig. 1a,b. Central pontine myelinolysis in a 41-year-old alcoholic woman with spastic paraparesis. MR scans show symmetric, batwing-like signal abnormality involving central portion of pons. Lesion appears homogeneous and sharply marginated and has no mass effect. On T1-weighted image (**a**) it is hypointense compared with normal white matter (but brighter than CSF), while on T2-weighted image (**b**) it is hyperintense. (Courtesy of Klaus Sartor and Marius Hartmann, Heidelberg)

locked-in syndrome. CPM should be suspected when an alcoholic patient with hyponatremia subacutely develops a pontine syndrome. The differential diagnosis includes multiple sclerosis, Binswanger's disease, progressive multifocal leukoencephalopathy, and basilar artery thrombosis.

Ancillary Tests

Magnetic resonance imaging (MRI) is more sensitive than computed tomography (CT) and can confirm the diagnosis of CPM. Patients usually have symmetrical, often bat-wing-shaped, partly confluent lesions in the center of the pons. These lesions are not space-occupying or contrast-enhancing (Fig. 1). Patients may also have abnormal

auditory and somatosensory evoked potentials. In patients recovering from CPM, evoked potentials may return to normal earlier than the pontine lesions seen on CT or MRI. CSF cell count and protein concentration are usually normal. Oligoclonal bands are not seen, although myelin basic protein levels may be increased.

Treatment and Prognosis

Hyponatremia can cause altered consciousness, myoclonic jerks, and seizures, and needs to be treated when present. In patients with severe hyponatremia (<110 mmol/l), especially those with chronic alcoholism, hyponatremia should be corrected slowly (not more than 0.5–2 mmol/l per hour). The risk of CPM is low if the daily increase in serum sodium concentration is less than 12 mmol/l. Once CPM has occurred, however, treatment is mainly supportive (for example, prophylaxis against deep venous thrombosis, pneumonia, and decubiti in immobilized patients and assisted ventilation in those with respiratory failure). Intravenous vitamin B_1 has not been shown to be beneficial. In the past, CPM was primarily a diagnosis made at autopsy. Today, because of better imaging techniques, such as CT and MRI, it is possible to diagnose CPM during life. Patients with mild CPM, diagnosed early, may have complete or partial recovery.

Suggested Reading

Adams RD, Victor M, Mancall EL (1959) Central pontine myelinolysis: a hitherto undescribed disease occurring in alcoholic and malnourished patients. Arch Neurol Psychiatr 81:154–172

Brunner JE, Redmond JM, Haggar AM, Kruger DF, Elias SB (1990) Central pontine myelinolysis and pontine lesions after rapid correction of hyponatremia: a prospective magnetic resonance imaging study. Ann Neurol 27:61–66

Laureno R (1983) Central pontine myelinolysis following rapid correction of hyponatremia. Ann Neurol 13:232–242

Lien YHH, Shapiro JI, Chan L (1991) Study of brain electrolytes and organic osmolytes during correction of chronic hyponatremia. Implications for the pathogenesis of central pontine myelinolysis. J Clin Invest 88: 303–309

Narins RG (1986) Therapy of hyponatremia. N Engl J Med 314:1573–1575

Norenberg MD, Papendick RE (1984) Chronicity of hyponatremia as a factor in experimental myelinolysis. Ann Neurol 15:544–547

Pfister HW, Einhäupl KM, Brandt T (1985) Mild central pontine myelinolysis: a frequently undetected syndrome. Eur Arch Psychiatr Neurol Sci 235:134–139

Sterns RH, Riggs JE, Schochet SS (1986) Osmotic demyelination syndrome following correction of hyponatremia. New Engl J Med 314:1535–1542

Stockard JJ, Rossiter VS, Wiederholt WC, Kobayashi RM (1976) Brainstem auditory-evoked responses in suspected central pontine myelinolysis. Arch Neurol 33: 726–728

Tien R, Arieff AI, Kucharczyk W, Wasik A, Kucharczyk J (1992) Hyponatremic encephalopathy: is central pontine myelinolysis a component? Am J Med 92:513–522

Chapter 81

Acute Obstructive Hydrocephalus

MARKUS S. VON HAKEN and ALFRED A. ASCHOFF

Introduction and History

In 1842, Magendie studied the anatomy of the meninges in the posterior fossa and spinal cord and postulated occlusion as a possible cause of hydrocephalus. Further work by Key and Retzius, published in their classic article in 1875, supported this concept. In 1881, Wernicke first described puncture of the ventricles (VP). After refinement of the surgical technique using specially designed atraumatic puncture needles, VP became a relatively safe and common procedure. For half a century, ventriculography with air or positive contrast media was the diagnostic method of choice to document ventricular enlargement and occlusive lesions. As a form of therapy, VP remained limited to emergencies, because its effects were only temporary and repeated puncture was associated with increased complications.

It was not until the 1930s that external ventricular drainage (EVD), especially after posterior fossa surgery, was developed. In 1949, the addition of a functional valve was made by Nulsen and Spitz, and drainage systems using such valves became commercially available in 1956. In the 1970s, ventriculoperitoneal or ventriculoatrial shunts became the standard treatment of hydrocephalus, replacing VP. Variations of EVD, such as continuous spinal drainage with indwelling catheters, finally led to the development of implanted subcutaneous reservoirs, which allows an intermittent on-demand drainage of ventricles or cystic lesions.

The clinical symptoms and signs of acute obstructive hydrocephalus include positional headache, vomiting, drowsiness, personality changes, and decreasing levels of consciousness. Some patients develop acute coma, oculomotor nerve paresis, and papilledema. Additional neurological symptoms depend on the underlying disease and may be variable.

Section Editor: Michael N. Diringer

Physiology of CSF Circulation

Secretion of CSF

Normally, 80–90% of the cerebrospinal fluid (CSF) is produced by the choroid plexus. Nonchoroidal sources of CSF include the cerebral parenchyma, the endothelial cells of the capillary vessels in the extracellular spaces, and ependyma. CSF production starts with an intracellular ultrafiltrate to which Na^+ and Cl^- are added by active transport via a membrane-bound Na^+-K^+ ATPase. Water passively follows the osmotic gradient. The average CSF production rate is 0.35–0.37 ml/min, or about 20 ml/h.

CSF production correlates with the volume of the brain, so that newborns (average brain weight 350 g) have one fifth the CSF production rate of adults. After 7 months, children have 50% the CSF production rate and after 4 years, 90% of the production rate. Therefore, CSF production reaches adult values early. The rate of CSF flow is relatively constant in all mammals (0.5%/min), so that CSF is exchanged at least four times daily.

CSF production depends to a certain extent on the perfusion pressure. It decreases with rising intracranial pressure (ICP) or with arterial hypotension. CSF secretion stops only at extreme values of ICP or hypotension. CSF production is decreased by serum hyperosmolarity, sympathetic stimulation, and ventriculitis. An increase in CSF secretion of up to 30% has been described after denervation of the sympathetic fibers and an increase of up to 100% can be attained by stimulation of cholinergic fibers and administration of cholera toxin. The latter effect is probably mediated by cyclic AMP.

Absorption of CSF

CSF flows through the foramen of Monro and the aqueduct and then exits from the fourth ventricle to the subarachnoid space, where it is absorbed by the arachnoid villi. To a smaller extent, CSF is also absorbed in the spinal nerve sheaths. In addition, there is a linear passive transport mechanism when the CSF pressure exceeds venous pressure by 2–8 cm H_2O.

Other ways that CSF is absorbed include via (a) the lymphatic system, (b) the cerebral parenchyma, (c) the choroid plexus, and (d) third spaces along cranial and spinal nerves and the central spinal canal. Lymphatic absorption plays the most important role. About 10–30% of CSF can be detected in lymph nodes of the neck when CSF is radioactively labeled. Clinically, swelling of the nasal mucosa is occasionally observed in patients with hydrocephalus. The choroid plexus has a relatively large absorption surface area and absorbs up to 10% of CSF.

Pathophysiology of CSF Circulation

Obstructive Cerebral Lesions and Risk for Hydrocephalus

Nearly all intracranial tumors and many of the developmental malformations, infections, postinflammatory processes, and vascular malformations can lead to hydrocephalus from *ob-*

struction of CSF pathways. The closer the lesions are to an anatomical isthmus (for example, the foramen of Monro, the aqueduct of Sylvius, and the fourth ventricle), the higher the risk of obstruction. Cysts near the foramen of Monro, tumors in the pineal region, and Dandy-Walker malformation are associated with a 90% or higher risk of hydrocephalus. *Communicating hydrocephalus* is caused by failure of resorption or by increased venous pressure in the sinuses.

Hypersecretory hydrocephalus is rare and occurs only in patients with plexus papilloma (and only in three fourths of these patients).

Many patients have *combined* causes for hydrocephalus. It is a common experience, that even after gross total resection of cerebellar tumors and thereby removal of the CSF pathway occlusion, approximately 20% of all patients still require shunting procedures. Possible reasons for this include intraoperative bleeding, high CSF protein, aseptic meningitis, or subclinical infections. Communicating hydrocephalus is the most common mechanism in these patients.

Although hydrocephalus following subarachnoid hemorrhage or spontaneous intracerebral hemorrhage accompanied by ventricular hemorrhage is often included under communicating hydrocephalus, partial or complete blockade of internal ventricular spaces can occur in addition to malabsorption. This can be demonstrated by measuring lumbar and ventricular pressures.

Dynamics of Acute Obstructive Hydrocephalus

As early as 1–2 h after cerebellar hemorrhage, a CT scan may show an obstructive hydrocephalus. The volume of the retained CSF then equals the production rate (20–40 ml/h). Often, the progression of hydrocephalus is much slower and depends on the development and the extent of the CSF pathway obstruction. The progression can be very slow, especially in patients with tumors of the cerebellopontine angle. In those with congenital stenosis of the aqueduct, the condition may be masked for decades until trauma or diagnostic lumbar puncture leads to symptomatic hydrocephalus. Colloid cysts near the foramen of Monro also may show rapid decompensation after a long asymptomatic interval. On the other hand, tumors located near the fourth ventricle can produce rapid decompensation within minutes, with an increase of hydrocephalic pressure and herniation of the cerebellar tonsils.

Treatment

Acute obstructive hydrocephalus is fully reversible if treated early. The longer the hydrocephalus and the increased ICP last, the more severe the resulting brain damage may be.

Medical

Occlusive hydrocephalus can be treated medically by decreasing the CSF production rate, reducing the size of the occlusion, reducing the perifocal edema of the lesion, by decreasing the ICP, and by using antimicrobial chemotherapy when indicated. The effects of medical treatment, however, are usually minor or of short duration and surgical intervention should follow immediately if possible.

Decreasing the CSF Production Rate. The production rate of CSF can be decreased by 20–50% by inhibiting the Na^+-K^+ ATPase within the choroid plexus cell with carboanhydrase inhibitors such as acetazolamide (Diamox). Higher doses or combination therapy do not further enhance this effect. Furosemide diuretics and corticosteroids also decrease CSF secretion to some extent.

Reducing the Size of the Occlusion. Medical debulking of occluding lesions is possible using corticosteroids (for example, in patients with intracerebral lymphomas). The use of bromocriptine in those with macroprolactinomas can result in an up to 50% reduction of tumor size in about 40% of patients within 3 weeks of treatment. Usually, these effects are too slow to prevent increases in ICP.

Reducing the Perifocal Edema of the Lesion and Decreasing the ICP. Treatment with dexamethasone and osmotic agents can relieve obstruction by decreasing brain swelling and perifocal edema in tumors. Most patients, especially those with cerebellar tumors, improve dramatically within 12–24 h. In many of them, hydrocephalus-related symptoms disappear.

Using Antimicrobial Chemotherapy when Indicated. Brain abscesses, empyemas, and cysts of parasitic origin can produce occlusion. Tuberculous meningitis often leads to postinflammatory adhesion at the level of the fourth ventricle. Antimicrobial chemotherapy therefore remains as important as drainage procedures and can decrease the size of an occluding lesion.

Radiotherapy

Germinomas of the pineal region or suprasellar ectopic germ cell tumors respond well to radiotherapy. Treatment with 10–20 Gy to the tumor often results in a significant shrinkage of the tumor volume. Intracavitary radiotherapy using stereotactically applied β-radiation (for example, 90 yttrium) can be used for occluding cysts of craniopharyngiomas. Recurrence of these cysts can be effectively inhibited by this method.

Surgical Intervention

The treatment of acute obstructive hydrocephalus should ideally be focused on the occluding lesion. The removal of the tumor, vascular malformation, hemorrhage, or cyst can avoid unnecessary shunting procedures for the patients.

EVD is the most important surgical method of treatment of urgent obstructive hydrocephalus caused by space-occupying lesions in the posterior fossa, such as hematomas, infarctions, or tumors. EVD is also widely used for all types of temporary hydrocephalus or when CSF cannot be drained immediately by an internal shunt (for example, after a subarachnoid hemorrhage, intraventricular hemorrhage, or ventriculitis). A common practice is to drain CSF and, after closure of the drainage, to measure the ICP and evaluate shunt dependency. If shunt dependency is proven, the CSF should be drained to low-pressure compartments or, in selected cases, an intrathecal bypass procedure should be performed. EVD also offers the possibility of measuring ICP, of collecting ventricular CSF, and of giving drugs intrathecally such as antibiotics, cytotoxic drugs, and fibrinolytic agents.

VP remains the basic therapy for occlusive hydrocephalus and is an essential part of every EVD and shunting procedure. This approach also remains the standard for stereotactic and endoscopic procedures. Today, the frontal or occipital site is preferred for puncture of lateral ventricles. The frontal approach has the advantage of landmarks that can be used for the burr hole (20–25 mm paramedian and 1–2 cm anterior to the coronal suture in adults) and the direction of the puncture. The average distances from brain surface to ependyma (40 mm) and to the foramen of Monro (60 mm) are relatively constant in adults. Recommendations for occipital burr holes vary significantly. The accuracy of the puncture can be improved by ultrasonography, intraoperative X-ray films, or the stereotactic approach.

Complications
of External Ventricular Drainage

Infection

Infection is a major complication of EVD. CSF leakage along the catheter may lead to potential catheter obstruction and increases the risk of infection from 5% to as high as 26%. An analysis of the data from 5037 EVD systems showed that 5.2% ($n = 263$) led to ventriculitis [8 deaths (0.2% of patients) occurred as a result of EVD system-related ventriculitis]. In patients with sanguineous CSF, signs of meningeal irritation, fever, CSF pleocytosis, and leukocytosis may occur without clinical evidence of ventriculitis. These signs are nonspecific. Positive bacterial cultures can often be obtained from EVD stopcocks and ports and can represent artificial contamination. Negative bacterial cultures can occur in patients who receive prophylactic antibiotics despite having a ventriculitis.

Infection rates in the literature vary from 0% to 50%. Careful handling of the EVD system significantly decreases the rate of infection. The risk of infection increases significantly with duration of the EVD and with the presence of sanguineous CSF. Other factors that increase the risk of infection include irrigation of the EVD system, multiple operations, increased ICP, treatment with corticosteroids, and patient age. Prospective double-blind studies of prophylactic antibiotics have not shown statistically significant differences in the infection rate.

Mechanical Complications

An EVD system consists of a silicone catheter, a stopcock, an adjustable drip chamber, a ventilation system, and a collection bag. Although not essential, sideports, three-way stopcocks, antireflux valves, and integrated pressure transducers are often helpful. The commercially available EVD systems are prone to a low bearing capacity due to construction faults. A break within an EVD system causes a sig-

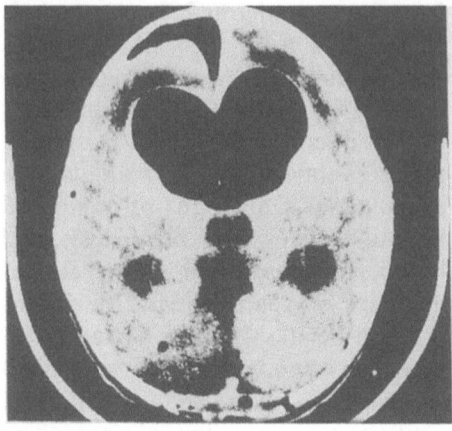

Fig. 1. Pneumatocephalus caused by overdrainage. This complication was recognized on the postoperative CT scan of a child with a pilocytic astrocytoma in the region of the collicular plate. The external ventricular drainage is not visualized on this scan, as the catheter tip is in the posterior occipital horn of the lateral ventricle

nificant loss of CSF and can lead to infection and tension pneumatocephalus (see Fig. 1). Usually, the required ICP limits are regulated by positioning the drip chamber higher or lower than the ventricles. If the drip chamber drops, an acute overdrainage may occur with life-threatening consequences. It is essential for the manufacturer to offer reliable adjustment systems. Draining bloody CSF in commercially available EVD systems must be done cautiously because the systems consist of too many stenoses (connectors, stopcocks) with an inner diameter less than 1.5 mm. Because there can be an accumulation of gas in the CSF collection bag, air ventilation is required. In the available systems, these ventilation filters are either missing or too small. Contact with saline results in occlusion of most (and with CSF nearly all) of the antimicrobial filter caps. Only four of 11 EVD sys-

tem valves tested at our institution showed sufficient, reliable properties. When the systems are in use for longer periods, the valve resistance can increase significantly. Therefore, we propose that the ICP and the hourly collected CSF be monitored simultaneously.

Complications of Surgery

About 10% of ventricular catheters are falsely placed. Using the frontal approach, penetration of the basal ganglia or the floor of the third ventricle can occur (see Fig. 2). Occasionally, the catheter is positioned in the mesencephalon or hypothalamus and, rarely, in the sylvian fissure. Using trigonal approaches, there is a risk for hemiparesis and aphasia. Occipital catheters may lead to impairment of visual fields and also have a risk for false placement in the thalamus or transverse fissure. Ventricular catheters in the posterior fossa are problematic because the orientation is difficult and a shift of the brain stem occurs secondary to collapse of the enlarged fourth ventricle. Lesions of the brain stem and fatal complications have been reported. Acute perioperative hemorrhages in the epidural, subdural, intracerebral (see Fig. 3), or ventricular spaces are dangerous complications of the procedure. In one large series, the incidence of perioperative hemorrhage was less than 1%. In neonates, the brain is especially vulnerable and the frequency of hemorrhage rises to 2.5%. In the treatment of acute hydrocephalus, the rapid relief of intraventricular pressure and the negative ventricular pressures in the upright position can cause life-threatening complications

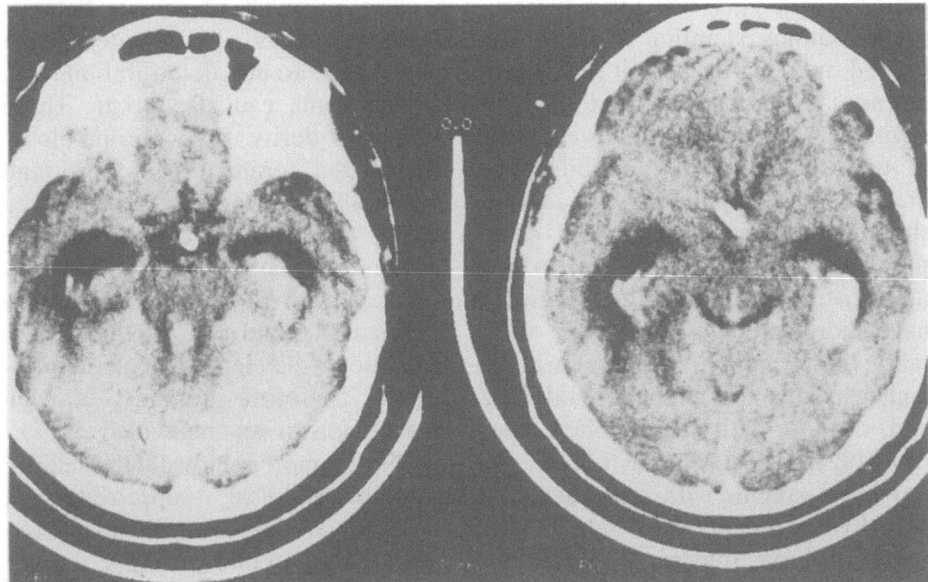

Fig. 2. External ventricular drainage was inserted following posthemorragic hydrocephalus. The ventricular catheter penetrated the floor of the third ventricle and the catheter tip came to lie in the prepontine cistern. No clinical symptomatology

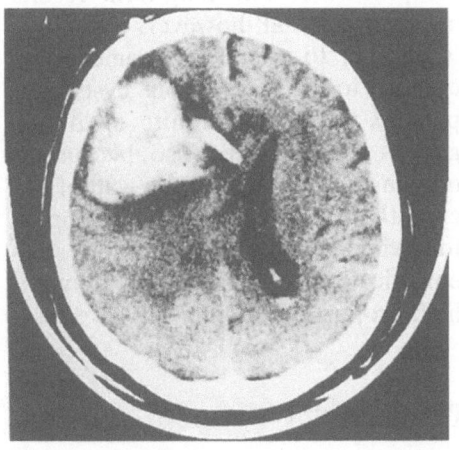

Fig. 3. Complicating intracerebral hemorrhage following intraoperatively uneventful ventricular puncture

including hemorrhage, tumor hemorrhage, rerupture of a nonclipped aneurysm, and transtentorial upward herniation.

Other Shunting Procedures

Intrathecal shunting procedures, including ventriculocisternostomy, recanalization of the cerebral aqueduct, and third ventriculostomy, as well as coagulation of the choroid plexus or extrathecal shunting procedures are not recommended for the emergency treatment of hydrocephalus and should be used only in selected, clinically stable patients.

Specific Problems in Selected Types of Obstructive Hydrocephalus

Posterior fossa Tumors

The introduction of corticosteroids significantly improved the outcome of patients with posterior fossa tumors. Precraniotomy shunting has also improved outcome because it provides a better preoperative condition. The risks of overdrainage, however, such as upward herniation and bleeding, are increased in patients who receive shunting. Patients with these complications should be managed in the neurocritical care unit. These patients have more infections, a higher mortality, more operative procedures, a higher incidence of shunt dependency, and, in those with medulloblastomas, probably more extraneural metastases. For most patients with acute obstructive hydrocephalus associated with posterior fossa tumors, preoperative corticosteroid and osmotherapy is sufficient as a first step. If there is no improvement after medical treatment or if the patient is at risk for postoperative cerebellar swelling, then we recommend an EVD perioperatively. A temporary EVD should be used (see Fig. 4), since most patients do not need a permanent shunt. This is also advantageous, as ICP can be measured intraoperatively and postoperatively and may be controlled by draining CSF. In addition, shunt dependency can be accurately evaluated. Precraniotomy shunts in patients with posterior fossa tumors are limited to selected cases where only partial resection or palliative surgery is planned. Shunts are inevitable when shunt dependency is proven postoperatively by increased ICP after the closure of the EVD system.

Colloid Cysts of the Foramen of Monro

Colloid cysts near the foramen of Monro are associated with hydroce-phalus in over 90% of patients. Patients characteristically have intermittent headaches. Acute deterioration with sudden coma can also occur. These symptoms derive from abrupt blockage of the foramen of Monro and eventually result in sudden death (see Fig. 5). The risk of acute obstruction of the foramen of Monro does not correlate with the size of the lesion. Even small colloid cysts less than 10 mm in diameter may lead to acute deterioration. Therefore, removal of even small lesions is recommended.

For tumor removal, the classic microneurosurgical approach is transcortical or interhemispheric-transcallosal. In most patients, a shunt can be avoided. There is a risk of hemiparesis and limbic lesions by trauma to the fornix. Stereotactic aspiration of cysts is associated with fewer complications. The long-term results are controversial, however, because it is difficult to completely remove the cysts or to aspirate viscous cysts, and patients frequently require open surgery as a second step. Also, because of ongoing secretion from the wall of the cyst, there is some risk of recurrence following aspiration. In addition, stereotactically treated patients have a high proportion of shunts.

Pineal Region Tumors

About nine of ten tumors of the pineal region produce hydrocephalus. Histologically, 75% are classified as germinomas. The rest are teratomas, pinealoblastomas, and others. Germinomas are extremly sensitive to radiotherapy and curative radiation is possible in most cases. Diagnosis is made by cytology, specific tumor

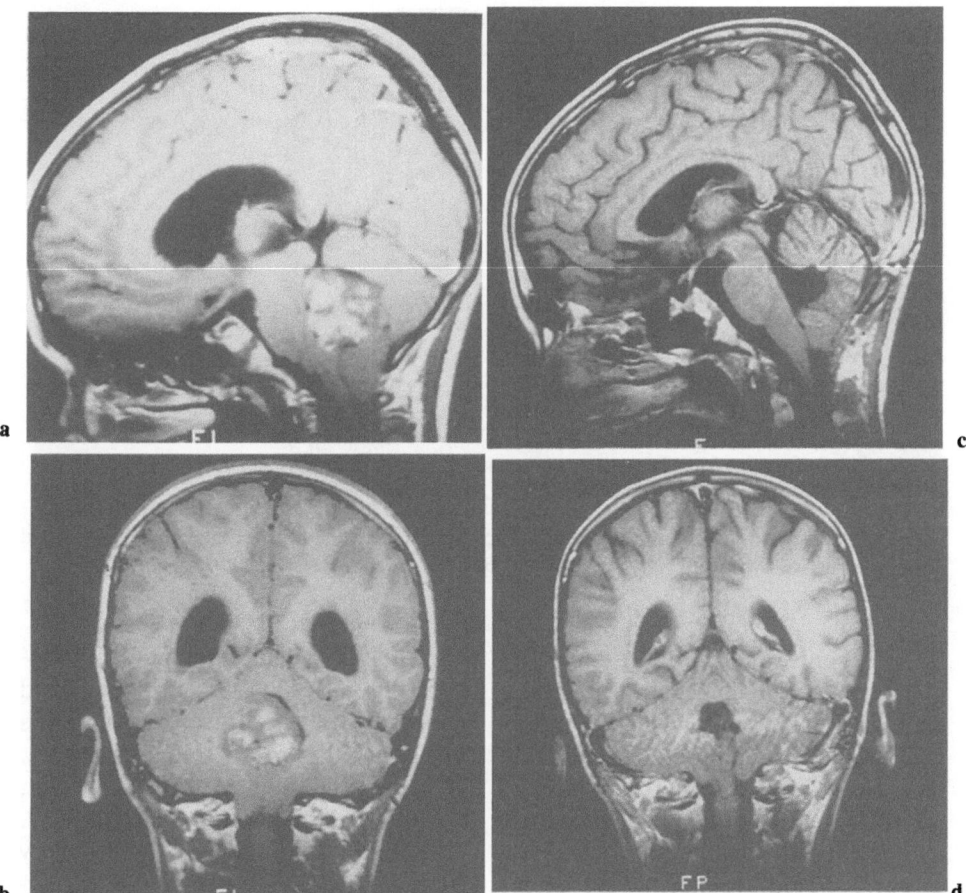

Fig. 4a–d. Medulloblastoma in a 10-year-old boy. Pre- (a,b) and postoperative (c,d) MRI scans demonstrate the clinically symptomatic, obstructive hydrocephalus prior to surgery. The gross total tumor removal and retrogression of hydrocephalus is visualized 3 months postoperatively. No shunt was necessary after removal of obstructing lesion and of the perioperative inserted EVD

markers (AFP, HCG), or stereotactic biopsy. As germinomas tend to shrink after treatment with 10 Gy, radiation therapy can be diagnostic. The CSF shows tumor cells in more than 60% of patients with colloid cysts. Metastatic spread by shunts is a serious danger, and the indication for a shunt should always be carefully reviewed in these patients.

Malformations of the Vein of Galen

The incidence of hydrocephalus in patients with aneurysms of the vein of Galen is almost 50%. Because the venous pressure is markedly increased, absorption of CSF is impaired. The incidence of hydrocephalus in small children is 71%, but it declines to 30% in adults. Shunting is dangerous in

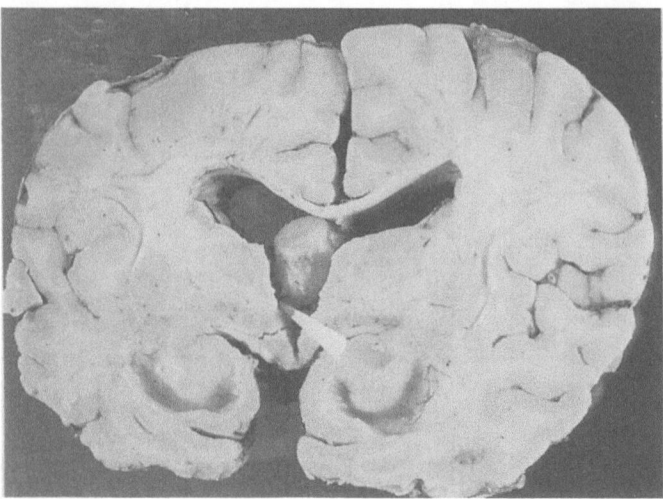

Fig. 5. Colloid cyst that led to sudden death. The abrupt blockade of the foramen of Monro caused acute, obstructive hydrocephalus. (Courtesy of Bernd Wowra, MD, Munich, Jerimany)

these patients, and there is a mortality of 10%. Venous congestion may be a contributing factor. If a shunt is inevitable, the ventricular catheter should be inserted from a frontal burr hole, a relatively high pressure level is recommended for the implanted valve, and surgery should be performed under antiseizure prophylaxis. The treatment of the malformation consists of a combination of interventional neuroradiological embolization and microneurosurgery.

Cerebellar Hemorrhage and Infarction

The treatment problems of cerebellar infarction and cerebellar hemorrhage are similar; therefore, they are often discussed together in the literature. Both lesions may produce occlusive hydrocephalus when they exceed 20 mm in diameter, especially when located in the midline. If the lesion is larger than 30 mm, obstruction almost always oc-

curs in adults. The frequency of hydrocephalus varies in the neurological and neurosurgical literature, but it occurs in about 50% of all treated patients. If ventricular hemorrhage is present, the hydrocephalus rate exceeds 90%. Although treatment strategies vary from center to center, large uncontrolled series suggest that surgery is efficacious and results in a high quality of life.

Patients with smaller infarctions or hemorrhages without CSF obstruction (Heros classification stage I) can be treated medically. Those in the intermediate Heros stage II, in which patients are responsive but have cranial nerve palsies (IV, VI, VII) and hydrocephalus, EVD should be performed to avoid open surgery. The EVD system should have a positive opening pressure of at least 20 cm of H_2O. If shunt dependency is proven, a definite shunt should be inserted after 8–14 days to avoid the increasing risk of ventriculitis.

For patients with cerebellar stroke, there are two treatment alternatives: evacuation of the hematoma and insertion of an EVD. Hematoma evacuation can decrease the pressure in the posterior fossa and leave the patient independent of a definite shunt (even if a EVD must temporarily be inserted).

Treatment only with insertion of an EVD is associated with a longer stay in the neurocritical care unit because of prolonged brain swelling and resorption of the hematoma. The frequency of a permanent shunt is higher.

For patients with Heros stage III, who are comatose, show signs of brainstem compression, neuroradiological evidence of quadrigeminal cistern compression and pathological evoked potential studies, the best therapy is neurosurgical decompression of the posterior fossa. This is usually combined with EVD. This operation clearly constitutes a neurosurgical emergency. A decompressive craniotomy of the posterior fossa, resection of the C-1 lamina, and a durapatch are performed. Visible infarcted tissue and cerebellar hemorrhage can additionally be evacuated.

EVD without decompressive craniotomy in Heros stage III is ineffective because compression of the brain stem is not eliminated. In our experience, EVD alone carries a significant risk of transtentorial upward herniation.

Dandy-Walker Malformation

The Dandy-Walker syndrome is a complex dysraphic malformation with cystic enlargement of the fourth ventricle; the vermis or cerebellum is dysplastic and the tentorium is cranially displaced. In about one fourth of patients the aqueduct is stenotic. In addition, the foramina of the fourth ventricle are usually obstructed.

The treatment recommendations for patients with the Dandy-Walker syndrome remain controversial. Some authors advocate a fenestrating intrathecal shunting procedure, while most advocate ventriculo-peritoneal shunts. The risk of decompensation remains extremely high. Because of the risk of transtentorial upward herniation, the mere shunting of one lateral ventricle should be avoided. If only the cyst is shunted and the aqueduct is not open, downward herniation can occur.

Obstructive-Malresorptive Hydrocephalus after Ventricular Bleeding and Subarachnoid Hemorrhage

The risk of development of early hydrocephalus increases with ventricular bleeding, tamponade of basal cisterns, vertebrobasilar or anterior communicating artery aneurysms, old age, and clinically poor grades on the Hunt and Hess scale (H&H). About 3% of patients with H&H grade I have ventricular enlargement on CT scan, while 42% of those with grade IV have enlargement. The incidence of hydrocephalus doubles in the first week after hemorrhage.

The treatment of early hydrocepalus involves some practical problems: (a) The content of blood in the CSF can be as high as 5 g/dl and blood clots can cause catheter obstruction; (b) the risk of infection is doubled when the CSF is sanguineous; (c) the rapid decrease of ICP by EVD can cause re-rupture of nonclipped aneurysms. The incidence of rebleeding varies significantly and is as high as 43% in the literature. Thus, the height of the drip chamber relative to the height of the foramen of Monro is very important. It should hang approximately 20 cm above the foramen of Monro to secure positive ICP and a constant resistance to the CSF drainage. The rate of implanted shunts following SAH ranges from 3% to 30%. Some authors suggest that EVD might promote shunt dependency. However, drainage is needed to rinse the clotted blood away and to free the basal cisterns. Most authors describe a low shunt frequency in their patients (ranging from 3% to 6.5%) and improvement of cerebral vasospasm by the use of EVD systems in patients with SAH. EVD systems are required to improve the treatment of hydrocephalus in SAH, and with correct handling, there is an acceptably low rate of complications. The drainage should be carefuly controlled.

Germinal-matrix Bleeding and Obstructive-Malabsorptive Hydrocephalus

Subependymal germinal-matrix bleeding occurs in 44–50% of children with very low birth weights. While the bleeding in Papile stages I and II has a good neurological outcome and very rarely leads to ventricular enlargement, Papile stages III and IV are associated with hydrocephalus in 25% of patients. Treatment of posthemorrhagic hydrocephalus with azetazolamide (Diamox) is controversial, and a significant beneficial effect has not been proven. Recent studies have shown that any effect is mild and

only temporary. Moreover, there are serious side effects from carbon dioxide retention that may cause an increase in ICP and nephrocalcinosis from electrolyte imbalance. Another treatment option is drainage by a subcutaneous reservoir, an EVD system, or a shunt. Generally, treatment is associated with a high risk of complications, as the body weight is low and the immune system is not sufficiently developed. Sanguineous CSF represents an additional risk for infection.

Timing of Interventions

For the managment of acute life-threatening hydrocephalus with *signs of transtentorial herniation*, a noncontrast CT scan should be performed immediately after intubation. In newborns, B-mode sonography is usually sufficient. All nonvital diagnostic procedures, such as administration of contrast medium for CT scan, MRI, evoked potential studies, or angiography, should be delayed. VP or EVD should be inserted as rapidly as possible. In emergencies, this is sometimes needed outside the operating room in order to save time. When a pre-existing burr hole is transcutaneously accessible using a Cushing cannula, this should be done, especially if the patient is deteriorating quickly. The peak pressure of ICP should initially be lowered to about 30–40 cm of H_2O, then cautiously and slowly to 15–20 cm of H_2O by releasing CSF. In the presence of space-occupying lesions in the posterior fossa or nonclipped aneurysms, the pressure should be relieved very cautiously. In many institutions dexamethasone is recommended at a dose of 1 mg/kg. Active osmotic substances can also be used in this situation, although the initial increase of volume in the presence of vasoparalysis may lead to an increase in ICP. After the emergency VP, it should be determined whether the cause of obstruction (for example, cerebellar hemorrhage) can be removed at the same time (that is, under the same anesthesia) without further endangering the patient.

In *noncomatose* patients with progressive disturbance of the level of consciousness and signs of increased intracranial pressure, the underlying disease should be evaluated carefully before surgery. In most patients with tumors, treatment with high-dose corticosteroids results in improvement and may help to delay the operation. For all patients, careful observation is recommended. If there is no improvement with medical treatment, an EVD or, if inevitable, a definite shunt should be considered. Special attention should be paid to loss of visual acuity, as irreversible blindness can occur (even after short-term increased ICP).

Conclusions

Removal of the occlusion remains the general aim in the treatment of occlusive hydrocephalus. In most patients the cause of obstruction of CSF pathways can be removed by the extirpation of tumors and malformations, removal of cysts, or decompressive craniotomies for cerebellar space-occupying lesions. In selected cases, medical treatment (for example, with lymphoma, macroprolactinoma) and specialized intensive therapy (for example, with cerebellar infarction and hemorrhage) may be successful. Radiotheraphy can result in marked reduction of tumor volume (for example, germinoma).

In emergencies, perioperatively, and for tumor surgery, EVD is the treatment method of choice. The risk of infection is minimal in the first few days and remains acceptable if the system is handled carefully. In those with shunt dependency after 7–14 days, the EVD should be replaced by a permanent shunt or changed to the contralateral side. Extrathecal shunts are associated with a high rate of complications and should be avoided whenever possible. The effect of drainage in shunts depends on the position of the patient; negative ICP may provoke hemorrhage. Space-occupying lesions in the posterior fossa can result in a transtentorial pressure gradient and can lead to transtentorial upward herniation. Nevertheless, primary shunts are indicated for palliative therapy.

Suggested Reading

Albright AL (1982) The value of precraniotomy shunts in children with posterior fossa tumors. Clin Neurosurg 30:278–285

Altman NR, Naidich TP, Braffman BH (1992) Posterior fossa malformations. AJNR 13: 691–724

Bogdahn U, Lau W, Hassel W, Gunreben G, Mertens HG, Brawanski A (1992) Continuous pressure-controlled, external ventricular drainage for treatment of acute hydrocephalus – evaluation of risk factors. Neurosurgery 31 (in press)

Chapman PH (1990) Hydrocephalus in childhood. In: Youmans JR (ed) Neurological surgery. Saunders, Philadelphia, pp 1236–1276

Choux M, Genitori L, Lang D, Lena G (1992) Shunt implantation: reducing the incidence of shunt infection. J Neurosurgery 77: 875–880

Davson H (1984) Formation and drainage of the cerebrospinal flud. In: Shapiro K, Marmarou A, Portnoy H (eds) Hydrocephalus. Raven, New York, pp 3–41

Drake JM, Sainte-Rose CH, Da Silva M, Hirsch JF (1991) Cerebrospinal fluid dynamics in children with external ventricular drains. Neurosurgery 28:242–250

Hirsch JF, Hoppe-Hirsch E (1988) Shunts and shunt problems in childhood. Advances and technical standards in neurosurgery, vol 16. Basel, Karger, pp 177–196

Matsumoto S, Tamaki N (eds) (1991) Hydrocephalus. Pathogenesis and treatment. Springer, Berlin-Heidelberg New York, pp 362–369

McComb JG (1983) Recent research into the nature of cerebrospinal fluid formation and absorption. J Neurosurg 59:369–383

McLaurin RL (1983) Disadvantages of the pre-operative shunt in posterior fossa tumors. Clin Neurosurg 30:286–292

Nulsen FE, Spitz EB (1952) Control of hydrocephalus by direct shunt from ventricle to jugular vein. Surg Forum 2:399–403

Pudenz RH (1981) The surgical treatment of hydrocephalus – an historical review. Surg Neurol 15:15–25

Pudenz RH, Foltz EL (1991) Hydrocephalus: overdrainage by ventricular shunts. A review and recommendations. Surg Neurol 35:200–212

Raimondi AJ (1987) Hydrocephalus. In: Raimondi AJ (ed) Pediatric neurosurgery. Springer, Berlin Heidelberg New York, pp 453–491

Sainte-Rose C, Hoffman HJ, Hirsch JF (1989) Shunt failure. Concepts Pediatr Neurosurg 9:7–20

Tronnier V, Aschoff A, Hund E, Hampl J, Kunze S (1991) Commercial external drainage sets: unsolved safety and handling problems. Acta Neurochir (Wien) 110: 49–56

Chapter 82

Parkinson's Disease

WERNER POEWE and WOLFGANG OERTEL

Akinetic Crisis

Definition

Parkinson's disease is a slowly progressive neurodegenerative disorder that can be associated with several important complications from the disease itself or from treatment of the disease (Table 1). Akinetic crisis, characterized by marked worsening of all motor symptoms, occurs in patients with advanced Parkinson's disease, although, it is usually precipitated by underdosing or withdrawal of levodopa (for example, during "drug holidays"), impaired gastrointestinal absorption of levodopa, or infection (Table 2).

Clinical Features

Akinetic crisis usually develops over days to weeks but can develop rapidly over the course of 24 h. Patients may be unable to stand or walk and may be completely immobilized. Speech may

Section Editors: Karl M. Einhäupl and Werner Hacke

be monotonous and unintelligible. Their extremities may be rigid and fixed in a flexed position and a continuous asymmetrical resting tremor may be present. Because they are often unable to eat or drink, patients often become dehydrated. There is a high incidence of urinary tract infections, deep venous thromboses, pressure sores, and pneumonia in patients with akinetic crisis. Hyperthermia can also occur, like that seen in neuroleptic malignant syndrome.

Treatment

When treating patients with akinetic crisis, possible precipitating causes should first be excluded, such as sepsis, pneumonia, ileus, or appendicitis. If akinetic crisis is the result of withdrawal of levodopa and is mildly to moderately severe, levodopa treatment should be restarted (orally or by dissolved tablet or opened capsule via nasogastric tube) at a lower dose than before and gradually increased to the previous dose over 1–2 days. If akinetic crisis is the result of underdosing of levodopa, the dose should be increased

Table 1. Acute exacerbations in Parkinson's disease ("Parkinson crisis")

Disease-related
Akinetic crisis
Related to drug withdrawal or drug-induced
Akinetic crisis
Malignant levodopa withdrawal syndrome
Off-period dysautonomia
Off-period dystonia
Drug-induced psychosis

Table 2. Conditions associated with "akinetic crisis" in Parkinson's disease

Primary underdosing of dopaminergic drugs
Withdrawal of antiparkinsonian medication ("drug holidays")
Secondary absorption failure
Swallowing difficulties
Gastrointestinal infections
Perioperative phases
Any severe infection

daily by 100 mg until a response is seen. Amantadine HCl can also be used in patients with mildly to moderately severe akinetic crisis, especially in those with difficulty swallowing or impaired gastrointestinal absorption. The dose is 200–400 mg intravenously daily (200 mg/500 ml). It is probably effective because of its moderate dopaminergic effect, although its NMDA-antagonistic properties may also play a part.

For patients with severe akinesia, levodopa can be given intravenously at a dose of 1–2 mg/kg per hour. Concomitant treatment with decarboxylase inhibitors, such as benserazide or carbidopa, is suggested for optimal efficacy, although this is not necessary in emergencies (must be given by nasogastric tube). Levodopa methyl-

ester (LDME) can also be used and can be given in smaller, more concentrated volumes (equivalent to 200 mg levodopa per milliliter). These intravenous preparations, which can also be given by nasogastric tube, are not commercially available yet and must be specially ordered from the pharmaceutical companies (levodopa from Hoffmann La Roche, Basel, Switzerland and LDME from Chiesi Pharmaceuticals, Milan, Italy).

Apomorphine can be given either by subcutaneous bolus injection or continuous s.c. infusion. When given by subcutaneous bolus injection, the dose is 2–5 mg. It is effective in 10–15 min and has a duration of up to 120 min (depending on the dose). When given as s.c. infusions, the rate of infusion should initially be 1–2 mg/h with increases of 0.5–1 mg/h every 12 h as needed. Potential side effects include nausea, vomiting, orthostatic hypotension, and bradycardia and other dysrhythmias. Concomitant treatment with domperidone may prevent some of the side effects; however, it may not be necessary in patients who have had dopaminergic therapy for many years. Domperidone can be given either 20 mg orally every 6–8 h (at least 12 h before apomorphine) or 60 mg orally 30–60 min before apomorphine (Table 3).

Malignant Levodopa Withdrawal Syndrome

Definition

Malignant levodopa withdrawal syndrome is a rare complication of levodopa therapy that occurs when the

Table 3. Management of akinetic crisis in Parkinson's disease

1. Ensure sufficient dopamine substitution
   (i) Enteral route:
       Oral levodopa (start with 100 mg q.i.d., 100 mg/day increments as necessary)
       Dispersible levodopa via nasogasatric tubes (as above)
   (ii) Parenteral route:
        Amantadine infusions (200 mg/500 ml once to three times daily; may be sufficient treatment in less severe cases when combined with oral levodopa)
        Apomorphine infusions s.c. (24 h pretreatment with 20 mg domperidone t.i.d.; 2 mg/h infusion rate over 12–24 h, 1 mg/h infusion rate increments)
        Levodopa infusions i.v. (5% glucose solutions with 125 mg levodopa/ 250 ml; infusion rates of 1–2 mg levodopa/kg per hour over 12–24 h)
2. Ancillary measures
   (i) Parenteral fluid with electrolyte plus calorie substitution
   (ii) Antithrombotic prophylaxis (low-dose heparin s.c.)
   (iii) Pneumonia prophylaxis

drug is abruptly stopped or when the dose is quickly reduced. It has also been reported with "drug holidays" and in patients with impaired gastro-intestinal absorption.

Clinical Features

Patients with malignant levodopa withdrawal syndrome have worsening of parkinsonian features within 48 h of the change in medication. They may appear to have akinetic crisis or neuro-leptic malignant syndrome. Physical findings include tachycardia, tachypnea, marked hyperthermia, and mental status changes such as disorientation, confusion, hallucinations, or somnolence. Laboratory findings may show markedly increased serum creatine kinase concentrations.

Treatment

Patients with Parkinson's disease who present with acute worsening of their symptoms with fever and tachycardia need neurocritical care. Other causes of fever and tachycardia should be excluded, such as infection, pulmonary embolism, and myocardial infarction. Patients should be treated with levodopa or LDME intravenously (or by nasogastric tube) or apomorphine. Amantadine HCl is rarely sufficient and should always be supplemented with levodopa or other dopamine agonists such as bromocriptine mesylate, lisuride, or pergolide mesylate. Patients should be started on the daily dose of levodopa or dopamine agonist that they were taking before. Dantrolene sodium may be considered for patients with markedly increased creatine kinase concentrations, although controlled trials have not yet evaluated its efficacy (Table 4).

Dopaminergic Psychosis

Definition

About 10%–20% of patients with Parkinson's disease develop confusion, hallucinations, and paranoid delusions during long-term treatment with dopaminergic drugs (levodopa or dopamine agonists). Confusion is dose-related and occurs more frequently with ergot agonists than levodopa. Other factors that may also

Table 4. Management of the malignant levodopa withdrawal syndrome

1. Substitute central dopamine
   200 mg/500 ml amantadine i.v. every 6 h plus oral levodopa or DA agonists (100–200 mg levodopa every 2–4 h; 5–10 mg bromocriptine or 0.2–0.4 mg lisuride or 0.25–0.5 mg pergolide every 6 h)
   Apomorphine infusions s.c. (see Table 3)
   Levodopa infusions i.v. (see Table 3)
2. General supportive measures
   Intravenous fluids, electrolytes, and calories
   Low-dose heparin
   Antibiotic prophylaxis
3. Whole-body cooling if fever >40°
4. Dantrolene sodium (in cases with marked creatine kinase elevations; start with 2.5 mg/kg i.v. infusion followed by 5–10 mg/kg/day i.v. as infusions or 4–5 bolus injections)

contribute to confusion include multi-infarct dementia from cerebrovascular disease and other causes of dementia (for example, diffuse Lewy body disease or Alzheimer's dementia).

Clinical Features

Vivid dreaming is often an early symptom reported by patients with dopaminergic psychosis. This can usually be controlled by reducing the dose. Some patients may develop paranoia and hallucinations and appear agitated and disoriented. They usually have tachycardia, sweating, and sometimes hypertension. Preexisting levodopa dyskinesis may become worse.

Treatment

Treatment of patients with dopaminergic psychosis consists of three main approaches. The first is the dose of the patient's medications. For patients treated with both levodopa and dopamine agonists, the latter should be reduced first (by at least 50% of the daily dose) or stopped. Other medications, such as anticholinergic agents and amantdine HCl, should also be gradually decreased or stopped. Clinicians must be cautious, however, because abrupt discontinuation of these medications can result in withdrawal syndrome and worsening confusion. The dose of levodopa should then be reduced to the minimum dose needed to control symptoms.

Secondly, neuroleptics can be used. Clozapine is the neuroleptic that is the least likely to worsen parkinsonian symptoms. It has an affinity for D_3 dopamine receptors, located in the projection areas of the mesocorticolimbic system, but has less D_2 dopamine receptor blocking activity than other classic neuroleptic drugs. Its efficacy for controlling dopaminergic psychosis is well established, and in most patients only a low dose is needed (12.5–25 mg/day). For those with more severe psychosis, clozapine can be started at doses of 50–150 mg/day in two to three divided doses. Because clozapine is associated with leukopenia and agranulocytosis (2–3 cases per 10000), weekly blood counts are necessary. Classic neuroleptic drugs (for example, haloperidol 3–10 mg) cause worsening of motor symptoms and a diminished response to dopaminergic drugs which may persist even after the neuroleptic is stopped. These agents should be avoided unless patients have severe refractory psychosis. Weak classic neuroleptics, such as sulpiride or pimozide, may be a compromise. Finally, general supportive care is important, including hydration, often a contributing factor

Table 5. Management of dopaminergic-induced psychosis in Parkinson's disease

---

1. Reduce antiparkinsonian drugs
   (i) Stop amantadine and/or anticholinergics
   (ii) Reduce (at least 50%) or stop ergot agonists
   (iii) Reduce levodopa to minimum effective dose
2. Add antipsychotic agents
   (i) Add clozapine (start with 12.5 mg nocte in mild cases; increase up to 100 mg/day in severe cases – weekly blood counts)
   (ii) Add classical neuroleptics (e.g., haloperidol 3–10 mg/day) (refractory paranoid psychosis only)
3. General measures to prevent complications
   (i) Oral or parenteral fluids
   (ii) Low-dose heparin (immobilized patients)
   (iii) Broad-spectrum antibiotics (immobilized febrile patients)

---

in elderly patients with confusion, deep venous thrombosis prophylaxis, and treatment of infections (Table 5).

Suggested Reading

Bittkau S, Przuntek H (1988) Chronic s.c. lisuride in Parkinson's disease – motor performance and avoidance of psychiatric side effects. J Neural Transm Suppl 27: 35–54

Critchley PH, Grlandas-Perez F, Quinn NP et al. (1988) Continuous subcutaneous lisuride infusions in Parkinson's disease. J Neural Transm 27:55–60

Frankel JP, Lees AJ, Kempster PA, Stern GM (1990) Subcutaneous apomorphine in the treatment of Parkinson's disease. J Neurol Neurosurg Psychiatry 53:96–101

Friedman JH, Lannon MC (1989) Clozapine in the treatment of psychosis in Parkinson's disease. Neurology 39:1219–1221

Friedman JH, Feinberg SS, Feldman RG (1984) A neuroleptic malignant-like syndrome due to L-dopa withdrawal. Ann Neurol 16:126–127

Kahn N, Freeman A, Juncos JL, Manning D, Watts RL (1991) Clozapine is beneficial for psychosis in Parkinson's disease. Neurology 41:1699–1700

Obeso JA, Luquin MR, Martínez Lage JM (1986) Intravenous lisuride corrects, oscillations of motor performance in Parkinson's disease. Ann Neurol 19:31–35

Oertel WH, Gasser T, Ippisch R et al. (1989) Apomorphine test for dopaminergic responsiveness. Lancet I:1262–1263

Poewe WH, Kleedorfer B, Wagner M et al. (1989) Side effects of subcutaneous apomorphine in Parkinson's disease. Lancet I:1084–1085

Poewe WH, Kleedorfer B, Wagner M, Schelosky L (1991) Continuous subcutaneous apomorphine infusions for fluctuating Parkinson's disease: long-term experience in 20 patients. Neurology 41 [Suppl 1]:172–173

Pollak P, Champay AS, Hommel M et al. (1989) Subcutaneous apomorphine in Parkinson's disease. J Neurol Neurosurg Psychiatry 52:544

Povlsen UJ, Noring U, Fog R, Gerlach J (1985) Tolerability and therapeutic effect of clozapine. Acta Psychiatr Scand 176–185

Scholz E, Dichgans J (1985) Treatment of drug-induced exogenous psychosis in parkinsonism with clozapine and fluperlapine. Eur Arch Psychiatr Neurol Sci 60–64

Sechi GP, Tanda F, Mutani R (1984) Fatal hyperpyrexia after withdrawal of levodopa. Neurology 34:249–251

Wolters EC, Hurwitz TA, Perpard RF, Calne DB (1989) An antipsychotic agent in Parkinson's disease? Clin Neuropharmacol 12:83–90

Chapter 83

Life-Threatening Hyperthermic Syndromes

ERNST F. HUND and FRANK LEHMANN-HORN

Neuroleptic Malignant Syndrome

Definition and Epidemiology

Several neurological disorders can be caused by treatment with neuroleptic drugs, including acute and tardive dyskinesia, tremor, akathesia, and parkinsonism. Neuroleptic malignant syndrome (NMS) is the rarest and most dangerous disorder, occurring in 0.5%–0.14% of patients taking neuroleptic drugs. It is twice as common in men and 80% of patients are younger than 40 years. NMS is usually associated with regular therapeutic doses of haloperidol and fluphenazine (the most potent and most commonly prescribed neuroleptics). Previous exposure is not a prerequisite. NMS can be caused by other neuroleptics, including those used to treat nausea and vomiting, dissociative diseases, Tourette's syndrome, Huntington's disease, and agitation, as well as by some antidepressants. It can also result

Section Editors: Karl M. Einhäupl and Werner Hacke

from withdrawal of dopaminergic drugs and may be identical to the malignant L-dopa withdrawal syndrome and acute akinetic crisis. In the past, death occurred in 25% of patients. The most common causes of death were pneumonia, hypotension, arrhymias, renal failure, and thromboembolism. Today, because of more widespread recognition and advances in supportive care, the mortality rate is approximately 10%.

Pathophysiology

The exact cause of NMS is not known, but a disturbance in central dopaminergic pathways has been postulated. Blockade of dopamine receptors in the basal ganglia results in enhanced muscle tone and hyperthermia. Blockade of receptors in the hypothalamus contributes to the hyperthermia because of impaired heat dissipation, and blockade in the spinal cord results in autonomic instability. Gamma-aminobutyric acid (GABA)-containing neurons, important in the nigrostriatal pathways, are also probably involved in the pathogenesis of NMS. Cholinergic mechanisms are not important; treatment with anticholinergic agents neither prevents NMS nor reduces the duration of symptoms or the mortality rate.

Clinical Features

The clinical hallmarks of NMS are hyperthermia, profuse sweating, and extrapyramidal signs such as muscle rigidity (Table 1). Most patients have fever ranging from 38 to 40°C (fever may be greater than 42°C). Patients may also have akinesia, tremor, chorea, and oculogyric crisis, but the presence of fever and profuse sweating distinguishes NMS from the common extrapyramidal side effects of neuroleptics. The full-blown syndrome usu-

ally develops over 24–72 h but it may develop as rapidly as within a few hours. Some patients, with severe muscle rigidity and decreased chest wall compliance, can develop respiratory failure. Rhabdomyolysis-induced renal failure can also occur. Hypotension and cardiac dysrhythmias from autonomic instability and hypovolemia from increased sweating may result in shock. Other patients may have changes in levels of consciousness, ranging from mild obtundation to stupor or coma, or may have catatonic behavior, mutism, and catalepsy. Underlying psychosis must be excluded in these patients.

Laboratory findings in patients with NMS are nonspecific and include leukocytosis (up to 30000/mm^3), increased creatine kinase (occasionally >10000 IU/l), abnormalities of liver injury tests, and electrolyte disturbances such as hypercalcemia. Results of cerebrospinal fluid · analysis are normal.

Several conditions can mimic NMS (Table 2). Heat stroke generally occurs in hot and humid weather. Patients with heat stroke, in contrast to those with NMS, have flaccid extremities and dry skin. Patients taking neuroleptic drugs, because of the anti-

Table 1. Clinical features of neuroleptic malignant syndrome (after Keck et al. 1989)

Fever
Extrapyramidal signs
  Lead-pipe muscle rigidity
  Cogwheeling
  Siallorrhea
  Oculogyric crisis
  Dyskinesia
  Tremor
Autonomic dysfunction
  Diaphoresis
  Pallor
  Hypertension
  Tachycardia
  Cardiac arrhythmia
  Incontinence
Alteration of consciousness
  Alert mutism or stupor
  Sopor or coma
Laboratory abnormalities (nonspecific)
  Elevation of creatine kinase (>1000 U/l)
  Leukocytosis (>15000/mm^3)
  Electrolyte disturbances (reflecting dehydration)
  Myoglobinuria (reflecting rhabdomyolysis)

Table 2. Differential diagnosis of neuroleptic malignant syndrome (after Guzé and Baxter 1985 and Olmsted 1988)

Heat stroke	Serotonin syndrome
Malignant hyperthermia	Strychnine poisoning
Viral encephalitis	Rabies
Central anticholinergic toxicity	Tetanus
Lethal catatonia	Stiff-man syndrome
Rhabdomyolysis from other causes	

Table 3. Differential features of hyperthermic syndromes

	Neuroleptic malignant syndrome	Malignant hyperthermia	Heat stroke	Central anticholinergic syndrome
Pathogenesis	Blockade of central dopamine receptors	Excessive calcium release into the myoplasm	Heat gain exceeds heat dissipation, brain edema	Anticholinergic toxicity
Offending agents	Neuroleptics, antidepressants, withdrawal of dopaminergic agents	Inhalational anesthetics, succinylcholine	None (but facilitated by drugs reducing heat loss)	Neuroleptics, anticholinergics, antiparkinsonian agents, opiates, antispasmodics, benzodiazepines
Time to onset after exposure	Variable	Seconds to minutes or hours	–	–
Sweating	Profuse	Profuse	Anhidrosis	Anhidrosis
Pupils	Normal	Normal	Constricted	Dilated
Muscle tone	Severe extrapyramidal rigidity	Severe muscle contraction	Flaccid	Normal
Genetic element	None	Autosomal dominant	None	None
Response to curare	Yes	No	–	–
Pharmacotherapy	Dopaminergic and GABAergic agents, dantrolene	Dantrolene	(Dantrolene ?)	Physostigmine

cholinergic effects, are predisposed to heat stroke (neuroleptic-related heat stroke). Malignant hyperthermia, an inherited myopathy (see below), and viral encephalitis can also present with fever and extrapyramidal signs. Patients with anticholinergic toxicity (see below) may appear similar to those with NMS. They are agitated and have absence of sweating, dilated pupils, dry mouth, urinary retention, and diminished bowel sounds. They do not, however, have muscle stiffness (Table 3). The serotonin syndrome also clinically resembles NMS. It is caused by overstimulation of brain stem and spinal cord serotinin receptors by serotonin agonists (fluvoxamine, fluoxetine HCl, clomipramine HCl) either alone or in combination with monoamine oxidase inhibitors.

Treatment

Patients with mildly to moderately severe NMS can usually be treated by reduction of the dose of the neuroleptic drug and the addition of anticholinergic drugs. In patients with marked severity, the neuroleptic drug should be stopped. Supportive treatment for hyperthermia, hypovolemia, electrolyte abnormalities, and respiratory failure should be provided and alkalinization of the urine should be done to prevent rhabdomyolysis-induced renal failure. Hemodialysis and hemofiltration do not remove protein-bound neuroleptics. Dopamine agonists such as amantadine HCl, bromocriptine mesylate, levodopa, and lisuride have been used successfully in the treatment of patients with NMS. Dantrolene sodium, a direct-acting muscle relaxant, can significantly shorten the duration of symptoms, and intravenous benzodiazepines, which can potentiate central GABA activity, have been effective in reversing catatonic and extrapyramidal features. Patients who do not respond to this therapy may respond to electroconvulsive therapy (Table 4).

In many patients with serious psychiatric diseases, it may not be possible to stop the neuroleptic drug. Patients should be completely recovered, however, before neuroleptics are restarted. Low doses of neuroleptics (preferable those of lower potency, such thioridazine or molindone) should be used.

Table 4. Management of advanced neuroleptic malignant syndrome and febrile catatonia

Discontinuation of neuroleptics and other drugs with anti-dopaminergic potency
Prompt institution of supportive medical care
Specific pharmacologic treatment:

Dopamine agonists:	
Amantadine	100 mg, b.i.d. or t.i.d.
Bromocriptine	5–30 mg/day
Levodopa/carbidopa	100–200/25–75 mg, q.i.d.
Lisuride	1–2 mg/24 h by subcutaneous infusion
GABA agonists:	
Benzodiazepines	lorazepam 1 mg b.i.d. to 5 mg q.i.d., orally or 1–2 mg i.v.
Muscle relaxants:	
Dantrolene:	100–600 mg/day orally, or 0.8–2.5 mg/kg i.v., q.i.d.
Electroconvulsive therapy	

Temperature and muscle tone should be monitored and creatine kinase measurements should be done daily for the first few days after restarting the drug.

Febrile Catatonia

The term "catatonia," first introduced by Kahlbaum more than a century ago, is usually associated with psychiatric disease, especially schizophrenia. Catatonic features can be seen in many diseases, however, and should be considered a sign rather than a specific entitiy (Table 5). Febrile or "lethal" catatonia is present when catatonia is associated with hyperthermia and autonomic dysfunction (tachycardia, sweating, labile blood pressure). It can often be difficult to distinguish febrile catatonia, schizophrenia-related catatonia, and NMS. Moreover, catatonia is a risk factor for NMS. In general, patients with

Table 5. Clinical features of catatonia

Psychosocial withdrawal:
  Negativism (patient refuses cooperation and
    faces away)
  Mutism (loss or refusal of all verbal output)
  Catatonic stupor
Psychosocial excitement:
  Catatonic furor
Motor signs:
  Catalepsy (maintenance of bizarre postures)
  Waxy flexibility (plastic increase in tone with
    a tendency to maintain unusual postures
    induced by the examiner)
  Stereotypies (uniform, not goal-directed
    movements)
  Mannerisms [goal-directed activities,
    performed in a bizarre way (unusual way of
    smoking, eating etc.)]
  Grimacing

febrile catatonia have less severe muscle stiffness and usually have a history of agitation; they may be uncooperative with treatment.

The best treatment for patients with febrile catatonia is not clear. Patients with early febrile catatonia have been successfully treated with neuroleptic drugs, whereas those at later stages usually do not respond and neuroleptic drugs should not be given. These patients should be treated according to the guidelines for treatment of NMS listed in Table 4.

Malignant Hyperthermia

Definition

Malignant hyperthermia (MH) is a potentially fatal myopathy that is similar to NMS. Patients with both disorders present with fever, muscle rigidity, tachycardia, and increased creatine kinase concentrations. There are important differences between them (Table 3). MH is triggered by inhalational anesthetics (usually halothane) and depolarizing muscle relaxants (usually succinylcholine) in genetically predisposed patients. In the past, 60% of patients died. Today, fewer than 7% of patients die, because of earlier recognition and effective treatment with dantrolene sodium.

Pathophysiology

MH is thought to be transmitted as an autosomal dominant trait in which calcium channels in the skeletal muscle triads have increased sensitivity to volatile anesthetics and depolarizing muscle relaxants. As a result, the intracellular concentration of calcium increases and a hypermetabolic state develops with increased oxygen consumption, metabolic acidosis, muscle contraction, hyperthermia, and rhabdomyolysis.

Clinical Features

Muscle rigidity usually begins minutes after the drug has been given, and in fulminant forms may develop in seconds. Patients may be difficult or even impossible to intubate. Unlike in NMS, nondepolarizing relaxants, such as pancuronium bromide and vecuronium bromide, are not effective in patients with MH. Other conditions that can mimic MH include sepsis, toxic shock syndrome, anoxic brain damage, pheochromocytoma, and thyroid storm. Muscle rigidity after anesthetics or depolarizing agents can also occur in Duchenne and Becker muscular dystrophy, some myotonias, and periodic paralysis. The diagnosis of MH can be confirmed by the in vitro contracture test. In this test, a muscle fiber, obtained at biopsy, is studied for its contraction properties when exposed to caffeine and halothane. Family members of patients and others at risk for MH (for example, those with King-Denborough syndrome and central core disease) should be screened for MH with this test and should carry an emergency card that identifies them as being at risk.

Treatment

When MH is suspected, volatile anesthetics should be immediately stopped and 100% oxygen should be given. Dantrolene sodium, which reduces intracellular calcium concentrations, should be given intravenously at a dose of 2.5 mg/kg of body weight (it is commercially distributed in 20-mg ampules). Some patients may need as much as 10 mg/kg before muscle relaxation occurs. Prophylactic dantrolene sodium is not helpful. Supportive measures such as treatment of acidosis and fluids to promote diuresis should also be provided (Table 6). In Germany, a hot-line service is available to provide information and a list of centers performing the muscle contracture test (telephone number 07131-482050).

Heat Stroke

Heat stroke (HS) is the most dangerous complication of high environmental temperatures and occurs when heat gain exceeds heat dissipation. HS occurs more commonly with high humidity and increased activity or excercise. Factors that predispose to heat stroke include old age, chronic disease, alcohol ingestion, skin disorders that interfere with heat loss, and the use of diuretics, anticholinergic agents, and neuroleptics (because of their anticholinergic effects) (see above).

HS commonly occurs among new military recruits undergoing basic training and novice long distance runners. On examination, patients have hyperthermia, mental status changes, hot, dry, flushed skin, and flaccid extremities, a feature that distinguishes heat stroke from NMS and malignant hyperthermia. Other findings on

Table 6. Management of acute malignant hyperthermia (adapted from Blanck and Humphrey 1990)

Stop all inhalation anesthetics and begin hyperventilation with 100% oxygen.

Administer dantrolene 1 mg/kg body weight i.v. Repeated doses are administered, titrated to heart rate, muscle rigidity, and temperature. Although 2 mg/kg is usually a successful dose, much higher doses may be needed (up to 10 mg/kg).

Administer bicarbonate according to blood gas analyses.

Monitor closely body temperature, urine output, serum potassium, calcium, and creatine phosphokinase levels, arterial blood gases, and clotting studies.

If arrhythmias do not respond to treatment of acidosis and hyperkalemia, 100–200 mg procainamide should be administered.

Start cooling of limbs and, if necessary, infuse cold solutions.

When the patient's condition has stabilized, dantrolene should be converted from intravenous to oral administration.

examination include constricted pupils, hyperventilation, and hypovolemia. Complications may include disseminated intravascular coagulation (DIC), rhabdomyolysis, renal failure, seizures, and shock.

Patients should be removed from the hot environment immediately and cooled to a core temperature of 39°C. Cooling is best done by surface cooling; iced gastric lavage is less effective. Volume status should be assessed by measurement of central venous pressure and hypovolemia should be corrected with isotonic saline. Careful measurements of urine output and serum electrolytes should be done. Pathological findings include brain edema and petechial hemorrhages in the brain, lungs, liver, and kidneys. Some studies have shown a benefit

when patients are given dantrolene sodium; however, definitive proof is lacking.

Central Anticholinergic Syndrome

Although most clinicians are aware of the peripheral side effects of anticholinergic drugs, the effects of blocking central anticholinergic pathways are often overlooked. Patients with central anticholinergic syndrome (CAS) can have agitation or depression. In the agitated form, patients have irritability, restlessness, confusion, hallucinations, disorientation, and motor hyperactivity (anticholinergic delirium). In the depressed form, they have decreased levels of consciousness ranging from somnolence to coma, motor hypoactivity, dysarthria, and disturbances of coordination.

Many centrally acting drugs have anticholinergic effects, such as neuroleptics, antidepressants, antispasmodics, antiparkinsonian agents, antihistamines, benzodiazepines, and opiates. Several eye drop preparations and over-the-counter sleep medications also have anticholinergic effects. Suicidal ingestion of belladonna preparations has also been reported as a cause of anticholinergic intoxication. Many of these drugs are combined. For example, patients in critical care units are routinely given large amounts of hypnotics, sedatives, and analgesics. CAS should be suspected if patients need excessive doses of sedatives or if they remain sedated after sedatives have been discontinued. Older patients and those with organic brain disease are at an increased risk of developing CAS.

The diagnosis of CAS is made clinically. The presence of peripheral anticholinergic signs may provide some confirming evidence (Table 7). The diagnosis is often difficult to make in patients in a critical care setting. The differential diagnosis includes hypertensive encephalopathy, intracranial hemorrhage, and encephalitis. Patients with alcohol or sedative withdrawal or intoxication with amphetamines or cocaine may also have tachycardia and fever. Other conditions include hypoglycemia, disturbances of water and electrolytes, sepsis, liver failure, renal failure, thyrotoxicosis, neuroleptic malignant syndrome, anemia, hypoxia, and respiratory or heart failure.

If CAS is suspected, all drugs with known anticholinergic properties should be decreased in dose or stopped. The diagnosis can be confirmed by infusion of physostigmine salicylate, a cholinesterase inhibitor, at a dose of 2 mg over 10 min. Another 2 mg may be given after 15–30 min. The symptoms will be relieved within seconds to minutes in patients with

CAS. Symptoms may recur, however, because of the drug's short half life. Patients should be given an additional 2 mg of physostigmine salicylate as a 24-h infusion. Side effects include cardiac dysrythmias, seizures, and signs of cholinergic crisis such as increased salivation, bladder and fecal incontinence, bowel hypermotility, and hypotension.

Suggested Reading

Barnes MP, Saunders M, Walls TJ, Saunders I, Kirk CA (1986) The syndrome of Karl Ludwig Kahlbaum. J Neurol Neurosurg Psychiatry 49:991–996

Blanck TJJ, Humphrey M (1990) Malignant hyperthermia. In: Breslow MJ, Miller CF, Rogers M (eds) Perioperative management. Mosby, St Louis, pp 394–403

Brede S, Dennhardt R (1991) Das zentrale anticholinerge Syndrom (ZAS) bei Intensivpatienten. Klin Wochenschr 69 (Suppl XXVI):89–94

Caroff SN (1980) The neuroleptic malignant syndrome. J Clin Psychiatry 41:79–83

Castillo E, Rubin RT, Holsboer-Trachsler E (1989) Clinical differentiation between lethal catatonia and neuroleptic malignant syndrome. Am J Psychiatry 146:324–328

Channa AB, Seraj MA, Saddique AA, Kadiwal GH, Shaikh MH, Samarkandi AH (1990) Is dantrolene effective in heat stroke patients? Crit Care Med 18:290–292

Ebadi M, Pfeiffer RF, Murrin LC (1990) Pathogenesis and treatment of neuroleptic malignant syndrome. Gen Pharmacol 21: 367–386

Fricchione GL (1985) Neuroleptic catatonia and its relationship to psychogenic catatonia. Biol Psychiatry 20:304–313

Fricchione GL, Cassem NH, Hooberman D, Hobson D (1983) Intravenous lorazepam in neuroleptic-induced catatonia. J Clin Psychopharmacol 3:338–342

Gelenberg AJ (1976) The catatonic syndrome. Lancet 1:1339–1341

Guzé BH, Baxter LR (1985) Neuroleptic malignant syndrome. N Engl J Med 313:163–166

Table 7. Signs and symptoms of anticholinergic toxicity

Peripheral	Central
Hyperthermia	Agitated confusion
Blurred vision	Hallucinations
Dry mucous membranes	Restlessness
Dry, flushed skin	Disturbed memory
Tachycardia	Aggression
Atrioventricular blocking	Diminished
Urinary retention	consciousness
Constipation	Coma
Decreased bowel sounds	

Hackl W, Mauritz W, Winkler M, Sporn P, Steinbereithner K (1990) Anaesthesia in malignant hyperthermia – susceptible patients without dantrolene prophylaxis: a report of 30 cases. Acta Anaesthesiol Scand 34:534–537

Hall RC (1982) Anticholinergic psychosis: differential dignosis and management. Psychosomatics 22:583–587

Harrison GG (1988) Dantrolene – dynamics and kinetics. Br J Anaesth 60:279–286

Kaufmann CA, Wyatt RJ (1987) Neuroleptic malignant syndrome. In: Meltzer HY (ed) Psychopharmacology: the third generation of progress. Raven, New York, pp 1421–1430

Keck PE, Pope HG, Cohen BM, McElroy SL, Nierenberg AA (1989) Risk factors for neuroleptic malignant syndrome. Arch Gen Psychiatry 46:914–918

Kline SS, Mauro LS, Scala-Barnett DM, Zick D (1989) Serotonin syndrome versus neuroleptic malignant syndrome as a cause of death. Clin Pharmacol 8:510–514

Kurlan R, Hamill R, Shoulson I (1984) Neuroleptic malignant syndrome. Clin Neuropharmacol 7:109–120

Lazarus A (1986) Treatment of neuroleptic malignant syndrome with electroconvulsive therapy. J Nerv Ment Dis 174:47–49

Lazarus A (1989) Differentiating neuroleptic-related heatstroke from neuroleptic malignant syndrome. Psychosomatics 30:454–456

MacLennan DH, Phillips MS (1992) Malignant hyperthermia. Science 256:789–794

Mann SC, Caroff SN, Bleier HR, Welz WKR, Kling MA, Hayashida M (1986) Lethal catatonia. Am J Psychiatry 143:1347–1381

Nelson TE, Flewellen EH (1983) The malignant hyperthermia syndrome. N Engl J Med 309:416–418

Olmsted TR (1988) Neuroleptic malignant syndrome: guidelines for treatment and reinstitution of neuroleptics. South Med J 81:888–891

Rodriguez ME, Luquin MR, Lera G, Delgado G, Salazar JM, Obeso JA (1990) Neuroleptic malignant syndrome treated with subcutaneous lisuride infusion. Mov Disord 5:170–172

Rosebusch P, Stewart T (1989) A prospective analysis of 24 episodes of neuroleptic malignant syndrome. Am J Psychiatry 146: 717–725

Rosenberg H (1988) Clinical presentation of malignant hyperthermia. Br J Anaesth 60: 268–273

Rosenberg MR, Green M (1989) Neuroleptic malignant syndrome. Review of response to therapy. Arch Intern Med 149: 1927–1931

Schneck HJ, Rupreht J (1989) Central anticholinergic syndrome (CAS) in anesthesia and intensive care. Acta Anaesthesiol Belg 40: 219–228

Shalev A, Hermesh H, Munitz H (1989) Mortality from neuroleptic malignant syndrome. J Clin Psychiatry 50:18–25

Slack T, Stoudemire A (1989) Reinstitution of neuroleptic treatment with molindone in a patient with a history of neuroleptic malignant syndrome. Gen Hosp Psychiatry 11:365–367

Sternbach H (1991) The serotonin syndrome. Am J Psychiatry 148:705–713

Stoudemire A (1982) The differential diagnosis of catatonic states. Psychosomatics 23:245–252

Susman VL, Addonizio G (1988) Recurrence of neuroleptic malignant syndrome. J Nerv Ment Dis 176:234–241

Torline RL (1992) Extreme hyperpyrexia associated with central anticholinergic syndrome. Anesthesiology 76:470–471

van Heerden PV, Collins CH (1989) Heat stroke – an uncommon presentation. Anaesthesia 44:660–662

Weinberger DR, Kelly MJ (1977) Catatonia and malignant syndrome: a possible complication of neuroleptic administration. J Nerv Ment Dis 165:263–268

White DAC, Robins AH (1991) Catatonia: harbinger of the neuroleptic malignant symdrome. Br J Psychiatry 158:419–421

White JD, Riccobene E, Nucci R, Johnson C, Butterfield AB, Kamath R (1987) Evaporation versus iced gastric lavage treatment of heat stroke: comparative efficacy in a canine model. Crit Care Med 15:748–750

| # Sleep Apnea Syndrome and Other Ventilatory Disturbances

MICHAEL P. BIBER and CHRISTOPH GARNER

Introduction and Definitions

Sleep apnea syndrome is characterized by recurrent cessations or substantial reductions of airflow in nose and mouth during sleep. In some patients the cessations (apneas) or reductions (hypopneas) occur because the upper airway is repeatedly sucked closed with inspiratory effort during sleep. In others, airflow may be reduced because of decreased ventilatory effort. Apneas and hypopneas with decreased or absent ventilatory effort are called non-obstructive or central, those with ongoing substantial effort obstructive. Sometimes, during an apnea there is initially no ventilatory effort, but then as the apnea continues ventilatory effort occurs before airflow resumes. This third type of apnea is called mixed. Often, patients with sleep apnea syndrome have more than one type of apnea. Commonly, both apneas and hypopneas occur in the same patient

Section Editors: Karl M. Einhäupl and Warner Hacke

during a typical sleep period. Hypoxia, hypercarbia, or increased ventilatory effort alone trigger arousals and associated resumptions of air flow. These arousals, even when they last only a few seconds, disrupt sleep architecture, contributing to the nonrestorative quality of sleep in patients with sleep apnea syndrome.

Clinical Features

Although all sleep apnea patients have an excessive number of apneas or hypopneas, sleep apnea syndrome is variable. The symptoms and complications depend not only on the number of ventilatory disturbances and the mechanism of airflow cessation but also on many other factors. For example, if many arousals are triggered by the breathing pauses, then drowsiness is likely to be proportionately severe. If the patient has substantial chronic obstructive lung disease with an abnormal baseline oxygen saturation, then each apnea or hypopnea will induce proportionately deeper drops in oxygen saturation. Generally, obstructive apneas are associated with greater oxygen desaturation and more dramatic variations in heart rate and blood pressure than nonobstructive apneas. Patients with ventricular irritability or marginal cardiac oxygenation will be excessively vulnerable to sleep-induced arrhythmias or cardiac ischemia.

While snoring, often loud, is an almost universal hallmark of untreated obstructive sleep apnea syndrome, in some patients who have undergone surgical procedures or who use dental appliances to increase the patency of their upper airway, snoring may be mild or absent despite the postoperative persistence of obstructions or increased upper airway resistance which disturbs sleep. Excessive drowsiness, often played down by patients, but often more accurately described by their observers, is common. This somnolence is largely attributable to the recurrent arousals and awakenings triggered by the ventilatory disturbance. These disruptions fragment sleep architecture, delaying the onset and reducing the amount of stage REM and slow wave sleep. Drowsiness is not only a major consequence of excessive apneas and hypopneas during sleep, it also exacerbates the breathing disturbance during sleep by raising the threshold of arousal, thereby prolonging the ventilatory pauses and deepening the oxygen desaturations.

Although sleep apnea syndrome is now believed to afflict up to 1% or more of the adult population, it was not defined in the medical literature until 1965. Despite the explosion of interest in sleep apnea in recent years and its association with cardiovascular complications, the prevalence and pathophysiology of the latter remain uncertain. Heart arrhythmias and blood pressure fluctuations often coincide with apneas, but there is as yet no convincing evidence that sustained hypertension is a consequence of sleep apnea syndrome except that obstructive sleep apnea may be a risk factor for sustained hypertension in young obese males. Obstructive apneas in severely affected patients do increase pulmonary artery pressure, promoting the development or exacerbation of cor pulmonale. Sleep apnea syndrome is a risk factor for brain and heart infarcts.

Aside from drowsiness and snoring, other symptoms of sleep apnea include restless sleep, occasionally with falls from bed during sleep, morning headaches, and, rarely, enuresis. The headaches may be cervicogenic, related to the excessive neck movements during sleep associated with sleep apnea syndrome. The excessive neck movements may irritate upper cervical spinal roots, causing pain within their cephalic dermatomes. Impaired vigilance and cognition are proportionate to the severity of the sleep apnea.

Signs of sleep apnea are quite variable. Roughly 50%–70% of adults with obstructive sleep apnea syndrome are obese. In some cases anatomic anomalies associated with upper airway narrowing are evident. These can include retrognathia, macroglossia, a shallow or crowded posterior oropharynx, a thick neck, or a deviated nasal septum. In young patients, especially children, the tonsils and adenoids may be enlarged. Snorers are more likely to be hypertensive than weight-, age-, and sex-matched controls. Sleep apnea syndrome may contribute to development of right- and left-sided heart failure. In patients with dilated cardiomyopathy and sleep apnea syndrome, effective nasal continuous positive airway pressure (CPAP) treatment improved left ventricular function.

Although awareness of sleep apnea syndrome has increased in recent years, inquiry about sleep symptoms and consideration of associated signs too often remains inadequate. Every patient with hypertension, heart failure, cardiac or cerebral ischemia, obesity, or snoring should be at least screened for sleep apnea syndrome by taking a relevant sleep history from the patient, and, if possible, an observer. The presence of suspicious signs, as noted above, warrants intensified investigation. Although history and signs alone may powerfully support the diagnosis of sleep apnea syndrome, ultimately polygraphic monitoring of the patient's sleep is required. Since the severity of apnea varies with body position, sleep stage, and time of day or night, diagnostic recording overnight is generally required. While documentation of pathologic ventilatory disturbances during a nap may be sufficient to confirm the diagnosis, a negative nap study does not preclude the diagnosis, especially if the recording does not include stage REM sleep with the patient supine.

Tests

A typical polygraphic sleep recording *includes electroencephalography* (EEG), chin muscle electromyography (EMG), and electro-oculography (EOG), which are required to stage sleep. In addition, airflow through nose and mouth, chest and ordinary ventilatory movements, and oxygen saturation are monitored continuously throughout the sleep period. Limb and body movements as well as sleep sounds are recorded with limb EMG and audio/video monitoring. This type of polysomnogram permits quantitative and qualitative characterization not only of breathing disturbances, but also of the impact of the ventilatory disturbance on sleep. Cardiac rhythm can be correlated with respiratory parameters. The association between body position and sleep stage with breathing disturbances can be documented. The contribution of not only breathing but also other monitored parameters such as movements, bruxism, snoring, seizures, somniloquy, and other sleep abnormalities can be defined.

Although polysomnographic criteria for the diagnosis of sleep apnea vary, most laboratories require at least five or ten apneas or hypopneas per hour of sleep. Other indices such as the maximum or mean fall in oxygen saturation are used to describe the severity of the syndrome.

Recently, devices for unattended monitoring of sleep have been promoted. These may consist only of a pulse oximeter and slow chart recorder or may record a number of polysomnographic channels. In some cases these unattended partial polysomnographic devices provide adequate screening for sleep apnea in the intensive care unit or elsewhere. However, if the recording is unattended special care must be taken to identify artifacts. Furthermore, if the device does not include channels to directly stage sleep (EEG, EMG, and EOG), then care must be taken to confirm that the patient actually slept during the recording. If the device monitors only ventilatory effort, airflow, oxygen saturation, and electrocardiogram (ECG), then the absence of sleep apnea syndrome should lead to further investigation if the patient is hypersomnolent or has symptoms and signs of a sleep disorder.

If obstructive sleep apnea is documented by physiologic monitoring then potentially remediable anatomic contributions to obstruction should be investigated. Direct inspection of the oral cavity to look for tongue enlargement, tonsillomegaly, or a shallow or crowded posterior oropharynx is necessary. The mandible and bite should be checked for retrognathia. Supine cephalometric X-rays and, more recently, three-dimensional computed tomography and magnetic resonance imaging of the upper airway may help to identify candidates for surgical widening of the upper airway.

Therapy

The treatment of sleep apnea syndrome should be individualized depending upon the severity of symptoms and likely complications as well as the physiologic and anatomic mechanism of the breathing disturbances. Patients with moderate or severe sleep apnea syndrome often benefit dramatically from use of nasal CPAP treatment. Success of CPAP treatment depends on adequate titration of CPAP to determine the minimum pressure required to minimize ventilatory distur-

bances and optimize sleep. Just as important is selection and fitting of the CPAP mask. With patient explanation and assistance some initially resistant patients can learn to tolerate and directly benefit from use of the cumbersome CPAP apparatus. In general, the more somnolent the patient is before treatment, the more likely it is that CPAP will be tolerated. When high CPAP pressures are required but the pressure itself disturbs sleep, then BiPAP, a machine which can deliver a higher pressure during inspiration than expiration, may be a better tolerated substitute.

When CPAP is not tolerated or ineffective for moderate or severe obstructive sleep apnea syndrome, other treatments must be considered according to the patient's individual circumstances. If soft tissues narrow the upper airway, uvulopalatopharyngoplasty may be warranted. Unfortunately, criteria to predict the outcome of these surgical procedures are still being developed. The best predictor may be three-dimensional display of airway volume constructed from computed tomographic or magnetic resonance images. Unfortunately, such imaging is expensive and only available at a very few sites. When mandibular and maxillary anomalies are defined, oral surgical procedures can be considered, but few centers can, at this time, provide the requisite expertise.

Oral appliances which are worn during sleep to advance the mandible or hold the tongue extended can reduce snoring and reduce upper airway obstructions during sleep. Unfortunately, few of these devices have been critically assessed in published reports. While these devices may provide adequate relief of snoring and upper airway obstructions, they are not risk-free. In some patients snoring is reduced, but pathologic apneas or increased upper airway resistance persist. These devices can provoke temporomandibular joint arthritis.

Obese patients with obstructive sleep apnea syndrome often benefit from weight reduction. Unfortunately, losing weight and then maintaining a reduced weight is extremely difficult, especially for middle-aged and older patients. Despite substantial weight loss sleep apnea can persist.

Mild sleep apnea, whether obstructive or nonobstructive, may respond at least minimally to treatment with certain medications. Certain antidepressants, such as protriptyline and trazodone, have a minimal beneficial effect. Medroxyprogesterone can be used as a ventilatory stimulant in selected men and postmenopausal women. However, like some tricyclic antidepressants, progesterone often causes or compounds partial impotence, so its use in young or middle-aged men should be cautious.

Nonobstructive sleep apnea usually does not respond adequately to conventional CPAP treatment. When treatment with drugs which stimulate ventilation is inadequate, other more invasive treatments may be required. Before these are instituted, medications which may be suppressing ventilation should be minimized or eliminated if possible. When inspiratory efforts are sufficient, BiPAP can be set to be triggered by these efforts. For patients with less adequate inspiratory effort, nasal BiPAP set to provide timed cycles of inspiratory and expiratory positive pressure can be used as a ventilator. In more severe cases intermittent positive pressure ventilation using a nasal mask can be effective. However, in some patients a ventilator or a diaphragmatic pacemaker must be used in conjunction with CPAP or tracheotomy to maintain a patent airway.

Differential Diagnosis

Many conditions treated in neurologic intensive care units predispose to ventilatory disturbances, especially during sleep. Brain infarcts, especially those involving ventilatory centers in brainstem, subarachnoid hemorrhage, subdural hematomas, mass lesions, and brain injuries may contribute to the development of sleep apnea. Cheyne-Stokes breathing can severely disrupt sleep architecture, causing sleep to be nonrestorative.

Polyradiculoneuritis or other causes of weakening of ventilatory muscles including muscular dystrophies and other myopathies can necessitate ventilatory support. In some cases use of patient-triggered BiPAP can substitute for or delay the use of a ventilator. Cervical cordotomies, especially bilateral, for relief of intractable pain can also trigger ventilatory failure necessitating ventilatory support. Familial dysautonomia has been documented as a cause of vocal cord paralysis necessitating prompt relief of obstruction via intubation or tracheotomy.

Sleep apnea syndrome can be caused by hypothyroidism and acromegaly. Conversely, it contributes to the encephalopathy which may be a consequence of these conditions. Alcohol, opiates, tranquilizers, hypnotics, antidepressants, anticonvulsants, antihypertensives, and drugs in other therapeutic categories may be sedating, mimicking, triggering, or exacerbating sleep apnea. Narcolepsy, idiopathic hypersomnolence, periodic limb movement disorder, depression, Kleine-Levin syndrome, and other disorders characterized by excessive sleepiness must be distinguished from sleep apnea syndrome.

In the intensive care unit hypersomnia must be distinguished from coma due to various causes, locked-in syndrome, vegetative state, akinetic mutism, and status epilepticus. Patients with hypersomnia show typical signs of physiologic sleep like yawning, spontaneous movements, and stretching. They can be awakened at least briefly and then, aside from sleepiness, have near baseline intellectual and cognitive capabilities. Metabolic workup, EEG, and neuroimaging may be required in some cases.

While sleep apnea can be a consequence of any condition which causes weakening of ventilatory muscles or upper airway adductors as well as a decrease in the level of consciousness (or increased threshold of arousal from hypoxemia, hypercarbia, or increased ventilatory effort because of increased upper airway resistance) sleep apnea may, in turn, exacerbate critical neurologic conditions. For example, somnolence attributable to sleep apnea may compound a decreased level of consciousness from any cause. Recurrent hypoxia due to sleep apnea may increase intracranial pressure and may worsen cerebral ischemia. Cardiac arrhythmias associated with sleep apnea may present additional risk.

Suggested Reading

Bedard MA, Montplaisir J, Richer F, Rouleau I, Malo J (1991) Obstructive sleep apnea syndrome: pathogenesis of neuropsychological deficits. J Clin Exp Neuropsychol 13:950–964

Biber MP (1988) Nocturnal neck movements and sleep apnea in headache. Headache 28:673–676

Cirignotta F, D'Allessandro R, Partinen M, Zucconi M, Christina E, Gerardi R, Cacciatore FM, Lugaresi E (1989) Prevalence of every night snoring and obstructive sleep apnoeas among 30–69 year old men in Bologna, Italy. Acta Neurol Scand 79:366–372

Diagnostic classification steering committee (1990) ICSD: international classification of sleep disorders. Diagnostic and coding manual. American Sleep Disorders Association, Rochester, Minnesota

Gislason T, Almqvist M, Eriksson G, Taube A, Boman G (1988) Prevalence of sleep apnea syndrome among Swedish men 30–69 years old estimated by a two-stage procedure. J Clin Epidemiol 41:571–576

Guilleminault C, Stoohs R (1991) Upper airway resistance syndrome. Sleep Res 20:250

Guilleminault C, Connolly S, Winkle R (1984) Cardiac arrhythmia and conduction disturbances during sleep in 400 patients with sleep apnea syndrome. Am J Cardiol 52:490–496

Hung J, Whitford EG, Parsons RW, Hillman DR (1990) Association of sleep apnea with myocardial infarction in men. Lancet 336: 261–264

Koehler U, Pomykaj T, Dubler H, Hamann B, Junkermann H, Grieger E, Lubbers C, Ploch T, Peter JH, Weber K et al. (1991) Sleep-related respiratory disorders and coronary heart disease. Pneumologie 45 [Suppl 1]:253–258

Koskenvou M, Kaprio J, Telakivi T, Partinen M, Heikkila K, Sarna S (1987) Snoring as a risk factor for ischaemic heart disease and stroke. Br Med J 294:16–19

Malone S, Liu PP, Holloway R, Rutherford R, Xie A, Bradley TD (1991) Obstructive sleep apnoea in patients with dilated cardiomyopathy: effects of continuous positive airway pressure. Lancet 338: 1480–1484

Millman RP, Redline S, Carlisle CC, Assaf AR, Levinson PD (1991) Daytime hypertension in obstructive sleep apnea. Prevalence and contributing risk factors. Chest 99:861–866

Ryan CR, Lowe AA, Fleetham JA (1991) Three dimensional upper airway computed tomo-graphy in obstructive sleep apnea. Am Rev Respir Dis 144:428–432

Saito T, Yoshikawa T, Sakamoto Y, Tanaka K, Inoue T, Ogawa R (1991) Sleep apnea in patients with acute myocardial infarction. Crit Care Med 19:938–941

Chapter 85

Pseudotumor Cerebri

Eric R. Eggenberger and Neil R. Miller

Definition and Epidemiology

Idiopathic intracranial hypertension and pseudotumor cerebri (PTC) are the terms most commonly applied to a clinical syndrome that is characterized by four major criteria: (a) increased intracranial pressure; (b) normal cerebrospinal fluid composition; (c) no evidence of a central nervous system mass lesion or hydrocephalus; and (d) a nonfocal neurological examination with the exception of papilledema with its potential visual sequelae and the occasional occurrence of abducens nerve palsies. Since the original description by Quincke in 1897, the syndrome has been known by many different names including otitic hydrocephalus, hypertensive meningeal hydrops, intracranial pressure without brain tumor, and benign intracranial hypertension.

PTC is rare, with an annual incidence among the general population of approximately one per 100 000 persons; however, among obese women between the ages of 20 and 44, the incidence increases to approximately 19 per 100 000 persons. The pathophysiology of PTC is unknown. Over 90% of PTC patients are obese and over 90% are women, with a mean age of 30 years at diagnosis. Numerous case reports linking various medications and PTC exist, implicating such agents as nitrofurantoin, vitamin A, isoretinoin, nalidixic acid, indomethacin or ketoprofen (with Bartter's syndrome), lithium, anabolic steroids, chlordecone (Kepone), amiodarone, tetracycline, psychotropics, and corticosteroid withdrawal. Many conditions ranging from endocrinopathies to the Guillain-Barré syndrome have been reported to be associated with PTC; however, no causal link has been established, and controlled studies have revealed significant associations only with obesity and recent weight gain. Many of the other reported conditions associated with PTC, such as menstrual irregularities, iron-deficiency anemia, pregnancy, and the oral contraceptive pill are common conditions among women of childbearing years and may represent chance occurrences.

Section Editors: Karl M. Einhäupl and Werner Hacke

Pathophysiology and Clinical Features

Increased intracranial pressure (ICP) produces the symptoms of PTC. In a prospective, controlled study of 50 PTC patients, headache was the most common initial symptom (94%), followed by transient visual obscurations (68%), pulsatile intracranial noises (58%), photopsia (54%), retrobulbar pain (44%), diplopia (38%) and visual loss (30%). Other investigators have reported similar findings.

The clinical signs of PTC are generally limited to the visual and oculomotor systems. Visual acuity is usually normal at the time of diagnosis, and is typically not affected until late in the course of the disease. Only 13% of PTC patients demonstrate visual acuity (VA) less than 20/20 upon initial evaluation. Visual fields, however, are often abnormal. Whether tested by kinetic or static perimetry, approximately 50–75% of PTC patients demonstrate significant visual field defects. Enlargement of the blind spot, resulting from swelling-induced peripapillary refractive error, is the most common defect. Other defects include paracentral scotomas, as well as both arcuate and altitudinal field loss. Constriction of the peripheral field may be present in chronic cases.

A unilateral or bilateral abducens nerve paresis occurs in approximately 10–20% of PTC patients. This is a nonlocalizing sign of increased intracranial pressure; other motility defects or cranial neuropathies are almost never seen, although oculomotor, trochlear, and facial nerve palsies, as well as skew deviation, have all been reported in isolated cases.

Papilledema is present in the vast majority of PTC cases and is no different in appearance from that resulting from any other cause of increased ICP. Disk swelling is usually bilateral and symmetric, but may be quite asymmetric or even unilateral. At presentation, one or both optic disks may exhibit a variety of changes, from blurred margins to circumferential disk elevation with obscuration of peripapillary retinal vessel segments caused by axon swelling, to the smooth dome-shaped elevation of chronic papilledema. The optic disks may be hyperemic or pale, and flame-shaped or splinter hemorrhages may be located at or adjacent to the disk margin. Cotton-wool spots may be present, as may hard exudate in the papillomacular bundle. When the ICP is elevated at the time of ophthalmoscopy, spontaneous venous pulsations are absent.

Ancillary Tests

Neuroradiology

Since PTC is a diagnosis of exclusion, neuroimaging is essential to rule out other causes of increased intracranial pressure. Computerized tomography is helpful in excluding mass lesions, hydrocephalus, or other causes of increased intracranial pressure; however, magnetic resonance imaging (MRI) has the advantage of increased sensitivity for dural sinus pathology and vascular malformations, making it the study of choice. Furthermore, MRI may reveal increased signal in the white matter, indicative of increased water content.

Cerebrospinal Fluid

Lumber puncture (LP) with intracranial pressure recording and cerebrospinal fluid examination is also necessary before the diagnosis of PTC can be made. It should be performed as soon as imaging studies confirm a morphologically normal brain. The intracranial pressure should be measured in the lateral decubitus position with the legs fully extended. Data obtained by Corbett and Mehta in an obese population suggest 250 mm of water as the upper range of normal intracranial pressure. It should be noted that PTC patients may have large variations in ICP. Thus, an isolated LP may reveal normal ICP in rare cases of PTC. Patients thought to have PTC but exhibiting normal ICP upon LP should undergo investigation for other causes of disk swelling. If no other explanation is found, repeat or serial LPs may be necessary to document intracranial hypertension. Complete cerebrospinal fluid (CSF) analysis should be obtained and must be entirely normal in order for a diagnosis of PTC to be made. An increased CSF protein concentration or the presence of cells in the CSF is incompatible with the condition and indicates a different etiology for the elevated ICP.

Management

PTC should be considered when one is evaluating a patient with complaints such as headache, transient visual obscurations, and diplopia, as well as when papilledema is detected. This syndrome is of importance to the clinician, not only because it represents a distinct etiology for these signs and symptoms and requires specialized treatment, but also because PTC is not necessarily a benign condition. Blindness or severe visual impairment occurs in approximately 25% of patients with PTC. Evidence has accumulated supporting the contention that PTC is a chronic disease, and intracranial pressure may remain elevated for many years despite the resolution of signs and symptoms. In addition, approximately 8% of PTC patients will suffer a recurrence of papilledema and symptoms after the apparent resolution of the syndrome. Thus, even for patients whose condition seems to resolve completely, long-term follow-up is essential.

PTC is best managed by a team approach utilizing the skills of the neurologist, ophthalmologist and neurosurgeon. Treatment must be individualized according to the clinical setting and patient status.

General Treatment

The initial management of asymptomatic patients without evidence of optic neuropathy includes education regarding the nature and potential complications of the condition, treatment of potential secondary causes, and a supervised weight-loss program for appropriate patients. Regular follow-up with attention to visual acuity, visual fields, oculomotor function, and ophthalmoscopic appearance is mandatory.

Patients without optic neuropathy whose only complaint is mild headache may be managed with non-narcotic analgesics in addition to the above measures. Severe headaches, especially episodic cephalgia similar to that of migraine, may respond to pharmacologic agents such as beta blockers, calcium-channel blockers, antidepressants, or ergot derivatives. Headaches more clearly related to increased intracranial pressure may respond to drugs such as acetazolamide, that lower ICP (see below). Patients with refractory, incapacitating cephalgia, even in the absence of visual signs or symptoms, may require surgical lowering of increased ICP.

Medical therapy to lower ICP may be appropriate in PTC patients who have mild visual deficits, such as minimal visual field defects without loss of color vision or visual acuity. Although there are no randomized prospective studies comparing the many options reported in the treatment of PTC, dehydrating agents constitute the most popular initial approach. The carbonic anhydrase inhibiter acetazolamide (Diamox) is the treatment of choice for most patients. Acetazolamide can be prescribed in doses from 1 to 4 g/day; however, side effects such as paresthesias, loss of libido, and anorexia often limit tolerable dosages to less than 1.5–2 g/day. Furosemide (Lasix) has been advocated as an alternative agent for those patients who cannot tolerate or do not respond to Diamox, or as adjunctive treatment for patients who respond incompletely to Diamox. When medical therapy is successful, evidence of decreased ICP in the form of resolution of headache and improvement of papilledema is usually apparent within about 2 weeks. Systemic steroid therapy, although used by many physicians in the past, is generally avoided because of concomitant fluid retention, systemic and intraocular hypertension, and multiple long-term adverse effects. Serial LPs may be used to lower ICP, but this treatment is often unsuccessful and is associated with reduced compliance over time. Other medical options remain anecdotal or limited by serious side effects. Because of the frequent association between PTC and sinus venous thrombosis, many scientists, especially in Europe, advocate heparin treatment for PTC patients until sinus venous thrombosis has been definitely ruled out by MRI.

Surgical Procedures

The presence of a significant optic neuropathy at initial presentation, or the development or progression of optic neuropathy despite optimum medical treatment, requires aggressive intervention. Several surgical procedures have been advocated in the treatment of patient with such dysfunction. The decision regarding which therapy to employ must be individualized, taking into account the advantages and disadvantages of each procedure; however, instituting these procedures before severe and possibly permanent visual dysfunction intervenes is essential.

Although subtemporal decompression was commonly used in the 1950s and 1960s, it has largely been abandoned because of the sequelae of seizures and cerebral infarction. CSF-diverting techniques employ the ventricular, cisternal, or spinal subarachnoid sites. Ventriculo- or cisternoperitoneal shunts are often technically difficult because the lateral ventricles in patients with PTC are not enlarged. Although cervical-peritoneal shunts have been employed in the past, shunts between the lumbar subarachnoid space and peritoneal cavity are relatively easy to insert and are a well-established method of achieving long-term control of intracranial pressure. Placement of a silastic lumboperitoneal shunt is currently the definitive procedure for restoring normal pressure in patients with PTC. Reports indicate that 65–100% of PTC patients experience resolution of symptoms, with stabilization or improvement of visual function following this procedure. Although the function of the shunt may be difficult to assess, and complications requiring shunt revision such as obstruction, infection, or symptoms of low pressure (e.g., postural headache and dizziness) occur in some patients, this procedure is one of the treatments of choice in PTC.

Optic nerve sheath fenestration (ONSF), first introduced by de Wecker in 1872, has been advocated as an alternative to lumboperitoneal shunting in the treatment of PTC. In this procedure, the surgeon creates one or more openings in the dural sheath of the orbital portion of the optic nerve, just posterior to the globe. Numerous reports documenting improved visual function and a relatively low rate of complications have been published. Following unilateral optic nerve sheath decompression, approximately 50% of patients experience relief of headache, and the same percentage of patients show improvement in contralateral visual field, papilledema, or both. The relative ease with which this procedure can be performed in the hands of a skilled ophthalmologist has led many to advocate ONSF as the initial surgical procedure in PTC. Nonetheless, the failure of ONSF to consistently lower ICP, the lack of long-term follow-up,

the potential for postoperative complications such as diplopia, pupillary dysfunction, and visual loss, and an approximately 20% failure rate indicate that the procedure has not been perfected to the point that it can be recommended as the procedure of choice. The exact mechanism of the success of ONSF is controversial, with some investigators favoring a filtering function of the fenestration, and others suggesting that postfenestration nerve sheath scarring prohibits the transmission of intracranial pressure to the optic nerves.

Since the swollen optic nerve requires increased perfusion pressures, surgical intervention should also be considered prophylactically under selected circumstances, such as in anticipation of potential hypotensive episodes (e.g., dialysis, or the administration of medications with antihypertensive effects). Similarly, protective intervention should be considered when accurate monitoring of visual function is not possible.

PTC associated with evidence of severe or rapidly progressive optic neuropathy is a neuro-ophthalmologic emergency. Untreated, these patients will become blind in a matter of days, and lost visual function can rarely be regained. The pathophysiology of visual loss in PTC is related to the transmission of elevated intracranial pressure to the optic nerve via its dural sheath. Increased pressure on the optic nerve produces disruption of axoplasmic flow and nerve conduction, and also carries the potential risk of secondary ischemia of the optic nerve caused by compression of its nutrient vessels. Thus, the treatment in these situations is directed at the urgent reduction of intracranial pressure, especially surrounding the optic nerves. In the neurocritical care setting, the initial treatment of increased intracranial pressure often includes elevation of the head of the bed (to improve venous return) and osmotherapy. In the PTC patient, these may be appropriate short-term measures in the setting of acute loss of visual function before a definitive procedure is performed. Attention should also be directed at minimizing co-existent risk factors for visual loss in PTC, with avoidance of blood pressure or intravascular volume extremes. Lumbar puncture is another option to quickly lower ICP while awaiting a more permanent treatment; however, the effects are short lived (hours) and repeat LPs become progressively more difficult and painful for the patient. On the other hand, a lumbar drain may be an effective means of rapidly achieving control of intracranial pressure for a relatively short period of time. This may allow the luxury of time while preserving visual function. Nevertheless, once it has been determined that urgent treatment of PTC is required, either a lumboperitoneal shunt or ONSF should be performed within 24–48 h.

Conclusion

The PTC syndrome remains a diagnosis of exclusion. Does the patient strictly adhere to the established PTC diagnostic criteria? Have all other reasonable explanations been excluded? These questions must be addressed prior to making treatment decisions.

When confronted with progressive visual loss in the setting of PTC, the neurocritical care specialist has several effective options for immediately lowering intracranial pressure. The two primary long-term surgical options in the treatment of PTC at the present time are the lumboperitoneal shunt and optic nerve sheath fenestration, each with unique advantages and disadvantages. The decision regarding which therapeutic option best suits a particular patient must be made on an individual basis.

Suggested Reading

Beatty RA (1982) Cervical-peritoneal shunt in the treatment of pseudotumor cerebri. Technical note. J Neurosurg 57:853–855

Billson FA, Hudson RL (1975) Surgical treatment of chronic papilledema in children. Br J Ophthalmol 59:92–95

Brourman ND, Spoor TC, Ramocki JM (1988) Optic nerve sheath decompression for pseudotumor cerebri. Arch Ophthalmol 106:1378–1383

Burde RM, Karp JS, Miller RN (1974) Reversal of visual deficit with optic nerve decompression in long-standing pseudotumor cerebri. Am J Opthalmol 77:770–772

Chutorian AM, Gold AP, Braun CW et al. (1977) Benign intracranial hypertension in Bell's palsy. N Engl J Med 296:1214–1215

Corbett JJ, Mehta MP (1983) Cerebrospinal fluid pressure in normal obese subjects and patients with pseudotumor cerebri. Neurology 33:386–388

Corbett JJ, Savino PJ, Thompson HS, Kansu T, Schatz NJ, Orr LS, Hopson D (1982) Visual loss in pseudotumor cerebri: follow-up of 57 patients from five to 41 years and a profile of 14 patients with permanent visual loss. Arch Neurol 39:461–474

Corbett JJ, Nerad JA, Tse DT, Anderson RL (1988) Results of optic nerve sheath fenestration for pseudotumor cerebri. The lateral orbitotomy approach. Arch Ophthalmol 106:1391–1397

Davies G, Zilkha KJ (1976) Decompression of the optic nerve in benign intracranial hypertension. Trans Ophthalmol Soc UK 96:427–429

de Wecker L (1872) On incision of the optic nerve in cases of neuroretinitis. Int Ophthalmol Congress Rep 4:11–14

Durcan FJ, Corbett JJ, Wall M (1988) The incidence of pseudotumor cerebri. Population studies in Iowa and Louisiana. Arch Neurol 45:875–877

Giuseffi V, Wall M, Siegel PZ, Rojas PB (1991) Symptoms and disease associations in idiopathic intracranial hypertension: a case-control study. Neurology 41:239–244

Gucer G, Viernstein L (1978) Long-term intracranial pressure recording in the management of pseudotumor cerebri. J Neurosurg 49:256–263

Gutgold-Glen H, Kattah JC, Chavis RM (1984) Reversible visual loss in pseudotumor cerebri. Arch Ophthalmol 102:403–406

Halpern JI, Gordon WH Jr (1981) Trochlear nerve palsy as a false localizing sign. Ann Ophthalmol 9:53–56

Herzau V (1978) Behandlung des Pseudotumor cerebri. In: Berneaud-Kotz G (ed) Versammlung des Vereins rheinisch-westfälischer Augenärzte. Zimmerman, Balve, pp 91–96

Johnston I, Besser M, Morgan MK (1988) Cerebrospinal fluid diversion in the treatment of benign intracranial hypertension. J Neurosurg 69:195–202

Kaye AH, Galbraith JEK, King J (1981) Intracranial pressure following optic nerve decompression for benign intracranial hypertension. Case report. J Neurosurg 55:453–457

Kellen RI, Burde RM (1987) Optic nerve decompression. Arch Ophthalmol 105:889

Kelman SE, Sergott RC, Cioffi GA, Savino PJ, Bosley TM, Elman MJ (1991) Modified optic nerve decompression in patients with functioning lumboperitoneal shunts and progressive visual loss. Ophthalmology 98:1449–1453

Kilpatrick CJ, Kaufman DV, Galbraith JEK et al. (1981) Optic nerve decompression in benign intracranial hypertension. Clin Exp Neurol 18:161–168

Knight RSG, Fielder AR, Feith JL (1986) Benign intracranial hypertension: visual loss and optic nerve sheath fenestration. J Neurol Neuro-surg Psychiatry 49:243–250

McCammon A, Kaufman HH, Sears ES (1981) Transient oculomotor paralysis in pseudotumor cerebri. Neurology 31:182–184

Merikangas JR (1978) Skew deviantion in pseudotumor cerebri. Ann Neurol 4:583

Moser FG, Hilal SK, Abrams G, Bello JA, Schipper H, Silver AJ (1988) MR imaging of pseudotumor cerebri. Am J Roentgenol 150:903–909

Pearson PA, Baker RS, Khorram D, Smith TJ (1991) Evaluation of optic nerve sheath fenestration in pseudotumor cerebri using automated perimetry. Ophthalmology 98:99–105

Quincke H (1897) Über Meningitis serosa und verwandte Zustände. Dtsch Z Nervenheilkd 9:149–168

Rosenberg M, Smith C, Beck R, Corbett J, Sergott R, Savino P, Schatz N (1989) The efficacy of shunting procedures in pseudotumor cerebri. Neurology 39 [Suppl 1]:209

Round R, Keane JR (1988) The minor symptoms of increased intracranial pressure: 101 patients with benign intracranial hypertension. Neurology 30:1461–1464

Rush JA (1980) Pseudotumor cerebri: clinical profile and visual outcome in 63 patients. Mayo Clin Proc 55:541–546

Sergott RC, Savino PJ, Bosley TM (1988) Modified optic nerve sheath decompression provides long-term visual improvement for pseudotumor cerebri. Arch Ophthalmol 106:1384–1390

Snyder DA, Frenkel M (1972) An unusual presentation of pseudotumor cerebri. Ann Ophthalmol 11:1823–1827

Spoor TC, Ramocki JM, Madion MP, Wilkinson MJ (1991) Treatment of pseudotumor cerebri by primary and secondary optic nerve sheath decompression. Am J Ophthalmol 112:177–185

Tomkins CM, Spalton DJ (1984) Benign intracranial hypertension treated by optic nerve sheath decompression. J R Soc Med 77:141–144

Wall M, George D (1987) Visual loss in pseudotumor cerebri. Incidence and defects related to visual field strategy. Arch Neurol 44:170–175

Wall M, George D (1991) Idiopathic intracranial hypertension (pseudotumor cerebri): a prospective study of 50 patients. Brain 114:155–180

Chapter 86

Stiff-Man Syndrome

HANS-MICHAEL MEINCK

Introduction

Stiff-man syndrome (SMS) is a motor disorder characterized by stiffness of the axial muscles and painful spasms or jerks. Although SMS is usually regarded as a neurological curiosity, life-threatening complications may occur. The most important complication is paroxysmal dysfunction of the autonomic nervous system, which can range from dilated pupils to severe hypotension and shock. Other complications, resulting from treatment with sedatives or antispastic agents, include ventilatory depression or rebound worsening of symptoms in patients having withdrawal.

Etiology and Epidemiology

Stiff-man syndrome is most likely an autoimmune disease. Antibodies against GABAergic neurons (possibly in the spinal cord) have been detected.

Section Editors: Karl M. Einhäupl and Werner Hacke

Although the disease is rare, the incidence may be greater than was once thought. SMS is diagnosed in our hospital in Heidelberg in about one patient per year (referral population about 1 million).

Diagnosis

The diagnosis of SMS is made clinically. Stiffness often develops insidiously over months or years and may continue to gradually worsen or remain essentially stable for decades. Deterioration occurs in 25% of patients and is characterized by attacks of severe stiffness and painful spasms. The spasms may occur spontaneously or may be triggered by a variety of external stimuli, such as sudden noises or a jolt to the bed, or internal stimuli, such as self-initiated movements or emotion. In some patients the spasms may be overlooked, as the joint movements are limited because of contraction of antagonist muscles. Moreover, with repeated stimulation, the spasms may habituate rapidly. Stiffness and spasms may be so severe that they result in skeletal abnormalities such as fixed lordosis. Some patients have a peculiar fear of walking over open spaces and are thought initially to have agoraphobia. Most often, the physical examination is normal except for brisk deep tendon reflexes, and patients are misdiagnosed as having psychiatric disorders. Nystagmus and other oculomotor abnormalities, proximal or distal muscle weakness, and Babinski's sign may occur.

The diagnosis of SMS can be confirmed by EMG. At baseline, a steady firing of normal motor units is seen. If an external stimulus, such as a loud noise or an electric shock, is suddenly delivered, the firing abruptly increases and then gradually decreases again over several seconds. The EMG pattern elicited from the trunk muscles is characteristic for the disease and consists of one to three bursts of activity with an onset latency of 50–80 ms. Burst activity in the antagonist muscles is synchronous, and is followed by desynchronized EMG activity (Fig. 1). The tonic motor firing, stiffness, and spasms diminish quickly or even stop with sleep (or general anesthesia) and small doses of intravenous benzodiazepines.

Neuroimaging studies can be helpful by excluding other causes of rigidity such as spinal cord or brainstem tumors. Analysis of cerebrospinal fluid (CSF) often shows oligoclonal bands, increased IgG levels (reflecting de novo IgG synthesis), and occasionally a mild lymphocytosis. There is an association with type-I diabetes mellitus, and antibodies against both pancreatic islet cells (PIC) and the GABA synthesizing enzyme glutamic acid decarboxylase (GAD)[1] are found in the sera and CSF of 50–60% of patients. An association with breast cancer has also been reported.

The differential diagnosis of patients presenting with muscle stiffness and spasms is summarized in Table 1. There appears to be a close clinical, electrophysiological, and immunological relationship between SMS and progressive encephalomyelitis with rigidity and myoclonus. This may be a malignant variant of SMS. Other conditions that can mimic SMS include axial dystonia, startle disease, neuromyotonia, rigid-spine syndrome, myositis fibrosa generalisata, polyneuropathy, vasculitis, borreliosis, multiple sclerosis, and acute disseminated encephalomyelitis.

Treatment

Treatment with benzodiazepines is effective in reducing the symptoms of most patients, although the required dose may vary widely (5–200 mg

---

[1] Requests for anti-GAD antibody testing may be addressed to:

Prof. P. DeCamilli
Dept. of Cell Biology
Yale University
295 Congress Ave.
New Haven, CT 06536-0812
U.S.A.
Fax (203) 787-3364

Prof. W. Oertel
Neurologische Klinik
Klinikum Großhadern
Marchioninistr. 15
81377 Munich
FRG
Fax (089) 7095-8883

Table 1. Differential diagnosis of disorders with stiffness, spasms, and acute autonomic disturbances

Diagnosis	Discriminating findings		
	Clinical	Ancillary	
Stiff-man syndrome (SMS)	Chronic; fluctuating axial muscle stiffness Generalized spontaneous and reflex spasms Paroxysmal autonomic disturbances Favorable response to subhypnotic benzodiazepines	Laboratory: EMG:	GAD/PIC autoantibodies Steady firing of motor units Spasmodic reflex myoclonus Reflex inhibition intact
Progressive encephalomyelitis with rigidity and myoclonus	Progressive course Largely identical with SMS plus brain stem symptoms Malignant variant of SMS?		No different from SMS CSF often normal
Tetanus	Initial trauma; monophasic course Lockjaw, trismus, risus Generalized spontaneous and reflex spasms Paroxysmal autonomic disturbances Favorable response to hypnotic benzodiazepines	Laboratory: EMG:	Tetanus toxin No or low tetanus autoantibodies Loss of reflex inhibition (silent period, jaw opening reflex)
Strychnine poisoning	Largely resembles tetanus	Laboratory: EMG:	Strychnine Resembles tetanus

GAD, Glutamic acid decarboxylase; PIC, pancreatic islet cells.

diazepam). Other drugs that may be effective are baclofen, valproic acid, and tizanidine. For patients who continue to have symptoms, intrathecal baclofen can be used. The results of treatment with plasmapheresis, corticosteroids, azathioprine, or high dose immunoglobulin infusions have been variable.

Autonomic Dysfunction

Autonomic dysfunction is the most important complication of SMS, and symptoms such as dilated pupils, tachycardia, hypertension, and sweat-

ing transiently occur in 75% of patients. Rarely, chronic symptoms such as fixed hypertension can occur. Patients may also have tachypnea and fever. Symptoms of autonomic dysfunction are usually closely associated with muscle spasms, even if the spasms are mild.

Patients who have frequent and violent spasms (status spasmodicus) may have severe autonomic dysfunction. They may eventually decompensate and become critically ill with bundle-branch block, heart failure, hypotension, shock, respiratory failure, coma, leukocytosis, and disseminated intravascular coagulopathy. Patients may be initially misdiagnosed as

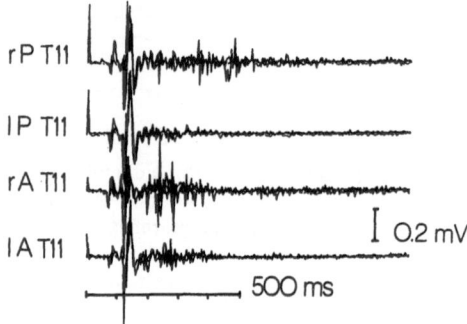

rP T11

lP T11

rA T11

lA T11

I 0.2 mV

500 ms

Fig. 1. Spasmodic reflex myoclonus in stiff-man syndrome, evoked by median nerve stimulation. Simultaneous electromyographic recording from the right (*r*) and left (*l*) paraspinal (*P*) and abdominal (*A*) muscles with needle electrodes. Three sweeps superimposed. Stimulus artifact at the onset of sweeps

having myocardial infarction (because of muscle spasm-related increases in creatine kinase), gram-negative sepsis, or acute intoxication (for example, from intrathecal baclofen). Clinically, the presence of muscle stiffness and spasms helps in distinguishing patients with acute exacerbation of SMS from those with other causes of shock or coma. The use of drugs such as clomipramine, reserpine, or benzodiazepine receptor blockers for diagnostic purposes ("provocation tests") can be dangerous.

Worsening of all symptoms and autonomic dysfunction can occur spontaneously and in patients having withdrawal from benzodiazepines or intrathecal baclofen, e.g., by equipment failure (for example, a broken pump or a leaking or displaced catheter). In the past decade, four of 20 patients with SMS whom we have been following have required neurocritical care and assisted ventilation. Three of these patients died from com-

plications of autonomic dysfunction, and in two of the patients, the autonomic dysfunction was precipitated by withdrawal of baclofen or diazepam, respectively. If equipment failure is suspected, a prompt inspection should be done. Instillation of X-ray contrast medium may be necessary to determine if the catheter is correctly positioned.

The pathophysiology of acute autonomic crises is unclear. Immune-mediated hypothalamic dysfunction has been suggested, but this does not explain the close relationship between autonomic dysfunction and motor symptoms. It is also possible that autonomic dysfunction results from the muscle spasms, or that both occur because of another, as yet unknown, reason. Treatment of acute autonomic dysfunction is similar to that associated with tetanus and includes cardiovascular and ventilatory support, the use of beta blockers, and the maintenance of metabolic equilibrium.

Suggested Reading

Lorish TR, Thorsteinsson G, Howard FM (1989) Stiff-man syndrome updated. Mayo Clin Proc 64:629–636

Meinck HM, Ricker K, Hülser PJ, Schmid E, Peiffer J, Solimena M (1994) Stiff-man syndrome: clinical, biochemical, and neuroimaging findings in eight patients. J Neurol 241:157–166

Mitsumoto H, Schwartzman MJ, Estes ML, Chou SM, la Franchise F, de Camilli P, Solimena M (1991) Sudden death and paroxysmal autonomic dysfunction in stiff-man syndrome. J Neurol 238:91–96

Whiteley AM, Swash M, Urich H (1976) Progressive encephalomyelitis with rigidity. Brain 99:27–42

Part IV

Neurological Manifestations of Internal Diseases

Part IV

The Presentation of Internal Disease

Chapter 87

Disturbances of Water and Electrolyte Balance

Ernst F. Hund, Hubert Böhrer, Eike Martin, and Daniel F. Hanley

Introduction

Total body water, which is distributed into the intracellular and extracellular compartments, makes up 50–60% of the body weight of the average adult patient. The intracellular compartment contains 60% of total body water, the extracellular compartment 40%. The extracellular compartment can be further subdivided into the intravascular and interstitial subcompartments, with the former containing approximately 3.5 l in the average adult patient (i.e., 4% of body weight). These fluid compartments are known to undergo dynamic changes depending on a multitude of factors such as solute or protein concentrations.

Mammalian cells maintain electrical potentials across membranes. These membrane potentials are achieved by creating an ionic imbalance, either via active transport of ions through the membrane or via diffusion of ions through the membrane as a result of a concentration gradient. Potassium is important for maintaining the resting membrane potential and for repolarization of excitable cells. Sodium plays an important role in the production of the action potential, whereas calcium sets the threshold of excitation.

Potassium

Total body potassium has been estimated at approximately 50 mmol/kg, and the large majority of this ion is located intracellularly, only 2% being in the extracellular compartment. Normal extracellular K^+ is 3.5–5.0 mmol/l, and intracellular K^+ is 150–160 mmol/l. Thus, the measurement of the serum potassium is a very poor guide to overall potassium status. The average adult's daily intake of potassium varies considerably, but in general it will be approximately 100 mmol. The kidney plays a central role in potassium homeostasis, whereas fecal excretion of K^+ normally is very small.

The potassium balance depends on a variety of mechanisms. Acid-base disturbances may cause K^+ shifts; e.g., in acidosis K^+ moves from the intracellular to the extracellular compartment in exchange for H^+. Insulin promotes the intracellular entry of potassium. Thus, insulin and glucose may be used to lower dangerously high serum potassium levels. Catecholamines such as epinephrine exert a biphasic effect on serum potassium levels. A short initial increase in serum K^+ is followed by a decrease caused by β_2-receptor stimulation, which enhances K^+ uptake by muscle and liver.

Hypokalemia is a reduction in serum potassium concentration and may arbitrarily be defined as a K^+ level ≤ 3.5 mmol/l. It is of interest to the intensivist because of its association with arrhythmias. Hypokalemia can be caused be an intracellular shift of K^+ that may occur with alkalosis, insulin therapy, or β-adrenergic stimulation. Gastrointestinal losses from diarrhea or vomiting can lead to hypokalemia. An increase in diuresis, especially due to furosemide or mannitol therapy, may also cause significant hypokalemia. Clinical signs and symptoms of hypokalemia include muscle weakness, paralytic ileus, neuropsychiatric disturbances, and cardiac abnormalities such as arrhythmias and increased sensitivity to digitalis.

The correct choice of management for the hypokalemic patient has to consider the rate of potassium loss. Hypokalemia occurring over hours or days may be more dangerous than hypokalemia occurring over weeks or months. In case of acute hypokalemia, K^+ should be replaced intravenously at a rate of up to 40 mmol/h using a solution containing 40–80 mmol/l. When correction of hypokalemia is done too rapidly, acute hyperkalemia may occur, which can result in cardiac arrest. When no emergency situation exists, potassium can be either substituted orally at a dosage of 40–120 mmol/d or given intravenously at a slow rate of 10 mmol/h.

Hyperkalemia can be defined as a serum K^+ level ≥ 5.5 mmol/l. One has to rule out factitious hyperkalemia from hemolysis, which may be associated with rapid withdrawal of blood through a small-bore needle. Hyperkalemia may be caused by rapid intravenous infusion of K^+ and acidosis. It commonly exists in renal failure because of decreased renal potassium excretion. Clinical features of hyperkalemia include muscle weakness and paresthesias. Most feared are cardiac abnormalities which may eventually lead to venticular fibrillation or cardiac arrest.

Treatment of hyperkalemia is initiated if there is an abrupt increase from normal to ≥ 6 mmol/l, or if electrocardiographic abnormalities occur. In an emergency situation, a bolus of calcium should be injected intravenously. A sodium bolus consisting of either $NaHCO_3$ or saline should also be administered to counteract the cardiac effects of K^+. If cardiac arrest has occurred, a third drug of choice would be epinephrine. A glucose-insulin infusion may be started. To avoid late-onset hypoglycemia, intravenous dextrose administration should be continued for several hours after the initial insulin and glucose are given. Loop diuretics such as furosemide are injected to enhance K^+ excretion. Ion-exchange resins may be administered orally or rectally to exchange Na^+ or Ca^{++} for K^+ in the gastrointestinal tract. When hyperkalemia is unresponsive to other measures, dialysis is indicated, with hemodialysis being superior to peritoneal dialysis. The insertion of a transvenous cardiac pacemaker may be necessary when atrioventricular block or severe bradycardia persists.

Calcium

The average normal adult body contains approximately 1000 g of calcium; 99% is found in the skeleton and 1% in tissues and in the extracellular compartment. Approximately 40% of plasma calcium is protein bound and thus does not participate in physiologic mechanisms. Of the remaining 60%, 10–15% exists as a diffusible nonionized fraction in a chelated form with bicarbonate, phosphate, and citrate; 45–50% is free ionized calcium, which accounts for most biologic activity. It is essential for cell membrane integrity, blood coagulation, and neuromuscular activity. There is a complex interplay between parathyroid hormone, calcitonin, and vitamin D which governs the level of ionized calcium. Normal values for serum ionized calcium range from 1.0 to 1.25 mmol/l versus 2.2 to 2.6 mmol/l for total serum calcium.

Hypocalcemia is characterized by a decrease in serum calcium concentration, which is most accurately reflected by low levels of ionized calcium. The fraction of ionized calcium is pH dependent; alkalosis can therefore reduce the serum calcium concentration. Rapid transfusion of whole blood or fresh-frozen plasma can cause ionized hypocalcemia through binding of ionized calcium by the citrate and thus precipitate hypotension and myo-cardial depression. In general, hypocalcemia is related to parathormone secretion and vitamin D synthesis. It can result from parathyroid insufficiency, which may be seen in an acquired form after neck surgery. Clinically, hypocalcemia is characterized by increased neuromuscular excitability, ranging from muscle spasms to acute tetany. Chvostek's and Trousseau's signs may be observed. The psychiatric symptoms, ranging from anxiety to psychosis, may be accompanied by cardiovascular abnormalities such as hypotension, arrhythmias, and QT and ST interval prolongation on the electrocardiogram.

Treatment of severe and symptomatic hypocalcemia consists of slow intravenous injection of calcium gluconate or calcium chloride; 10–20 ml of a 10% solution are commonly used. Additional calcium may be infused if symptoms persist. An oral calcium preparation can be administered in asymptomatic hypocalcemia, with additional supplementation of vitamin D.

Hypercalcemia is defined by an elevation of the serum calcium concentration. It may be associated with a variety of clinical conditions such as hyperparathyroidism and malignancy. The clinical features include fatigue, nausea and vomiting, and mental confusion. Signs and symptoms of hypercalcemic crisis, which is the most severe manifestation of hypercalcemia, are dehydration, renal failure, and coma. Management of hypercalcemia aims at eliminating calcium from the body. The intravascular volume is repleted with intravenous fluids, and intravenous boluses of furosemide are added to increase diuresis. In refractory cases, the administration of the chemotherapeutic agent mithramycin, calcitonin, or diphosphonates may be necessary. The addition of steroids may also be useful.

Sodium and Water

Sodium and water homeostasis is regulated by several separate feedback loops using both humoral and neuronal pathways. High-pressure (aortic) and low-pressure (atrial) baroreceptors sense blood volume and pressure and modulate vascular tone, ADH release, and the juxtaglomerular apparatus function via autonomic nerves. Sodium balance, and thus blood volume, is also influenced by the reninaldosterone system, which is activated by renal hemodynamics and the renal tubules' sodium concentration as well as cardiac natriuretic factors (which are released according to atrial stretch). Water balance, in turn, is regulated by osmotically driven ADH release. Thus, different mechanisms are at work at the same time for maintenance of sodium and water homeostasis.

Sodium salts (mainly as chloride, to a lesser degree as sodium bicarbonate and phosphate) are the main electrolytes of the extracellular fluid and account for more than 90% of its osmolality. Since water quickly crosses cell membranes to dissipate osmotic gradients, movement of sodium ions is rapidly followed by water shifts. The close interrelation of sodium and water shifts has important impacts. For example, hyponatremia does not simply indicate sodium depletion, but rather an excess of "free water". With the exception of hyperosmolar hyponatremia, a condition found after admin-istration of mannitol or in uncontrolled diabetes mellitus, hyponatremic states are accompanied by intracellular volume gain due to shifting of water towards the higher intracellular sodium concentration. Conversely, hypernatremic states always result in intracellular volume contraction. By contrast, isotonic volume changes affect only extracellular spaces.

Isotonic Volume Depletion

A combined deficit of sodium and water in the proportion present in the extracellular compartment leads to isotonic volume depletion. Although often equated with dehydration, the latter term should be reserved to describe pure water depletion resulting in plasma hypertonicity (see below). Inadequate fluid intake and abnormal renal or extrarenal losses are the main reasons for isotonic volume depletion (Table 1).

Inadequate Intake. Physiological thirst mechanisms can be impaired for various reasons. Also, a person's ability to supply himself or herself with fluids may be reduced. As a clinical rule, such elderly persons admitted to the hospital should be checked for possible volume depletion. In the intensively treated patient, fluid administration may be inadequate with respect to fluid losses, especially when not adapted for elevated body or environmental temperatures.

Extrarenal Losses. Loss of gastrointestinal fluids and abnormal sweating are the most common causes of extrarenal volume depletion. Since gastric and intestinal fluids contain significant

Table 1. Common causes of isotonic volume depletion

A Inadequate fluid intake
 1. Impaired thirst mechanisms (old age, hypothalamic lesions)
 2. Impaired ability to maintain adequate fluid intake (altered mentation, coma, tetraparesis, endotracheal intubation)
 3. Inadequate fluid administration, especially in the critically ill patient
B Extrarenal losses
 1. Gastrointestinal (diarrhea, vomiting, gastric suction, fistulas, abdominal sequestration)
 2. Insensible losses via the skin and lungs (fever, high ambient temperatures, hyperventilation)
 3. Skin (sweating, wounds, burns)
C Renal losses
 1. Polyuric kidney diseases
 2. Diuretics
 3. Osmotic diuresis (mannitol, sorbitol, diabetic glucosuria)
 4. Endocrine (adrenal or anterior pituitary insufficiency)

amounts of potassium and either hydrogen ion or bicarbonate, hypokalemia and metabolic acidosis or alkalosis, respectively, are often associated with gastrointestinal fluid loss. Secondary activation of the renin-aldosterone system further aggravates hypokalemia. Volume may also be lost by sequestration of fluids into an obstructed or infarcted gut or into the abdominal cavity in patients with cirrhosis. Disorders associated with autonomic disturbances, such as delirium, neuroleptic malignant syndrome, or Guillain-Barré syndrome, can cause sweating severe enough to result in volume depletion. Elevations of body or environmental temperatures will increase both sensible and insensible losses via the lungs and skin. Extended damage to the skin (large wounds, decubitus, burns) also can entail significant fluid losses.

Renal Losses. Abnormal renal losses are due mainly to polyuric renal failure, prolonged administration of diuretics (including mannitol and sorbitol for control of elevated ICP), and intrinsic osmotic diuresis (uncontrolled diabetes mellitus). Rarely, Addison's disease or hypoaldosteronism due to anterior pituitary insufficiency are responsible for depleted volumes. Renal losses driven by impaired renal sodium reabsorption may eventually lead to hyponatremia (see below).

The clinical features of isotonic volume depletion are those of plasma and extracellular volume contraction. The skin turgor is decreased, the oral mucous membranes are dry, and sweating is absent. Resting tachycardia, postural or recumbent hypotension, and, ultimately, frank shock are characteristic signs of hypovolemia and occur according to the amount of fluid lost. Laboratory examination reveals an increase in hematocrit and in the concentrations of plasma proteins, plasma creatinine, and blood urea nitrogen. Urinary sodium concentration may be used to differentiate extrarenal from renal losses. With renal losses, urinary sodium will exceed 20 mmol/l, whereas with extrarenal losses sodium is efficiently spared by the kidney, with the result of an oliguria of less than 10 mmol sodium per liter.

Isotonic volume depletion is treated by an immediate increase of enteral or parenteral fluid administration. When losses continue, careful fluid balancing with monitoring of the CVP is necessary to determine the amount of fluids needed, especially when the patient is not able to respond to an increased sensation of thirst because of coma, tetraparesis, or mechanical ventilation. In patients with concomitant left ventricular dysfunction, Swan-Ganz catheterization is a useful means of avoiding fluid overload.

Hyponatremia

As outlined above, hyponatremia indicates that body fluids are diluted. According to the extracellular volume state, hypovolemic, normovolemic, and hypervolemic hyponatremia can occur (Table 2).

Hypovolemic Hyponatremia. In patients with volume depletion, especially in forms caused by renal sodium loss, hyponatremia may accompany volume depletion. In such cases,

Table 2. Common causes of hyponatremia

A Hypovolemic hyponatremia
1. See forms with primary sodium loss listed in Table 1
2. Salt-depleting kidney diseases
3. Cerebral salt wasting
B Hypervolemic hyponatremia
1. Congestive heart failure
2. Liver cirrhosis
3. Nephrotic syndrome
4. Infusion of hypotonic or salt-free glucose solutions
C Hyponatremia without overt hypo- or hypervolemia
1. Syndrome of inappropriate ADH secretion (SIADH)
2. Endocrine (adrenal insufficiency, hypothyroidism)
3. Severe psychogenic polydipsia
4. Redistribution of plasma water: hyperglycemia, mannitol
5. Factitious: hyperlipidemia, hyperproteinemia

hyponatremia is usually of minor importance and reponds well to corrections of the volume deficit. For the occasional symptomatic patient (i.e., confusion, lethargy, seizures) with a serum sodium level below 120 mmol/l, some of the replacement fluids should be given as hypertonic saline until the sodium concentration has reached 125 mmol/l. Above this level, isotonic solutions are given. When hyponatremia is due to cerebral salt wasting, a condition now being more frequently recognized in patients with subarachnoid hemorrhage, sodium and water depletion is more vigorously treated. For details see Chap. 87.

Hypervolemic Hyponatremia. In edematous states such as congestive heart failure, liver cirrhosis, and nephrotic syndrome, hyponatremia is a regular finding despite an increase of the total body sodium content. The reason for this seemingly paradoxical finding is unclear, but one possible explanation has been that the "effective" plasma volume is lowered, thereby reducing glomerular filtration and increasing tubular sodium reabsorption. Volume-mediated stimulations of ADH and the renin-aldosterone system then exaggerate sodium and water gain. Hyponatremia occurring in these conditions is usually of minor significance, as the clinical performance of the patient is determined merely by the underlying condition. Fluid intake should be restricted to 1000–1500 ml per day, and loop diuretics are given under careful monitoring of the serum sodium level to reduce fluid overload. The administration of hypertonic solutions is contraindicated, since edematous patients already have an excess of total body sodium. Serial patient weights are particularly helpful for diagnosis and to assess response to treatment.

Normovolemic Hyponatremia. In patients without a history or signs of either volume depletion or overload, water diuresis may be impaired by nonosmotic stimulation of hypophysial ADH secretion or by autonomous ADH release from malignant or nonmalignant lung tissue (see Chap. 87). Other causes of hyponatremia, including adrenal insufficiency, hypothyroidism, and, rarely, psychogenic polydipsia, must be excluded. In patients receiving osmotically active solutes for control of ICP, plasma sodium is diluted by the water shift induced by these agents. The same is true in patients with hyperglycemia. Plasma osmolality, which is diminished in other types of hyponatremia, will be elevated in such circumstances. In patients with severe hyperlipidemia or hyperproteinemia, hyponatremia is purely artifactual, since significant parts of any plasma volume taken for analysis will be replaced by lipids or proteins, respectively. Plasma osmolality will be normal in this type of hyponatremia.

Hypernatremia

Hypernatremia indicates a deficit of body water relative to sodium content. The clinical features are similar to those observed in hyponatremia and appear to be attributable to dehydration of brain cells. For a clinical approach, hypernatremia is classified as due to pure water loss, to combined water and sodium loss (with water loss out of portion to sodium loss), and to excessive *sodium retention* (Table 3). Pure water loss may be renal or extrarenal.

Table 3. Common causes of hypernatremia

A Pure water loss
1. Renal (central or nephrogenic diabetes insipidus)
2. Extrarenal (insensible losses via skin and lungs)
B Combined water and sodium loss
1. Renal (osmotic diuresis combined with inadequate water intake)
2. Extrarenal (excessive sweating)
C Inadequate sodium gain
1. Excessive sodium administration (e.g., hypertomic solutions or salf-containing solutions)
2. Adrenal hyperfunction (hyperaldosteronism, Cushing's syndrome)
3. Exogenous steroids

Insensible losses via the skin and lungs may reach several liters per day, especially in patients with fever, increased respiration, autonomic dysfunction, or extensive burns. Renal water losses are due mainly to central diabetes insipidus (DI), which may rapidly cause hypertonic hypovolemia when the patient is unable to increase fluid intake. Urinary volumes of patients with head trauma or neurosurgical procedures must therefore be closely monitored to avoid this complication. Other causes of DI include neoplastic, granulomatous, and vascular lesions to the hypothalamus. Rarely, hydrocephalus and ventricular cysts may be the cause of DI. DI often complicates evolving or manifest brain death. Rapid recognition and treatment is necessary to avoid vascular collapse. Urine osmolality characteristically is very low in DI, whereas the high urine output associated with volume overload, osmotic diuresis, or administration of diuretics has a much higher tonicity, usually in the range of plasma osmolality. Similarly, hypernatremia can occur in patients with osmotic diuresis who are unable to complain of thirst or to maintain fluid intake. Examples may be the patient with diabetic coma and the neurocritical patient placed on a high-protein feeding causing urea diuresis (Note: osmotic agents, by their dilutional effect, cause hyponatremia, so that normo- and hypernatremia occurring in these circumstances strongly indicate water depletion). Excessive sweating also tends to produce hypernatremia, since sweat is poor in sodium. Excessive sodium retention can result from administration of large amounts of hypertonic solutions or of salt-containing intravenous antibiotics, from adrenal hyperfunction, and from exogenous steroids.

Hypernatremia should be corrected slowly because of the lag of cerebral cellular osmoles behind plasma osmoles. With rapid replacement of plasma water, cerebral edema and intracranial hypertension can be exacerbated. Hypotonic solutions must not necessarily be used, since in hypernatremia even 0.9% saline is hypotonic in relation to the hypertonic plasma. When volume depletion with circulatory insufficiency is predominant, vigorous treatment with normotonic saline is mandatory. When central diabetes insipidus is the cause, s.c. or i.v. administration of 2–5 units of aqueous vasospressin or 1–5 µg of its analogue desmopressin (DDAVP) will effectively reduce water diuresis, thereby decreasing the serum sodium concentration. When hypernatremia is due to excessive sodium gain, hypotonic saline (0.45%) may be used to replace, in part, additional water deficits.

Syndrome of Inappropriate Secretion of ADH

A surprisingly large number of neurological patients have disturbances of sodium and water homeostasis that manifest as hyponatremia. If neither the signs of hypervolemia nor volume depletion are present, SIADH is usually assumed to account for this abnormality. The diagnostic criteria for SIADH include a high urine sodium concentration (more than 20 mmol/l) in the presence of hyponatremia, a urine osmolality that exceeds serum osmolality, and the absence of other conditions known to produce hyponatremia (Table 4). When measured, serum levels of ADH are inappropriately high in relation to the actual serum osmolality. In fact, serum levels of ADH should be virtually undetectable in sera with osmolalities below 270 mOsm/l. A variety of different conditions are known to be associated with SIADH, acting by either tumorous ADH release, reduced left atrial pressure, or direct hypothalamic irritation (Table 5). For the neurointensivist, inflammatory CNS diseases, subarachnoid hemorrhage, and drug-induced SIADH are most important. In Guillain-Barré syndrome, non-osmotic secretion of ADH may be provoked by various mechanisms, including cardiovascular instability, pain, emotion, and resetting of the ADH osmostat due to inflammatory impairment of afferent pathways.

The treatment of true SIADH is volume restriction and maintenance of adequate salt intake. Daily fluid intake is reduced to 1000–1500 ml, allowing water losses to exceed intake and serum sodium concentration to rise. In symp-

Table 4. Cerebral salt syndromes

	Na_{serum}	Na_{urine}	$Osmo_{serum}$	$Osmo_{urine}$	Total body water
SIADH	↓	>20	↓	$>Osmo_{serum}$	↑
Cerebral salt wasting	↓	>20	↓	?	↓
Diabetes insipidus	↑	<10	↑	very low	↓

Table 5. Common causes of SIADH

A. Malignant neoplasm with autonomous ADH
   release
      Oat-cell carcinoma of the lung
      Hodgkin's disease
B. Nonmalignant pulmonary diseases
      Tuberculosis
      Chronic emphysema
      Pneumothorax
C. CNS diseases
      Subarachnoid hemorrhage
      Central venous thrombosis
      Encephalitis
      Meningitis
D. Drugs
      Vincristine
      Carbamazepine
      Tricyclic antidepressants
E. Various
      Positive pressure ventilation
      Stress (pain, emotion)
      Exogenous administration of ADH
      Guillain-Barré syndrome

tomatic patients, hyponatremia is more aggressively treated until the serum sodium reaches 125 mmol/l. This can be achieved by administering 100-ml boluses of a 3.0% sodium solution over 1-h intervals. The increase of the serum sodium level should not exceed 2 mmol/l per hour to avoid hypernatremia and its potential complications such as central pontine myelinolysis. When a concentration of 125 mmol/l is achieved, volume restriction as described above will be sufficient for further increase of the serum sodium level.

Cerebral Salt Wasting

Hyponatremia frequently complicates subarachnoid hemorrhage (SAH). Although often attributed to SIADH, sodium balance studies and direct measurements of blood volume demonstrated volume depletion and renal sodium loss in most SAH patients, a finding not consistent with ADH excess. These patients appear to suffer from salt wasting rather than from SIADH. The pathophysiology of this so-called cerebral salt wasting is not understood very well, but it may include release of natriuretic factors and disturbances of the central regulation of sodium homeostasis. The concept of cerebral salt wasting has altered the therapeutic approach to SAH. To account for sodium and water wasting, ample amounts of sodium and volume are administered instead of volume being restricted. This regimen has been shown to reduce the incidence of cerebral infarction from vasospasm. More recently, fludrocortisone 0.2–0.4 mg/day has been added to this therapy.

Cerebral salt wasting is not unique to patients with SAH. It has also been reported in brain tumors, carcinomatous meningitis, and head trauma. Differentiation of cerebral salt wasting from SIADH can be a difficult task in clinical routine. Routine laboratory parameters are not very helpful, and

Table 6. Clinical conditions known to produce disturbances of water and electrolyte homeostasis

Water

Retention	Loss	References
Hyperosmolality	Increased respiration	Anderson et al. (1985)
Hypovolemia	Excessive sweating	De Fronzo and Thier (1980)
Arterial hypertension	Diarrhea	Diringer et al. (1989)
SIADH	Insufficient ADH	Narins (1986)
Exogenous ADH	Osmotic diuresis	
	Renal insensitiviy to ADH	

Sodium

Retention	Loss	References
Glucocorticoid excess	Diuretics	Arieff (1993)
Mineralocorticoid excess	Hypocortisolism	Brown (1993)
Congestive heart failure	Hypoaldosteronism	
Liver cirrhosis	Hypothyroidism	
Nephrotic syndrome	Salt-depleting nephritis	
Pregnancy	Cerebral salt wasting	
Hypovolemia		
Arterial hypertension		

Potassium

Increase	Decrease	References
Renal failure	Polyuria	Freedman and Burkart (1991)
Hypoaldosteronism	Hyperaldosteronism	Williams (1991)
Potassium-sparing diuretics	Loop diuretics	
Acidosis	Alkalosis	
Hemolysis	Diarrhea	
Rhabdomyolysis	Vomiting	

Calcium

Increase	Decrease	References
Hyperparathyroidism	Parathyroid insufficiency	Davis and Attie (1991)
Vitamin D intoxication	Vitamin D insufficiency	Zaloga (1991)
Malignancies	Renal failure	
Thiazide diuretics	Hypoalbuminemia	
Sarcoidosis	Acute pancreatitis	
Immobilization	Transfusion of citrated blood	

ADH levels are high in both of these syndromes. However, careful assessment of the volume status is probably the most reliable feature. Weight loss of more than 1 kg/day or signs of volume depletion in the presence of deteriorating hyponatremia favor the diagnosis of cerebral salt wasting.

Table 6 gives an overview of clinical conditions that affect water and electrolyte balance.

Suggested Reading

Anderson RJ, Chung H-M, Kluge R, Schrier RW (1985) Hyponatremia: a prospective analysis of its epidemiology and the pathogenetic role of vasopressin. Ann Intern Med 102:164–168

Arieff AI (1993) Management of hyponatremia. Br Med J 307:305–308

Brown RG (1993) Disorders of water and sodium balance. Postgrad Med 93:231–234 and 239–240 passim

Davis KD, Attie MF (1991) Management of severe hypercalcemia. Crit Care Clin 7: 175–190

DeFronzo RA, Thier SO (1980) Pathophysiologic approach to hyponatremia. Arch Intern Med 140:897–902

Diringer M, Ladenson PW, Borel C, Hart GK, Kirsch JR, Hanley DF (1989) Sodium and water regulation in a patient with cerebral salt wasting. Arch Neurol 46:928–930

Freedman BI, Burkart JM (1991) Hypokalemia. Crit Care Clin 7:143–153

Narins RG (1986) Therapy of hyponatremia: does haste make waste? N Engl J Med 314:1573–1575

Nelson PB, Seif SM, Maroon JC, Robinson AG (1981) Hyponatremia in intracranial disease: perhaps not the syndrome of inappropriate secretion of antidiuretic hormone (SIADH). J Neurosurg 55:938–941

Robertson GL, Aycinena P, Zerbe RL (1982) Neurogenic disorders of osmoregulation. Am J Med 72:339–353

Sterns RH (1987) Severe symptomatic hyponatremia: treatment and outcome. Ann Intern Med 107:656–664

Sterns RH, Riggs JE, Schochet SS Jr (1986) Osmotic demyelination syndrome following correction of hyponatremia. N Engl J Med 314:1535–1542

Wijdicks EFM, Vermeulen M, ten Haaf JA, Hijdra A, Bakker WH, van Gijn J (1985) Volume depletion and natriuresis in patients with a ruptured intracranial aneurysm. Ann Neurol 18:211–216

Williams ME (1991) Hyperkalemia. Crit Care Clin 7:155–174

Zaloga GP (1991) Hypocalcemic crisis. Crit Care Clin 7:191–200

| **Renal Diseases**

G. Bryan Young

Acute Uremic Encephalopathy

Clinical Features

Although the clinical manifestations of acute uremia are not specific or diagnostic in themselves, the combination of hyperventilation, encephalopathy, and myoclonus should strongly suggest that diagnosis. Acute renal failure is most commonly caused by ischemia from shock, but nephrotoxic agents, myoglobinemia, thrombotic thrombocytopenic purpura, and other etiologies may be operative. These in themselves have neurological and other clinical and laboratory features. In general, the more acute the development of uremia, the more florid the encephalopathy.

Early mental status changes include lethargy and irritability, followed by inattention, disorientation, and confusion. Lucid periods may occur. While most patients are subdued, delirium with hallucinations, restlessness, and sleep disturbance may precede stupor or coma, especially if uremia develops very acutely. Catatonia has rarely been described.

Amaurosis was described in the older literature, but it may have been related to hypertensive encephalopathy (see below), rather than to uremia per se. Other cranial nerve palsies are rare. In uremia seizures are usually generalized convulsions, although focal seizures may occur as a manifestation of a metabolic encephalopathy. If they are persistently focal, one should consider a structural lesion.

Motor abnormalities include tremor, myoclonus, and asterixis. Myoclonus is probably more prominent than in most metabolic encephalopathies. It may be multifocal or action induced (by active movement) myoclonus. Tetany is common. Focal signs such as hemiparesis are common; they may switch sides and resolve with dialysis. Like seizures, if they remain on the same side, or are poorly responsive to therapy of uremia, a structural lesion should be strongly considered. Limb wasting, especially in the vastus medialis muscle, and muscle tenderness are common. Uremic neuropathy is rare in acute uremia but common in chronic renal failure.

Section Editor: Daniel F. Hanley

Differential Diagnosis

Hypertensive encephalopathy (HE) is the main condition which simulates acute uremic encephalopathy. In HE one commonly finds seizures and focal neurological signs in association with renal impairment. Differentiating features include: papilledema with retinal hemorrhages removed from the disk, elevated protein in the cerebrospinal fluid (CSF), and a more dynamic, fluctuating course and less severe renal impairment in HE as compared with acute renal failure (ARF).

Septic encephalopathy (SE) is part of the systemic inflammatory response syndrome. Impairment of consciousness, hyperventilation, and renal impairment are common in severe SE. However, evidence of acute systemic inflammation is present and renal impairment is usually insufficient to produce coma.

Other conditions which may cause encephalopathy and metabolic acidosis include diabetic ketoacidosis, anoxia, circulatory failure, or certain exogenous toxins such as methanol, ethylene glycol, formaldehyde, salicylates, paraldehyde, and formaldehyde. These conditions can usually be diagnosed if they are considered.

Ancillary Tests

Electroencephalography. The electroencephalogram (EEG) reflects the acuteness and severity of the uremia. The features do not differ, except in degree, from those found in chronic renal failure. Sustained diffuse, nonfocal slowing of background rhythms, especially the occipital rhythm, and superimposed, bisynchronous bursts of high-voltage slow waves in either the anterior or posterior head are the most common features. Generalized epileptiform activity is seen in 25% of acutely uremic children, but it is rate in adult uremics. Improvement in the EEG follows treatment of the renal failure with dialysis or renal transplantation.

Clinical Chemistry. Renal function is by definition abnormal. Oliguria is always present in the initial stages of acute renal failure. Serum creatinine commonly increases by 40–80 μmol/l per day, but with fever or trauma increase can be up to 160–400 μmol/l per day. Hyperkalemia, hyperphosphatemia, hypocalcemia, and metabolic acidosis are common. If water intake is not controlled, dilutional hyponatremia may occur. Hypermagnesemia may occur if the patient is taking magnesium compounds. Examination of the urinary sediment is of great value in determining the cause or mechanism of the renal failure (e.g., glomerular disease vs pre- or postrenal failure).

Pathogenesis

Since the encephalopathy is reversible with dialysis therapy, the acute uremic syndrome must be due to a dialyzable chemical that is normally excreted by the kidney but retained in renal failure. There is no consensus on the identity of the uremic neurotoxin or its mechanism of action. There are a number of chemical candidates, including urea itself, guanidine and related compounds, phenols, aromatic hydroxyacids, amines, various peptide "middle molecules", *myo*-inostiol, parathormone, and amino acid imbalance. Since each of these has a toxic effect on the nervous system, it seems unlikely that there is just one toxin, and it is likely that they all play a role. Further work needs to be done to demonstrate causation, using the criteria suggested by Massry (1985).

The mechanism of action of uremic neurotoxins is also uncertain. Possibilities include: depression of transketolase in the nervous system; disturbed energy metabolism; altered sodium transport across neuronal membranes; increased blood-brain permeability in uremia, leading to exposure of the neurons and glia to chemicals normally excluded; increased aluminum concentration in the brain (short of dialytic encephalopathy) with its various effects (see below); increased calcium and decreased magnesium in the brain. These could in turn produce dysfunction by altering neuronal chemical transmission, the balance of neurotransmitters and synaptic function, and enzyme inhibition and by impairing axonal transport.

Treatment

The first step in treating acute uremic encephalopathy is to determine the cause of the renal failure and to remedy those causes which are potentially reversible. This includes the exclusion and correction of obstructive uropathy, prerenal factors such as hypovolemia, and vascular and hematological disorders. In some cases dialysis for the removal of nephrotoxins (e.g., ethylene glycol) is indicated. An attempt should be made to establish urine flow by ensuring adequate blood volume and the use of diuretics. Management of nitrogen, water, and electrolyte balance with appropriate clinical and biochemical monitoring and maintenance of adequate nutrition to prevent further protein catabolism are all necessary. Dialysis therapy is necessary or mandatory when acute uremic encephalopathy is present or if hyperkalemia, acidosis, or fluid overload cannot be managed conservatively.

Seizures, usually brief generalized convulsions, reflect severe renal failure or sudden electrolyte changes. They may also reflect an etiology, e.g., ethylene glycol or thrombotic thrombocytopenic purpura, which directly affects the brain and the kidney, or a complication of treatment, e.g., penicillin therapy. Prophylaxis against seizures is usually not necessary, but when they occur, the cause should be identified and treated and an appropriate anticonvulsant given. Phenytoin is useful, since it can be given parenterally and is not metabolized to a biologically active substance. Protein binding of phenytoin is altered in uremia and the free (unbound) concentration in the serum should be monitored. Standard doses are usually indicated and tolerated. Phenobarbital is largely cleared through the kidney, so dosage adjustments have to be made for the reduced clearance. Valproic acid, like phenytoin, is displaced from plasma proteins, and its free fraction should be measured. Carbamazepine may cause hyponatremia and is available only in tablet form; it is not suitable for acute renal failure and seizures. Status epilepticus is uncommon. When it occurs, it should be managed in the standard fashion (see Chap. 66).

Dysequilibrium Syndrome

Dialysis dysequilibrium refers to a set of clinical features which appear during or just following a dialysis procedure.

Clinical Features

In the mildest form, the syndrome consists of headache, nausea, vomiting, restlessness or drowsiness, and muscle cramps. In moderate cases the patient has disorientation, somnolence, asterixis, and myoclonus. In severe cases the patient may have an organic psychosis, stupor, coma, or generalized convulsions. Although all ages are affected, the very old and very young are especially susceptible. Some cases end in death, either from neurological or from cardiac causes.

Ancillary Tests

Electroencephalography. Encephalopathic patients typically show bursts of medium- to high-voltage bisynchronous slow waves, usually <3 Hz. The ongoing background shows different degrees of slowing, reflecting the degree of obtundation. Quantitative EEG may provide a more sensitive means of detecting early slowing of EEG frequencies during dialysis (Arieff et al. 1978).

Neuroradiology. La Greca et al. (1982) found a consistent reduction by 20–30% in brain parenchymal density as measured by Hounsfield units on CT, comparing patients before and after dialysis. These changes occurred more rapidly with conventional hemodialysis than with the use of polyacrylonitrile membranes. Even with this density change, there was no evidence of significant brain swelling, i.e., no significant reduction in size of ventricles or subarachnoid space.

Pathophysiology

The osmotic concentration gradients between cerebral tissues and plasma may play a major role in the pathophysiology of the dialysis dysequilibrium syndrome. In a dog model, the concentration gradient was greatest 30–60 min after the onset of rapid hemodialysis. The equilibration time for the osmolality difference between brain and plasma was approximately 1–3 h. Swelling (increased water content) was 75% in the white matter and 50% in the gray matter. This, along with the above density measurements in CT, would support a net shift of water from the plasma into brain cells, as the osmolality of the plasma drops more acutely with the onset of dialysis. The osmolutes in brain tissue are higher in concentration than those in plasma during the initial phase of dialysis. There is some "lag time" before adjustments in brain osmolality can occur, partly by diffusion of some of these osmotically active particles, including urea, from the brain into the extracellular spaces and into the cerebrospinal fluid (CSF) and plasma.

Osmotic water shifts from plasma into brain cells may not be the whole explanation for the syndrome. A reduction in cortical potassium and intracellular acidosis in the brain have been reported. The mechanism for the acidosis is uncertain, but it may relate to increased production of organic acids in the brain.

Prevention and Treatment

The syndrome can be prevented by preventing the rapid osmotic shift from plasma to brain. This can be accomplished by using slower flow rates for dialysis, or by increasing the osmolality in the dialysate by the addition of urea, sodium, mannitol, or glycerol. More recently, it has been found that hemofiltration has a lower incidence of dysequilibrium syndrome and fluid balance disturbances than does hemodialysis.

Progressive Dialysis Encephalopathy

Clinical Features

The manifestations of progressive dialysis encephalopathy (PDE) include an initial speech disturbance, involuntay motor phenomena, gait disturbance, and other mental and neurological features. The major clue to the diagnosis of PDE is the above constellation of features in a patient with chronic renal failure who is receiving what should be adequate dialysis therapy (e.g., thrice weekly). PDE is commonly associated with vitamin D-resistant osteomalacia with a tendency for fractures and a severe, refractory, non-iron-deficient, microcytic, hypochromic anemia.

The speech disturbance is usually among the first signs of PDE. It is found in the course of illness in over 93% of cases. Characteristically, there is a decrease in the fluency of speech. Speech becomes effortful; this may take the form of a nonfluent aphasia, in which effortful, low-output speech is associated with word-finding problems and difficulty in repeating oral speech. Word-finding difficulty may dominate the picture; patients may use word substitutions. Comprehension is relatively preserved, but it may be impaired, along with other signs of dysfunction of the posterior speech center such as perseveration and paraphasic errors. Dysarthria and stammering are also common. Some patients have been described as having speech apraxia, in which the tongue fails to make contact with the alveolar ridge or hard palate. Syllables may be ommitted. Speech becomes slowed in order to be expressed more clearly. Writing is often slow and laborious, with omissions and misspellings. The finding of speech and language problems is often helpful in differentiating early dialytic encephalopathy from other metabolic encephalopathies.

Motor phenomena include myoclonus, asterixis, and gait disturbance. Myoclonus tends to affect the upper limbs in the early stages but thereafter becomes multifocal. The face may be involved. The myoclonus may be stimulus sensitive in some patients, brought on by movement or external stimuli such as light, sound, or startle. Asterixis, or a drop in postural tone, occurs in advanced cases of PDE. Grimacing and athetoid movements, indicating extrapyramidal dysfunction, have been described in a few patients. Upper limb ataxia is occasionally present to a marked degree. Focal motor signs are rare. Gait disturbance, a prominent and early feature, may take the form of a frank ataxia or an apraxia, the latter with small steps and difficulty initiating walking. Seizures are common in the late phases of the disease; they are mainly generalized tonic-clonic in type but may be myoclonic.

Behavioral changes appear early but may be subtle and nonspecific. Apathy, inappropriate behavior, attitude alterations, depression, and paranoia have all been described. Daytime somnolence and directional disorientation may be seen. These features are not uncommon in patients with chronic renal failure, but the *change* in mental status should make one consider PDE in such patients. In children the syndrome may be more acute and florid and consists of ataxia, myoclonus, seizures, dementia, and bulbar features (Foley et al. 1981).

Differential Diagnosis

PDE can occasionally be confused with other complications of dialysis: subdural hematoma, Wernicke's encephalopathy, dialysis dysequilibrium, and other disturbances of fluids and electrolytes including hypercalcemia (Rivera- Vasquez et al. 1980). Other diagnoses to consider include: drug intoxication, especially with benzodiazepines; depressive psychosis; degenerative conditions such as Alzheimer's disease or senile dementia of the Alzheimer type; Creutzfeldt-Jakob disease; and focal or multifocal brain disease of ischemic, neoplastic, or inflammatory nature.

Ancillary Tests

Electroencephalography. The EEG is the principal investigative test for PDE. The combination of the clinical setting of deterioration despite what should be adequate dialysis frequency, clinical

syndrome, and characteristic EEG features establishes the diagnosis. The most common EEG feature is intermittent bursts of frontally predominant rhythmic delta (<4 Hz), especially >50 in a 20-min recording. The bursts of slow waves must be differentiated from drowsy patterns in elderly patients. Sometimes these are associated with triphasic waves, which can be a helpful diagnostic feature. More specific, herhaps, is the presence of bursts of irregular, poorly stereotyped generalized spike-and-wave activity (Fig. 1).

Serum aluminum is a very rough and unsatisfactory test for PDE; PDE has been described in patients with serum aluminum levels ranging from 15 to $>1000\,\mu g/l$ ($550-37\,000$ nmol/l), but the average is $150\,\mu g/l$ (5500 nmol/l). Serum aluminum levels of $<50\,\mu mol/l$ (1833 nmol/l) are not likely to be associated with PDE, but they do not exclude the diagnosis.

The deferoxamine (DFO) infusion test is a more sensitive measure of the body's aluminum burden. DFO is infused at 40 mg/kg. Levels of serum aluminum $>200\,\mu g/l$ ($7333\,\mu mol/l$) are highly correlated with aluminum-associated osteomalacia and would also support the diagnosis of PDE. It should be noted, however, that the DFO infusion test lacks specificity, in that patients with renal osteodystrophy may have similar changes.

Pathology

The brain in PDE has not shown consistent neuropathological abnormalities. Usually, the brain is macroscopically and microscopically normal or similar to brains of patients with chronic renal

DROWSY   40 yrs

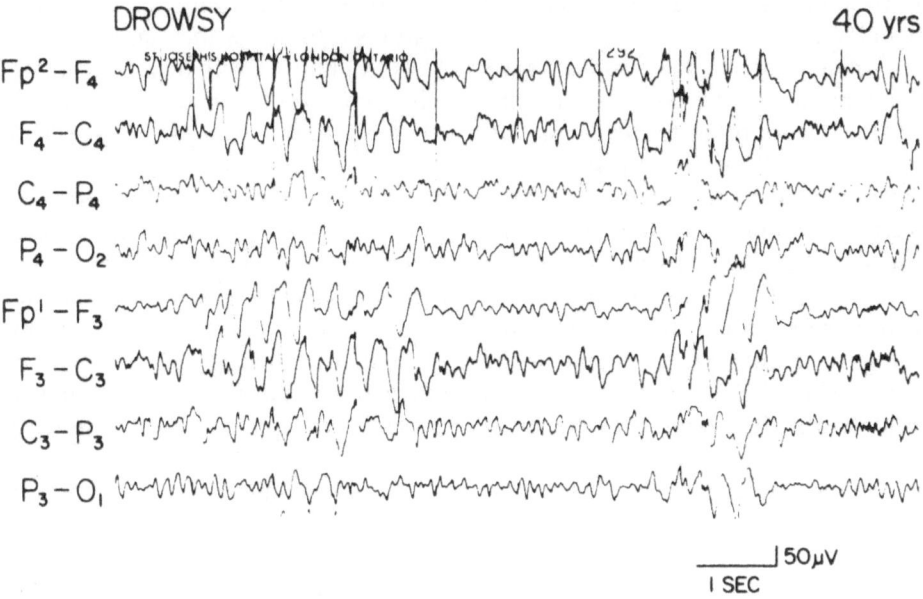

Fig. 1. EEG of a 40-year-old man with early progressive dialysis encephalopathy. Bursts of poorly stereotyped spike-and-wave activity mixed with slow frequency waves are accentuated in the anterior head. (From Bolton and Young 1990)

failure. Some pathological findings are of interest, however. A reduction in cerebellar Purkinje cells is said to be the most common abnormality; it is possible that this may correlate with the gait disturbance. Spongy change, with vacuoles in neurons, neuronal processes, and astrocytes have occasionally been found in the superficial layers of the cerebral cortex (Winkelman and Ricaniti 1986). Of greater interest, however, is the presence of neurofibrillary degeneration and/or senile plaques, similar to those found in Alzheimer's disease. These features do not appear to be merely the coincidental occurrence of Alzheimer's disease in dialyzed uremic patients: the clinical features were characteristic of PDE; the distribution of the pathological changes in the brain was atypical for Alzheimer's disease;

the neurofibrillary material more closely resembled that produced experimentally with aluminum toxicity than that found in Alzheimer's disease; and the intraneuronal aluminum was mainly intracytoplasmic rather than intranuclear, the opposite of Alzheimer's disease. Although this finding is uncommon, it does give support to the diagnosis of aluminum-mediated neurotoxicity.

Pathogenesis

There is strong epidemiological and clinical evidence that PDE is related to neurotoxicity from aluminum. Early "epidemics" of PDE occurred in certain centers, sparing others. It was shown that the geographical distribution correlated with elevated aluminum in the water supply in the areas of higher incidence. With control of the aluminum concentration in the dialysate, such epidemics are thing of the past, although sporadic cases still occur.

In comparison with other diseases, in PDE the brain shows significantly higher aluminum levels. There are a number of mechanisms by which aluminum could impair neuronal functions: binding with adenosine triphosphate, interference with phosphate transfer, interference with calcium uptake and utilization, altered neurotransmitter function, altered microtubular transport, effects on RNA and DNA metabolism.

A syndrome similar to PDE has been noted in humans poisoned with aluminum in industry, and mental and motor deficits have been produced in experimental animals exposed to aluminum. It has also been possible to reverse early PDE by removing aluminum from the dialysate or to arrest the disease, at least in some cases, with DFO, which chelates the aluminum from the brain. Furthermore, as mentioned, PDE has a strong association with aluminum-induced osteodystrophy.

Prevention and Treatment

Prevention has been effective; it is mandatory to monitor aluminum concentrations in the dialysate. Aluminum-containing oral antacids have almost certainly been a source of aluminum poisoning in some patients with chronic renal failure; many centers are now switching to calcium carbonate as a phosphate-binding antacid. Monitoring of serum levels of aluminum is of limited value, but, in general, if serum levels are well above 50 μg/l (1800 μmol/l), it is worth taking steps to prevent PDE and dialysis osteomalacia.

Benzodiazepines can transiently reverse the clinical features of PDE, suggesting that there is dysfunction of the gamma amino butyric acid (GABA) or benzodiazepine receptors in the brain. Benzodiazepines are not curative.

Treatment should be begun as soon as PDE is diagnosed, the earlier the better. In early PDE, removal of aluminum exposure via dialysate and oral intake is mandatory. DFO administration is the most definitive step in the management of established PDE. Substantial improvement may occur in about 70% of patients, and at least stabilization may occur in many as well. Symptomatic management of seizures with phenytoin or other antiepileptic drugs is sometimes required.

Suggested Reading

Arieff AI, Massry SG, Barrientos A, Kleeman CR (1973) Brain, water and electrolyte metabolism in uremia: effects of slow and rapid hemodialysis. Kidney Int 4:177–187

Arieff AI, Massry SG, Barrientos A, Kleeman CR (1978) Brain, water and electrolyte metabolism in uremia: effects of slow and rapid hemodialysis. Kidney Int 4:177–187

Bolton CF, Young GB (1990) Neurological complications of renal disease. Butterworths, Boston, pp 12–30, 44–48, 171–200

Cartier F, Chatel M, Allain P (1981) Aluminum toxicity in renal failure. In: Zurukzoglu W, Papadimitriou M, Pyrpasapoulos M et al. (eds) Proceedings of the 8th international congress of nephrology. Karger, Basel, pp 1022–1029

Chadwick D, French AT (1979) Clinical, biochemical and physiological factors distinguishing myoclonus responsive to 5-hydroxytryptophan, tryptophan plus a

monoamine oxidase inhibitor, and clonazepam. Brain 100:455–487

Chaptal J, Passouant P, Puech P (1954) Sur la
forme hypertenive des glomerulonephrites
de l'enfant. Arch Fr Pediatr 11:192

Chokroverty S, Gandhi V (1982) Electroence-
phalograms in patients with progressive
dialytic encephalopathy. Clin Electroencephalogr 13:122–127

Crapper DR, Dalton AJ (1973) Alterations in
short-term retention conditioned avoidance
acquisition and motivation following
aluminum-induced neurofibrillary degeneration. Physiol Behav 10:925–933

Foley CM, Polinski MS, Gruskin AB et al.
(1981) Encephalopathy in infants and
children with chronic renal disease. Arch
Neurol 38:656–658

Gilliland KG, Hegstrom RM (1963) The effect
of hemodialysis on cerebrospinal fluid pressure in uremic dogs. Trans Am Soc Artif
Intern Org 1:408–411

Hughes JR, Schreeder MT (1980) EEG in dialysis encephalopathy Neurology 30:1148–
1154

Jack R, Rabin PL, McKinney TW (1983–1984)
Dialysis encephalopathy: a review. Int J
Psychiatry Med 13:309–326

Jacob JC, Gloor P, Elwan OH et al. (1965)
Electroencephalographic changes in chronic
renal failure. Neurology 15:419–429

Kennedy AC, Linton AL, Luke RG, Renfrew S
(1963) Electroencephalographic changes
during haemodialysis. Lancet 1:408–
411

LaGreca G, Biasioli S, Chiaramonte S et al.
(1982) Studies of brain density in hemodialysis and peritoneal dialysis. Nephron
31:146–150

Lederman RJ, Henry CE (1978) Progressive
dialysis encephalopathy. Ann Neurol 4:
199–204

Locke S, Merrill JP, Tyler HR (1961) Neurological complications of acute uremia. Arch
Intern Med 108:519–530

Lowenstein DH, Simon RP (1992) Antiepileptic
drugs useful in status epilepticus. In:
Faingold CL, Fromm GH (eds) Drugs for
control of epilepsy: actions on neuronal
networks involved in seizure disorders.
CRC Press, Boca Raton, pp 513–525

Massry SG (1985) Current status of the role of
parathyroid hormone in uremic toxicity.
Contrib Nephrol 49:1–11

O'Hare JA, Callaghan NM, Murnaghan DJ
(1983) Dialysis encephalopathy: clinical,
electroencephalographic and interventional
aspects. Medicine (Baltimore) 62:129–141

Olthof CG, de Vries PM, Kouw PM, De PL,
Gerlag PG, Schneider H, Donker AJ
(1992) The recovery of fluid balance after
hemodialysis and hemofiltration. Clin
Nephrol 37:135–139

Pappius HM, Oh JH, Dossetor JB (1966) The
effects of rapid hemodialysis on brain tissues
and cerebrospinal fluid of dogs. Can J
Physiol Pharmocal 45:129–147

Parkinson IS, Ward MK, Kerr DNS (1979) Frac-
turing dialysis osteodystrophy and dialysis
encephalopathy: an epidemiological survey.
Lancet 1:406–409

Port FK, Johnson WJ, Klass DW (1973) Prevention of dialysis dysequilibrium syndrome by
the use of high sodium concentration in the
dialysate. Kidney Int 3:327–333

Rivera-Vasquez AB, Noriega-Sanchez A,
Ramirez-Gonzalel R, Martinez-Maldonaldo
M (1980) Acute hypercalcemia in haemodialysis patients: distinction from "dialysis
dementia". Nephron 25:243–246

Scholtz C, Swash M, Gray A et al. (1987)
Neurofibrillary degeneration in dialysis
dementia: a feature of aluminum toxicity.
Clin Neuropathol 6:93–97

Wakim KG (1969) The pathophysiology of the
dialysis dysequilibrium syndrome. Mayo
Clin Proc 44:406–429

Winkelman MD, Ricanati ES (1986) Dialysis
encephalopathy: neuropathological aspects.
Hum Pathol 17:823–833

Chapter 89

Hepatic Coma

KARIN WEISSENBORN, LUIS MARSANO, ANNA MAE DIEHL, and KLAUS KUNZE

Definition

Hepatic encephalopathy (HE) arises as a complication in fulminant hepatic failure (FHF) as well as in chronic liver failure. Initially it is characterized by minor mental and personality changes and discrete cognitive impairment. With progression there are prominent motor abnormalities, as well as increasing loss of consciousness until deep coma is present.

Because of its dramatic course and high mortality, FHF patients usually require intensive care. FHF denotes the acute onset of major hepatic dysfunction in the absence of known previous liver disease, with the development of hepatic encephalopathy occurring within 8 weeks after the initial symptoms. The main causes of FHF are viral hepatitis, side effects of drugs, and toxins (Table 1). In continental Europe as well as the USA, viral hepatitis accounts for up to 80% of the cases of FHF. The most frequent cause is hepatitis B, followed by hepatitis C, and simultaneous in-fection with hepatitis B and delta agent. In Great Britain, FHF from acetaminophen poisoning is as frequent as that from viral hepatitis. Rare, but worth mentioning because of special therapeutic aspects, is FHF after *Amanita* mushroom ingestion as well as FHF in Wilson's disease.

Compared with FHF, where the encephalopathy is one of the cardinal features, in chronic liver disease coma episodes are quite rare. Conn observed episodes of HE in five of 100 patients with cirrhosis without, but in 25 of 100 cirrhotics with clinical signs of portal hypertension. HE of chronic liver disease usually develops more slowly than in FHF. However, progression from early HE to deep coma may also occur within hours, irrespective of therapy. ICU management is required only in higher grade HE (III–IV).

Pathophysiology

Despite decades of intensive research, the pathophysiology of HE has not been clarified. It has also not been

Section Editor: Michael N. Diringer

Table 1. Etiology of FHF

Viruses	All hepatotropic	50–80%
Drugs	Halothane	30–50%
	Acetaminophen	
	INH	
Toxins	CCl$_3$	5%
	Amatoxin	
	Phosphorus	
Ischemia	Budd-Chiari	5–10%
	shock syndrome	
Diverse	Wilson's disease	5–10%
causes	Reye syndrome	
	Fatty liver of pregnancy	

Table 2. Pathophysiology of hepatic encephalopathy

A. Neurotoxins
  Ammonia metabolism (-intoxication)
  Short- and medium-chain fatty acids
  Mercaptans
  Phenols
B. Altered neurotransmission
  Neurotransmitter hypothesis
  – Alteration of serotoninergic and
    glutaminergic neurotransmission
  – False neurotransmitters
  Benzodiazepine-like substances

resolved whether or not the pathophysiology of HE due to FHF and to chronic hepatocellular failure differ in a fundamental way. Today, both are considered to be of multifactorial etiology. The main causes seem to be the impairment of the functional metabolism of astrocytes and neurons due to the effect of neurotoxins like ammonia, mercaptans, phenols, and short- and middle-chain fatty acids on the one hand, and changes in the neurotransmitter status with predominance of the inhibitory neurotransmission on the other hand. Decreased energy metabolism in HE is probably the result of decreased energy demand, rather than the cause of HE (Table 2).

Now, as before, hyperammonemia is considered to be the main cause of HE. Ammonia is primarily generated from the digestion of dietary protein and the metabolism of circulating glutamine in the small intestine. The intestinal bacterial metabolism of nitrogenous substances, like food proteins and urea, which has diffused into the lumen of the intestines is another essential source of ammonia.

Ammonia detoxification occurs primarily in the liver, where the ammonia is metabolized mainly to urea but also to glutamine. In healthy people plasma ammonia levels are regulated within a narrow range. In hepatic diseases, however, as a result of a disturbance in urea and glutamine synthesis, hyperammonemia occurs and is often exacerbated by catabolism and electrolyte disturbances.

Reduction in ammonia detoxification may be caused either metabolically or hemodynamically. A combination of both is usual, with the metabolic component leading in FHF and the hemodynamic in cirrhosis. Thus encephalopathy in cirrhotics is often named portosystemic encephalopathy (PSE).

Since about 47% of the ammonia present in arterial blood is extracted in one passage through the brain, hyperammonemia inevitably leads to raised cerebral ammonia levels. In the brain ammonia detoxification takes place predominantly in the astrocytes via the amination of glutamate to glutamine. This pathway seems to be significant in the development of HE.

Inhibition of the glutamine synthesis in rats stopped the deleterious course of experimental hepatic coma induced by lethal doses of ammonia.

The toxic effect of ammonia has not yet been clarified. In addition to inhibition of the Na^+-K^+-dependent ATPase and an impairment of Cl^- extrusion from postsynaptic neurons, the disturbance of the glutamatergic neurotransmission has recently been considered to be important.

Like ammonia, mercaptans, phenols and short- and medium-chain fatty acids accumulate in hepatic failure. With regard to the pathogenesis of HE, however, they seem to be of minor importance. The levels of all these substances observed in either animal experiments or patients with HE are far below those known to induce coma. On the basis of experiments by Zieve and co-workers, it is assumed that these substances act synergistically with ammonia in the development of HE. Phenols for example reduce the amount of ammonia needed for the induction of coma by about 25%.

More recently, changes in neurotransmission have been discussed as pathophysiological factors in HE. It is assumed that there is an imbalance between excitation and inhibition, with predominance of the latter. This may be caused by changes in the catecholamine and indole metabolism, as well as by alterations in glutamatergic and GABAergic neurotransmission. A detailed presentation of the recent findings in this field is far beyond the scope of this article. The interested reader is encouraged to read review articles by Butterworth (1992) or Weissenborn (1992). As they have some influence on therapeutic approaches, however, two aspects are briefly mentioned here.

A characteristic finding in cirrhotics is an imbalance between the aromatic (AAA) and branched-chain plasma amino acids (BCAA), with increased levels of the AAA and decreased BCAA. With regard to these changes in the plasma amino acid pattern in cirrhotics, Fischer and Baldessarini (1971) developed their hypothesis of "false neurotransmitters". It is based on the following train of thought: Amino acids compete for the same carrier system at the blood-brain barrier, and the transport depends on concentrations. The consequence of altered plasma amino acid balance is that the concentration of the AAA in the brain increases and that of the BCAA decreases. The raised concentration of tryptophan in the brain then leads to an increase in the synthesis of serotonin and thus intensifies inhibitory neurotransmission. The raised level of phenylalanine inhibits the hydroxylation of tyrosine to dopa, thus inhibiting the biosynthesis of dopamine and noradrenaline. As a result of the inhibition of the usual pathway, tyrosine and phenylalanine are metabolized via an alternative route to phenylethanolamine and octopamine. Both substances bind to the catecholamine receptor but have only a small catecholaminergic effect. Thus, according to this theory, HE can be seen as a consequence of an increase in the inhibitory serotonergic neurotransmission with a concomitant reduction of catecholaminergic neurotransmission.

The basis of this hypothesis – the imbalance of plasma amino acids – applies only to liver cirrhosis. In FHF there is an extreme increase of all plasma amino acids. The postulated pathomechanism, in addition, was also not confirmed in chronic HE. There are several studies which demonstrate that the cerebral synthesis of catecholamines is not impaired in PSE. Studies on the metabolism of tryptophan or serotonin are inconsistent. In most of them there are some indications of an increased serotonin turnover. There is some doubt, however, about the meaning of this finding for HE, since no correlation is found between the grade of HE and the turnover of serotonin. At present the synthesis of the potent neurotoxin and NMDA-receptor agonist quinolinic acid as the second metabolic pathway of tryptophan seems to be more interesting. The significance of this substance for the pathogenesis of HE, however, has not been clarified.

Currently the impairment of glutamatergic neurotransmission with HE is the major focus of research. The reuptake of glutamate as well as aspartate from the synaptic cleft was shown to be reduced in HE. Moreover, a down-regulation of glutamate binding was found. The prolonged stay of the transmitters in the synaptic cleft is thought to be an explanation for the mood changes in patients with HE, while the lowered reuptake is assumed finally to lead to a depletion of the pool, resulting in lethargy and coma.

While, on the one hand, these findings lead to the assumption that the excitatory neurotransmission might be impaired in HE, there are several results which make increased GABA tone in HE probable. Experimental results in animals indicate that a yet unidentified substance might be induced in FHF, which works as a benzodiazepine-receptor agonist and thus causes an increased GABA tone. By application of GABA- or benzodiazepine-receptor antagonists, HE in experimental FHF was improved. Later on benzodiazepine-like substances were detected in cerebrospinal fluid (CSF), plasma, urine, and saliva of patients with HE in acute and chronic liver failure. The benzodiazepine-like activity in the plasma correlated with the grade of HE. Thus, it was assumed that the GABA-benzodiazepine receptor complex may be important in the pathogenesis of HE. This hypothesis was supported by reports of the successful therapy of acute and chronic HE by benzodiazepine antagonists in man. Meanwhile, however, some failures in therapy have been reported too, so that the significance of an increased GABA tone in the pathophysiology of HE remains unclear.

Fulminant Hepatic Failure

Clinical Course

In FHF the hepatic encephalopathy may occur even in the first few days after the onset of the liver disease. Sometimes cerebral symptoms precede the first symptoms of liver disease by hours. There are reports that the first symptoms of the disease include extreme irritability, anxiety, and agitation, which may precede increasing jaundice and the typical hepatic fetor. Many patients initially complain about uncharacteristic symptoms like epigastric trouble, loss of appetite, nausea, and vomiting. With progression there are changes in initiative and mood and disturbances of the sleep pattern. Especially young patients with an acute course of the disease sometimes present with initial restlessness and anxiety, followed by confusion or delirium with increased psychomotor activity and grimacing. In less acute cases sluggishness may be the predominant symptom.

Fluctuating but differently expressed psychopathological findings predominate in the early phases, whereas in the late phases of the disease brain-stem signs and coma prevail. The encephalopathy begins with rather nonspecific signs such as irritability, anxiety, and agitation changing to signs of multifocal cerebral dysfunction such as disturbances of memory, concentration, mood, and affect, finally evolving to confusion, delirium, and coma. These signs are increasingly accompanied by motor dysfunction such as restlessness, grimacing, flapping tremor, or myoclonus. A very early sign of decompensation of motor (sensorimotor-) skill is a change in handwriting. A check of handwriting should be included in early clinical evaluations. During the clinical progression tendon reflexes in legs and arms are exaggerated, muscle tone increases, and Babinski's signs may develop. Brain-stem reflexes are generally preserved up to the last stages, especially pupillary light reflexes. This is important for excluding other types of coma. The loss of oculovestibular reflexes in the last stages is associated with a bad outcome. Different types of pathological nystagmus and eye muscle pareses do not belong to HE (but to Wernicke's encephalopathy). In some cases focal neurological deficits, e.g., hemiparesis, may develop, but in these cases particularly other causes for the focal signs have to be excluded very carefully.

As the brain stem is especially involved in HE, respiration disturbances are found early during the clinical course. During development of coma exaggerated reflexes and increased muscle tone change to flaccid tetraparalysis without reflexes.

In 10–30% of the patients cerebral (epileptic) fits develop, and it is assumed that hypoglycemia, found in about 40% of the cases, plays the major role. Depending on the clinical symptoms, several stages of HE are distinguished (Table 3).

One of the cardinal complications of FHF is cerebral edema, which can be expected in up to 80% of the patients. Cerebral edema is the most frequent direct cause of death in FHF. Usually it develops within some hours. In some cases, however, an abrupt increase of intracranial pressure may be observed. A number of mechanisms, including the influx of fluid into the brain caused by damage to the blood-brain barrier, as well as the direct damage of the brain cells and the dilatation of cerebral vessels, have been suggested to explain the cerebral edema of FHF.

By clinical assessment an increase of intracranial pressure may not easily be differentiated from advanced HE, as many of the more typical signs of increased intracranial pressure such as papilledema, hyperventilation, vomiting, and bradycardia may occur late or be absent. Loss of the oculovestibular and pupillary reflexes, decerebrate posturing, and focal or generalized epileptic seizures may indicate cerebral edema.

Since therapeutic efforts often come too late, when there is clinical evidence of brain-stem compromise, monitoring of the EEG or a con-

Table 3. Staging of hepatic encephalopathy

Grade	Consciousness	Intellect	Behavior	Motor	Psychometric
0–I	Normal	Normal	Normal	Normal	Poor performance
I	Inverted sleep pattern, insomnia, hypersomnia	Short attention span, low perception, impaired calculation	Mood changes, anxiety/apathy, irritability, monotonous voice	Incoordination, poor handwriting, tremor	Prolonged
II	Slow response, lethargy	Poor memory, disorientation for time	Decreased inhibitions, disobedience, inappropriate behavior	Asterixis, ataxia, dysarthria, expressionless face, hyper-reflexia	Very prolonged
III	Confusion, delirium, paranoia, semi-stupor	Disorientation for place, incoherent, amnesia, unable to compute, perseverations	Bizarre behavior, anger, paranoia	Hyper-reflexia, nystagmus, Babinski's signs, rigidity, muscle twitching, yawning, sucking, blinking, incontinence, hyperventilation	Unable to perform
IV	a) Coma arousable to pain; b) coma – unresponsive	None	Absent	Decorticate/decerebrate posture, dilated pupils	Unable to perform

tinuous measurement of the intracranial pressure by extradural pressure transducers is recommended. It should be mentioned, however, that such extradural pressure transducers can be safely placed only in patients with a Quick score of more than 40% and more than 40 000 thrombocytes.

Focal or generalized seizures occur in FHF, not only as a consequence of cerebral edema but also as a complication of the frequently arising hypoglycemia caused by a decreased metabolism of insulin, as well as by impaired gluconeogenesis.

Another frequent and severe complication of FHF is bleeding from the upper gastrointestinal tract (in 50%). It results from gastric ulcers as well as from coagulopathy caused by a decrease in the synthesis of the coagulation factors and abnormal platelet production and function. Whether disseminated intravascular coagulation plays a role in the bleeding diathesis associated with FHF is yet unclear.

A number of forms of renal dysfunction are seen in FHF. "Functional renal failure" (hepatorenal syndrome) is the most frequent type. It appears to be a result of intense renal vasoconstriction mediated by one or more circulating vasoactive substances as yet not identified. The morphological structure of the kidneys is not damaged. Characteristically, in functional renal failure the urine sodium concentration is below 20 mmol/l while the urine is hyperosmolar. The hepatorenal syndrome is reversible, in principle. With normalization of liver function the function of the kidneys improves, too.

Other causes of renal dysfunction in FHF are prerenal azotemia and acute tubular necrosis. The prerenal azotemia is usually related to hypovolemia, for example, due to gastrointestinal hemorrhage, ascites, or over-vigorous diuresis. As in hepatorenal syndrome, the urine is hyperosmolar and the sodium excretion decreased. In contrast, in acute tubular necrosis an isosmolar urine with high sodium concentration is found. Granulated casts indicate significant tubular damage.

Even without renal dysfunction a derangement of the acid-base homeostasis must be expected in FHF. Respiratory alkalosis is the most common form of acid-base disturbance and is probably caused by a direct stimulation of the respiratory center by unidentified substances accumulating in liver failure. Vomiting, gastric aspiration, and hypokalemia may result in metabolic alkalosis, while a depression of the respiratory center related to increased intracranial pressure can lead to respiratory acidosis. An increase of serum lactate caused by impaired peripheral perfusion and decreased lactate metabolism by the liver results in metabolic acidosis.

In 80% of the patients with FHF a significant systemic hypotension with the systolic blood pressure below 80 mmHg is observed. In many cases hypotension may be explained by hemorrhage, cardiac or respiratory complications, or the effect of therapeutic interventions like extracorporeal perfusion. However, in 60% of the cases such causes are not present. Hypotension in FHF is characterized by peripheral vasodilatation, relative bradycardia, and normal cardiac output. Pulmonary wedge pressure and central venous pressure are normal. Factors thought to be responsible for the hypotension are endotoxinemia and increased intracranial pressure, as well as increased capillary permeability. The result is tissue hypoxia and lactic acidosis.

Diagnostic Procedures

The symptoms of encephalopathy seen in FHF are nonspecific. Any other metabolic or toxic coma may present with similar clinical signs. Medical history, the results of the clinical examination, the obligatory hepatic fetor, and characteristic laboratory findings support rapid diagnosis. Typical laboratory findings are maximal increase of serum bilirubin as well as serum transaminases; an increase of the prothrombin time, the partial thromboplastin time, and thrombin time; decreased serum glucose, choline esterase, and albumin levels; an increase in plasma ammonia and serum lactate; and acid-base derangements. Serum transaminases may normalize with extensive liver cell necrosis.

Evaluation of bilirubin, transaminases, BUN, and creatinine should be performed once daily, that of electrolytes, glucose, and coagulation factors every 4–6 h. Serum glucose should be controlled immediately in deterioration of consciousness.

Specific etiologies of liver failure should be identified by serologic tests (IgM anti-HBc, anti-HBc, HBV-DNS, HBs-AG, IgM anti-HAV, IgM anti-HDV, anti-HCV). If there are any indications of acetaminophen intoxication plasma levels should be determined. In FHF of unknown origin serum copper should also be examined.

In view of the extremely bad prognosis of acute on chronic liver disease, cirrhosis should be excluded by ultrasound; if present, transplantation should be considered soon.

In the case of acute deterioration of consciousness, besides hypoglycemia and cerebral edema, intracranial bleeding (cerebral hemorrhage as well as subdural hematoma) resulting from the coagulopathy must be considered and should be excluded by cranial computer tomography (CCT).

Follow-up examinations should be performed, not only clinically but also electroencephalographically. In higher grade encephalopathy the EEG usually shows a significant slowing of the general activity, as well as characteristic 2–3/s waves, predominantly in the frontal and temporal leads. In the individual case EEG parallels the clinical course. Continuous EEG monitoring may be of special value, since the EEG is thought to be able to indicate an increase of ICP by further slowing. In specialized units where the facility exists, direct ICP monitoring with an extradural pressure transducer can be employed after correction of any coagulopathy.

In general, the patients should be admitted to the intensive care unit as soon as the diagnosis is made. Transfer to a specialized center with the capacity for liver transplantation should be facilitated whenever possible.

It is not useful to define a rigid monitoring system for patients with FHF. In each patient, however, hemodynamic monitoring by a Swan-Ganz catheter and arterial line should be performed. An exact balance of fluid intake and excretion is essential. Arterial blood gases must routinely be checked. Some clinicians advocate daily cultures of biological fluids, since the usual signs of sepsis may be absent in the patient with FHF.

Therapy

The main therapeutic aspects in FHF are replacement of fluid, glucose, electroytes, and coagulation factors, reduction of plasma ammonia, and management of the increased ICP. Usually, the patients are nourished parenterally by infusion of 20–40% glucose solutions. Fructose, sorbit, and xylitol are contraindicated. The use of amino acid solutions is disputed, since the levels of plasma amino acids are elevated in FHF and additional amino acids might increase ammonia production. The infusion of fat is also not advisable.

To reduce the formation and resorption of toxic substances in the intestines resulting from gastrointestinal bleeding or intestinal protein metabolism, retention enemas with 250 ml of lactulose in 750 ml electrolyte solution are recommended. Additionally, neomycin in a daily dose of 3×2 g is administered.

The coagulopathy should be corrected by the infusion of fresh-frozen plasma (FFP). The resulting fluid overload may be treated by plasma exchange or diuretics. The risk of an adult respiratory distress syndrome (ARDS) that complicates repeated intravenous infusion of FFP is reported to be avoided by infusion of the plasma into the femoral artery. Plasma exchange with 3–4 l FFP is recommended daily until the Quick score is no longer under 25% or the patient is awake. In the case of hemorrhage necessitating transfusion, fresh blood should be used. In thrombopenia of less than 50 000/mm^3 thrombocytes must be given.

Sustained hypotension with systolic blood pressure of less than 90 mmHg should initially be treated by volume, with simultaneous control of the central venous as well as the pulmonary wedge pressure. In case of no response, dopamine is used.

Since gastrointestinal bleeding is the second most common cause of death in FHF, prophylaxis for gastric ulcers with H$_2$-antagonists is essential in these patients. Administration of H$_2$-antagonists significantly reduces the frequency of GI hemorrhage in FHF. Moreover, it was observed that ranitidine may reduce the ICP by about 10–15 mmHg.

The recommended therapy for cerebral edema, however, is the administration of a 20% solution of mannitol (1 g/kg body weight) as bolus if the ICP exceeds 30 mmHg for more than 5 min. If there is no facility for continuous ICP monitoring 100 ml of 20% mannitol should be given each hour. In the case of renal failure or lack of response mannitol is contraindicated. Steroids are ineffective.

In the past there were several approaches to providing artificial hepatic support. The results were disappointing. With regard to the coagulopathy, necessitating the administration of FFP, as well as to the electrolyte and body fluid disturbances, however, plasma exchange and hemodialysis are recommended.

Despite the maximal supportive care, 80–90% of patients with FHF die. The fatal outcome of the disease seems to be averted by liver transplantation. It is suggested that liver transplantation might improve survival rates to 60–65%. In spite of these impressive data, the indication for transplantation should be considered carefully. Survival in FHF varies between 5 and 40%. In those patients who survive restitution of hepatic parenchyma and liver function is almost complete. On the other hand, long-term follow-up studies after transplantation in FHF are lacking. Moreover, transplantation requires life-long immunosuppression.

Thus, research today is focused on the definition of prognostic factors in FHF. Patients with Wilsons's disease presenting as FHF and patients with Budd-Chiari syndrome and FHF are thought to be good candidates for liver transplantation. In the other patients, mainly age and initial response to supportive therapy influence the decision. Transplantation should be considered especially in those cases with rapid deterioration of the neurological status, a decrease of factor V below 20%, patient's age above 40 years or less than 11 years, plasma bilirubin >300 μmol/l, and liver disease with known high mortality (halothane hepatitis, hepatitis C, simultaneous hepatitis B and D infection, acute on chronic liver disease). Today there are no valid guidelines for transplantation in FHF.

Specific Therapeutic Interventions

Specific therapeutic interventions are needed in FHF caused by acetaminophen intoxication or *Amanita* mushroom ingestion. About 10 g of acetaminophen induces liver necrosis. First symptoms of liver disease occur 48 h after ingestion of the drug. Initial therapy includes gastric lavage and forced diarrhea to eliminate substance not yet resorbed. Additionally, N-acetylcysteine is administered, which binds and inactivates the acetaminophen metabolites; in adults initially a rapid infusion of 150 mg/kg body weight diluted with a glucose solution

should be given. Another 50 mg/kg body weight should be infused within the next 4 h and an additional 100 mg/kg during the following 16 h.

Liver failure with *Amanita* mushroom ingestion also occurs after 48 h. It is accompanied by renal failure. Therapy consists in repeated gastric lavage, forced diuresis and diarrhea, enemas, and the ingestion of activated charcoal. The toxin's absorption by the liver is counteracted by the administration of penicillin G (1 000 000 IU/kg body weight/day for 3 days). Additionally, charcoal hemoperfusion is recommended.

HE in Chronic Liver Disease

Clinical Course

Acute episodes of encephalopathy are more frequent in patients with chronic liver disease than in those with FHF. Because it is caused by the portocaval bypass, HE in these patients is called portosystemic encephalopathy. The clinical symptoms of PSE generally resemble those of HE in FHF. It should be mentioned, however, that the irritability and anxiety seen especially in young patients with FHF are rare in PSE, and that epileptic seizures are usually not a symptom of PSE. Cerebral edema also is rare in PSE and was found at autopsy in only 10–30% of the patients who died in hepatic coma caused by cirrhosis.

PSE usually develops more slowly than encephalopathy in FHF. Disturbances of the sleep-wake cycle, discrete personality changes often noticed only by family members, and minimal cognitive deficits not detectable by clinical examination are the initial symptoms. They are followed by changes of the patient's initiative, psychomotor retardation, and flattening of affect. Later on, as in FHF, loss of orientation, neuromuscular symptoms like flapping tremor, ataxia, dysarthria, hyper- or hyporeflexia, extrapyramidal symptoms, signs of pyramidal tract lesions, grasping, sucking and increasing loss of consciousness leading to coma can be observed (Table 3).

A special type of PSE has recently been defined. It is called subclinical or latent encephalopathy and is characterized by psychometrically or neurophysiologically evident impairment of cerebral function without clinical symptoms of encephalopathy. This special type of HE will not be further discussed here, since it is not important with regard to intensive care.

Diagnostic Procedures

Diagnosis of PSE is usually evident from medical history, characteristic symptoms of cirrhosis, and the typical laboratory findings. Difficulties may arise in patients with moderate liver dysfunction in whom a PSE episode is set off by gastric hemorrhage or excessive protein ingestion while clinical signs of liver disease are missing. In these cases the diagnosis of PSE cannot be made before other causes of organic psychosis have been excluded and laboratory examinations, including the measurement of ammonia and methionine, are performed.

If there is an acute or subacute deterioration of consciousness in cirrhotics the presence of intracranial hemorrhage, especially of a chronic subdural hematoma, must be con-

sidered. Thus, CCT should be performed. On the other hand, other metabolic causes like hypo- or hyperglycemia, acid-base and electrolyte disturbances, or uremia have to be ruled out. In alcoholics a withdrawal syndrome or Wernicke-Korsakoff syndrome should be considered.

Diagnosis is usually based on the clinical and laboratory findings. Often an EEG is additionally performed. However, it does not really facilitate diagnosis because the slowing and even the characteristic frontal 2–3/s waves are not specific for HE but can also be seen in several other, especially metabolic, diseases.

Therapy

Most of the PSE episodes occur as a consequence of dietary mistakes, gastrointestinal hemorrhage, infection, alkalosis, or hypokalemia with diuretic therapy or administration of sedatives. In several cases the elimination of the causative factor is sufficient for the reversal of PSE (Fig. 1). If no trigger can be identified, additional measures for the reduction of the production and resorption of ammonia have to be instituted. As the most frequent cause of a "spontaneous" PSE episode is a limited protein tolerance, it is sensible first to prescribe a protein-free diet for several days and then slowly increase the protein intake again from approximately 20 g/day, increasing by 10 g/day weekly, up to at least 50 g/day, then if possible 60–70 g/day. If the protein tolerance is limited to below 60 g/day it can be improved by the use of vegetable instead of animal protein. However, in fact, a wholly vegetarian diet is not usually accepted by the

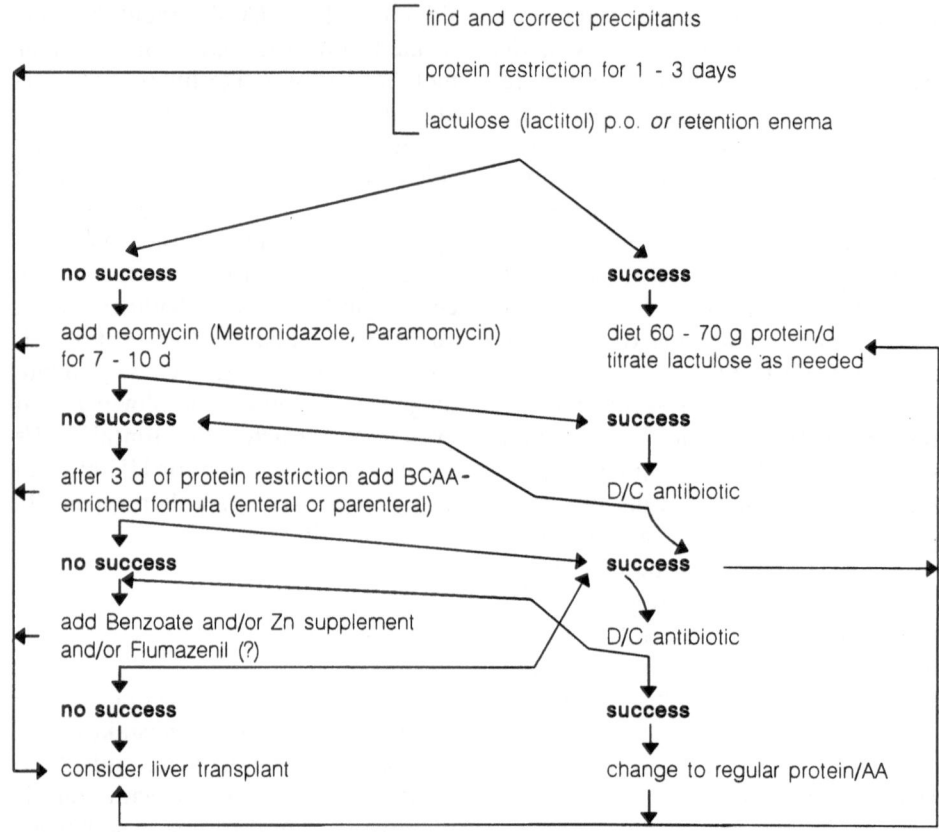

find and correct precipitants

protein restriction for 1 - 3 days

lactulose (lactitol) p.o. *or* retention enema

no success

add neomycin (Metronidazole, Paramomycin) for 7 - 10 d

success

diet 60 - 70 g protein/d
titrate lactulose as needed

no success

after 3 d of protein restriction add BCAA-enriched formula (enteral or parenteral)

success

D/C antibiotic

no success

add Benzoate and/or Zn supplement and/or Flumazenil (?)

success

D/C antibiotic

no success

consider liver transplant

success

change to regular protein/AA

Fig. 1. Treatment of HE of chronic liver failure

patients because of flatulence and repletion. Alternatively, the protein may be replaced in part by a mixture of BCAAs, which can produce a positive nitrogen balance to approximately the same order of magnitude as a corresponding amount of food protein without precipitating HE.

Simultaneous with protein restriction, lactulose (or lactitol) is prescribed which significantly reduces the intestinal ammonia synthesis and thereby leads to a drop in plasma ammonia levels. The drug is given orally in doses which produce two to three soft stools a day. Administration of 60–150 ml lactulose or 10–40 g

lactitol is usually required. As in FHF, initially retention enemas with lactulose can also be given.

If with lactulose no satisfactory result is achieved, 2 g of neomycin three times a day are administered. Both substances are potent in reducing plasma ammonia levels. Because of fewer side effects lactulose is preferred to neomycin. By combining both drugs an additive effect is achieved. Metronidazole or paramomycin have been used instead of neomycin. However, today there are no controlled studies on their efficacy.

Recently there have been new approaches to PSE therapy such as the administration of BCAA, zinc sulphate or acetate, sodium benzoate or phenylacetate, ornithin-aspartate and benzodiazepine antagonists. The use of these new measures is still disputed.

Because of their relation to new concepts of the pathophysiology of HE the therapeutic attempts with benzodiazepine-receptor antagonists like flumazenil will be discussed. There are predominantly case reports and uncontrolled studies on the use of flumazenil in HE. A synopsis of these reports showed that about two thirds of the patients improved after the administration of flumazenil – at least for minutes or hours. A recent controlled study, however, did not show any effect. The evaluation of benzodiazepine-receptor antagonists in HE therapy is complicated by the fact that most patients have been treated with benzodiazepines a short time before the PSE episode occurs. In cirrhotics, however, benzodiazepine metabolites persist for up to 2 months. It may be assumed, therefore, that the therapeutic success with flumazenil is, on the whole, based on the antagonization of previously applied benzodiazepines. Spectacular improvements in HE are reported in patients with evidence of prior use of benzodiazepines. Thus flumazenil could find a therapeutic niche in the reversal of PSE precipitated by benzodiazepines.

Flumazenil is given intravenously. There are no rules for the initial dose. Reported are single doses of 0.2–0.3 mg given every 1–3 min for a total dose of 2 mg, as well as an infusion of 2 mg in 15 min. In case of a response the infusion should be continued with a dose of 0.4–1 mg/h. Duration and dosage are determined by the clinical response.

The prognosis of PSE episodes is infinitely better than that of FHF. Usually patients with cirrhosis do not die of PSE but of gastrointestinal bleeding, cardiovascular complications, renal failure, or infections. Nevertheless, PSE has prognostic relevance, since 1 year after the first PSE episode only 50%, and 5 years after only 20% of the patients are still alive.

Suggested Reading

Bansky G, Meier PJ, Riederer E, Walser H, Ziegler WH, Schmid M (1989) Effects of the benzodiazepine-receptor antagonist flumazenil in hepatic encephalopathy in humans. Gastroenterology 97:744–750

Basile AS, Skolnick P, Jones EA (1991) Benzodiazepine-receptor ligands and hepatic encephalopathy: electrophysiological and neurochemical studies. In: Bengtsson F, Jeppsson B, Almdal T, Vilstrup H (eds) Progress in hepatic encephalopathy and metabolic nitrogen exchange. CRC Press, Boca Raton, pp 131–136

Bengtsson F (1991) Round-table discussion on brain monoamines: some personal reflections. In: Bengtsson F, Jeppsson B, Almdal T, Vilstrup H (eds) Progress in hepatic encephalopathy and metabolic nitrogen exchange. CRC Press, Boca Raton, pp 233–239

Bergeron M, Pomier Layrargues G, Butterworth RF (1989a) Aromatic and branched-chain amino acids in autopsied brain tissue from cirrhotic patients with hepatic encephalopathy. Metab Brain Dis 4:169–176

Bergeron M, Reader TA, Pomier Layrargues G, Butterworth RF (1989b) Monoamines and metabolites in autopsied brain tissue from cirrhotic patients with hepatic encephalopathy. Neurochem Res 14:853–859

Bernau J, Rueff B, Benhamou JP (1986) Fulminant and subfulminant liver failure: definitions and causes. Semin Liver Dis 6:97–106

Brunner G (1991) Diagnose und Therapie des fulminanten Leberversagens. Internist (Berl) 32:256–261

Butterworth RF (1992) Pathogenesis and treatment of portal-systemic encephalopathy: an update. Dig Dis Sci 37:321–327

Conn HO, Lieberthal MM (eds) (1979) The hepatic coma syndrome and lactulose. Williams and Wilkins, Baltimore

Fischer JE, Baldessarini RJ (1971) False neurotransmitters and hepatic failure. Lancet 2: 75–80

Grüngreiff K, Wolf G, Schmidt W, Franke D, Kleine FD (1991) High-affinity uptake of transmitter glutamate (GLU) in brain tissue with reference to hepatic encephalopathy (HE). Z Gastroenterol 29 [Suppl 2]:95–100

Hindfelt B, Plum F, Duffy TE (1977) Effect of acute ammonia intoxication on cerebral metabolism in rats with portocaval shunts. J Clin Invest 59:386–396

Hütteroth TH, Meyer zum Büschenfelde KH (1988) Akutes Leberversagen. In: Schuster HP, Schölmerich P, Schönborn H, Baum PP (eds) Intensivmedizin. Innere Medizin, Neurologie, Reanimation, Intoxikationen. Thieme, Stuttgart, pp 281–292

Manns MP (1991) Akutes Leberversagen: Definition, Ätiologie, klinisches Bild und Prognose. Z Gastroenterol [Verh] 26:7–9

Martin P, Pappas SC (1990) Fulminant hepatic failure. Dig Dis 8:128–151

Morgan MY (1991) The treatment of chronic hepatic encephalopathy. Hepatogastroenterology 38:377–387

O'Grady JG, Gimson AES, O'Brien CJ, Pucknell A, Hughes RD, Williams R (1988) Controlled trials of charcoal hemoperfusion and prognostic factors in fulminant hepatic failure. Gastroenterology 94:1186–1192

Zieve L (1984) Role of synergism in the pathogenesis of hepatic encephalopathy. In: Capocaccia L, Fischer JE, Rossi-Fanelli F (eds) Hepatic encephalopathy in chronic liver failure. Plenum, New York, pp 15–23

Weissenborn K (1992) Recent developments in the pathophysiology and treatment of hepatic encephalopathy. In: Shields R (ed) Baillieres clinical gastroenterology: portal hypertension, vol 6 (3). Baillière Tindall, London, pp 609–630

Chapter 90

Neurological Symptoms Associated with Endocrine Diseases

CHRISTIAN WÜSTER and DANIEL F. HANLEY

Diabetes Mellitus

Diabetic Ketoacidosis

Definition

Diabetic ketoacidosis is often the first manifestation of previously undiagnosed diabetes mellitus. In patients with known diabetes it may be due to inadequate exogenous insulin. This deficiency might be exaggerated by various precipitating factors such as infection, surgery, gastrointestinal disease with persisting nausea, myocardial infarction, stroke, or glucocorticoid treatment. In some patients ketoacidosis occurs due to dietary insults, poor compliance, or inadequate patient education.

Pathophysiology

Diabetic ketoacidosis is due to acute insulin deficiency leading to increased lipolysis from adipose and protein breakdown from muscle tissues. The resulting aminoacids and free fatty

acids will be hepatically metabolized to ketones and this is followed by metabolic acidosis. This effect is potentiated by the increased concentrations of anti-insulin hormones such as corticosteroids, catecholamines, glucagon, and growth hormone. Insulin deficiency also leads to a diminished peripheral utilization of glucose and ketones. The hyperglycemia leads to glucosuria, hyperosmolarity, and intravascular volume depletion. Severe hyperosmolarity (>330 mosmol) is closely correlated with the degree of coma.

Signs and Symptoms

Patients usually present with a history of polyuria, polydipsia, polyphagia, and recent weight loss. These symptoms are aggravated by marked fatigue, nausea, vomiting, and anorexia. Patients slowly lose consciousness. This varies from slight drowsiness to profound lethargy; deep coma is rare. The rapid, deep respiration of Kussmaul is pathognomonic. The "fruity" odor of acetone on the breath strongly suggests the diagnosis. On examination the patient shows signs of dehydration,

---

Section Editor: Daniel F. Hanley

Table 1. Typical laboratory findings in patients with acute complications of diabetes

	Diabetic ketoacidosis	Hyperglycemic nonketotic coma	Hypoglycemia	Lactic acidosis
Glucose (mg/dl)	300–600	800–1200	<40	40– > 300
Sodium (mmol/l)	120–130	125–135		
Potassium (mmol/l)	>4.5	>4.5	Normal	Normal
Bicarbonate (mmol/l)	<10	>15	Normal	<10
Osmolality (mosmol/kg serum water)	<320	>330	Normal	Normal
pH	<7.2	Normal	Normal	<7.2
Ketones (mmol/l)	8– > 15	Normal	Normal	Normal
Lactate (mmol/l)	Normal	Normal	Normal	>6

and sometimes tachycardia and hypertension. The typical laboratory values are shown in Table 1. Glycosuria, ketonuria, hyperglycemia, ketonemia, low arterial blood pH, and low plasma bicarbonate should help to make the diagnosis. The differential diagnosis is that of any coma, especially of hypoglycemia, which is solved in an emergency by the intravenous administration of glucose. This will rapidly wake up the hypoglycemic patient, but will not alter serum glucose or the prognosis of the ketoacidotic or hyperosmolar patient.

Treatment

Treatment is always on the intensive care unit because of the possibility of acute cardiovascular complications (e.g., ventricular fibrillation) due to fast intra- and extracellular electrolyte exchange, which also involves cardiac cells. Furthermore, cerebral edema and cardiac shock have to be avoided.

The general lines of treatment are as follows:

Central venous catheter, or, in the case of cardiovascular collapse, a Swan-Ganz catheter, several peripheral intravenous infusion sites to insure fluid replacement; gastric intubation with aspiration of gastric secretions; an indwelling bladder catheter.

Fluid replacement. Usually 4–5 l have to be replaced within the first 4–5 h, possibly faster, according to central venous or pulmonary arteric pressure. When blood glucose reaches 250 mg/dl, fluids should be given as 5% glucose in order to prevent hypoglycemia and cerebral edema, which could result from to rapid decline of blood glucose.

Insulin. Bolus: 0.3 IU/kg body weight regular insulin i.v. Continously: 0.1 IU/kg/h i.v.; if blood glucose falls less than 10% in the first hour, give another bolus and increase continuous dose.

Regular monitoring of blood pressure, pulse, ECG, blood gases, respiration rate, electrolytes, glucose, and routine blood chemistry.

Potassium. After initiation of insulin and fluid treatment and normalization of acidosis, a potassium influx from the extracellular space into cells is initiated, which is followed by a fast drop in extracellular potassium. Substitution should be carried out by a continuous independent infusion pump at a rate of 5–20 mmol/h and should start when serum levels are still above 4.5 mmol/l. The premature administration of potassium before insulin has begun to act may cause fatal hyperkalemia, while later, when insulin is acting, failure to administer potassium may lead to fatal hypokalemia in potassium-depleted patients. Monitoring of T-waves on the ECG can be useful, as flattened T-waves may be a sign of hypokalemia.

Sodium bicarbonate. 50 mmol should be given when blood pH is below 7.1.

Phosphate substitution is necessary when serum phosphate is below 0.5 mmol/l; about 50 mmol potassium or sodium phosphate solution should be given over 8 h; hypocalcemia may develop, but tetany is rarely seen.

Prognosis

Adequate treatment with insulin, fluids, and potassium have significantly reduced the mortality associated with diabetic ketoacidosis. However, if ketoacidosis is complicated by other diseases, such as cardiovascular pathologies, it still can be a cause of death, especially in elderly people. In these patients the mortality rate may be as high as 5%–10%. Danger may result from missing signs and changes in a patient's condition during treatment, such as failure to improve in mental status, continued hypotension with minimal urine flow, or prolonged ileus (which may suggest infarction of mesenteric arteries). Patients with known diabetes mellitus should be trained in measuring ketonuria and taught to take adequate action in case of persisting ketonuria, especially when vomiting develops.

Hyperosmolar, Nonketotic Diabetic Coma

Definition and Pathophysiology

This is the typical complication of type 2 noninsulin-dependent diabetes mellitus (NIDDM) in the elderly. It most frequently occurs in the case of intercurrent diseases, where hepatic glucose production is increased due to secondary stress hormones. The fluid intake is usually diminished, leading to a decrease in extracellular fluid and plasma volume. This results in a decreased capacity to excrete glucose in the urine as urine volume falls. Due to intracellular dehydration, central nervous system dysfunction develops, leading to further impairment of fluid intake. The presence of even small amounts of insulin is believed to prevent the development of ketosis by inhibiting lipolysis in adipose tissues.

Signs and Symptoms

The predominant signs in nonketotic diabetic coma are weakness, polyuria, and polydipsia, which develop slowly over several days. Patients often have a history of reduced fluid intake, sometimes due to other, often more severe illness such as pneumonia or abdominal abscess. Myocardial infarctions, stroke, or acute pancreatitis can also be accompanied by this event.

On examination the patient shows signs of severe dehydration up to overt shock with hypotension and tachycardia. The neurological deficit may be mild with lethargy and confusion, but may also lead to frank coma. Severe hyperglycemia is the leading laboratory finding, with glucose levels ranging between 800 and 2000 mg/dl. Dehydration is usually not acccompanied by disturbances of serum sodium concentrations, but in severe cases hypernatremia can develop, producing serum osmolalities of 280–295 mosmol/l. Acidosis may also be present, but is usually not due to ketosis (cf. urine analysis), but rather results from lactic acidosis (see below).

Treatment

This follows the same lines as in diabetic coma due to ketoacidosis. Fluid replacement is the predominant task and should consist of 4–6 l i.v. in the first 8–12 h. This should be monitored by central venous pressure or pulmonary artery pressure using a Swan-Ganz catheter in patients with cardiac insufficiency. In the state of hyperglycemia, 0.9% saline is given; if hypernatremia is present this should be 0.45%. After blood glucose levels of around 250 mg% are reached, we change to 5% glucose infusions. Oral fluids are encouraged when patients become conscious again.

Less insulin and less potassium is required in the nonketotic patient. Fifteen international units of regular insulin should be given as an intravenous bolus and 0.1 IU insulin/kg per hour intravenously thereafter, according to the blood glucose level, which should fall by 10% per hour.

Prognosis

The search for the precipitating event of metabolic derangement is important: chest X-rays, blood and urine cultures, analysis of cardiac enzymes, and ECG, as well as determination of serum amylase and careful examination of the abdomen are important. The underlying diseases and the increased age of the patients are the reasons for the higher mortality associated with this form of diabetic coma.

Lactic Acidosis

Definition and Pathophysiology

This complication is often present in acidotic diabetics with or without mild ketosis. Excessive plasma lactate (>6 mmol/l) is characteristic and can develop due to tissue hypoxia (overproduction of lactate), hepatic failure (diminished removal), or circulatory shock (overproduction and no removal). Patients are usually severely ill. Several drugs can induce lactic acidosis: phenformin, salicylates, sodium nitroprusside, fructose, sorbitol, ethanol, and other substances.

Signs and Symptoms

The predominant sign is hyperventilation and mental confusion; in secondary cases of severely ill patients the signs of the underlying disease are present. Plasma glucose is often only mildly elevated, plasma bicarbonate and arterial pH are low; an anion gap (sum of bicarbonate and chloride minus sodium) is usually present. Hyperphosphatemia may be due to lactic acidosis.

Treatment

Treatment of underlying disease is the main task. Early intubation and respiration, adequate fluid replacement, and antibiotic treatment are important. The plasma pH should be kept above 7.2 by intravenous administration of sodium bicarbonate, which, however, often does not influence the outcome.

Hypoglycemia

Definition and Pathophysiology

Symptoms usually develop when the plasma glucose level drops below 45 mg/dl, in elderly patients with reduced cerebral blood supply; central nervous system glycopenic manifestations can develop at slightly higher plasma glucose levels. This is also true of patients with chronic hyperglycemia due to poorly controlled diabetes mellitus.

Differential Diagnosis

Hypoglycemia is divided into fasting and nonfasting states, fasting hypoglycemia occurring with or without hyperinsulinemia. Nonfasting or reactive hypoglycemia is often alimentary in patients with rapid gastric emptying, after gastric surgery, or with liver insufficiency. Hyperinsulinemia is present in patients with insulinoma, after an overdose of sulfonylurea or insulin treatment, or in the rare disorders of autoimmune hypoglycemia. Normal insulin levels may be present in fasting states of hypoglycemia due to renal or hepatic disorders, in hypocortisolism, alcohol abuse, or non-

pancreatic tumors. Asymptomatic hypoglycemia may be seen during prolonged fasting, strong exercise, or pregnancy. Laboratory artefacts have to be excluded. With fasting for up to 72 h blood glucose does not fall below 55 mg/dl in normal men, but may fall as low as 30 mg/dl in healthy women.

Signs and Symptoms

The consequences of central nervous system glycopenia and subsequent adrenergic symptoms are summarized in Table 2. Adrenergic symptoms usually develop first in acute hypoglycemia, followed by confusion, lethargy, unresponsivess, and, occasionally, seizures or focal signs. Signs and symptoms can often be confused with those of alcohol or other intoxications. However, Whipple's triad is characteristic of hypoglycemia:

1. Signs and symptoms of hypoglycemia

Table 2. Signs and symptoms of hypoglycemia

CNS glycopenia:
  Impaired ability to concentrate
  Headache
  Confusion
  Lethargy
  Transient ischemic attack
  Coma
  Drowsiness
  Convulsions
  Seizures
  Hemiparesis
Adrenergic symptoms:
  Aggression
  Anxiety
  Palpitations
  Sweating
  Hunger
  Tremor
  Tachycardia
  Pallor

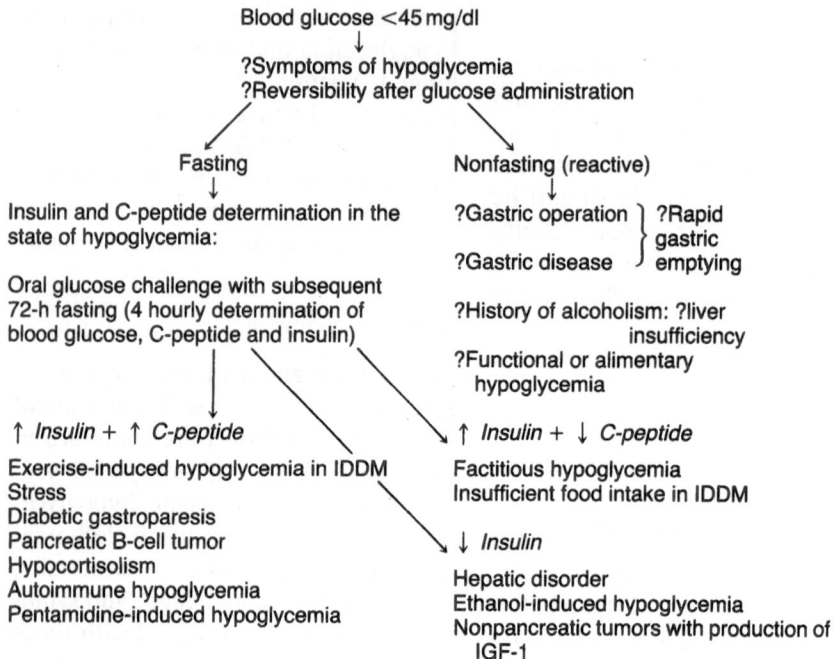

Blood glucose <45 mg/dl
↓
?Symptoms of hypoglycemia
?Reversibility after glucose administration

Fasting
↓
Insulin and C-peptide determination in the
state of hypoglycemia:

Oral glucose challenge with subsequent
72-h fasting (4 hourly determination of
blood glucose, C-peptide and insulin)

↑ Insulin + ↑ C-peptide
Exercise-induced hypoglycemia in IDDM
Stress
Diabetic gastroparesis
Pancreatic B-cell tumor
Hypocortisolism
Autoimmune hypoglycemia
Pentamidine-induced hypoglycemia

Nonfasting (reactive)
↓
?Gastric operation ⎫ ?Rapid
                    ⎬ gastric
?Gastric disease   ⎭ emptying

?History of alcoholism: ?liver
                          insufficiency
?Functional or alimentary
   hypoglycemia

↑ Insulin + ↓ C-peptide
Factitious hypoglycemia
Insufficient food intake in IDDM

↓ Insulin
Hepatic disorder
Ethanol-induced hypoglycemia
Nonpancreatic tumors with production of
IGF-1

Fig. 1. Differential diagnosis of hypoglycemia. IDDM, Insulin-dependent diabetes mellitus

2. An associated plasma glucose level of below 45 mg/dl
3. Reversal of symptoms after glucose administration

The latter point is the reason why an intravenous injection of glucose can be tried in emergency situations of coma of unclear origin. The diagnostic procedure is shown in Fig. 1.

Treatment

Hypoglycemia is reversible by glucose administration of any route. If glucose is not available, 1 mg glucagon i.m. or i.v. can be injected, but this is probably a rare situation. The glucagon treatment has no advantage over glucose. Urgent action is required as prolonged hypoglycemia causes permanent brain damage or even death. Table 3 shows the various possibilities for treatment of the hypoglycemic patient. Symptoms of hypoglycemia usually reverse within minutes after glucose administration. Afterwards, diagnostic procedures should be carried out according to the schema in Fig. 1.

Adrenocortical Insufficiency

Definition and Pathophysiology

Adrenocortical insufficiency (AI) is characterized by lack of glucocorticoid and mineralocorticoid secretion from the adrenal glands. Primary AI (Addison's disease) is mainly caused by autoimmune antibodies against adrenal tissues (80% of cases) or tuberculosis (20% of cases). Other

Table 3. Treatment of hypoglycemia due to various causes

Underlying disorder	Cause of hypoglycemia	Mode of action
Insulin-dependent diabetes mellitus	Inadequate food intake	Oral glucose
	Exercise	Oral glucose
	Overdose of insulin	20%–40% Glucose i.v. + subsequent monitoring
Noninsulin-dependent diabetes mellitus	Overdose of sulfonylurea	20%–40% Glucose i.v. + subsequent monitoring
Factitious hypoglycemia	Overdose of insulin in suicidal intention	Glucose i.v., psychotherapy
Pancreatic B-cell tumor (insulinoma)	Overproduction of endogenous insulin including C-peptide	Regular oral meals or glucose, operation, diazoxide
Ethanol-induced hypoglycemia	Glycogen stores depletion after fasting	Glucose i.v. Banting cure
Nonpancreatic tumors	Nonsuppressible insulin-like activity	Operation
Reactive hypoglycemia	Postgastrectomy or functional alimentary	Several small meals at short intervals

rare causes include adrenal hemorrhage and infarction, fungal infections, radiation therapy, surgical adrenalectomy, hemochromatosis, sarcoidosis, amyloidosis, metastatic disease, AIDS, enzyme inhibitors (metyrapone, aminoglutethimide, trilostane), cytotoxic agents (mitotane, o,p'-DDD) or congenital defects (enzyme or receptor defects).

Autoimmune disease is often associated with other immune disorders causing the polyglandular failure syndrome (PGF). The combination of AI with primary hypothyroidism due to Hashimoto's thyroiditis is called Schmidt's syndrome. Diabetes mellitus, ovarian failure leading to secondary amenorrhea, testicular failure, and hypoparathyroidism may be other features of PGF. Autoantibodies against parietal cells or intrinsic factor may be present in 30% and 9% of cases, respectively, and may be associated with macrocytic anemia. Secondary AI is caused by pituitary failure and will be discussed below. ACTH-suppressive long-term glucocorticoid treatment with subsequent rapid withdrawal may also be a cause of secondary AI. Relative hypoadrenalism may occur in those patients with inadequate substitution due to increased requirements in situations with concomitant severe diseases such as pneumonia or myocardial infarction.

Signs and Symptoms

These are mainly caused by cortisol deficiency and include weakness, fatigue, anorexia, abdominal symptoms such as nausea and vomiting, hypotension, and hypoglycemia. Mineralocorticoid deficiency results in renal loss of sodium and retention of potassium, leading to dehydration and hypotension. Clinical features vary according to the duration of onset of AI. Chronic AI is mainly associated with weakness, fatigue, weight loss, and abdominal symptoms. Due to hypersecretion of ACTH, hyperpigmentation of the skin, especially of handlines and around the nipples, are striking features in primary AI. Acute AI (Addison's crisis) is characterized by neurological symptoms up to frank coma, hypotension and shock, dehydration and volume depletion, abdominal symptoms, and hypoglycemia. This is an emergency situation and requires rapid actions as untreated it leads to death. Relative AI with increased cortisol requirements is often missed and not properly identified and treated as Addison's crisis.

Diagnostic Procedures

Hyperkalemia and hyponatremia combined with low blood pressure are classical signs, but are rare in the acute crisis. This emergency condition is often only diagnosed on the basis of the history of previous chronic glucocorticoid substitution or treatment. In newly diagnosed primary AI, only the clinical experience of the physician and subsequent low serum cortisol and high ACTH levels allow the diagnosis. In suspected AI, measurement of serum cortisol concentrations 30 and 60 min after exogenous ACTH administration (rapid ACTH stimulation test) may be required to confirm the diagnosis and to distinguish between primary and secondary AI. To exclude decreased ACTH reserve, metyrapone or insulin-hypoglycemia testing or stimulation with corticotrophin-releasing hormone may be necessary. Regular

monitoring of patients with primary AI to optimize dosing should include an exact history, measurements of blood pressure, electrolytes, and resting serum ACTH as well as serum renin (after 1 h bedrest).

Treatment

Addison's crisis:

100 mg hydrocortisone in 250 ml NaCl 0.9% i.v. in 30 min every 6 h.
Reduce to 75–80 mg hydrocortisone every 6 h when patient is clinically stable.
Rehydration with 5% glucose i.v. if necessary.
Treatment of underlying diseases.

Maintenance therapy:

Hydrocortisone: 15–20 mg p.o. in the morning, 10 mg at 2 p.m. and possibly 5 mg in the evening; alternatively cortisone acetate: 25 mg morning, 12.5 mg afternoon.
Fludrocortisone: 0.05–0.2 mg p.o./day according to blood pressure.
Supply of emergency card.
Dose adjustment: viral infection: up to 50 mg hydrocortisone; examination or other psychic stress: up to 75–100 mg h./day; operation: 50 mg hydrocortisone in 250 ml NaCl 0.9% in 30 min i.v., thereafter 50–100 mg hydrocortisone in 50 ml NaCl 0.9% i.v. in 12 hours via perfusion pump for 2–3 days peri- and postoperatively.

Thyroid Diseases

Hypothyroidism

Definition and Pathophysiology

Hypothyroidism is due to deficiency of thyroid hormones. In most cases it is of primary origin, with Hashimotos' thyroiditis being the most common cause. In this disorder thyroid destruction is due to lymphocytic inflammation and thyroid microsomal autoantibodies. Other types of thyroiditis are more rare. Both radioactive iodine treatment and surgical thyroid operations may finally lead to hypothyroidism. Rare causes are iodine deficiency or excessive iodine intake, goitrogens such as lithium, and antithyroid drugs, or, very rarely, inborn errors of thyroid hormone synthesis. Secondary hypothyroidism is discussed below under Hypopituitarism. Peripheral resistance to thyroid hormone due to receptor defects is extremely rare and only seen in a handful of families all over the world. Thyroid hormone deficiency involves all tissues due to accumulation of glycosaminoglycans subsequent to their decreased turnover and degradation.

Signs and Symptoms

In newborn infants, cretinism is the striking feature. This is characterized by mental retardation, short stature, puffy appearance of face and hands, deaf-mutism, and pyrimidal tract signs. Later on, respiratory insufficiency, jaundice, poor feeding, hoarse cry, and marked retardation of bone maturation may develop. In older children symptoms may be similar but not as severe. In adults, only one of the many systems influenced by thyroid hormones may be involved. Common features are coldness, weight gain, constipation, dry hair, tiredness, puffy hand and face, and a dull and apathetic appearance. Cardiomegaly with overt cardiac failure and low voltage in ECG are cardiovascular signs. Anemia is often present and may be due to concomitant pernicious anemia, folate or iron deficiency, and impaired hemoglobin synthesis. The central nervous system demonstrates signs of thyroid hormone deficiency, including inability to concentrate, lethargy, or chronic fatigue. Muscle cramps, muscle weakness, or paresthesias may be present.

Diagnosis

Elevated serum TSH levels are characteristic of primary hypothyroidism. Peripheral blood concentrations of T_3 and T_4 are low or decreased. The combination of low T_3 and low TSH is suggestive of the diagnosis of secondary hypothyroidism due to pituitary disease (see below). A pitfall in the diagnosis of hypothyroidism is elderly patients who are severely ill (in intensive care). Due to decreased peripheral conversion of T_4 to T_3, serum T_3 concentrations are low in almost every patient on the intensive care unit. This can also affect T_4 levels in very critically ill patients, which might be due to a decrease in thyroid hormone binding, and resulting in rapid clearance of T_4 from the blood. However, free T_3 and TSH levels are usually normal and demonstrate the intrinsic euthyroidism of these patients. In patients with high TSH and low T_3, if thyroid antibodies are positive and thyroid ultrasound shows the typical appearance of low echoresonance, the diagnosis of Hashimoto's thyroiditis can be made and life-long replacement therapy with thyroid hormones can be started. The finding of a neck scar is suggestive of postablative hypothyroidism, which should also lead to lifelong thyroxine replacement. TRH testing is only necessary in patients with low TSH and pituitary disease to test for the hypothalamopituitary axis. If there is a negative response after TRH administration, but peripheral T_3 and T_4 levels are high, a radioactive iodine scan should be performed in order to exclude toxic nodular goiter.

Treatment

The intravenous administration of $400-500 \mu g$ L-thyroxine as a bolus injection is indicated in patients with myxedema coma on the intensive care unit with life-threatening complications such as hypothermia (below 35°C rectally) or bradyarrhythmia. For bradycardia, a pacemaker is usually required. Alveolar hypoventilation, leading to CO_2 narcosis, needs to be treated by assisted ventilation. Fluid balance should be carefully monitored; often severe dilutional hyponatremia is present and requires hypertonic saline infusions. External warming may cause vascular collapse, therefore it is usually enough to prevent further heat loss. A significant increase in body temperature can be seen after L-thyroxine administration, so body temperature can be used to monitor the effectiveness of L-thyroxine treatment. If secondary hypothyroidism is suspected, an additional 100 mg hydrocortisone i.v. should be given. Oral L-thyroxine treatment should be con-

tinued as soon as the patient is able to take drugs orally.

Prognosis

Prognosis of myxedema coma is poor, although survivals have been reported. Survival depends on how early adequate treatment is initiated, and how well the underlying disease problems (e.g., infections, cerebral diseases) can be managed. As intravenous administration of large doses of L-thyroxine in older patients can cause relative coronary artery insufficiency, heart failure, or arrhythmias, this type of treatment should be reserved for critical patients only. In all other cases, a slow oral replacement starting with $12.5 \mu g$ L-thyroxine p.o. with increasing doses ($12.5 \mu g$/week) should be tried. L-thyroxine has a half-life of $7-8$ days, thus it only needs to be given once weekly. Absorption is best when it is given 30 min before breakfast and $60\%-80\%$ of most other preparations are absorbed. In adults, replacement doses usually required are between $50-200 \mu g$/day. In patients with primary hypothyroidism, the dose of L-thyroxine is monitored by serum TSH measurement. A TSH-suppressive treatment with TSH below 0.05 mU/l is not required, unless the underlying disease is a thyroid carcinoma. In children, the dose should be $4-6 \mu g$/kg body weight per day.

Thyrotoxicosis

Definition and Pathophysiology

Thyrotoxicosis is usually due to thyroid hormone overproduction from Graves' or Basedow's disease or from a toxic nodular or diffuse goiter. Thyrotoxic crisis is frequently induced by iodine administration after radiological examinations with contrast medium or after long-term treatment with iodine-containing drugs such as the antiarrhythmic drug amiodarone (Cordarex). Iodine-induced thyrotoxicosis very often leads to overt crisis. It is very difficult to treat and has a poor prognosis. Rare causes are thyrotoxicosis factitia after ingestion of large doses of L-thyroxine, seen in psychiatric patients, or in young women with anorexia. During thyroiditis usually only mild hyperthyroidism is seen.

Graves' or Basedow's disease is characterized by the occurrence of multiple thyroid stimulating autoantibodies. If these are also causing inflammation and swelling of the eye muscles, patients develop endocrine orbitopathy with typical eye changes such as proptosis, chemosis, or double vision. Toxic goiters are characterized by the presence of one or multiple "hot" nodules producing thyroid hormone without being regulated by the TSH feedback mechanism. Diffuse toxic goiters without nodules and without the presence of autoantibodies are difficult to distinguish from antibody-negative Graves' disease.

Signs and Symptoms

Thyrotoxicosis is characterized by typical symptoms such as tachycardia, nervousness, sleeplessness, hyperkinesia, tremor, weight loss, hyperdefecation, excessive sweating, and the preference for cold. In younger patients this full clinical picture together with a large goiter with a thrill on palpation and a bruit ("Non-nensausen") on auscultation makes the diagnosis. The presence of eye symptoms is often a key sign.

In older patients only one or two of the above-mentioned symptoms is usually present and the diagnosis is often missed. In patients with atrial fibrillation, thyrotoxicosis should always be excluded as the cause since atrial fibrillation due to hyperthyroidism is associated with a high rate of arterial embolism. Patients with concomitant heart disease are especially threatened by hyperthyroidism. However, thyrotoxic crisis is most often seen in these patients after coronary artery angiography, or due to treatment with amiodarone. The patient's neck should be examined using ultrasound and a radioiodine scan if nodules are present. In thyrotoxicosis crisis treatment is started without the results of these additional investigations.

Laboratory Diagnosis

Increased serum levels of T3 and/or T4 with suppressed TSH concentrations are suggestive of hyperthyroidism. If total T3/T4 is measured, a normal TBG concentration should exclude the possibility of increased binding protein due to estrogen intake, pregnancy, or liver disease. Therefore the measurement of free T3/T4 is used more frequently, although these radioimmunoassays are not always robust enough to be relied upon exclusively. TSH measurements can be used for screening. This should be done especially in cardiac patients to detect latent hyperthyroidism. TSH measurements detect compensated situations with peripheral euthyroidism, but not toxic nodules, which may require prophylactic treatment before iodine

exposure in angiography. If hyperthyroidism is diagnosed, measurement of
thyroid autoantibodies should follow.
This can usually be performed from
the same blood sample.

Treatment

The goal is blockade of thyroid hormone synthesis and action. Treatment
of thyroxicosis crisis is summarized in
Table 4.

The treatment with antithyroid
drugs is usually effective. The indication for intravenous administration
depends on the severity of the underlying disease and the compliance of the
patient. Methimazole (10–40 mg/day)
or carbimazole (5–30 mg/day) are the
drugs most often used.

Side effects are agranulocytosis
(occurrence ≤1%), therefore regular
monitoring of hematology values is
necessary. Increases in liver enzyme
concentrations can be seen, although
alkaline phosphatase may be increased

Table 4. Treatment of thyrotoxicosis crisis

Medical
  2–4 Ampoules (80–160 mg) methimazole
    (Favistan) i.v.
  3 × 15 Drops Lugols' solution (6 mg
    iodine/day) p.o.
  β-Blocker (e.g., propranolol) according to
    pulse and left ventricular function
  100 mg Prednisolone i.v.
  Sedation with diazepam or haloperidol
  Fluid substitution (using central venous
    pressure measurements)
  High caloric intake i.v.
  Cooling to reduce body temperature
  Anticoagulation
Surgical
  In patients resistent to conservative measures
  In iodine-induced thyrotoxicosis
  In patients with frequent relapses
Removal of thyroid hormones
  Dialysis plasmapheresis

due to the thyrotoxicosis itself. Skin
rashes frequently occur but regress
after drug withdrawal. In this case an
alternative drug is propylthiouracil,
of which usually 50–400 mg p.o./day
is required.

In severe cases, in patients with
frequent relapses, and in patients with
large goiters, high-dose iodine treatment may be necessary. Due to the
acute Wolff-Chaikoff effect (inhibition
of organic binding), and due to the fact
that high doses of iodine inhibit hormone release, this is a effective way
of treatment. However, surgical treatment is usually required about 10 days
after initiation of this treatment,
otherwise iodine-induced thyrotoxicosis can develop which may then be
difficult to control.

In critically ill patients, surgical
treatment should be considered early.
Indications include (1) resistance to
medical treatment; (2) iodine-induced
thyrotoxicosis; (3) large goiters; (4)
frequent relapses. The risks of surgical
intervention in the state of overt thyrotoxicosis are multiple: (1) danger of
malignant arrhythmias at onset of
narcosis; (2) profuse bleeding in
Graves' or Basedow's goiters; (3) prolonged duration of operation. Therefore euthyroidism is usually required
in the noncritically ill patient with
goiter.

Radioactive iodine therapy is usually recommended for older patients
after a euthyroid state is reached with
conservative antithyroid hormone
treatment. This will induce shrinkage
of the thyroid, and bring about euthyroidism within 6–10 weeks. In patients
with large goiters several large doses
may be required, and therefore surgical
treatment should also performed when
tracheal compression is present.

Prognosis

The prognosis of hyperthyroidism is good. However thyrotoxicosis crisis is still lethal in 20% of all patients encountering this serious complication.

Hypopituitarism

Definition and Pathophysiology

The deficiency of pituitary hormones is characteristic for this event. It can occur chronically or acutely. Patients will present with signs of the deficiency of peripheral hormones from glands controlled by pituitary stimulation. The reasons for pituitary insufficiency are multiple and are listed in Table 5.

Signs and Symptoms

Hypothyroidism and secondary adrenal insufficiency have been discussed above. Additional symptoms are those of hypogonadism, with amenorrhoea in females, loss of libido, and impotence; symptoms can exist, especially in men, for many years. Galactorrhea may be present in patients with large prolactinomas. The only symptom of prolactin deficiency is failure of post partum lactation. This typically presents in women with Sheehan's syndrome.

The main symptom of growth hormone deficiency is growth retardation in children up to the age of epiphyseal closure. In adults, the *syndrome of growth hormone deficiency* has only recently been recognized. It is characterized by increased fatigability, adiposity, mental symptoms up to frank depression, and diminished quality of life. Pituitary-insufficient patients seem to suffer more often from hyperlipidemias, with consequent increased prevalence of arteriosclerosis. Mortality is increased and life expectancy shortened even if substitution therapy with L-thyroxine, hydrocortisone, and sex steroids is given. An increased prevalence of osteoporotic fractures has been described in these patients. Hypopituitary crisis is usually characterized by a long absence of thyroid and adrenal hormones with symptoms of a combination a myxedema coma and Addison's crisis.

Table 5. Causes of hypopituitarism

Tumors or adenomas
  Hormonal active or nonactive pituitary
    tumors – craniopharyngiomas
  Metastases
  Meningiomas, gliomas, epidermoid tumors,
    etc.
Infarction
  Post partum (Sheehan's syndrome)
  Pituitary apoplexy
Granulomatous disease
  Sarcoidosis
  Histiocytosis X
Head injury
Iatrogenic
  Surgery
  Radiation
Idiopathic
Infections
  Tuberculosis
  Fungal

Diagnosis

The diagnosis of hypopituitary crisis is made mainly on a clinical basis; blood can be drawn for later determination of peripheral hormones such as cortisol and T3/T4. However, treatment is initiated before the results of hormone tests are received. In nonurgent cases, the stimulation tests for ACTH and cortisol, TSH, LH/FSH, prolactin, and growth hormone are conducted by the administration of the respective hypothalamic releasing hormones. Furthermore, if radiological examination (MRI/CT) reveals pituitary disease showing a large tumor (>10 mm), the diagnosis of pituitary insufficiency is more likely.

Treatment

This follows the general lines given for the treatment of myxedema and adrenal insufficiency (see above). Substitution of sex hormones as well as growth hormone are only important outside of the intensive care unit in specialized endocrine out-patient departments, where patients are best followed up.

Chapter 91

Blood Diseases and Neurologic Symptoms

Gregory J. del Zoppo and Richard Hermann

Alterations in microvascular flow caused by hyperviscosity or thrombosis can lead to neurological symptoms. Sustained reduction in flow may produce permanent central nervous system injury. Chronic hematologic disorders which may produce hyperviscosity syndromes include multiple myeloma and Waldenström's macroglobulinemia. More ominous, because of their abrupt and potentially catastrophic onset, are the microvascular thrombotic disorders thrombotic thrombocytopenic purpura and hemolytic uremic syndrome. Prompt recognition that the neurological findings are of hematologic origin is necessary for reversal of symptoms.

Thrombotic Thrombocytopenic Purpura

Definition

Thrombotic thrombocytopenic purpura (TTP) is a microvascular disorder

Section Editor: Michael N. Diringer

which may present with a spectrum of findings from mild symptoms with thrombocytopenia to severe disease with a fatal outcome. While the pentad of thrombocytopenic purpura, microangiopathic hemolytic anemia, renal dysfunction, a spectrum of fluctuating neurologic abnormalities, and fever may typify the disorder, initial presentation can involve any of these features alone or in combination. Neurologic findings may span the spectrum of symptoms from headache, mild paresthesias, hemiparesis, hemisensory defects and aphasia, to coma. Laboratory findings include hemolytic anemia with decreased red cell life span, thrombocytopenia with a decreased platelet survival time, and increased fibrin degradation products with a relatively normal fibrinogen turnover. Reticulocytosis, an elevated serum lactate dehydrogenase (LDH) concentration, and unconjugated hyperbilirubinemia invariably accompany those findings. Normal prothrombin time (Quick) and activated partial thromboplastin time studies distinguish TTP from disseminated intravascular coagulation (DIC). Proteinuria, hematuria, or an increased blood urea nitrogen (BUN) concentration indicates renal involvement, most common in hemolytic uremic syndrome.

Pathogenesis

While the pathogenesis of TTP is not known, the presence of hyaline arteriolar occlusions and capillary platelet-fibrin thrombi suggests a thrombotic microvascular process. Biopsies of the gingiva, bone marrow, and lymph node may demonstrate microvascular thrombi, but occlusion of small vessels may also occur in the myocardium, brain, and abdominal viscera. The presence of such thrombotic lesions is not pathognomonic for TTP or hemolytic uremic syndrome.

Mechanisms suggested to underlie TTP include the presence of a platelet-aggregating factor; the absence of an inhibitor to platelet-aggregating factor; decreased large molecular weight von Willebrand factor multimers; toxic, infectious, or immune-mediated endothelial injury; diminished endothelial prostacyclin (PGI_2) production; or other abnormalities of small blood vessels. TTP may be an isolated condition or associated with infectious mononucleosis, influenza vaccination, *Mycoplasma pneumoniae* infections, acute pancreatitis, pregnancy, eclampsia, autoimmune disorders (e.g., systemic lupus erythematosus, polyarteritis nodosa, and Sjögren's syndrome), circulating immune complexes, oral contraceptives, penicillin and penicillamine, dysfibrinogenemia, or cirrhosis. This implies that multiple processes may lead to microvascular platelet thrombus formation and erythrocyte fragmentation. Endothelial cell damage may account for most of the clinical features of the syndrome, but the nature of any primary endothelial injury is still unknown.

Mortality from unrecognized and untreated TTP is high, particularly during pregnancy. Increased BUN and creatinine, as in hemolytic uremic syndrome, are significant indications of a poor outcome. With currently recommended therapeutic approaches, reported remission rates for TTP may approach 60%–80%. Clinical improvement, including resolution of neurological symptoms, is accompanied by an increase in platelet count, decrease in serum lactate dehydrogenase, and resolution of the microangiopathic hemolytic anemia.

Therapy

Treatment is empirical and multifactorial, consisting of plasma infusions/exchange transfusions, antiplatelet agents, immunosuppressive agents, and transfusions of red cells and platelets. The latter (platelet transfusions) are reserved for life-threatening situations.

Transfusions. Packed red cell transfusions may be required for severe or symptomatic anemia. Although transfusions of type-specific random donor platelets have been recommended, they may augment the rapid platelet consumption and decreased platelet survival. Hence, platelet transfusions are not recommended unless life-threatening hemorrhage develops. Alternatively, plasma infusions or plasma exchange transfusions may effect an improvement in platelet count and produce clinical remission in some patients.

Plasma Infusions/Exchange Transfusions. Plasma infusions with 2–3 l fresh frozen plasma or plasma exchange transfusion should be initiated upon diagnosis. A recent prospective randomized trial has demonstrated that plasma exchange is more effective than plasma infusion in eliciting a positive response (platelet count) for up to 6 months. The possible presence of circulating toxic substances or immune complexes, or the absence of a "plasma factor" in which TTP patients are deficient, has been suggested to explain the success of these approaches. Plasma infusion may induce remission in 60%–70% of patients. A clinical response with an increase in the platelet count may occur within 48–72 h following the infusion of 6–8 units per day of fresh frozen plasma. For patients who fail to respond to plasma infusions or have a limited tolerance to large plasma infusion volumes, exchange transfusion with 2–3 l plasma or plasmapheresis with equivolume replacement should be initiated. Response rates may be 80%. Exchange transfusions or plasma infusions should be continued until a clinical remission is achieved. Infusion therapy must be individualized, as remission may be achieved with as little as 2 units infused, and relapse may occur despite continued plasma administration or exchange. Limitations of plasma infusion include (1) the hazards of a large plasma volume load, (2) the time necessary to produce a clinical response, and (3) lack of response. For these reasons, exchange transfusion may be the initial approach.

Adjunctive Therapy with Antiplatelet Agents. Antiplatelet and immunosuppressive agents are usually employed as adjunctive therapy. The combination aspirin/dipyridamole may induce remission when administered alone or in combination with other modalities. Aspirin (100–3600 mg/day) and dipyridamole (150–1600 mg/day) have been associated with a variety of clinical responses. Despite conflicting data, antiplatelet agents are generally combined with plasma infusion or exchange therapy when TTP is suspected or confirmed. Doses recommended are aspirin 325 mg and dipyridamole 75 mg, given together as a combination every 8 h. Sulfinpyrazone (800 mg/day in divided doses) has been used alone or with aspirin or dipyridamole, but it has not been proven that this agent is a suitable alternative to the more widely used combination aspirin/dipyridamole. We note that remission induction by sole use of antiplatelet agents is unusual. Therefore, we remain doubtful about the utility of this approach alone and recommend the use of antiplatelet agents as an adjunct to plasma infusion.

Dextran infusions have been used as an adjunct in the initial treatment of TTP; however, the contribution of this agent to a beneficial outcome has not been proven. Serious hemorrhage occurred in patients receiving large amounts of dextran, but remission has been achieved in some patients receiving corticosteroids and dextran 70.

Intravenous infusion of prostacyclin (PGI_2) has been used in occasional patients who failed to respond to plasma infusion or exchange transfusion with other antiplatelet agents. The several reports of long-term infusions in refractory patients are of historical interest. An initial PGI_2 infusion dose rate of 4 ng/kg min for 24 h, with dose escalation at hourly intervals thereafter, was used in one successful outcome. Diastolic hypotension and tachycardia occur at high dose rates.

Adjunctive Therapy with Immunosuppressive Agents. The possibility that TTP may be the clinical equivalent of the generalized Shwartzman reaction has supported the adjunctive use of systemic corticosteroids. Clinical response has been reported in 67% of TTP patients receiving high-dose corticosteroids and antiplatelet agents, with or without dextran, heparin, or splenectomy, in one retrospective survey. Other immunosuppressive agents, including vincristine, azathioprine, and 6-mercaptopurine have been employed in TTP, but their individual utility has not been proven.

Other Approaches. Despite earlier enthusiasm, there appears little evidence that splenectomy offers any advantage. Therefore, the added risk of splenectomy may not be justified. It is possible that the benefit previously noted was related to the volume of plasma and blood transfused at operation.

Heparin and warfarin are contraindicated in TTP because full-dose anticoagulation with heparin has been associated with increased mortality. Because of significant theoretical risks and lack of supportive evidence for benefit, thrombolytic agents are not used in TTP.

Maintenance Therapy. Plasma infusions or intermittent plasma exchange may be required in some patients to prevent relapse. Maintenance therapy with aspirin/dipyridamole may be appropriate in certain patients. Doses should be those used during initial therapy. Because there are no studies which have prospectively verified either approach, their use (with or without corticosteroids) should be individualized. Successful maintenance therapy is associated with persistent elevation of platelet count, hematocrit, and large von Willebrand factor multimers.

General Considerations

When a diagnosis of TTP is suspected, high-dose prednisone and aspirin/dipyridamole should be started. Plasma infusion and/or exchange transfusion may be indicated at this time. Serial infusion of 6–8 units fresh frozen plasma should be given as tolerated by the patient's plasma volume status, or plasmapheresis with plasma exchange transfusion of one plasma volume equivalent per day is recommended. Exchange transfusion should be performed daily as tolerated for up to 2 weeks. Whole blood exchange transfusion may be substituted if plasmapheresis is not available; however, the latter is preferable. Should a combination of plasma exchange transfusion, antiplatelet agents, and corticosteroids fail to lead to clinical improvement, immunosuppressive agents (e.g., vincristine, azathioprine) may replace corticosteroids. Finally, in patients refractory to the above maneuvers, dextran therapy may be considered. Splenectomy, anticoagulants, and thrombolytic agents are not recommended. Once remission is attained, maintenance therapy with antiplatelet agents may be necessary. Intermittent plasma infusions or plasma exchange transfusion may be required in some patients. One recent report has suggested that salvage of refractory TTP with splenectomy, corticosteroids, and dextrans may be effective.

Hyperviscosity Syndromes of Paraproteinemia

Introduction

Hyperviscosity syndromes result from paraproteinemias which accompany multiple myeloma, Waldenström's macroglobulinemia, and certain examples of chronic lymphocytic leukemia.

Plasma cell neoplasms, in addition to producing symptomatic paraproteinemia and hyperviscosity, may elicit neurologic abnormalities of varying severity by a number of mechanisms, including hypercalcemia, compression of cerebral tissues by calvarial tumors or intracranial plasmacytomas, meningeal myelomatosis, spinal cord compression, and/or peripheral neuropathies. Cranial nerve palsies arise from meningeal involvement by myeloma. Sensorimotor polyneuropathy may result from amyloid deposition, and symptoms confined to one peripheral nerve (root) may appear secondary to compression by osteosclerotic bone lesions or plasmacytomas.

The management of hypercalcemia is addressed in Chap. 90. The overall management of plasma cell neoplasms is beyond the scope of this section and has been amply addressed in a number of standard textbooks. This section will be concerned with the consequences of paraproteinemia.

Pathogenesis

Hyperviscosity syndromes secondary to paraproteinemias may present a spectrum of symptoms from diffuse headache, ataxia, gait abnormalities, visual disturbances to somnolence, obtundation, or coma. Visual disturbances may include blurred vision, diplopia, or frank visual loss. Here, retinal hemorrhages, exudates, and/or papilledema may accompany tortuosity and segmental dilatation ("sausaging" or "box-carring") of the retinal veins. Accompanying the cerebral symptoms are diffuse slow-wave abnormalities often documented on electroencephalography which are related to serum viscosity. While hyperviscosity syndromes are related to the intravascular concentration of paraproteins produced by cells of the B-cell lineage, the severity of the syndrome depends upon the type of immunoglobulin expressed and its concentration. For instance, myeloma proteins of the IgA or the IgG_3 type may undergo polymerization and are more likely to cause hyperviscosity, particularly at plasma concentrations above 5.0 gm/dl. Macroglobulinemia marked by IgM levels as low as 3.0 gm/dl may be associated with symptoms of hyperviscosity. It is well recognized that a threshold of relative plasma viscosity exists, usually around 4, beyond which hyperviscosity symptoms may be observed. In addition, a linear correlation between viscosity and plasma volume has been shown, where an increase in plasma viscosity results in plasma volume expansion. This has important consequences for therapy and reinforces the danger of inappropriate transfusion in these disorders, which may lead to cardiopulmonary compromise. It should be recognized that the primary symptomatic association in these syndromes is with elevated viscosity, which may not correlate directly with immunoglobulin level, although rapid reduction in immunoglobulin level may be warranted to relieve symptoms.

Associated effects of persistent elevated monoclonal immunoglobulin levels in multiple myeloma may include amyloidosis and its various targets, renal insufficiency, and viral or bacterial infections. In contrast, renal compromise is unusual in Waldenström's macroglobinemia, although the effects of amyloidosis are similar to that of multiple myeloma.

The most common neurological manifestations are polyneuropathies which may include mononeuritis multiplex, isolated mononeuropathies, and sensory or sensorimotor polyneuropathies. Presentation of polyneuropathy is more common with macroglobulinemia (up to 20%) than with plasma cell neoplasms (<1%). In the latter cases, elevated monoclonal immunoglobulin levels have most commonly involved IgM – more often than elevations of IgG – less commonly IgA, and, as an unusual occurrence, light chain components. The pathological lesion consists of various combinations of axonal degeneration and segmental demyelination. With IgM disease, the mechanism is autoimmune against peripheral nerve myelin sheaths.

An unusual central nervous system manifestation of macroglobulinemia, Bing-Neel disease, follows from multifocal cerebral demyelination with axonal degeneration, which may be accompanied by perivascular accumulation of characteristic lymphoplasmacytoid cells and IgM. Symptoms of this manifestation may be responsive to treatments for the hyperviscosity syndrome.

Therapy

Treatment for symptoms of hyperviscosity is directed at reduction of the increased plasma monoclonal immunoglobulin by plasmapheresis. If not already undertaken, treatment of the underlying neoplastic clone should be initiated.

Plasmapheresis. Treatment for manifestations of the hyperviscosity syndrome requires plasmapheresis to decrease the circulating abnormal levels of symptom-producing IgA, IgG, or IgM. In the latter case, use of this technique may be effective because of the predominantly intravascular compartmentalization of IgM. An acceptable regimen for acute reduction of immunoglobulin is to replace one (plasma) volume over 2–3 days for IgG gammopathies and more frequently for IgM gammopathies. A single volume plasmapheresis may acutely reduce IgG levels by 60%, which will not be sustained because of the extravascular distribution of this immunoglobulin type. Multiple plasmaphereses may be necessary. For macroglobulinemia associated with hyperviscosity syndromes, less frequent initial plasmapheresis will be required. It is not necessary to reduce the plasma viscosity to normal.

Chemotherapy. The use of cytoreductive therapy for the acute management of plasma cell and lymphoplasmacytoid cell proliferative disorders producing hyperviscosity syndromes is beyond the scope of this text, and the reader is referred to a recent work by Wells on the subject (see Suggested Reading). If the patient is not already under treatment and has not been found to be refractory, several courses of action are possible. For multiple myeloma, single-agent treatment with melphalan, corticosteroids, cyclophosphamide, or vincristine, or combination therapy with melphalan/prednisone (MP), melphalan/cyclophosphamide/BCNU/ prednisone (MCBP), vincristine/mel-phalan/BCNU/prednisone (VMBP), vincristine/BCNU/adriamycin/pred-nisone (VBAP), or melphalan/pred-nisone/cyclophosphamide/BCNU/ vincristine (the M2 protocol) may be offered. The combination vincristine/ adriamycin may be offered to primarily resistant patients or those in relapse. There is a suggestion that the addition of interferon to some established regimens may produce improved response in multiple myeloma. For Waldenström's macroglobulinemia, single-agent therapy with cyclophos-phamide, chlorambucil, or melphalan has found favor, although multi-agent therapy with the M2 regimen, VAD, or BCNU with adriamycin produce responses. Alternative approaches using high-dose corticosteroids, 2'-deoxycoformycin, or interferon are under scrutiny. In either disorder, the therapy should be tailored to the severity of the clinical manifestations and previous responses, taking into account the expected side effects of the multi-agent regimens for resistant disease. It should be remembered that cure of either disorder generally is not possible. For young patients allogenic bone marrow transplantation may be the only possibility for cure.

Maintenance Therapy. Serial plas-maphereses may be required to control symptoms of hyperviscosity, and, if the status of the underlying cellular disorder remains unchanged, may be quite successful. Generally, a combination of plasmapheresis and cytore-ductive therapy will be required.

General Considerations

As noted, plasmapheresis is the initial approach to central nervous system manifestations of hyperviscosity. Therapy should involve plasmaphere-sis of one plasma volume every 2–3 days for monoclonal IgG disorders, and one plasma volume every 1–3 days for monoclonal IgM disorders. Correlation of plasma viscosity with clinical symptoms should dictate the frequency of plasmapheresis.

Suggested Reading

Amir J, Krauss S (1973) Treatment of thrombotic thrombocytopenic purpura with antiplatelet drugs. Blood 42:27–33

Amorosi EL, Karpkin S (1977) Antiplatelet treatment of thrombotic thrombocytopenic purpura. Ann Intern Med 86:102–106

Aster RH (1985) Plasma therapy for thrombotic thrombocytopenic purpura: Sometimes it works, but why? N Engl J Med 312:985–987

Atkins JN (1985) Platelet-aggregating factor in thrombotic thrombocytopenic purpura. Ann Intern Med 102:560–561

Aul C, Scharf RE, Königshausen T, Schneider W (1985) Thrombotisch-thrombozyto-penische purpura. Klin Wochenschr 63: 123–132

Beaufils M, Beaufils H, Lucsko M, Chapman A, Gu'edon J (1975) Late streptokinase therapy in thrombotic microangiopathy: a case study. Clin Nephrol 4:160–163

Birgens H, Ernst P, Hansen MS (1979) Thrombotic thrombocytopenic purpura: treatment with a combination of antiplatelet drugs. Acta Med Scand 205:437–439

Blitzer JB, Granfortuna JM, Gottlieb AJ et al. (1987) Thrombotic thrombocytopenic purpura: treatment with plasmapheresis. Am J Hematol 24:329–339

Bonomini V, Vangelista A, Frascà G (1984) A new antithrombotic agent in the treatment of acute renal failure due to hemolytic-uremic syndrome and thrombotic thrombocytopenic purpura. Nephron 37:144–144

Breckenridge RL Jr, Solberg LA, Pineda AA, Petitt RM, Dharkar DD (1982) Treatment of thrombotic thrombocytopenic purpura with plasma exchange, antiplatelet agents, corticosteroid, and plasma infusion: Mayo Clinic experience. J Clin Apheresis 1:6–13

Budd GT, Bukowski RM, Lucas FV, Cato AE, Cocchetto DM (1980) Prostacyclin therapy of thrombotic thrombocytopenic purpura. Lancet 2:915–915

Bukowski RM (1982) Thrombotic thrombocytopenic purpura: a review. Prog Hemost Thromb 6:287–337

Byrnes JJ (1981) Plasma infusion in the treatment of thrombotic thrombocytopenic purpura. Semin Thromb Hemost 7:9–14

Cuttner J (1980) Thrombotic thrombocytopenic purpura: a ten-year experience. Blood 56:302–306

Del Zoppo GJ (1987) Antiplatelet therapy in thrombotic thrombocytopenic purpura. Semin Hematol 24:130–139

Del Zoppo GJ, Harker LA (1987) Thrombotic thrombocytopenic purpura. In: Bayless TM, Brain MC, Cherivak RM (eds) Current therapy in internal medicine 2. Decker, Ontario, p 378

Eckel RH, Crowell EB Jr, Waterhouse BE, Bozdech MJ (1977) Platelet-inhibiting drugs in thrombotic thrombocytopenic purpura. Arch Intern Med 137:735–737

Fahey JL, Barth WF, Solomon A (1965) Serum hyperviscosity syndrome. JAMA 192:464

FitzGerald GA, Maas RL, Stein R, Oates JA, Roberts J (1981) Intravenous prostacyclin in thrombotic thrombocytopenic purpura. Ann Intern Med 95:319–322

Giromini M, Bouvier CA, Dami R, Denizot M, Jeannet M (1972) Effect of dipyridamole and aspirin in thrombotic microangiopathy. Br Med J 1:545–546

Glas-Greenwalt P, Hall JM, Panke TW, Kant KS, Allen CM, Pollak VE (1986) Fibrinolysis in health and disease: abnormal levels of plasminogen activator, plasminogen activator inhibitor, and protein C in thrombotic thrombocytopenic purpura. J Lab Clin Med 108:415–422

Gordon LI, Kwaan HC, Rossi EC (1987) Deleterious effects of platelet transfusions and recovery thrombocytosis in patients with thrombotic microangiopathy. Semin Hematol 24:194–201

Gresele P, Arnout J, Deckmyn H, Vermylen J (1985) Combining antiplatelet agents: potentiation between aspirin and dipyridamole. Lancet I:937–938

Guelpa G, Trono D, Audetat F, Hochstrasser D (1986) Purpura thrombotique thrombocytop'enique trait'e par la prostacycline: a propos de deux observations. Schweiz Med Wochenschr 116:647–651

Holdrinet RSG, Namdar Z, Haanen C (1988) Thrombotic thrombocytopenic purpura: clinical course and response to therapy in twelve patients. Netherlands J Med 33:113–132

Isbister JP (1981) Plasma exchange in the management of hyperviscosity syndromes. Bibl Haematol 47:228

Jaffe EA, Nachman RL, Merskey C (1973) Thrombotic thrombocytopenic purpura – coagulation parameters in twelve patients. Blood 42:499–507

Jobin F, DelÅge J-M (1970) Aspirin and prednisone in microangiopathic haemolytic anaemia. Lancet II:208–210

Joneau M, Cordonnier C, Vernant J-P, Touzet C, Sobel A (1985) How many plasma exchanges to cure thrombotic thrombocytopenic purpura? Scand J Haematol 34:157–159

Kaplan BS, Proesmans W (1987) The hemolytic uremic syndrome of childhood and its variants. Semin Hematol 24:148–160

Kelton JG, Moore J, Santos A, Sheridan D (1984) Detection of a platelet-agglutinating factor in thrombotic thrombocytopenic purpura. Ann Intern Med 101:589–593

Kennedy SS, Zacharski LR, Beck JR (1980) Thrombotic thrombocytopenic purpura: analysis of 48 unselected cases. Semin Thromb Hemost 6:341–349

Kwaan HC (1987) Miscellaneous secondary thrombotic microangiopathy. Semin Hematol 24:141–147

Kwaan HC (1987) Introduction: thrombotic microangiopathy. Semin Hematol 24:69–70

Kwaan HC (1987) Clinicopathologic features of thrombotic thrombocytopenic purpura. Semin Hematol 24:71–81

Kwaan HC (1987) Role of fibrinolysis in thrombotic thrombocytopenic purpura. Semin Hematol 24:101–109

Kyle RA (1989) Monoclonal gammopathies and the kidney. Annu Rev Med 40:53

Lerner RG, Rapaport SI, Meltzer J (1967) Thrombotic thrombocytopenic purpura: serial clotting studies, relation to the generalized Shwartzman reaction, and remission after adrenal steroid and dextran therapy. Ann Intern Med 66:1180–1190

Lian EC-Y, Mui PTK, Siddiqui FA, Chiu LLS (1983) Purification and some properties of a protein obtained from normal human plasma which inhibits the platelet aggregation induced by thrombotic thrombocytopenic purpura plasma. Thromb Res 33:69–76

Lian EC-Y (1987) Pathogenesis of thrombotic thrombocytopenic purpura. Semin Hematol 24:82–100

Lian EC-Y, Siddiqui FA (1985) Investigation of the role of von Willebrand factor in thrombotic thrombocytopenic purpura. Blood 66:1219–1221

Machin SJ (1984) Thrombotic thrombocytopenic purpura. Br J Haematol 56:191–197

MacKenzie MR, Lee TK (1977) Blood viscosity in Waldenstrom's macroglobulinemia. Blood 49:507

McGrath MA, Penny R (1976) Paraproteinemia: blood hyperviscosity and clinical manifestations. J Clin Invest 58:1155

Moake JL, Byrnes JJ, Troll JH et al. (1985) Effects of fresh-frozen plasma and its cryosupernatant fraction on von Willebrand factor multimeric forms in chronic relapsing thrombotic thrombocytopenic purpura. Blood 65:1232–1236

Moake JL, Rudy CK, Troll JH et al. (1985) Therapy of chronic relapsing thrombotic thrombocytopenic purpura with prednisone and azathioprine. Am J Hematol 20:73–79

Murgo AJ (1987) Thrombotic microangiopathy in the cancer patient including those induced by chemotherapeutic agents. Semin Hematol 24:161–177

Murphy WG, Moore JC, Kelton JG (1987) Calcium-dependent cysteine protease ac-tivity in the sera of patients with thrombotic thrombocytopenic purpura. Blood 70: 1683–1687

Myers TJ, Wakem CJ, Ball ED, Tremont SJ (1980) Thrombotic thrombocytopenic purpura: combined treatment with plasmapheresis and antiplatelet agents. Ann Intern Med 92 (Part 1):149–155

Nalbandian RM, Henry RL (1980) A proposed comprehensive pathophysiology of thrombotic thrombocytopenic purpura with implicit novel tests and therapies. Semin Thromb Hemost 6:356–390

Petitt RM (1980) Thrombotic thrombocytopenic purpura: a thirty year review. Semin Thromb Hemost 6:350–355

Pini M, Manotti C, Megha A, Poli T, Potì R (1982) Normal prostacyclin-like activity and response to plasma exchange in thrombotic thrombocytopenic purpura: report of 2 cases. Acta Haematol 67:198–205

Pisciotta AV, Gottschall JL (1980) Clinical features of thrombotic thrombocytopenic purpura. Semin Thromb Hemost 6:330–340

Remuzzi G, Zoja C, Rossi EC (1987) Prostacyclin in thrombotic microangiopathy. Semin Hematol 24:110–118

Revell P, Slater NGP (1992) Antiplatelet therapy in thrombotic thrombocytopenic purpura (letter). Lancet 340:851–852

Rock GA, Shumak KH, Buskard NA et al. (1991) Comparison of plasma exchange with plasma infusion in the treatment of thrombotic thrombocytopenic purpura. N Engl J Med 325:393–403

Rosove MH, Ho WG, Goldfinger D (1982) Ineffectiveness of aspirin and dipyridamole in the treatment of thrombotic thrombocytopenic purpura. Ann Intern Med 96:27–33

Ruggenenti P, Remuzzi G (1991) Thrombotic microangiopathies. Crit Rev Oncol Hematol 11:243–265

Savona S, Nardi MA, Lennette ET, Karpatkin S (1985) Thrombocytopenic purpura in narcotics addicts. Ann Intern Med 102:737–741

Scheithauer BW, Rubinstein LJ, Herman MM (1984) Leukoencephalopathy in Waldenström's neuroglobulinemia. J Neuropathol Exp Neurol 43:408

Schneider PA, Rayner AA, Linker CA, Schuman MA, Liu ET, Hohn DC (1985) The role of splenectomy in multimodality treatment of thrombotic thrombocytopenic purpura. Ann Surg 202:318–322

Scully RE, Mark EJ, McNeely WF, McNeely BU (1988) Case report. N Engl J Med 318:1047–1057

Scully RE, Mark EJ, McNeely WF, McNeely BU (1990) Case report. N Engl J Med 323:1050–1061

Shepard KV, Bukowski RM (1987) The treatment of thrombotic thrombocytopenic purpura with exchange transfusions, plasma infusions, and plasma exchange. Semin Hematol 24:178–193

Siddiqui FA, Lian EC-Y (1985) Novel platelet-agglutinating protein from a thrombotic thrombocytopenic purpura plasma. J Clin Invest 76:1330–1337

Siddiqui FA, Lian EC-Y (1988) Platelet-agglutinating protein P37 from a thrombotic thrombocytopenic purpura plasma forms a complex with human immunoglobulin G. Blood 71:299–304

Taft EG, Baldwin ST (1981) Plasma exchange transfusion. Semin Thromb Hemost 7:15–21

Thompson CE, Damon LE, Ries CA, Linker CA (1992) Thrombotic microangiopathies in the 1980s: clinical features, response to treatment, and the impact of the human immunodeficiency virus epidemic. Blood 80:1890–1895

Tuddenham EGD, Bradley J (1974) Plasma volume expansion and increased serum viscosity in myeloma and macroglobulinemia. Clin Exp Immunol 16:169

Weiner CP (1987) Thrombotic microangiopathy in pregnancy and the postpartum period. Semin Hematol 24:119–129

Wells R (1970) Syndromes of hyperviscosity. N Engl J Med 183:183

Wiernik PH, Canellos GP, Kyle RA et al. (1991) Neoplastic diseases of the blood, 2nd edn. Churchill Livingstone, New York

Wu KK, Hall ER, Rossi EC, Papp AC (1985) Serum prostacyclin binding defects in thrombotic thrombocytopenic purpura. J Clin Invest 75:168–174

Zacharski LR, Walworth C, McIntyre OR (1992) Antiplatelet therapy for thrombotic thrombocytopenic purpura. N Engl J Med 285:408–409

Zimmerman SE, Smith FP, Phillips TM, Coffey RJ, Schein PS (1982) Gastric carcinoma and thrombotic thrombocytopenic purpura: association with plasma immune complex concentrations. Br Med J 284:1432–1434

Chapter 92

Systemic Immunologic Diseases Affecting the Nervous System

PATRICIA M. MOORE and PETER BERLIT

Background and Immunologic Mechanisms

A variety of systemic immunologic diseases affect the nervous system; these include the connective tissue diseases and the vasculitides. Immunologically mediated diseases result from several distinct mechanisms; knowledge of the predominant pathogenic mechanism in specific diseases aids the physician in appropriate diagnosis and treatment. Antibody-mediated disorders may result from direct interaction of the antibody with the target (such as anti-acetylcholine receptor antibodies and the acetylcholine receptor) or through indirect means (such as immune complex formation, deposition in the vasculature, and resultant inflammation). Cell-mediated diseases typically result from interaction of antigen-specific lymphocytes with the target and secondary recruitment of nonspecific cells via cytokines. An overlap between antibody- and cell-mediated diseases is well established.

Section Editor: Thomas P. Bleck

It is clinically useful, after recognizing the primary mechanism of disease, to consider whether the neurologic abnormalities appear early or late in the course of the disease. In the latter circumstance, complications of therapy such as infection, toxicity of medication, or metabolic abnormalities may play a central role in the neurologic abnormalities (Table 1).

Definition of Diseases

Systemic autoimmune diseases affecting the nervous system are typically divided into two large groups: the connective tissue diseases and the vasculitides. Although the division is based on clinical and histologic features, an overlap is recognized, as some patients with the connective tissue diseases have a prominent component of vascular inflammation and, likewise, patients with vasculitis may develop arthralgias, fever, and nonspecific parameters of systemic inflammation. Most of the disorders described here are idiopathic – currently without an identifiable cause.

Table 1. Systemic immunologic diseases presenting as acute neurologic disease

Systemic lupus erythematosus (SLE)
Mixed connective tissue disease (MCTD)
Sjögren's (PSS)
Rheumatoid arthritis (RA)
Systemic sclerosis (SSC)
Polyarteritis nodosa (PAN)
Churg-Strauss angiitis (CS)
Wegener's granulomatosis (WEG)
Lymphomatoid granulomatosis (LG)
Secondary vasculitides (2°v)
Hypersensitivity vasculitis (HS)

In the group of vasculitides, however, there is a specifically identified category of secondary vasculitis. This distinction is important clinically, because optimal treatment should be focused on the underlying cause, be it infectious, toxic, or neoplastic.

Acute neurologic abnormalities may occur as primary manifestations of disease, thus presenting a diagnostic challenge, or they may occur after a diagnosis of systemic inflammatory disease has been made. In the first case the physician must maintain a high index of suspicion for these groups of diseases and use appropriate serologic, angiographic, and histologic studies. When acute neurologic abnormalities occur in the context of a previously diagnosed autoimmune disease, identifying the pathophysiology and appropriate treatment is more complex. The physician must reexamine the underlying diagnosis as well as identify secondary complications including infections (from the immunosuppression), toxins (from medications such as corticosteroids and anti-hypertensives), and metabolic abnormalities (from organ dysfunction such as renal failure).

Acute central nervous system manifestations of these systemic immunologic diseases are most often encephalopathies, seizures, subarachnoid hemorrhage, visual loss, and stroke. Acute peripheral nervous system abnormalities are typically polyradiculopathies, extensive mononeuropathies, mononeuropathy multiplex, and sensory neuropathy. Table 2 shows the relative occurrence of these clinical features in the disorders discussed here.

Connective Tissue Diseases

Systemic lupus erythematosus (SLE) is a multisystem inflammatory disease characterized by prominent circulating autoantibodies and immune complexes. SLE most frequently affects the skin, kidneys, musculoskeletal system, and nervous system. The mechanism of tissue damage, however, differs in the kidneys and in the nervous system. Glomerulonephritis results primarily from immune complex deposition with secondary inflammation.

Neurologic abnormalities develop from several acute and chronic mechanisms. Acutely, seizures and encephalopathies may result from direct autoantibody-mediated effects on neurons as well as from the secondary conditions of infections, toxins (usually medications), and metabolic derangements. Chronically, degenerative changes in the blood vessels (from chronic low levels of circulating immune complexes and/or possibly antiphospholipid antibodies) and cardiac emboli appear to produce many of the focal neurologic abnormalities. Both

Table 2. Types of neurologic abnormalities occurring with systemic immunologic disease

	SLE	MCTD	PSS	SSC	RA	PAN	CS	Weg	LG	HS	2°
Encephalopathy	+++	+	+	–	–	++	++	+	++		+++
Seizures	+++	+	+	–	–	++	++	+	+	+	+++
Subarachnoid hemorrhage	+	–	+	+	+	+	+	+	+	++	++
Hypertensive crisis	++	–	–	+	–	++	+	+	+		
Hypothalamic changes (DI)	+	–	+	–	–	++		++			
Myelopathies	+	–	–	–	++	++	++	+	+		++
Extensive mononeuropathies	+	+		–	+	++	+	++	+		++
Autonomic changes	+	–	–	–	–	–	–	–	–	–	–
Polyradiculopathies (Guillain-Barré)	++	–	+	–	–	–	–	–	–	–	–
Sensory neuropathies	+	–	++	–	–	–	–	–	–	–	–

DI, Diabetes insipidus; for other abbreviations, see Table 1.

diagnostically and therapeutically, these differences are important. The MRI, CT scan, angiography, and cerebrospinal fluid analysis may be abnormal for a variety of reasons and may not identify the primary pathologic process. Thus, neuro-SLE results from a number of mechanisms; clinical judgement and experience, not a specific diagnostic test, are crucial to patient care.

Mixed connective tissue disease (MCTD) is probably a clinical subset of SLE; MCTD is characterized by high titers of a distinct autoantibody to a ribonuclease-sensitive extractable nuclear antigen, the ribonucleoprotein (RNP). The pattern of neurologic abnormality appears more restricted than in SLE. Aseptic meningitis predominates; trigeminal neuropathy, moncneuropathy multiplex, psychosis, and seizures occasionally occur.

Sjögren's disease affects primarily women and is the second most common rheumatic disorder. Characteristic features are the xerophthalmia and xerostomia resulting from lymphocyte-mediated destructive infiltration of the salivary and lingual glands, leading to diminished or absent mucosal secretions. The disease may be restricted to oral and ocular secretions or it may run a frank lymphoproliferative course. Although the cellular infiltrates are striking and important in diagnosis, both cell- and antibody-mediated mechanisms may contribute to visceral involvement. Patients may develop interstitial pulmonary fibrosis, renal tubular acidosis, and Hashimoto's thyroiditis. A variety of autoantibodies occur in Sjögren's. Most clearly disease associated is the anti-Ro; the target is a small cytoplasmic ribonucleoprotein.

Neurologic abnormalities occur in 10–32% of patients with Sjögren's syndrome; the most frequent are peripheral neuropathies and cranial neuropathies. Trigeminal neuropathy, the most common mononeuropathy in autoimmune diseases, typically presents as dysesthesias and hypesthesias in more than one division of the trigeminal nerve. The pathogenesis of the neuropathies appears to be vasculitis, based on histologic abnormalities in several series. Central nervous system abnormalities also occur; the exact incidence and pathogenesis are under investigation. A venulitis is suggested but not verified. MRI abnormalities are apparent but do not always correlate with clinical disease. Aseptic meningitis, seizures, myelopathies, or subarachnoid hemorrhage occur occasionally.

Rheumatoid arthritis, a chronic progressive disease affecting and deforming the joints, rarely affects the nervous system directly but can cause serious neurologic abnormalities secondary to atlantoaxial subluxation (resulting in a myelopathy). Less severe but nevertheless debilitating are the more frequent compression mononeuropathies. Rarely, the brain parenchyma may be affected by vasculitis.

Systemic sclerosis (SSC) or scleroderma, a generalized disorder of connective tissue characterized by fibrosis and degenerative changes in the skin, synovium, digital arteries, and in the parenchyma and small arteries of the gastrointestinal tract, lungs, heart, and kidneys, is variably severe and progressive. Although the most striking histologic feature of SSC is the widespread overgrowth of connective tissue, there are many inflammatory and vascular changes resembling those in other connective tissue diseases. Neurologic abnormalities in SSC are unusual. Cranial neuropathies occur in about 4% of patients. Rarely, a systemic vasculitis may affect the central nervous system.

The Vasculitides

The systemic necrotizing vasculitides are a group of diseases sharing certain features, including widespread inflammation and necrosis of blood vessels. Distinction among these disorders is based upon characteristic clinical and histologic features. The common denominator of tissue injury in all is ischemia. Occasionally, cytokines, edema, and granulomas may contribute to tissue injury.

Polyarteritis nodosa (PAN) is a multisystem disease of small and medium-sized muscular arteries. Typically, the lungs are spared. Hypertension occurs in more than half of the patients. Neurologically, abnormalities of the peripheral nervous system, present in 50–60% of patients, appear early, while central nervous system abnormalities usually occur after the diagnosis is established. Of note to acute-care physicians is the fact that patients may present with hypertension and an encephalopathy. It is important to remember that the diagnosis is not hypertensive encephalopathy; both conditions result from the vasculitis. Appropriate treatment is not restricted to lowering the blood pressure; it must also address the vascular inflammation.

Churg-Strauss angiitis, distinctive for a pulmonary involvement and a peripheral eosinophilia, has a small-vessel predominance. Clinically, peripheral neuropathies usually represent the multiplex type and encephalopathies are more typical than in PAN.

Wegener's granulomatosis is characterized by granulomatous vasculitis of the respiratory tract with or without glomerulonephritis. Initial symptoms are commonly related to the upper respiratory tract. Neurologic abnormalities result both from contiguous extension of the necrotizing granulomas and from the systemic vasculitis. Contiguous extension of the granulomas results in cranial neuropathies in the middle and posterior fossa. The occasional diabetes insipidus also appears to result from local spread of disease. The peripheral neuropathies more clearly result from the systemic vasculitis.

Lymphomatoid granulomatosis is an unusual vasculitis affecting the skin, lungs, and nervous system. A destructive, pleomorphic mononuclear infiltrate involves both arteries and veins; these infiltrating lymphocytoid and plasmacytoid cells transform to neoplasia in up to 50% of patients. Both the central and peripheral segments of the nervous system are affected.

Hypersensitivity vasculitis is the most common vasculitis. Primarily a venulitis of the skin, this group of disorders includes drug-induced allergic vasculitis, Henoch-Schönlein purpura, cutaneous vasculitis, post-infectious vasculitis, and some cases of mixed cryoglobulinemia. Neurologic abnormalities are not common with the hypersensitivity vasculitides (<10%), with the exception of serum sickness, which has a higher incidence of brachial plexopathy, encephalopathy, and seizures. Subarachnoid hemorrhage and stroke have been reported with Henoch-Schönlein purpura.

Vasculitis associated with malignancy, infection, and toxins may result in neurologic abnormalities and is increasingly recognized as an important cause of neurologic diseases. This reactive vasculitis may mimic the idiopathic disorders. Care in diagnosis is important to avoid immunosuppressing a patient who has an underlying infection causing inflammatory vascular disease. Similarly, vasculitis from neoplasia or toxins should be directed at removing the underlying cause.

Diagnostic Considerations

Clues to an associated vasculitis or connective tissue disease reside in the presence of clinical or subclinical visceral disease. The presence of abnormal renal function, casts, or sediment in a fresh urine specimen, or an abnormal creatinine clearance should be vigorously pursued. Cutaneous lesions, retinal vascular changes, and hematologic abnormalities provide clues to a multisystem disease. The physician then determines if the processes are associated with autoantibodies or cellular infiltration. Autoantibody-mediated diseases typically have serologic abnormalities supporting a diagnosis (Table 3); cell-mediated diseases may remain undiagnosed without biopsy. Histologic information is invaluable, both to confirm antibody-mediated changes and to diagnose cell-mediated injury, as well as to investigate the occurrence of underlying disorders such as neoplasia or infection.

Treatment

Treatment of the vasculitides and the connective tissue diseases depends upon (a) identifying and removing any underlying infectious or toxic disorders and (b) the judicious use of corticosteroids and immunosuppressive agents. While usage is empirical, most guides suggest using an adequate initial dosage to achieve the goal (reduce immune complex deposition, reduce proteinuria, minimize serosal inflammation), then reducing the dosage to the lowest dose which will maintain the remission. Treating the neurologic abnormalities is similar, except that the physicians should distinguish between those neurologic abnormalities which are part of the acute immunologic injury and those which may be consequences of chronic disease. For example, an acute stroke which results from thrombosis of a degenerative vasculopathy or cardiac embolus does not require corticosteroid therapy. Also, some manifestations of neuro-SLE or other disorders with high levels of circulating immune complexes or autoantibodies may respond to plasmapheresis.

Immunosuppression is safer if a physician organizes specific goals and limitations of the medications. Some medications may have side effects not unlike the disease the physician is treating. For example, corticosteroids may cause a toxic psychosis but are used to treat neuro-SLE; cyclophosphamide may depress the bone marrow, but the medication is useful in hematologic abnormalies in SLE. Thus, the physician needs to outline the clinical responses anticipated, serologic and other laboratory para-

Table 3. Diagnostic considerations to aid in correct diagnosis

Disease	Organs involved	Serologic	Angiographic	CSF	MRI	Biopsy	Other
SLE	Skin, kidneys, blood, other	++ ANA, anti-DNA anti-Sm	–	+/–	+/–	++	
MCTD	Joints, muscle, esophagus	++ anti-RNP	–	+/–	+/–	++	
Sjögren's	Salivary glands	anti-Ro	–	+/–	+	++	
Rheumatoid arthritis	Joints	Immune complexes Rheumatoid factor	–	–	–	– –	(cervical spine X-rays) (EMG/NCV)
SSC	Skin, esophagus	+	–	–	–	++	
PAN	Kidneys, skin	+/–	++	+/–	+/–	++	
Churg-Strauss	Lungs	+/–	+/–	+/–	+/–	++	
Wegener's	Respiratory, kidneys	cANCA	+/–	+/–	+	++	
Lymphomatoid	Skin, lungs	+/–	+/–	+/–	+/–	++	
Hypersensitivity vasculitis	Skin	+	–	–	–	++	
Secondary vasculitis	May be only brain	+/–	+	+	+	++	

meters of disease (e.g., ANA, anti-DNA, immune complexes, complement, EEGs, MRI scans) to be monitored regularly, as well as potential complications of medications, including infections.

Suggested Reading

Bonfa E, Golcmbek SJ, Kaufman LD et al. (1987) Association between lupus psychosis and anti-ribosomal P protein antibodies. N Engl J Med 317:265–271

Citron BP, Halpern M, McCarron M et al. (1970) Necrotizing angiitis with drug abuse. N Engl J Med 283:1003–1011

Ellis SG, Verity MA (1979) Central nervous system involvement in systemic lupus erythematosus: a review of neuropathologic findings in 57 cases, 1955–1977. Semin Arthritis Rheum 8:212–221

Hietaharju A, Yli-Kerttula U, Hakkinen V, Frey H (1990) Nervous system manifestations in Sjögren's syndrome. Acta Neurol Scand 81:144–152

Hoffman GS, Kerr GS, Leavitt RY et al. (1992) Wegener granulomatosi: an analysis of 158 patients. Ann Intern Med 116:488–498

Johnson RT, Richardson EP (1968) The neurological manifestations of systemic lupus erythematosus: a clinical-pathological study of 24 cases and review of the literature. Medicine (Baltimore) 47:337–369

Kissel JT, Rammohan KW (1991) Pathogenesis and therapy of nervous system vasculitis. Clin Neuropharmacol 14(1):28–48

Lazaro M, MaldonadoCccco JA, Catoggio LJ, Babini SM, Messina OD, Morteo OG (1989) Clinical and serologic characteristics of patients with overlap syndrome: Is mixed connective tissue disease a distinct clinical entity? Medicine (Baltimore) 68:58–65

Miller DH, Ormerod IEC, Gibson A, du Boulay EPGH, Rudge P, McDonald WI (1987) MR brain scanning in patients with vasculitis: differentiation from multiple sclerosis. Neuroradiology 29:226–231

Moore PM, Immune mechanisms in the primary and secondary vasculitides. J Neurol Sci 93:129–145

Moore PM, Cupps TR (1983) Neurological complications of vasculitis. Ann Neurol 14: 155–167

Moore PM, Fauci AS (1981) Neurologic manifestations of systemic vasculitis. A retrospective and prospective study of the clinicopathologic features and reaponses to therapy in 25 patients. Am J Med 71: 517–524

Moore PM (1989) Lisak RP (1990) Multiple sclerosis and Sjögren's syndrome: a problem in diagnosis or in definition of two disorders of unknown etiology. Ann Neurol 27:586

Rumbaugh CL, Bergeron RT, Fang HCH, McCormick R (1971) Cerebral angiographic changes in the drug abuse patient. Radiology 101:335–344

Winfield JB, Shaw M, Silverman LM, Eisenberg RA, Wilson HA III, Koffler D (1983) Intrathecal IgG synthesis and blood-brain barrier impairment in patients with systemic lupus erythematosus and central nervous system dysfunction. Am J Med 74:837–844

Chapter 93

Neurologic Complications in Organ Transplantation

FRIEDRICH VON ROSEN and THOMAS P. BLECK

Introduction

Transplantations of kidney, liver, bone marrow, heart, pancreas, and lung are established treatment for end-stage organ failure and otherwise fatal hematologic malignances. Liver and bone marrow transplantations are also performed in some hereditary disorders of metabolism that, if untreated, lead to severe neurologic compromise such as in Wilson's disease, tyrosinemia, adrenoleukodystrophy, or metachromatic leukodystrophy.

Neurologic symptoms and disorders can be divided into (a) complications of preexisting diseases (e.g., arteriosclerosis in heart or pancreas recipients) or of the operative procedure; (b) sequelae of metabolic disorders (e.g., hepatic coma); (c) sequelae of immunosuppression (infections and lymphoma); and (d) neurotoxic side effects of drugs. While metabolic encephalopathies and opportunistic infections are common in all acute-stage organ recipients, the other complications are more

---

Section Editor: Thomas P. Bleck

specific to particular types of transplant (Table 1).

Clinical Features

Most life-threatening neurologic complications arise in the acute phase of transplantation, when the patients are very sick, clinical presentation is non-diagnostic, and the possibility of neurologic examination is limited. In intensive care patients with impaired consciousness due to sedation or a known metabolic encephalopathy (e.g., hepatic encephalopathy), central nervous system (CNS) complications will only become apparent when they cause a worsening of coma, focal or generalized motor seizures, motor asymmetry, pupillary signs, or oculomotor signs not compatible with sedation alone (skew deviation, ocular bobbing). Muscle relaxation leaves only pupillary function to the clinical observer and should be avoided if possible.

In patients with a normal neurologic baseline, CNS complications are heralded by nonspecific symptoms such

Table 1. Complications typically related to transplantation of particular organs

Kidney:	Hypertensive encephalopathy
	Neuropathy of femoral and lateral cutaneous femoral nerve
Liver:	Brain edema with increased intracranial pressure before and during transplantation for fulminant hepatic failure
	Cyclosporin neurotoxicity
	Intracranial hemorrhage in coagulation failure
	Central pontine and extrapontine myelinolysis
	early after transplantation
	Aspergillosis
	Brachial plexus injury
Heart:	Brain infarcts early after operation
	Global anoxic brain damage
	Meningitic syndrome following OKT3 treatment
	Cyclosporin neurotoxicity
	Central nervous system lymphoma
Bone marrow:	Intracranial hemorrhage during thrombocytopenia
	Bacterial infection
	Aspergillosis
	Viral infections with herpes viruses
	Leukoencephalopathy
	Thalidomide-induced neuropathy
	Slowly developing dementia, cerebellar syndrome
Lung, heart-lung:	Air embolism
	Same complications as heart transplantation

as subtle changes in consciousness, frank delirium, psychosis, headache, visual disturbances, or seizures. Any of these signs in an organ transplant recipient should prompt a careful search for CNS infection, septicemia, metabolic derangements, or drug neurotoxicity. Table 2 lists the differential diagnosis of common neurologic symptoms in transplant patients.

Ancillary Tests

The diagnostic workup of a transplant recipient with neurologic symptoms includes a careful neurologic examination, an inspection for fever, hypertension, coagulation disorders, renal function, and serum ammonia, sodium, magnesium, glucose and cyclosporin levels. Computed tomography (CT) or magnetic resonance imaging (MRI) should be carried out to look for signs of brain edema, intracranial hemorrhage or infarction, abscesses, granuloma, pontine demyelination, and confluent white matter lesions. The cerebrospinal fluid (CSF) should be analyzed, including by appropriate microbiologic investigations (Gram, India ink, and acid fast stain; culture for bacteria und fungi; polymerase chain reaction for viruses of the herpes group). Pulmonary infection with *Aspergillus*, *Nocardia*, or *Cryptococcus* should be looked for.

Table 2. Differential diagnosis of common neurologic symptoms in organ transplant patients

Symptoms	Underlying pathology	Risk factors, causes
Acute coma	Intracranial hemorrhage	Thrombopenia (BMT, LTP), bleeding diathesis (LTP, BMT), aspergillosis
	Embolism (air, thrombus)	Lung fistula (lung TP), endocarditis (marantic endocarditis in BMT), other cardiac embolic source
	Status epilepticus (convulsive or nonconvulsive)	Secondary to metabolic disorders, drug toxicity, intracranial infections, or vascular events
Progressive worsening of consciousness	Metabolic encephalopathy	Hepatic encephalopathy (graft dysfunction in LTP), uremia (LTP, HTP), hyponatremia (LTP), hypomagnesemia, etc.
	Drug toxicity	Cyclosporin (LTP > other organs); acyclovir, ganciclovir (both rare); sedatives, etc.
	Intracranial infection	Meningitis with or without meningitic syndrome caused by common nosocomial agents, *Listeria*, *Cryptococcus*; encephalitis with CMV, HSV, VZV; cerebritis or abscesses with *Aspergillus*, *Toxoplasma*, *Nocardia*, *Mucor*
	Myelinolysis (central pontine and extrapontine)	Following hyponatremia and/or rapid serum sodium changes in LTP (rarely KTP)
Not waking up	Diffuse anoxic brain damage	Secondary to brain edema in fulminant hepatic failure before or during LTP; operative complication in HTP and lung TP
	Drug toxicity	Prolonged paralysis, sedation hangover, severe cyclosporin neurotoxicity
	Myelinolysis	See above
	Intracranial hemorrhage	See above
	Embolism	See above
Focal neurologic signs (hemiparesis, aphasia, cortical blindness, etc.)	Vascular events	See above
	Intracranial infections (abscess, cerebritis)	*Aspergillus*, *Nocardia*, *Toxoplasma* slowly developing in PML
	Drug neurotoxicity	Cortical blindness in cyclosporin neurotoxicity
Seizures	Drug-induced	Cyclosporin, antibiotics (more common in uremia)
	Metabolic disorders	Uremia, hypo- or hypernatremia, hypomagnesemia, hypocalcemia, hepatic failure, mixed derangements
	Intracranial infections due to vascular events	See above See above
Meningitic syndrome	Infectious meningitis	Bacteria (early after BMT), *Listeria*, *Cryptococcus*, *Candida*
	Aseptic meningitis	OKT3 neurotoxicity (HTP)

Table 2. *Continued*

Symptoms	Underlying pathology	Risk factors, causes
Headache	Meningeal irritation drug-induced	See above OKT3, cyclosporin
Paralysis (tetraplegia ± muscle wasting)	Drug-induced	Prolonged action of muscle relaxants, myopathy caused by muscle relaxants plus steroids
	Acute neuropathy	Critical illness polyneuropathy; Guillain-Barré syndrome
Cerebellar syndrome, tremor	Drug-induced	Cyclosporin, antiepileptics
	Metabolic encephalopathy	Hepatic or uremic
	Infections	Viral encephalitis (herpes group), *Legionella*
	Degenerative (?)	Late stage after BMT

Transplants: BMT, Bone marrow transplantation; LTP, liver transplantation; HTP, heart transplantation; KTP, kidney transplantation; TP, transplantation. Other abbreviations: CMV, cytomegalovirus; HSV, herpes simplex virus; VZV, varicella-zoster virus; PML, progressive multifocal leukoencephalopathy.

Common Types of Complication

CNS Infections

CNS infections occur in 5%–10% of organ transplant recipients, with a mortality of 40%–77% directly related to these infections. The incidence has decreased with changes in immunosuppressive regimens, particularly since the introduction of cyclosporin, and is probably further diminishing with the advent of selective bowel decontamination and preventive treatment with fluconazole, acyclovir, and cytomegalovirus (CMV) hyperimmune globulin in high-risk groups.

Abscesses are caused by *Aspergillus* species, *Toxoplasma gondii*, *Nocardia asteroides*, or staphylococci. Less common agents are *Mucor* or *Rhizopus*, *Candida*, *Cladosporium trichoides* and *Klebsiella pneumoniae*.

Meningitis can be due to *Listeria*, *Cryptococcus*, gram-negative bacteria (especially early after bone marrow transplantation), *Pneumococcus*, or *Staphylococcus*. Rarely meningitis is caused by fungi such as *Aspergillus*, *Candida*, Phycomycetes, *Coccidiodes immitis*, and *Pseudallescheria boydii*.

Encephalitis is usually caused by herpes simplex virus (HSV), varicella-zoster virus (VZV), or cytomegalovirus (CMV).

Fungal infections most commonly occur in severely ill patients within the first 2 months after transplantation. Aspergillosis is the most aggressive of the fungal diseases. The usual portal of entry is the lung (rarely, the skin or lymph nodes), and the agent spreads hematogenously to the brain. Ten to fifty percent of pulmonary infections disseminate to the brain, causing rapidly expanding necrotic areas (Fig.

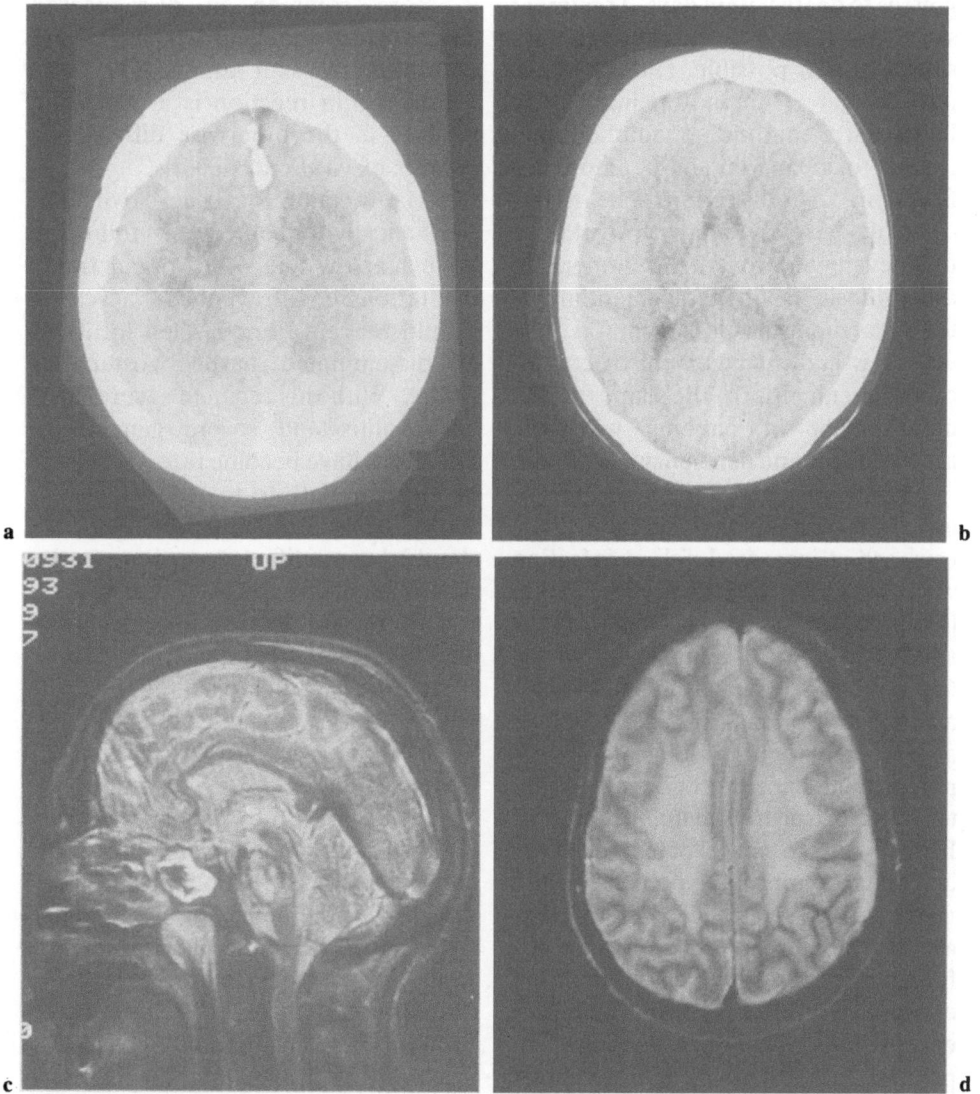

Fig. 1a–d. Computed tomographic (CT) and MRI scans of common complications in transplant recipients. **a** CT scan of multifocal central nervous system aspergillosis in a liver recipient. **b** CT scan of diffuse brain swelling in a 23-year-old woman with fulminant hepatic failure prior to transplantation. **c** Sagittal MRI scan of a 61-year-old liver recipient demonstrating central pontine myelinolysis. **d** Leukencephalopathy in a 19-year-old man 2 years after bone marrow transplantation for treatment of acute lymphoblastic leukemia. The patient demonstrated tetraspasticity, ataxia, and mild dementia

1a–c). Thrombosis of medium-sized vessels and hemorrhagic infarctions are caused by intravascular spread. The prognosis of aspergillosis is grave: 94% of bone marrow and 75% of liver transplant patients with pulmonary aspergillosis died; brain involvement in disseminated infections usually progresses to death within days. Treatment should comprise reduction of immuno-suppression if possible, and high-dose intravenous amphotericin. The liposomal preparation of amphotericin is less toxic and might be more efficient in CNS infection. The newer conazole derivatives have not yet been fully evaluated for the treatment of aspergillosis. Brain involvement in systemic candidiasis is less common. The diagnosis and management of crypto-coccal meningitis is the same as the management in patients with the acquired immune deficiency syndrome.

Viral infections. Organ recipients, especially those receiving bone marrow, are at increased risk of infection with viruses of the herpes group [Epstein-Barr virus (EBV), HSV 1 and 2, CMV, VZV, human herpesvirus 6] caused by de novo infection or re-activation of latent virus. CMV causes aseptic meningitis, subacute ence-phalitis, and chorioretinitis in addition to severe extracerebral manifestations; EBV is a rare cause of encephalitis, cerebellar symptoms, psychosis, and myelitis; HSV-1 and HSV-2 can cause aseptic meningitis and subacute or fulminant brainstem or generalized encephalitis (different from the limbic encephalitis in immunocompetent patients, see Chap. 44). Herpes zoster has been described in 5% of kidney, up to 20% of heart, and up to 50% of bone marrow transplant patients; the median time after transplantation is 4–5 months. Cutaneous dissemination and visceral spread are common when treatment is delayed, and the likeli-hood of postherpetic neuralgia is in-creased to 18%–24%. VZV can also cause transverse or ascending myelitis, cerebral large-vessel arteritis, and severe encephalitis. VZV encephalitis

is more common in disseminated cutaneous zoster and appears some days after the skin lesions. The poly-merase chain reaction is a promising method in the otherwise difficult di-agnosis of viral encephalitis.

Many centers give acyclovir pro-phylactically for some weeks following bone marrow and other organ trans-plantations. Intravenous acyclovir should be reinstituted when localized or disseminated herpes zoster de-velops. With this regimen severe HSV encephalitis and severe generalized infections have become rare. Acyclovir may accumulate to toxic levels in the setting of renal dysfunction. The dose should be modified according to the creatinine clearance.

Table 3 summarizes the pathology, diagnosis, and treatment of the most common CNS infections.

CNS Lymphoma

Organ transplant recipients are at in-creased risk of lymphoproliferative diseases and malignant lymphoma, especially when high-dose immuno-suppressants or multiple agents ("quadruple therapy") are used. Primary B-cell lymphoma of the CNS occurs in approximately 2% of heart or liver recipients and 1% of kidney recipients. Lymphoma of the CNS was more common before cyclosporin was introduced. EBV genome can be demonstrated in the majority of lymphomas.

Primary lymphomas of the CNS are often located in deep brain struc-tures, sometimes lining the ventricles or involving the corpus callosum. They are multifocal in 25%–50% of cases; the CT appearance is usually isodense

Table 3. Summary of pathology, diagnosis, and treatment of the most common infections of the central nervous system in organ transplant recipients

Agent	Pathology	Diagnosis	Treatment
Parasite			
Toxoplasma gondii	Multifocal necrotizing encephalitis	Serology (low sensitivity), brain biopsy	Clindamycin or sulfadiazine plus pyrimethamine
Fungi			
Candida	Meningitis, abscess (rare)	*Candida* in blood culture or multiple body fluids, CSF microscopy, CSF culture	Amphotericin B (liposomal ?)
Aspergillus species	Hemorrhagic encephalitis, abscesses, granuloma (rare)	CT lesion plus diagnosis of *Aspergillus* infection in the lung (culture of tracheal aspirate)	Amphotericin B, liposomal amphotericin B, itraconazole?
Cryptococcus	Subacute or chronic meningitis	CSF microscopy (India ink) and culture, CSF antigen assay	Fluconazole, amphotericin B
Bacteria			
Common nosocomials	Meningitis (often without meningeal reaction), abscess (rare)	CSF microscopy (Gram stain) and culture	Appropriate antibiotics
Listeria	Meningitis, (brainstem) encephalitis or meningoencephalitis	CSF microscopy (Gram stain) and culture	Ampicillin (plus aminoglycoside), alternative trimethoprim-sulfmatiaxal
Nocardia	Brain abscess (single or multiple)	Gram stain and acid fast stain of tracheal aspirate; stereotactic biopsy of abscess	Sulfisoxazole or tmp/smx, surgical abscess drainage
Viruses			
Varicella-zoster virus	Nodular encephalitis, angiitis of large intracerebral arteries	Serology, PCR	Acyclovir i.v.
Cytomegalovirus	Diffuse (nodular) encephalitis	Early antigen in body fluids, CSF PCR	Ganciclovir
Herpes simplex virus	Encephalitis (focal limbic or atypical)	MRI and EEG in typical cases, CSF antibodies (late); PCR	Acyclovir i.v.
JC virus	Subacute multifocal demyelinating encephalopathy	MRI suggestive, serology not helpful, PCR (?)	No known treatment; reduction of immunosuppression?

CSF, Cerebrospinal fluid; CT, computed tomography; PCR, polymerase chain reaction; MRI, magnetic resonance imaging; EEG, electroencephalograpy; tmp/smx.

to mildly hyperdense (rarely hypodense), and the contrast enhancement homogenous. Diagnosis is sometimes made by CSF immunocytology, but in the majority of patients typical CT features or a stereotactic brain biopsy allow the diagnosis to be made.

Neurotoxicity of Immunosuppressants

Cyclosporin causes a fine, rapid tremor in 20%–55% of patients, headache in up to 20%, and mild distal axonal neuropathy with distal paresthesias in some. Severe cyclosporin neurotoxicity has been reported in up to 35% of liver transplant patients, in 4% of bone marrow or heart recipients, and rarely in kidney recipients, with a higher incidence in children. It presents most commonly with seizures, acute cerebellar ataxia, or visual and mental impairment, progressing to cortical blindness, coma, or tetraparesis in severe cases. Serum cyclosporin levels are within therapeutic limits in most patients. The diagnosis of cyclosporin neurotoxicity remains a diagnosis of exclusion; nevertheless, it should be suspected when the patient has developed arterial hypertension and CT or MRI show white matter signal changes in the parieto-occipital region (Fig. 2). All symptoms or signs of cyclosporin neurotoxicity should clear after reduction or discontinuation of treatment with the drug, though individual case reports have described permanent sequelae. For the treatment of headache alone a trial of low-dose propanolol may be warranted.

OKT3, a monoclonal anti-CD3-antibody, is used to prevent and reverse graft rejection following heart, liver, and kidney transplantation. Approximately 10% of patients receiving OKT3 develop aseptic meningitis characterized by fever, headache, delirium or obtundation, and mild or moderate pleocytosis, mimicking CNS infection. The use of OKT3 may increase the risk of lymphoma.

High-dose steroids can cause delirium, manic or paranoid behavior, and insomnia.

Neurotoxic side effects with obtundation or coma due to acyclovir and ganciclovir have occasionally been reported in bone marrow transplant patients with renal impairment.

Seizures and Management of Seizures

Focal or generalized seizures occur in 10%–25% of transplant recipients. They can be the initial manifestation of intracranial infections, vascular complications, intracranial lymphoma, central pontine myelinolysis, metabolic encephalopathy, or cyclosporin neuro-

---

Fig. 2a–f. White matter changes due to treatment with cyclosporin in a 40-year-old man with immuno-suppression after liver transplantation. Initial axial MR images ((a) proton density-weighted image, (b) T2-weighted image, (c) T1-weighted image after IV administration of paramagnetic agent), obtained after the patient developed right hemiparesis, aphasia and seizures, show extensive signal abnormalities in both parietooccipital regions, left more than right, without abnormal enhancement. Lesions involve predominantly white matter but include cortex. d–f Corresponding images obtained 1 month later after discontinuation of cyclosporin show marked regression of the abnormalities. (Courtesy of Klaus Sartor and Marius Hartmann, Heidelberg)

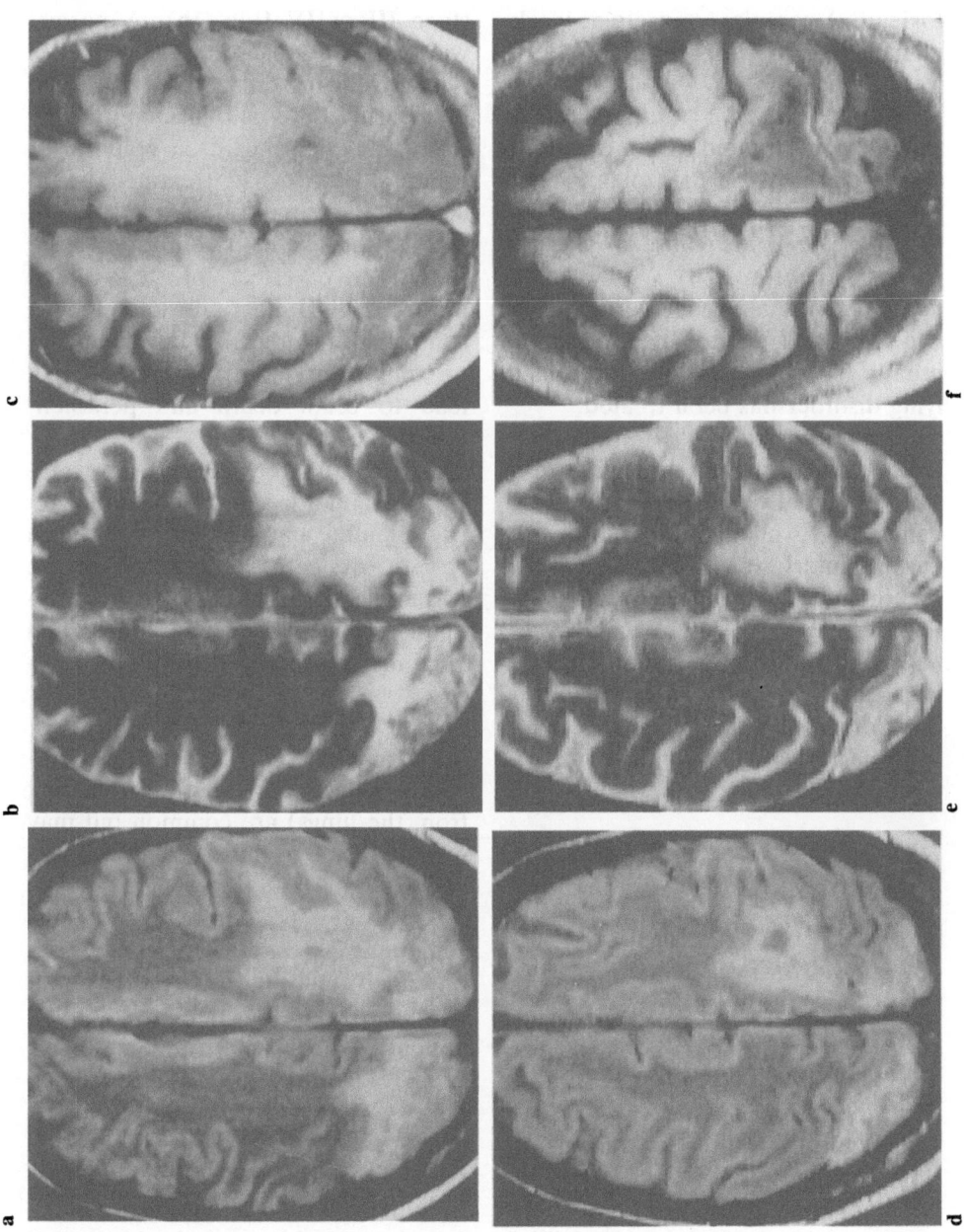

toxicity. A complete neurologic work-up including CT or, preferably, MRI is warranted.

Serial seizures or status epilepticus should be terminated with intravenous benzodiazepines (midazolam, diazepam, lorazepam) or barbiturates. When seizures are caused by cyclosporin neurotoxicity, hypomagnesemia, metabolic disorders, or hypertension, maintenance therapy is usually not required once the underlying disorder has been treated.

Valproic acid and, to a lesser extent, carbamazepine and phenytoin are potentially hepatotoxic. Carbamazepine, phenytoin, and phenobarbital interfere with the metabolism of immunosuppressant drugs. Its seems therefore prudent to give clonazepam or phenobarbital to liver transplant patients, while recipients of other organs might also be treated with valproic acid (no intravenous preparation available).

Special Aspects of Transplantation of Particular Organs

Liver

Though chronic end-stage liver disease is the indication for liver transplantation in most patients, transplantation is increasingly undertaken for the treatment of fulminant hepatic failure, defined as the development of encephalopathy within 8 weeks after the onset of hepatic symptoms. Cytotoxic brain edema with increased intracerebral pressure (ICP) occurs in more than 50% of patients in fulminant hepatic failure with hepatic encephalopathy

stage III or IV (Fig. 1b). A normal width of CSF spaces in a CT scan does not preclude increased ICP. ICP should be measured pre- and intraoperatively in these patients with an epidural or subdural device. The treatment of increased ICP should be aggressive, including the use of barbiturates, since the positive effect of ICP-guided treatment has been documented in controlled studies. Untreated or treatment-refractory increases in ICP lead to brain death and persistent vegetative state.

Approximately 20% of liver recipients and a larger proportion of retransplanted patients suffer from a variety of combinations of severe metabolic disorders, severe coagulopathy, multiple organ failure, and systemic infections in the early postoperative phase. Metabolic encephalopathies, central pontine myelinolysis, intracranial hemorrhages, and intracranial infections (usually originating from the lungs) are common but may go undetected in these heavily sedated and often paralyzed patients.

Central pontine myelinolysis, sometimes accompanied by extrapontine demyelination, has been found at autopsy in up to 10% of liver transplant patients dying during the acute stage (Fig. 1c) and rarely in renal transplant patients. Central pontine myelinolysis is associated with perioperative hyponatremia and rapid changes of serum sodium levels. Data on clinical manifestations and prognosis of central pontine myelinolysis in liver transplant patients are lacking. A brachial plexus injury with protracted recovery has been described in up to 6% of liver recipients.

Bone Marrow

Prior to transplantation patients are conditioned with 10–15 Gy whole body irradiation and chemotherapy including high-dose cyclophosphamide. During the neutropenic and thrombocytopenic phase following bone marrow transplantation (median time to engraftment 28 days) the patient is kept in an isolated environment. Bacterial (gram-negative), viral, and fungal infections are common during granulocytopenia. Bacterial meningitis can present without meningism; the CSF commonly shows no or only mild pleocytosis.

Subarachnoid and intracerebral spontaneous hemorrhages occur in severely thrombopenic patients, usually before engraftment. Hematoma evacuation should be undertaken early when mass effect causes a progressive impairment of consciousness. Ischemic infarctions were found in 4% of patients dying after bone marrow transplantation, caused by bacterial endocarditis or nonbacterial thrombotic endocarditis. Disseminated CMV and VZV infections due to reactivation or infection via graft cells were very common in bone marrow recipients before prophylactic administration of acylovir and CMV hyperimmune globulin became routine.

Cyclosporin neurotoxicity was reported in 4% of bone marrow recipients in one study, in most cases reversible. Optic disc edema due to cyclosporin was seen in eight patients in one series. Secondary CNS malignancies are rare in bone marrow transplantation, while leukemic recurrence is a real threat in patients transplanted for acutely lymphocytic patients (up to 13%, even higher risk in recipients of autologous bone marrow with prior CNS involvement).

A considerable number of bone marrow recipients develop mild dementia, a cerebellar syndrome, and/or pyramidal tract signs months to years after bone marrow transplantation (Fig. 1d). An acute parkinsonian syndrome associated with MRI white matter changes has been described. With the exception of radiation, the risk factors and causes of leukoencephalopathies have not been investigated. Bone marrow recipients treated with thalidomide for chronic graft versus host disease are at risk of severe sensory neuropathy.

Heart

Cerebrovascular disorders following heart transplantation were described in 9% of patients followed for an average of 18 months. Global ischemic brain damage, embolic infarctions, and intracranial hemorrhages caused by the transplantation procedure itself were seen in 2.3%. Ischemic strokes, transient ischemic attacks, and, less commonly, intracranial hemorrhages developed later in 6.7%. Only one-third were causally related to the transplantation, including embolic infarcts following right ventricular endomyocardial biopsy and infarcts caused by aspergillosis, while the rest were probably related to generalized arteriosclerosis.

Vigorous immunosuppressive treatment following heart transplantation leads to signs of neurotoxicity in 10%–20% of patients in the postoperative period. OKT3, given within the first 2 weeks, provokes a meningeal syndrome with fever, cognitive dysfunction, and aseptic pleocytosis in 10%, which has to be differentiated from bacterial, viral, and fungal infections. Cyclosporin neurotoxicity is often manifested by seizures alone, but can also lead to visual disturbances, stupor, and white matter changes on MRI, the syndrome commonly seen in liver recipients.

Infectious complications usually caused by the opportunistic agents listed above occur in 4%–10% of patients. Non-Hodgkin B-cell-lymphoma develops in up to 4% of patients. It may appear as early as 1 month after the transplantation.

Lung

Experience with lung and heart-lung transplantation is still limited. Air embolism due to a bronchial fistula has been described. Patients treated with extracorporeal CO_2 removal for early postoperative lung failure are at risk of intracranial hemorrhage. The incidence of bacterial, fungal, and CMV infections of the lung is high during the acute phase, with potential hematogenous spread to the CNS. Side effects of high-dose immunosuppression and lymphoma are probably common.

Kidney

The kidney is by far the most commonly transplanted organ. The operative procedure itself is usually well tolerated; most patients do not need intensive care. Subclinical CNS damage due to longstanding uremia and underlying conditions (connective tissue diseases, diabetes, hypertension) cause an increased vulnerability of the brain to metabolic and vascular complications. Cerebrovascular events occured in 8.6% of kidney transplant patients followed for a median of 4.3 years. The occurrence of thrombembolic events was highest in the first 6 months following transplantation. *Listeria, Cryptococcus*, and *Aspergillus* account for 90% of nonviral CNS infections in kidney recipients. Herpes zoster occurred in 5% of patients within 5 years, while aseptic meningitis and subacute encephalitis caused by viruses of the herpes group were found occasionally. HSV and VZV infections can cause a nodular brainstem or generalized encephalitis; polymerase chain reaction might be helpful in early diagnosis. Seizures caused by uremia, cyclosporin, or a combination of factors are common, but severe cyclosporin neurotoxicity is rare.

Pancreas

Pancreas and kidney-pancreas recipients are usually suffer from advanced diabetic complications including atherosclerosis, arterial hypertension, and diabetic neuropathy. The high incidence of cerebrovascular events following transplantation is therefore probably not related to the transplantation itself. Diabetic neuropathy improves slightly in the years following successful pancreas transplantation.

Suggested Reading

Adair JC, Woodley SL, O'Connell JB, Call GK, Baringer JR (1991b) Aseptic meningitis following cardiac transplantation: clinical characteristics and relationship to immunosuppressive regimen. Neurology 41:249–252

Adair JC, Call GK, O'Connell JB, Baringer JR (1992) Cerebrovascular syndromes following cardiac transplantation. Neurology 42:819–823

Adams HP, Dawson D, Corrman TJ (1986) Stroke in renal transplant recipients. Arch Neurol 43:113–115

Andrykowski MA, Altmaier EM, Barnett RL, Burish TG, Gingrich R, Henslee-Downey PJ (1990) Cognitive dysfunction in adult survivors of allogenic marrow transplantation: relationship to dose of total body irradiation. Bone Marrow Transplant 6: 269–276

Bale JF Jr (1984) Human cytomegalovirus infection and disorders of the central nervous system. Arch Neurol 41:310–320

Bamborschke S, Wullen T, Huber M, Neveling M, Baldamus CA, Korn K, Jahn G (1992) Early diagnosis and successful treatment of acute cytomegalovirus encephalitis in a renal transplant recipient. J Neurol 239: 205–208

Boon AP, Adams DH, Buckels J, McMaster P (1990) Cerebral aspergillosis in liver transplantation. J Clin Pathol 43:114–118

Britt RH, Enzmann DR, Remington JS (1981) Intracranial infections in cardiac transplant recipients. Ann Neurol 9:107–119

Canalese J, Ginson AES, Davis C, Mellon PJ, Davis M, Williams R (1982) Controlled trial of dexamethasone and mannitol for the cerebral edema of fulminant hepatic failure. Gut 23:625–629

Castaldo P, Statta RJ, Wood RP, Markin RS, Patil KD, Shaefer MS, Langnas AN, Reed EC, Li S, Pillen TJ, Shaw BW Jr (1991) Clinical spectrum of fungal infections after orthotopic liver transplantation. Arch Surg 126:149–156

Conti DJ, Rubin RH (1988) Infection of the central nervous system in organ transplant recipients. Neurol Clin 6:241–260

De Groen PC, Aksamit AJ, Rakela J, Forbes GS, Krom RA (1987) Central nervous system toxicity after liver transplantation. The role of cyclosporine and cholesterol. N Engl J Med 317:861–866

Diener HC, Ehninger G, Schmidt H, Stab U, Majer K, Marquardt B (1991) Neurologische Komplikationen nach Knochenmarkstransplantation. Nervenarzt 62: 221–225

Estol CJ, Lopez O, Brenner RP, Martinez AJ (1989) Seizures after liver transplantation:

a clinicopathologic study. Neurology 39: 1297–1301

Estol CJ, Pessin MS, Martinez AJ (1991) Cerebrovascular complications after orthotopic liver transplantation: a clinicopathologic study. Neurology 41:815–819

Ferreiro JA, Robert MA, Townsend J, Vinters HV (1992) Neuropathologic findings after liver transplantation. Acta Neuropathol Berl 84:1–14

Forbes A, Alexander GJM, O'Grady JG (1989) Thiopental infusion in the treatment of intracranial hypertension complicating fulminant hepatic failure. Hepatology 10: 306–310

Ganem G, Kuentz M, Bernaudin F, Gharbi A, Cordonnier C, Lemerle S, Karianakis G, Vinci G, Rochant H, Lebourgeois JP, Vernant JP (1989) Central nervous system relapses after bone marrow transplantation for acute lymphoblastic leucemia in remission. Cancer 64:1796–1804

Gilmore RL (1988) Seizures and antiepileptic drug use in transplant patients. Neurol Clin 6:279–296

Hall WA, Martinez AJ, Dummer JS, Griffit BP, Hardesty RL, Bahnson HT, Lunsford (1989) Central nervous system infections in heart and heart-lung transplant recipients. Arch Neurol 46:173–177

Hoogerbrugge PM, Brouwer OF, Fischer A (1991) Bone marrow transplantation for metabolic diseases with severe neurological symptoms. Bone Marrow Transplant 7 [Suppl 2]:71

Hotson JR, Enzman DR (1988) Neurologic complications in cardiac transplantation. Neurol Clin 6:349–365

Katirji MB (1989) Brachial plexus injury following liver transplantation. Neurology 39: 736–738

Lidofsky SD, Bass NM, Prager MC, Washington DE, Read AE, Wright TL, Ascher NL, Roberts JP, Scharschmidt BF, Lake JR (1992) Intracranial pressure monitoring and liver transplantation for fulminant hepatic failure. Hepatology 16:1–7

Lockman LA, Sung JH, Krivit W (1991) Acute parkinsonian syndrome with demyelinating leukoencephalopathy in bone marrow transplant recipients. Pediatr Neurol 7: 457–463

McManus RP, O'Hair DP, Schweiger J, Beitzinger J, Siegel R (1992) Cyclosporine-associated central neurotoxicity after heart transplantation. Ann Thorac Surg 53: 326–327

Patchell RA, White CL, Clark AW, Beschorner WE, Santos GW (1985) Neurologic complications of bone marrow transplantation. Neurology 35:300–306

Patchell RA (1988) Primary central nervous system lymphoma in the transplant patient. Neurol Clin 6:297–304

Polo JM, Fábrega E, Casafont F, Farinas MC, Salesa R, Vázques A, Berciano J (1992) Treatment of cerebral aspergillosis after liver transplantation. Neurology 42:1817–1819

Reece DE, Frei-Lahr DA, Shepherd JD, Dorovini-Zis K, Gascoyne RD, Graeb DA, Spinelli JJ, Barnett MJ, Klingemann HG, Herzig GP (1991) Neurologic complications in allogenic bone marrow transplant patients receiving cyclosporin. Bone Marrow Transplant 8:393–401

Schuchter LM, Wingard JR, Plantagosi S, Burns WH, Santos GW, Saral R (1989) Herpes zoster infection after autologous bone marrow transplantation. Blood 74:1424–1427

Shibata D (1992) PCR diagnostics of herpesvirus-group infections. Ann Med 24: 221–224

Vazques de Prada JA, Martin-Duran R, Garcia-Monco C, Calvo JR, Olalla JJ, Gonzalez-Vilchez F, Gutierrez JA (1990) Cyclosporine neurotoxicity in heart transplantation. J Heart Transplant 9:581–583

Weiner LP (1989) Virus diseases in immunocompromised hosts. In: McKendall RR (ed) Handbook of clinical neurology, vol 12. Elsevier, Amsterdam, pp 467–487

Wszolek ZK, Aksamit AJ, Ellingson RJ, Sharbrough FW, Westmoreland BF, Pfeiffer RF, Steg RE, de Groen PC (1991) Epileptiform electroencephalographic abnormalities in liver transplant recipients. Ann Neurol 30:37–41

Chapter 94

Cardiac Care in Critically Ill Neurological Patients

JOHANNES BRACHMANN, LAURIE MOORE, and HANS PETER SCHUSTER

Hypertension

Introduction

The upper limits of normal for systolic and diastolic blood pressures are 140 and 90 mmHg, respectively. Repeated measured values above 150 mmHg systolic or 90 mmHg diastolic must be considered hypertension. Chronic hypertension is implicated in ischemic heart disease, atherosclerotic vascular disease, renal failure, and stroke. Although the most common form of hypertension, essential hypertension, is of unknown etiology, secondary causes of hypertension include renal and renovascular disease, endocrine disorders (Cushing's syndrome, Conn's syndrome, pheochromocytoma, or carcinoid), obesity, and pregnancy. A thorough evaluation of hypertensive patients is indicated. An overview is given in Table 1.

Neurological causes of hypertension include elevated intracranial pressure (via tumor, encephalitis, or inadequate ventilation producing

respiratory acidosis), spinal cord trauma, familial dysautonomia, sleep apnea, acute porphyria, and Guillain-Barré syndrome. Hypertension in patients with neurological disease is frequently associated with increases in sympathetic nervous activity. For instance, autonomic hyperreflexia can be triggered in patients with high chronic spinal cord injuries. These brief episodes of hypertension can be episodic and profound. They are caused by the release of norepinephrine from storage vescicles below the level of cord transection. In the absence of inhibitory influences from higher centers, any stimulus for sympathetic stimulation can produce profound vasoconstriction and a reflex bradycardia. Similar acute hypertensive episodes are seen with Landry-Guillain-Barré neuropathy and bulbar poliomyelitis. Electroconvulsive therapy can produce a pronounced hypertensive response associated with the intense sympathetic stimulation.

It is important to distinguish hypertensive encephalopathy from hypertension caused by a neurological disorder (e.g., intracranial hypertension, Table 2). In hypertensive en-

Section Editor: Daniel F. Hanley

Table 1. Recommended basic diagnostic procedures in hypertension (Modified from Deutsche Liga zur Bekämpfung des hohen Blutdruckes e.V. 1992)

History	family history of hypertension, stroke, myocardial infarction renal disease	genetic predispostion
	pregnancy complications	
	cardiac disease	
	alcohol/ovulation inhibitor	
	hypertensive crisis/duration of hypertension	pheochromocytoma
	smoking habits	
Physical examination	repetitive blood-pressure measurements	
	overweight	cushing syndome
	auscultation: heart, carotids	carotid stenosis, vitium cordis
	blood pressure differences arm (right/left)/foot	aortic coarctation, peripheral vascular disease
	abdominal bruit	renal artery stenosis
Urine	protein	
	sediment	renal disease
	glucose	
Laboratory blood	creatinine	
	potassium	hyperaldosteronism, saline diuresis, laxative
	glucose, uric acid, triglyceride cholesterol (HDL:LDL)	
Additional diagnostic procedures	electrocardiogram	
	sonography: aorta, kidney	aortic aneurysm, renal disease, adrenal tumor
If diastolic pressure is >105 mmHg	blood pressure protocol	white – coat syndrome
	angiography of renal arteries	renal artery stenosis
	exercise test	coronary heart disease
	echocardiography	malignant hypertension
	fundoscopy	left ventricular hypertrophy
	endocrinological tests	endocrine hypertension

cephalopathy, a smooth and rapid reduction of mean arterial blood-pressure (MABP) must be accomplished in an intensive care setting. When arterial hypertension is secondary to high intracranial pressure (ICP; the Cushing response) reduction in blood pressure must be done with extreme caution as the hypertension may be a physiological attempt to maintain cerebral perfusion pressure (CPP; MABP-ICP=CPP). For this reason, in the comatose patient with severe hypertension it is optimal to monitor ICP prior to reducing MABP.

General recommendations, including weight reduction, sodium limitation, and avoidance of alcohol are appropriate for long-term control of hypertension, but obviously they are not options in the intensive care unit. For long-term management of hypertension initial monotherapy is attempted using either beta blockers,

Table 2. Features that help to distinguish hypertensive encephalopathy from cerebral events (from Thompson 1989)

Diagnosis	Onset speed	Signs	Consciousness	Headache	Optic fundi
Hypertensive encephalopathy	Days	Nausea, vomiting, seizure	Clear but progressive obtundation	Severe, hours to days	Hemorrhages, exudates, papilledema common
Cerebral hemorrhage	Quick	Dense fixed loss	Coma soon manifest	Sudden, severe	±Subhyaloid hemorrhage
Cerebral embolus	Quick	Varying	Sleepy	Mild	Retinal emboli
Cerebral infarct	Minutes to hours	Fixed paresis or plegia	Sleepy	None	–
Subarachnoid bleeding	Quick	Stiff neck, cranial nerve palsies	Alert to coma	Sudden, "worst ever"	±Subhyaloid hemorrhage

diuretics, calcium-channel blockers, or angiotensin-converting enzyme (ACE) inhibitors. If unsuccessful, combination therapy may be attempted. In any individual patient the response to antihypertensive therapy cannot be fully predicted, but it can be expected that the full pharmacological effect will take 2–4 weeks. Interventional studies have demonstrated favorable results with the combination of diuretics and beta blockers. Concurrent medical conditions may modify specific drug recommendations as demonstrated in Table 3. In the setting of acute ischemic stroke, subarachnoid hemorrhage, or spontaneous intracerebral bleeding, some modifications in the management of hypertension will apply. Please refer to Chaps. 5, 56, 57.

Hypertensive Crisis

The hypertensive crisis is defined as an excessive increase in blood pressure producing clinical symptoms such as encephalopathy, pulmonary edema, myocardial ischemia, or aortic dissection. Hypertensive encephalopathy is characterized by papilledema, retinal hemorrhage, visual blurring, dizziness, or a change in mentation. Persistent diastolic pressure exceeding 130 mmHg is often associated with acute vascular damage. The hypertensive crisis is a medical emergency requiring immediate intensive therapy. Table 4 lists circumstances which require rapid control of blood pressure. It must be mentioned that any patient with an acute increase of blood pressure above 200/120 mmHg, although presenting with unspecific symptoms only, may develop life-threatening hypertensive crisis within a short period of time. Patients with acute increase of arterial blood pressure should therefore be treated like patients with hypertensive crisis.

Therapy of Hypertensive Crisis

In a hypertensive crisis, immediate reduction of blood pressure is necessary

Table 3. Antihypertensive therapy in specific clinical conditions

Condition	Therapy
Coronary artery disease	Preferably beta blockers and calcium antagonists
Left ventricular hypertrophy	ACE inhibitors, beta blockers, calcium antagonists
Heart failure	Diuretics and ACE inhibitors
Renal failure	Preferably loop diuretics such as furosemide; ACE inhibitors in combination with potassium-saving diuretics may cause hyperkalemia!
Chronic obstructive lung disease	Preferably calcium antagonists, ACE inhibitors, and lung postsynaptic alpha-1-blockers; betablockers contraindicated
Diabetes mellitus	Restrictive use of nonselective beta blockers and diuretics
Hyperuricemia	Restrictive use of diuretics
Pregnancy	Beta-1-selective receptor blockers and alpha-methyl-dopa
Elderly patients	Preferably diuretics and calcium antagonists

Table 4. Conditions requiring immediate control of blood pressure (modified from Kaplan 1986, p 386)

Neurological emergencies
  Cerebrovascular
  Hypertensive encephalopathy
  Intracerebral hemorrhage
  Subarachinoid hemorrhage
Cardiac emergencies
  Acute aortic dissection
  Acute left ventricular failure
  Myocardial ischemia
Other emergencies
  Postoperative bleeding
  Severe epistaxis

to avoid end-organ failure or death. Because of the ease of administration, the therapy of first choice may be sublingual nifedipine, 5–10 mg, or nitroglycerine, 0.8 mg/capsule or 0.4 mg/aerosol (1–3 per acute administration). These may be administered while invasive monitoring is instituted. The minimum required is placement of an arterial line for continuous MABP monitoring. Some form of central access is also appropriate in this setting. If the patient is in frank congestive heart failure as a result of the increased afterload, or if the volume status of the patient is unclear, placement of a pulmonary arterial catheter (PAC) is helpful for medical management of these patients. In addition to measuring left-sided filling pressures, the PAC will allow for actual measurement of systemic vascular resistance (afterload), data of obvious importance. If these initial pharmacologic maneuvers are inadequate, as they frequently are, clonidine (0.075–0.15 mg subcutaneously or intravenously), hydralazine (2–20 mg i.v. incrementally), labetolol (5 mg increments i.v. titrated to effect – not available in

Germany), or urapidil (25 mg increments i.v. titrated to effect) may be attempted. If all these procedures are ineffective, nitroprusside may be administered. Because of its rapidity of onset and short half-life of action, administration of nitroprusside must be monitored very carefully to avoid severe depression in blood pressure. In addition, intoxication due to generation of toxic metabolites is possible. Furthermore, as a direct vasodilator, nitroprusside may increase ICP in patients with abnormal intracranial compliance. As nitroprusside produces a reflex tachycardia, esmolol, a beta-1 selective antagonist with a half-life of 9 min, is a rational addition to therapy. An alternative to nitroprusside can be trimethophan, although rapid tachyphylaxis is common with this drug. In patients with pheochromocytoma phentolamine (5–10 mg i.v.) is the drug of choice.

Goals of therapy in this setting include the rapid return of MABP to within the range of cerebral autoregulation, which for most individuals is a MABP between 60 and 150 mmHg, systolic blood pressure below 170 mmHg, and diastolic pressure below 110 mmHg. MABP should not be reduced by more than 15–20% in the first hour or two of therapy. Hypotension must be avoided in these patients as the lower physiological limit of cerebral autoregulation is unknown for any given individual, particularly in the patient with chronic hypertension where the autoregulatory curve may be "shifted to the right". Furthermore, if there are changes in mentation, an increase in ICP secondary to hemorrhage or edema and the CPP must be considered and ideally monitored. As

blood pressure returns toward a normal range, patients previously intensely vasoconstricted may require volume replacement, particularly in the setting of early renal failure. A pulmonary artery catheter may be helpful in the management of these critically ill patients. Finally, a cause for the hypertensive crisis must be sought and treated appropriately (Table 1).

Cardiomyopathies

Introduction

Most cardiomyopathies are idiopathic. Those due to coronary artery disease, or associated with other known disease processes are termed secondary cardiomyopathies. For example, several neuromuscular diseases are associated with a progressive cardiomyopathy, as indicated in Table 5. Cardiomyopathies are defined by three functional classifications. A dilated cardiomyopathy is characterized by ventricular dilatation and contractile dysfunction. An hypertrophic cardiomyopathy demonstrates an inappropriate and frequently asymmetric left ventricu-

Table 5. Neuromuscular causes of cardiomyopathy (modified from Wynne and Braunwald 1992, p 1395)

Duchenne muscular dystropy
Facioscapulohumeral muscular dystrophy
Limb-girdle dystrophy of Erb
Myotonia dystrophica
Friedreich's ataxia
Kearns-Sayre syndrome
Nemaline cardiomyopathy
Multicore cardiomyopathy

ADAPTIVE PACING DURING
SUSTAINED VENTRICULAR TACHYCARDIA

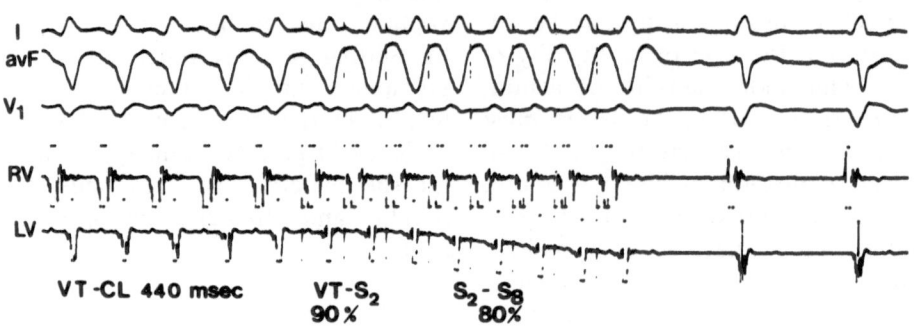

Fig. 1. Adaptive pacing during sustained ventricular tachycardia. Rate-adaptive pacing for termination of sustained ventricular tachycardia using temporary pacing

lar hypertrophy. Finally, a restrictive cardiomyopathy is characterized by impaired diastolic filling of the ventricle, which impairs stroke volume. Frequently, these three functional categories overlap, producing characteristics of each clinically.

Dilated Cardiomyopathy

Patients with dilated cardiomyopathy clinically present with symptoms of left-sided heart failure (paroxysmal nocturnal dyspnea, orthopnea, fatigue and weakness, and evidence of systemic or pulmonary emboli). On physical examination the patient may demonstrate cardiomegaly, jugular venous distension, hepatic enlargement, an S_3 gallop, and mitral regurgitation. The chest X-ray may demonstrate cardiac enlargement and evidence of pulmonary venous congestion. The electrocardiogram frequently demonstrates a tachycardia (an attempt to maintain cardiac output in the setting of a low stroke volume), frequent premature atrial and ventri-

cular contractions, ST segment and T-wave abnormalities, and perhaps an interventricular conduction delay. Left- or right-sided heart catheterization will demonstrate a poor cardiac output with an elevated left ventricular end diastolic pressure (LVEDP).

The vast majority of dilated cardiomyopathies are idiopathic or result from ischemic heart disease. Other more unusual causes include infections, toxins, metabolic, postgestational, or infiltration (e.g., amyloid) problems, and neuromuscular disease.

Primary therapy for the patient with a dilated cardiomyopathy includes afterload reduction and diuresis. ACE inhibitors have been successful in improving the quality of life and prognosis in these patients. Because of the high incidence of emboli, to prevent systemic embolic events secondary to impaired ventricular wall motion, anticoagulation should be considered. In acute congestive failure afterload reduction should be combined with inotropic support as necessary. Depending on the underlying cause of the cardiomyopathy, prognosis is poor in these patients, and cardiac transplantation is the only curative treatment at present.

Hypertrophic Cardiomyopathy

The classic example of a hypertrophic cardiomyopathy is termed asymmetric septal hypertrophy (ASH, previously termed idiopathic hypertrophic subaortic stenosis, or IHSS). In contrast to patients with aortic valvular disease, patients with ASH have a dynamic obstruction to ventricular outflow, which can vary based on the contractile state of the heart and LVEDP. Clinical symptoms include dyspnea, angina pectoris, syncope, and sudden death. On physical examination patients have mild cardiomegaly, an apical systolic thrill, and a systolic murmur, which increase with a valsalva maneuver (which effectively decreases venous return and LVEDP, therefore increasing the obstruction). The electrocardiogram demonstrates left atrial enlargement and left ventricular hypertrophy. Abnormal Q waves can also be seen. Echocardiography demonstrates ASH and systolic anterior motion of the mitral valve. Endomyocardial biopsy demonstrates marked myocardial hypertrophy and disorganization.

Most cases of ASH are idiopathic, though frequently a family history of sudden death can be obtained, as the syndrome can be transmitted as an autosomal dominant trait. A similar clinical picture is seen in patients with Friedreich's ataxia.

Calcium channel antagonists and beta blockers can reduce outflow obstruction by reducing myocardial contractility. These may also reduce the mortality, possibly by reducing malignant arrhythmias. Dehydration is obviously dangerous in these individuals. Surgical myotomy to reduce obstruction and implantable defibrillators are used as necessary. Cardiac transplantation has been employed in specific circumstances.

Restrictive Cardiomyopathy

As the pathophysiology of restrictive cardiomyopathies results in increased resistance to ventricular filling, clinical symptoms include dyspnea, fatigue, and peripheral edema. Physical examination will demonstrate mild cardiomegaly and S_3 or S_4 gallop, hepatomegaly, ascites, and jugular distension. At the bedside, this cardiomyopathy may be difficult to distinguish from a restrictive pericarditis. An electrocardiogram demonstrates low-voltage, interventricular conduction delays and atrioventricular conduction delays. An echocardiogram reveals increased left ventricular wall thickness, reduced or normal left ventricular dimensions, and normal systalic function.

Restrictive cardiomyopathies are caused by infiltrative processes, including amyloidosis, sarcoidosis, hemochromatosis, glycogen deposition, and neoplastic invasion. Management, if possible, of the primary disease process is paramount in halting the progression of this cardiomyopathy. Symptomatic control of heart failure with diuretics and afterload reduction, as well as management of arrhythmias, is done as needed. Again, with end-stage disease cardiac transplantation is the only curative option.

Prognosis is variable and depends on the underlying disease process.

Arrhythmias

Introduction

Conduction disturbances are very common in neurological patients, particularly in the setting of acute head injury or subarachnoid hemorrhage. Arrhythmias are due to both alterations in the autonomic nervous system and structural changes in the myocardium. Conduction disturbances are also common in patients with chronic neuromuscular disease, as indicated in Table 6.

Table 6. Neuromuscular diseases with known involvement of the myocardium and/or the conduction system (modified from Rettig et al. 1986)

- Muscular dystrophies
- Myotonia dystrophica
- Friedreich's ataxia
- Charcot-Marie-Tooth disease
- Facioscapulohumeral muscular dystrophy
- Limb-girdle dystrophy of Erb
- Kearns-Sayre syndrome
- Multicore cardiomyopathy

In the acute neurointensive setting, electrocardiographic changes are commonplace. In subarachnoid hemorrhage, hemodynamically significant arrhythmias are also common, providing a further reason why these patients should be monitored in the ICU setting. Serum and urine catecholamine levels are markedly elevated following subarachnoid hemorrhage, possibly contributing to the high incidence of electrocardiographic changes and distinctive pathology on autopsy, where focal areas of myocardial necrosis are seen. Rather than being a harbinger of cardiac death, in these patients cardiac manifestations probably represent a more severe underlying neurological injury. These cardiac manifestations need to be monitored and managed aggressively. However, in patients without a prior history of cardiac disease, it is the neurological process that needs to be managed primarily, and surgery should not necessarily be delayed because of electrocardiographic changes.

In the setting of chronic neuromuscular disease, a different management approach must be undertaken. Standard evaluation of the neuromuscular patient with syncopal symptoms should include a standard electrocardiograph and a 24-h holter-ECG

Table 7. Lown classification of cardiac arrhythmias (modified from Lown and Wolff 1971)

Grade	Rhythm disturbance
I	Occasional, isolated ventricular premature beats ($<30/h$)
II	Frequent ventricular premature beats ($>1/min$ or $30/h$)
III	Multiform ventricular premature beats
IV	Repetitive multiform ventricular premature beats
	a) couplets
	b) salvos

Table 8. Therapy schemes for bradycardias or bradyarrhythmias

Sinus bradycardia	Temporary atropine i.v.; in symptomatic patients (congestive heart failure or low cardiac output) as a reŝult of sinus bradycardia, atrial and/or ventricular temporary or permanent pacing (pacemaker therapy) is required
Sinus pause or sinus arrest	Pacemaker therapy if symptomatic
Sinus atrial exit block	Pacemaker therapy if symptomatic
Hypersensitive carotid sinus syndrome	Pacemaker therapy if symptomatic
Sick sinus syndrome	Pacemaker therapy if symptomatic
Atrioventricular dissociation with idioventricular rhythm	Pacemaker therapy if symptomatic

employing the Lown classification (Table 7). If life-threatening arrhythmias are discovered or a high level of suspicion is present, invasive electrophysiological studies are indicated.

Therapy

Both tachyarrhythmias or bradyarrhythmias may lead to significant hemodynamic compromise. Significant bradyarrhythmias include sinus bradycardia, atrial fibrillation with low ventricular rate, atrioventricular blockade, sick sinus syndrome, and a hypersensitive carotid sinus. These syndromes may be treated acutely pharmacologically or with temporary transcutaneous or transvenous pacing. Following evaluation, a permanent pacemaker can be placed if necessary. Particular patients with Guillain-Barré syndrome may require either insertion of a temporary pacemaker for short-term treatment or a permanent pacemaker for long-term treatment of severe bradycardias. Therapy for bradyarrhythmias is described in Table 8.

Tachyarrhythmias are divided into supraventricular and ventricular be-cause of significant differences in therapy. The most common supraventricular tachyarrhythmias include sinus tachycardia, supraventricular tachycardia, atrial flutter or fibrillation, AV nodal reentrant rhythms, paroxysmal tachycardia, and AV reentrant tachycardia seen with Wolff-Parkinson-White syndrome. Supraventricular tachycardias can be acutely treated by drugs, electrical overdrive pacing, cardioversion, or ablative procedures. To prevent recurrence of supraventricular tachyarrhythmias, long-term therapy with antiarrhythmic drugs or curative catheter ablation may be useful.

Ventricular tachyarrhythmias include frequent ventricular premature complexes, accelerated idioventricular rhythms, monomorphic or polymorphic ventricular tachycardia, and ventricular fibrillation. Ventricular flutter or fibrillation causing cardiac arrest requires immediate defibrillation using energy levels of 200–400 joules. In stable hemodynamic conditions, sustained ventricular tachycardias may be terminated by intravenously administered antiarrhythmic drugs or by different modes of ventricular overdrive pacing in

Table 9. Therapy of supraventricular arrhythmias

Sinus nodal reentrant tachycardia	Carotid sinus massage, β-blocking agents, calcium antagonists (verapamil, diltiazem)
Premature atrial complexes	Commonly do not require therapy unless symptomatic, β-blockers (sotalol), quinidine, propafenone
Atrial flutter	Carotid sinus massage, digitalis, calcium antagonists or β-blockers to reduce ventricular rate, cardioversion with low energies (<50 joules) or rapid atrial overdrive pacing if duration less than 48 h and history of atrial fibrillation is ruled out; antiarrhythmic drugs (class III and class IA, IC) to prevent recurrence
Atrial fibrillation	If duration less than 48–72 h cardioversion (if hemodynamically unstable regardless of duration), drugs – digitalis, calcium antagonists or β-blockers for reducing ventricular rate in combination with antiarrhythmic drugs, [quinidine (IA), propafenone (IC), sotalol or amiodarone (III)] using electro-cardiographic monitoring; if duration longer than 48–72 h anticoagulation for 3 weeks before elective cardioversion and 2–4 weeks after reversion to sinus rhythm is mandatory; antiarrhythmic drug therapy to prevent recurrence (class III and class IA, IC)
Atrioventricular (AV) nodal reentrant tachycardia	Vagal maneuvers (carotid sinus massage), digitalis, calcium antagonists (verapamil or diltiazem), β-blocking agents (sotalol with additional class-III action), adenosine, catheter ablation
Accessory atrioventricular pathways, WPW (Wolff-Parkinson-White syndrome)	*Acute therapy*: ajamalin i.v., procainamide i.v., overdrive pacing, β-blockers (sotalol); *Long-term therapy*: class III and class IA,C antiarrhythmic drugs, catheter ablation; if atrial fibrillation verapamil and digitalis are contraindicated

patients with temporary pacemakers (Fig. 1). Therapy schemes for treatment of ventricular and supraventricular tachycardias are presented in Tables 9 and 10. Ventricular tachyarrhythmias are treated with antiarrhythmic drugs, overdrive pacing, and electric defibrillation. If these measures are not successful, an implantable defibrillator may be necessary.

Antiarrhythmic drugs have variable effects on the cardiac action potential due to different effects on ion channels and receptors. A classification of antiarrhythmic drugs according to Vaughan Williams is given in Table 11. The most significant side effect of all antiarrhythmias is their proarrhythmic potential. This proarrhythmic effect lead to excessive mortality in the CAST trial using IC drugs in asymptomatic patients with ventricular ectopy following myocardial infarction.

Other significant side effects of antiarrhythmic drugs include negative inotropy, conduction disturbances, specific intestinal disorders, allergies, lupus erythematosis (procainamide), pulmonary fibrosis, hyper- and/or hypothyroidism, corneal deposits (amiodarone), gingival hyperplasia (diphenylhydantoin), cholestasis (ajamalin), and neurological symptoms (mexiletine, lidocaine).

Table 10. Therapy of ventricular arrhythmias

Ventricular premature beats	Commonly no therapy required including nonsustained; if symptomatic, acute therapy with lidocaine under ECG monitoring; chronic therapy with class III and class IA,C antiarrhythmic drugs; programmed stimulation in CHD and nonsustained VT for determination of antiarrhythmic therapy
Sustained ventricular tachycardia (>30 s)	If hemodynamically unstable cardioversion, intravenous lidocaine, ajmaline or procainamide; if refractory, amiodarone i.v.; prevention of recurrence with class-III (sotalol, amiodarone) and class-IA, class-IC antiarrhythmic drugs, determined by programmed electrical stimulation; automatic implantable cardioverter defibrillator; catheter-/surgical ablation
Ventricular fibrillation ventricular flutter	Immediate nonsynchronized defibrillation (200–400 joules); prevention of recurrence with class-III (sotalol, amiodarone) and class-IA, class-IC antiarrhythmic drugs, determined by programmed electrical stimulation; automatic implantable cardioverter defibrillator
Torsade de pointes	Temporary ventricular pacing; isoproterenol to maintain a rate of 90/min until pacing is possible; intravenous lidocaine occasionally effective; K^+, Mg^{++} increase to maximum normal values; antiarrhythmic drugs that prolong QT interval (class IA and III) are contraindicated

Table 11. Vaughan Williams' classification of antiarrhythmic drugs according to their electrophysiological effects on the action potential (modified from Vaughan Williams 1984 and Task Force of Working Group on arrhythmias of European Society of Cardiology 1991)

Class I	Drugs with direct membrane action (Na^+-channel block)
Class Ia	Depression of action potential upstroke, slow conduction, prolongation of repolarization (quinidine, procainamide, disopyramide)
Class Ib	Little effect on upstroke in normal tissue, depression of upstroke in abnormal fibers, shortening of repolarization (lidocaine, mexiletine, diphenylhydantoin, morizicine)
Class Ic	Marked depression of upstroke depolarization, marked slowing of conduction, slight effect on repolarization (flecainide, propafenone, encainide, ajmalin, prajmalin)
Class II	β-receptor blocking agents
Class III	Drugs which prolong repolarization (amiodarone, sotalol), potassium channel blockers
Class IV	Calcium channel-blocking drugs (verapamil, diltiazem, gallopamil)

Conduction Disturbances Caused by Neurologic Drug Therapy

In addition to class-I A and class-III agents, the phenothiazin and tricyclic antidepressants can produce QT prolongation with life-threatening torsade de pointes. Central nervous system conditions (cerebrovascular accident, subarachnoid hemorrhage, head injury) can cause acquired adrenergic syndromes with QT prolongation and malignant arrhythmias. In these cases ventricular premature contractions frequently occur, but severe arrhythmias may be observed in about 15% of the patients.

Summary

In summary, cardiovascular disease is commonly seen in conjunction with neurological disease. This presents two problems for the clinician. First, the autonomic nervous system is frequently disrupted with neurological injury, resulting in cardiovascular dysfunction. Therefore, treating the cardiovascular manifestations without consideration of the underlying neurological illness may result in suboptimal therapy. Second, treatment of the cardiovascular manifestations may have unexpected effects on the neurological condition of the patient. It is this close relationship between the neurological and cardiovascular systems that makes the management of these patients both interesting and challenging. Both systems must be considered when determining the principal management of these critically ill patients.

Suggested Reading

Braunwald E et al. (eds) (1987) Harrison's principles of internal medicine, 11th edn. McGraw-Hill, New York

Burch GE, Myers R, Abildskev JA (1954) A new electrocardiographic pattern observed in cerebrovascular accidents. Circulation 9:719–723

Carruth JE, Silverman ME (1980) Torsade de point: atypical ventricular tachycardia complicating subarachnoid hemorrhage. Chest 78:886–888

CAST Investigators (1989) Preliminary report – effect of encainide and flecainide on mortality in a randomized trial of arrhythmia suppression after myocardial infarction. N Engl J Med 321:406–412

Ciraulo D, Lind L, Salzman C et al. (1978) Sodium nitroprusside treatment of ECT-induced blood pressure elevations. Am J Psychiatry 135:1105

Deutsche Liga zur Bekämpfung des hohen Blutdruckes e V (1992) Empfehlung zur Hochdruckbehandlung in der Praxis und zur Behandlung hypertensiver Notfälle, 10th edn. Heidelberg, pp 5–6

Estanol BV, Marin OSM (1975) Cardiac arrhythmias and sudden death in subarachnoid hemorrhage. Stroke 6:382–386

Fromer M, Brachmann J, Block M, Siebels J, Hoffmann E, Almendral J, Ohm OJ, den Dulk K, Coumel P, Camm J, Touboul P (1992) Efficacy of automatic multimodal device therapy for ventricular tachyarrhythmias as delivered by a new implantable pacing cardioverter defibrillator. Circulation 86:363–374

Hall, Schmidt, Wood (1992) Principles of critical care. McGraw-Hill, New York

Hammer WJ, Lussenhop AJ, Weintraub AM (1975) Observations on the electrocardiographic changes associated with subarachnoid hemorrhage with special reference to their genesis. Am J Cardiol 59:427–433

Hersch C (1961) Electrocardiographic changes in head injuries. Circulation 23:853–860

Hugenholtz PG (1962) Electrocardiographic abnormalities in cerebral disorders. Report of six cases and review of the literature. Am Heart J 63:451–461

Kaplan NM (1986) Clinical hypertension, 4th edn. Williams and Wilkins, Baltimore

Kupersmith J (1993) Long QT syndrome. In: Singer I, Kupersmith J (eds) Clinical manual of electrophysiology. Williams and Wilkins, Baltimore, pp 156–158

Lee YC, Sutton FJ (1984) Concomitant pulses and U wave alternans associated with head trauma. Am J Cardiol 55:851–852

Liberatore MA, Robinson DS (1984) Torsades de pointes: a mechanism for sudden death associated with neuroleptic drug therapy? J Clin Psychopharmacol 4(3):143–146

Lown B, Wolff M (1971) Approaches to sudden deaths from coronary heart disease. Circulation 44:130–142

Marion DW, Segai R, Thompson ME (1986) Subarachnoid hemorrhage and the heart. Neurosurgery 18(1):101–106

Naftchi NE Tuckman (1989) Hypertensive crises in spinal man. Am Heart J 97:537

Rettig G, Stober T, Sen S (1986) Disorders of the central nervous system and cardiac arrhythmias. Z Kardiol 75 [Suppl 5]: 57–64

Sen S, Stober T, Burger L et al. (1984) Recurrent torsades de pointes-type ventricular tachycardia in intracranial hemorrhage. Intensive Care Med 10:263–2643

Shoemaker WC, Ayres S, Grenvik A, Holbrook PR, Thompson WL (1989) Textbook of critical care. Saunders, Philadelphia

Task Force of the Working Group on arrhythmias of the European Society of Cardiology (1997) The Sicilian gambit. Eur Heart J 12:1112–1131

Thompson WL (1989) Hypertensive urgencies and emergencies. In: Shoemaker et al. (eds) Textbook of critical care, 2nd edn. Saunders, Philadelphia, pp 391–412

Vaughan Williams EM (1984) A classification of antiarrhythmic action reassessed after a decade of new drugs. J Clin Pharmacol 24:129–147

Wynne J, Braunwald E (1987) The cardiomyopathies and myocaritides. In: Braunwald E et al. (eds) Harrison's principles of internal medicine, 11th edn. McGraw-Hill, New York, pp 998–1004

Wynne J, Braunwald E (1992) The cardiomyopathies and myocardites: toxic, chemical, and physical damage to the heart. In: Braunwald E (ed) Heart disease. A textbook of cardiovascular medicine, 4th edn. Saunders, Philadelphia, pp 1394–1450

Zipes DP (1992) Specific arrhythmias: diagnosis and treatment. In: Braunwald E (ed) Heart disease. A textbook of cardiovascular medicine, 4th edn. Saunders, Philadelphia, pp 628–666

Subject Index